PRIMARY CARE
GERIATRICS

PRIMARY CARE GERIATRICS

A Case-Based Approach

Richard J. Ham, M.D.
Director, West Virginia University Center on Aging
Professor of Geriatric Medicine and Psychiatry
Professor, Blanchette Rockefeller Neurosciences Institute
Robert C. Byrd Health Sciences Center
West Virginia University
Morgantown, West Virginia

Philip D. Sloane, M.D., M.P.H.
Elizabeth and Oscar Goodwin Distinguished Professor of Family Medicine
Co-Director, Program on Aging, Disability and Long-Term Care
Cecil G. Sheps Center for Health Services Research
University of North Carolina
Chapel Hill, North Carolina

Gregg A. Warshaw, M.D.
Martha Betty Semmons Professor of Geriatric Medicine
Professor of Family Medicine
Office of Geriatric Medicine
University of Cincinnati College of Medicine
Cincinnati, Ohio

Marie A. Bernard, M.D.
The Donald W. Reynolds Chair in Geriatric Medicine
Professor and Chairman
Reynolds Department of Geriatrics
University of Oklahoma College of Medicine
Associate Chief of Staff, Geriatrics and Extended Care
Oklahoma City Veterans Affairs Medical Center
Oklahoma City, Oklahoma

Ellen Flaherty, Ph.D., A.P.R.N., B.C.
Adjunct Clinical Professor
New York University College of Nursing
Director of Quality Improvement
Village Care of New York
New York, New York

Fifth Edition

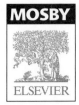

MOSBY

ELSEVIER

1600 John F. Kennedy Blvd.
Ste 1800
Philadelphia, Pennsylvania 19103-2899

Primary Care Geriatrics: A Case–Based Approach

ISBN-13: 978-0-323-03930-7
ISBN-10: 0-323-03930-8

NOTICE

Knowledge and best practice in this field are constantly changing. As new research and experience broaden our knowledge, changes in practice, treatment and drug therapy may become necessary or appropriate. Readers are advised to check the most current information provided (i) on procedures featured or (ii) by the manufacturer of each product to be administered, to verify the recommended dose or formula, the method and duration of administration, and contraindications. It is the responsibility of the practitioner, relying on their own experience and knowledge of the patient, to make diagnoses, to determine dosages and the best treatment for each individual patient, and to take all appropriate safety precautions. To the fullest extent of the law, neither the Publisher nor the Editors assumes any liability for any injury and/or damage to persons or property arising out or related to any use of the material contained in this book.

The Publisher

Library of Congress Cataloging-in-Publication Data
Primary care geriatrics : a case-based approach / [edited by] Richard J. Ham ... [et al.]. – 5th ed.
   p. ; cm.
 Includes bibliographical references and index.
 ISBN-13: 978-0-323-03930-7
 ISBN-10: 0-323-03930-8
  1. Geriatrics–Case studies. I. Ham, Richard J.
 [DNLM: 1. Geriatrics. 2. Case Reports. 3. Primary Health Care. WT 100 P952 2007]
RC952.7.P75 2007
618.97–dc22

2006043836

Acquisitions Editor: Rolla Couchman
Developmental Editor: Karen Lynn Carter
Project Manager: Bryan Hayward

Working together to grow
libraries in developing countries

www.elsevier.com | www.bookaid.org | www.sabre.org

ELSEVIER   BOOK AID International   Sabre Foundation

Printed in United States of America

Last digit is the print number: 9   8   7   6   5   4

In memory of my parents, John and Eileen Ham, and of Lawrence J Frankel, who died in 2004 at 100 years of age, pioneer of exercise in old age as the means to "be alive as long as you live".

RJH

To my parents, Walter and Grace Heddesheimer, and my in-laws, Aaron and Janice Itkin, who have taught me much about what matters as one ages.

PDS

To my wife, Martha Capps Warshaw

GAW

To my children, Lisa Therese Jenkins and Michael Lee Jenkins

MAB

To my grandmothers, Gertrude Campbell Hain and Mary Mullane Flaherty.

EF

My thoughts on old age...

A gift for old age is to be able to delight in comfort.
Bed, bath, food, drink. To enjoy the simple and immediate.

Acknowledge one's disabilities—then try to forget them.

For our children we must be brave, happy–looking, and interesting.
They will never see you as you are but
as you were. It is only to old friends that one can speak
frankly.

Nothing works properly – our bodies are unreliable.

I just hope I die before I lose my independence.

If there is life after death, I shall be most interested.
I don't know what, if not. Well, I shall be happy to just finish.

Think of us sometimes (the best bits).
Think of us on our birthdays and play for me, Richard.

Eileen Ham (1920-2001), in a notebook found after her death

And death shall have no dominion.
Dead men naked they shall be one
With the man in the wind and the west moon;
When their bones are picked clean and the clean bones gone,
They shall have stars at elbow and foot;
Though they go mad they shall be sane,
Though they sink through the sea they shall rise again;
Though lovers be lost love shall not;
And death shall have no dominion.

Dylan Thomas (1914-1953), from And Death Shall Have No Dominion

CONTRIBUTORS

Tarannum Alam
Multicampus Program in Geriatric Medicine and
Gerontology and Veterans Administration Greater
Los Angeles Healthcare System
Geriatric Research, Education, and Clinical Center
University of California, Los Angeles School of
Medicine
Los Angeles, California
VA Sepulveda Ambulatory Care Center
Geriatric Research, Education and Clinical
Center (11E)
North Hills, California

Cathy A. Alessi
Multicampus Program in Geriatric Medicine and
Gerontology and Veterans Administration Greater
Los Angeles Healthcare System
Geriatric Research, Education, and Clinical Center
University of California, Los Angeles School of
Medicine
Los Angeles, California
VA Sepulveda Ambulatory Care Center
Geriatric Research, Education and Clinical
Center
North Hills, California

Neil B. Alexander, M.D.
Mobility Research Center
Professor
Division of Geriatric Medicine
Department of Internal Medicine
Institute of Gerontology
University of Michigan
Ann Arbor VA Health Care System
Director
Geriatric Research Education and Clinical Center
Ann Arbor, Michigan

Kyle R. Allen, DO
Associate Professor of Internal Medicine
and Clinical Family Medicine
Northeastern Ohio Universities College of Medicine
Rootstown, Ohio
Chief, Division of Geriatric Medicine
Medical Director, Post Acute/Senior Service Line
Summa Health System
Akron, Ohio

Kristin M. Alline, M.D.
Geriatrician
Quality Geriatric Care
Rutherford, North Carolina

Michael J. Anderson, Pharm.D.
Director of Clinical Programs and Education
Ovations Pharmacy Solutions
Minnetonka, Minnesota

Lodovico Balducci, M.D.
Professor of Oncology and Medicine
Interdisciplinary Oncology Program
University of South Florida
Tampa, Florida

Karlene K. Ball, Ph.D.
Department of Psychology
University of Alabama at Birmingham
Birmingham, Alabama

Steve Bartz, M.D., FAAFP, R.Ph.
Family Medicine Residency Program
Mercy Health System
Janesville, Wisconsin

Douglas B. Berkey, DMD, MPH, MS
Professor, Department of Applied Dentistry
University of Colorado at Denver and Health
Sciences Center
School of Dentistry
Aurora, Colorado

Jeremy Boal, M.D.
Associate Professor of Medicine and Geriatrics
The Mount Sinai School of Medicine
New York, New York

Lucy Bonnington, PAC
Department of Dermatology
Norristown Dermatology
Plymouth Meeting, Pennsylvania

Malaz A. Boustani, M.D., MPH
Assistant Professor of Medicine and Scientist
Indiana University Center for Aging Research
Regenstrief Institute, Inc.
Indianapolis, Indiana

Sally L Brooks, M.D.
National Medical Director
Ovations Pharmacy Solutions
West Chester, Ohio

Kenneth Brummel-Smith, M.D.
Charlotte Edwards Maguire Professor and Chair
Department of Geriatrics
Florida State University College of Medicine
Tallahassee, Florida

Amna Buttar, M.D.
Clinical Assistant Professor of Medicine
Indiana University Center for Aging Research
Indianapolis, Indiana

James W. Campbell, M.D., MS, AGSF
Professor of Family Medicine
CASE School of Medicine
Chair, Department of Family Medicine and Geriatrics
The MetroHealth System
Cleveland, Ohio

Alvah R. Cass, M.D., S.M.
Associate Professor
Vice Chair and Director of Research
Department of Family Medicine
The University of Texas Medical Branch
Galveston, Texas

Charles A. Cefalu, M.D., MS
Professor and Chief, Section of Geriatric Medicine
Department of Family Medicine
LSU Health Science Center
New Orleans, Louisiana

Heather B. Congdon, Pharm.D, CACP, CDE
Assistant Professor of Clinical Pharmacy
West Virginia University Health Sciences Center
Martinsburg, West Virginia

David V. Espino, M.D.
Professor and Deputy Chairman
Family and Community Medicine
University of Texas Health Science Center
San Antonio, Texas

Laura Esslinger
Senior Director of Development
and Government Affairs
Evercare
Maitland, Florida

Maria Fedor, M.D.
Broward General Medical Center
Department of Emergency Medicine
North Broward Hospital District
Ft. Lauderdale, Florida

Karen Funderburg, MS, RD/LD
Assistant Professor
Chairman, Department of Nutritional Sciences
The University of Oklahoma Health Sciences Center
College of Allied Health
Oklahoma City, Oklahoma

Allon Goldberg, PT, Ph.D.
Assistant Professor
Department of Health Care Sciences
Program in Physical Therapy
Wayne State University
Detroit, Michigan

Nathan E. Goldstein, M.D.
Hertzberg Palliative Care Institute and
The Brookdale Department of Geriatrics and Adult
Development
The Mount Sinai School of Medicine
New York, New York
The Bronx-New York Harbor Geriatric Research,
Education, and Clinical Center
Bronx, New York

Anne Gunderson, ANP
College of Nursing
University of Illinois at Chicago
Chicago, Illinois

Richard J. Ham, M.D.
Director, WVU Center on Aging
Professor of Geriatric Medicine and Psychiatry
Professor, Blanchette Rockefeller Neurosciences
Institute
Robert C. Byrd Health Sciences Center
West Virginia University
Morgantown, West Virginia

Arthur E. Helfand, DPM
Professor Emeritus
Department of Community Health, Aging,
and Health Policy
Temple University School of Podiatric Medicine
Temple University School of Medicine
Philadelphia, Pennsylvania

Cynthia Holzer, M.D., CMD, AGSF
Director, Geriatric Education
Roger Williams Medical Center
Providence, Rhode Island
Assistant Professor of Medicine
Boton University School of Medicine
Boton, Massachusetts

Jamal Islam, M.D., MS
Assistant Professor
Director of Sponsored Clinical Trials
Department of Family Medicine
University of Texas Medical Branch
Galveston, Texas

Jerry Johnson, M.D.
Professor of Medicine
Geriatric Medicine Division
University of Pennsylvania
Philadelphia, Pennsylvania

Karin Johnson, DO, OD
Assistant Professor
Geriatrics Division
Department of General Medicine, Geriatrics
and Palliative Care
University of Virginia
Charlottesville, Virginia

Larry E. Johnson, M.D., Ph.D.
Associate Professor
Departments of Geriatric Medicine and Family and
Preventive Care
University of Arkansas for Medical Sciences
Little Rock, Arkansas
Medical Director
Nursing Home Care Unit
Central Arkansas Veterans Healthcare System
North Little Rock, Arkansas

Richard King, M.D., Ph.D.
Senior Resident
Department of Neurology
Massachusetts General Hospital
Boston Massachusetts

Clifford Y. Ko, M.D., MS, MSHS
Associate Professor
Department of Surgery
David Geffen School of Medicine
University of California Los Angeles
Los Angeles, California

J. Eugene Lammers M.D., MPH
Medical Director
Center for Geriatric Medicine
Clarian Health/Methodist Hospital
Indianapolis, Indiana
Clinical Professor of Medicine, Adjunct
Indiana University School of Medicine
Indianapolis, Indiana

Timothy J. Lewis, M.D.
Assistant Professor
Division of General Internal Medicine
University of Cincinnati College of Medicine
Cincinnati, Ohio

Anna Loengard, M.D.
Assistant Professor of Geriatrics
The Brookdale Department of Geriatrics and Adult
Development
The Mount Sinai School of Medicine
New York, New York

Robert J. Luchi
Professor of Medicine, Chief, Geriatric Section
Director, Huffington Center on Aging
Baylor College of Medicine
Houston, Texas
Associate Chief of Staff for Geriatrics
and Extended Care
Houston VA Medical Center
Houston, Texas

Scott L. Mader, M.D.
Clinical Director, Rehabilitation and Long Term
Care Division
Portland VA Medical Center
Associate Professor of Medicine
Oregon Health and Science University
Portland, Oregon

Vincent Marchello, M.D., CMD
VP, Medical Affairs
Metropolitan Jewish Health System
Medical Director
Metropolitan Jewish Geriatric Center
Brooklyn, New York
Assistant Professor of Medicine
Department of Medicine
Mount Sinai School of Medicine
New York, New York

Jennifer L. Martin, Ph.D.
Multicampus Program in Geriatric Medicine and
Gerontology and Veterans Administration Greater
Los Angeles Healthcare System
Geriatric Research, Education, and Clinical Center
University of California, Los Angeles School
of Medicine
Los Angeles, California
VA Sepulveda Ambulatory Care Center
Geriatric Research, Education and Clinical
Center
North Hills, California

Marlene J. Mash, M.D.
Department of Dermatology
Norristown Dermatology
Plymouth Meeting, Pennsylvania

Migy K. Mathew, M.D.
Assistant Professor of Geriatric Medicine
The Donald W. Reynolds Department
of Geriatric Medicine
University of Oklahoma Health Sciences Center
Oklahoma City, Oklahoma

Marcia L. McGory, M.D.
Resident Surgeon
Department of Surgery
David Geffen School of Medicine
University of California Los Angeles
Los Angeles, California

David R. Mehr, M.D., MS
Professor
Department of Family Medicine
University of Missouri-Columbia
Columbia, Missouri

Kurt P. Merkelz, M.D.
Medical Director
VITAS Healthcare of Texas, L.P.
Houston, Texas

R. Sean Morrison, M.D.
Professor
Department of Geriatrics and Adult Development
Professor
Department of Medicine
The Mount Sinai School of Medicine
New York, New York

Laura Mosqueda, M.D.
Director of Geriatrics
Professor of Family Medicine
Program in Geriatrics
University of California, Irvine—School of Medicine
Orange, California

Charles P. Mouton, M.D., MS
Professor and Chair
Department of Community Health and Family
Practice
Howard University College of Medicine
Washington, D.C.

Aman Nanda, M.D.
Assistant Professor of Medicine
Brown Medical School
Providence, Rhode Island

Yuri Nakasato, M.D.
Assistant Professor of Geriatrics and Rheumatology
The Donald W. Reynolds Department of Geriatric
Medicine
University of Oklahoma Health Sciences Center
Oklahoma City, Oklahoma

Konrad C. Nau, M.D.
Associate Dean, Eastern Panhandle Clinical Campus
Associate Professor, Department of Family Medicine
Robert C Byrd Health Sciences Center
West Virginia University
Harper's Ferry, West Virginia

Bonny Neyhart, M.D.
Clinical Professor
Department of Family and Community Medicine
University of California, Davis
Sacramento, California

Neil J. Nusbaum, J.D., M.D., FACP, FACHE
Professor and Chair
Department of Medicine
University of Illinois College of Medicine
Rockford, Illinois

Zachary Palace, M.D.
Attending Physician
The Hebrew Home for the Aged at Riverdale
Riverdale, New York

Jane F. Potter, M.D.
Harris Professor of Geriatric Medicine
Chief, Section of Geriatrics and Gerontology
Department of Internal Medicine
University of Nebraska Medical Center
Omaha, Nebraska

Steven Record, OD
Director, Low Vision Center
University of Virginia
Charlottesville, Virginia

Barbara Resnick, Ph.D., CRNP, FAAN, FAANP
Professor
University of Maryland School of Nursing
Baltimore, Maryland

Deborah W. Robin, M.D.
Assistant Professor of Medicine
Vanderbilt University Medical Center
Nashville, Tennessee

Carlos A. Salazar, M.D.
Senior Fellow in Geriatrics
Baylor College of Medicine
Houston, Texas

Robert C. Salinas, M.D.
Assistant Professor
Department of Family and Preventive Medicine
The University of Oklahoma College of Medicine
Oklahoma City, Oklahoma

Diana C. Schneider, M.D.
Assistant Professor of Family and Internal Medicine
Medical Director, LAC+USC Adult Protection Team
Keck School of Medicine at USC
Los Angeles, California

Sonia R. Sehgal, M.D.
Assistant Clinical Professor
Internal Medicine and Geriatrics
University of California, Irvine
Irvine, California

Banu Sezginsoy, M.D.
Assistant Professor
Department of Geriatric Medicine
The Donald W. Reynolds Department of Geriatric
Medicine
University of Oklahoma Health Sciences Center
Oklahoma City, Oklahoma

Richard V. Sims
Associate Professor of Medicine and Chief
Geriatrics Section
Birmingham VA Medical Center
Birmingham, Alabama

Amrit Singh
Assistant Professor
Department of Family Medicine and Program
on Aging
University of North Carolina
Chapel Hill, North Carolina

Richard Slevinski, M.D.
President, Emergency Learning and Resource Center
EMS Medical Director (Retired)
State of Florida
Pace, Florida

Philip D. Sloane, M.D., MPH
Elizabeth and Oscar Goodwin Distinguished
Professor of Family Medicine
Co-Director, Program on Aging, Disability and
Long-Term Care
Cecil G. Sheps Center for Health Services Research
University of North Carolina
Chapel Hill, North Carolina

Mary Beth Slusar
Doctoral Candidate in Sociology
Ohio State University
Columbus, Ohio

Barbara J. Smith, Ph.D., RDH, MPH
Assistant Professor
Department of Periodontics and Oral Medicine
University of Michigan School of Dentistry
Ann Arbor, Michigan

William D. Smucker, M.D., CMD
Associate Director
Family Practice Residency Program
Summa Health System
Akron, Ohio
Professor
Family Medicine
Northeastern Ohio Universities College of
Medicine
Rootstown, Ohio

Monica Stallworth, MA, M.D., MPH, CMD
Faculty, Harvard Division on Aging
Harvard Medical School
Boston, Massachusetts
Geriatrician
Department of Medicine
The Cambridge Hospital
Boston, Massachusetts
Medical Director
Neville Centre at Fresh Pond Rehabilitation
and Nursing
Cambridge, Massachusetts

Kenneth K. Steinweg, M.D.
Professor of Family Medicine
Director, Geriatric Division
Brody School of Medicine
East Carolina University
Greenville, North Carolina

Lorraine M. Stone, M.D., MSPH
Fellow in Geriatric Medicine
Duke University Medical Center and Veterans Affairs
Medical Center
Durham, North Carolina

Mark A. Stratton, PharmD, BCPS, CGP, FASHP
Professor of Pharmacy
Herbert and Dorothy Langsam Endowed Chair
in Geriatric Pharmacy
University of Oklahoma Health Sciences Center
Oklahoma City, Oklahoma

George E. Taffet, M.D.
Associate Professor of Medicine
Department of Geriatrics
Baylor College of Medicine
Houston, Texas

Heather M. Titman
Fellow, Geriatric Medicine
Department of Internal Medicine
University of Nebraska Medical Center
Omaha, Nebraska

Ingrid H. Valdez, DMD
Director
Geriatric Dentistry
Veterans Affairs Medical Center
Denver, Colorado

Janice Weinhardt, MSN, APRN, BC
Clinical Nurse Specialist
Stroke Center
Summa Health System
Akron, Ohio

Douglas C. Woolley, MD, MPH, AGSF, CMD
Delos Smith Professor of Community Geriatrics
Department of Family and Community Medicine
Kansas University School of Medicine
Wichita, Kansas

Jonelle E. Wright, Ph.D., RN
Associate Professor of Research
The Donald W. Reynolds Department
of Geriatric Medicine
University of Oklahoma College of Medicine
Oklahoma City, Oklahoma
Clinical Scientist
Research and Development
Veterans Affairs Medical Center
Oklahoma City, Oklahoma

Kathy Wright, MSN, APRN, BC
Advanced Practice Nurse
STEPS CARE Trial
Health Services Research and Education Institute
Summa Health System
Akron, Ohio

Robert A. Zorowitz, M.D., MBA, FACP, AGSF
Medical Director, Post-Acute Service
Health Net of the Northeast, Inc.
Shelton, Connecticut

Preparing this fifth edition has once again demonstrated how fast the field of geriatric medicine is moving forward. The basic purpose of the book remains the same: to teach those health professionals practicing primary care (physicians, nurse practitioners, physician assistants), the currently recommended approaches to the problems elders and their carers face, to disease prevention and health promotion, and to the reduction and postponement of morbidity and dependency, using a case-based text, with the patients and families cast in the settings of primary care - the office, the emergency room, the hospital, the nursing home, and the patient's own place: home, the best place to get a realistic impression of how the person's life really is, and how the patient, family and carers are handling the difficulties they face.

All the authors and editors in this new edition are, as before, experienced in clinical primary care, yet also prepared to take an evidence-based approach, utilizing the best possible evidence for all recommendations.

It is great to welcome two further editors to the team in Marie Bernard, whose enthusiasm for "our" book attracted us, and who has been zealous in keeping to deadlines and guidelines, and has shepherded in a large number of new authors and subjects, and Ellen Flaherty, our lively nursing colleague, who has similarly been responsible for new authors, new subjects and fresh approaches.

Recognizing that physician assistant and advance practice nursing students and practitioners have been using this book since its first edition, we made the decision this time to use the word "clinician" in the case materials and text, clarifying that it is not only physicians who practice primary care in our increasingly complex and diverse health care system, as we all attempt to make good health care accessible to all Americans.

Regarding terminology, it is possible that a few uses of the word "providers" have slipped through the editorial process, but we have tried to avoid that term. That it is useful, there is no doubt. But the concept of "providing" health care like a measured commodity, when in fact all realize that the interaction between clinician/prescriber and patient/family is far more complex than that—a negotiation of sorts, with recommendations made by one or more professionals and considered and acted upon (or not) by the other; a partnership devoted to the objective of improved health, bringing different perspectives and responsibilities to each situation.

Our patients are changing, as the cohorts we serve move forward in time. Our oldest patients experienced the Second World War and I still enjoy some reminiscences of the rather flatter areas of my home country where the "Yanks" came and helped us out with their planes, their enthusiasm, their supplies, and their lives. And I still treasure a few of the remaining "GI Brides" who fell for all of that American charm and immigrated (as, later, I did with my family) to a land with a very different set of opportunities than Europe presented at that time. For those of us who love old people because of the history they represent, this movement forward in time is very intriguing. The music and events of the past that evoke their youth and young adulthood, or their "best" time, is gradually moving forwards. And the expectations of younger family members (we Baby Boomers) are a powerful influence on changing the patterns of care, and the expectations of what medical care should be able to do, or should not attempt.

For me, the originator of this book, these last few years have been an immersion in the issues and challenges facing rural elders, now that I am relocated to West Virginia. I have come full circle: I was originally recruited to the Midwest, to Springfield, Illinois, to a medical school founded in order to address the shortage of primary care physicians in rural southern Illinois, where many counties had no doctor, or, at best, had a doctor clearly destined to retire or die on the job imminently, and counties where the only primary health care professional was a chiropractor. Since the majority of us in medicine, nursing and all of the other professions that it takes to create comprehensive care of elders still tend to gather round hospitals and therefore in more urban settings (and certainly we academics do), it is too easy to assume the availability of services generally found in well organized urban and suburban settings (like meals on wheels, day care, respite services, visiting nurses). In rural America (and all states have some rural elders) such resources simply may be unavailable - out of the question for an individual who wants to stay in their own home in their own community. Also, Americans in general had barely begun to discover the "obesity epidemic" when the evidence became clearer and firmer that obesity predisposes not only to type 2 diabetes, the illness that accounts for so much of our health care spending, but also that obesity and diabetes between them represent risk factors for the illness that has dominated my life clinically: Alzheimer's disease and the other progressive dementias.

These past few years have continued to emphasize healthy lifestyles and preventive approaches, so that those of us who survive into old age will approach it in as good shape as we can. But we all know that we are more excited (at least the media make us more excited) about the dramatic interventions after the event than the more ordered, anticipatory and careful, but less exciting (more dull!) efforts that we must make to exercise right, eat right, and make a good social effort to have a network of people we care for and care about, and a sense of purpose to drive us and keep us going on our journey through life. The system we work in and its incentives, and we ourselves as individuals, must constantly look beyond the immediately presented situation to see the "big picture" of our patient's future, and recognize the often quite mundane or small-scale, individualized recommendations or interventions which will make a profound difference to that future.

In addressing rural health care, other issues like health literacy and the unique vocabulary, assumptions, expectations and so forth that characterize yet another culture that has not been incorporated into our medical education efforts, are becoming better defined. Cultural competency is seen to involve not only race, ethnicity, education, religion, language, communication etc, but also location and the history behind each and every individual's unique personality, knowledge and beliefs.

Those familiar with the book will note that we have retained the literary (and sometimes patient or family initiated) quotations at the start of each of the three units. We have encouraged the use by our authors of those short highlights and aphorisms that have the quality of "pearls", the pearls of wisdom that the pioneering teacher-clinicians like Osler used in teaching their accumulated clinical wisdom: ("Listen to the patient, he is telling you the diagnosis" - which I like to change to "Listen to the family, they are telling you the diagnosis" - and "pneumonia: the old man's friend").

Our publishers have once again risen to the challenge of implementing a book that is a bit more complex to assemble than more conventional texts. The intermingled cases and the pearls, boxes, tables and figures, the pre and post tests and the objectives, have - by adding color and using different fonts - become easier to differentiate from the text, so that the book can be used for reference as well as a programmed, self-paced, straight-through read and learning experience. As I wrote in the Preface to the last edition, we have tried to produce "not a biblical text with everything in it, but a practical clinical guide to the most germane issues and approaches, which, if well learned and consistently applied, would improve the *enjoyment* of geriatric medical practice by all clinicians, and would improve the care of the older patients and families whom we serve."

A significant change has been the addition of the CD, under the authoritative leadership of Phil Sloane, who has been editing this text almost as long as I have! The use of the CD enables us to access video and illustrative material, as well as more extensive references, guidelines and appendices than could be included in the book without excessively increasing its size and cost.

As before, our cases, most of them completely rewritten, continue to emphasize the relative passivity of the most needy of our patients, the ones who will *not* push forward and make an appointment and come and see us, but will worry their family, or possibly just neighbors and friends, good Samaritans and fellow church goers, enough to get them medical attention. The actual recognition of the insidiously progressive chronic problems of old age is still a "hit and miss" affair, and very often the route to a thorough investigation is in fact devastating illness which perhaps could have avoided (or at least its effects could have been minimized) if the person had already been established in the care of a primary clinician who knew how to "ask the right questions" and "watchfully wait."

The energy of all of our editors has resulted in a more sweeping revision to the text than ever before: we have still divided the book into three units, but with modified titles, allowing us to put some of the major illnesses into that second unit with the "geriatric giants" – the syndromes that dominate the clinical picture and help to define the clinical approaches needed, and reserving the third section for (mostly) organ-system-specific issues, and discrete areas of care (such as chronic pain, the older adult driver, maltreatment). Of the fifty-two chapters, forty-five are complete rewrites with new authors. Syncope and delirium are now separated out into their own chapters.

It is always tempting, in the context of a Preface to a book like this, revised every few years as it is, to comment on the changes in the political scene. In view of public payment for health care services for the old and disabled, it is a public concern, and thus a political issue, as to who will pay for what and the priorities to be given to which aspects of health care. The American Geriatrics Society, of which we are all proud members, has been working hard on the CPT codes for the chronic care of the multiply ill complex patient, and we would urge all our colleagues to continue to support such efforts at making the Medicare system more reflective of the needs of our patients and of the efforts that all of us who specialize in providing health care for elders make every day. (One day, we may get paid for all that telephone - and now email - work!)

The current fiscal and political crises challenge all of us to get involved and stay involved, to make our voices, knowledge and opinions heard by those who try to lead us. Decisions and policies still too often reflect the depth of ignorance of what it is like to be old, what the real needs are of our elders, and how to improve health and reduce dependency of "our" patients and their families, both right now and in the future as we Baby Boomers age - with our different expectations and demands!

For those new to this book, we have retained the "Introduction: How to use this book" section, and we hope that a new generation - and many returning visitors to our pages - will enjoy what we have written, and find it useful as they struggle to ensure that all their older patients get the best, most comprehensive and thoughtful management that can be achieved.

We are already thinking about the next edition. Let us know what you think - and please continue to enjoy the uniqeness and fascination of each and every one of the wonderful elders whom we all care about so much.

Richard J Ham MD

June 6, 2006

ACKNOWLEDGMENTS

I am delighted that my wife Joanna helped me appear better read than I am, in selecting the mostly new quotations on the section title pages. Wit *and* wisdom is rare among health professionals – and if you really appreciate old people, you surely would enjoy (and benefit) from the insights of the great authors (when you find the time!). I will be eternally grateful for the tolerance and patience of all the editors, especially Phil Sloane, as I struggled in a difficult year to complete my share of the work; and of course we could not have done this without the cheerful and intelligent help of the Elsevier team: Rolla Couchman, Jeff Somers, Karen Carter, Bryan Hayward and others!

RH

Special thanks to Sang-Hyun Lee, MD, PhD, for his insightful and substantial contribution to the editing of selected chapters and to preparation of the CD-ROM.

PS

I greatly appreciate the support and dedication of the faculty and staff of the Donald W. Reynolds Department of Geriatrics at University of Oklahoma. Without their help my contributions, and those of our faculty who wrote chapters for this text, would not have been feasible.

MAB

I wish to acknowledge the wisdom shared with me by my patients and their families during thirty years of clinical practice. I would also like to thank my colleagues at the University of Cincinnati Academic Health Center for their dedication to educating the next generation of clinicians to care for older adults. I also wish to acknowledge the ongoing assistance of Sharon Harding with the many tasks that went into the preparation of this book.

GW

A Note on Level of Evidence Ratings

Where A through D ratings are used, they correspond (as appropriate) to:

A, evidence from well-designed meta-analysis, or well-done synthesis reports such as those for the Agency for Healthcare Policy and Research or the American Geriatrics Society; *B*, evidence from well-designed controlled trials, both randomized and nonrandomized, with results that consistently support a specific action; *C*, evidence from observational studies or controlled trials with inconsistent results; *D*, evidence from expert opinion or multiple case reports.

A, supported by one or more high-quality randomized clinical trials (RCTs) in an appropriate population, without contradictory evidence from other clinical trials; *B*, supported by one or more high quality non-randomized cohort studies or low-quality RCTs; *C*, supported by one or more case series and/or poor-quality cohort and/or case–control studies; *D*, supported by expert opinion and/or extrapolation from studies in other populations and/or settings; *X*, the preponderance of evidence supports the treatment being ineffective or harmful.

INTRODUCTION

This book is described as having a "case-based approach." Although many other texts of geriatric medicine have appeared since our first edition, this book is still unique in its approach. We hope that you will find it an enjoyable way not only of acquiring skills and knowledge concerning geriatric health care, but also of experiencing the *enjoyment* that the editors and authors of this book all share as they assist their elderly patients and families to make the best of the many challenges that life and society have handed them.

Our book is designed on the assumption that learning medicine from real cases is much more vivid, practical, memorable, and meaningful than reading fact-filled texts. In most of the chapters, the initial presentation, progress, and management of illustrative cases are integrated into the text. As you, the reader, work through the cases, the text reviews the illnesses and syndromes exemplified by them. The text itself is completely updated and generally takes a problem-oriented approach. We have tried to exemplify, or to "role model," in general, the optimal approaches to the many situations and syndromes that fill our text. Not all the cases are managed correctly; where things should have been done better, the case discussion says so: after all, it is the cases where we could have done better from which we learn most.

We have attempted to maintain a problem-oriented approach, although the necessity of having individual chapters on individual diseases has forced us to vary our approach somewhat; still, a problem-oriented approach is implied. After all, this is an important principle of geriatric medicine: focus on the problems as they affect the patient's life, define them, figure out all the diagnoses and influences that cause them, prioritize them, and address them. Thus we hope that at the end of each chapter our readers will have a refreshing and up-to-date fund of knowledge, some of the skills needed to apply the information to future cases,

and a sense of the current consensus on treatment, its intensity, and breadth. This is all based on the principle that Professor Brocklehurst and others have espoused: that involvement breeds enthusiasm and that enthusiasm is what we must feel as health professionals for our elderly patients and what we must communicate to those around us.

In organizing and writing this text, we have used the approach we would use for a midday case conference in a primary care training program. A resident or student might present the opening part of a particular case. A faculty member or visitor would be available to cover the topic concerned. After the initial presentation, the faculty person would stop and comment on the mode of presentation and the considerations going through his or her mind at that point. Then the case would continue with extra details. After further specific comments on the case, more broad and general comments, amounting to a formal presentation regarding the main syndrome or problem illustrated by the patient, would be given. At the end, to give a sense of completion, the resolution of the case would be presented, with some closing comments about the application of the generic material to that particular situation. It is to this ideal, "case-based" approach that we have devoted ourselves. By using real cases, we hope that practicality and application of the material are immediately seen and dryness is avoided.

The chapters are all similarly organized. There are formal objectives so that the reader will know what we wish to achieve in each chapter. There are pretest and posttest questions (as well as study questions after the cases in the text) to stimulate creativity and active learning. The pretests and posttests are not formally validated and are not intended to be used as quantitative assessments of knowledge. In general, the posttest is more rigorous than the pretest. If the reader has trouble with the pretest, he or she certainly needs to read the chapter. If the reader has trouble with the posttest, he or she needs to read it again. But the main objective of the questions is to encourage involvement.

Generally, the next item in the chapter is the first part of one case (or several). All are identified by a fictitious name, and all were real patients (sometimes modified to illustrate certain points). The opening case descriptions are followed by study questions, which are questions the health care professional should be asking at that point in the presentation of the patient.

Following these initial parts of the case(s), the text begins. It is typographically differentiated from the cases, so that it can be easily referred to separately for later review and reference. In the clinical chapters (16 onwards), we have tried to use a consistent format, with four main sections: (1) Prevalence and Impact; (2) Pathophysiology and Risk Factors; (3) Differential Diagnosis; and (4) Management. Where necessary, each condition within a chapter is described using this set of subheadings, but in general these are the only main sections of each chapter. We felt this would make it easier for our readers to use the chapters for reference, by making it easier to find specific content. The text alternates with the cases but is organized to stand alone as well.

In general, we have tried not to have more than two cases in progress at once—it would get confusing. Occasionally the cases are mere vignettes, but often the cases progress over months and sometimes many years (as in the chapters on dementia and on normal aging). The cases in this book, as in primary care practice, are seen in many sites—the emergency room, the hospital, the nursing home, the office, the home, and elsewhere in the community.

Each chapter has a brief summary of the main principles or content and their significance from the perspective of primary care practice, and each chapter ends with posttest questions and references (which include authoritative reviews to facilitate further reading).

The book is divided into three units. The first outlines the principles of geriatric primary care and the characteristics of older people from which these principles arise. The second provides detailed, case-based approaches to the major geriatric syndromes and conditions. The third section is more of a potpourri of common conditions and situations that we believed required separate consideration. This is not a fully comprehensive textbook. We gave much thought to what should be excluded, since this book is not intended to be encyclopedic. We believe that application of the principles outlined in Unit I and demonstrated in Units II and III to *any* condition presenting in an older patient would result in better care.

Although the first edition of this book was originally based on materials for medical students, it would be a rare medical student who would graduate knowing everything in this text. All four prior editions were widely used in primary care residency training programs, in the training of nurse practitioners and physician assistants, and by many other health professionals in training. It has also been useful, gratifyingly for us, to our peers: faculty in academic geriatric programs and practicing physicians, who, on a daily basis, face the challenge of providing optimal geriatric care and education despite the limitations of our system and of our societal response to those in need. We know of others, including clergy and other non–health care professionals, who have enjoyed and learned from the book; this is good, since many other individuals (not all health professionals) are essential to an effective team. Even so, the language of the book is directed toward clinicians in primary care practice and training i.e. physicians, physician assistants and advance practice nurses and nurse practitioners – all those with the power to prescribe the many aspects of management, investigation and activity that, when well addressed by an informed and caring team of health professionals, will help elderly patients and those who care for and about them, in the last decades of their lives.

We hope that you enjoy this book and that you will find it refreshing, "different," and a practical way to learn or update your knowledge of geriatric health care.

Preparing already for the sixth edition, we always appreciate suggestions, comments, and ways in which this text can be improved.

Richard J. Ham, M.D.

CONTENTS

Principles and Practice

If I'd known I was gonna live this long, I'd have taken better care of myself!
— EUBIE BLAKE (1883–1983), *jazz pianist and composer, on reaching his 100th birthday*

It is not by muscle, speed or physical dexterity that great things are achieved, but by reflection, force of character, and judgement; in these qualities old age is usually not only not poorer, but is even richer.
— CICERO (106–43 BC) *in On Old Age, VI*

Nothing ages like happiness.
— OSCAR WILDE (1854–1900), *in An Ideal Husband, Act One*

To live effectively, with a real purpose and not merely to exist, you must be active, interested, involved – both physically and mentally.
— LAWRENCE J FRANKEL (1904–2004), *exercise in old age pioneer; in Be Alive as Long as you Live"*

The soul is born old but grows young – that is the comedy of life
And the body is born young and grows old – that is life's tragedy.
— OSCAR WILDE (1854–1900), *in A Woman of No Importance, Act One*

I was so much older then, I'm younger than that now.
— BOB DYLAN (b 1941), *in "My Back Pages"*

To get back my youth I would do anything in the world, except take exercise, get up early, or be respectable.
— OSCAR WILDE (1854–1900), *in The Picture of Dorian Gray, Chapter 19*

All that the young can do for the old is to shock them and keep them up to date

— GEORGE BERNARD SHAW (1856–1950), *in "Fanny's First Play"*

Oh, to be seventy again!

— GEORGES CLEMENCEAU, *French statesman, noticing a pretty girl on the Champs d'Elysee on his 80th birthday.*

At 90, they seem to bring you breakfast every hour...

— CHRISTOPHER FRY (b 1907), *English playwright*

Devoting one's life to keeping well is one of the most tedious of ailments.

— DUC FRANCOIS DE LA ROCHEFOUCALD (1630–1680)

It is better to wear out than to rust out.

— BISHOP GEORGE HORNE, *in an 18th century sermon*

———

Caring for Older Patients and an Aging Population

Kenneth Brummel-Smith and Anne Gunderson

OBJECTIVES

Upon completion of this chapter, the reader will be able to:

- Describe the demographic changes resulting from the aging population of the United States.
- Explain how demographic changes occurring among rural population, minorities, and women will affect health care.
- Discuss primary care as it pertains to geriatrics.
- Describe two features that make up the foundation of geriatric medicine.
- Describe the newest trends and programs in geriatric care.

● There is wide diversity in health and function among adults age 65 years and over.

The percentage of Americans who are older than 65 years is the highest it has ever been. While many older people are in good health, the portion of elders with serious medical conditions or functional problems is higher than any other age group. This book is designed to provide you with the necessary knowledge to provide excellent care for the healthy and the ill older adult.

The assignment of an individual to the "geriatric" age group is arbitrary. Historically, retirement was linked to reaching the age of 65 years; however, the fact is that most 65-year-old Americans are as fit and active as adults in their 50s. While it is also true that Medicare coverage begins at age 65, medical care utilization does not start to rise dramatically until after age 75.

There is wide diversity in health and function among adults age 65 and over. At no time in the human lifespan are individuals more different from one another. People over age 65, especially those 85 and over, have had a long time to accumulate changes in life experiences, physiologic insults, and illnesses. Although there are important demographic facts one should be aware of when caring for older persons, one must remain acutely aware that each older person is an individual and that general predictions on the basis of population norms may not always apply.

POPULATION DEMOGRAPHICS

In 2003, nearly 36 million people age 65 and over live in the United States, accounting for more than 12% of the total population. In the last 100 years, the population aged 65 and over grew from 3 million to 35 million. By 2050, the population over age 65 will approach 90 million people[1] (Fig. 1-1). Although there are large numbers of older people in all communities, many are concentrated in certain portions of the country, primarily Florida, Arizona, and the midwestern United States. In one county in North Dakota, 35% of the population is age 65 and over. In one county in Florida (charlotte), 37% of the population is over age 65.[2] This increase in numbers will affect the practice of every medical specialty and every type of care provider. It will also have significant effects on the society at large.

Women make up 58% of those over age 65 and almost 70% of those over 85. The percentage of women who are widows rises significantly after age 70[3] (Fig. 1-2). Most men who are older are married, and if care is needed, it is usually provided by the man's spouse. Such is not the case with older women, who tend to rely on their daughters or daughters-in-law. For the present cohort of women age 85 and older, their daughters (age 60 or so) were raised at a time when women were socialized to be caregivers. When the baby boom generation reaches old age in 2010, it is likely that daughters will have been raised to work outside the home. They may be less available to serve as caregivers, creating a large need for formal caregivers in the community.

A common myth in America is that older people are "dumped" into nursing homes. In reality, 85% of all informal care is provided by the family.[4] Families go to great trouble to provide for their loved ones, often limiting or quitting jobs or even incurring severe financial difficulties. Some 9 million Americans provide caregiving services, and approximately 40% of these caregivers are also employed full-time in other jobs. On average, caregivers spend approximately 24 hours a week providing supportive services.[5] It is usually only after the family has become exhausted by caregiving demands, or fatigued by disturbing symptoms such as severe behavioral disturbances seen in some patients with dementia, that families consider nursing home admission.

● Older Americans are becoming increasingly more ethnically diverse.

Caregiving experiences vary among ethnic groups. Nursing home utilization, for instance, is much more common among frail whites than other ethnic groups. Blacks, Asians, and Hispanics all have lower rates of nursing home utilization even at similar levels of dependency. In part this may reflect increased availability of caregivers in some ethnic groups. In some cultures it is less common for middle-aged women to

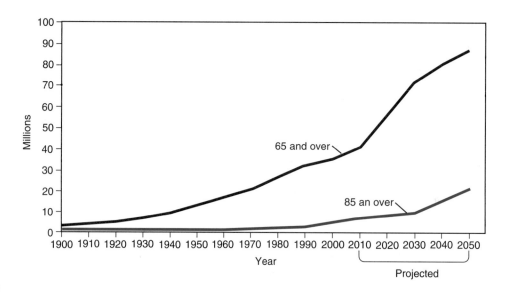

FIGURE 1-1

Number of people age 65 and over, by age group, selected years 1900 to 2000 and projected 2010 to 2050. *(Redrawn from U.S. Census Bureau, Decennial Census and Projections, 2000.)*

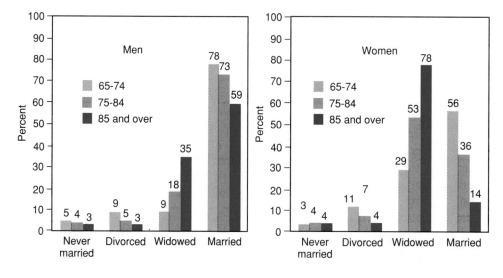

FIGURE 1-2

Marital status of the population age 65 and over, by age group and sex, 2003. *(Redrawn from U.S. Census Bureau, Current Population Survey, Annual Social and Economic Supplement, 2004.)*

continue working outside the home; therefore, they are more available to provide caregiving. In addition, some ethnic groups tend to have larger families, which increases the "pool" of potential caregivers.[6]

The older population is also becoming ethnically diverse. By 2050 the percentage of elders who are white will fall by over 20%, while the percentage of blacks will increase by 50%, and Asians and Hispanics will triple[7] (Fig. 1-3). As these changes ensue, clinicians will need to understand the varied cultural practices and beliefs of their patients, from the use of traditional therapies to differences in the approach to end-of-life care.

RURAL ELDERS

Eighteen percent of the rural population is age 65 and older versus 15% of the urban population. Rural elderly living on farms are more likely than urban elderly to be married and living with their spouse. Approximately 71% of rural elderly ages 60 to 74 are married, compared with 66% of urban elderly. By age 75, the likelihood of living alone is slightly higher among rural (nonmetropolitan) elderly (51% versus 48%). While rural elderly are more likely to own their homes, their homes are of lesser value and in poor condition. In addition, rural elders have limited access to health

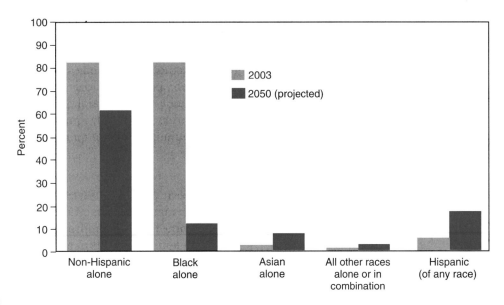

FIGURE 1–3

Population age 65 and over, by race and Hispanic origin, 2003 and projected 2050. *(Redrawn from U.S. Census Bureau, Population Estimates and Projections, 2004.)*

care, and transportation problems are more severe.[8] These limitations affect rural elders' use of health care services, especially owing to limited access to health maintenance visits and preventive care. Instead, because of the difficulties accessing preventative care, rural elders are more likely to wait until medical situations have reached a crisis stage to be treated.

● Social Security income has provided the largest share of income for older Americans since the early 1960s.

ECONOMICS OF AGING

Since 1974, the proportion of elders who live in poverty has declined. By 2002, only about 10% live in poverty and 28% are in the low-income group. While the decline in poverty rates is certainly positive, it must be remembered that socioeconomic factors have significant effects on health care and service utilization. Fortunately for some, the proportion living in the high-income group has increased in the last 30 years, from 18% in 1974 to 26% in 2002.

Social Security income has provided the largest share of income for older Americans since the early 1960s. Income from pensions and assets is declining, while income from earnings from savings in increasing. Pension income has had a major shift, from defined benefit plans to defined contribution plans (such as 401K plans). The percentage of income that Social Security provides individuals varies markedly with total income. For those in the lowest fifth of income, Social Security provides 83% of total income, while for those in the upper fifth it provides only 20% of the total income[9] (Fig. 1-4).

● Only 5% of Americans age 65 and over reside in an institutional setting.

DEMOGRAPHY AS IT AFFECTS HEALTH CARE

Why are there so many older people now? A common misconception is that better medical care for adults is extending older people's lives. In reality, the main cause of the increasing numbers of elders is that childhood mortality has been significantly reduced in the past century. In 1900, the average life expectancy at birth was only 47 years. Almost one-quarter of the population died before reaching age 10. Now life expectancy at birth is over 77 years for men and 80 years for women.[10] Changes in public health—cleaner water, better nutrition, less poverty, improved prenatal care, and childhood immunizations—have all but eradicated childhood mortality. In addition, changes in public safety measures, such as worker safety laws and the use of automobile safety belts, have lowered the mortality risk of middle ages. Finally, Americans are smoking less, which reduces later mortality as well.

However, mortality in later life is also declining. Deaths from heart disease and cerebrovascular disease, the number one and number three causes of death, have been declining for over a quarter-century. Hence, life expectancy at age 65 and 85 has risen slightly in the past century. The average 65-year-old woman can expect to live almost 20 more years, while the average 85-year-old man can expect 5 more years[11] (Fig. 1-5).

Another important change during the past century is the leading causes of death. Before the 1940s, infections

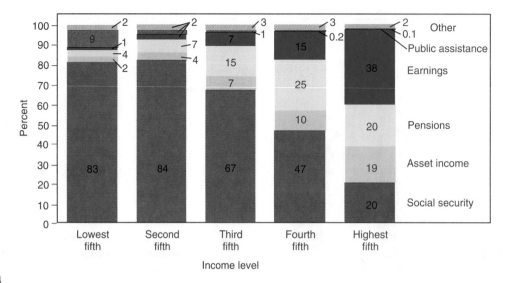

FIGURE 1-4

Sources of income for the population age 65 and over, by income quintile, 2002. *(Redrawn from U.S, Census Bureau, Current Population Survey, Annual Social and Economic Supplement, 2004.)*

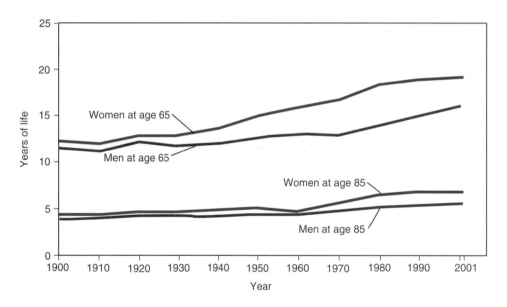

FIGURE 1-5

Life expectancy at ages 65 and 85, by sex, selected years 1900 to 2001. *(Redrawn from Centers for Disease Control and Prevention, National Center for Health Statistics, National Vital Statistics System, 2004.)*

and trauma were major causes of death. Now it is chronic diseases: heart disease, cancer, stroke, Alzheimer's disease, diabetes, and others. In addition, older people are living so long that sensory impairments are extremely common. Almost 50% of men have difficult hearing, 20% have problems seeing, and almost a third have no natural teeth. Memory impairment is also common, with about 10% of people over 65 having some problems with memory and over one-third of those over age 85 having moderate problems with memory.[12] Other "geriatric syndromes" are also common (Box 1-1). Finally, the older population has a high rate of

Box 1–1	Common Geriatric Syndromes

Falls
Urinary incontinence
Confusion
Immobility
Sleep disorders
Fatigue
Weight loss

depression, affecting about as many as 20% of the population. Clinicians providing primary care to older persons must be skillful in managing chronic conditions, provide resources and interventions for sensory impairment, properly diagnose and manage dementia and other geriatric syndromes, and be adept at caring for mental health problems.

Many people fear losing the ability to live independently as they age. Fortunately, because of the above-mentioned reduction in cardiovascular and cerebrovascular diseases, as well as better management of chronic conditions, disability rates are falling. Only about 20% of elders have some level of disability, which is lower than the 25% that were disabled in 1984.[13] Most of these older adults are only mildly disabled, with limitations of instrumental activities of daily living (e.g., shopping or cooking) or one or two activities of daily living (e.g., bathing, ambulation, or toileting). Only 5% of the older population resides in an institutional setting.[14] Functional limitations become more common in adults age 75 and over, and attention to functional problems is one of the distinguishing characteristics of quality geriatric care.

> ● The expectations and needs of the baby boomers will dramatically change the future of long-term care.

CHANGES IN LONG-TERM CARE AND THE INFLUENCE OF THE BABY BOOMERS

Long-term care refers to a broad range of supportive medical, personal, and social services needed by individuals who are unable to meet their basic living needs for an extended period of time. These services may be delivered at home by family, by visiting health care agencies, or within institutions. In many states, alternative settings of long-term care are growing rapidly, such as assisted-living facilities and elder care communities (see Chapters 11 and 12).

The baby boomer generation is expected to be unlike prior generations. They are used to being in charge, were raised during the information age, and are likely to not accept the status quo of their grandparents. To accommodate expectations and the changing needs of the next generations, the health care system will need to undergo a transformation. One of the greatest shifts in long-term care culture is currently occurring within the nursing home setting.

Nursing homes are an integral component of the broad array of long-term care services available to elderly Americans and are a part of the primary care continuum. Traditionally, however, the nursing home industry has received a tremendous amount of negative attention in well-documented cases of poor quality of patient care. To combat the negative perceptions of the public, many nursing homes are undergoing a culture change. This shift focuses more attention on the needs of the residents, improvement of patient care, and the creation of a more homelike environment. To accomplish this culture shift, many nursing homes have aligned with academic medical centers, allied health agencies, and community hospitals.

In addition to the challenge of improving perceptions of the industry, nursing homes are combating a shortage of staff available to provide direct patient care and reductions in reimbursement from funding sources such as Medicare and Medicaid. Given the high incidence of chronic health needs in old age and the increasing numbers of older adults projected in the future, costs of long-term care are one of the most critical and controversial policy issues facing our nation. The baby boomers' expectations and needs will have a tremendous impact on the future of long-term care.

PROVIDERS OF GERIATRIC CARE

Formal health care services for older persons are provided by many different types of providers. All clinicians see older persons; even pediatric clinicians assist older persons when they see children brought in by grandparents. Hence, there is ample justification to expect all health care providers to have substantial geriatrics training. A description of geriatric care provided by each member of the multidisciplinary team is beyond the scope of this chapter so our attention will be turned to care provided by primary care providers: physicians, nurse practitioners (NPs), and physician assistants (PAs).

> ● Successful primary care for the frail/complex older adult is based both on a special knowledge set and on a philosophy of care.

PRIMARY CARE

Primary care providers are those clinicians who provide first-contact services that are of a continuous and comprehensive nature. In addition, the primary care provider also serves to coordinate the often complex network of other specialty care providers. Specialty care providers, such as those in ophthalmology and orthopedics, may have practices in which the majority of their patients are elders, but they would not be considered primary care geriatric providers because the services are focused and condition specific. The primary care provider is prepared to address the complete range of patient needs, from routine health promotion and disease prevention to chronic disease care, transient hospitalization, long-term care, and end-of-life care.

Older persons have higher rates of health care utilization than do younger people. Usually about 20% of a family physician's practice and 30% of an internist's practice involve visits by older persons.[14] Because most older people are reasonably healthy, especially those in the 65- to 74-age group, the practice of providing primary care in many practices is often conducted in a manner similar to that used with younger persons. However, when providing care to frail elders and those with multiple, interacting complex medical problems, a different approach is required.

Some family physicians, internists, NPs, and PAs choose to specialize in caring for older persons. Additional training in a fellowship program may lead to recognition of this special skill set with a certification. The American Geriatrics Society recognizes geriatricians as providing both primary care and consultative services.[15] The percentage of older patients in the practices of such providers may be as high as 100%. However, because of relatively low Medicare reimbursement rates and "adverse selection" (such practices have very high percentages of very frail and complex elders who require a great deal of care), clinicians usually are involved in other activities such as being medical directors of nursing homes or geriatric service line directors for hospitals.

The approach to providing primary care to the frail/complex older adult is based both on a special knowledge set and on a philosophy of care. The knowledge set extends beyond the basic aspects of proper diagnosis and treatment of medical maladies. It encompasses how diseases present differently in old age and how different conditions interact with one another to make treatment much more complex. Because medications play such an important role in the medical management of disease and because they can present many risks in old age, an up-to-date knowledge of changes seen in pharmacodynamics and pharmacokinetics is necessary. In addition, strategies for reducing polypharmacy are used. Finally, knowledge of rehabilitation is needed as many of the common diseases affect the older person's ability to function.

> ● Treatment decisions should be evaluated in terms of the potential benefit of enhancing or maintaining function versus the potential risk of causing a loss of independence.

Geriatrics as a Philosophy of Care

Just as important as the specialized knowledge base is an understanding of the philosophical basis of geriatric care. In younger adults, reducing premature mortality is the chief objective. As people age, especially after age 75, maintaining independent functioning becomes a much greater concern than is mortality for most people. In some studies, the fear of death among older adults falls below reported fears of becoming dependent on others for daily care needs, being a burden on their family, or having to go to a nursing home. Almost a third of elders report they would rather die than live permanently in a nursing home. Every intervention, or a decision not to intervene, should be evaluated in terms of its potential benefit of enhancing or maintaining function versus the potential risk of causing a loss of independence.

This philosophical approach can affect every decision made in medical care with an older person. In deciding to treat hypertension, a condition that itself causes no functional impairment but if untreated can lead to one of the most serious causes of loss of function (a stroke), one must consider the effects of the prescribed medications on daily living or whether the cost of the drug could impair the person's ability to spend needed money on other important aspects of life, such as food or transportation costs. In caring for an older person with dysphagia after a stroke, a consultant may speak of the insertion of a percutaneous enterostomal gastric (PEG) tube as a "minor procedure." In some older persons, such continued nutritional support may be just what is required to assist them through a period of decreased intake so they can participate in rehabilitation and recover lost function. But in individuals with such serious deficits that they are not likely to recover independent function, the very same treatment may not be desired at all.

> ● The diversity in experiences and desires among older adults makes it unlikely that clinicians can accurately predict a patient's approach to treatment decisions.

Ethical Decision Making

The functional approach to geriatric care is intricately tied to ethical decision making. There is much that we *can* do in medicine, but the key question in geriatric care is what we *should* do. The primary care geriatric clinician needs to be skillful in discussing such questions with older patients. The vast diversity in experiences and desires seen in older persons makes it unlikely that clinicians can accurately decide in advance what a patient will request. Studies have shown that physicians, nurses, social workers, and even family members have no better than a chance likelihood of correctly predicting what medical decisions an elderly person will make. The only way to determine the patient's desires is to ask the patient, if he or she understands (see Chapter 8).

On one hand, some may see this requirement as a stumbling block in the complex process of trying to provide care to older persons. On the other hand, some may view it as an opportunity to enhance one of the most important functions we all desire—the right to control our own destiny. Many of the losses associated with advanced age can not be corrected. If an older adult remains cognitively intact, even after becoming physically dependent, the ability to make a personal choice about the care received provides an important level of independence and control.

This approach requires an understanding of the patient's values. Different people may have markedly different values regarding health care choices and interventions. One individual may view the development of a serious condition as a special opportunity to allow loved ones to care for him or her. Another may view the very same condition as an extreme burden on the family. Geriatric clinicians need to be aware of their own values toward disease and disability. If not aware, the clinician risks the possibility of communicating a lack of acceptance of, or even disfavor with, the patient's choices.

Patient-centered Care

Patient-centered care is fundamental to primary care geriatrics (Box 1-2). The clinician can utilize the questions in the acronym *FIFE* to explore the meaning and impact of changes in the patient's life:

F = Feelings, especially specific fears and hopes—"Do you have any specific fears or concerns that we should know about?" "What hopes do you have?"

I = Ideas about what is going on—"What do you think is the main problem?" "What do you think needs to be done?"

F = Function, specifically impact on functioning—"How is your illness affecting daily activities?" "Are there things you want to do that you cannot do?"

E = Expectations—"What are your expectations—of the disease process, of yourself, of others, of caregivers, of me?"[16]

Box 1–2	Components of Patient-Centered Care

Exploring the disease and the illness experience
Understanding the whole person
Finding common ground regarding management
Incorporating prevention and health promotion
Enhancing the doctor/patient relationship
Being realistic

Working with older persons provides the geriatric clinician with the opportunity to develop greater self-awareness about many facets of life. Most clinicians do not share the conditions that they treat in their patients. Oldage, as Maurice chevalier said, "is not so bad, when you consider the alternatives." When caring for older persons, one has the opportunity to witness how people cope with repeated adversities, how families come to the aid of their loved ones, how certain people delve deep into spiritual realms to sustain them, and how one can lead a fulfilling and dignified life in the face of disease or disability.

● Ageism is the unfair judging of elderly adults simply because of their advanced age.

RECOGNIZING AND AVOIDING AGEISM

Older individuals are affected in unique ways by the combined effects of the normal aging process, disease processes, lifestyle, and environment.[17] Perceptions regarding the aging process and providing care for the elderly population vary from individual to individual. Many Americans are prejudiced against elders in multiple ways, and health care providers may be also share these beliefs. Ageism refers to the unfair judging of elderly adults simply because of their advanced age. This stereotyping can be so prevalent in society that it is almost invisible, but it can perpetuate negative attitudes that influence behaviors.[18,19] Reversible causes of problems such as memory loss, incontinence, and immobility are often overlooked because of a misconception that they are an unavoidable part of aging. Evidence exists to suggest that the lack of appropriate care for elderly has eroded the quality of care provided to older Americans.[20]

Caring for older persons, however, is one of the most challenging and exciting areas of health care, combining the biological, psychological, and social changes associated with aging. Working with older patients gives geriatric health care providers the opportunity to make a difference in the lives of the patients and their families and can be extremely rewarding for the provider. Geriatricians have the highest rate of satisfaction among all medical specialists.[21] The aging of America provides an impetus and opportunity to confront ageism or knowledge deficits in geriatric care that will positively impact the care of all older Americans.

● Effective care of the older adult is highlighted by collaboration between multiple health care providers.

FUTURE TRENDS

Collaborative Practice

Effective care of the older adult is highlighted by collaboration between multiple health care providers. The geriatric team is often a collaborative effort between a physician, NP, PA, social worker, psychologist, and various therapy specialties. In particular, NPs and PAs play a vital role in primary care for the older adult population. In a collaborative practice, there is a shared responsibility and accountability for the care of patients.

Collaboration includes both independent and cooperative decision making based on the training and ability of the practitioner. The need for trust and interdependence as a key to the success or failure of the partnership cannot be overemphasized.[22] Often collaborative practice will be seen in the form of a comprehensive geriatric assessment team, a geriatric consultant team, or a collaborative practice agreement that is individualized and agreed on between a NP and physician. Collaborating geriatric NPs and physicians have been shown to deliver high-quality primary care to frail nursing home residents, individuals in ambulatory care facilities, and individuals in hospitals.[23]

The numbers of NPs and PAs in training and in practice have increased dramatically. There is ongoing legislative activity in many states to expand the scope of practice for nonphysician providers and to ensure federal payment policy. The benefits of collaborative practice include improved access to care, reduction of costs for service, improved patient satisfaction, increased productivity, and improved quality of care.

Preventive Care

There is a long-standing myth that older adults do not respond to efforts that maintain or restore health; however, research has shown that health promotion and disease prevention activities are beneficial at any age. There is valid and justifiable argument that attention to health promotion activities can prevent, delay, and manage many chronic illnesses; decrease health care expenditures; and improve quality of life for older adults (see Chapter 5).

Modern health care demands early detection and prevention of illness and injury through functional rehabilitation, education, and the promotion of healthier lifestyles. Through the use of preventative care, outside of a traditional medical model, it is possible to promote a lifelong continuum of care. Health educators, fitness trainers, and elders can work together to improve quality of life, reduce risk of re-injury after trauma, and reduce overall health care costs. In this setting, physical therapists, athletic trainers, exercise physiologists, and nutritionists might work together as a team to develop an individualized program of rehabilitation, fitness, and preventive medicine. Areas of prevention might include heart disease, low back injury prevention, smoking cessation, and healthy eating and weight management.

> ● The current health care system is poorly designed to support clinicians in their efforts to care for patients with chronic diseases.

Chronic Disease Self-Management

The term chronic disease management (CDM) describes a system of care designed to improve patient outcomes and reduce costs associated with long-term, ongoing illnesses. A chronic care delivery model identifies the essential elements of a health care system that encourage high-quality chronic disease care. These elements are *the community*, *the health system*, *self-management support*, *delivery system design*, *decision support*, and *clinical information systems*. Attention to each element fosters productive interactions between informed patients who take an active part in their care and providers with resources and expertise.[24] The model can be applied to a variety of chronic illnesses, health care settings, and target populations.

The current health care system is poorly designed to support clinicians in their efforts to care for patients with chronic diseases. Also, patients with chronic conditions generally are not taught how to care for their own illnesses. During spring 2004, the Center for Medicare and Medicaid Services (CMS) released a request for proposal (RFP) inviting health care organizations to bid on chronic care improvement pilot projects. For the first time, outside of managed care, Medicare will provide coverage of disease assessment and care management for eligible Medicare beneficiaries. Many challenges to implementation have arisen and the program is still not in full demonstration at this time.

Improving the treatment of chronically ill patients begins with identifying high-risk patients. Priority chronic conditions include diabetes, asthma, congestive heart failure, coronary artery disease, and depression. Disease control and outcomes depend to a significant degree on the effectiveness of patient education and successful self-management. Effective self-management support includes acknowledging the patients' central role in their care, one that fosters a sense of responsibility for their own health. By using a collaborative approach, providers and patients work together to define problems, set priorities, establish goals, create treatment plans, and solve problems.[25] Educating and managing older patients with chronic conditions may be an effective way to improve outcomes and reduce health care costs.

Special Programs for Organizing, Funding, and Providing Geriatric Care

The complexity involved in providing comprehensive geriatric care has led to the development of a number of special programs to improve quality and reduce risks. Programs exist to provide comprehensive care to frail elders in order to prevent hospital and nursing home admission, to optimize care across different health care settings, and to enhance the quality of care (and reduce costs) of nursing home patients.

PROGRAM OF ALL-INCLUSIVE CARE OF THE ELDERLY

An example of a managed, capitated approach to improving the care for the frail elderly is the Program of All-inclusive Care of the Elderly (PACE). PACE was initiated by On Lok in San Francisco in the late 1970s. This comprehensive care program was designed to prevent placement of frail elders in nursing homes. In 1988, Congress approved a series of replication projects around the United States. By 1997, enough evidence and experience showed that the program was worth sustaining, and it was approved as a Medicare benefit by Congress. As of 2006, 41 PACE programs across the United States were caring for approximately 8000 "participants."

To be eligible for PACE enrollment, one must have been judged by the state long-term care system to be "nursing home eligible" and must be eligible for Medicare and Medicaid or willing to pay the Medicaid rate. Nursing home eligibility essentially is a functional dependency measurement, although the actual tool used to make the assessment varies by state. If the person chooses to enroll, he or she receives all of necessary care from the PACE program and pays no additional fees or copayments.[26]

An essential ingredient of the program is the integration of health care finances and health care services. The program serves as both the insurer and the provider. Primary care, home care, rehabilitation, day care, transportation, hospice care, mental health care, and pharmaceuticals are usually provided by the PACE interdisciplinary team. The program contracts with specialists, hospitals, laboratories, radiology providers, and nursing homes to provide those services, although usually it is the PACE primary care providers and other team members who deliver the professional care in those sites as well.

As opposed to multidisciplinary care, in which different care providers see the patient and communicate on paper or by electronic means, PACE provides interdisciplinary care. The team members regularly assess the participants (usually every 4 to 6 months), meet as a team and discuss care plans, and then meet with the participant and the family to reach final agreement. This regular, comprehensive review by a team is critical to preventing problems whenever possible and treating them early when prevention does not work.

PACE programs primarily focus on functional problems. Under traditional Medicare reimbursement requirements, providers caring for patients receiving rehabilitation services must be able to show that patients improvement in function. In frail patients, however, their chronic conditions may be resistant to rehabilitation interventions that are able to demonstrate such improvements. Rehabilitation designed to prevent decline (or maintain functional status) is not covered under traditional Medicare. Because PACE programs receive a capitated payment, they are able to apply resources to maintain the participants function without fear of not being reimbursed.

The two highest cost medical care components are hospital and nursing home care. PACE programs are able to expand the range of covered services and offer close patient oversight by reducing the utilization of these inpatient services. This is accomplished through effective use of preventive measures, early identification of treatable problems, and alternative methods for providing medical interventions that are effective but cost lower than hospital admission. For instance, a participant might receive daily antibiotic therapy in the clinic for an uncomplicated pneumonia. A participant may be admitted directly to a nursing home for a short rehabilitation stay. A participant attending the day health center for socialization may be noticed by an aide to "be acting funny" and then can be evaluated immediately in the adjacent clinic by the primary care clinician.

Another important feature of PACE care is regular attention to advance care planning. All PACE sites offer advance care planning and prospectively discuss the participants' wishes. In one study, such a process resulted in participants receiving the care they desired and not getting care they didn't want (cardiopulmonary resuscitation, artificial nutrition, and intravenous fluids) in 84% to 96% of cases.[27] In contrast, the SUPPORT study of hospitalized patients in academic medical centers demonstrated that less than 50% of persons received desired care despite an intervention designed to inform treating physicians of those wishes.[28]

Some concerns have been raised about prospective, capitated care. The obvious moral dilemma is the risk that the program will withhold needed care to save money (or make a profit). The concern is understandable but does not appear to be occurring. A large study of a matched population of PACE enrollees and a group who were found eligible for enrollment but chose to remain in a fee-for-service environment showed higher rates of satisfaction, better functional outcomes, more time spent in the community, more provision of rehabilitation aides, lower hospitalization rates, and a lower mortality rate in the PACE participants.[29] In addition, because the national disenrollment rate is less than 2%, it is unlikely that PACE programs are withholding desired care from their participants.

CARE TRANSITIONS

PACE and similar programs are currently available to a very small percentage of older adults. However, the principles of care developed in these innovative systems can be borrowed for wider use. Unfortunately, a common experience in the care of older persons in regular medical care settings is movement across different care sites without a single team that knows the person and follows him or her at each site. A patient may be admitted from home to the hospital, be discharged to a rehabilitation facility, then need a period of nursing home care, and finally return to home with home care services. The episode of care will involve four separate assessments, often without adequate communication between sites. The American Geriatrics Society produced a position paper on the necessary requirements for effective management of transitions in care[30] (Box 1-3).

Better communication can be facilitated by a standardized assessment instrument that is part of an electronic health record. Except in some systems, such as Kaiser Permanente or the Veterans Health Administration, such a development is still likely years away. The University of Colorado has developed a paper-based system that is managed by the patient or family.[31] This model is based on the fact that while

providers may change from site to site, the patient is the one constant across all transitions. Similar to the principles described above in chronic disease self-management training, having the patient educated and "in charge" will likely lead to fewer medication problems, more assurance of completion of treatments, and fewer mistakes. Studies are being conducted to measure the effectiveness of the program.

NURSING HOME–BASED PHYSICIAN–NURSE TEAMS

Nursing home–based primary care teams, comprised of physicians and NPs (or PAs), are used to manage complex patients in the skilled nursing facility.[32] The main goal of the care is to provide early recognition and intervention for those conditions that can be safely treated in the facility. Similar to PACE, cost savings from lower hospitalization rates are used to pay for increased primary care services delivered "at the bedside." Family meetings are held frequently to discuss care and provide deeper discussion into patient's wishes. End-of-life care can be more effectively coordinated, and advance directives can be completed. Large health maintenance organizations (HMOs) such as Kaiser piloted such teams. Another option that was available in 16 states in 2005 is EverCare.[33] EverCare is a commercial managed Medicare plan that contracts with CMS to provide HMO and preferred provider organization (PPO) care for nursing home residents. The use of NPs to provide improved continuity of care and intensive services in the nursing home is central to the EverCare model.

COMPREHENSIVE PRIMARY CARE

Some nonacademic health care systems have established comprehensive primary care geriatric practices.[34] The PeaceHealth Senior Health and Wellness

---

Box 1-3   Components of Effective Care Transitions

- Communication between the sending and receiving clinicians regarding:
  - A common plan of care
  - A summary of care provided by the sending institution
  - The patient's goals and preferences (including advance directives)
  - An updated list of problems, baseline physical and cognitive functional status, medications, and allergies
  - Contact information for the patient's caregiver(s) and primary care practitioner
- Preparation of the patient and caregiver for what to expect at the next site of care
- Reconciliation of the patient's medication prescribed before the initial transfer with the current regimen
- A follow-up plan for how outstanding tests and follow-up appointments will be completed
- An explicit discussion with the patient and caregiver regarding warning symptoms or signs to monitor which may indicate that the condition has worsened, plus the name and phone number of whom to contact if any of these occur

Center (SHWC) in Eugene, Oregon, provides primary care coordinated by geriatricians and an interdisciplinary office practice team that addresses the multiple needs of geriatric patients. This hospital outpatient clinic focuses on the care of frail elders with multiple interacting chronic conditions and management of chronic disease in the healthier older population. Based on the Chronic Care Model,[35] the SHWC strives to enhance coordination and continuity along the continuum of care, including outpatient, inpatient, skilled nursing, long-term care, and home care services. It uses a patient-centered approach to identify service needs. The model emphasizes team development, integration of evidence-based geriatric care, site-based care coordination, longer appointment times, utilization of an electronic medical record across care settings, and a prevention/wellness orientation. This collection of services addresses the interrelationships of all senior issues, including nutrition, social support, spiritual support, caregiver support, physical activity, medications, and chronic disease. The founders of this innovative program have developed a business model that attempts to improve access and quality of care to seniors in a mostly noncapitated health care setting, as well as attempts to remain financially viable.

SUMMARY

The aging of the population will mean that all primary care clinicians will spend a significant portion of their time providing care to older persons. Clinicians must be aware that the "older population" is very diverse and each patient is likely to present with special needs and challenges. Geriatric care involves both a specific knowledge base and a particular approach to problems. The foundation of that approach is attention to the patient's functional capabilities and an appreciation for the ethical questions that underlie all medical decisions. Because of the complexity involved in caring for this diverse population, interdisciplinary teams and special programs are often necessary.

References

1. U.S. Census Bureau. Dicennial Census and Projections. Washington, DC: U.S. Census Bureau, 2000.
2. U.S. Census Bureau. Population Estimates. Washington, DC: U.S. Census Bureau, 2002.
3. U.S. Census Bureau. Current Population Survey: Annual Social and Economic Supplement. Washington, DC: U.S. Census Bureau, 2004.
4. Administration on Aging. National Family Caregiver Support Program, Department of Health and Human Services, http://www.aoa.gov/prof/aoaprog/caregiver/carefam.asp, accessed 3/28/05.
5. Anderson G and Horvath J. The Growing Burden of Chronic Disease in America. Public Health Reports. 119(3): 263-270. 2004
6. Wallace SP, Levy-Storms L, Kington RS, Andersen RM. The persistence of race and ethnicity in the use of long-term care. J Gerontol B Psychol Sci Soc Sci. 1998;53(2):S104-12.
7. U.S. Census Bureau. Population Estimates and Projections. Washington, DC: U.S. Census Bureau, 2004.
8. Ham RJ, Goins RT, Brown DK. West Virginia University Center on Aging, 2003, www.hsc.wvy.edu/coa/.
9. U.S. Census Bureau. Current Population Survey: Annual Social and Economic Supplement. Washington, DC: U.S. Census Bureau, 2004.
10. Centers for Disease Control and Prevention [CDC], National Center for Health Statistics. Bethesda, MD: National Vital Statistics System, CDC, 2004.
11. Centers for Disease Control and Prevention, National Center for Health Statistics, National Vital Statistics System, 2004. Federal Interagency Forum on Aging-Related Statistics. Older Americans 2004: Key Indicators of Well-being. Washington, D.C.: U.S. Government Printing Office. November 2004.
12. Health and Retirement Study, 2004. Federal Interagency Forum on Aging-Related Statistics. Older Americans 2004: Key Indicators of Well-being. Washington, D.C.: U.S. Government Printing Office. November 2004.
13. Centers for Disease Control and Prevention [CDC], National Center for Health Statistics. Bethesda, MD: National Vital Statistics System, CDC, 2004.
14. U.S. Department of Health and Human Services, Public Health Service. National Ambulatory Medical Care Survey: 1998 Summary, Vital and Health Statistics no. 315, July 19, 2000.
15. Burton JR, Solomon DH. Geriatric medicine: a true primary care discipline. J Am Geriatr Soc 1993;41:459.
16. Gray GR. Teaching patient-centered care. Fam Med 2002;34:644-645.
17. Matteson MA and McConnell ES. Gerontological Nursing. Philadelphia: W.B. Saunders Company, 1988.
18. Grant LD. Effects of ageism on individual and health care providers' responses to healthy aging. Health Soc Work. 1996;21(1):9-15.
19. Tomkowiak J, Grunderson A. When Patients Teach Their Doctor: A Curriculam for Geriatric Education. Educational Gerontology 2004;30(9):785-790.
20. Alliance for Aging research. Medical Never-Never Land: ten Reasons Why American is Not Ready for the Upcoming Age Boom. Washington, D.C. 2002.
21. Leigh JP, Kravitz RL, Schembri M, Samuels SJ, Mobley S. Physician career satisfaction across specialties. Arch Intern Med. 2002;162(14):1577-84.
22. Shires BW, Spector PM. The clinical nurse specialist and psychiatrist in joint practice. Perspect Psychiatr Care. 1993;29(4):21-4.
23. Mezey M and Ebersole P. The Future of Geriatric Medicine: A National Crisis Looms. Geriatric Nurses Vital to Care. Aging Today. http://www.asaging.org/at/at-220/Nurses.html. Accessed 3/25/05.
24. Wagner EH. Chronic disease management: what will it take to improve care for chronic illness? Eff Clin Pract. 1998;1(1):2-4.
25. Bodenheimer T, Lorig K, Holman H, Grumbach K. Patient self-management of chronic disease in primary care. JAMA. 2002;288(19):2469-75.
26. Eng C, Pedulla J, Eleazer PG, McCann R, Fox N. Program of All-Inclusive Care of the Elderly (PACE): an innovative model of integrated geriatric care and financing, J Am Geriatr Soc 1997;47:25-29.
27. Lee MA, Brummel-Smith K, Meyer J, Drew N, London M. Physician Orders for Life-Sustaining Treatment (POLST): outcomes in a PACE Progrram. J Am Geriatr Soc 2000;48:1219-1225.
28. The SUPPORT Principal Investigators. A controlled trial to improve care for seriously ill hospitalized patients: the Study to Understand Prognoses and Preferences for Outcomes and Risks of Treatments (SUPPORT), JAMA 1995;74:1591-1598.
29. Bodenheimer T. Long-term care for frail elderly people: the On Lok model. N Engl J Med 1999;341:1324-1328.
30. Coleman EA, Boult C. Improving the quality of transitional care for persons with complex care needs: Position statement of the American Geriatrics Society Health Care Systems Committee. J Am Geriatr Soc 2003; 51:556-557.
31. Coleman EA. Falling through the cracks: challenge and opportunities for improving transitional care for persons with continuous complex care needs. J Am Geriatr Soc 2003;51:549-555.
32. Farley DO, Zellman G, Ouslander JG, Reuben DB. Use of primary care teams by HMOs for care of long stay nursing home residents. J Am Geriatr Soc 1999;139-144.
33. Kane RL, Flood S, Bershadsky B, Keckhafer G. Effect of an innovative medicare managed care program on the quality of care for nursing home residents. Gerontologist 2004;44:95-103.
34. Stock R, Reece D, Casario L. Developing a comprehensive interdisciplinary senior health practice. J Am Geriatr Soc 2004;52:2128-2133.

CHAPTER 2

Clinical Implications of Normal Aging

Monica Stalworth and Philip D. Sloane

OBJECTIVES

Upon completion of this chapter, the reader will be able to:

- Describe the major biologic theories of aging and their effects on observed phenomena of human aging.

- Discuss and give examples of the following principles of aging: frailty, functional reserve, and the distinction between usual and successful aging.

- Identify and discuss common changes that occur with age in the following systems: musculoskeletal, skin, cardiovascular, respiratory, gastrointestinal, central nervous, special senses, and endocrine.

PRETEST

1. Which one of the following signs of aging occurs earliest in most adults?
    a. Difficulty reading fine print without glasses
    b. Inability to stay up all night and work the next day
    c. Radiologic evidence of osteoarthritis of the spine
    d. Intense awareness that life is limited ("midlife crisis")
    e. Fixed wrinkling around the mouth

2. Which of the following statements is true about individuals at age 80 years?
    a. Vibratory sensation is equally reduced in distal and proximal joints.
    b. More than half of older persons report trouble sleeping at night.
    c. Renal perfusion is 75% to 80% of its value at age 30 years.
    d. Fewer than half of couples have been affected by death or disability of one or both spouses.

3. Which one of the following symptoms referable to the urogenital system is commonly reported by older women?
    a. Increased vaginal mucus
    b. Reduced urinary frequency
    c. Vaginal bleeding
    d. Incontinence

Aging is a process of gradual and spontaneous change, resulting in maturation through childhood, puberty, and young adulthood and then decline through middle and late age. Senescence is the process by which the capacity for cell division, growth, and function is lost over time, ultimately leading to an incompatibility with life; that is, the process of senescence terminates in death. Aging has both the positive element of development and the negative element of decline. Senescence refers only to the degenerative processes that ultimately make continued life impossible.

In both aging and senescence, many physiologic functions deteriorate, but normal decline is not usually considered the same as ailment. Mild cognitive changes do occur with progressive aging and are considered normal; however, cognitive decline consistent with dementia, although usual in late life, is considered an illness.

Martha Hilliard Robinson (Part I)

CHILDHOOD AND YOUNG ADULTHOOD

Martha Hilliard Robinson was born on January 10, 1898, in the small rural community of Tarboro in eastern North Carolina. She had three older brothers, and her father owned a hog farm. Taking unusually well to "book learning," she was the first member of her family to complete high school. After graduation, Martha persuaded her father to allow her to attend Roth School of Nursing in Durham, North Carolina.

In the wave of patriotism after war was declared, Martha enlisted as an army nurse. She was sent to Base Hospital Number 165, north of

Paris. There she met her first husband, Gerald Anthony Hilliard, a 27-year-old army physician from Raleigh who "had a gift for putting anyone at ease." Martha and Dr. Hilliard fell in love in France but decided to postpone marriage. Martha did not want to anger her father, who was furious that she had enlisted in the army without his permission.

In 1918 Martha returned to Roth to complete her nursing education, and Dr. Hilliard resumed his appointment at Rex Hospital in Raleigh. They were married in 1920. Martha then worked for a private physician in Raleigh until she had a child, Gerald Junior. Thirteen months later, Jeremiah was born, and 2 years later, Martha had a third child, Rachel. Understandably, she did not consider returning to work. Her primary job was that of wife and homemaker, and wives of prominent physicians were expected to stay at home to care for the family.

Martha's life changed suddenly when Gerald Anthony Hilliard was killed on a rainy night in 1932. He had been returning home from the hospital when his car collided with a milk wagon, killing him instantly. Martha was 35 years old with three school-age children. Her father insisted that she move back to the family homestead in Tarboro, where she remained for 4 years. With her mother available to help care for the children, Martha resumed her nursing career by taking a part-time job in a local physician's office.

In 1936 Martha applied for a staff nurse position at Roth Hospital because she "believed in what Roth was doing." Roth provided nearly three fourths of all free bed-care furnished to the destitute sick white citizens of Durham County (there was a separate black hospital at that time). Three months after Martha began working at Roth, her children joined her.

During 1936 Martha met her second husband, Benjamin Robinson, III, an attorney. She had retained his services because of a problem with her first husband's death benefit. She was determined that the government not reduce her widow's pension, especially because she had three dependent children. She and Benjamin Robinson were married in 1939 and remained together until his death in 1981, when Martha was 83.

STUDY QUESTION

1. How would knowledge of Mrs. Robinson's early life history have assisted a physician in providing sensitive, appropriate care for an acute illness at age 90 years?

There is increasing evidence that the black box we have referred to as "biologic aging" is composed of genetic factors and many types of environmental exposures. Some of the most potentially modifiable elements are those attributable to disuse or insufficient exposure to certain kinds or intensities of physical stressors during the course of the life span. Preventive actions targeting community-dwelling frail older people will be increasingly important with the growing number of very old and, thereby also frail, people.

Traditionally, the aging process, including the development of physical frailty toward the end of life, has been considered to be physiological and inevitable. Recently, it has become evident that stereotypes of aging as an irreversible process of decline and loss are not correct. The overarching goal should be "an increase in years of healthy life with a full range of functional capacity at each stage of life" (Table 2-1). Such a compression of morbidity can often be achieved through lifestyle measures, but a number of aspects of the aging process invite the development of "routine" medical intervention programs in order to setback the aging process and to permit us to live for a longer period in a relatively intact state.

● Functional problems in the elderly often have multiple causes.

| Table 2–1 | Life Expectancy and Number of Remaining Years Free of Dependency in Activities of Daily Living |||

Age, Years	Life Expectancy[a], Average		Disability-Free Years Remaining	
	Men	Women	Men	Women
65-69	13	20	9	11
70-74	12	16	8	8
75-79	10	13	7	7
80-84	7	10	5	5
≥85	7	8	3	3

[a]For independent noninstitutionalized elderly men and women in Massachusetts. Longevity and disability-free longevity are surprisingly long and must be incorporated into treatment decisions. All figures rounded to nearest year.

From Katz S, Branch LG, Branson MH, et al: Active life expectancy, *N Engl Med* 309:1218-1824, 1983.

A physician seeing Mrs. Robinson for an episode of pneumonia or diverticulitis at age 92 years might not immediately appreciate the independence and self-reliance that she has demonstrated through her earlier life experiences. Her background in nursing, if known by her physician, would call for a more sophisticated level of communication about her illness than would be used with a poorly educated former laborer, for example.

Martha Hilliard Robinson *(Part II)*

At age 46, Martha Robinson told her new family physician, Dr. Hensley, that she was worried about "getting decrepit." Dr. Hensley took each complaint seriously; Mrs. Robinson liked that. When his evaluation was complete, he explained each concern in language she understood, reassured her that her general health was excellent, and told her what she could do to stay healthy.

He explained that the bright red spots on her abdomen, which had become prominent over the past 10 years, were benign cherry angiomata clumps of blood vessels that commonly arise when a patient is in his or her 30s or 40s. He explained that the wrinkles around her eyes were normal by age 40; he called them "smile marks." He advised her, however, to avoid sun exposure, which accelerates wrinkling. He explained that her occasional right knee pain was osteoarthritis that had set in early because that knee had been injured playing baseball as a teenager. Finally, he explained that her problems reading fine print were also normal and caused by the lens of each eye losing its ability to change shape. He advised her to be fitted for reading glasses.

USUAL VERSUS SUCCESSFUL AGING

There is substantial disparity in the effects of aging on healthy individuals, with some persons exhibiting extensive alteration in physiological functions with age and others little or none. It has been suggested that it might be useful to differentiate between *usual* and *successful* patterns of aging.[1] Genetic factors, lifestyle, and societal investments in a safe and healthful environment are important aspects of successful aging. Normal aging includes the collective set of diseases and impairments that characterize aging for many of the elderly. Successful (healthy) aging refers to a process by which deleterious effects are minimized, preserving function until senescence makes continued life impossible. The concept of successful aging is that aging is not necessarily accompanied by debilitating disease and disability. For example, the elderly may be able to avoid the complications of vascular disease, even while the circulatory system continues to age, by controlling blood glucose levels and body fat percentage.

Centenarians are persons who have escaped major common diseases, cancers included, and have reached the extreme limits of the human life span. Thus, they are the best example of successful aging. Demographic and epidemiological studies indicate that frequency and mortality for cancer level off at around 85 to 90 years of age, followed by a plateau, or even a decline, in the last decades of life. It is reasonable to infer that centenarians are people endowed with an atypical resistance to cancer. The genetic basis of this situation is poorly understood.

Relatively early in Mrs. Robinson's adulthood, occasional osteoarthritic pain developed in her right knee, which had been injured when she was a teenager. That joint became an important source of physical impairment later in life.

Frailty

Age-related disability is characterized by generalized weakness, impaired mobility and balance, and poor endurance (Box 2-1). In the oldest old, this state is

---

BOX 2-1 Frailty Syndrome

Outcomes

Prolonged or repeated hospitalizations	Prolonged or limited recoveries

Proximate causes

Multiple comorbid conditions	Falls/fractures

Intermediate causes

Loss of organ system reserve	Prolonged reaction time
	Loss of strength
Polypharmacy	Poor vision
	Osteoporosis

Initial causes

Changes in endocrine function

called physical frailty, which is defined as a state of reduced physiological reserves associated with increased susceptibility to disability. Clinical correlates of physical frailty include falls, fractures, impairment in activities of daily living, and loss of independence. It is hypothesized that a rapid decline of functional condition may follow even minor perturbations of physiological homeostasis in frail persons. The same perturbation would cause only negligible or transient illness in a healthy person. Interventions for disability prevention are considered most likely to be cost-effective when targeted to frail older persons.

Loss of muscle strength is a significant factor in the process of frailty. Muscle weakness can be caused by aging of muscle fibers and their innervation, osteoarthritis, and chronic debilitating diseases. A sedentary way of life and decreased physical activity and disuse are also important determinants of the decline in muscle strength. In a study of 100 frail nursing home residents (average age, 87 years), lower-extremity muscle mass and strength were closely related. Supervised resistance exercise training (for 45 minutes three times per week for 10 weeks) doubled muscle strength and significantly increased gait velocity and stair-climbing power.[2] This demonstrates that frailty in the elderly is not an irreversible effect of aging and disease but can be reduced and perhaps even prevented. Prevention of frailty can be achieved by exercise.

> ● The organ system usually associated with a particular symptom is less likely to be the source of that symptom in older individuals than in younger ones.

Martha Hilliard Robinson
(Part III)

Mrs. Robinson was at the peak of her professional career at age 60. She had moved to Raleigh to become dean of the College of Nursing at Mercy Hospital. She recognized that her stamina had diminished, however, and she became fatigued particularly during out-of-town business trips. Routines had become important to maintain her energy. She exercised daily, and she was always in bed by 9:30 p.m. She also noticed trouble reading in dim light and was frequently bothered by knee pain, especially when walking long distances or on stairs.

During the decade that followed, Mrs. Robinson's knee continued to be her biggest health problem. She stopped using the stairs, moved to a one-story house, changed her evening walks to avoid a downward

grade, and frequently had pain at night. She took increasing doses of acetaminophen, occasionally with codeine, for pain. She began using a cane whenever she went outside the house. Her daily walks were replaced by swimming three times a week at the neighborhood pool.

At age 68, Mrs. Robinson saw Dr. Hensley because of vaginal bleeding after intercourse. He prescribed an estrogen cream, and the problem soon resolved. She was now retired and traveled frequently with her husband, Benjamin.

At age 72, she was placed on a diuretic for elevated blood pressure, which she attributed in part to her husband's heart attack the previous year.

STUDY QUESTIONS

1. To what extent are the above changes noted by Mrs. Robinson likely to be attributed to normal aging?
2. To what extent are the above changes noted by Mrs. Robinson likely to be attributed to disease?
3. To what extent are the above changes noted by Mrs. Robinson likely to be attributed to disuse or deconditioning?
4. List 10 environmental adjustments that may enhance the independence of an older person with severe osteoarthritis of the knee.

MAINTENANCE OF HOMEOSTASIS

Because of decreased physiological reserve, older patients frequently develop symptoms at an earlier stage of their disease. Homeostatic strain caused by onset of a new disease often leads to symptoms associated with a different organ system, compromised by subclinical disease. For example, heart failure may be precipitated by mild hyperthyroidism, cognitive dysfunction by urinary tract infection, and nonketotic hyperosmolar coma by mild glucose intolerance.

Drug side effects can occur in older adults with drugs and drug doses unlikely to produce side effects in younger people. For instance, a sedating antihistamine (e.g., diphenhydramine) may cause confusion, digoxin may induce depression, and over-the-counter sympathomimetics may precipitate urinary retention in men with mild prostatic obstruction.

The predisposition to develop symptoms at an earlier stage of disease or with medication use is often offset by two factors. First, symptoms may present soon after if there is functional inadequacy in another system. Ischemic heart disease or congestive heart failure may not cause symptoms as early in patients whose mobility is compromised by arthritis. Second, because debility is accepted as normal for our older population and disability and illness are accepted as normal consequences of aging, the elderly are less likely to seek attention until symptoms become disabling. Therefore, any symptom, particularly with a change in functionality, must be taken seriously and evaluated swiftly.

> ● Drug side effects can occur with drugs and drug doses unlikely to produce side effects in younger people.

THEORIES OF BIOLOGIC AGING

Aging clearly occurs at dissimilar rates for different species and at different rates among individuals. By inference it appears that aging must be genetically controlled, at least to some extent. Both within and between species, lifestyle and exposures may alter the aging progression. Most gerontologists consider senescence as a group of degenerative entropic processes linked only by the fact that they occur over time. Some theories of aging address what controls these processes and why the controls exist as they do. Other theories of aging focus on the issues of whether senescence is more programed, rather than random entropy, thus offering some advantage for a species. For instance, senescence may have evolved to increase the rate at which adaptive mutations are introduced.

Cellular and Molecular Aging

Cells lose their capacity to divide over time unless they become cancerous. This limit to cellular replicative competence (Hayflick's limit or phenomenon) can be demonstrated in fibroblasts removed from the umbilical cord of newborns and cultured in vitro. Fibroblasts removed from aged persons tend to divide a lesser number of times. Telomeres are stretches of DNA at the end of chromosomes that act as handles by which chromosomes are moved in the course of the telophase of meiosis. Telomeres are irrevocably shortened each time a cell divides. When the telomeres become too short, the cell can no longer divide. In transformed (e.g., cancerous) cells, the enzyme telomerase lengthens telomeres after telophase. The telomeres of transformed cells do not shorten after each division, and thus, the cells become immortal, dividing far beyond Hayflick's limit.

Necrosis and apoptosis

Cell death may occur by necrosis or apoptosis. Necrosis is due to physical or chemical insults (e.g., metabolic inhibition, ischemia) that overwhelm normal cellular progression and make the cell nonviable. In necrosis, loss of ion gradients across the cell membrane leads to an incursion of calcium and other ions, which initiates proteolysis and break down of the organelle membranes. Necrosis is an entirely entropic event due to loss of the cell's capacity to transform external energy.

In contrast, apoptosis is a decidedly regulated, orderly process by which a cell in effect commits suicide. The stimulus for apoptosis is a physiologic sign or a very mild insult. A significant feature of apoptosis is the fragmentation of the cell's DNA, produced by a regulated activation of deoxyribonuclease. However, numerous other biochemical processes that also lead to cell death are concurrently induced. Apoptosis is vital for normal growth and remodeling. Apoptosis has been thought to contribute to several age-related ailments, including Alzheimer's disease. Whether age-related cell death is due primarily to necrosis or to apoptosis affects whether aging is considered the outcome of entropic processes (if due primarily to necrosis) or of comparatively simpler, more regulated processes.

Three theories of aging that remain actively investigated, include[3]:

"Free Radical" Theory

This theory proposes that an entropy-producing agent—free radicals—gradually disrupts cellular macromolecular constituents. Theoretically, free radicals, generated during oxidative phosphorylation, can variously alter macromolecules, mainly through oxidation. Evidence suggests that oxidative injury increases with age. Certain oxidized derivatives of nucleotides from DNA amplify in frequency.

"Glycosylation" Theory

This theory proposes that glycosylation can create modified proteins that accumulate and cause dysfunction with aging. Experimental evidence that rats on low calorie diets have lower blood glucose levels, accumulate fewer proteins, and may live longer lends some theoretical support for this theory.

Ultraviolet Light–Induced DNA Damage

This theory proposes that the ability to repair ultraviolet (UV) light damage to DNA may be related to life span.

Martha Hilliard Robinson
(Part IV)

Two months after her 78th birthday, Mrs. Robinson fell and broke her right wrist. She had been taking the garbage out to the compost pile in her backyard (a habit from her childhood days on the farm). It was dark, and she did not notice a piece of gravel on the uneven ground. "My ankle twisted, and I wasn't able to catch myself," she explained. Thinking back, she remembered that she had tripped several other times in the backyard since purchasing the house 14 years before, but this was the first time she had fallen.

Dr. Hensley felt that the accident might be a result of normal aging changes, but he followed up the incident with a thorough health evaluation. He noted that Mrs. Robinson had difficulty performing tandem gait but could maintain a standing position with her eyes closed (Romberg's test). Her heart, lungs, and kidneys were fine. Her right knee was considerably larger than the left knee, without an effusion, and a 10-degree flexion contracture was evident. Quadriceps, hip abductors, and hip extensors were all weak on the right side.

Laboratory test results included a hematocrit of 41%, a blood urea nitrogen of 14 mg/dl, a creatinine of 1.1 mg/dl, and a cholesterol level of 234 mg/dl. Radiograph of her right wrist showed moderate osteoporosis and a displaced Colles' fracture. Her audiogram showed bilateral high-frequency hearing loss, consistent with presbycusis.

Although he could not be certain that her severe knee osteoarthritis had caused Mrs. Robinson's fall, Dr. Hensley believed that it was the major treatable contributing factor. He arranged for her to see an orthopedic surgeon about a knee replacement. Several months later, Mrs. Robinson had the surgery. She worked hard to regain her strength and mobility during postoperative rehabilitation. By 6 months after surgery, her knee mobility and strength were markedly improved and she was pain free.

STUDY QUESTION

1. When an elderly patient is noted to have a functional problem such as weakness, recurrent falls, incontinence, or confusion, what general approach should the physician use to identify the relative contributions of disease, disuse, and normal aging to the problem?

COMMON LABORATORY TESTS AND AGING

Distinguishing true physiologic effects of aging from disease and disuse has also proven difficult in the area of laboratory testing. It appears, however, that most laboratory values change little, if at all, in normal healthy elderly. These include hematocrit, white cell count, electrolytes, calcium, thyroxine (T_4), and thyroid-stimulating hormone (TSH). Notable exceptions are postprandial blood sugar, serum cholesterol in women, sedimentation rate, and serum tri-iodothyronine, or T_3 (because peripheral thyroxine [or T_4] is converted at lower rates in the elderly). Brain natriuretic peptide (BNP) level is a relatively new laboratory test used primarily in management of congestive heart failure. BNP tends to have higher levels in the elderly primarily owing to underlying renal insufficiency. Renal adjustments for several frequently used laboratory tests need to be adjusted at higher baseline levels owing to age-related renal function decline seen in the elderly.[4]

ORGAN SYSTEM CHANGES WITH AGING

Table 2-2 summarizes selected age-related changes and their physiologic consequences.

Skin Changes

The most visible signs of aging consist of changes in the skin and hair. Wrinkling, sagging of subcutaneous support, hair loss and graying, and a variety of benign and malignant skin conditions increase with frequency as individuals age. Many such changes occur more rapidly in fair-skinned persons and are accelerated by sun exposure.[5] Although the pace varies, the sequence of changes is relatively uniform: sagging of lateral aspects of the eyebrows, wrinkling of the forehead, horizontal skin lines at the lateral canthus of the eye, sagging of the tip of the nose, perioral wrinkling, and fat absorption of the buccal and temporal areas. Microscopic changes visible in aged skin include epidermal thinning, degeneration of the elastic fibers providing dermal support, thickening of collagen fibers in the dermis (often with pseudoscar formation), reduction in the numbers of sweat and sebaceous glands, and reduction in skin flow because of diminished vascularity.

Case Discussion

Mrs. Robinson's fall illustrates the principle that functional problems in the elderly tend to have multiple causes. Physiologic studies demonstrate that dark adaptation declines with age, so Mrs. Robinson's vision was somewhat impaired as she walked to the compost pile. Furthermore, reaction times are slower, so she probably had more difficulty righting herself when she lost her balance. In addition, a disease process, osteoarthritis of the knee, had caused further impairment, leading to

Table 2–2 | Selected Age-Related Changes and their consequences

Organ/System	Age-Related Physiologic Change[a]	Consequences of Age-Related Physiologic Change	Consequences of Disease, Not Age
General	↑Body fat ↓Total body water	↑Volume of distribution for fat-soluble drugs ↓Volume of distribution for water-soluble drugs	Obesity
Eyes/ears	Presbyopia Lens opacification ↓High-frequency acuity	↓Accommodation ↑Susceptibility to glare Need for increased illumination	Blindness
Endocrine	Impaired glucose homeostasis ↓Thyroxine clearance (and production) ↑ADH, ↓renin, and ↓aldosterone ↓Testosterone ↓Vitamin D absorption and activation	↑Glucose level in response to acute illness ↓T_4 dose required in hypothyroidism Osteopenia	Diabetes mellitus Thyroid dysfunction ↓Na^+, ↑K^+ Impotence Osteomalacia, fracture
Respiratory	Decreased cough reflex ↓Lung elasticity and ↑chest wall stiffness Decreased DL_{CO}	Microaspiration Ventilation/perfusion mismatch and ↓PO_2 Decreased resting PO_2	Aspiration pneumonia Dyspnea, hypoxia Dyspnea
Cardiovascular	↓Arterial compliance and ↑systolic BP →LVH ↓β-Adrenergic responsiveness ↓Baroreceptor sensitivity and ↓SA node automaticity	Hypotensive response to ↑HR, volume depletion, or loss of atrial contraction ↓Cardiac output and HR response to stress Impaired blood pressure response to standing, volume depletion	Syncope Heart failure Heart block
Gastrointestinal	↓Hepatic function ↓Gastric acidity ↓Colonic motility ↓Anorectal function	Delayed metabolism of some drugs ↓Ca^{2+} absorption on empty stomach Constipation	Cirrhosis Osteoporosis, vitamin B_{12} deficiency Fecal impaction Fecal incontinence
Hematologic/ immune system	↓Bone marrow reserve (?) ↓T-cell function ↑Autoantibodies	 False-negative PPD response False-positive rheumatoid factor, antinuclear antibody	Anemia Autoimmune disease
Genitourinary	Vaginal/urethral mucosal atrophy Prostate enlargement	Dyspareunia, bacteriuria ↑Residual urine volume	Symptomatic UTI Urinary incontinence; urinary retention
Musculoskeletal	↓Lean body mass, muscle ↓Bone density	Functional impairment Osteopenia	 Hip fracture
Nervous system	Brain atrophy ↓Brain catechol synthesis ↓Brain dopaminergic synthesis ↓Righting reflexes ↓Stage 4 sleep Impaired thermal regulation	Benign senescent forgetfulness Stiffer gait Body sway Early awakening, insomnia Lower resting temperature	Dementia, delirium, depression Parkinson's disease Falls Sleep apnea Hypothermia, Hyperthermia

T_4 indicates thyroxine; ADH, antidiuretic hormone; PO_2, partial pressure of oxygen (artery); DL_{CO}, diffusion capacity of carbon monoxide; BP, blood pressure; LVH, left ventricle hypertrophy; SA, sinoatrial; PPD, purified protein derivative; UTI, urinary tract infection.

[a]Changes generally observed in healthy elderly subjects free of symptoms and detectable disease in the organ system studies. The changes are usually important only when the system is stressed or other factors are added (e.g., drugs, disease, or environmental challenge); they rarely result in symptoms otherwise.

localized muscle atrophy and a mild contracture. One other physiologic factor certainly contributed to her injury: reduced bone mass in the wrist from osteoporosis. Despite all these physiologic limitations, Mrs. Robinson did well until an environmental factor, a stone on uneven ground, created a challenge to her physiologic reserves. Because of the multiple factors just cited and probably because of others as well, Mrs. Robinson was unable to prevent an injurious fall.

Aging and the Heart

In the resting aging heart, there are largely no alterations of systolic function, with preserved ejection fraction and stroke volume. The resting heart rate is unchanged or only minimally reduced with aging; cardiac output is also preserved. Aging alters cardiac responsiveness to β-adrenergic stimuli. Both the catecholamine- or exercise-induced increases in heart rate and myocardial contractility are definitely blunted in elderly subjects. Thus, for cardiac output to be increased in proportion to the body's metabolic needs despite inadequate contractile and chronotropic reserves, the aging left ventricle mainly engages the Frank-Starling mechanism.[6] It has been suggested that the heart of the elderly behaves like a younger heart subjected to beta-blocker treatment.

Several cardiovascular features of the elderly most likely depend on aging, but often impaired performance also results from various combinations of subclinical cardiovascular or noncardiovascular illnesses, for example, thyroid dysfunction, diabetes, and borderline hypertension. The situation is further complicated because age-related changes by no means consist of a uniform and generalized structural degeneration.

Aging and the Lung

A variety of physiologic changes in the lung with normal aging can lead to a decline in forced expiratory volume (FEV) and forced expiratory vital capacity (FVC), as well as an increase in residual volume. These changes result from reduced elasticity, decreased lung mass, chest wall stiffness, and decreased respiratory muscle strength. Airway ciliary action and the cough are less effective, increasing the risk for pulmonary infection.

Case Discussion

Of the laboratory values obtained by Mrs. Robinson's physician, the hematocrit is clearly normal and should not change with age. The creatinine is in the high-normal range for that laboratory test. The test value probably represents significant reduction in creatinine clearance because creatinine clearance generally needs to be reduced by about half before the creatinine rises. Mrs. Robinson's serum cholesterol of 234 mg/dl is probably normal, given the rise in median cholesterol with age seen in healthy women. The relative importance of cholesterol values in older adults, particularly women, remains controversial.

Aging and the Kidney

In cross-sectional studies, creatinine clearance declines at a rate of 10 ml per decade. However, longitudinal studies have demonstrated that this decline is highly variable within older subgroups.[7] The use of medications with primary renal excretion requires caution in the very old. The older kidney demonstrates decreased sodium excretion and conservation, as well as decreased concentrating capacity.

Aging and the Gastrointestinal System

The older stomach has mild decrease in stomach acid production. Colonic contractions are less effective and contribute to symptoms of constipation. The liver size is decreased, as is liver blood flow. The CYP3A subfamily of the cytochrome P450 system is critical to the hepatic metabolism of many medications (e.g., calcium channel blockers, statins, benzodiazepines). CYP3A activity may be reduced by up to 50% in some older adults. These changes may lead to clinically significant changes in drug metabolism.

Martha Hilliard Robinson (Part V)

During her annual physical examination at age 84 by Dr. Hensley, Mrs. Robinson expressed concern about not being able to sleep. "I'm in bed by 9:00 p.m., read until 10:00 p.m., and generally fall asleep," she said. "But by 2:30 a.m. I'm likely to be awake. Often, but not always, I go to the bathroom. Then, if I fall asleep, I wake up again at 4:30 or 5:00 a.m. If only I could get a complete night's sleep!" With probing, Dr. Hensley was able to get Martha to talk about her husband's death of a stroke 8 months earlier. After determining that she was undergoing a normal adjustment to loss of a spouse, Dr. Hensley reassured her. He discussed the normal pattern of responses after losing a spouse. He also reviewed the physiology of sleep and emphasized that her sleep pattern was normal.

At a later visit, Mrs. Robinson expressed concerns about her memory. "I can't remember the names of people I ought to know—people I just met; people in church," she stated. "I find myself writing notes to remember what to buy, even if I'm only going to the store for three or four items. I'm worried I might have Alzheimer's disease. What do you think, doctor?"

STUDY QUESTIONS

1. How can a primary care physician effectively differentiate between benign forgetfulness and early dementia?
2. Is sleep disturbance normal or abnormal in older persons?

Aging and the Musculoskeletal System

Without regular physical exercise, usual aging will result in a loss of muscle fibers and a decrease in muscle mass. Decreasing bone mass occurs in both men and women. Osteoarthritis is associated with age, and by age 40 years, many adults have osteoarthritic changes visible in radiographs of the cervical spine. However, not every older person is equally affected, and in individuals not every joint is equally affected. Age-related physiologic changes combine with other factors to determine the extent of symptomatic disease.

> ● Functionally significant aging changes are especially common in the urinary, musculoskeletal, and neurologic systems and in the special senses.

Aging and the Endocrine System

Postprandial glucose tolerance is impaired with age (increased by 10 mg/dl per decade). Nocturnal growth hormone peaks are lost, and there is a marked decrease in dehydroepiandrosterone (DHEA). Aging of women starts with slow decreases of ovarian steroid production, followed by unexpected and almost complete termination of sex hormone production at menopause. Men do not experience universal absolute gonadal failure. Testicular androgen production declines gradually, with significant individual variability along with the aging course. There are multiple factors influencing testosterone levels in elderly men: genetics, environment, and socioeconomic state (diet, hygiene). Older men will experience a prolonged refractory period for erections. Men and women will experience reduced intensity of orgasms.

Aging and the Immune System

Aging is associated with a decline in cell-mediated immunity. The thymus gland atrophies with a loss of thymic hormones. These changes result in more nonresponders to vaccines and decreased delayed-type hypersensitivity. There is a decreased production of antibodies to specific antigens by B cells.[8]

Martha Hilliard Robinson (Part VI)

For her 90th birthday, Mrs. Robinson was interviewed for a feature by a reporter from the Durham Morning Star. An independently wealthy widow, Mrs. Robinson had donated an undisclosed sum of money to the Roth School of Nursing. At the interview her white hair was pulled back into a thin, neat bun; her posture was stooped; and she walked with the assistance of a four-pronged cane. She wore a hearing aid and an eye bandage, having recently undergone laser surgery on her left eye. Nevertheless, she continued to live alone in her one-story home, receiving homemaker services 3 hours a day. Her daughter, 15 miles away, assisted with transportation and shopping. A visiting nurse was coming daily to check on her eye but would discontinue services soon. The interviewer, a journalism graduate student from a local small college, had gone to considerable length to prepare for the interview. She had learned that Mrs. Robinson was somewhat hard of hearing and bothered by bright lights. She also knew that Mrs. Robinson preferred a morning interview, generally taking a nap and then visiting with friends in the afternoon.

"Based on your own experience," the interviewer asked, "is it better to let things go or to keep as active as possible?"

"A little of both, I guess," responded Mrs. Robinson. "I'm not as active as I used to be, but I still do as much as I feel able. I guess I'd say I pace myself. I'm an early riser, take my pills, do a few exercises, and have breakfast. Morning is my work time for shopping, writing letters, paying bills, seeing the doctor, or being interviewed by you. Two mornings a week I go to the senior center, where I'm in a bridge group. We use large-print playing cards."

Aging and the Nervous System

There is small decrease in brain mass with age, with an associated loss of neurons. Normal aging is associated with scattered neurofibrillary tangles and senile plaques, but in smaller numbers than seen in Alzheimer's disease. There is some slowing of central processing and reaction time, resulting in more difficulty recalling facts. In the peripheral nervous system, there is a decrease in vibratory sensation, especially in the feet. Changes in autonomic regulation result in a decrease in sweat production, resulting in an increased core temperature required to start sweating.[9]

Sensory Changes

VISION

Beginning in early adulthood, the ability of the lens to accommodate for near-vision gradually diminishes. Eventually the eye is no longer able to change the shape of the lens enough to focus on near objects, such as fine print. This gradual loss of lens elasticity, which is the most common age-related eye problem, is called presbyopia. By their 40s, most adults require reading glasses. By age 55 nearly all persons have great difficulty focusing on close objects without glasses.[10]

HEARING

Hearing loss is the third most common chronic condition in older adults. High-frequency hearing loss (presbycusis) is the most common form in this population. This type of hearing loss decreases the ability to interpret speech, which can lead to communication difficulties, increased isolation, and depression. Although most hearing loss in older adults is sensorineural, cerumen impaction and chronic otitis media may be present in up to 30% of this population.

SMELL AND THIRST

Smell detection decreases by 50%, resulting in changes in taste as well. Older adults retain the taste of sweetness but report a decline in the detection of saltiness. There is a decrease in the recognition of thirst.

Case Discussion

Healthy aging, as exemplified by Martha Hilliard Robinson, involved preparation, adaptation, and good fortune. Mrs. Robinson prepared for a healthy old age by adopting good health habits early in life. She did not overeat, did not smoke, exercised regularly, got plenty of sleep, married, and raised a family. Her lifestyle during older years involved routines of exercise, eating, rest, productive work, and socializing. All of these factors have been linked to longevity. Furthermore, she managed to enter old age relatively well off economically; the well-to-do live longer and remain healthier than the impoverished.

Despite entering old age with superior health habits and economic resources, Mrs. Robinson needed to adjust successfully to a variety of losses. She retired, her husband became ill and died, and she suffered from osteoarthritis, osteoporosis, and hearing impairment. In her case, successful adaptation involved being able to give up some activities and continue others. Thus she was able to continue to find meaning in life despite limitations and losses. She maintained a strong faith in God and a close attachment to her family, drawing strength from these in difficult times.

STUDY QUESTION

1. Mrs. Robinson had many advantages that helped her age gracefully. Identify some of the problems that a less advantaged person might face and what physicians can do to provide assistance in addressing each.

● Death and dying are a normal part of aging.

Martha Hilliard Robinson *(Part VII)*

At age 92, Mrs. Robinson suffered a stroke, which left her aphasic and unable to use her right hand. After rehabilitation, she was able to walk with a cane. She moved in with her daughter, whose care was supplemented by home health nursing. She died of pneumonia at age 94.

CASE DISCUSSION

Those like Mrs. Robinson, who have led a long, full life, often face death unafraid. Indeed, it is the period of dependency and disability that often accompanies the final years that older persons most often fear because it is often a difficult time for the older person and his or her family. Mrs. Robinson was fortunate to have a supportive daughter and physician and to die in relative comfort at home.

SUMMARY

Older Americans are not straightforwardly categorized. Their requirements and preferences are diverse and becoming more dissimilar. A useful appraisal of this population need not take an inordinate amount of time or occur as a single event to effectively prevent, or at least delay, many of their major causes of morbidity and mortality. Most functional loss later in life is related to specific disease processes and not to aging itself. Greater stress on disease prevention, as opposed to disease management, through appropriate screening, immunization, and healthy behaviors and lifestyle choices can significantly retard disability and death.

References

1. Rowe JW, Kahn RL. Successful aging. Gerontologist 1997;37:433-440.
2. Fiatarone MA, O'Neill EF, Ryan ND, et al. Exercise training and nutritional supplementation for physical frailty in very elderly people. N Engl J Med 1994;330:1769-1775.
3. Miller RA. When Will the biology of aging become useful? future landmarks in biomedical gerontology. J Am Geriatr Soc 1997;45:1258-1267.
4. Dybkaer R. Relative reference values for clinical, chemical, and haematological quantities in "healthy" elderly people. Acta Med Scand 1981; 209:1-9.

5. Gilchrest BA. Skin aging and photoaging. Dermatol Nurs 1990;2:79-82.
6. Lakatta EG. Cardiovascular regulatory mechanisms in advanced age. Physiol Rev 1993;73:413-467.
7. Lindeman RD, Tobin J, Shock NW. Longitudinal studies on the rate of decline in renal function with age. J Am Geriatr Soc 1985;33:278-285.
8. Fietta A, Merlini C, Dos Santos C, Rovida S, Grassi C. Influence of aging on some specific and nonspecific mechanisms of the host defense system in 146 healthy subjects. Gerontology 1994;40:237-45.
9. Kokmen E, Bossemeyer RJ, Barney J, Williams WJ. Neurological manifestations of aging. J Gerontol 1977;32:411-419.
10. Carter TL. Age-related vision changes: a primary care guide. Geriatrics 1994;49:37-42.

POSTTEST

1. Which of the following normal aging changes contributes to impaired night driving skills among 80-year-old individuals?
a. Reduced dark adaptation
b. 19% decrease in foot reaction time compared with young adults
c. 70% reduction in light reaching the retina
d. Reduced ability to hear approaching sirens
e. All of the above

2. Which one of the following statements is false about individuals aged 65 to 70 years?
a. Reported happiness is greater than at any other age.
b. Percentage of body fat is greater than at age 20.
c. They report less independence and more financial worries than do younger adults.
d. Sexual activity is correlated with physical health.

3. All of the following are true about normal aging except which one?
a. Established routines often constitute a helpful adjustment to aging.
b. Sensory impairments limit many older persons' ability to make friends.
c. Major disability is uncommon among older persons.
d. Worrying about memory loss is more often a symptom of normal aging than of Alzheimer's disease.

4. Mr. Carter, an 80-year-old retired engineer, is active in a bridge club, the local church, and a daily exercise class. His wife, on the other hand, spends the majority of her time either watching television (during cold days) or sitting on the front porch (during warm days). Which one of the following is false about this couple?
a. Mrs. Carter exemplifies the disengagement theory of successful aging.
b. Mr. Carter exemplifies the activity theory of successful aging.
c. Mr. Carter is likely to live longer than Mrs. Carter.
d. The continuity theory could apply to either spouse.

PRETEST ANSWERS
1. b
2. b
3. d

POSTTEST ANSWERS
1. b
2. c
3. c
4. c

Illness and Aging
Richard J. Ham

OBJECTIVES

Upon completion of this chapter, the reader will be able to:

- Describe typical ways in which the presentation of acute illness is modified in older patients, including cognitive and functional change as presentations.

- Recognize that some changes still widely accepted as "normal" in fact represent treatable or preventable illnesses (e.g., osteoporosis, memory loss, and joint pain), and how this influences presentation and management of chronic illnesses causing disability in old age.

- Define the multiple factors that inhibit presentation of older individuals for health care.

- Describe methods to improve communication both with and about older individuals, especially at times of change in the site of care.

- Outline how to reduce deconditioning, dysmobility, and immobility resulting from illness in old age, especially in the hospitalized or institutionalized patient.

- Describe the principles of prioritizing multiple concurrent problems of differing types.

PRETEST

1. Which of the following is *not* a characteristic presentation of illness in old age?
   a. Depression without sadness
   b. Infectious disease without leukocytosis
   c. Fever without cause
   d. Apathetic thyrotoxicosis
   e. Myocardial infarction without chest pain

2. Which one of the following statements is false concerning ways in which clinicians might "harm" older persons?
   a. The half-life of many medications is prolonged in healthy older people.
   b. Twenty percent of hospitalizations of older people are prolonged by a major adverse advent.
   c. Follow-up to assess the effect of prescriptions is often lacking.
   d. Communication between clinicians about patients often excludes consideration of the patient's functional level.
   e. Premature mobilization after illness increases fall risk.

3. Which one of the following aspects of a dependent older person has *not* been demonstrated to be a major stressor of the caregiving family member?
   a. The patient's ingratitude
   b. The use of multiple medications
   c. The patient's being awake at night
   d. The physical dependency of the patient

4. A 69-year-old black woman who works full-time and lives with her daughter has a lesion that she fears is cancerous. Four problems are defined at her brief visit. Which problem takes the highest priority?
   a. Blood pressure of 175/90
   b. Demonstrable stress incontinence
   c. Hearing difficulties: the patient can manage one on one
   d. The brown nevus on her anterior chest that has remained unchanged for several years

5. A 75-year-old woman is taking amitriptyline, isophane insulin suspension, digoxin, and a thiazide diuretic and has established diagnoses of congestive heart failure with left bundle branch block, diabetes mellitus, and depression. Which one of the following statements concerning the interactions between her diagnoses and treatments is *false?*
   a. The thiazide predisposes her to digoxin toxicity.
   b. The amitriptyline may be the cause of the bundle branch block.
   c. The hyperglycemia may be worsened by the diuretic.
   d. The digoxin predisposes her to the risk of hypoglycemia.

6. Which *one* of the following statements concerning family members and the care of elderly patients is *false?*
   a. The clinician is obligated to carry out noninvasive investigations if demanded by the health care proxy.
   b. An individual named as health care proxy has the right to refuse treatment on behalf of the patient, if the patient cannot understand.
   c. In the absence of a health care proxy, the family has no right to refuse treatment on the patient's behalf.
   d. Disturbed nights head the list of patient characteristics that stress caregivers.

- Understand the dangers of having multiple prescribers for one patient.
- Appreciate that health promotion and maintenance of function must be incorporated into illness management.
- Understand the roles, problems, and utility of the family and other surrogates in the care of elderly patients.
- Appreciate how to manage the family, other caregivers, and community support systems efficiently in diagnosis and management.
- Define the factors increasing family and caregiver stress and the methods to relieve them.
- Describe the range of housing alternatives to be considered and the principles of organizing placement when an elder has to relocate.
- Understand the influence of the environment on the presentation and management of illness in old age.
- Outline the principles of decision making about intensity of treatment and other ethical aspects of elderly care.
- Describe the rationale for clinician involvement in the design of public policy.
- Outline the principles and characteristics of good primary care of elders.

OVERVIEW

The changes that usually occur with increasing age, the way society treats the old, and the way individuals view themselves as they age combine to modify the ways in which illnesses present and the methods that health care professionals must employ for optimal management. Generalizations about older people as patients are difficult to make; people become more unique as they age, so each individual situation must be carefully assessed. However, issues and characteristics are sufficiently frequent and recurrent in the elderly patient (e.g., hearing loss or mobility problems) that approaches generically designed to fit those characteristics are appropriate. Doctors' offices and the approaches of their staff need to be modified to take these common characteristics into account, while not patronizing relatively well elders by assuming difficulties where they do not exist.

Rather than the traditional "investigate, diagnose, treat, and cure" sequence and the usual one-on-one relationship with the patient, the clinician to the older patient must integrate the family members and others who frequently have differing perceptions than the patient; indeed, *their* concerns (and supporting them in their caring roles) may be more meaningful than direct face-to-face care of the patient, especially with the frail. The patient's ability to function and the long-term consequences of many concurrent factors, illnesses, treatments, and their interactions must all be taken into account.

The view of what is normal (and acceptable) in old age and what is unacceptable or treatable is changing. Osteoporosis is the best example of an illness that used to be regarded as a normal aging change, and which is now regarded as a treatable illness, preventable to a degree, with implications for lifelong preventive measures. Exercise, nutrition, and personal habits can influence the bone mass, and therefore the symptomatology of many older women and men. Most current elders tend to tolerate symptoms that nowadays represent treatable disease. Clinicians and their staff must be alert and actively seek such nonpresented, treatable illnesses.

Robert Olsen

Robert Olsen is a 76-year-old man who lives on his own. He is brought to you by a community social service worker, who was called to the house by neighbors because of the weight loss and self-neglect they had observed in this isolated, elderly man as he puttered around in his garden. On formal testing, his mental status is normal, but his limited mobility (secondary to degenerative joint disease), hearing loss, diminished visual acuity, and urinary incontinence are clinically obvious, with apparent weight loss, dehydration, and undernutrition.

CASE DISCUSSION

Mr. Olsen typifies the isolated older individual who tolerates slowly increasing difficulties, the functional effects of which will ultimately be difficult to correct even though the "treatment" is medically simple. Major efforts will need to be made in this case to institute appropriate therapy to try to improve Mr. Olsen's mobility, investigate and control his incontinence, and improve his nutrition. After what has probably been several years of silence, it is unlikely that efforts to get him to use a hearing aid will be successful. If he later needs care in a skilled nursing facility, his hearing loss will be especially isolating.

NONPRESENTATION WHEN ILL

The health care system is built around simple assumptions that are often incorrect for elderly patients. The first assumption is that patients have to present in the first place to declare that they have a symptom or something that is worrying them and seek the doctor's help. Yet most of the disabling, chronic conditions of old age tend to have an insidious onset and symptoms so common in old age that for centuries the conditions have been regarded as a normal part of aging. It is not just older adults who may have these assumptions, but also their dependents (including the caregivers and adult children who might encourage them to seek health care). Older adults are viewed as often having hearing loss; difficulties with memory; shortened stature; aches and pains in the bones, muscles, and joints; and various other changes. However, hearing loss is preventable to a degree and treatable to a large extent. Progressive memory loss in old age is generally caused by Alzheimer's disease, an illness for which stabilizing treatment is now available and many treatment approaches can reduce its effects. Osteoporosis is the cause of the loss of height and of most bone pain in old age and is a predisposing factor to hip fracture—one of the devastating acute events of the elderly (one in three women, and one in six men who live to be 90, the frailer of whom will die as a result. However, this illness is not only treatable after the event with bone-strengthening medications, but also to a large degree, preventable by dietary and exercise measures and lifestyle changes; these need to be instituted in adolescence to be effective—there is truly a lifetime perspective to the prevention of this condition! Osteoarthritis, the most common chronic condition in the world, is not a normal aging change. Rather, it is the result of changes in the joints, which can often be relieved and prevented by proper attention to gait and asymmetry and by medical management, including medications, physical therapy, and surgical procedures. Even with all this knowledge, the clinician frequently sees an older person who has been receiving medical care, and yet whose osteoporosis, for example, has never been addressed or even considered, until a crush fracture or a devastating hip fracture draws attention to it. Thus nonpresented, chronic symptomatology may ultimately be acutely damaging or fatal, and even before it is, it will contribute to decline and disability, with drab and dreadful consequences for many as they grow older.

Clinicians are trained to start the write-up of the patient's history with the abbreviation *c/o*, meaning *complains of*. Patients are expected to "complain" and thus attract medical attention. However, many older individuals simply do not do this. Despite the fact that views on the treatability of many chronic illnesses are changing, many individuals still have denial, ignorance, fear, and negativity about aging; this can lead some older persons to tolerate problems believing them to be "normal aging". The cultural barriers to declaring mental symptoms, such as depression or memory loss, contribute to the underuse of mental health services by older patients and the under-recognition of these common syndromes. Some symptoms are embarrassing "private" issues, like urinary incontinence; since infancy, most people have been trained to regard it as shameful to wet oneself, and yet here is a syndrome that devastates the lives of many, especially women, and not necessarily the elderly alone. Thus, there are multiple explanations for why symptoms of treatable illnesses may not be presented to the clinician. The clinician, therefore, must modify the approach to the older patient and cannot afford to wait until the patient mentions symptoms. The clinician must review for symptoms and, when reviewing systems, must ask specific questions about the common problems, and should make observations that will enable him or her to see if the patient is having a painful time moving, or cannot hear, or is for some reason tolerating something that might be treatable. Preappointment questionnaires (encouraging family members to contribute, so that they can report on aspects the patient may deny or be unaware of) and a review of symptoms during the physical examination are two useful ways to ensure that everything gets covered.

> ● The art of geriatric medicine includes asking the right questions.

Studies in Scotland decades ago demonstrated the extent of untreated illness among older individuals, even when access to health care is exemplary (in that case, by the well-publicized development of the National Health Service after World War II).[1] Illnesses that were tolerated despite being treatable included mental disturbance, depression, diabetes, anemia, and malnutrition, as well as lesser problems such as earwax buildup producing deafness, and dental and podiatric problems. A number of such characteristic "hidden illnesses" are summarized in Box 3–1.

THREE MODIFIED PRESENTATIONS OF ACUTE ILLNESS

Virginia Tsadlick

Virginia Tsadlick, an 82-year-old nursing home resident, falls twice during the day. She has previously been functioning well, with no problems with gait or balance. She eats less supper than

---

Box 3-1 "Hidden" Illnesses in Older Adults

- Depression
- Hearing loss
- Incontinence
- Dementia
- Musculoskeletal stiffness
- Dental problems
- Falling
- Poor nutrition
- Alcoholism
- Sexual dysfunction
- Osteoporosis
- Osteoarthritis

---

usual but has normal vital signs, both that evening and the following morning. The following afternoon her blood pressure is found to be very low, and she is transferred to the emergency room, where abnormal bowel sounds and an abdominal x-ray examination lead to a diagnosis of perforated diverticulum; she is septic and hypotensive from peritonitis. At no time does she have abdominal tenderness or abdominal pain.

Harold Robinson

Harold Robinson is a 76-year-old man who lives a comfortable retired life with his wife in a self-contained small house with a small garden that is his major hobby and pastime. He complains of fatigue, saying that he lacks energy to carry out his normal functions. His mood appears fine, and at a glance he looks quite well. However, on physical examination he has marked cardiomegaly, rales at both bases, and other signs suggestive of congestive heart failure (CHF). He denies any history of dyspnea, nocturnal coughing, or orthopnea.

Donna Wilkinson

Donna Wilkinson is an 83-year-old woman cared for by her disabled sister. Her main problem has been an ongoing progressive dementia. Over a period of 24 hours, she develops respiratory symptoms and a cough that sounds productive, although no sputum is seen. An in-home chest x-ray examination is performed less than 24 hours after her symptoms start; it is reported as clear. Within

another 24 hours, she has overt physical signs of right lower lobe consolidation, tachypnea, and a temperature of 103°F. She has to be hospitalized, at which time a diagnosis of right lower lobe pneumonia is made. After a stormy hospital course, she recovers.

In the elderly, an abrupt change in functional status is a vital sign of potential illness.

> People become more unique as they age, so their symptoms and how they perceive them are inevitably different.

NONSPECIFIC PRESENTATION

Severe acute or significant chronic illness in older individuals often presents with vague, nonspecific, or seemingly trivial symptoms. Typical signs and symptoms may be absent or delayed. The brain is especially vulnerable to the effects of illness (and of treatment), and so an ill-defined change in cognition or mood may be the nonspecific sign of illness. Typical nonspecific symptoms that may represent specific illnesses in old age are summarized in Box 3–2. The onset of such symptoms, either abruptly or over a matter of days, should alert the clinician to the possibility of a developing acute illness.

Premonitory falls are falls occurring as a "prodrome" to a developing illness. An older individual who has a new onset of falling or confusion, or any of the other symptoms listed in Box 3–2, should be observed for the development of acute illness. An abrupt change in functional status of any kind (e.g., ceasing to go shopping) should similarly be regarded as a sign of potential physical or mental illness (especially depression).

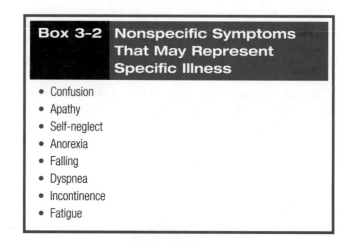

Box 3-2 Nonspecific Symptoms That May Represent Specific Illness

- Confusion
- Apathy
- Self-neglect
- Anorexia
- Falling
- Dyspnea
- Incontinence
- Fatigue

PRESENTATION IN THE "WRONG" ORGAN SYSTEM

The brain is an especially vulnerable organ, so that a change in mental status is one of the most frequent presenting symptoms of acute illness in older patients. However, certain illnesses frequently present in an organ systems remote from those primarily affected because of the limited reserve of several organ systems. Thyroid disease, although it can present in typical fashion, often presents symptomatically with cardiac, gastrointestinal, or cerebral symptoms. Cardiovascular presentations, secondary to the lack of reserve of the aged cardiovascular system, are often presentations (or concurrent complications) of other illnesses, especially if there is an increased hemodynamic state, as with hyperthyroidism or an acute infection. Sometimes aggressive diuretic treatment for CHF is continued for years or for life on the assumption of cardiac disease, when in fact the state of CHF was induced by intercurrent illness; thus, once the precipitating illness is resolved, the CHF may not need such vigorous continuing management.

TYPICAL ALTERED PRESENTATIONS

A number of altered presentations of disease in the elderly occur so frequently that they may be regarded as syndromes for which clinicians should be alert (Box 3–3).

Depression without Sadness

Major depression in an older individual may involve little overt dysphoria (sadness); often, apparent mental confusion dominates the clinical picture, demonstrating the vulnerability of the brain to an illness that is increasingly viewed as physical in nature. This phenomenon is generally referred to as the *dementia syndrome of depression*. In other elders with major

---

Box 3-3	**Typical Altered Presentations of Specific Illnesses in Older Adults**

- Depression without sadness
- Infectious disease without leukocytosis, fever, or tachycardia
- Silent surgical abdomen
- Silent malignancy ("mass without symptoms")
- Myocardial infarction without chest pain
- Nondyspneic pulmonary edema
- Apathetic thyrotoxicosis

---

depression, somatic symptoms dominate; often the individual focuses on something that is somewhat uncomfortable or troublesome and so it is tempting for the clinician to focus on the physical finding or apparent physical explanation and miss the underlying depression that made the person overaware of the somatic symptom he or she mentions. It must also be said that depression in the lay sense (i.e., sadness and "blueness" of mood) is often present and relatively neglected because of assumptions such as "wouldn't you be depressed in that situation?" In fact, because most depression in old age occurs in association with physical illness, clinicians who are not alert to the possibility of depression will miss it because there is usually plenty of other nonpsychiatric medical illness continuing on, upon which they can focus their energy. Although it may be masked, the sadness of the depression is often (but not always) found to be present if it is carefully sought.

Mass without Symptoms

Sometimes a malignant mass that is found on routine physical examination, especially in the gastrointestinal tract, has produced remarkably little functional impairment such as bowel disturbance. This is sometimes secondary to lesions located in clinically "silent" parts of the bowel (e.g., the ascending colon), but it may be secondary to reduced neuronal sensitivity in the gastrointestinal tract itself or reduced central awareness.

Silent Infectious Disease

Often an older patient has sepsis without leukocytosis, fever, or tachycardia. In pneumonia, chest x-ray examination results may be normal. Many clinicians believe that the radiologic changes are delayed in old age. Possibly the radiologic appearance of pneumonia only manifests when associated dehydration is corrected.

Silent Surgical Abdomen

The normal sequence of localized tenderness and pain, leading to generalized tenderness and pain as local peritonitis spreads and generalizes, is often greatly modified. The patient may have tachypnea and pneumonia-like symptoms or vague mental or urinary symptoms, without anything specifically pointing to the acute abdominal problem itself. Clinicians must be familiar with the conditions likely to produce an abdominal catastrophe in old age. Ischemic colitis (mesenteric insufficiency) may produce only vague but persistent, nonspecific bowel disturbance or even more general symptoms like anorexia or fatigue until completion of the thrombotic process or embolization to the bowel leads to ischemia and ultimately gangrene of the bowel, which is a life-threatening situation. Presentation of other major abdominal problems such as appendicitis and cholecystitis, the most common cause of acute abdominal conditions in old age, can be remarkably clinically silent.

Myocardial Infarction without Chest Pain (Silent Myocardial Infarction)

A proportion of acute myocardial infarctions (MIs) in older individuals is clinically silent, with no chest pain or other symptoms to aid in identification; they are found only later on routine or preoperative electrocardiograms (ECGs). Other MIs involve symptoms other than chest pain.[2] Again, the clinician should be alert to the elderly individual who has a history of several days of vague illness, perhaps with a little exercise intolerance or nausea, and should obtain an ECG and cardiac enzyme levels; such a patient may well "rule in."

Nondyspneic Pulmonary Edema

The patient with nondyspneic pulmonary edema exhibits definite signs of CHF but does not subjectively experience dyspnea, paroxysmal nocturnal dyspnea, or coughing; instead the patient has vague symptoms or none at all. Unfortunately, if this condition is not corrected, the ultimate morbidity and mortality are the same as in the more symptomatic patient. This phenomenon may be partially explained by reduced sensation and partially by self-limitation of activity—the patient keeps within limits of exercise tolerance that are insidiously reduced and thus perhaps unnoticed.

Apathetic Thyrotoxicosis

Much hyperthyroid disease (and most hypothyroid disease) presents the typical clinical picture. The syndrome known as apathetic thyrotoxicosis involves tiredness and slowing down caused by hyperthyroidism. The syndrome is sufficiently well recognized to be considered one of the classic "altered presentations" of illness in old age.[3] The "opposite" is also observed; hypothyroid patients may demonstrate agitation and confusion rather than tiredness and slowing down.

WHY ACUTE PRESENTATION IS MODIFIED IN OLD AGE

Altered central processing is one factor in the modification of acute presentation in old age; it can be caused by reduced cognitive status as a result of the direct effect on the brain of the illness itself or by preexisting (perhaps previously unrecognized) dementia. Some individuals, because of *negativity* about what is likely to happen to them with increasing age, tolerate or ignore symptoms, limiting their activities if necessary, and accept the symptoms as "old age." Tolerance of an insidious onset of disability is understandable, yet this same negativity is also often seen when more acute changes occur. Some health professionals, lacking an adequate explanation of various phenomena, will attribute symptoms to old age; this encourages patients and their family members to do likewise. *Fear*, not only of illness but also of its treatment (e.g., hospitalization or placement in an institution), is often a factor. These factors may lead to *denial*. Actual *ignorance* of the significance of bodily changes may be an issue. Neuronal degeneration causes reduction of *peripheral sensitivity*, reducing sensation and awareness. Many elders suffer unrecognized *depression*; this common treatable illness creates negativity, reducing the individual's initiative to seek medical care. Medical illnesses themselves, especially if chronically progressive, are associated with being prone to depression (often with guilt and low self-esteem), creating a spiral of decline.

Case Discussions

Ms. Tsadlick has the characteristic presentation of a silent acute abdomen with vague, nonspecific symptoms and normal vital signs, even just a few hours before impending collapse. This is a life-threatening situation.

The case of Mr. Robinson exemplifies the classic insidious presentation of nondyspneic pulmonary edema: a patient of clear mental status who lacks specific symptomatology and demonstrates a rather vague symptom for which the differential diagnosis is wide. He could be suffering from depression or a number of medical illnesses. Finding signs of CHF is not sufficient in a presentation such as this. One generic rule in geriatric medicine is that individual signs and symptoms often have multiple causes. Thus, proper investigation of a previously well-functioning individual like Mr. Robinson must include attention to the many other potential causes of fatigue. Laboratory tests should be carried out, with organ-specific testing if any symptoms point to a specific organ system. Depression should be seriously considered, even while treatment is initiated for the CHF itself.

Ms. Wilkinson shows classic delay in the development of objective radiologic evidence, although she is clinically in clear need of medical attention. (The white blood cell count may have been normal, too, had it been obtained.) Her case emphasizes the importance of observation over time, the need to record changes in signs and symptoms, and the necessity to act on them (sometimes with empirical treatment) and on clinical suspicions, rather than relying only on exclusionary laboratory and radiologic data.

COMMUNICATION PROBLEMS

The Patient

Hearing loss is common in old age. Many clinicians fail to take the time or do not organize the lighting needed to facilitate the lip reading on which many older individuals rely for full comprehension. The clinician must be in a well-lit area and on the same level as the patient, with the clinician and patient looking full into each other's face. In old age, environmental noise (universally present in emergency rooms and in many medical offices) diminishes auditory acuity. Further, under the stress of a medical visit when ill, even without dementia, many elders find their concentration reduced.

The preserved social facade of patients with dementia frequently misleads health professionals; the patient may appear to be (and may actually be) both registering and understanding information but may be failing to memorize or process it. For this reason, informal or even formal screening for impaired cognitive status should be carried out whenever impaired cognition is suspected at all. Individuals with unrecognized cognitive deficits are likely to be placed at unnecessary risk. Neither the family nor the clinician might realize that the patient cannot, rather than will not, comply. Even in younger, unimpaired individuals, remarkably little information is actually learned and retained by patients during their interactions with their clinicians. Reinforcement, written reminders, and the family (if available) can increase compliance and understanding in the management of forgetful patients, old or young.

The Family

The necessary involvement of family caregivers also produces communication problems; the family will have their own anxieties to address and will often have more to say privately about the patient than they would ever say in the patient's presence. Family members are frequently the means of implementing the management plan. Good communication involves both giving time to family members and other caregivers away from the patient and giving sufficient time to the patient, whose autonomy and input must be respected. It is up to the patient, if competent, to decide what is to be done; some family members "take over" too soon. Others deny problems and expose vulnerable individuals to unnecessary risk.

Once good communication with the family is in process, the primary care clinician is in a much better position to address complex ethical issues such as resuscitation, tube feeding, and other aspects of the intensity of treatment.

The Team

Communication between health professionals about elders is a special skill. The ability to work as a team (which will often never meet face to face), using and interacting with a wide range of health professionals—often by telephone and fax—is essential to good care. Clinician-to-clinician communication can be problematic. Elderly patients often have several clinicians involved in their care. Who is "in charge"? The primary care clinician should be in charge, but there is sometimes competition for this role. Many organ-specific specialists take on primary care roles for patients with whom they are involved. This happens partly because of the shortage of primary care clinicians. When several clinicians are involved, one of them should be declared the primary care clinician, or "personal clinician," the others being limited to specific roles.

Relocation

Special communication skills must be used when a patient transfers from one care setting to another; this often involves an entirely new set of health professionals. Communication must include the medications (including the reasons for prescription, the "target symptoms" or other purpose for each, suggested follow-up plans to assess their utility, and when to stop them); current formal diagnoses and functional problems, with an impression of the speed of change; other therapeutic interventions that have been helpful; social and other health professional services already involved (including the names of the agencies and, if possible, the individuals involved); the patient's insight into his or her problems; and the patient's interests and ethnic, cultural, and religious background. Objective measurements, numeric if possible, of such areas as mental status, activities of daily living (ADLs) and instrumental ADLs (IADLs), the range of movement in degrees, and exercise tolerance by distance, should be used whenever possible so that change can be appreciated and acted upon.

William Henry

William Henry is an 80-year-old man who has been led to believe that he has been brought to your office for a routine physical. He describes himself as "well," having a little difficulty moving around, but otherwise not needing attention. You have a pleasant conversation with him about his activities in World War II. After a physical examination, you find him to be a delightful old man. You are then surprised to receive an emotionally charged phone call from the man's son, who had felt constrained from speaking in front of his father. The son gives a history of tolerating more than a year of multiple late-night phone calls from his father, who lives alone, gets confused, and suffers hallucinations at night. In fact, he has been brought back by the police more than once after being found walking around outside, inadequately dressed, at night.

CASE DISCUSSION

This case dramatically illustrates the difference between the patient's and the family's perceptions. Mental status screening in this case would have revealed considerably more impairment than the brief interview, which by focusing not on current events but on events in the past, entirely missed the patient's deficits and needs. Better communication, with the son describing the problems by phone to the office staff, could have prevented the misunderstanding and delay.

Ethel Harrington

Ethel Harrington is an 82-year-old lady. She has been transferred from an assisted living facility after a fall and head injury. Seen in the emergency room, she is confused and combative and can barely make her needs known. Her problem list includes the word "dementia," and it is unclear what her current medications are. Her family members are out of state and not currently available for comment. They rarely see her. The aide at the facility is unfamiliar with Ms. Harrington, having started her job only on this shift. Ms. Harrington is too agitated for an x-ray examination or a computed tomography scan, so laboratories are obtained and she is observed for 2 to 3 hours. She abruptly undergoes full cardiopulmonary

arrest and is resuscitated and intubated, absent any specific directive. The next day, her family contacts the hospital, complaining about the resuscitation, which runs counter to advance directives that were on file at the first facility but were not forwarded with the patient. Ms. Harrington is extubated and dies. An autopsy shows a subdural hematoma.

CASE DISCUSSION

This situation is a diagnostic and management mess. The clinician is obligated to do perhaps more than would be done if he or she knew how poor the situation had been before. The clinician may do less than should be done if incompetence and disability are assumed based on where the patient lives or the circumstances of the patient being found; for example, "found on the floor" at a facility for homeless men may carry inappropriate implications about the likely status of the patient. This patient was in fact a highly functioning patient with dementia, and the change following the head injury was very striking, had anyone been able to draw attention to it. More aggressive approaches based on knowledge of the patient's changed status may have saved her. She was both underinvestigated and then, too late, overtreated as a result of the poor communication between the facility and the hospital in the first place.

DYSMOBILITY

Dysmobility includes a wide range of problems: instability, gait disturbance with poor balance, falling and its consequences (including loss of self-confidence, i.e., fear of falling), partial immobility (with assistance being needed for transfers), and being bed-bound or at least chair-bound. Dysmobility can follow a progressively downward spiral over weeks to months for older individuals, in whom the consequences of immobility are many and severe and include life-threatening conditions, conditions that increase morbidity, and conditions that cause potentially permanent disability such as flexion contractures (Box 3–4).

> ● "Why is this patient in bed?"—Marjorie Warren, pioneer geriatrician, 1940s, Britain.

DECONDITIONING

Hospitals and nursing homes are still described by the number of beds they have. Marjorie Warren's question to her junior clinicians still needs to be asked.

Box 3-4	Consequences of Immobilization

Stiffness, contractures

Loss of muscle strength

Confusion, sensory loss, depression

Dependence, institutionalization

Instability, loss of confidence

Dehydration, electrolyte imbalance

Malnutrition

Osteoporosis

Thrombosis: arterial and venous, pulmonary embolism

Pneumonia, atelectasis

Hypothermia

Pressure areas, pressure sores

Urinary retention, urinary incontinence, urinary tract infection, calculi

Constipation, fecal impaction, fecal incontinence

Deconditioning refers, in part, to the underuse and consequent loss of musculoskeletal strength and suppleness and of coordinated balancing and righting reflexes. This is familiar to anyone who has suddenly been immobilized for a few days by an intercurrent illness or surgery; in an older person, deconditioning occurs much faster. Recovery from such deconditioning is prolonged or incomplete in many older persons, and the consequences may be severe: falling and injury, loss of confidence, further immobility, and even a continuing downhill spiral of deterioration that can be difficult to stop. Cardiovascular deconditioning, as well as consequences of immobility like constipation and impaction, dehydration, and anorexia, all complicate the clinical picture. Patients are often temporarily immobilized while under the care of specialized clinicians (e.g., perioperatively and while in intensive care). Efforts to maintain range of motion, to physically get the patient out of bed, to continue weight-bearing exercises, and to keep the patient moving around and breathing deeply must be vigorously maintained. Encouraging all of this is one of the most vital functions of the general clinician in the specialized or tertiary care setting.

William Wilkinson

William Wilkinson is a 73-year-old patient of yours who was hospitalized for urosepsis while he was on vacation out of town. He had previously been independently mobile, although he had morning stiffness of both hips. Before hospitalization, he had regular bowel movements, and his morning habit of walking around the house both helped this and helped to move bronchial secretions that "sat on his chest" overnight. (He suffered from chronic obstructive pulmonary disease [COPD].) Septic and unwell in a tertiary care hospital, he was initially given intravenous therapy and antibiotics; however, fecal impaction with fecal incontinence rapidly developed, and Mr. Wilkinson became confused and developed a persistent, nonproductive cough. His son, alarmed at this rapid deterioration, was instrumental in initiating respiratory and physical therapy. However, Mr. Wilkinson's bowel habits, hips, and chest are still problems for him, 2 months after hospitalization. He describes this experience to you as "the worst thing that has ever happened to me."

CASE DISCUSSION

This case demonstrates a relatively minor range of complications; at least the patient is on the road to recovery. The much more depressing scenario of patients suffering virtually all the consequences listed in Box 3-4 can be seen in any tertiary care hospital any day of the week.

MULTIPLICITY OF PROBLEMS

Frequently an older individual's management is complicated by several ongoing chronic conditions and their medical treatment, together with superimposed acute illness or illnesses. Added to these multiple diagnoses are the various unique psychosocial and environmental factors that influence function, behavior, and management.

The primary care clinician should be ideally positioned to be the coordinator when multiple systems are impaired; this may involve coordinating the efforts of several organ specialists, often on an ongoing basis. The principle of restricting prescription of medications to only one clinician or one pharmacy could reduce duplicate prescribing, overprescribing, and drug–drug or drug–disease interactions.[4] *Setting priorities* becomes a necessary skill. Clinicians are often tempted to treat the problem that is easiest to treat, which often means a prescription of a medication. However, this may not be the most important problem in functional terms (which is probably what matters most to the patient and family members). An immediate or ongoing threat to life may take precedence, although the patient may not appreciate the significance of the situation; for example, the patient will not

---

Box 3-5   Contents of Problem List for Elderly Patient

Formal diagnoses with an indication of functional severity if appropriate (e.g., generalized osteoarthritis, painful but ambulatory)

Syndromic problems that require a specific therapeutic plan (e.g., falling or instability)

Contributory life events (e.g., recent bereavement with date)

Living circumstances (e.g., "lives alone")

Any history of continuing significance (e.g., suicide attempt, hysterectomy)

Certain medications (e.g., anticoagulants)

Numerically measurable items, when available (e.g., ejection fraction of less than 15%, Mini-Mental Status Examination score of 12/30)

Family history of alcoholism, depression, or suicide.

---

go to the hospital, even after sustaining an acute syncopal episode out in the community. To set priorities, the primary clinician must, over the first one or two visits to the office, evolve a comprehensive *problem list*. This list should include not only formal diagnoses, but also broader symptom complexes that do not fall into traditional diagnostic categories (such as falling or instability) but that nonetheless require a management plan in and of themselves. The problem list must also include contributory psychosocial features (e.g., recent bereavement), factors in the living circumstances (e.g., lives alone), and any special characteristics that may be crucial to the patient and his or her illness management. Such a problem list can be consulted so that attention to even one individual problem will efficiently and appropriately take into account the other factors. A well-organized, current problem list can ensure a coordinated approach. Such a problem list also aids communication at times of transition from one clinical site to another (Box 3–5).

Kathleen Travis

Kathleen Travis is an 81-year-old patient who is brought by her grandson to initiate primary care with you. He is concerned about the number of medications she is on and about her rather depressed state of mind. He and his wife give most of the history. At your request, they have brought all the medications that they could find in her drug cupboard.

Kathleen has lived for years in the same ranch-style house with three of her sisters, the last of whom died several months ago. On an average day she is

"bored," but she avoids going out. For 4 weeks her right arm has been aching, a constant and dull pain. She has previously suffered chronic low back and neck pain, and she currently has stiffness in multiple joints. She takes her medications sporadically. Ms. Travis uses eye drops and medication for glaucoma and sees an ophthalmologist; she cannot see well enough to watch the television or read. She has a long-standing prescription from another clinician for acetaminophen with codeine (Tylenol #3), which she takes for her aches and pains. She also has a diuretic (hydrochlorothiazide) that she takes most days for her swollen ankles. She has some 6-year-old nitroglycerine tablets, a prescription from 2 years ago for the antidepressant doxepin, and a similarly aged prescription for L-thyroxine, which she claims to "not need." She has been having problems sleeping for several months, and three or four times a week she takes diphenhydramine (Benadryl) 25 to 50 mg to help her sleep. She wakes often, frequently with pain in her back or arm, and she generally has to get up to urinate more than once in the night. She is constipated and gets very tired on the few occasions she visits with her family. Physical examination confirms her poor visual acuity and shows that her mental status is good, at least on screening. She is almost impacted with feces on rectal examination. She has signs suggestive of slight CHF with cardiomegaly, as well as kyphoscoliosis, restricted neck movements, and diminished range of motion of her shoulders and hips. Her muscle tone is poor. She walks with an unsteady gait and becomes dizzy on movement of her neck.

CASE DISCUSSION

Ms. Travis's problem list includes recent symptoms but is dominated by major ongoing problems and by several prescribed medications that she is taking intermittently. She has signs of depression and must be investigated for hypothyroidism, osteoporosis, and osteoarthritis. Osteoporosis is a particular hazard because Ms. Travis lives alone, has an unsteady gait, and is at risk of falling and, therefore, fracture (which would probably be the beginning of the end). Because she did not choose to come to see you, it is important to obtain her input and involve her. She, her grandson, and you must set priorities for her safety. The problem list will assist in this process.

Her medications include drugs that suggest diagnoses of hypothyroidism, depression, and coronary artery disease having been entertained by some clinician in the past. Ms. Travis currently takes a constipating pain reliever that may be making her more depressed, and uses an over-the-counter sleep aid that is known to produce confusion and lethargy the next day in many individuals, especially if there is some Alzheimer's disease present. Some of her current symptoms may be truly iatrogenic or the result of neglected medical conditions that were addressed in previous years. Her ophthalmologist, who is the clinician whom she has seen most frequently in the past few years, must be included in the planning. Ms. Travis may well need to continue several medications for some of the conditions already hinted at; these medications must be coordinated through you to avoid problems.

THE NEED FOR MULTIDISCIPLINARY MANAGEMENT

There are many reasons why other health care disciplines (and disciplines outside the health care field) must be made available for the ongoing management of elderly patients. Elderly patients commonly are affected by multiple conditions, which may necessitate the input of other clinicians such as dentists, podiatrists, and organ-specific clinicians such as nephrologists and cardiologists who may need to follow the patient on a long-term basis. Most clinicians believe that they understand the relative roles of the doctor and the nurse, but the power of the social worker to integrate the limitations, capabilities, and financial aspects of our chaotic health care system with the family's own potential and problems and the individual's autonomy and function is less well understood. Medical, pharmaceutical management will be confounded by the psychosocial factors if those factors are not professionally addressed.

The real potential to reduce disability once present and to prevent it in a proactive way lies in the input of several other professionals, and particularly occupational and physical therapy services. Many clinicians underestimate the power of physical therapy to reduce discomfort and improve function. Many times the physical therapist is needed for proper prescription and fitting of walking aids; yet walking aids are often not suggested, and the patient may resist them. The potential for an occupational therapist to improve daily function, the quality of life, and, in particular, the safety of the patient (e.g., by expert input into home safety modifications) is underused (and underavailable).

The multidisciplinary approach is also needed to take advantage of today's knowledge of the preventability of many of the disabilities of old age. Good exercise, good nutrition, and a sense of purpose could be described as the three essentials of enjoyable, successful old age. Yet most clinicians hesitate to recommend exercise to older, frailer individuals and need professional backup to implement such a program. Clinicians may lack the time for the detailed nutritional counseling and ongoing educational efforts that are necessary if an inadequate diet is to be modified into something nutritionally dense and effective in maintaining the patient's strength and resistance. The power of social programs to give the patient a sense of purpose (and often contribute to exercise and nutrition) must not be understated either. The clinician must be able to direct a person to these resources with enthusiasm and persistence. Only by such a multidisciplinary approach can clinicians have an effect on the sometimes apparently inexorable progression of disability in elders.

The multidisciplinary team includes the caregiving family. In some situations (especially progressive dementias), the caregiving family member is probably the most consistent member of the team, the one person who will follow the patient all the way through many relocations and living arrangements. This team generally will not meet together, but will need to communicate well by such methods as fax, phone, letter, and email. Simply copying records between the different disciplines is valuable in itself. If the family member is an important member of the team, then with the patient's permission the family member should receive at least some of the most important parts of the record and recommendations each time the patient is seen or each time changes are made.

Unfortunately, many clinicians are not trained to be "team players." Many individuals see the doctor as being the only answer to the problems. By working together, the various disciplines can come to appreciate one another's strengths and limitations.

> ● Three essentials for a successful old age: good exercise, good nutrition, and a sense of purpose.

UNMET PREVENTIVE AND HEALTH PROMOTION NEEDS

The health care system, society, the financing of health care, and societal attitudes all seem directed toward providing care *after* illness strikes. This approach is too limited to optimally address health care needs of the elderly. Once the crisis, the illness, or the problem requiring hospitalization is an established fact, irrevocable changes may be taking place already, and the spiral of decline may be beginning. However, risk factors can be identified at routine health care visits. Once problems are identified, a proactive, preventive approach can (and must) be used. This approach goes far beyond the traditional cancer-related, cardiovascular and gynecologic care that is delivered to many educated individuals in their middle age; yet even cancer screening is underemphasized in the elderly population.[4]

> ● In older adults, it is not enough to merely provide care *after* illness strikes.

The prevention of needless disability and functional decline and thus the postponement of dependency is a key principle of geriatric medicine. Musculoskeletal problems that will irrevocably worsen must be addressed, even if they are currently tolerable. Rather than withdrawing from activity to avoid falling, the progressively immobilized or dysmobile patient should be exercising to increase capacity and keep going. The clinician must develop the attitude of continually looking ahead both negatively and positively from the presented situation, asking questions such as, "What would you do if you became ill while alone at home?" "How would you contact help?" "How do you currently get food?" "How will this patient look 6 months from now?" "What else could this person be doing or enjoying?"

> ● When prescribing medication, you should define the target symptoms or signs and schedule a follow-up visit to assess effectiveness.

POLYPHARMACY

Polypharmacy is a term generally used to imply the overprescription of multiple concurrent medications. Often the problem results from *reflex prescribing*—that is, responding with a medication prescription to each of many presented problems. Many chronic problems of old age are improved by medication, but nonmedication therapies should be considered first or at least concurrently. The risk of drug–drug and drug–disease interactions increases with the number of prescriptions. When more than one clinician is prescribing, duplicate prescription can occur; confusion between generic and proprietary names can contribute to this situation (e.g., taking Lasix and furosemide together).

Another major factor in polypharmacy is *failure to follow up* on the effectiveness and potential side effects of medications and on the continuing need for prescribing them. Clinicians are often hesitant to stop medications, fearing that an already fragile patient will come to further harm. This most often occurs when a patient transfers clinicians (e.g., following nursing home or hospital transfer). The high incidence of iatrogenic illness[5–7] makes it good practice for the cli-

nician to not prescribe anything without a review of all existing medications (including complementary and over-the-counter medications) and always to define and record the anticipated effect of prescriptions. With the target symptom(s) or sign(s) defined, follow-up can allow the medication's effectiveness to be judged. Numeric, or at least objective, measurements should be used wherever possible: measuring sadness on a validated scale, measuring range of motion in degrees, measuring joint circumference with a tape measure, numerically scoring mental status, using a pain scale and recording functionality as objectively as possible.[8]

Changing *pharmacodynamics* with increasing age make many older individuals either more susceptible to side effects at a given dose or responsive to lower doses than would be used in younger patients. Many medications have an increased half-life in older individuals and exert their effects over a longer time, for good and ill. Knowing the patient's renal function when renally excreted drugs are prescribed is a help. The traditional phrase is "start low, go slow"; however, sometimes clinicians make the mistake of failing to raise the dose (slowly) to therapeutic levels.[8] Quite often, elderly patients are chronically given too small a dose, especially of antidepressants and pain relievers.

> ● Start low, go slow—but go!

The psychotropic medications (those given deliberately to affect brain function or mood) require special attention. Family members and patients are often extremely suspicious, fearing adverse outcomes that are mercifully much more rare nowadays, given the advances in pharmaceutical specificity. With these medications it is more important than usual to define the "target symptoms" and have the family and patient realize what is likely to be achieved, thus involving them in reporting whether success is accomplished or not. The wise clinician avoids investing too much "ego" in what should always be regarded as a therapeutic trial in most of the situations in which effects are sought on the elderly brain.

To avoid the confusion of having several clinicians prescribing for one patient, all prescriptions should be routed through the primary clinician. But patients establish links with organ-specific specialists, and routing all prescriptions through one office can lead to communication errors. If there must be several clinicians, the patient or family should at least be encouraged to use one pharmacist. Most pharmacists have more capability to be alert to potential interactions than most clinicians. If several clinicians must prescribe for one patient, they must communicate with each other.

> ● One clinician/one pharmacist: the key to safe prescribing.

When any change in prescription is anticipated, indeed at all medical visits, it is wise to review all medications. Many potent medications are now available over the counter, including nonsteroidal antiinflammatories, H_2 blockers, and allergy medications. Patients have access to prescriptions over the Internet. The growth in alternative medicines, more properly called *complementary medicines*, is welcomed by patients and families because it gives them a sense of control. In fact, this trend is exposing many people to not only the risk of wasting financial resources, but also the possibility of using pharmaceutical substances in an uncontrolled environment (e.g., St. John's wort is a "real" antidepressant and should not be mixed with others); unfortunately, many patients and families are secretive about their personal medication habits.

A useful geriatric medical technique is the "paper or plastic bag" test, in which either a family member or a visiting health professional brings in *all* the medications found in the house, including the spouse's medication, other "borrowable" medications, all herbal and other over-the-counter medications, and any outdated prescriptions. This technique can be extraordinarily revealing and is particularly recommended in making the initial evaluation of a patient new to a clinician's practice.

> ● Use the "plastic bag test" to find out *all* the medicines a patient could be taking!

William Powers

William Powers is a 72-year-old man who is a new patient to you. He is a heavy smoker who has had symptomatic COPD for nearly 10 years. After several hospitalizations for exacerbations, including at least one episode with complicating CHF, he is now taking many medications. He is taking an antihypertensive medication and an antidepressant that he began taking 2 years ago for urinary frequency. He has been sleeping badly, and he has been taking some phenobarbital that his late wife used to take to help her sleep when she was terminally ill with cancer. Last year on vacation, during some hot days in Florida, he became dizzy and faint and was started on cyclizine. He has continued using it because it calms him, and he believes that it dries some of his chest secretions. He still gets a little dizzy on standing. His son has come with him to your office and has brought a large bag of medications: hydrochlorothiazide, prescribed at 50 mg daily; potassium chloride, 20 mEq/day; albuterol inhaler, two puffs four times a day and every 2 hours if needed; docusate, twice daily; digoxin, 0.25 mg/day; imipramine, 50 mg each night; terbutaline, 5 mg three times a day; meclizine, 12.5 mg three times a day; phenobarbital, 60 mg at bedtime; an over-the-counter sinus medication containing an antihistamine, a decongestant, and acetaminophen; and some diphenhydramine hydrochloride (Benadryl) for sinus congestion and to help Mr. Powers sleep.

CASE DISCUSSION

It is unlikely that most of these medications are really needed long term. It is unknown if Mr. Powell's COPD is responsive to the bronchodilators, which may be contributing to his anorexia and insomnia. Mr. Powell could be depressed. He is taking several medications that could produce depression, as well as an antidepressant in low dose, essentially given for its side effect (for his urinary frequency, which may be made worse by the diuretics he is on). In fact, Mr. Powell takes several medications with anticholinergic side effects in any one day, which could be affecting his thinking, motivation, and balance. He lacks current signs of CHF yet continues on CHF treatment. He is taking digoxin in a fairly high maintenance dose with no clear indications, which also could be contributing to his anorexia.

Chronically taken barbiturates interfere with sleep. Polypharmacy may be Mr. Powell's number one problem.

IATROGENESIS

"First, do no harm" is the beginning of the Hippocratic oath. Whereas the term *iatrogenesis* is usually equated with clinicians harming patients by the prescribing of medication, the potential to cause harm goes beyond this.

Relocation of elderly individuals can cause great disruption, precipitating confusion and falling, anorexia, and even malnutrition. Primary care clinicians must act as advocates for their patients to reduce to the minimum the effects of the often multiple relocations older individuals must frequently undergo, especially when ill.

> ● Relocate and hospitalize elders in daylight if possible to reduce "relocation stress."

Hospitalization is hazardous to an older person's health: around 20% of older individuals' hospitalizations are prolonged by major adverse events.[5–7] These events include nosocomial infections; falls, accidents, and other trauma; problems with pressure sores and other consequences of the relative immobility of hospitalization; and delirium, depression, and medication side effects. The primary care clinician has a vital role in shortening and appropriately planning hospital stays and in assisting nursing and medical colleagues to respond behaviorally and environmentally to the needs of the individual elderly patient. All health professionals have a role in "reducing the harm."

MULTIPLE CAUSES FOR EACH PROBLEM

Clinicians are generally thrilled when they find a convincing medical explanation for a patient's symptoms, particularly if the cause had seemed elusive. The problem in old age is that each symptom, each syndrome, and each problem is liable to have multiple contributory factors; it is often impossible to work out which is the most important. The danger is that clinicians "medicalize" the situation too much and go for the medically treatable factor, ignoring "softer" contributors. A good example is the syndrome of falling; most falls are the result of the interaction of multiple factors (e.g., lighting and flooring), and preventing a fall from happening again (which may be life saving for the patient) depends on paying attention to all factors, not just the "medically" obvious ones. The same applies to several chronic syndromes, such as incontinence and dementia, in which there are frequently several contributory factors. Even though it is recognized that Alzheimer's disease underlies most progressive dementias in old age, secondary factors are often missed (e.g., vascular disease, prior alcoholism, and maybe depression, as well as the Alzheimer's disease). With urinary incontinence, if elective surgery is about to be undertaken, the fact that multiple other causes may be contributing will lead to disappointment or at best incomplete relief if a surgical approach is not preceded by a thorough medical workup.

> ● Each separate symptom often has *multiple* causes in elders.

Harold Steinkampf

Harold Steinkampf is a 75-year-old patient of yours with mild cognitive impairment. He saw another clinician in your group a week ago because of persistent agitation while staying temporarily with his daughter following lens implants for cataracts; haloperidol, 0.5 mg three times a day, was prescribed. You are called by the emergency room clinician. Harold has been taken there after a fall in the night; he had been found on the floor in the dark between his bedroom and the bathroom. He has a subcapital fracture of the right femur with displacement which urgently needs internal fixation and pinning. He is known to have ischemic heart disease, and he is taking hydrochlorothiazide, 50 mg/day, for hypertension. The emergency room clinician has found that Mr. Steinkampf is in atrial fibrillation, which had not previously been known to the family.

STUDY QUESTIONS

1. There are many factors to consider in the workup for an apparent fall. What factors are already identified as predisposing in this case?
2. What steps could have been taken to prevent this fall in the first place?

CASE DISCUSSION

Like most falls in elders, Mr. Steinkampf's was caused by the interaction of multiple factors. His agitation, the unfamiliar place, possibly the nocturia that made him get up in the first place, potential orthostasis, the darkness, and the recent prescription of a tranquilizer, which may have reduced his attention and potentially added to his orthostasis, are all contributors, along with variation in his visual acuity following the recent surgery. This AF, if new, means he needs to be "ruled-out" for an MI (myocardial infarct); this would be a bad time to operate if he had just sustained one! And, clearly, some of this was forseeable and preventible.

FUNCTIONAL STATUS: LOSING IT, MAINTAINING IT, RECORDING IT

When each medical problem of an elderly patient is defined, the functional implications must also be assessed. Knowing the functional implications helps set priorities for treatment in the multiply impaired individual.

When functionality is defined objectively, better communication about a person's baseline status can take place when the patient is transferred to other health professionals, as may occur with hospitalizations and relocation or other placement. Decline may be overlooked; the potential for recovery may be underestimated or overestimated without such information. The already functionally impaired person may be exquisitely sensitive to even a slight change. For example, a seemingly minor podiatric problem developing in an individual who is already barely able to make it to the bathroom will render that individual wholly dependent for essential functions. Recognizing that function is of such overriding importance affects all medical, environmental, and social decision making for older individuals.

> ● Good care of the acutely ill patient is impossible unless the functional baseline is known.

The term *instrumental activities of daily living* (*IADLs*) is now favored to describe the detailed daily living functions that are instrumental to life. These include not the self-care skills, but the daily more complex functions such as handling finances, collecting personal tax information, preparing a meal, shopping, driving or otherwise accessing transport, and so forth. The term *ADLs* is reserved for personal self-care skills: the ability to groom oneself, dress oneself, bathe, handle toileting and be continent, and ambulate and transfer. Measurable scales are available to record these functions and their relative impairment.[9]

Description of elderly patients and diagnosis of their conditions should always be made in functional terms. It is truly ageist to describe an individual only in terms of chronologic years. To improve communication and to avoid assumptions made on the basis of the patient's age, all health professionals should become used to quickly characterizing a person's level of function. Anecdotal incidents of individuals being treated differently because of a typographic error on the record of their chronologic age emphasize the dangers of such assumptions.

> ● Age in and of itself is never a criterion for medical decision making; function is.

MODIFIED SPEED OF RECOVERY

Some physiologically "young" older patients recover as quickly as younger individuals from acute illness and disability; however, as a general rule, recovery from illness is prolonged by several factors in the elderly, especially the more physically frail or passive. Many clinicians underestimate the rehabilitation potential of elderly patients or assume that progressive decline after a major event is inevitable. With today's emphasis on short hospitalization and the desirability of the most rapid recovery possible, there is the danger of prematurely deciding that an individual has

already "reached a plateau" and will not recover further. The primary care clinician may have to advocate for such a patient. There must be an active search for factors that might be inhibiting the road to recovery such as unrecognized dementia or depression or unaddressed pain. Short-term rehabilitation (STR) is an excellent concept, but relocation and the fact that it often involves using a nursing home setting can be negative. Although it may be impossible to rehabilitate to full independence, rehabilitation to close to the previous level of function should normally be the aim. (This is why the previous level of function needs to be known and recorded before hospitalization!) Recording overall functional status (ADLs and IADLs) at intervals ensures that very slow change over time can be appreciated as the individual shifts from one level and site of care and one set of health professionals to another. Although a slow downward spiral of function does happen in many individuals with multiple problems, decline should be neither assumed nor anticipated. Recovery after anoxic brain damage, for example, may take a long time and perhaps be incomplete, but the patient may well end at a less dependent level than originally predicted. This sometimes results in patients initially being placed at a higher level of care than they need in the long term.

IMPORTANCE OF THE ENVIRONMENT

It is astonishing how inappropriate our living environments are for life at any age. But with increasing age, both "normal" changes and age-associated illnesses interact with the environment in ways that can be extremely negative. Poor lighting and poor signage each make it impossible for people to find their way. Noise pollution (a bane of today's society) often takes the form of background noise and makes the partially hearing-impaired individual unable to comprehend conversations. Clutter and complications in the environment increase the likelihood of falling, fearfulness, and inability to get around. Familiar, convenient, well-lit surroundings with the right acoustics could improve the functionality of all individuals, especially as they age. Ironically, the settings in which clinicians assess patients are frequently appalling environments in relation to these characteristics, and the situation is compounded by the anxiety that many individuals feel in a clinical setting. Clinicians are frequently asked to assess a person's cognitive capabilities (and functional capacity) in conditions very unlike those in which the person lives. This is why the home circumstances must be assessed, or at least known about, for decisions to be made about home safety and the appropriateness of the environment to which a patient's discharge is planned. Doctors' offices are not designed for older patients either. Tables are too high, even dangerous, and the corridors may be threatening, lacking the handholds that should be on the walls.

The environment of nursing homes is unspeakably inappropriate in many cases. It is well known that a calming, quiet, soothing environment with healthy reminiscences, well-lit, warm and welcoming, and homelike, really does help to calm behavioral and emotional disturbances in those with and without dementia. So why are nursing homes designed to look like rather unwelcoming convenience stores? Where are the carpeting and drapes? Why does everyone need to be harassed by loud alarms that are intended only to alert nurses to patients in danger? Clinicians should speak out, rather than merely respond with increasing doses of psychotropic medications for patients who may in part be merely suffering from the chronic disruption of an aggressive and noisy environment.

● Do not try to medicate a patient into tolerating a bad environment !

INVOLVEMENT OF FAMILY

When or if an older patient seeks care is greatly influenced by family members or other caregivers. The increased dependency of many frail elders creates a parallel to the relationship between the parent and child. Just as the manifestations and reactions to illness in a child are influenced by the parental response, so it often is with illness in the more dependent older person. Just as the implementation of management in a child generally depends on the parent, guardian, or some other caregiver, so it also does with the older patient. In certain situations the family member or caregiver must be trained to be therapeutically skilled, especially when behavioral techniques are required, as in the patient with dementia (Box 3–6).[10]

It is often necessary to work through surrogates or family members at times when life-or-death decisions about the intensity of treatment need to be made. This is in part a result of the frequent impairment of the patient's cognition (either long term from a dementing illness or short term as the effect of illness, relocation, or treatment). Even when the elderly patient is clearly competent, family members and other concerned caregivers who are aware of the vulnerability of elderly people and of the problems they face feel bound to be involved. Dealing with families, using their energy, and training them to become part of the team are some of the most important skills of the health professional helping an older patient. It is up to the clinician to set the tone for family involvement from the outset.

It is crucial to identify and agree on a single family member who will be the family spokesperson.

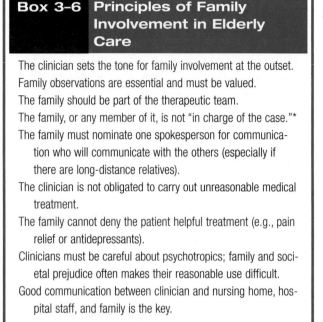

Box 3-6 Principles of Family Involvement in Elderly Care

The clinician sets the tone for family involvement at the outset.

Family observations are essential and must be valued.

The family should be part of the therapeutic team.

The family, or any member of it, is not "in charge of the case."*

The family must nominate one spokesperson for communication who will communicate with the others (especially if there are long-distance relatives).

The clinician is not obligated to carry out unreasonable medical treatment.

The family cannot deny the patient helpful treatment (e.g., pain relief or antidepressants).

Clinicians must be careful about psychotropics; family and societal prejudice often makes their reasonable use difficult.

Good communication between clinician and nursing home, hospital staff, and family is the key.

*If a family member is the health care proxy or named as having the durable power of attorney for health care (if the patient cannot participate), he or she is to act then as the patient, not as the clinician.

This can help, but not entirely prevent, the familiar syndrome of the "long-distance" family member who often disagrees with the intensity of treatment endorsed by the local family members in a patient unable to make his or her own decisions. Recognition of the powerful caring feelings of such an individual and efficiently maintaining contact with him or her (perhaps by mailing this person a copy of your notes, with the patient's permission) can help.

● Try to identify *one* primary caregiver or family spokesperson.

Salvatore Diballo

Salvatore Diballo is a 78-year-old patient who comes under your care following his transfer to the nursing home from an assisted living facility because of behavioral disturbances with which the first facility could not cope. Mr. DiBallo is a sociable man who speaks only Italian. The nursing home staff tell you that Mr. DiBallo's son objects to his father being described as "demented," and has ordered that no psychotropic medications be given without his specific consent and involvement. Within the first 24 hours of his admission, the patient physically assaults another patient (a wandering old lady who came into his room) and subsequently an aide who approaches him to assist him with bathing. He does not appear to be in any pain, and he ambulates freely. He will not allow a close physical evaluation, however. You review the records and find that his diagnosis of dementia is fairly well established, with a convincing history from other family members of progressive decline in mental function over a period of several years. There are notes to the effect that this patriarchal man was always short tempered, but that he has become more so as his dementia has progressed. Unable to contact the son and faced with an aggressive patient and an anxious nursing home administration, you initiate treatment with divalproex and intermittent lorazepam. With the first dose of lorazepam, he falls into a deep sleep. The son visits and complains to the nursing home administration and to the Health Department that his father has been "drugged."

STUDY QUESTIONS

1. How could the son's misperceptions have been avoided?
2. Has Mr. Diballo been overtreated?
3. Does the son have the right to control the treatment of his father?

CASE DISCUSSION

This is a sad situation of familial hostility to "the system," as well as a demonstration of denial by the son. Clearly, some straight talk with the son is needed. The son needs to recognize that the father has dementia, for otherwise his father would have to be held responsible for his antisocial actions—actions that are in fact explicable on the basis of his dementia, and of course forgivable, but in need of treatment. The son also needs to realize that his father cannot be accommodated without medication approaches, that oversedation is a likely side effect of dose titration during the acute phase of his father's agitation, and that the side effect will reverse. The possibility of controlling the behavior without even making the patient sleepy should be explained (many families do not realize this). In this case, the son is actually not the health care proxy, and therefore his rights are fairly restricted. If he were the health care proxy, he would have the right to be very directive about treatment; even in that case, however, the safety of other patients and

the humane management of his own father could override the son's power as proxy.

Ann Southard

Ann Southard is a patient with advanced dementia. She is in considerable discomfort from time to time from an old, ununited hip fracture. Ms. Southard is depressed and weeps to herself during the day. Whenever her family comes, she complains that she is in pain. You have a long discussion with two daughters of eight children, and both daughters express the desire that their mother be allowed to "die peacefully," since her life is currently so miserable. However, the patient is not terminal, is physically robust, even overweight, and still eats well. She can make her needs known and can clearly express her mood, which is one of resignation and depression.

STUDY QUESTIONS

1. The family members are trying to be humane, but are they giving up too soon?
2. How should the clinician redirect this family's concern into making a good plan for the future care of their mother?

CASE DISCUSSION

In this case the family members are perhaps overestimating the terminal nature of their mother's condition. They are underestimating the treatability of depression and the fact that her complaints of pain may be linked to her depression. Ms. Southard should be treated with an antidepressant and concurrently with adequate pain relievers. Efforts beyond the pharmaceutical should be made to improve physical comfort by mobilizing her if possible and by local physical therapy techniques to relieve pain. Management should focus on doing what can be done to relieve her while planning reasonably what to do for the future in the event that she should become acutely ill. Discussion with the family centers on what would be done should she become sick again (the patient has had recurrent urinary tract infections and has had a septic condition twice; both times she was saved from the brink with intravenous antibiotics and hospitalization, occasions which the daughters describe as "horrific" because their mother became so agitated in the hospital setting). One of the daughters is the health care proxy, so she has the right to make decisions, as her mother is unable to fully perceive her situation. Orders are written that should she become acutely ill, "comfort care" measures only will be taken. During the next 10 months or so, increasing doses of opiates are used for pain relief, and antidepressants are used with some effect on her underlying sadness. An abrupt episode of hypotension heralds a swinging febrile illness with temperatures up to 105°F and some cloudiness of the urine. The probability of urosepsis is high, but the patient is by now almost comatose and remains hypotensive. Even with oxygen, saturations cannot be brought above the mid-80s. Increasing doses of opiates, continuous oxygen, and tepid bathing are used to increase her comfort and bring her fever down, along with acetaminophen suppositories. The family gathers from far and near for a moving vigil at her deathbed. She dies peacefully, surrounded by family members, who clearly believe that they have done the right thing by allowing her to die of an acute illness when her overall situation was distressing and uncomfortable for her and when she did not have a quality of life she would choose to prolong.

A principle demonstrated throughout this book is that family members should be used and if possible, incorporated as part of the therapeutic team. However, family members need to recognize that they are not directing the management of the case. An exception to this may occur when the patient has appointed a health care proxy or has a durable power of attorney for health care; in this situation the family member or other surrogate is really acting as the patient and therefore has the same right to refuse treatment as any competent patient. However, even in such instances the health care team may have reached consensus about a certain direction of management, and a family member may disagree. Although every effort should be made to understand the family member's point of view, health care professionals are not obligated to (and ethically should not) carry out medically inappropriate investigations or treatments, especially treatments that may harm or distress the patient. Nor are clinicians obligated to deny the patient the potential benefit of medications, such as antidepressants or analgesics. Because negative images of older patients "drugged and incapable" are widespread, psychotropic medications are a problem for some families. Clinicians may find themselves in opposition to family members who would prefer to see the patient alert and frightened, rather than calm yet less attentive. Whereas the clinician must listen to the family and staff in assessing the effect of each situation or dose change, the therapeutic window for drugs in many older patients is narrow. It is best to prepare the family by mentioning the possibility of oversedation during the dose titration of psychotropics that are intended to calm.

> ● When tranquilizers are used, the alternatives are not "alert" versus "drugged," but "frightened" versus "calm."

Families and health care professionals alike often do not realize that unless there is a legal authority (health care proxy or durable power of attorney), the rights and obligations of family members are limited. It is clearly undesirable to have to act against family members' wishes; however, this may be necessary at times. Before such issues become contentious, the clinician would be wise to involve colleagues, other health professionals, ethics committees, hospital administration, and even legal counsel. Especially in nursing home and hospital sites, such disagreements sometimes reach a crisis before it is realized that no one has actually spent time with the family member to find out what is creating the misdirected advocacy.

In the nursing home and sometimes in the hospital, the clinician may not have a long history of knowing the family and patient. In both sites the bonding between a health professional and a family member may have occurred with a nurse or social worker, rather than the clinician. Good communication between these professionals and the clinician is then essential.

> ● In the case of a health care proxy or durable power of attorney, the family member or surrogate can act as the patient but does not act as the clinician.

George Heilenkampf *(Part I)*

George is a long-term nursing home patient of yours who is kyphotic, dependent, and immobilized. For several weeks he has been overtly depressed and uninterested. He has been weeping, refusing food, and even refusing his medications and pulling off his oxygen. Thinking he might be depressed, you initiate sertraline (Zoloft) with strikingly good effect, and virtually all the target symptoms respond. His niece, whom you have never met, sees him 4 weeks later. She is shocked to find him on a psychotropic medication and insists that it be stopped. She believes that her uncle is "different" than he used to be and that the medication is interfering with his mind.

STUDY QUESTIONS

1. How would you justify the medication to the niece?
2. Does the niece actually have the right to insist on the medication being stopped?

George Heilenkampf *(Part II)*

Despite explanations of the treatment and the lack of an official proxy, Mr. Heilenkampf's niece insists on the medication being withdrawn. Following discussion with the nursing home administration, it is decided to temporarily discontinue the medication; but you insist that it will be restarted should his symptoms break through again. The trial period without the medication commences and all the symptoms return. When you call to describe this to the niece, she mentions that he was previously on an antidepressant following a suicide attempt and that she had suppressed both facts in giving the history when he was first admitted to the facility because she feared that he would be treated differently if the facility staff members thought he was "mentally ill" or a suicide risk.

STUDY QUESTIONS

1. What common misapprehensions and prejudices are revealed here?
2. Was it right to withdraw Mr. Heilenkampf's medication even though everyone on the team knew that it had been effective?

CASE DISCUSSION

It was convincingly demonstrated to the niece that the medication was a necessity, and she did not have the right to interfere. The withdrawal of a potentially helpful medication when there was adequate record that the patient had responded well to it and was not suffering side effects was inappropriate. Further discussion would have revealed the niece's unreasonable, although common, prejudices and embarrassment about her uncle's "mental" history. The stigma of mental illness is an issue for many family members, and it can interfere profoundly with treatment and contribute to misunderstandings.

FAMILY STRESSES

The role of the family or other caregiver is stressful; situations often continue over years, many times involving increasing dependency. The primary care clinician's role in enhancing the caregiver's coping and behavioral skills must be balanced by an active approach to preventing and relieving these stresses.[11,12]

Characteristics of the dependent patient that are especially stressful include disturbed nights, aggressive or abusive behavior by the patient, physical dependence on the caregiver for ADLs, incontinence, and ingratitude. This last characteristic incorporates a range of behaviors that are not necessarily under the patient's conscious control.

Factors in the caregiver that increase the caregiver's stress include the caregiver's own frailty, alcoholism or other emotional problems, other stressful responsibilities, and poor health.

The burden of caregiving frequently lands on one individual, even when there are multiple family members. The primary caregiver is often a woman who generally has many other responsibilities, including job and family.

The primary care clinician must be familiar with and recommend the vital resources known to improve quality of life and provide respite for the caregiver: day care programs for the patient (both social and medical, as appropriate to the intensity of the patient's needs), senior centers, nutrition programs, transportation, legal and management services, in-home respite (e.g., "granny-sitting," home aides, and volunteers), and short-stay respite programs (short admissions of up to 2 weeks to long-term care facilities). If these options are not locally available, clinicians should encourage local initiatives to develop such services.

PLACEMENT: GETTING THE LEVEL OF CARE RIGHT

The issue of appropriate placement and housing is in part a clinical decision, and doctors must be involved. Yet many clinicians are relatively inexperienced in what the different "levels of care" mean and what their implications are for the patient and the family.

Assisted Living

The terminology for the different types of housing alternatives varies from state to state. In general, however, assisted living (also known as board and care, adult homes, retirement communities, and other names) generally implies a setting in which a person must have a fair degree of personal independence but will need help, perhaps progressively, for certain aspects of daily life, such as transportation and obtaining and preparing food. Generally, an assisted living facility is not financed by any insurance system but is a self-pay situation for the family or patient. Assisted living represents one of the fastest-growing parts of the health care industry in this country today. Although an individual may be safer in such an environment and certainly may gain from the social companionship, better nutrition, and supervision of medications that might take place in that setting, the loss of one's own home and the dignity and independence of the home must be weighed against the advantages. Some patients welcome such a setting, relieved of the stresses of managing a household or a home. Others welcome it because they are lonely. Many more resist, often out of morbid, primitive fears associated with nursing homes.

Assisted living facilities are a resource limited to those who can afford them. A danger of using such a facility is the premature use of the patient's financial resources, while the patient is still relatively independent. If skilled nursing placement is likely in the future because of progressive underlying disease or disability, it may be desirable to keep a proportion of the person's estate available for that purpose so that the choices of placement when skilled care (i.e., a nursing home) is needed will not be restricted. Other individuals work hard to achieve Medicaid eligibility, "spending down" resources to make themselves technically poor enough for Medicaid (ironically, our country's main payor for nursing home care, even though it was designed to provide health care for the poor and needy). Clearly, making such decisions involves financial expertise. Also, since the decisions about such housing alternatives must be made on the basis of the patient's prognosis, the clinician should be involved at least in assessing what that prognosis is. The presence of a progressive illness such as Alzheimer's disease, versus the relative recoverability of an individual temporarily disabled from surgery or a stroke, would obviously make a difference in such planning.

Home Care

Continuing to live at home with increasing home care services is an alternative, but the actual availability of home health aides is a current crisis in this country because of the fact that the system underpays them and society undervalues them. There is no career structure, and people do not last long in the job. As a result, these aides go elsewhere and get higher pay. Private arrangements to garner aide support for dependent individuals carry risks, yet because agencies supplying such aides are generally run for profit, there is more expense involved. Once an individual needs

more than about 8 hours of aide service per day, this option becomes more expensive than institutional care because of the high costs of home care services. However, an individual may be much better settled in the familiarity and comfort of his or her own home environment. These issues of where the more frail and dependent elder should live in our society are burning current issues in the political and social climate. Ironically, an individual eligible for Medicaid and still able to live at home has access to a pleasing range of home care services (which still nonetheless depends on the recruitment of the personnel to actually do the job).

Nursing Homes

Although many assisted living facilities allow the patient or family to buy more and more services, so that a very dependent person can continue to live in the same environment, the most dependent of the elderly population (unless enormous personal and financial resources can be brought to bear to keep the person at home) cannot be accommodated in other than a *nursing home* setting—that is, a skilled nursing facility (SNF). An individual who needs skilled care will be quite dependent for his or her daily functions, possibly with some continence issues, or will have a regular need for medical treatments and be in need of sufficient assistance with self-care skills (ADLs) that he or she could *not* be accommodated in an assisted living setting designed for people who can generally walk to meals or get there themselves. The environment of nursing homes is generally institutional, hospital-like, and not homelike, even though it will become the home of someone placed there for the long term. Hopefully, pressure by boomers on behalf of their parents and elders will ultimately improve the general environment of nursing homes: smaller and more "home-like" is the aim. The mix of patients is very broad: many have dementia, but some have good cognition and physical frailty. There will also be some much younger patients in this setting. Whereas the physically frail often welcome such placement because of the relief and sense of safety, others do not welcome placement and would prefer a life of slight risk, valuing their independence. Decisions clearly need to be individualized. Rural elders tend to be placed sooner, due to the difficulties of accessing home care. There is also much prejudice against nursing homes that is inappropriate: a person may be safer and better accommodated in a nursing home than in an unsafe house (even though it is "home"). The illegality of a hospital discharging a patient to an unsafe location, considering the person's needs, remains a major factor in making hospitalization a major route to nursing home placement for older individuals.

FINANCIAL CONCERNS AND PUBLIC POLICY

Although the health care of older persons consumes a large proportion of public spending on health care, at least half of health care costs are still direct expenses to the elderly themselves or to their families. Older people may avoid health care or at least not fill prescriptions, fearing their own impoverishment or the impoverishment of their family after they have gone. The welcomed prescription drug benefit (Medicare Part D) has been seriously compromised by its complexity; too many choices!

Because health care for the old is publicly financed, changing policies regarding payment for services and limitations on these payments are issues for everyone. All health professionals can and must provide strong input into policy development.[13,14]

The cost of good comprehensive health care is high. As a person becomes more dependent, increasing the use of professional time from a variety of disciplines is justified; this might postpone the period of maximal dependency, including long-term institutional care, which still forms the closing chapter of many older persons' lives (at considerable public expense).

Medicaid, although designed to provide medical care for the truly poor (and the American poverty line is drawn very low, relative to other Western countries), has become the main source of payment for nursing home care. It therefore has been naturally tempting for families to make their loved one Medicaid eligible (i.e., poor enough to qualify for Medicaid) by divesting themselves of their estates in different ways. Obviously, this is antisocial and counterproductive to the whole system in many ways. However, some would argue that such families are only gaining access to their tax dollars for services that (in the opinion of some) might properly be covered by a beneficent system.

Because Medicare is federally funded, and because Medicaid is influenced by federal funding and implemented at the state level, there are many opportunities for clinicians to have useful input into the policies and their implementation at all levels. The clinician's primary duty must be to his or her individual patient in ensuring that the patient gets a fair share of the resources available; however, the role of the clinician as an advocate for reasonable public policy is also significant. Clinicians and all other health professionals must be advocates for change in the health care system, to encourage payment for and development of the health care services that will fit the characteristics of old persons when ill and the patterns of illness and disability that can be anticipated. At present, our payment system is based on old-fashioned principles of "reactive" medical practice, not the preventive, proactive approach that elderly patients need.

ETHICAL ISSUES

Humanitarian and financial concerns, issues of intensity of treatment and of resuscitative efforts, and how much, how invasively, and how expensively to investigate and manage medical problems in older individuals are among the core ethical issues in geriatric medical care.

The central principle of the patient's autonomy as the prime decision maker in health care must always be maintained and acknowledged. Yet in the old, the cognitive impairment so frequently accompanying illness necessitates substituted judgments, leading to the necessity of legal steps such as power of attorney, health care proxy, and different types of advance directives. Much of this effort is directed at preventing unnecessary and sometimes inappropriate life-prolonging modes of care for the individual. However, the issue is not as simple as merely omitting expensive aspects of care. Often, an expensive intervention that would appear to be "high tech" may in fact be palliative and reduce the person's dependency on others for some considerable time.

Every decision in an older person's medical management must be coordinated with the patient's known wishes, the clinician's knowledge of how medically worthwhile the procedure or intervention is (information that is often difficult to obtain accurately), and other factors. It must be remembered that competence is task specific (i.e., the patient may be competent to take part in some decisions, yet not able to take part in others that are more complex). For the clinician to make a positive contribution to this process, he or she must have full knowledge of the patient and family, based on a comprehensive assessment.

SUMMARY OF PRINCIPLES OF GERIATRIC PRIMARY CARE

The principles of geriatric primary medical care flow naturally from the characteristics of older persons and the prevalence of the major chronic and acute diseases. Older individuals lacking a family member or other advocate require the advocacy of professionals: community social services, the primary care clinician, volunteers, and others. Yet elders have the right to refuse this help, and skill is required to properly comprehend an individual's competence. For example, living alone is not without risk, although it may be what the patient wants. If so, it is up to the professionals involved to do everything possible to make things safe, even if there is risk. The following principles of geriatric primary care should be observed. Practicing clinicians using this text may wish to compare these principles with their own practices.

PRINCIPLES OF PRIMARY CARE

- *Accessibility:* This includes the physical ability of the patient to get in to see the health care professional, with home visitation available as an alternative. Good telephone access is also necessary.
- *Comprehensiveness:* All involved health professionals must be comfortable handling not only physical and social problems, but also sexual, psychologic, fiscal, and ethical problems. Health professionals must be familiar with the range and roles of other professional services.
- *Coordination:* This extends to the coordination of not only other health professional disciplines, but also nonhealth professionals, such as those concerned with housing, legal and financial issues, and tax liability.
- *Continuity:* This is often challenging. Ideally, the same primary care clinician and health care team care for the patient in the various clinical sites. Especially during some hospitalizations or with long-term care facility placement, the primary clinician may have to take a secondary role in medical care of the patient; continuity must then be achieved by good communication.
- *Accountability:* This principle is vital because the frailty of many older people can lead to the inability to be assertive in obtaining care. Health professionals must take responsibility (while never overlooking the autonomy of the patient) in following up on prescriptions and plans. (This includes scheduling follow-up visits and calling or even visiting "no-shows" if they are frail or at high risk.)

The characteristics of old people when ill mandate the following principles of geriatric care:

PRINCIPLES OF GERIATRIC CARE

- *Asking the right questions:* In general with the elderly patient, it is not enough to see what the individual's concerns are. The clinician must ask the right questions about functionality and symptoms that must be addressed, even if the patient does not mention the symptoms or realize their significance.
- *Clinical alertness:* The clinician should look for subtle changes in mental status and function so that an anticipatory approach is achieved and emergent acute illness is identified early.

- *Advocacy:* The clinician's role sometimes extends beyond accountability, since the patient often needs a health care professional to act as advocate through the complexity of the system. This may involve the clinician in shared control of decision making, including the sharing of such control with fiscal managers.
- *Integration of the family's and other caregivers' roles:* The family is part of the team, and may even at times "lead" the team, but must be well trained and informed. The family can sometimes be adversarial.
- *Emphasis on function:* Maintaining physical and psychosocial function if at all possible, including during hospitalization, is an important principle. Health professionals must be aware of their patient's functional level, objectively measure and record it, and always work to maintain or regain it.
- *Accurate diagnosis:* Recognition that several diagnoses may contribute to one symptom or problem, making it necessary to hunt for contributory medical illnesses and other problems (environmental, behavioral, familial, psychologic) in all cases.
- *Serial observation:* Using *time* to assess the diagnosis and function, rather than relying on the acute care technique of comprehensive tests at a specific point in time. This involves tolerating ambiguity on occasion; "watchful waiting" is too low key for many professionals and families, but it is often the best approach.
- *Recognition that even a good intervention may produce harm:* Elders should not be denied the many benefits of modern medical management simply to avoid potential side effects. Careful follow-up is the safety net to discover unexpected problems.
- *Setting of clear goals, identifying target symptoms, and organizing good follow-up:* Everyone (especially the clinician) needs to know what the intervention (e.g., prescription, relocation, or procedure) is intended to do, and the follow-up process should establish whether these objectives are achieved or not.
- *Pursuit of the noncompliant or no-show patient:* Follow-up visits in elders should be scheduled. If patients fail to keep appointments, it may be a sign that they are ill or have not realized the importance of their visit. The clinician and staff must be aggressive at maintaining follow-up, which often becomes neglected, to the patient's (and society's) cost.
- *Allowing sufficient time for recovery of function:* It is appropriate to hurry patients out of the hospital before *full* recovery, but the primary care clinician and community services must then ensure that further recovery is facilitated.

- *Postponement of dependency:* A central principle of geriatric medicine, postponement of dependency also makes postponement of institutionalization possible. A multidisciplinary effort must be made to maintain individuals in the familiarity and dignity of their home surroundings for as long as possible. This must not be done at too high a cost to the functioning and financial status of the caregivers and their families.

- *Communication:* Ongoing, clear communication with the patient, the family, and all others involved, especially at times of transfer from one level of care to another, is vital. Communication must use "functional" language.

SUMMARY

The special characteristics of many older patients and of their responses to treatment and other interventions mandate significantly different approaches to their care than have become the standard for younger adults. In particular, the clinician and family have a much greater role in ensuring safety and good health care because older patients frequently cannot advocate for themselves.

References

1. Williamson J, et al. Old people at home: their unreported needs. Lancet 1117, 1965.
2. Barsky AJ, et al. Silent myocardial ischemia: is the person or the event silent? JAMA 264(9):1132, 1990.
3. Nordyke RA, Gilbert FI, Harada ASM. Graves' disease: influence of age on clinical findings, Arch Intern Med 148(3):626, 1988.
4. U.S. Preventive Services Task Force. Guide to Clinical Preventive Services, 2005. Agency for Healthcare Research and Quality, DMMS, 2005.
5. Lehmann LS, Puopolo AL, Shaykevich S, Brennan TA. Iatrogenic events resulting in intensive care admission: frequency, cause, and disclosure to patients and institutions. Am J Med 118(4):409, 2005.
6. Jahnigen D, et al. Iatrogenic disease in hospitalized elderly veterans. J Am Geriatr Soc 30(6):387, 1982.
7. Classen DC, et al. Adverse drug events in hospitalized patients: excess length of stay, extra costs, and attributable mortality. JAMA 277(4):301, 1997.
8. Rochon PA, Gurwitz JH. Prescribing for seniors: neither too much nor too little. JAMA 282(2):113, 1999.
9. Gallo JJ, et al. Handbook of Geriatric Assessment. 3rd ed. Rockville, Md.: Aspen, 1999.
10. Ham RJ. Evolving standards in patient and caregiver support. Alzheimer Dis Assoc Disord 13(suppl 2):S27, 1999.
11. Torti FM, Gwyther LP, Reed SD, Friedman JY, Schulman KA. A multinational review of recent trends and reports in dementia caregiver burden. Alzheimer Dis Assoc Disord 18(2):99, 2004.
12. Rabins PV, Mace NL, Lucas MJ. The impact of dementia on the family. JAMA 248(3):333, 1982.
13. Ball RM. Public-private solutions to protection against the cost of long-term care. J Am Geriatr Soc 38:156, 1990.
14. Schneider EL, Guralnik JN. The aging of America: impact on health care costs. JAMA 263(17):2335, 1990.

POSTTEST

1. Which one of the following is not a typical nonspecific presentation of illness in old age?
   a. Self-neglect
   b. Headache
   c. Falling
   d. Anorexia
   e. Fatigue

2. Even when access to health care is good, symptoms that have been shown to be disproportionately *not* presented to clinicians include all except which one of the following?
   a. Falling
   b. Depression
   c. Deafness
   d. Nocturia
   e. Incontinence

3. Which one of the following has *not* been demonstrated to be a consequence of immobilization?
   a. Osteoporosis
   b. Venous thrombosis
   c. Insomnia
   d. Pressure sores
   e. Instability

4. Which one of the following statements concerning illness in old age is false?
   a. Depression can be diagnosed in the absence of sadness.
   b. Peritonitis often fails to localize in acute appendicitis.
   c. CHF, once it occurs, rarely resolves.
   d. One-third of MIs in old age are asymptomatic.
   e. Peripheral sensitivity is reduced.

5. A 75-year-old man has diagnoses of prostatism, constipation, depression, CHF, and allergic rhinitis. He regularly takes furosemide, amitriptyline, dioctyl, and an over-the-counter hay fever medication. Which one of the following is false?
   a. Three of his four medications will increase the need for the dioctyl.
   b. The over-the-counter preparation may worsen three of his five diagnoses.
   c. Only two of his medications increase the risk of acute retention of urine.
   d. He is at risk of orthostasis from three of the medications.
   Questions 6 and 7 relate to the following patient:
   A 79-year-old woman who lives in the country with her retired farmer husband, age 92, comes to your office for the first time. She has not been seen by any clinician for 3 years, but she has continued to take the following long-term medications, generally renewed by telephone. She brings them in a paper sack at your request: furosemide, 40 to 80 mg/day (the dose varying depending upon how much ankle swelling she has); potassium chloride (Slow-K), three times a day; hydrochlorothiazide/triamterene (Dyazide), 50 mg/day; cyclizine (Antivert), 25 mg three times a day; oxybutynin (Ditropan), 5 mg three times a day; amitriptyline, 50 mg at night; phenobarbital, 30 to 60 mg at night as needed for sleep; and digoxin, 0.25 mg/day.
   Her husband asks for her to be seen because she has been dizzy on standing for over a year and has fallen three times in the past 2 weeks, although without injury. She is chronically short of breath on exertion and has some stress incontinence. He describes her as very nervous, often "down" in mood, and tired. She wakes frequently in the night.
   On examination, she is a little confused. Her pulse is regular and there are no signs of CHF. However, her blood pressure is 125/80 sitting and 90/60, with dizziness, on standing.

6. Which one of the following statements relating to the above patient is false?
   a. Four of her existing medications could be contributing to her feelings of depression.
   b. Phenobarbital is probably making her sleep worse.
   c. Digoxin should not be discontinued because her CHF is not controlled.
   d. Ankle swelling is an unreliable indicator of diuretic need.

7. Which one of the following plans of action, in addition to having the patient seen by the visiting nurse at her home in 2 days and by the clinician in the office in 2 weeks, represents the best course of action for the patient?
   a. Obtain an ECG and a serum potassium level, and immediately stop all potentially hypotensive medications.
   b. Stop *all* the medications and prescribe elastic support hose to increase the venous return and reduce orthostasis.
   c. Stop the diuretics and doxepin, but retain the cyclizine and oxybutynin because she still has symptoms that they may be relieving.
   d. Stop all the medications and photograph the contents of her paper bag of medications in anticipation of a formal complaint about her prior clinician.

PRETEST ANSWERS

1. c
2. e
3. b
4. b
5. d
6. a

POSTTEST ANSWERS

1. b
2. d
3. c
4. c
5. c
6. c
7. a

Initial Assessment
Kenneth K. Steinweg

OBJECTIVES

Upon completion of this chapter, the reader will be able to:

- Describe the physical office characteristics that address the special needs of older patients.
- Understand how to assess a new complex older patient in the office

- Understand the importance of overall function, including activities of daily living (ADLs) and instrumental activities of daily living (IADLs).
- Outline the review of systems as it pertains to older patients, with attention to geriatric syndromes.
- Describe the characteristics of an initial office-based physical examination of the older patient, including attention to specific key physical examination findings and observations.
- Understand the principles of the comprehensive problem list and its use in office-based care.
- Describe the concept of transitional care and the concerns associated with these types of transfers.

PRETEST

1. Which one of the following is an instrumental activity of daily living rather than an activity of daily living?
   a. Bathing
   b. Dressing
   c. Toileting
   d. Shopping
   e. Ambulation

2. When seeing older patients, concerns about which one kind of symptoms should trigger mental status testing?
   a. Behavioral changes
   b. Apathy
   c. Memory difficulties
   d. Concerns about judgment
   e. All of the above

3. You are examining a new patient, an older male, in your office. Which of following physical examination findings are you not expecting to find and will trigger further investigations in this patient?
   a. Presbycusis
   b. Cataracts
   c. S_4 on cardiac examination
   d. Small testes
   e. Enlarged smooth prostate

Performing an evaluation of an older patient can be a daunting but satisfying experience. These patients come with extensive life histories, prior relationships, values established in a different generation than those caring for them, and unique family situations. They often have multiple comorbidities, complex medication regimens, and a different spectrum of symptoms and medical conditions than younger patients. In addition, they require attention to specific issues, such as function and cognition, which require special assessment tools. All these issues require an integrated and logical process that results in a unique synthesis and priority setting for each patient. Not all older patients are medically complex, but many will be. Above all, adequate evaluation requires patience and an organized approach.

Millie Lipton, *Part 1*

Your new patient is Millie Lipton, a 79-year-old woman who will be coming to your office to establish care. Her daughter, Michele, has scheduled the appointment and will accompany her. Mrs. Lipton has moved to your area 2 weeks ago from another state to be close to her daughter following the death of her husband a year ago. She lives in an independent apartment only blocks away from her daughter, who is an English professor at a local university.

STUDY QUESTIONS

1. How should a primary care office be organized so as to best address the needs of elderly patients such as Mrs. Lipton?
2. How should the routine history and physical examination of an elderly patient such as Mrs. Lipton differ from that of a younger adult?
3. What should be done beforehand to ensure that the initial visit goes well?

PREVISIT PREPARATION

A successful office assessment is a significant challenge and requires previsit preparation, a proper office focus, excellent medical records, attention to aspects of care that are different in older patients, and follow-up visits to finish incomplete business. Above all, flexibility in the approach to the patient as the history and physical examination unfolds is necessary to meet both patient and physician expectations. It is unreasonable to expect to do everything on the first visit. Instead, a reasonable expectation of the first visit is to establish a relationship with the patient, fully understand the priorities for care, and develop a plan for follow-up visits.

> ● An optimal assessment is a significant challenge and requires previsit preparation, a proper office focus, excellent medical records, attention to aspects of care that are different in older patients, and follow-up visits.

Appropriate previsit preparation can streamline the collection of essential information and reduce frustration for patient, family, and health care provider alike. Our office requires prior medical records be obtained before appointments will be made. Before this requirement, the availability of past medical records was below 50%, resulting in incomplete documentation and provision of care. Even with this requirement, records are often incomplete and require additional requests after the first visit. An alternative method would be to use an extensive questionnaire, to be completed at home before the office visit; Box 4-1 outlines the essential elements of such a questionnaire.

Use of an electronic medical record (EMR) is now considered essential to quality medical care of older patients.[1] The frequent use of the emergency departments, hospital, specialty consultants, and nursing homes by older patients requires the timely transfer of this essential health information. EMRs have numerous advantages over the paper medical record, and the time spent in loading essential health information before and during this first visit is worthwhile. Some of this information gathering can be done by the office staff or by the physician at the time of the initial interview. An explanation of the EMR and its advantages to the patient is important. Interacting with the computer, the patient, and the family in a way that is complementary is an important skill and need not detract from the quality of the visit.

Insist that your patients or their families bring their medications with them for each visit, not just the first visit. Recent or frequent medication changes are often not remembered or recalled accurately, and medications prescribed by multiple providers are often not contained in the medical record. The use of generic and trade names of medications are often confusing to patients and can result in taking duplicates or other self-administration errors.[2]

PROPER OFFICE FOCUS

Ideally, a clinical setting for older patients will take their special needs into consideration. This would include office design and construction, patient flow to allow for transportation and mobility devices, and attention to specific physical and physiologic characteristics of these patients.

Preparation for caring for older patients begins outside of the examination room. There are many special

---

Box 4-1   Suggested Items for a Geriatric Preappointment Questionnaire

1. Patient name, address, and date of birth
2. Family members/caregivers and proximity (including whom to contact in emergencies)
3. Who lives with the patient? Does the patient live alone?
4. Nature of home
5. Name, address, and phone number of current/recent physicians and pharmacy
6. Current medical problems
7. Current medications, including over-the-counter and complementary remedies
8. Past medical problems
9. Past operations and surgeries
10. Past fractures or other accidents
11. Past hospitalizations
12. Mental health history
13. Family history
14. Recent laboratory studies and X-rays
15. A review of systems to include questions about sexuality, continence, falling, mood, and memory loss, as well as dyspnea, chest pain, other pain, mobility problems, and organ system review
16. Personal history of alcohol, smoking, and illicit drug use
17. Recent health maintenance or screening procedures
18. Specifics about cancer screening
19. Immunization history
20. Description of meals and drinks on a typical day
21. Exercise on a typical day
22. Driving history
23. Services already provided in the home
24. Special arrangements made for emergency contact such as "life line"
25. Patient identification or emergency bracelet worn

characteristics that need to be considered in approaching the facility. Among these are parking, ease of entry, wheelchair access, and interior design. Once inside your office, pleasant personnel who are familiar with working with older frail patients and their families will make a favorable impression and put the patient at ease. Examination room size will need to be adequate to accommodate a third person in addition to the patient and physician, as many older patients are accompanied by spouses, their children, or caregivers, whose input and assistance is often helpful. There are many additional environmental considerations in caring for older patients; these are summarized in Box 4-2.

Scheduling should allow for patients to be seen at the time of their appointment. It is reasonable to expect patients to arrive 15 minutes before their appointment time, but it is then incumbent that they be seen at their appointment time or shortly thereafter. Many of the conditions that afflict older patients make it difficult for them to wait long periods of time, and often their caregiver will have similar or pressing issues. If the patient cannot be seen within 20 minutes of their appointment, they should be given an explanation and estimation of when they will be seen.

Finally, adequate time should be allowed for the initial visit. Most patients will require a full 50 minutes to complete the first visit, and often this will still not be enough time. Scheduling new patient appointments early in the morning or first thing in the afternoon will often allow uninterrupted time. In any case, protected time needs to be planned to meet the goals of the first visit: establishing a relationship with the patient, understanding the priorities for care, and developing a plan for follow-up visits.

Millie Lipton, *Part 2*

You have 10 pages of old medical records on Mrs. Lipton. Her previous primary care physician's records include a medication list, diagnoses, and recent heath maintenance activities. You identify the following:

Past Medical History: hypertension, coronary artery disease with stent placement 10 years ago, hyperlipidemia, osteoarthritis of the cervical spine, and Alzheimer's disease

Medications: aspirin 81 mg/day, calcium 500 mg/day, pravastatin 40 mg hs (bedtime), donepezil 10 mg hs, amlodipine 5 mg/day

Past Surgical History: bilateral cataract extractions, hysterectomy, cholecystectomy

Health Maintenance: two negative pap smears and two normal mammograms in the past 3 years and an unremarkable physical examination in the preceding year

Laboratory work, done approximately 1 year ago, reveals a normal complete blood count (CBC),

---

Box 4-2 Characteristics of an Ideal Office for Older Patients	
Exterior and access • Well-lit parking and sidewalks • Oversized parking spaces • Minimize grade changes • Easy access and proximity • Wheelchair accessible • Handicapped spaces for parking • Proper sidewalk maintenance • Covered walkway/driveway for inclement weather • Automatic doors • Signage with large letters and numbers **Interior** • Simple "way-finding" and patient traffic flow • Signage with large letters and numbers • Use of color change to mark borders (e.g., between wall and floor) • Adequate lighting (i.e., brighter than usual) • Sound-absorbent materials to dampen noise	• Temperature is warm and stable throughout the facility • Waiting area large enough to accommodate wheelchairs, walkers, and family members • Halls and ramps free of clutter • Rails along hallway walls • Levers instead of door knobs • Minimal background noise (including little or no background music) • Bathrooms that are wheelchair accessible and equipped with grab bars, raised toilet seats, and wheelchair-accessible sinks **Examination Room** • Entrance wide enough to accommodate wheelchairs, walkers, and gurneys • Large enough to accommodate family members (i.e., one or more extra chairs) • Electric examination tables (that can be raised and lowered) • Computer located in a convenient place for physician use

Modified from American Geriatrics Society Health Care Systems Committee. Ambulatory Geriatric Clinical Care and Services: American Geriatric Society Position Statement, The American Geriatrics Society, New York, 2000. Adapted from Brennenman, KS. The Office Visit. In Practical Ambulatory Geriatrics, 2nd ed. (Yoshikowa TT, Cobbs EL, Brummel-Smith K, eds.), Mosby-Year Book, St. Louis, 1998.

CHEM-7, and thyroid-stimulating hormone (TSH). The lipid profile is excellent with a total cholesterol of 188, low-density lipoprotein (LDL) of 98, and high-density lipoprotein (HDL) of 45, and you assume that these were obtained while she was on her lipid-lowering medication.

Your office nurse tells you that Mrs. Lipton is accompanied by her daughter.

CASE DISCUSSION

The case of Mrs. Lipton illustrates the beginning of a typical new elderly patient visit in a busy clinic setting. An important task of the initial visit is to understand the patient's context in regard to this visit. As is often the case, a change in the patient's situation has occurred (the death of her husband). Just as important is why and how the decision was made that the patient should leave her home, friends, and social supports of 40 years to live near her daughter. Clearly there are some important issues here, and an appropriate opening comment will help in beginning to understand this decision: "Welcome to our office, how is it that you came to live in our town?"

The presence of the daughter in the room is also important. An additional person in the examination room is common in the care of older patients and often signifies some loss of independence, concern that certain topics or issues will not be addressed, or cognitive impairment in the patient. The agenda of this family member will also need to be understood and addressed.

THE INTERVIEW AND HISTORY

Taking the time to review the old medical record before stepping into the examination room is important for many reasons. It will aid in understanding the issues that are about to confront you, identify gaps in the information that will need to obtained, and assist in the task of priority setting. It will help in establishing baseline information in the five domains of care in assessing older patients: mental health, physical health, functional abilities, social supports, and economic resources. Just as importantly, reviewing the records before starting the visit demonstrates interest, preparation, and concern.

> ● A complete initial assessment of older patients will require the evaluation of five domains: mental health, physical health, functional abilities, social supports, and economic resources.

The introduction and history is often a substantial portion of the first visit. Usually the vast majority of diagnoses and their associated assessment and plan are derived from this comprehensive history. Its components are listed in Box 4-3. It is recommended that the patient remain fully clothed and comfortable during the initial interview. This is encouraged because of the time required for history taking and because older patients do not tolerate environmental extremes. During the subsequent short period of time necessary to prepare the patient for the physical examination, you can update the medical record, fill out paperwork, respond to messages, or conduct other office activities.

The examination room should be conducive to a good interview, with a quiet environment and the patient and physician sitting close to one another. Many older patients have a degree of hearing impairment. Patients with hearing impairment use lip reading to facilitate their understanding of what is said. Therefore, the physician should ask which side is best for hearing and sit face-to-face to enhance eye contact.

Although family members can be extremely important in providing additional and corroborative information and in assisting in the implementation of your diagnostic and treatment plans, the presence of another person in the examination may not be what the patient prefers. Office staff will need to be attuned to this situation and an opportunity created during vital sign determination or another office routine for the patient to be briefly separated from those accompanying them to ascertain the patient's wishes in a tactful way. This brief intervention will also help in understanding the reason for the desired presence of the additional person.

Medications should be reviewed on the first and every subsequent visit.[2] Noting discrepancies in dose and in additional prescription and nonprescription

---

Box 4–3 Components of the History of the Older Patient

- History of current problems
- Past medical history
- Past surgical history
- Medication review
- Social history
- Family history
- Caregiver status
- Review of symptoms and systems, including geriatric syndromes
- Specialty physicians currently involved in care
- Functional history: activities of daily living (ADLs) and instrumental activities of daily living (IADLs)
- Current use of community resources

medications taken is common, so this review is one of the first things to be accomplished. Often a medication will indicate a missing diagnosis, and inquiry regarding the reason for its use is very helpful.

ASPECTS OF DISEASE PRESENTATION UNIQUE TO OLDER PATIENTS

Several aspects of disease presentation are characteristic of geriatric medicine and, therefore, are worthy of note here. They include the occurrence of multiple conditions, the vague and nontraditional presentation of disease, the frequent occurrence of certain syndromes as presenting symptoms, and the presence of certain diseases that are largely unique to the older population.

Multiple Medical Conditions

The typical older patient usually has several medical conditions, such as arthritis, lung, and heart disease. Figure 4-1 displays the most common conditions that affect older patients. Study of this figure suggests that most patients will have at least two, and many will have three or more, chronic conditions. Accurately capturing and recording these conditions is a major component of the initial visit. As an example, Figure 4-2

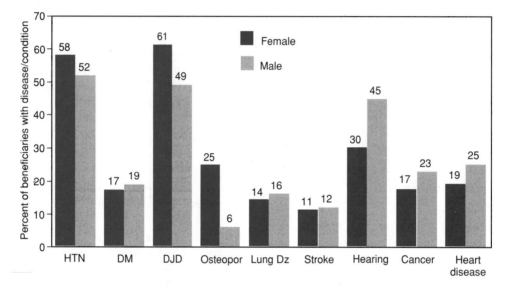

FIGURE 4–1

Medicare beneficiaries' self-reported diseases and chronic conditions, by sex, 2000. *(Modified from Centers for Medicaid and Medicare Services, Office of Research, Development, and Information. Data from the Medicare Current Beneficiary Survey [MCBS] 2000. Access to Care File.)*

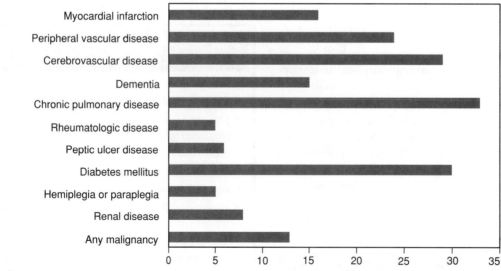

FIGURE 4–2

Percentage of heart failure patients with comorbid diseases. *(Redrawn from Zhang JX, Rathouz PJ, Chin MH. Comorbidity and the Concentration of Healthcare Expenditures in Older Patients with Heart Failure, J Am Geriatr Soc 51:476-482, 2003.)*

provides a glimpse of the comorbid conditions that often accompany patients who have congestive heart failure. Because of this frequent presence of multiple comorbid conditions, a routine geriatric office visit is complex, requiring tracking of clinical and laboratory data for each condition.

Vague, Ill-Defined Symptoms

It is not uncommon for older persons to present with vague, often puzzling symptoms such as "weakness," "not feeling right," or "losing energy." While such symptoms in older patients are nonspecific and difficult to interpret, they often represent new functional deficits that reflect a new illness or condition. These symptoms may be the only manifestation of classic conditions with more typical signs and symptoms in younger patients (e.g., pneumonia, worsening heart failure, urinary tract infection).

Collections of Symptoms Called Geriatric Syndromes

Some collections of symptoms are so common that they have been labeled *geriatric syndromes;* examples include mental status changes, urinary incontinence, falls, and dizziness (Box 4-4). Often, the development of a geriatric syndrome represents the loss of specific functional capacities caused by multiple pathologies in multiple organ systems.[3] These syndromes commonly occur in older patients and now have defined evidence-based approaches to assessment and treatment. The first step in treatment is recognition that one of these syndromes exists and then initiation of the appropriate approach. Geriatric syndromes can be integrated in the review of systems, if desired, but they must often be explicitly sought for in the overall evaluation.

Exclusive Disease Entities

Certain disease entities occur almost exclusively in older patients, such as hip fracture, Parkinson's disease, and polymyalgia rheumatica (see Box 4-4). These geriatric-specific conditions are common, and health care providers need to be comfortable in caring for them in the office setting. Many will involve the use of specialists, for example, hip fractures, but the ongoing long-term management will fall to the primary care provider. Often, involvement of consultants requires frequent written and oral communication, so office systems need to facilitate both forms of communication and to ensure that the results are part of the medical record.

Millie Lipton, *Part 3*

With the old medical records in hand, you start reviewing the medications she has brought with her. You sit facing the patient and note that she is articulate about her past medical history. She uses a week-long daily pill dispenser that her daughter helps to set up at the beginning of each week. As you review her medication bottles, you notice that the doses on the medication labels for donepezil (5 mg/day) and pravastatin (20 mg hs) are half of what the old medical records indicate. The other medications are correct as recorded in the old medical records.

The patient does not know the details of the change in dosage of pravastatin or the donepezil. After a glance from the patient, the daughter mentions that she thought there was some diarrhea and fecal incontinence with the higher dose of the donepezil that resolved on the lower dose. Otherwise the patient is knowledgeable about her

---

Box 4-4 **Conditions that Commonly Occur in Older Patients**	
Classic Geriatric Syndromes	**Geriatric-Specific Disease Entities**
• Dementia	• Osteoporosis
• Delirium	• Alzheimer's disease
• Urinary incontinence	• Stroke
• Falls and gait abnormalities	• Hip fracture
• Behavioral changes	• Polymyalgia rheumatica and/or temporal arteritis
• Weight loss	• Parkinson's disease
• Dizziness	• Pressure sores
• Poor nutrition or feeding impairment	• Macular degeneration
• Sleep disorders	• Sexual dysfunction
	• Gonadal failure in men

medications. You are impressed with her ability to give a past medical history, particularly in light of her "Alzheimer's" history and the fact that she is on donepezil.

You note that she was evaluated by a neurologist 9 months ago for some kind of memory problem— "cognitive impairment." You mention "mild cognitive impairment," and she agrees with the term as does her daughter. She mentions that the examination was performed at a university hospital near her former home but cannot remember the physician's name. She does recall having lots of laboratory work done and a brain scan. Her daughter confirms that all this occurred. After further questions, you request that the daughter help in obtaining those medical records, and make a note to complete a mini-mental status examination at the next visit.

CASE DISCUSSION

There is a clear indication to assess cognition soon. In addition, there appears to be a discrepancy in the diagnosis. The primary care medical record indicates the patient has Alzheimer's disease, and the patient and daughter agree with the term mild cognitive impairment provided by the neurologist. Obtaining her prior neurological evaluation will be critical. In either case, Mrs. Lipton carries a diagnosis that warrants being followed carefully and may represent the beginning phase of a disease causing brain failure that will progress over time. If there are constraints to doing a cognitive assessment on today's visit because of more pressing issues, then a follow-up appointment very shortly is certainly indicated.

ASSESSMENT OF COGNITIVE STATUS

Mental status evaluation of the older patient holds a special area of emphasis and concern in geriatrics. Cognitive deficits, mood disorders, and other behavioral disturbances are common in older patients. Even seasoned health care providers can be misled by patients who retain their social skills while memory, judgment, executive function, and orientation become severely impaired. There is ample evidence that cognitive impairment is not recognized in older patients and depression often missed (Fig. 4-3).

Therefore, health care providers should be attuned to any reference by the patient, caregiver, or family member to memory loss, behavioral change, or reduced function, because any of these may herald the onset of early cognitive impairment, depression, or other serious mental health illness. Thus, *your first-line screening* should be any concern about cognition, behavior, or judgment. This should prompt the selection and administration of an appropriate objective screening tool.

> ● Any concern about cognition, behavior, or judgment should prompt mental status testing.

The prevalence of dementia and Alzheimer's disease rises exponentially with age, doubling every 5 years after age 65.[4] Overall prevalence is about 2% between the ages of 65 and 74, 8% from 75 to 84, and 30% for ages 85 and over.[5] Although routine mental status screening is not recommended for the general

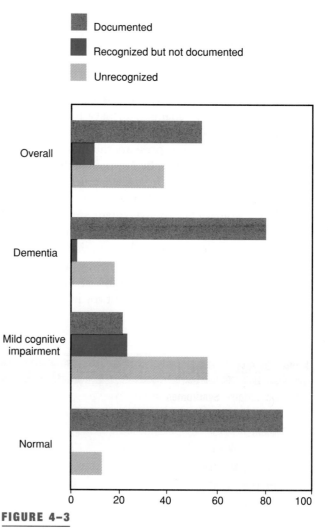

FIGURE 4-3

Detection of cognitive impairment. *(Redrawn from Chodosh J, Petitti DB, Elliott M, et al. Physician Recognition of Cognitive Impairment: Evaluating the Need for Improvement. J Am Geriatr Soc 52:1051-1059, 2004.)*

population,[6] screening should be triggered by any suggestion of cognitive difficulty. In practice, many healthy persons in their 60s and early 70s will not require much inquiry, but as age advances a higher proportion may warrant routine informal screening to ensure nothing is overlooked.

Cognitive screening can be either informal or formal. The *clock drawing test* and the *set test* are two tests that can be used for rapid screening. To administer the clock drawing test, the patient is requested to draw a clock face with numbers on a blank piece of paper, and to place the large hand and small hand at the time indicated by the examiner.[7,8] The time selected should involve separate number locations for each hand, such as "10 minutes after 11" or "1:45." This is a test not only of visuospatial ability but also of motor execution, attention, language comprehension, and numerical ability. Although there are several formal scoring systems for this exercise, any significant distortion or difficulty is important. This is only a screening test, and concerning results must be confirmed by other forms of testing and history taking.

The *set test*, sometimes referred to as the *category fluency test*, is particularly helpful in assessing patients with low formal education levels that the mini-mental state examination (MMSE) can not reliably be used to test.[9,10] To administer the set test, the older person is asked to name as many items as they can in each of four sets or categories. The four sets are fruits, animals, colors, and towns. This test examines a number of cognitive domains including language, executive function, and memory. The best score is 10 in each set, for a maximum score of 40. A score of less than 15 is abnormal. In addition, set naming "red flags" are the inability to stay on track with the correct category, naming fewer than 10 objects in a minute, and/or repeating objects early in the naming process. Both of these informal screening tools can be administered before the beginning of the office visit by office staff with proper training.

Another red flag for possible cognitive impairment is a patient's poor performance on the instrumental activities of daily living, discussed in depth later in this chapter. These complex mental tasks are very sensitive to executive dysfunction and hence early dementing illness. New problems with finances and medication use are concerning symptoms and should automatically prompt a thorough mental status screening.

One final caveat, regarding a patient with a newly discovered abnormal mental status screening, is that these patients are often oblivious to their deficits. Often, they will indicate quite emphatically that they are independent in their activities of daily living (ADLs) and instrumental activities of daily living (IADLs) when this is not the case. If cognitive impairment is suspected, a reliable observer will need to be found who can give an accurate assessment of the patient's functional levels.

For patients with concerning signs or symptoms of cognitive impairment or whose screening test is worrisome, there are several assessment tools available for use in more formal cognitive screening. The most frequently used and validated mental status screening instrument is the MMSE.[11] It tests several areas of cognitive function and provides a convenient score for assessment and later comparison; furthermore, since it has been widely used for 2 decades, its meaning and limitations are well understood by professionals working with older persons. It has several drawbacks:

- It requires some experience.
- It can elicit a negative reaction among patients who object to being "tested."
- Its cutoff (23 of 30 correct) misses many patients with mild cognitive impairment and early dementia.
- The score interpretation must be adjusted for educational level (by lowering the cutoff as much as four points for persons with less than a 12th-grade education, and six points for those with less than an 8th grade education.)
- Administration may be difficult in the face of severe visual or hearing impairment.
- Patients who do not give it their full effort (especially depressed patients) may be improperly labeled as impaired.

Many of these limitations apply to other cognitive status tests as well, so the MMSE remains a commonly used evaluation tool. Ideally, a primary care geriatrician should be familiar with several other cognitive evaluation tools and should choose which tests to use depending on the patient.

In many situations, patients will present with worrying behavioral, cognitive, or functional changes that are suggestive of early dementing illness but the screening tests mentioned earlier will not be conclusive. For these patients, referral for formal neuropsychological testing is very helpful and is indicated. The neuropsychological examination permits objective assessment of cognitive function using standardized tests of cognitive abilities, memory, attention and concentration, orientation to time, language, and sensory-motor ability. The evaluation can be used to verify the presence or absence of a cognitive dysfunction and aid in the differential diagnosis. The early symptomatic phase of Alzheimer's disease can be indistinguishable on clinical office examination from normal aging but can be identified by detailed neuropsychological testing. Further details on cognitive assessment can be found in Chapter 16.

Contrary to prior assumptions, the incidence of major depression among older patients in the community is approximately the same as in other age groups, averaging approximately 3%. However, subsyndromal depression affects over twice that many, with estimates ranging from 8% to 15% of community-dwelling elderly.[12] In a primary care practice setting of older patients, the prevalence was 5.6%, with another 7.9% with probable or masked depression.[13] Depression is much higher in medically ill populations in hospitals and nursing homes, reaching as high as 25%. This is a complex illness and can be a primary problem, related to medical illnesses such as Alzheimer's disease, Parkinson's disease, and stroke, or can be a reaction to medical problems. Its presence should be looked for and treated because there can be serious consequences to unrecognized depression: increased morbidity, suicide, and decreased quality of life. In addition, depression can affect performance on mental status testing, so the clinician should be astute to the subtle signs of depression and should be familiar with the diagnostic criteria and screening tests for this condition. One of the most gratifying experiences in geriatrics can be the successful treatment of a patient with depression, resulting in improvement in relationships, function, and quality of life. More in Chapter 17.

M i l l i e   L i p t o n , *Part 4*

Mrs. Lipton has done well since moving to your town. She has settled into her apartment and can operate most of the appliances well, including the microwave and oven. She does need some help with paying bills, and her daughter's phone number is written on her home phones. Mrs. Lipton no longer has a laundry routine, allowing her dirty clothes to accumulate. She requires prompting to wash her dirty clothes, something new for her. She does not drive because she admits she does not know anything about the town and its roads. Her daughter confides that her mother does have problems with executive function. Mrs. Lipton does not notice running low on food and therefore does not plan to go shopping. Likewise, if the phone or television is not working, she will not make any attempt to get them fixed. She seems puzzled about what to do, and this is of concern to her daughter. Mrs. Lipton will not initiate any shopping requests, but will gladly go with her daughter if offered the chance. She is fully functional at home regarding her ADLs (Fig. 4-4).

CASE DISCUSSION

Assessment of functional status, in particular the patient's ability to perform everyday tasks, is a critical part of the evaluation of all elderly patients. In the case of Mrs. Lipton, you will need to differentiate what she can do herself from what her daughter does for her, and to identify areas where her function is failing and additional support may be needed. In Mrs. Lipton's case, her loss of some executive function, and consequently IADLs (Fig. 4-5), means that she meets the full criteria for dementia, not just mild cognitive impairment. Her problems extend beyond just memory impairment. At a scheduled follow up visit (soon), formal MMSE and specific questions to assess for Alzheimer's Disease are vital. The diagnosis of this needs to be discussed in an appropriate and tactful manner.

ASSESSMENT OF FUNCTIONAL STATUS

Assessing and understanding functional ability is critical to caring for older patients. Functional ability is critical to maintenance of independence and quality of life. In caring for older patients, knowing the diseases that afflict an individual is only one part. Indeed, disease care is sometimes far less important than maximizing the function of individuals. As Figure 4-6 demonstrates, functional loss is common in older patients.

Here are some of the reasons why function is so important:

- Functional loss is a final common pathway for many clinical problems in older patients. Despite this, health care providers often do not recognize functional disabilities in their patients.[14] Therefore, functional assessment becomes a central focus in the initial assessment and care of the older patient.

- Change in functional status is an important presenting symptom in older patients. An acute illness or the decompensation of a known medical problem such as heart or lung disease will usually be accompanied by a functional decline. Knowing the prior functional status enables the provider to immediately recognize an emerging illness that is presenting as functional change.

- Being aware of patient function helps with the prioritization of problems and establishment of the goals of therapy. Restoration of function is an important goal for patients and should also be for

The physical self-maintenance scale (PSMS) activities of daily living			
Patient's Name _____ **Date** _____			
Rated by _____			
Numbers 1 through 5 in each category represent worsening states of function. Choose the number that best describes the patient's functional status. Scores in all six categories should then be totaled. The higher the final score, the greater the degree of impairment.			
			Score
A. Toileting	1. Cares for self at toilet completely, no incontinence.		
	2. Needs to be reminded or needs help in cleaning self, or has rare (weekly at most) accidents.		
	3. Soiling or wetting while asleep more than once a week.		
	4. Soiling or wetting while awake more than once a week.		
	5. No control of bowels or bladder.		
B. Feeding	1. Eats without assistance.		
	2. Eats with minor assistance at mealtimes and/or with special preparation of food, or help in cleaning up after meals.		
	3. Feeds self with moderate assistance and is untidy.		
	4. Requires extensive assistance for all meals.		
	5. Does not feed self at all and resists efforts of other to feed him/her.		
C. Dressing	1. Dresses, undresses, and selects clothes from own wardrobe.		
	2. Dresses and undresses self with minor assistance.		
	3. Needs moderate assistance in dressing or selection of clothes.		
	4. Needs major assistance in dressing, but cooperates with efforts of others to help.		
	5. Completely unable to dress self and resists efforts of others to help.		
D. Grooming (neatness, hair, nails, hands, face, clothing)	1. Always neatly dressed, well groomed, without assistance.		
	2. Grooms self adequately with occasional minor assistance, e.g., shaving.		
	3. Needs moderate and regular assistance or supervision in grooming.		
	4. Needs total grooming care, but can remain well groomed after help from others.		
	5. Actively negates all efforts of others to maintain grooming.		
E. Ambulation	1. Goes about grounds or city.		
	2. Ambulates within residence or about one block distance.		
	3. Ambulates with assistance of (check one) a ( ) another person, b ( ) railing, c ( ) cane, d ( ) walker, e ( ) wheelchair-gets in and out without help, f ( ) wheelchair-needs help getting in and out.		
	4. Needs total grooming care, but can remain well groomed after help from others.		
	5. Actively negatives all efforts of others to maintain grooming.		
F. Bathing	1. Bathes self (tub, shower, sponge bath) without help.		
	2. Bathes self with help getting in and out of tub.		
	3. Washes face and hands only, but cannot bathe rest of body.		
	4. Does not wash self but is cooperative with those who bathe him/her.		
	5. Does not try to wash self, and resists efforts to keep him/her clean.		
			TOTAL SCORE
Score	1. Can perform the task without any help 2. Can manage the activity with some reminding, prompting, or minor assistance 3. Needs moderate assistance 4. Requires major assistance and support 5. Is totally dependent		

FIGURE 4-4

The physical self-maintenance scale (PSMS) activities of daily living. (*Modified from Assessment of Older People: Self-Maintaining and Instrumental Activities of Daily Living, Gerontologist 9:179, 1969.*)

Functional activities questionnaire (instrumental activities of daily living)				
Patient's Name: _____				
Informant's name: _____				
Date:_____ Interviewer:_____				
INSTRUCTIONS				
Place a check mark under the column that best describes the patient's ability to perform the tasks listed below: 3 - Completely unable to perform task 2 - Requires assistance 1 - Has difficulty but accomplishes task, or has never done, but the informant feels could do task with difficulty 0 - Normal performance, or has never done task, but the informant feels the patient could do the task if necessary				
	(3 points)	**(2 points)**	**(1 point)**	**(0 points)**
1. Writing checks, paying bills, balancing a checkbook				
2. Assembling tax records, business affairs, or papers				
3. Shopping alone for clothes, household necessities, or groceries				
4. Playing a game of skill; working on a hobby				
5. Heating water, making a cup of coffee, turning off the stove				
6. Preparing a balanced meal				
7. Keep track of current events				
8. Paying attention to, understanding, or discussing a TV show, book, or magazine				
9. Remembering appointments, family occasions, holidays, and medications				
10. Traveling out of the neighborhood, driving, arranging to take buses				
POINTS PER COLUMN				
			Total points	_____

FIGURE 4–5

Functional activities questionnaire (instrumental activities of daily living). *(Redrawn from Pfeffer RI, Kurosaki TT, Harrah CH, Chance JM, Filos S. Measurement of Functional Activities in Older Adults in the Community, J Gerontol 37:323, 1982.)*

the clinician. At the conclusion of a visit, functional losses should be high on your follow-up agenda.

- Loss of independence in one or more key functions often signals the need for involvement of other members of the health care team, such as physical therapists and occupational therapists. Careful consideration should be given to involve-

ment of these professionals as soon as functional loss is identified.

- Appreciation of functional status, therefore, holds a central position in the assessment and care of older patients.

● Measuring, preserving, and nurturing functional status is at the core of quality geriatric medicine.

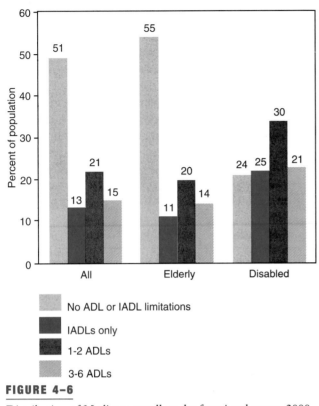

FIGURE 4-6

Distribution of Medicare enrollees, by functional status, 2000. *(Modified from Centers for Medicaid and Medicare Services, Office of Research, Development, and Information. Data from Medicare Current Beneficiary Survey [MCBS] 2000. Access to Care File. June 2002 Edition. C Section III.B.2. Page 4.)*

Because of its importance, functional status should be elicited during the history and parts of it confirmed during the physical examination. There are several readily administered questionnaires or templates in the EMR that can capture and track the status of ADLs[15] and IADLs.[16]

ADLs play a central role in the independence of older patients and are now generally used to describe basic self-care skills. There are a number of different assessment instruments that evaluate these functions, and the physical self-maintenance scale (PSMS) is one of them (see Fig. 4-4). ADLs are part of the "language of geriatrics" because they are used in many different care settings to evaluate and recommend treatment older patients. It is a fundamental evaluation tool for rehabilitation in nursing homes, rehabilitation centers, and home health care to name a few areas. The assessment of ADLs is also an integral part of admission evaluation and ongoing care in assisted-living facilities. For those who care for older patients, it is a required "language."

> ● Much can be learned about a patient's functional status by observing the patient move about the office and examination room.

IADLs are the other essential component of the language of geriatrics. Unlike ADLs, IADLs are complex mental processes that are required for independent living. Executive function and judgment must be used to accomplish them. Executive functions deal with planning, organizing, sequencing, and performing complex tasks. It is not surprising then, that patients with early cognitive impairment will often manifest themselves first with difficulties in IADLs. This will become apparent clinically, for example, when patients are having difficulty with remembering medication regimens and whether they have even been taking their medications. Another common scenario is worsening difficulty in financial matters, such as forgetting to pay bills or exceptional errors in financial affairs. The functional activities questionnaire (FAQ) is one of several recommended IADL instruments (see Fig. 4-5). Because of its sensitivity to cognitive impairment, reviewing a patient's IADLs in cases of suspicious cognitive impairment will often uncover severe deficits that family members have been handling for some time. Many times in early dementing illness, a patient's MMSE will be in the normal range, but their new difficulty in IADLs will alone be enough to establish the diagnosis of serious degenerative brain disease. ADL and IADL assessments do not take very long. Answers about medication administration, driving, finances, phone use, and shopping can be quickly obtained. Functional status, however, in cases of patients with suspected cognitive impairment must be confirmed by another person in addition to the patient.

> ● Patients with cognitive impairment are usually oblivious to their IADL deficits. Their IADL status needs to be confirmed by a reliable observer.

Millie Lipton, *Part 5*

Mrs. Lipton was married for 57 years before the death of her husband from melanoma. She has two daughters and a son. The eldest daughter, Michele, is with her today. Michele made the arrangements for Mrs. Lipton to move here and set up today's appointment. The daughters and son have agreed informally on this arrangement and that Michele will manage the patient's affairs locally.

Mrs. Lipton completed graduate school in business and worked for 30 years as a bookkeeper for a small business. She has never smoked. Her use of alcohol was always rare, confined to social situations, and she has not used any alcohol since her husband died. Mrs. Lipton's father died of heart disease, and her mother's cause of death is unknown. She has two brothers who are already deceased, from Parkinson's disease and heart disease.

EXPANDED SOCIAL AND FAMILY HISTORY

The social and family history should concentrate on the strengths and weaknesses of family support. The majority of older patients will have a period of dependency in their later years, and knowing the family resources available to provide support is critical to providing optimal care. This requires the addition of several topics to the usual social history assessment when evaluating older patients (Box 4-5).

The family medical history is relatively less important because hereditary risks have usually manifested themselves by old age. However, patients often have strong feelings about the circumstances of their parent's death and may have concerns that their health events in later years will parallel those of parents or other family members. Therefore, knowing this information may help you understand some of their emotions, questions, and behaviors.

Millie Lipton, *Part 6*

Mrs. Lipton's review of systems indicates that her appetite is good and her weight has been stable. She sleeps well at night with only occasional awakening. She has had a recent eye examination. She acknowledges her hearing loss, and it has been evaluated in the recent past. She has not had any chest pain in years, and her cholesterol was monitored regularly by her former clinician with adjustments in her medication. She has had no respiratory or gastrointestinal symptoms. She has frequent stiffness of her hands and knees that responds to acetaminophen. She denies incontinence and falls.

She has had regular annual examinations that have included mammograms, pap smears, and stool Hemoccult testing. She had a full colonoscopy 7 years ago. Immunization status, however, is unclear. The flu season is approaching, and she does not remember ever having a pneumonia vaccination. The records that accompany her do not indicate this immunization either.

THE IMPORTANCE OF THE REVIEW OF SYSTEMS

The review of systems goes beyond the history of present illnesses and past history and uses direct

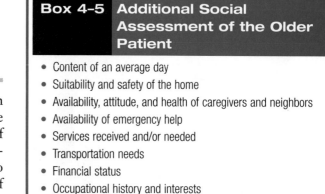

Box 4–5 Additional Social Assessment of the Older Patient

- Content of an average day
- Suitability and safety of the home
- Availability, attitude, and health of caregivers and neighbors
- Availability of emergency help
- Services received and/or needed
- Transportation needs
- Financial status
- Occupational history and interests

questions to ensure that all systems are adequately covered. This review is particularly important in examining older patients because of the large number of hidden illnesses and geriatric syndromes that are often not mentioned owing to embarrassment, ignorance that something can be done, or fear of a negative impression. Box 4-6 lists geriatric-specific topics to include in a review of systems. For a new patient appointment, the review of systems can often be highly productive in setting priorities for care and follow-up visits.

Box 4–6 Geriatric-Specific Topics to Include in a Review of Systems

General
- Weight change
- Sleep quality
- Depression
- Hearing loss
- Alcoholism
- Falls

Genitourinary
- Incontinence
- Sexuality
- Nocturia

Neurologic
- Confusion
- Memory loss

Musculoskeletal
- Prior fractures
- Range of motion of joints
- Pain

Modified from Ham RJ. Geriatrics I, monograph 89, Home Study Self-Assessment Program, Kansas City, MO, American Academy of Family Physicians, Leewood, KS, 1986.

A well-structured systems review is a way to ensure that all necessary background information is covered, and the review should include a thorough documentation of health maintenance activities in the past. For example, in reviewing the eye history, the time of the last eye examination is important to note because of the high incidence of eye disease in older patients. The exact details of these measures are often not well remembered, and old medical records are invaluable in tracing the details.

Millie Lipton, *Part 7*

You leave the room for a short period of time to update your EMR with what you have learned while your nursing staff prepares Mrs. Lipton for her physical examination. Her daughter does not leave the room and remains behind.

Her temperature is 37.0°F, blood pressure 155/90 mm Hg, pulse 72 and regular, respirations 16, weight 123 pounds. The daughter reports that her mother has never weighed much more than this.

As you return to the examination room to begin, you have already noted during the history portion of the examination that her hearing is impaired. You needed to sit directly in front of Mrs. Lipton for her to understand what you were saying, and you continue this method during the examination, always facing her when speaking. In addition to the hearing loss, the examination of the head reveals mild hair thinning. Her lenses are very clear, reflecting the prior cataract surgery, but the age-related small pupils in both eyes makes your retinal examination incomplete. Fortunately, as you comment on this, her daughter mentions that she has had a recent eye examination and things were fine. Mrs. Lipton's oral hygiene is excellent.

The neck examination reveals excellent carotid upstrokes and no bruits. Her thyroid is normal on examination. Her chest examination reveals a mild kyphosis and reinforces your concern about possible osteoporosis and perhaps compression fractures. The lung examination is remarkable for bilateral dry crackles at the bases only but is otherwise clear. Cardiac examination reveals a very regular rhythm with an occasional extra systole, a normal point of maximal impulse (PMI), and a soft II/VI systolic ejection murmur at the aortic area and apex without radiation elsewhere. Her breast examination reveals redundant skin with homogenous breast tissue.

Mrs. Lipton's abdominal examination is unremarkable, with normal bowel sounds and no organomegaly or bruits. Her pelvic examination reveals vaginal atrophy and the absence of a cervix or uterus. No masses are felt in her adnexa. Rectal examination reveals good sphincter tone, and her stool is Hemoccult negative.

Examination of her joints only reveals mild enlargement of her distal interphalangeal joints with excellent range of motion. Her feet do not have any deformities, and she has good pulses in her lower extremities.

You leave the room to allow her to get dressed. When you return later, you walk her through the "timed get up and go test," which she does very easily and quickly, meeting the standards of the test.

CONDUCT OF THE PHYSICAL EXAMINATION

The conduct of the history taking has already given you considerable opportunity and cues to the issues regarding the physical examination. The astute clinician catalogs these findings as they reveal themselves. The general appearance of the patient, quality and loudness of the voice, and robustness of the handshake are clues. Observing the patient walk to the examining room and/or transfer from a chair to the examining table gives additional information on functional ability.

Once the patient is comfortable, a critical place to start the physical examination is the vital signs. All are important indicators of well-being, especially in the older patient. Abnormalities such as weight loss, an irregular pulse, or mild tachypnea have important implications. It is not unusual for the blood pressure to be elevated when a new patient is seen in a strange environment; so elevated readings should be rechecked. Blood pressure should be taken in the supine position after at least 10 minutes of rest and then immediately after and 3 minutes after standing. Orthostatic hypotension, defined as a drop of 20 mm Hg in systolic blood pressure, rises rapidly with advancing age and is a common finding in those over the age of 85.[17]

If excellent medical records accompany the patient, the physical examination may ironically be relatively unrewarding in regard to new findings. There are, however, specific geriatric physical examination findings and observations that are often missed unless the examiner looks for them. Many of these are listed in Box 4-7.

Box 4-7	Important Specific Physical Examination Findings to Note in Older Patients
Eyes	Cataracts
	Retinal abnormalities
	Visual acuity
Ears	Hearing evaluation
	Removal of wax if necessary
Mouth	Condition of teeth and gums
	Ability to eat
	Remove dentures if present
Head and neck	Premalignant and malignant skin lesions (usually seen in the most sun-exposed area)
	Thyroid evaluation
	Elevated neck veins
	Range of motion of the cervical spine
	Auscultation of the carotids
Chest	Kyphosis and/or scoliosis
	Dry crackles in the lung bases
Breast examination	Remember that breast cancer can occur in the very old
Cardiovascular	Regularity of rhythm
	Presence of an S_4 is common
	Atrial and ventricular ectopy
	Systolic murmurs are common
	Arterial pulses in extremities (especially legs and feet)
Abdomen	Liver edge below the right costal margin
	Palpable enlarged aorta
	Abdominal bruit
	Rectal examination that reveals fecal impaction
Genitourinary	*Male:* small testes, prostatic enlargement, and/or nodularity
	Female: cystocele, rectocele, and uterine descent; adnexal masses in an older women is considered malignant until proven otherwise
Skin	Concerning skin lesions
	Gait abnormalities
Musculoskeletal	Motor asymmetry
	Range of motion of each major joint
	Fine finger movement
Lower extremities	Hygiene
	Condition of the toenails
	Presence of edema
Nervous system	Balance and cerebellar testing (see Box 4-8)

A few of these areas merit some additional discussion. Vision and hearing screening are important, given the high prevalence of impaired vision and hearing among older patients. These conditions lead to subsequent functional loss. Visual impairment was predictive of mortality over 10 years, and combined impairment had the highest risk of 10-year functional decline.[18] Annual eye examinations by eye specialists should be encouraged, owing to the high incidence of silent diseases such as glaucoma and macular degeneration. Hearing deficits are more readily discernible and can be assessed by using the whisper test or an audioscope equipped with tone testing.[19] In Mrs. Lipton's case, her hearing impairment was obvious and her vision was just recently evaluated.

The chest can be difficult to examine because the rib cage is often fixed owing to the changes of aging. Diaphragmatic breathing plays a much more important role in respiratory function in older patients for this reason. Breath sounds may be more difficult to hear, and often dry crackles can be heard at the bases that do not imply serious pathology.

The cardiac examination in the older patient will often have some findings. Atrial and ventricular ectopy of a benign nature are common and do not imply an ominous prognosis.[20] A split second heart sound, with inspiration increasing the split, is a normal finding in older patients. An S_4 heart sound is common among older patients without cardiac disease, but an S_3 is always suggestive of congestive heart failure.

Another common cardiac finding is the presence of systolic murmurs in many older patients. Benign murmurs in older patients will typically be an ejection type murmur that is soft (grade 2/6 or less) and heard best at the base and possibly at the apex. These murmurs probably represent turbulence over sclerotic aortic valves. If the murmur is concerning, some patients may merit further evaluation with an electrocardiograph (ECG) and echocardiography. Because left ventricular enlargement has a serious prognosis, careful physical examination for cardiac size is important and, if found, warrants further diagnostic studies.

The nervous system permeates the entire body, so it is not surprising that neurologic changes are extensive in older patients. There is still considerable disagreement among experts regarding normal versus abnormal neurological changes associated with aging. The prevalence of several neurologic findings not associated with disease increases with age. These include elements of cranial nerve function, extrapyramidal function, and some primitive reflexes.[21] Box 4-8 outlines many of

these manifestations. Because all of these changes are present in only a minority of patients, the challenge is deciding when a change is associated with a new disease process and is abnormal enough to merit workup, or deciding the change is a manifestation of normal aging.

The musculoskeletal system is the source for many common complaints in older patients. Gait and balance testing should be a part of all initial examinations of all older adults. This can be as simple and unobtrusive as the get up and go test.[22] This test was subsequently modified to the timed get up and go test,[23] in which the time taken to perform the test is measured and used as a score. A more in-depth discussion of gait and balance testing is in Chapter 18. Observation of the patient while he or she performs this simple evaluation can be very revealing.

Millie Lipton, *Part 8*

As Mrs. Lipton is getting dressed, you begin to organize your thoughts. You make the following assessment and plan in the EMR.

1. Hypertension Control: not controlled today; reassessed for now, will follow and re-evaluate.
2. Cognitive Impairment: will assist the daughter in obtaining records of the evaluation performed to date; will re-assess her cognitive function with an MMSE next visit. Impression,

---

Box 4–8 Common Neurologic Changes in Older Patients

All percentages in parentheses are for subjects 85 years and older. For younger persons, the percentages are less.

Cranial nerve function: eye signs
Unequal pupils (11%)
Diminished reaction to light and near reflex (9%)

Auditory
Hearing loss for higher tones

Olfactory
Diminished olfactory sensitivity
Extrapyramidal function
Abnormal gait (20%)
Increased rigidity and tone in the legs (22%)
Flexion posture
Diminished reaction time
Decreased arm swing (29%)

Motor
Tremor (17%)
Increased muscle tone in legs (22%)
Diminished muscle strength in legs and arms (5%)
Spontaneous movement decrease (14%)

Sensory
Diminished vibratory sense distally (21%)
Proprioception preserved
Mild increase in threshold for light touch, pain, and temperature

Reflexes
Diminished or absent ankle jerks (15%)
Romberg abnormal (14%)

Pathologic reflexes present
Snout (32%)
Grasp (28%)
Root (13%)

Data from Sirven JI, Mancall E. Neurologic Examination of the Older Adult. In Sirven J, Malamut B, eds. Clinical Neurology of the Older Adult (Sirven J, Malmut B, eds.), Lippincott Williams and Wilkins, Philadelphia, 2002. Data from Odenheimer GL, Funkensetin JJ, Beckett L, et al. Comparison of Neurologic Changes in "Successful Aging" Persons versus the Total Aging Population. *Arch Neurol* 51:573-580, 1994.

because she has both memory loss and mild functional loss, is that she probably has early Alzheimer's disease.

3. Advance Directives: introduced the concept today because she has not established any. Give handout on living will and durable power of attorney.

4. Lipids: will obtain fasting lipids before her next visit on the present dose of pravastatin to establish whether this is an adequate dose.

5. Possible Osteoporosis: her low weight and age are risk factors. She is ambulatory, and her life expectancy is such that she would benefit from treatment. Will change her calcium supplementation to begin Ca 500 mg + 200 IU Vitamin D tablets by mouth (PO) three times a day; will also add a multivitamin with 400 IU of vitamin D. Will discuss the need for bone mineral density testing on the next visit.

6. Health Maintenance: immunization status is unclear, and my office assistant will call the previous doctor to ascertain Pneumovax and flu vaccination; will give tetanus booster today.

7. Coronary Artery Disease: no symptoms in years; will get a baseline ECG on the next visit, as none are included in her medical records.

Mrs. Lipton will return for an extended appointment for these assessments in approximately 2 weeks.

SYNTHESIS

Often, at the completion of the initial assessment, your top priority is not making new diagnoses but maximizing the medical management of the conditions that have already been identified. Many of the chronic conditions encountered in older patients have corresponding evidence-based guidelines and will need treatment changes. Certainly, the discovery of a new geriatric syndrome is satisfying and opens doors for new treatment, but clarification of medications and meeting disease-specific standards of care are more common accomplishments of the first visit. Finally, there will be a number of past investigations or specialty medical records that will need to be obtained to complete the patient's records.

At the conclusion of the initial visit, it is important to review your goals for this visit: establishing a relationship with the patient (and family if necessary), fully understanding the priorities of care, and developing a plan for follow-up visits. Ask yourself if these have been met.

ORDERING LABORATORY WORK

There are no evidence-based protocols for deciding appropriate laboratory studies in older patients. What each individual patient requires will depend to a great extent on the laboratory history included in prior medical records and the comorbid conditions that accompany each patient. There are, however, well-described, disease-specific laboratory tests. Finally, there may be symptoms elicited during the review of systems that will trigger studies. Therefore, what is ordered at the time of an initial visit for any given patient is a unique response to these many factors.

ATTENTION TO THE CAREGIVER

Older patients often require the assistance of a caregiver, and that person will often attend clinic visits with your patient. In most cases this is a welcome and important circumstance. Caregivers can often provide important clues to subtle changes or problems with medications. In patients with cognitive impairment, the caregiver is often the source of the most reliable information regarding how well the patient is doing. It is important in these situations to ask the caregiver if they have any questions or concerns.

The more dependent the patient, the more demands are placed on the caregiving setting and, depending on the arrangements, on the individual caregiver. In these situations, the astute clinician will realize the importance of the caregiver to the well-being of the patient and will assess the level of stress and difficulty experienced. The role of caregiving has negative psychological effects and can result in anger, depression, anxiety, and frustration.[24] Maintaining caregiver health, therefore, is important to the stability of the care setting in preventing institutionalization. The assessment of the patient, therefore, extends in many cases to the caregiver.

Millie Lipton, *Part 9*

In Mrs. Lipton's family situation, her daughter has employment responsibilities during the day that limit her ability to be with Mrs. Lipton full-time. There will come a time during Mrs. Lipton's Alzheimer's disease when she should not be alone. There are several ways of handling this situation, but closer observation of Mrs. Lipton will most likely be needed in the future. A discussion with the daughter about this issue at a subsequent visit should occur soon. You note this issue in your problem list as number 8, planning for caregiving as the disease progresses.

USE OF THE HEALTH CARE TEAM

Geriatrics by its very nature is multidisciplinary, and good geriatric care is team care. Your clinic nursing staff will play a critical role in collecting and assessing patients and their caregivers. Indeed, your office staff will often be the first to alert you to a change in a patient. Other important team members include home health nurses, physical and occupational therapists, and hospice personnel. Communicating with these professionals will enhance the care you provide and will often provide insights from home visits that are not available to you. Medicare benefits are generous for care provided in these areas, and patients often benefit from early intervention. Consultation with one of these disciplines should be obtained if there is a remote chance your patient will benefit from their skill and assessment.

SUBSEQUENT OFFICE VISITS

It is rare that a new older patient with their multiple medical problems and medication issues will not need some kind of follow-up soon after their first visit to establish care. For this reason it is important to have a scheduling system that takes that into account. This complexity also requires a way to capture the complete synthesis generated on a first visit for use on subsequent visits. Accurate problem lists and medication lists are essential. EMRs excel in this regard for a number of reasons. Every prescription ever written can be easily tracked. Problem lists and medication lists can be added to each clinical encounter. Relevant past medical and social history can be reviewed and added at a click of a button. Past clinical assessments are instantly available and, if done with a comprehensive approach, will make the follow-up visit seamless.

In beginning a subsequent office visit, it is best to prepare by looking at the prior note for recommendations about follow-up and, when beginning the interview, inquire if the patient has any issues that he or she wishes to discuss to be sure agenda items are addressed. Finally, a brief review of the entire problem list and health maintenance activities will often yield additional items that need attention.

Millie Lipton, *Part 10*

While awaiting her next appointment with you, Millie Lipton falls in her new apartment and sustains a displaced femoral neck fracture. She is admitted to the orthopedic service in your hospital and undergoes a hemiarthroplasty. Her postoperative course is complicated by a delirium for several days and a urinary tract infection associated with foley catheter placement. On the seventh day, her mental status is improved and she is transferred to the rehabilitation center in your hospital. She spends a total of 4 weeks there and is now ambulatory with a rolling walker and ready for discharge. Her daughter is concerned about her mother living alone during much of the day at the time of discharge, and she leaves a phone message for you to call her about these concerns. The daughter has investigated a local assisted-living facility and wonders if you think that is a good idea. Mrs. Lipton's physical and occupational therapy will continue through home health at the assisted-living facility.

Although you were aware that Mrs. Lipton was admitted for her hip fracture and subsequently transferred to the rehabilitation center, you are not aware of the details of her hospitalization and subsequent rehabilitation stay. Her daughter provides the name of the physician (Dr. Wilson) caring for Mrs. Lipton in the rehabilitation center, and you begin the task of obtaining the hospital discharge summaries and initiating an attempt to contact Dr. Wilson about this patient's current status. Dr. Wilson faxes the rehabilitation discharge summary to your office. An extended hospital discharge follow-up appointment is scheduled with you in your office the day after she is discharged.

Mrs. Lipton arrives with her daughter in your office several days later. She is ambulating with a rolling walker. Vital signs are as follows: temperature 97°F, blood pressure 98/70 mm Hg, pulse 88, respirations 16, and weight 112 pounds. The patient appears to be unfamiliar with your office and does not remember her previous visit. The medication list from the assisted-living facility includes the following: multivitamin daily, amlodipine 5 mg PO daily, pravastatin 20 mg hs, and aspirin 81 mg PO daily. You note that she is not on donepezil or any calcium or vitamin D supplementation.

STUDY QUESTIONS

Mrs. Lipton's clinical situation has changed considerably and has become much more complex. It is clear that she will require extensive re-evaluation and very close follow-up. What would you recommend be done regarding these new and ongoing issues:

1. Mental status (should medications for Alzheimer's disease be restarted?)
2. Weight loss and related nutrition
3. Goals of home health physical and occupational therapy
4. Blood pressure management (Should her medications be cut back? What laboratory work should be requested?)
5. Lipid management (Does she need it given her weight loss?)
6. Advanced directives (What are her expectations?)
7. Osteoporosis (Should she be evaluated and/or treated?)

TRANSITIONAL CARE USE BY OLDER PATIENTS

In the later years of life, the majority of older patients experience care at multiple sites and situations as their medical conditions become more numerous and complex.[25] Use of assisted-living facilities, nursing homes, inpatient rehabilitation centers, and home health are examples of common sites in the continuum of care. Transitional care is defined "as a set of actions designed to ensure the coordination and continuity of health care as patients transfer between locations or different levels of care within the same location."[26] Changes in the needs of patients drive the use of these different levels of care, and each site has distinct goals and objectives. Because transitions are associated with a number of identified problems, recommendations have been developed to improve the quality of care during this time (Box 4-9). It is important that the primary care provider be aware of the uses of these care sites as they occur, the circumstances that precipitated their use, and the associated medical changes.

> ● Changes in the site of care for older patients often signals significant changes in health or function. At such times, it is important to understand the issues that precipitated the change and to modify goals and objectives of care.

A transitional care follow-up visit is generally complex and tends to require extensive time and a comprehensive approach, much like a new patient visit. Different levels of care (e.g., hospital, rehabilitation center, home care) all have different goals and objectives for care and associated complexity. Communication between providers at and across each level is critical.

> ● Transitional care follow-up is often very complex. Patients will need to be assessed and reassessed as they move from one care site to another.

Box 4-9 Recommendations to Improve the Quality of Transitional Care

1. Clinical professionals must prepare patients and their caregivers to receive care in the next setting and actively involve them in decisions related to the formulation and execution of the transitional care plan.
2. Bidirectional communication between clinical professionals is essential to ensuring high-quality transitional care.
3. Policies should be developed that promote high-quality transitional care.
4. Education in transitional care should be provided to all health care professionals involved in the transfer of patients across settings.

From Coleman EA, Boult C. The American Geriatric Society Health Care Systems Committee. Improving the quality of transitional care for persons with complex care needs. *J Am Geriatr Soc* 51:556-557, 2003.

Millie Lipton: *Case Discussion*

This case illustrates a number of important issues and problems in caring for older patients when transferred between care settings. There is a continued need for ongoing assessment and reassessment to look for the development of new problems and changes in old ones. It addition to the identified problems during the first visit (early Alzheimer's disease, hypertension, and possible osteoporosis), several new problems have developed related to a single event, her hip fracture. As is typically the care in older patients, many of these problems are interrelated. The patient experienced an acute delirium postoperatively, no doubt predisposed to by her suspected dementia and a subsequent urinary tract infection from a foley catheter. Her weight loss reflects poor oral intake over a considerable period of time, as she is now 6 weeks after the fracture. Nutrition is, thus, a new problem, and an evaluation and intervention plan is needed. Her blood pressure is low, perhaps related to her weight loss and poor oral intake; so her blood pressure medication should probably be stopped. With the known gastrointestinal side effects of nausea and diarrhea associated with donepezil, should restarting this medication be delayed until better weight gain is established?

Her hip fracture, advanced age, female sex, and low weight make osteoporosis likely. She is not on adequate oral calcium or vitamin D, and she will most likely require a bisphosphate. Because you estimate her life expectancy to be at least 4 years and she continues to be ambulatory, bone mineral density testing should probably be done to establish a baseline. Finally, the hip fracture is a considerable functional setback, and you will need to assess her carefully, and on an ongoing basis, for pain and function. Physical and occupational therapy need to continue and be monitored to ensure that she reaches, and your learn what is, her maximal benefit.

ASSESSMENT IN THE HOME, HOSPITAL, AND NURSING HOME

While patients seen in the hospital, nursing home, or at home have unique care settings with very different characteristics, assessment of the same five domains of care is required. Often, one aspect of patient care will take priority at times, but the other domains require monitoring and may deteriorate without careful attention.

Such is the case with hospital care. It is often precipitated by an acute serious medical problem that rightly consumes considerable attention. Worsening congestive heart failure, pneumonia, falls with fractures, or chronic obstructive pulmonary disease (COPD) exacerbation are all good examples. However, hospital admissions with these types of problems are often associated with functional decline and medication changes that require their own interventions and monitoring, and comorbid conditions cannot be forgotten. Good care requires a comprehensive understanding of the patient's characteristics in each of the five domains of care before admission and then carefully following each domain's special problems. Discharge planning begins on the day of admission.

Most nursing home admissions are transfers from acute care hospitals, and the issues discussed earlier are often transferred to this setting for identification, assessment, and treatment. For example, approximately one-quarter of all transfers to nursing homes from hospitals are associated with a change in mental status and will need to be followed and addressed.[27] A comprehensive assessment involving the five domains is again essential: mental health, physical health, functional abilities, social supports, and economic resources.

Unlike hospitals and nursing homes, which tend to have standardized staff and procedures, home care is always unique. Often the patient is surrounded by concerned and attentive family, and home is the environment that the patient prefers. But in addition to careful coordination with home health care professionals, the primary care provider needs to instruct and encourage the family caregivers. Often these family members lack basic patient assessment skills. Realistic expectations need to be given to the family in terms of what can be accomplished at home, especially if there is an acute medical change.

An irony of these different levels in the continuum of care—nursing homes, hospitals, and home care—is that you will often find the same kind of patient at each level. Many times these patients will have different expectations regarding the availability or desire for aggressive diagnostic procedures or treatment, *but the basic assessment skills required of the clinician are the same.* Careful adaptation of treatment decisions to the care environment and optimization of care is different in each setting.

● Regardless of the care setting, the same basic geriatric assessment skills are required to provide optimal care.

SUMMARY

Assessment of an older patient is a complex and often challenging experience. By focusing on limited goals for this first visit, using standard geriatric principles and excellent medical record-keeping, having a logical approach to the patient, and remaining flexible, both the patient and the health care provider can come away from this first encounter with a feeling of satisfaction and confidence that the goals of this initial visit have been met. Subsequent encounters will need to build on this experience, following the priorities outlined in previous visits, using an evidence-based, problem-oriented approach and being attentive to new problems and events that affect one or several of the five domains of care. Patients transitioning through different levels in the continuum of care require constant assessment and reassessment.

References

1. Ambulatory Geriatric Clinical Care and Services. American Geriatric Society Position Statement. American Geriatric Society Health Care Systems Committee. 2000. http://www.americangeriatrics.org/products/position-papers/ambultry.shtml.
2. Knight EL, Avorn J. Quality indicators for appropriate medication use in vulnerable elders. Ann Intern Med. 2001;135:703-710.
3. Tangororang GL, Kerins GJ, Besdine RW. Clinical approach to the older patient: an overview. In Geriatric Medicine, 4th ed. (Cassel CK, Leipzig RM, Cohen HJ, Larson EB, Meier DE, eds.). New York: Springer, 2003.
4. Jorn AF, Korten AE, Henderson AS. The prevalence of dementia: a quantitative integration of the literature. Act Psychiatr Scand 1987;76:465-479.
5. Graves AB, Kukull WA. The epidemiology of dementia. In Handbook of Dementing Illnesses (Morris JC, ed.). New York: Marcel Dekker, 1994.
6. U.S. Preventive Services Task Force. Screening for dementia: recommendation and rationale. Ann Intern Med. 2003;138:925-926. http://www.preventiveservices.ahrq.gov.
7. Cahn D, Salmon D, Monsch A. Screening for dementia of the Alzheimer's type in the community: utility of the Clock Drawing Test. Arch Clin Neuropsychol 1996;11:529-539.

8. Wolf-Klein GP, Silverstone FA, Levy AP, et al. Screening for Alzheimer's disease by clock drawing. J Am Geriatr Soc 1989;37:730-734.
9. Issacs B, Akhtar AJ. The set test: a rapid test of mental function in old people. Age Ageing. 1972;1:222-226.
10. Issacs B, Kennie AT. The set test as an aid to the detection of dementia in old people. Br J Psychiatry 1973;123:467-470.
11. Folstein MF, Folstein SE, McHugh PR: Mini-mental state: a practical method for grading the cognitive state of patients for the clinician, J Pshchiatr Res 1975;12:186.
12. Blazer DG. Is depression more frequent in late life? An honest look at the evidence. Am J Geriatr Psychiatry 1994;2:193-198.
13. Barrett JE, Barrett JA, Oxman TE, et al. The prevalence of psychiatric disorders in primary care practice. Arch Gen Psychiatry 1988;45:1100-1106.
14. Calkins DR, Rubenstein LV, Cleary PD, et al. Failure of physicians to recognize functional disability in ambulatory patients. Ann Intern Med 1991;114:451.
15. Lawton MP, Brody EM: Assessment of older people: self-maintaining and instrumental activities of daily living. Gerontologist 1969;9:179.
16. Pfeffer RI, Kurosaki TT, Harrah CH, Chance JM, Filos S. Measurement of functional activities in older adults in the community. J Gerontol 1982;37:323.
17. Oowi WL, Barrett S, Hossain M, et al. Patterns of orthostatic blood pressure change and their clinical correlates in a frail elderly population. JAMA 1997;277:1299-1304.
18. Reuben DB, Mui S, Damesyn M, et al. The prognostic value of sensory impairment in older persons. J Am Geriatr Soc 1999;47:930-935.
19. Lichtenstein MJ, Bess FH, Logan SA. Validation of screening tools for identifying hearing-impaired elderly in primary care. JAMA 1988, 259:2875-2878.
20. Fleg JL, Kennedy HL. Long-term prognostic significance of ambulatory electrocardiographic findings in apparently healthy subjects more than 60 years of age. Am J Cardiol 1992;70:748-751.
21. Odenheimer GL, Funkensetin JJ, Beckett L, et al. Comparison of neurologic changes in "successful aging" persons vs the total aging population. Arch Neurol 1994;51:573-580.
22. Mathias S, Nayak US, Isaacs B. Balance in elderly patients: the "get up and go" test. Arch Phys Med Rehabil 1986;67:387-389.
23. Podsiadlo D, Richardson S. The timed "up & go": a test of basic functional mobility for frail elderly persons. J Am Geriatr Soc 1991;39:142-148.
24. Schulz R, O'Brienn AT, Bookwala J, Fleissner KK. Psychiatric and physical morbidity effects of dementia caregiving prevalence, correlates, and causes. Gerontologist 1995;35:771.
25. Murtaugh CM, Litke A. Transitions through postacute and long-term care setting: patterns of use and outcomes from a national cohort of elders. Med Care 2002;40:227-236.
26. Coleman EA, Boult C. The American Geriatric Society Health Care Systems Committee. Improving the quality of transitional care for persons with complex care needs. J Am Geriatr Soc 2003;51:556-557.
27. Marcantonio ER, Simon SE, Bergmann MA, Jones RN, Murphy KM, Morris JN. Delirium Symptoms in Post-Acute Care: Prevalent, Persistent, and Associated with Poor Functional Recovery. J Am Geriatr Soc 2003;51:4-9.

POSTTEST

1. You are assessing a new patient's functional status. Which item below is *not* an activity of daily living?
   a. Eating
   b. Grooming
   c. Using the phone
   d. Dressing
   e. Ambulation

2. An 81-year-old new patient presents with objective memory complaints, and trouble handling financial matters and has gotten lost driving in his hometown. He has a college education. You perform an MMSE with a score of 27/30. To better evaluate this patient's mental status, the appropriate thing to do is
   a. Perform a clock test
   b. Perform a set test
   c. Refer for formal neuropsychological testing
   d. Repeat the MMSE next visit

3. Functional assessment plays a central role in caring for older patients because of which one?
   a. Functional changes are common and are often the final common pathway for many illnesses
   b. Functional changes may be the presenting symptom of a new medical problem
   c. Functional loss helps to set priorities for assessment and care
   d. Functional loss should trigger the immediate use of other health care disciplines for therapeutic interventions to restore function
   e. All of the above

4. In people 80 years or older, which condition listed below is the most common?
   a. Urinary incontinence
   b. Degenerative joint disease
   c. Diabetes mellitus
   d. Coronary artery disease
   e. Alzheimer's disease

5. The term *geriatric syndrome* refers to all of the following conditions *except*:
   a. Urinary incontinence
   b. BPH
   c. Falls
   d. Mental status changes
   e. Weight loss

6. Reasonable goals for the initial office evaluation of an older patient include all of the following *except*:
   a. Performing a complete physical examination
   b. Medication review
   c. Functional assessment
   d. Establishing a relationship with the patient
   e. Determining priorities of care

7. Aspects of disease presentation that are characteristic of older patients include all of the following *except*:
   a. Multiple medical conditions that often interact
   b. Related more to "hidden" effects than medication effects
   c. Vague, ill-defined presenting symptoms rather than traditional symptoms for specific diseases
   d. The common presentation of a "geriatric syndrome" representing a specific new medical problem
   e. The presence of diseases almost unique to elders

8. Among the patient-related symptoms listed below, early cognitive impairment from Alzheimer's disease is most likely to become apparent to health care providers by
   a. Medication errors
   b. Difficulty with bathing
   c. Frequent complaints about memory
   d. Urinary incontinence
   e. Difficulty with details of their remote medical history

PRETEST ANSWERS

1. d
2. e
3. d

POSTTEST ANSWERS

1. c
2. c
3. e
4. b
5. b
6. a
7. b
8. a

Health Maintenance, Exercise, and Nutrition

Barbara Resnick

OBJECTIVES

Upon completion of this chapter, the reader will be able to:

- Define the purpose of health promotion and disease prevention in older adults.
- Describe an appropriate immunization schedule for older adults.
- Describe three lifestyle modifications that can prevent disease.
- Describe the relevant relationship between nutrition and nutritional status and health.
- Delineate the use of prophylactic medication on cardiovascular, musculoskeletal, and cancer prevention.
- State appropriate cancer screening guidelines for older adults
- Plan strategies for putting prevention into practice by identifying facilitators and motivational techniques.

PRETEST

1. Even though older adults are less likely to get counseled for smoking cessation, they have which of the following:
    a. The same quit rates as younger individuals, with approximately 70% of smokers who want to quit and 46% making some attempt each year at quitting.
    b. The same quit rates as younger individuals, with approximately 50% of smokers who want to quit and 46% making some attempt each year at quitting.
    c. The same quit rates as younger individuals, with approximately 40% of smokers who want to quit and 60% making some attempt each year at quitting.
    d. Much higher quit rates than younger individuals.

2. In contrast to self-report questionnaires, clinical laboratory procedures provide objective evidence of problem drinking with the most useful laboratory tests including which one of the following:
    a. Complete blood count (CBC)
    b. Gamma-glutamyl transpeptidase (GGT), and carbohydrate-deficient transferrin (CDT)
    c. Blood alcohol levels
    d. All of the above

3. The modified food pyramid for mature (70+) adults was modified to include which of the following:
    a. It now has eight 8-ounce glasses of water.
    b. A flag was added to the top of the pyramid to remind older adults that they may not be getting adequate protein, fiber, and calcium.
    c. Complex carbohydrates are in a new position at the top of the pyramid, and the refined carbohydrates moved to the bottom.
    d. The proteins with saturated and partially hydrogenated fats should be at the bottom of the pyramid.

ESSENTIALS OF HEALTH PROMOTION FOR AGING ADULTS

Health promotion is the science and art of helping people change their lifestyle to move toward a state of *optimal health*, defined as a balance of physical, emotional, social, spiritual, and intellectual health.[1] The purpose of health promotion and disease prevention is to reduce the potential years of life lost in premature mortality and to ensure better quality of remaining life. As Americans live longer, it is suggested that health promotion activities are all the more important for older adults because these individuals will have more years to benefit from preventive services.

Health promotion activities include the use of immunizations to prevent the occurrence of acute problems such as influenza and pneumonia, risk factor reduction through lifestyle modifications such as smoking cessation or regular physical activity, and the prophylactic use of medication to prevent cardiovascular disease or prevent musculoskeletal disorders. In addition, health promotion includes screening to facilitate the early identification of disease so that treatment can be initiated. Most important among these is the screening for malignancies.

There are multiple guidelines for health promotion activities available for clinicians as well as patient-specific information to help individuals decide what type of health promotion activities they want to engage in. The decisions about whether or not to adhere to these guidelines are often difficult for the older individual or the individual with power of attorney (POA) to make. Guidelines for overall health screening decisions[2] can help direct clinicians and the patient or POA in this decision process. An individualized approach is critical when working with older individuals in the area of health promotion and should drive the decision process.

Mrs. W

Mrs. W is an 81-year-old white female with a known history of Parkinson's disease, hypertension, irritable bowel disease with a lactose intolerance, urinary incontinence, hypothyroidism, glaucoma, alcohol abuse with no alcohol intake for 25 years, and regular nicotine use with a one-half pack per day history of 50 years. She currently lives in a senior high-rise and is independent with personal care activities, although she gets help with medication set up into a weekly pill box, and while she fixes her own breakfast, she has her two other meals in the cafeteria or facility dining room. Her weight has been relatively stable, with a consistent body mass index (BMI) of 29.2.

Mrs. W is very concerned about her health and very fearful of future health impairments. She goes for regular screenings, including routine colonoscopies, annual mammograms, pap tests, and dermatological evaluations, all of which have been negative. She reports that she is unable to tolerate aspirin, calcium, and any of the bisphosphonates because of associated diarrhea. She has made some attempts to cut back and/or stop smoking but has been unable to do so. She does not exercise regularly. She is, however, very interested in learning about ways to improve her health and prevent problems, although she acknowledges that she does not always follow through with what is suggested. Her medications include the following: Sinemet 25/100 twice daily (bid), Norvasc 10mg every day (qd), Lomotil up to 12 a day as needed, and intermittently Detrol 4 mg qd.

STUDY QUESTIONS

1. What interventions might you implement to help Ms. W's quality of life?
2. How would you prioritize your interventions?
3. What motivational strategies would you use to help Ms. W change her behavior in challenging areas such as smoking cessation and exercise?

PREVENTION OF DISEASE

Immunizations

Table 5-1 provides an overview of recommendations for immunizations for older adults. The U.S. Advisory Committee on Immunization Practices and the Centers for Disease Control currently recommend that all older adults be immunized against influenza annually and that they receive at least one pneumococcal vaccination.[3] All high-risk older adults (as defined in Table 5-1) should receive an additional pneumococcal vaccination 5 years or more after their first immunization. Older adults should receive a one-time revaccination for pneumonia if they were initially vaccinated more than 5 years previously and were less than 65 years of age at the time of the initial vaccination.[4] Compliance with recommended immunization guidelines has improved,[5] although the goal set in Healthy People 2010 of 95% adherence to immunization has not been met. To facilitate compliance the federal government in 2002 approved standing orders for annual influenza vaccinations and pneumococcal pneumonia vaccination for older adults in institutional settings and home health agencies for all Medicare and Medicaid beneficiaries. At this point in time, however, Medicare does not cover tetanus immunizations as there are only about 50 cases reported each year in the United States, although half of these are in people over the age of 65.[6]

Table 5-1	Recommended Immunizations for Older Adults	
Vaccine	**Ages 50 to 64**	**Ages 65 and older**
Tetanus, diphtheria	One dose every 10 years	One dose every 10 years
Influenza	Annual	Annual
Pneumococcal	One dose	One dose[a]

[a]Revaccinate once after 5 years if the individual has a history of immunodeficiency, leukemia, or lymphoma; has a known malignancy; is on alkylating agents or antimetabolites; has known leakage of cerebrospinal fluid; has had radiation or large amounts of corticosteroids; or has known renal failure, asplenia, or HIV infection. One-time revaccination is recommended for those older than 65 years who were vaccinated more than 5 years earlier and were younger than 65 at the time of the initial vaccination.

Risk Factor Reduction through Lifestyle Behaviors

SMOKING CESSATION

> ● Even though older adults are less likely to get counseled for smoking cessation, they have the same quit rates as younger individuals, with approximately 70% of smokers who want to quit and 46% making some attempt each year at quitting.

Older smokers carry the greatest burden of smoking-related disease and associated health care costs.[7] Older adults may be particularly resistant to quitting, may have had a long history of unsuccessful quit attempts, may have a longer history of addiction, and may believe that they have lived this long smoking and thus see little benefit in quitting. Although there is some support to indicate that quitting smoking even after age 65 can increase years of life,[8] it may be more important to focus on the potential improvement in quality of life with smoking cessation. Even though older adults are less likely to get counseled for smoking cessation,[8] they have the same quit rates as younger individuals, with approximately 70% of smokers who want to quit and 46% making some attempt each year at quitting.[9,10] Clinicians working with older adults should certainly attempt to address smoking cessation and encourage individuals, regardless of age, to consider this as a way to improve overall health status.

The most commonly used model to promote individual smoking cessation is Prochaska's transtheoretical model of change.[11] Individuals are evaluated and encouraged to proceed through the following stages: precontemplation, contemplation, preparation, action, and maintenance. The Agency for Healthcare Research and Quality recommends a comprehensive guideline that includes a brief intervention described as the five A's: ask, advise, assess, assist, and arrange follow up,[7] which has been noted to be successful in encouraging smoking cessation.

Pharmacological interventions for smoking cessation are also an option and are known to augment behavioral interventions. There is currently an ongoing demonstration project, The Medicare Stop Smoking Program,[12] sponsored by the Centers for Medicare and Medicaid Services, that is comparing reimbursement for provider counseling alone versus provider counseling and nicotine replacement therapy. The findings from this demonstration project will provide important information related to combined use of medications and behavioral interventions for smoking cessation with older adults.

PREVENTION OF POLYPHARMACY

> ● When working with older adults, attempts should be made to simplify drug regimens, and medications should be reviewed at each provider–patient interaction.

Polypharmacy is the use of more medications than are clinically needed or indicated. Older adults are particularly at risk for polypharmacy because of multiple comorbidities and the risk of seeing multiple health care providers. The best way to prevent polypharmacy is to avoid unnecessary medication use and attempt to implement behavioral interventions as a first line of treatment. Specifically, dietary interventions, exercise, stress management, and behavioral management techniques will often be sufficient if implemented and adhered to. Moreover, combining behavioral interventions with medications may allow for lower drug dosages to be used. Clinicians should also make certain to be very clear about drug use instructions and provide both verbal and written accounts of how to use the medication. Drug regimens should be simplified, and medications should be reviewed at each provider– patient interaction.

ALCOHOL USE

According to the 2000 National Household Survey on Drug Abuse, 5.6% of people 65 years of age or older engaged in binge drinking during the previous month, 1.6% engaged in heavy alcohol use, and 0.5% were alcohol dependent.[13] More than 2 million people 65 years of age or older had some sort of alcohol problem. Clinical studies estimate that 15% of men and 12% of women are high-risk drinkers based on the definitions provided by the National Institute on Alcohol Abuse and Alcoholism[14] (Table 5-2). Hospitalized patients and those in institutional settings are also likely to have alcohol problems.[15-18] About two-thirds of elderly alcoholic patients started drinking at a young age, and late-onset drinking accounts for the remaining one-third of elderly persons who abuse alcohol.[19] Late-onset drinkers tend to have a higher level of education and income than do those who started drinking at a younger age.[19] Stressful life events, such as bereavement or retirement, may trigger late-onset drinking in some, but not all, persons.

SCREENING FOR ALCOHOL USE/ABUSE

> ● Laboratory procedures provide objective evidence of problem drinking. The most useful laboratory tests to confirm alcohol-abuse problems in older adults are gamma-glutamyl transpeptidase (GGT), mean corpuscular volume (MCV), and carbohydrate-deficient transferrin (CDT).

Table 5–2	Recommendations Related to Alcohol Intake
Risk Classification	**Definition**
Low-risk drinking	• No more than one drink per day[a] and a maximum of two drinks on any drinking occasion. This is a moderate level of alcohol intake. • CAGE score of zero. • No evidence of dysfunction related to drinking (physical, psychological, or social). • Not using medications that interact adversely with alcohol or have conditions that alcohol may trigger or worsen.
At-risk drinking	• On average: more than one drink per day, more than seven drinks per week, or more than three drinks on heavier drinking occasions. • CAGE score of more than zero. • Evidence of drinking-related dysfunction. • Using alcohol and medications in combinations that might interact adversely. • Using alcohol and having conditions that may be triggered or worsened by alcohol.
Alcohol abuse	*Abuse:* More than one of the following criteria met, and has never met criteria for dependence: • Recurrent drinking resulting in the failure to fulfill major obligations at work or in the home (less applicable to older adults who may have fewer obligations). • Recurrent drinking in situations where it is physically hazardous. • Recurrent alcohol-related legal problems (older adults uncommonly have these problems). • Continued drinking despite persistent or recurrent social problems caused or worsened by alcohol (older adults may not realize these problems are related to drinking).
Alcohol dependence	*Dependence:* More than three of the following criteria met: • Tolerance, or requiring more alcohol to get "high" (older adults may have problems with even low intake due to increased sensitivity to alcohol and higher blood alcohol levels). • Withdrawal, or drinking to relieve/prevent withdrawal (older adults who develop dependence may not develop physiological dependence). • Drinking in larger amounts, or for a longer period of time than intended (older adults may have increased cognitive problems as a result of alcohol use and may not be able to monitor intake). • Persistent desire to drink, or unsuccessful efforts to cut down or control drinking. • A lot of time spent in activities necessary to obtain or use alcohol or recover from effects. • Important occupational, social, or recreational activities given up or reduced owing to drinking (older adults may have fewer activities, making detection of problems more difficult). • Drinking continues despite knowledge of persistent/recurrent physical or psychological problems likely to be caused or worsened by alcohol (older adults may not know or understand that problems are related to use, even after medical advice).

[a]One drink is equivalent to 12 ounces of beer; 1.5 ounces of 80 proof alcohol; or 5 ounces of wine. Based on the National Institute on Alcohol Abuse and Alcoholism and the American Geriatrics Society Guidelines. (American Geriatrics Society. Position Statement: Clinical Guidelines for Alcohol Use Disorders in Older Adults. AGS Clinical Practice Committee. http://www.americangeriatrics.org/products/positionpapers/alcohol.shtml.)

Two types of alcoholism-screening instruments are available: self-report questionnaires and clinical laboratory tests. Screening instruments vary in their ability to detect different patterns and levels of drinking and in the degree of their applicability to specific subpopulations and settings. The CAGE (Box 5-1) questionnaire[20] is commonly used among clinicians. When used with older adults, it has reported sensitivities ranging from 43% to 94% for detecting alcohol abuse and alcoholism.[21] The CAGE questionnaire is well suited to busy primary care settings because it poses four straightforward yes/no questions. It may fail, however, to detect low but risky levels of drinking and often performs less well among women and minority populations.

LABORATORY TESTS FOR ALCOHOL ABUSE

In contrast to self-report questionnaires, clinical laboratory procedures provide objective evidence of problem drinking. The most useful laboratory tests to confirm alcohol-abuse problems in older adults are GGT, MCV, and CDT.[23] The serum GGT determination is one of the most widely used laboratory tests. This hepatic enzyme is elevated in patients who use alcohol excessively.[24] MCV also has been used as a marker of heavy alcohol consumption, although it is less sensitive than is the GGT level and should not be used alone to indicate alcohol abuse. CDT tests are

Box 5-1	CAGE Questionnaire

Alcohol dependence is likely if the patient gives two or more positive answers:

C: Have you ever felt you should CUT down your drinking?

A: Have people ANNOYED you by criticizing your drinking?

G: Have you ever felt bad or GUILTY about your drinking?

E: Have you ever had a drink first think in the morning to steady your nerves or get rid of a hangover (EYE-opener)?

available to screen for excessive alcohol consumption. Four to seven drinks per day for at least 1 week can significantly elevate CDT levels in patients with alcoholism.[25] CDT seems to be useful as a first-line biological marker to confirm or disprove suspected alcohol misuse. High CDT and GGT is indicative of alcohol dependence, whereas high CDT with a GGT below normal is evidence of alcohol abuse.[23] The accuracy of these markers is affected by various factors such as nonalcoholic liver damage, use of medications or drugs, and by metabolic disorders.[26]

HEALTH BENEFITS AND RISKS OF ALCOHOL USE

The signs and symptoms associated with alcohol abuse in the older adult are numerous and include the same spectrum of physical, behavioral, and psychological problems that can be found in younger individuals. Conversely, however, a number of health benefits have been associated with drinking alcohol at low-risk levels. Specifically, there is evidence to suggest that one to two standard drinks has a positive effect on lipid metabolism,[27-30] results in decreased mortality following a myocardial infarction,[31] decreases risk of developing congestive heart failure,[32] and lowers risk of ischemic stroke in the young-old (60 to 69 years of age).[33,34] In several large epidemiological studies,[35-38] findings have suggested that moderate alcohol use was not associated with cognitive decline and individuals who abstained from alcohol reported worse physical health than those who drank alcohol.[38-40]

EVIDENCE-BASED INTERVENTIONS FOR ABSTINENCE FROM ALCOHOL

Older adults who do engage in treatment to abstain from alcohol have been noted to have substantially better outcomes and are more likely to complete treatment compared with younger adults.[42] Unfortunately, no known published studies have been done to consider the impact of these interventions with cognitively impaired older adults. For impaired individuals it is not certain that cognitive behavioral interventions are effective. Structured interventions, however, that remove access to alcohol and provide alternative activities can be very effective in preventing ongoing high-risk alcohol intake in these individuals.[17] This requires a strong interdisciplinary team approach and must include support from family and friends.

Pharmacological treatments have not traditionally played a major role in the long-term treatment of older alcohol-dependent adults. Until recently disulfiram (Antabuse) was the only medication approved for the treatment of alcoholism, but it was seldom used in older patients because of concerns about adverse effects.

In 1995, the opioid antagonist naltrexone (ReVia) was approved by the U.S. Food and Drug Administration for the treatment of alcoholism and was found to be safe and effective in preventing relapse and reducing the craving for alcohol in older adults.[43] Acamprosate, which was approved for use to the treatment of alcohol abuse in July 2004, has likewise been used effectively with older adults.[44]

Physical Activity

> ● For healthy, asymptomatic adults of any age, the U.S. Preventive Services Task Force (USPSTF) does not recommend any type of cardiac screening (electrocardiogram, exercise test) before the initiation of physical activity. For sedentary older people who are asymptomatic, low-intensity physical activity can be safely initiated regardless of whether or not an older person has had a recent medical evaluation.

A substantial body of scientific evidence indicates regular physical activity can bring dramatic health benefits to older adults (Table 5-3). Physical activity allows older individuals to increase the likelihood that they will extend years of active independent life, reduce disability, and improve their quality of life in mid-life and beyond.[45,46]

GUIDELINES FOR PHYSICAL ACTIVITY

The specific amount of exercise needed to achieve the desired benefit varies based on individual goals and capabilities. Combining recommendations from the American College of Sports Medicine (ACSM),[47] the Centers for Disease Control and Prevention (CDC),[48] and the National Institutes of Health (NIH),[49] clinicians should recommend that older adults engage in 30 minutes of physical activity most days of the week, and this activity should incorporate aerobic activity (walking, dancing, swimming, biking), resistance training, and flexibility. Exercises can be done individually or in group settings depending on the individual's preference, cognitive ability, and motivational level.

GUIDELINES FOR SCREENING BEFORE EXERCISE

Despite the relatively low risk of cardiovascular events with low- or moderate-intensity exercise or physical activity,[50] guidelines from national organizations such as the ACSM[51] and the American Heart Association (AHA)[52] have traditionally recommended that adults over age 40 have some type of screening done before starting a physical activity program. There is no single evidence-based strategy recommended.[53-55]

| Table 5-3 | Health Benefits of Physical Activity for Older Adults |

Health Issue	Treatment Strategy	Evidence-Based Support	Comments
Cardiovascular health[136-138]	Increasing physical activity with aerobic activity	A	• Improves myocardial performance • Increases peak diastolic filling • Increases heart muscle contractility • Reduces premature ventricular-contractions • Improves blood lipid profile • Increases aerobic capacity • Reduces systolic blood pressure • Improves diastolic blood pressure • Improves endurance • Improves muscle capillary blood flow
Body composition[139,140]	Increasing physical activity with aerobic activity	A	• Decreases abdominal adipose tissue • Increases muscle mass
Metabolism[141]	Increasing physical activity with aerobic activity	A	• Increases total energy expenditure • Improves protein synthesis rate and amino acid uptake into the skeletal muscle • Reduces low-density lipoproteins • Reduces cholesterol/very low density lipoproteins • Reduces triglycerides • Increases high-density lipoproteins • Increases glucose tolerance
Bone health[142]	Increasing physical activity with weight-bearing exercise	A	• Slows decline in bone mineral density • Increases total body calcium, nitrogen
Psychological well-being[143-145]	Increasing physical activity through aerobic activity	A	• Improves perceived well-being and happiness • Decreases levels of stress-related hormones • Improves attention span • Improves cognitive processing speed • Increases slow wave and rapid eye movement sleep • Provides sense of accomplishment • Decreases anxiety and improves overall mood
Muscle weakness and functional capacity[146-149]	Increasing physical activity through resistance and balance training	A	• Reduces risk of musculoskeletal disability • Improves strength and flexibility • Reduces risk of falls • Improves dynamic balance • Improves physical functional performance
Preventing falls and fear of falling[150-154]	Increasing physical activity through resistance, aerobic and balance exercise	A	• Decreases falls and fear of falling

Ideally the purpose of screening is to (1) minimize cardiac risk while allowing the individual to achieve the maximum benefit from physical activity,[56] (2) identify medical problems that should be used to modify the activity program, and (3) identify functional impairments that the activity program will address.[57] Based on results of the screening, individuals may be required to see their primary clinicians and/or have a "sign off" on a screening form before being allowed into exercise programs. This type of safety screen has been used to stratify individuals by risk for cardiovascular events and to establish the need for more extensive testing such as an exercise treadmill test or thallium treadmill.

Requiring screening for older adults who simply want to engage in low- to moderate-level lifestyle activities such as walking or gardening may, however, be a deterrent to initiating or maintaining any physical activity. For healthy, asymptomatic adults of any age, the USPSTF[60] does not recommend any type of cardiac screening (electrocardiogram, exercise test) before the initiation of physical activity. For sedentary older people who are asymptomatic, low-intensity physical activity can be safely initiated regardless of whether or not an older person has had a recent medical evaluation.

PHYSICAL ACTIVITY PROGRAMS ACROSS ALL LEVELS OF CARE

For general health and well being, a well-rounded physical activity program should include endurance, strength, balance, and flexibility.[61] Endurance-related physical activity refers to continuous movement that involves large muscle groups and is sustained for a minimum of 10 minutes. Examples of endurance activity include biking, swimming, walking, and lifestyle activities that incorporate large muscle groups. Strength-related activity refers to increasing muscle strength by moving or lifting some type of resistance, such as weights or elastic bands, at a level that requires some physical effort.

The amount of resistance recommended and number of repetitions will vary for each individual and muscle group. In general, one to three sets of 10 to 12 repetitions are regarded as the optimal amount for increasing muscle strength. Resistance exercises, or strength training, should not be performed on consecutive days to give the muscles time to recover between sessions. Flexibility-related activity facilitates greater range of motion around the joint. These exercises should be performed a minimum of 2 days a week. Balance is the ability to maintain control of the body over the base of support so as to avoid falling. Static balance is the ability to maintain balance without moving, whereas dynamic balance is the ability to move without loosing balance or falling.

Nonambulatory patients can likewise engage in physical activity. In fact, it is these individuals who are most likely to benefit the most from an exercise program. Muscle weakness and atrophy are probably the most functionally relevant and reversible aspects to exercise in nonambulatory older adults, and attempting to reverse these deficits can have a major impact on function and quality of life.

Maintaining Optimal Nutritional Intake

● Evaluating food intake in older adults is particularly important as inadequate intake can result in weight loss and loss of muscle mass, which may result in decreased strength and power, decreased walking speed, and impaired balance and a decline in activity.

AGE-RELEVANT REQUIREMENTS

The first change in the Modified Food Pyramid for Mature (70 or older) adults (Fig. 5-1) was to add a new foundation to the pyramid of eight 8-ounce glasses of

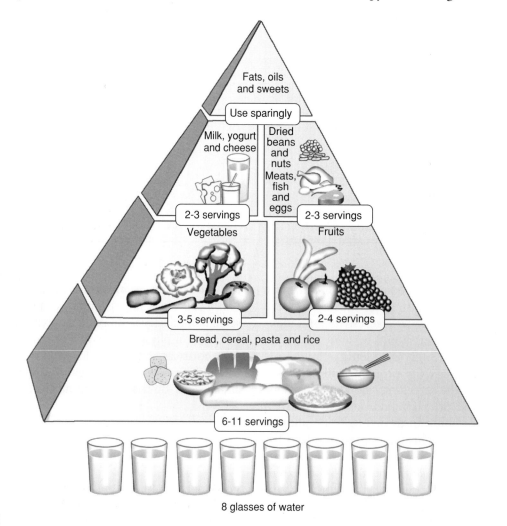

FIGURE 5-1

Food pyramid. Although the information illustrated provides generalized guidelines applicable to most older individuals, in April 2005 the U.S. Department of Agriculture released new food guide pyramids that are individualized, based on age, sex, and activity. *(Redrawn from http://www.MyPyramid.gov.)*

water[62]. In addition, a flag was added to the top of the pyramid to remind older adults that they may not be getting adequate calcium, vitamin D, and vitamin B_{12} and that supplements may be needed. Haber[63] recommends further revisions in this pyramid so that the complex carbohydrates are moved to the bottom of the pyramid and the refined carbohydrates are moved to the top of the pyramid and eaten sparingly. In addition, proteins with saturated and partially hydrogenated fats should be at the top of the pyramid and eaten sparingly, and the monounsaturated and polyunsaturated omega-3 fats moved down lower on the pyramid. Fish, beans, nuts, vegetable oils, and similar products should be consumed in greater amounts than red meat, butter, and refined carbohydrates.

For older adults it is particularly important to consider nutritional health because of the impact that nutrition can have on functional performance. Inadequate food intake can result in weight loss and loss of muscle mass, which may result in decreased strength and power, decreased walking speed, and impaired balance and a decline in activity.[64-66] Calcium, vitamin D, magnesium, and phosphorus have been associated with structural and muscular function.[65,66] Attempts should be made to reach recommended levels of these nutrients.

WATER

Water is essential for lubrication of the joints; transport of nutrients and salts; hydration of the skin, eyes, nose, and mouth; removal of waste products; regulation of body temperature; and promotion of adequate blood volume. Inadequate hydration can result in constipation, fatigue, hypotension, hyperthermia, dizziness, breathing difficulties, and irregular heartbeat. Fluids are best taken in the form of water, juice, or milk; alcohol, caffeinated tea and coffee, and soft drinks have a diuretic effect and therefore raise fluid level more modestly.

FATS

Saturated fats can raise blood cholesterol and increase the risk of heart disease. A 2002 Institute of Medicine[67] report recommended that 20% to 35% of total calories should be from fat, 45% to 65% from carbohydrates, and 10% to 35% from proteins. A simple technique to determine the number of allowable grams of fat per day can be calculated by dividing the individual's ideal weight in half and allowing that number of grams of fat. Monounsaturated fats, such as olive oil, are the best type of fat as they lower low-density lipoprotein (LDL) but leave the high density lipoprotein (HDL) intact. Polyunsaturated fats, such as sunflower, corn, and soybean oils, appear to lower LDL and HDL.

FIBER

Fiber is the indigestible residue of food that passes through the bowel and is eliminated in the stool. It is a natural laxative, adds bulk to stool, absorbs water, and reduces the amount of time that stool is in the bowels. It is currently recommended that older adults increase dietary fiber intake so that there are 14 g of dietary fiber per 1000 calories consumed.[68] Ideally fiber intake should include cereal fibers and be consumed with sufficient fluid intake (64 ounces daily).

PROTEIN

Proteins form antibodies that help the body to resist disease and enable the growth and repair of body cells. Complete proteins contain the eight essential amino acids that are needed and can be found in foods such as fish, dairy products, and eggs. Protein should make up 12% to 20% of the total calories in the diet. It is not unusual for older adults who are acutely ill to decrease protein intake and become protein deficient. Supplements can be used to augment dietary intake as described in Chapter 27, "Malnutrition and Feeding Problems."

MICRONUTRIENTS: VITAMINS AND MINERALS

Micronutrients (vitamins and minerals) are particularly important to overall health in older adults. Increasing fruit and vegetable intake to five servings daily optimizes the intake of vitamins A, C, and E and potassium. B_{12} intake is generally adequate, although older adults should be encouraged to increase the intake of the crystalline form of vitamin B_{12}, which is found in fortified foods such as whole-grain breakfast cereals. Vitamin D intake is generally below recommendations, which are currently for 1000 IU daily.[69] Supplementation is generally needed as recommended amounts of vitamin D are not easily obtained in foods and there is less opportunity for older adults to make vitamin D in the skin. Water-soluble vitamins (C and eight of the B vitamins) are excreted in urine, although adverse effects can still result from exceeding the upper-level recommendations. The surplus fat-soluble vitamins (A, D, E, and K) are stored in body tissue, and excessive amounts can become toxic.

ASSESSMENT OF NUTRITIONAL HEALTH AND APPROACH TO OBESITY

There are several useful tools to help guide individuals and/or caregivers in the evaluation of the nutritional health of an older individual. The Determine Your Nutritional Health check list (see Chapter 27) is a simple measure that allows individuals to establish if they are in good nutritional health or if they are at moderate or high risk of insufficient nutritional intake. It is estimated that one-third of homebound older adults are overweight. Older adults, therefore, should be screened for obesity as per the USPSTF recommendations.[71] Obesity has an impact on mobility and overall function,[72] as well as being a risk factor for coronary heart disease and other chronic conditions.[73,74] BMI, calculated as weight in kilograms divided by height in meters squared, is a reliable and valid measure to identify adults who are at increased risk for mortality and morbidity owing to overweight and obesity. Overweight individuals are defined as those who have a BMI of 25 to 29.9 kg/m^2. Obesity is defined as a BMI of 30. The BMI, however, is age dependent and does not account for body fat distribution. Older adults at high risk of excess weight are likely to be underestimated because many have excess body fat that is counteracted by a loss of muscle mass with age.

The most effective interventions for weight loss in older adults combine nutritional education, diet, and exercise counseling with behavioral strategies. Recent studies have demonstrated that there was little difference in the degree of weight loss achieved between individuals who used low-carbohydrate versus low-fat diets.[75] For individuals who have hypertension and are overweight, the Seventh Report of the Joint National Committee on Prevention, Detection, Evaluation, and Treatment of High Blood Pressure (JNC-7)[76] suggests that clinicians counsel patients to adhere to salt-restricted diets, increase physical activity, and decrease alcohol consumption. The Dietary Approaches to Stop Hypertension (DASH) eating plan is commonly recommended as this diet consists of fruits, vegetables, whole grains, low-fat dairy products, poultry, and fish.[77]

PROPHYLACTIC MEDICATION USE

Prevention of Cardiovascular Disease

> ● Unfortunately, despite the evidence that oral anticoagulation with warfarin is the most effective prevention of stroke caused by atrial fibrillation, older adults are less likely to be provided with this treatment option. When addressing anticoagulation for these individuals, consideration should be given to quality-of-life issues and the need for ongoing monitoring of blood work, as well as underlying disease and lifestyle issues.

Clinical trials remain the cornerstone for guiding providers as to what treatment options are provided to older individuals regarding prevention of cardiovascular disease. The "ABC" format (antiplatelet agents/anticoagulation, blood pressure control, cholesterol management) has been used to best summarize findings and organize recommendations.

ANTIPLATELET AGENTS

Aspirin inhibits the cyclooxygenase enzyme involved in the production of thromboxane, a factor that promotes platelet aggregation. Two meta-analyses[78,79] support the importance of aspirin therapy in the prevention of cardiovascular disease in dosages of 75 to 325 mg of aspirin daily. Daily aspirin decreases mortality as well as the number of cardiovascular events.[80, 81] In patients with no established cardiovascular disease, low-dose aspirin (75 to 81 mg) should be recommended. If the individual has documented cardiovascular disease, the benefit of low-dose aspirin is anticipated to be even greater. Aspirin use is known, however, to increase the risk of gastrointestinal irritation owing to the antiplatelet and gastric mucosal effects,[82] and cotherapy with a proton pump inhibitor (PPI) is an effective preventive option.[83] Clopidogrel inhibits platelet activation by blocking the binding of adenosine diphosphate to its receptor on the platelet surface. As shown in several randomized trials,[84,85] clopidogrel should be recommended in place of aspirin in patients who are intolerant or resistant to the effects of aspirin.

The use of warfarin or aspirin in older adults with a known history of atrial fibrillation to prevent stroke should likewise be addressed. Please see the chapter titled "Cerebral Vascular Disease" for an extensive discussion of warfarin management. As with other health prevention interventions, the patient needs to be aware of the risk versus benefit to treatment and the implications of accepting or rejecting treatment options. Unfortunately, despite the evidence that oral anticoagulation with warfarin is the most effective prevention of stroke caused by atrial fibrillation,[86,87] older adults are less likely to be provided with this treatment option[87,88] (see Chapter 38). Consideration should be given to quality-of-life issues such as the trauma of ongoing monitoring of blood work, as well as underlying disease and lifestyle issues. If a decision to treat with warfarin is made, optimal anticoagulation in the range of 2.0 to 3.0 international ratios (INR) should be the goal. The risk for intracranial hemorrhage was reported to increase for those 85 years of age or older when the INR ranged from 3.5 to 3.9. The risk of intracranial hemorrhage at INRs of less than 2.0, however, was not different from the risk of hemorrhage at INRs of 2.0 to 3.0.[89]

BETA-BLOCKERS

Beta-blocker use has been recommended to prevent first events of nonfatal myocardial infarction in patients with high blood pressure since 1989.[90] Beta-blocker use has also been noted to be effective as secondary prevention of a myocardial infarction and can lead to a 19% to 48% decrease in mortality and up to a 28% decrease in reinfarction rates.[91] Older adults may need to be started on a lower dose than recommended in the younger adult population owing to normal physiologic changes that increase the risk of low cardiac output and bradycardia. In diabetic patients, beta-blockers can impair glucose control, leading to hypoglycemia, and blood glucose levels should be monitored regularly in these individuals. In patients with decompensated heart failure, beta-blocker use can lead to further cardiac depression, and drugs need to be initiated at low doses. Likewise, beta-blockers can induce bronchospasm in patients with chronic obstructive pulmonary disease or asthma, although use of cardioselective beta-blockers and albuterol can minimize these effects.

The only absolute contraindications to beta-blockers are severe bradycardia, preexisting sick sinus syndrome, second- and third-degree atrioventricular block, severe left ventricular dysfunction, active peripheral vascular disease with rest ischemia, or reactive airway disease so severe that airway support is required.[91] As with other prophylactic medications, beta-blockers and the benefit versus risk ratio should be addressed with all older adults or their health care POA.

STATINS

The Adult Treatment Panel III (ATPIII) of the National Cholesterol Education Program (NCEP) established current recommendations based on a review of five randomized, controlled clinical trials. Overall, the statins seem to be most helpful in patients who have underlying cardiovascular disease.[92,93] It should be recognized, however, that although there were some older adults in these trials, very few of the participants were older than 70 years of age. In high-risk persons, treatment should be aggressive, and the recommended LDL cholesterol (LDL-C) goal should be less than 100 mg/dl and ideally could drop to an LDL-C goal of less than 70 mg/dl. Moreover, when a high-risk patient has high triglycerides or low HDL cholesterol (HDL-C), consideration can be given to combining a fibrate or nicotinic acid with a LDL-lowering drug. For moderately high-risk persons (2 or more risk factors and 10-year risk 10% to 20%), the recommended LDL-C goal should at least be less than 130 mg/dl. In addition to drug treatment, all individuals at high or moderately high risk for coronary heart disease who have lifestyle-related risk factors (e.g., obesity, physical inactivity, elevated triglycerides, low HDL-C, or metabolic syndrome) should be encouraged to engage in appropriate lifestyle modifications.

Prevention of Musculoskeletal Disorders

> ● It is never too late to initiate healthy habits that will augment musculoskeletal health as one ages. This is best done by incorporating exercise into daily activities and adding optimal calcium and vitamin D intake.

Although prevention of musculoskeletal disorders ideally should begin in childhood and young adulthood, it is never too late to initiate healthy habits that will augment musculoskeletal health as one ages. This is particularly true with regard to osteoporosis and degenerative joint disease. Osteoporosis by definition is a bone density that is 2.5 or more standard deviations below the young-adult peak bone density. Osteopenia, defined as 1 to 2.5 standard deviations below the young-adult peak bone density, is a weakening of the bones that, if left untreated, will likely progress to osteoporosis. The USPSTF recommends that routine screening for osteoporosis begin at age 65 for all women.[94] It is not clear, however, how often individuals should go through screenings and/or when such screening should be terminated.

Exercise is central to prevention of osteoporosis[95-97] and is one of the most effective nonpharmacologic treatments for osteoarthritis, particularly osteoarthritis of the knee.[98-100] Well-conditioned muscle and muscular balance are needed to withstand physical activity such as walking, provide joint stability, and support function and independence. Muscular conditioning can be achieved through well-designed exercise programs, specifically, long-term walking,[101] isokinetic quadriceps exercise,[102,103] high- and low-intensity bicycling,[104] aquatic exercise classes,[105,106] and tai chi.[107]

In addition to exercise, dietary and pharmaceutical interventions are effective in maintaining and improving bone density. The bisphosphonates alendronate and risedronate, the selective estrogen-receptor modulator raloxifene, the anabolic agent parathyroid hormone, and, most recently, strontium ranelate are beneficial in terms of reducing vertebral fractures owing to osteoporosis. The bisphosphonates and hormone replacement therapy (HRT) have been reported to reduce hip fractures in community-dwelling women, and calcium plus vitamin D has been reported to reduce fractures in elderly people in institutions. Evidence for the antifracture efficacy of calcitonin, fluoride, and anabolic steroids is insufficient to justify their use.

CALCIUM AND VITAMIN D

The nutritional needs for optimizing bone health can be met by a diet that is high in fruits and vegetables (five or more servings per day), that is adequate in protein but moderate in animal protein, and that includes dairy or calcium-fortified foods. For those individuals in whom there is inadequate calcium intake from diet, supplemental calcium can be used. Supplemental or dietary calcium should be spread out throughout the day so that a total intake of 1200 to 1500 mg is achieved, with 500 mg or less being consumed at each meal to optimize absorption. The upper limit for calcium supplementation is 2500 mg per day.[108] Calcium unfortunately is a difficult mineral to absorb, and some foods actually inhibit calcium absorption, including spinach, green beans, peanuts, and summer squash. In addition, high levels of protein, sodium, or caffeine result in higher levels of excretion of calcium in the urine and thus should be avoided. Calcium citrate is better absorbed than is calcium carbonate and does not need to be taken with food.

In all individuals older than 70 years, vitamin D intake of at least 600 IU per day (up to 1000 IU per day) and an upper limit of 2000 IU per day is recommended to enhance the absorption of calcium, as well as strengthen bones and decrease the risk of fracture.[69,109,110] Dosage options of 100,000 IU every 4 months have been reported to decrease the risk of first fracture among older males and females living in the community.

BISPHOSPHONATES

Bisphosphonates for the prevention and management of older adults with osteoporosis are recommended. Decisions regarding the use of bisphosphonates should be based on the individual's comorbidities, lifestyle, cognitive factors, and personal preferences. Adherence to the treatment protocol for safe and effective use of bisphosphonates may be another challenge for older individuals. Once-a-week treatment options for the bisphosphonates generally facilitate adherence, although some patients find that medication used once a week is more difficult to remember and adhere to than is daily administration.[111] Future options for bisphosphonate use will likely include once-a-year infusions.[112]

SELECTIVE ESTROGEN RECEPTOR MODULATORS

Estrogen replacement is no longer indicated for the prevention or management of osteoporosis.[113] Selective estrogen receptor modulators (SERMs) are a new generation of estrogen-like drugs, sometimes referred to as "designer estrogens." SERMS have a different chemical structure and do not actually contain estrogen, nor are they considered hormones.

Raloxifene, for example, is a SERM that preserves bone density but is not associated with estrogen risk factors such as uterine or breast cancer. Tamoxifen was the first SERM developed but has only been noted to weakly increase bone mineral density (BMD) so is not used for treatment or prevention of osteoporosis.[114] SERMS may cause hot flashes and blood clots at a risk comparable to that of estrogen. They are not recommended, therefore, in individuals who have a known history of thromboembolic disease.

PARATHYROID HORMONE

The mechanism of action related to bone health of teriparatide, or parathyroid hormone, is unique in that it possesses anabolic properties and therefore builds bone. Since the approval of teriparatide in the United States in 2002, a great deal of interest regarding its use in osteoporosis has developed. Teriparatide has been studied in men, postmenopausal women with osteoporosis, and drug-induced osteoporosis (specifically corticosteroid-induced osteoporosis). The data available from various clinical trials demonstrate an increase in both BMD and bone mineral content (BMC) with the use of teriparatide compared with placebo.[115] Teriparatide is recommended as an alternative to traditional therapies, as long as there is scheduled monitoring for adverse effects such as hypercalcemia and urinary calcium excretion.

GLUCOSAMINE AND VITAMIN D

Glucosamine in dosages of 1.5 g per day and vitamin D are the only prophylactic treatments currently recommended to prevent osteoarthritis. Although it is not clear what dosage of supplemental vitamin D is needed, it has been shown that adequate blood levels may help in delaying the onset of hip osteoarthritis and in decreasing the risk of progression of knee osteoarthritis.[116] In addition, glucosamine has been noted to demonstrate some effectiveness in the prevention and management of osteoarthritis. In a recent Cochrane review of 13 randomized controlled trials,[117] glucosamine was noted to be effective and safe in osteoarthritis.

CANCER SCREENING

● Determining whether an older adult should undergo screening depends on several key factors: the risk of the disease, the benefit of screening, the implications of not screening, and if treatment is an acceptable option.

There are numerous published recommendations for cancer screening for older adults and specific guidelines for Medicare coverage for the recommended screening tests. Determining whether an older adult should undergo screening depends on several key factors: the risk of the disease, the benefit of screening, the implications of not screening, and if treatment is an acceptable option. Strict adherence to guidelines for all older adults, however, can result in unnecessary stress and burden to the individual.[118] Decisions about screening should be individualized, so that the potential benefit and burden can be assessed by patient, POA and clinician.

Breast Cancer Screening

Breast cancer screening guidelines from several organizations differ as to when to stop screening, the frequency of screening, and whether to include clinician breast examination or breast self-examination in the guideline. The USPSTF,[119] for example, recommends that mammography screening cease at age 70, although the American Geriatrics Society[120] (AGS) advises discontinuation at age 85. Although breast self-examination is not a definitive screening technique for breast cancer, given the ease of administration it serves as a useful first step and can be helpful in determining the need for further screening.

Colon Cancer Screening

Consistently the published guidelines recommend that individuals 50 years of age and older undergo annual colon cancer screening. Given that 90% of all cases of colon cancer occur after age 50, all older adults are at risk. Individuals with additional risk factors (i.e., a personal or familial history of adenomatous polyps, colon cancer, or inflammatory bowel disease) should be targeted for screening and follow-up. Screening for bowel cancer is particularly focused on identifying premalignant adenomatous polyps. It is believed that this type of polyp will progress from an adenoma to cancer over a 5- to 10-year period. Screening for colon cancer, therefore, has a particular advantage in that it is more likely to prevent the occurrence of bowel cancer rather than just identify disease once it is present.

There is no single "best" test to screen for colon cancer so four options are provided: fecal occult blood test (FOBT), a flexible sigmoidoscopy, colonoscopy, and double-contrast barium enema. New approaches to screening include screening for DNA mutations. DNA is a useful marker because it is not degraded during passage through the gastrointestinal tract and is excreted in the stool. Ongoing research is needed

before this type of screening goes into widespread use. Moreover, it may be burdensome for the patient both in terms of the cost ($500 to $700) and the stool collection process. Virtual colonoscopy is another new technique using computer programing. Ongoing studies are likewise needed to determine the cost/benefit of this type of testing over traditional colonoscopy.

Cervical and Prostate Cancer Screening

USPSTF,[119] AGS,[120] and American Cancer Society[121] (ACS) all recommend against screening older women for cervical cancer if they have had negative tests in the past and have no risk factors for cervical cancer. Older women who have never had a prior pap test should be screened until there are two negative tests. There are no consistent recommendations regarding screening for prostate cancer. The ACS[121] recommends a digital rectal examination (DRE) and prostatic-specific antigen (PSA) test annually for all men older than 50. Men who have a first-degree relative with prostate cancer or individuals who have urinary symptoms should be considered high risk and testing should be encouraged. Combining DRE with a PSA has been noted to be more effective than either test alone.[122]

PUTTING PREVENTION INTO PRACTICE

Despite evidence to support the benefit of participating in health promotion activities and cancer screening among older adults, adherence to these recommendations remains low.[123] Unfortunately, adherence rates to guideline-based health promotion activities are often equated with the quality of care the individual is receiving. There are, however, some major pitfalls to that assumption. When caring for an older adult, it is possible that the sample audited should not be screened based on patient preferences or clinician judgment. With older adults an individualized approach is essential. Health promotion and disease prevention opportunities should be addressed with each patient or individual with POA and outcomes geared toward immediate benefit. Another barrier to adherence to health promotion activities is that these practices are generally not strongly supported by our health care system. Over 95% of the annual health care budget goes to medical care, and less than 5% is allocated to improve health behaviors and prevent disease. There are, however, many techniques that can be used to optimally implement prevention guidelines into practice and increase adherence to health promoting behaviors and activities.

Facilitators for Implementation of Prevention Practices

PROFESSIONALS AND RESOURCES

> ● Utilizing an interdisciplinary team and advances in technology can help put prevention-focused activities into practice.

Numerous studies have demonstrated the positive effect clinicians can have on the health behavior of their patients,[124-126] and there is an increasing awareness that addressing health promotion activities with patients is important and useful. Clinicians, however, do not need to do all of the health promotion activities themselves. There are many available resources to facilitate the process and to provide patients with appropriate information. Moreover, there are case managers in local aging service organizations and social workers, nurses, and discharge planners in institutional settings that can help connect older patients to appropriate benefits and services.

There are strong evidence based guidelines available to help direct health promotion activities and examples of effective programs and practices that have successfully implemented these guidelines. Moreover, there is some financial support from Medicare for patient education related to health promotion services as well as Medicare reimbursement for recommended screenings. Increasingly, medical schools as well as educational programs for other types of health care providers recognize the importance of health promotion and disease prevention, and this information is being incorporated into traditional coursework.[127] In particular, there is a need to focus education on communication skills to facilitate behavior change.[128] This opens an exciting opportunity for team approaches to education and integration of knowledge from psychology and other specialty areas. The use of technology is another important tool to help providers put prevention into practice. Easy access to guidelines through Web-based information as well as a plethora of health information for patients can greatly ease implementation of guidelines. Although the majority of older adults may not own and use computers regularly, there is a growing cadre of older individuals who use computers and are able to communicate with health care providers in this way. Health care providers can refer older patients who are computer literate to appropriate Web pages for health promotion educational material and/or print this material to give to individuals and families.

PATIENT FACILITATORS

> ● Maximizing participation in health promotion activities among older adults is best done by using a multidimensional framework, as is afforded by social cognitive theory and the theory of self-efficacy.

Working with older adults to engage in health promotion activities and, in some cases, to change lifelong behaviors can be challenging. There are many known patient barriers to these activities, including a lack of understanding of the benefits and an assumption that with increased age there is no point to good health behaviors and prevention, lack of resources that generally include money and/or easy access to services, and never being told by their clinician what health promotion activities to consider engaging in.[127,129,130] Older adults can, however, change behavior.[131-133] Maximizing participation in health promotion activities among these individuals is best done by using a multidimensional framework, as is afforded by social cognitive theory and the theory of self-efficacy. This theory suggests that the stronger the individuals' efficacy expectations, the more likely they will initiate and persist with a given activity.[134] Efficacy expectations include both self-efficacy, which is the belief in one's ability to organize and execute a course of action, and outcome expectations, which are the beliefs that if a certain behavior is performed there will be a certain outcome. Efficacy expectations are dynamic and are both appraised and enhanced by four mechanisms: (1) performance accomplishment; (2) verbal persuasion; (3) role-models, or seeing like individuals perform a specific activity; and (4) physiological or affective states such as pain, fatigue, or anxiety associated with a given activity.

MOTIVATING YOUR PATIENTS TO ENGAGE IN HEALTH PROMOTION ACTIVITIES: THE SEVEN STEP APPROACH

Based on prior research and using the theory of self-efficacy, a seven-step approach (Box 5-2) was developed to help motivate older adults to engage in health behaviors. The steps include (1) education, (2) assessment of need for health promotion activity, (3) goal identification, (4) elimination of barriers, (5) exposure to role models, (6) verbal encouragement, and (7) ongoing verbal reinforcement and rewards. It is particularly important to establish the barriers to engaging in the behavior and working with the individual to eliminate those barriers.

Box 5-2 Seven Steps to Motivating Older Adults to Engage in Healthy Behaviors

Step 1: Educate

To facilitate learning, give information in multiple formats: an interactive lecture, a written handout, and videotape. Repeat the information and reinforce it both informally in one-on-one conversations with patients and formally in teaching programs.

Step 2: Assess Needs

Evaluate the individual to establish his or her need to participate in a given health promotion/disease prevention activity:

- Conduct physical examination, including health history
- Review prior screenings
- Evaluate barriers to engaging in the behavior (e.g., fear, no access, too old)

Step 3: Identify Goals

Set realistic goals and let the patient know exactly in what behavior to engage:

- Walk daily for 30 minutes
- Decrease to three cigarettes a day
- Avoid all desserts

Step 4: Eliminate Barriers

Aggressively attempt to eliminate the barriers associated with a given activity.

Step 5: Provide Role Models

Provide examples of successful patients who have changed health behaviors and noted benefits.

Step 6: Supply Verbal Encouragement

At the next encounter, make sure to ask the patient about his or her health behaviors, and provide verbal encouragement toward any positive change.

Step 7: Continue Verbal Reinforcement and Rewards

At each visit, continue to address health promotion behaviors and provide the patient with positive reinforcement as well as other rewards of interest to the patient. Rewards may include anything from a hug from a staff member for improved blood pressure or weight, to a prize once a certain weight is achieved, and so on.

SUMMARY

Older adults vary with regard to their willingness to engage in health-promoting activities. With age there seems to be less interest in engaging in health promotion activities for the purpose of lengthening life, and greater interest in engaging in these activities only if they improve current quality of life.[135] It is important, therefore, to approach health promotion activities with older adults by using an individualized approach. The goal of each professional engaged in health care of older individuals is to provide these individuals with information about each health promotion activity and with the risks and benefits associated with each, and to help them engage in activities that will optimize health and overall quality of life.

References

1. Green L, Kreuter M. Health Promotion Planning: An Educational and Environmental Approach, 2nd ed. Mountain View, CA: Mayfield, 1991.
2. American Geriatrics Society: Health screening decisions for older adults: AGS Position Paper. J Am Geriatr Soc 2003;27:3.
3. Bridges CB, Harper SA, Kukuda K, et al. (2004). Prevention and control of influenza Recommendations of the Advisory Committee on Immunization Practices. MMWR Recomm Rep 2004;52(RR-8):1-34.
4. Centers for Disease Control and Prevention: Influenza and pneumococcal vaccination levels among adults aged 65 or over in the United States 1998. JAMA 1998;280:1818-1819.
5. Daniels NA, Nguyen TT, Gildengorin G, et al. Adult immunization in university-based primary care and specialty practices. J Am Geriatr Soc 2004;52:1007-1012.
6. Tetanus and Diphtheria Health Threats. www.theallineed.com/health/tetanus_diphtheria_health_threats.htm.
7. U.S. Department of Health and Human Services. Healthy people 2000. Washington, DC: US Government Printing Office, 1991.
8. Houston TK, Allison JJ, Person S, Kovac S, Williams OD, Kiefe CI. Post-myocardial infarction smoking cessation counseling: associations with immediate and late mortality in older Medicare patients. Am J Med 2005; 118:269-275.
9. Hyland A, Li Q, Bauer JE, Giovino GA, Steger C, Cummings KM. Predictors of cessation in a cohort of current and former smokers followed over 13 years. Nicotine Tob Res 2005;6:S363-S369.
10. U.S. Public Health Service. A clinical practice guideline for treating tobacco use and dependence: a U.S. public health service report. JAMA 2000; 283:3244-3254.
11. Prochaska JO, DiClemente CC. Stages and processes of self-change in smoking: toward an integrative model of change. J Consult Clin Psych 1983; 51:390-395.
12. Arday DR, Lapin P, Chin J, Preston JA. Smoking patterns among seniors and the Medicare stop smoking program. J Am Geriatr Soc 2002;50:1689-1697.
13. Office of Applied Studies. Summary of Findings from the 1999 National Household Survey on Drug Abuse. Rockville, MD: Substance Abuse and Mental Health Services Administration, 2000.
14. National Institute on Alcohol Abuse and Alcohol. The Physicians' Guide to Helping Patients with Alcohol Problems, publication no. 95-3769. Bethesda, National Institutes of Health, 2004.
15. Crawford MJ, Patton R, Touquet R, et al. Screening and referral for brief intervention of alcohol-misusing patients in an emergency department: a pragmatic randomized controlled trial. Lancet 2004;64:1334-1339.
16. Klein WC, Jess C. One last pleasure? Alcohol use among elderly people in nursing homes. Health Soc Work 2004;27:193-203.
17. Resnick B. Alcohol use in a continuing care retirement community. J Gerontol Nurs 2003;29:22-29.
18. Resnick B, Perry D, Applebaum G, et al. The impact of alcohol use in community-dwelling older adults. J Community Health Nurs 2003;20:135-145.
19. Oslin DW. Late-life alcoholism: issues relevant to the geriatric psychiatrist. Am J Geriatr Psychiatry 2004;12:571-583.
20. Ewing J. Detecting alcoholism; the CAGE questionnaire. JAMA 1984; 252:1905-1907.
21. Hinkin CH, Castellon SA, Dickson-Fuhrman E, et al. Screening for drug and alcohol abuse among older adults using a modified version of the CAGE. Am J Addict 2001;10:319-326.
22. Saunders JB, Aasland OB, Babor TF, et al. Development of the Alcohol Use Disorders Identification Test (AUDIT): WHO Collaborative Project on Early Detection of Persons with Harmful Alcohol Consumption-II. Addiction 1993;88:791-804.

23. Schwan R, Albuisson E, Malet L, et al. The use of biological laboratory markers in the diagnosis of alcohol misuse: an evidence-based approach. Drug Alcohol Depend 2004;74:273-279.

24. Allen JP, Litten RZ. Screening instruments and biochemical screening tests. In Principles of Addiction Medicine. 2d ed. (Graham AW, Schultz TK, Wilford BB, eds.). Chevy Chase, MD: American Society of Addiction Medicine, 1998.

25. Golka K, Sondermann R, Reich SE, et al. Carbohydrate-deficient transferrin (CDT) as a biomarker in persons suspected of alcohol abuse. Toxicol Lett 2004;151:235-241.

26. Chen J, Conigrave KM, Macaskill P, Whitfield JB, Irwig L, on Behalf of the World Health Organization and the International Society for Biomedical Research on Alcoholism Collaborative Group. Combining carbohydrate-deficient transferrin and gamma-glutamyltransferase to increase diagnostic accuracy for problem drinking. Alcohol 2003;38:574-582.

27. Lussier-Cacan S, Bolduc A, Xhignesse M, et al. Impact of alcohol intake on measures of lipid metabolism depends on context defined by gender, body mass index, cigarette smoking, and apolipoprotein E genotype. Arterioscler Thromb Vasc Biol 2002;22:824-831.

28. Gaziano J, Buring J, Breslow J, et al. Moderate alcohol intake increased levels of high-density lipoprotein and its subfractions and decreased risk of myocardial infarction. N Engl J Med 1993;329;1829-1834.

29. Klatsky A, Armstrong M, Friedman G. Alcohol and mortality. Ann Intern Med 1992;117:646-654.

30. Pitsavos C, Makrilakis K, Panagiotakos DB, et al. The J-shape effect of alcohol intake on the risk of developing acute coronary syndromes in diabetic subjects: the CARDIO2000 II Study. Diabet Med 2005;22:243-248.

31. Mukamal KJ, Jadhav PP, D'Agostino RB, et al. Alcohol consumption and hemostatic factors: analysis of the Framingham Offspring cohort. Circulation 2001;104:1367-1373.

32. Abramson J, Williams S, Krumholz H, et al. Moderate alcohol consumption and risk of heart failure among older persons. JAMA 2001;285:1971-1977.

33. Djousse L, Pankow JS, Eckfeldt JH, et al. Relation between dietary linolenic acid and coronary artery disease in the National Heart, Lung, and Blood Institute Family Heart Study. Am J Clin Nutr 2001;74:612-619.

34. Palmer AJ, Fletcher AE, Bulpitt CJ, et al. Alcohol intake and cardiovascular mortality in hypertensive patients: report from the Department of Health Hypertension Care Computing Project. J Hypertens 1994;13:957-964.

35. Leroi I, Sheppard JM, Lyketsos CG. Cognitive function after 11.5 years of alcohol use: relations to alcohol use. Am J Epidemiol 2002;156:747-752.

36. Reid IR, Brown JP, Burckhardt P, et al. Intravenous zoledronic acid in postmenopausal women with low bone mineral density. N Engl J Med 2002;346:653-661.

37. Schinka JA, Vanderploeg RD, Rogish M, et al. Effects of the use of alcohol and cigarettes on cognition in elderly adults. J Int Neuorpsychol Soc 2002;8:811-818.

38. Blow FC, Barry KL. Older patients with at-risk and problem drinking patterns: new developments in brief interventions. J Geriatr Psychiatry Neurol 2000;13:115-123. Review.

39. Nelson HD, Helfand M, Woolf SH, et al. Screening for postmenopausal osteoporosis: a review of the evidence for the U.S. Preventive Services Task Force. Ann Intern Med 2002;137:529-541.

40. Resnick B. Alcohol use in a continuing care retirement community. J Gerontol Nurs 2003;29:22-29.

41. Moore A, Hays R, Greendale G, et al. Drinking habits among older persons: findings from the NHANES I epidemiologic follow up study (1982-1984). J Am Geriatr Soc 1999;47:412-416.

42. Oslin DW, Pettinati H, Volpicelli JR. Alcoholism treatment adherence: older age predicts better adherence and drinking outcomes. Am J Geriatr Psychiatry 2002;10:740-747.

43. Garbutt JC, West SL, Carey TS, et al. Pharmacological treatment of alcohol dependence: a review of the evidence. JAMA 1999;281:1318-1325.

44. Pelc I, Ansoms C, Lehert P, et al. The European NEAT program: an integrated approach using acamprosate and psychosocial support for the prevention of relapse in alcohol-dependent patients with a statistical modeling of therapy success prediction. Alcohol Clin Exp Res 2002;26:1529-1538.

45. Atienza A. A review of empirically-based physical activity program for middle-aged to older adults. JAPA 2001;9(Suppl):S38-S55.

46. U.S. Department of Health and Human Services. Physical Activity and Health: A Report of the Surgeon General. Washington, DC: U.S. Department of Health and Human Services, 2001.

47. American College of Sports Medicine: The Recommended Quantity and Quality of Exercise. Available at: http://www.acsmmsse.org/pt/re/msse/positionstandards.htm. Accessed March, 2006.

48. National Institutes on Aging. Exercise: A Guide from the National Institutes on Aging. h ttp://www.nia.nih.gov/exercisebook/index.htm.

49. National Institutes on Aging. Exercise: A Guide from the National Institutes on Aging. http://www.nia.nih.gov/exercisebook/index.htm.

50. Morey MC, Sullivan RJ. Medical assessment for health advocacy and practical strategies for exercise initiation. Am J Prevent Med 2003;25(3 suppl):204-208.

51. American College of Sports Medicine Position Stand and American Heart Association. Recommendations for cardiovascular screening, staffing, and emergency policies at health/fitness facilities. Med Sci Sports Exerc 1998;30:1009-1018.

52. American Heart Association Recommendations for cardiovascular screening, staffing, and emergency policies at health/fitness facilities. Med Sci Sports Exerc 1998;30:1009-1018.

53. Olds T, Norton K. Pre-Exercise Health Screening Guide. Champaign, IL: Human Kinetics; 1999.

54. Shephard RJ. Does insistence on medical clearance inhibit adoption of physical activity in elderly? JAPA 2000;8:301-311.

55. Gill TM, DiPietro L, Krumholz HM. Role of exercise stress testing and safety monitoring for older persons starting an exercise program. JAMA 2000;284:342-349.

56. Balady GJ, Chaitman B, Driscoll D, et al. Recommendations for cardiovascular screening, staffing, and emergency policies at health/fitness facilities. Med Sci Sports Exerc 1998;30:1009-1018.

57. Bean JF, Vora A, Frontera WR. Benefits of exercise for community-dwelling older adults. Arch Phys Med Rehabil. 2004;85(Suppl 3):S31-42.

58. Canadian Society for Exercise Physiology. Gloucester, Ontario: PAR-Q & You, 1994.

59. Chisholm DM, Collis ML, Kulak LL, et al. Guide to Clinical Preventive Services, 2nd ed. Washington, DC: U.S. Preventive Services Task Force, 1975.

60. U.S. Department of Health and Human Services. Promoting physical activity: A guide for community action. Bethesda, MD: Centers for Disease Control and Prevention, National Center for Chronic Disease Prevention and Health Promotion Division of Nutrition and Physical Activity, 1999.

61. Robert Wood Johnson Foundation. National blueprint for increasing physical activity for adults 50 and older. JAPA 2001;9(Suppl):S5-S12.

62. Reinventing the Food Pyramid for Older Adults. Available at: http://www.nutrition.tufts.edu/magazine/1999fall/pyramid.html. Accessed march, 2006.

63. Haber D. Health Promotion and Aging, 3rd ed. New York: Springer, 2004.

64. Ferrari CK. Functional foods, herbs and nutraceuticals: towards biochemical mechanisms of healthy aging. Available at: http: //www.ncbi.nlm.nih.gov/entrez/query.fcgi?cmd=Retrieve&db=pubmed&dopt=Abstract&list_uids=15547316&query_hl=3&itool=pubmed_docsum. Biogerontology. 2004; 5(5):275-89. Accessed March, 2006.

65. Janssen HC, Samson MM, Verhaar HJ. Vitamin D deficiency, muscle function, and falls in elderly people. Am J Clin Nutrit 2002;75:611-615.

66. Zamboni M, Zoico E, Tosoni P, et al. Relation between vitamin D, physical performance, and disability in elderly persons. J Gerontol A Biol Med Sci 2002;57:M7-M11.

67. IOM Report on Fats: Report on Dietary Reference Intakes for Trans Fatty Acids. www.iom.edu/report.asp?id=5410.

68. IOM Report on Dietary Fiber Dietary Reference Intakes for Energy, Carbohydrate, Fiber, Fat, Fatty Acids, Cholesterol, Protein, and Amino Acids www.iom.edu/report.asp?id=4340.

69. U.S. Department of Agriculture. Dietary Guidelines for Americans. www.Health.gov/dietaryguidelines/.

70. Mininutritional assessment sensible aging: using nutrient-dense foods and physical exercise with the frail elderly. Nut Today 2001;36:202-207.

71. www.Preventive services.ahrq.gov.

72. Fields S, Nicastri C. Health Promotion/disease prevention in older adults: an evidence-based update. Clin Geriatr 2004;12:18-26.

73. Daviglus ML, Stamler J, Pirzada A, et al. Favorable cardiovascular risk profile in young women and long-term risk of cardiovascular and all-cause mortality. JAMA 2004;292:1588-1592.

74. Field AE, Coakley EH, Must A, et al. Impact of overweight on the risk of developing common chronic disease during a 10-year period. Arch Intern Med 2001;161:1581-1586.

75. Stern L, Iqbal N, Seshadri P, et al. The effects of low carbohydrate versus conventional weight loss diets in severely obese adults: one year follow up of a randomized trial. Ann Intern Med 2004;140:778-785.

76. Chobanian AV, Bakris GL, Black HR, et al. The seventh report of the joint national committee on prevention, detection, evaluation and treatment of high blood pressure: the JNC 7 report. JAMA 2003;289:2560-2572.

77. Appel IJ, Champagne CM, Harsha DW, et al. Effects of comprehensive lifestyle modification on blood pressure control: main results of the PREMIER clinical trial. JAMA 2003;289:2083-2093.

78. Antiplatelet Trialists Collaboration. Secondary prevention of vascular disease by prolonged antiplatelet treatment. BMJ 1988;296:320-331.

79. Antiplatelet Trialists' Collaboration. Collaborative overview of randomized trials of antiplatelet therapy, I: prevention of death, myocardial infarction, and stroke by prolonged antiplatelet therapy in various categories of patients. BMJ 1994;308:81-106.

80. Eidelman RS, Hebert PR, Weisman SM, et al. An update on aspirin in the primary prevention of cardiovascular disease. Arch Intern Med 2003;163:2006-2010.

81. U.S. Preventive Servies Task Force. Aspirin for the primary prevention of cardiovascular events: Recommendation and rationale. Ann Intern Med 2002;136:157-160.

82. Kimmey MB. Cardioprotective effects and gastrointestinal risks of aspirin: maintaining the delicate balance. Am J Med 2004;117 (Suppl 5A):72S-78S.

83. Pilotto A, Franceschi M, Leandro G, et al. Proton-pump inhibitors reduce the risk of uncomplicated peptic ulcer in elderly either acute or chronic users of aspirin/non-steroidal anti-inflammatory drugs. Aliment Pharmacol Ther 2004;20:1091-1097.

84. Hirsh J & Bhatt DL. Comparative benefits of clopidogrel and aspirin in high-risk patient populations: lessons from the CAPRIE and CURE studies. Arch Intern Med 2004;164:2106-2110.

85. Woodward M, Lowe GD, Francis LM, et al. CADET Study Investigators: a randomized comparison of the effects of aspirin and clopidogrel on thrombotic risk factors and C-reactive protein following myocardial infarction: the CADET trial. J Thromb Haemost 2004;2:1934-1940.

86. Johnson CE, Lim WK, Workman BS. People aged over 75 in atrial fibrillation on warfarin: the rate of major hemorrhage and stroke in more than 500 patient-years of follow-up. J Am Geriatr Soc 2005;53:655-659.

87. Pusser BE, Robertson SL, Robinson MD, Barton C, Dobson LA. Stroke prevention in atrial fibrillation: are we following the guidelines? N C Med J 2005;66:9-13.

88. Jones M, McEwan P, Morgan CL, Peters JR, Goodfellow J, Currie CJ. Evaluation of the pattern of treatment, level of anticoagulation control, and outcome of treatment with warfarin in patients with non-valvar atrial fibrillation: a record linkage study in a large British population. Heart 2005;91:472-477.

89. Fang MC, Chang Y, Hylek EM, et al. Advanced age, anticoagulation intensity, and risk for intracranial hemorrhage among patients taking warfarin for atrial fibrillation. Ann Intern Med 2004;141:745-752.

90. Psaty BM, Lumley T, Furberg CD, et al. Health outcomes associated with various antihypertensive therapies used as first-line agents: a network meta-analysis. JAMA 2003;289:2534-2544.

91. Aronow WS. Management of the elderly person after myocardial infarction. J Gerontol A Biol Med Sci 2005;59:1173-1185.

92. Grundy SM, Cleeman JI, Merz CN, et al. Implications of recent clinical trials for the National Cholesterol Education Program Adult Treatment Panel III Guidelines. Circulation 2004;110:227-239.

93. Walsh JM, Pignone M. Drug treatment of hyperlipidemia in women. JAMA 2004;291:2243-2252.

94. Nelson H, Helfand M, Woolf SH, Allan JD. Screening for postmenopausal osteoporosis: a Review of the evidence for the U.S. Preventive Services Task Force. Ann Intern Med 2002;137:529-541.

95. Hagberg JM, Zmuda JM, McCole SD, et al. Moderate physical activity is associated with higher bone mineral density in postmenopausal women. J Am Geriatr Soc 2001;49:1411-1417.

96. Kaptoge S, Welch A, McTaggart A, et al. Effects of dietary nutrients and food groups on bone loss from the proximal femur in men and women in the seventh and eighth decades of age. Osteoporos Int 2003;14:418-428.

97. Blanchet C, Giguere Y, Prud'homme D, et al. Leisure physical activity is associated with quantitative ultrasound measurements independently of bone mineral density in postmenopausal women. Calcif Tissue Int 2003;73:339-349.

98. Deyle GD, Henderson NE, Matekel RL, et al. Effectiveness of manual physical therapy and exercise in osteoarthritis of the knee: a randomized controlled trial. Ann Intern Med 2000;132:173-181.

99. Suomi R, Collier D. Effects of arthritis exercise programs on functional fitness and perceived activities of daily living measures in older adults with arthritis. Arch Phys Med Rehabil 2003;84:1589-1594.

100. de Jong Z, Munneke M, Zwinderman AH, et al. Is a long-term high-intensity exercise program effective and safe in patients with rheumatoid arthritis? Results of a randomized controlled trial. Arthritis Rheum 2003;48:2415-2424.

101. Dias RC, Dias JM, Ramos LR. Impact of an exercise and walking protocol on quality of life for elderly people with OA of the knee. Physiother Res Int 2003;8:121-130.

102. Quilty B, Tucker M, Campbell R, et al. Physiotherapy, including quadriceps exercises and patellar taping, for knee osteoarthritis with predominant patello-femoral joint involvement: randomized controlled trial. J Rheumatol 2003;30:1311-1317.

103. Seguin R, Nelson ME. The benefits of strength training for older adults. Am J Prev Med. 2003;25(Suppl 2):141-149.

104. Mangione KK, McCully K, Gloviak A, et al. The effects of high-intensity and low-intensity cycle ergometry in older adults with knee osteoarthritis. J Gerontol A Biol Med Sci 1999;54:M184-M190.

105. Foley A, Halbert J, Hewitt T, et al. Does hydrotherapy improve strength and physical function in patients with osteoarthritis—a randomized controlled trial comparing a gym based and a hydrotherapy based strengthening programme. Ann Rheum Dis 2003;62:1162-1167.

106. Spencer AC, Kinne S, Belza BL, et al. Recruiting adults with osteoarthritis into an aquatic exercise class: strategies for a statewide intervention. Arthritis Care Res 1998;11:455-462.

107. Song R, Lee EO, Lam P, et al. Effects of tai chi exercise on pain, balance, muscle strength, and perceived difficulties in physical functioning in older women with osteoarthritis: a randomized clinical trial. J Rheumatol 2003;30:2039-2044.

108. Food and Nutrition board of the Institute of Medicine recommendations for Vitamin D. Available at: http://www.iom.edu/CMS/3788.aspx. Accessed March, 2006.

109. United States Department of Health and Human Services and Agriculture. Agriculture Dietary Supplement Fact Sheet: Vitamin D. Available at: http://www. ods.od.nih.gov/factsheets/vitamind.asp. Accessed March, 2006.

110. Trivedi DP, Doll R, Khaw KT. Effect of four monthly oral vitamin D3 (cholecalciferol) supplementation on fractures and mortality in men and women living in the community: randomized double blind controlled trial. BMJ 2003;326:469.

111. Resnick B, Wehren L, Orwig D. Reliability and validity of the self-efficacy and outcome expectations for osteoporosis medication adherence. Orthop Nurs 2003;22:139-147.

112. Reid IR, Brown JP, Burckhardt P, et al. Intravenous zoledronic acid in postmenopausal women with low bone mineral density. N Engl J Med 2002;346:653-661.

113. Writing Group for the Women's Health Initiative Investigators. Risks and benefits of estrogen plus progestin in healthy postmenopausal women. JAMA 2002;288:321-333.

114. Zidan J, Keidar Z, Basher W, et al. Effects of tamoxifen on bone mineral density and metabolism in postmenopausal women with early-stage breast cancer. Med Oncol 2004;21:117-121.

115. Quattrocchi E, Kourlas H. Teriparatide: a review. Clin Ther 2004;26: 841-854.

116. McAlindon TE. Osteoarthritis. In Handbook of Clinical Nutrition and Aging (Bales CW, Ritchie CS, eds.). Totowa, NJ: Humana Press; 2004.

117. Towheed TE, Anastassiades TP, Shea B, et al. Glucosamine therapy for treating osteoarthritis: Issue 3. Chichester, UK: John Wiley & Sons, Ltd. Available online at www.cochrane.org/cochrane/resabstr/ab002946.htm.

118. Walter L, Covinsky K. Cancer screening in elderly patients: a framework for individualized decision making. JAMA 2000;285:2750-2756.

119. Preventive Serivces Task Force Mammography Screening Guidelines. Available at: http://www.cdc.gov/id/. Accessed March, 2006.

120. The American Geriatrics Society—Position Paper: Breast Cancer. Available at: http://www.americangeriatrics.org/products/positionpapers/brstcncr.shtm 1. Accessed March 2006.

121. American Cancer Society Guidelines. Available at http://www.cancer.org/docroot/PED/content/. Accessed March 2006.

122. Murphy GD, Byron DP, Pasquale D. Underutilization of digital rectal examination when screening for prostate cancer. Arch Intern Med 2004;164:313-316.

123. Infeld DL, Whitelaw N. Policy initiatives to promote healthy aging. Clin Geriatr Med 2002;18:627-642.

124. Humair JP, Buchs CR, Stalder H. Promoting influenza vaccination of elderly patients in primary care. Fam Pract 2002;19:383-389.

125. Petrella RJ, Koval JJ, Cunningham DA, et al. Can primary care doctors prescribe exercise to improve fitness? The Step Test Exercise Prescription (STEP) project. Am J Prev Med 2003;24:316-322.

126. Zimmerman RK, Nowalk MP, Bardella IJ, et al. Physician and practice factors related to influenza vaccination among the elderly. Am J Prev Med 2004;26:1-10.

127. McMenamin SB, Schmittdiel J, Halpin HA, et al. Health promotion in physician organizations: results from a national study. Am J Prev Med 2004;26:259-264.

128. Hudon E, Beaulieu MD, Roberge D. Canadian Task Force on Preventive Health Care. Integration of the recommendations of the Canadian Task Force on Preventive Health Care: obstacles perceived by a group of family physicians. Fam Pract 2004;21:11-17.

129. Resnick B. Alcohol use in a continuing care retirement community. J Gerontol Nurs 2003;29:22-29.

130. Anis NA, Lee RE, Ellerbeck EF, et al. Direct observation of physician counseling on dietary habits and exercise: patient, physician, and office correlates. Prev Med 2004;38:198-202.

131. Mossavar-Rahmani Y, Henry H, Rodabough R, et al. Additional self-monitoring tools in the dietary modification component of The Women's Health Initiative. J Am Diet Assoc 2004;104:76-85.

132. Toobert DJ, Strycker LA, Glasgow RE, et al. Enhancing support for health behavior change among women at risk for heart disease: the Mediterranean Lifestyle Trial. Health Educ Res 2002;17:574-585.

133. Brassington GS, Atienza AA, Perczek RE, et al. Intervention-related cognitive versus social mediators of exercise adherence in the elderly. Am J Prev Med 2002;23(Suppl):80-86.

134. Bandura A. Self-Efficacy: The Exercise of Control. New York: W.H. Freeman; 1997.

135. Resnick B. Health promotion practices of the older adult. Public Health Nurs 2000;17:160-168.

136. Corvera-Tindel T, Doering LV, Gomez T, et al. Predictors of noncompliance to exercise training in heart failure. J Cardiovasc Nurs 2004;19:269-277.

137. Pescatello LS, Guidry MA, Blanchard BE, et al. Exercise intensity alters postexercise hypotension. J Hypertens 2004;22:1881-1888.

138. Thompson PD, Buchner D, Pina IL, et al. American Heart Association Council on Clinical Cardiology Subcommittee on Exercise, Rehabilitation, and Prevention; American Heart Association Council on Nutrition, Physical Activity, and Metabolism Subcommittee on Physical Activity. Exercise and physical activity in the prevention and treatment of atherosclerotic cardiovascular disease: a statement from the Council on Clinical Cardiology (Subcommittee on Exercise, Rehabilitation, and Prevention) and the Council on Nutrition, Physical Activity, and Metabolism (Subcommittee on Physical Activity). Circulation 2003;107:3109-3116.

139. Tager IB, Haight T, Sternfeld B, et al. Effects of physical activity and body composition on functional limitation in the elderly: application of the marginal structural model. Epidemiology 2004;15:479-493.

140. Grant S, Todd K, Aitchison TC, et al. The effects of a 12-week group exercise program on physiological and psychological variables and function in overweight women. Public Health 2004;118:31-42.

141. Okura T, Nakata Y, Tanaka K. Effects of exercise intensity on physical fitness and risk factors for coronary heart disease. Obes Res 2003;11:1131-1139.

142. Gold DT, Shipp KM, Pieper CF, et al. Group treatment improves trunk strength and psychological status in older women with vertebral fractures: results of a randomized, clinical trial. J Am Geriatr Soc 2004;52:1471-1478.

143. Mummery K, Schofield G, Caperchione C. Physical activity dose-response effects on mental health status in older adults. Aust N Z J Public Health 2004;28:188-192.

144. Bourret EM, Bernick LG, Cott CA, et al. The meaning of mobility for residents and staff in long-term care facilities. J Adv Nurs 2002;37:338-345.

145. Resnick B, Spellbring AM. Understanding what motivates older adults to exercise. J Gerontol Nurs 2000;26:34-42.

146. Baum EE, Jarjoura D, Polen AE, et al. Effectiveness of a group exercise program in a long-term care facility: a randomized pilot trial. J Am Med Dir Assoc 2003;4:74-80.

147. Brach JS, VanSwearingen JM, FitzGerald SJ, et al. The relationship among physical activity, obesity, and physical function in community-dwelling older women. Prev Med 2004;39:74-80.

148. Chu KS, Eng JJ, Dawson AS, et al. Water-based exercise for cardiovascular fitness in people with chronic stroke: a randomized controlled trial. Arch Phys Med Rehabil 2004;85:870-874.

149. Sherrington C, Lord SR, Herbert RD. A randomized controlled trial of weight-bearing versus non-weight-bearing exercise for improving physical ability after usual care for hip fracture. Arch Phys Med Rehabil 2004;85:710-716.

150. Suomi R, Collier D. Effects of arthritis exercise programs on functional fitness and perceived activities of daily living measures in older adults with arthritis. Arch Phys Med Rehabil 2003;84:1589-1594.

151. Liu-Ambrose TY, Khan KM, Eng JJ, et al. Both resistance and agility training increase cortical bone density in 75- to 85-year-old women with low bone mass: a 6-month randomized controlled trial. J Clin Densitom 2004;7:390-398.

152. Lord SR, Castell S, Corcoran J, et al. The effect of group exercise on physical functioning and falls in frail older people living in retirement villages: a randomized, controlled trial. J Am Geriatr Soc 2004;51:1685-1692.

153. Schoenfelder DP, Rubenstein LM. An exercise program to improve fall-related outcomes in elderly nursing home residents. Appl Nurs Res 2004;17:21-31.

154. Sherrington C, Lord SR, Finch CF. Physical activity interventions to prevent falls among older people: update of the evidence. J Sci Med Sport 2004;7(Suppl):43-51.

Web References

National Institutes on Aging. Exercise: A Guide from the National Institutes on Aging. http://www.nia.nih.gov/exercisebook/index.htm.

Dietary guidelines for Americans. USDA. http://www.Health.gov/dietaryguidelines/.

Preventive Health Care Services. http://www.Preventiveservices.ahrq.gov.

POSTTEST

1. The U.S. Advisory Committee on Immunization Practices and the Centers for Disease Control currently recommend that:
   a. All older adults be immunized against influenza annually and that they receive at least one pneumococcal vaccination.
   b. All high-risk older adults should receive an additional pneumococcal vaccination 5 years or more after their first immunization.
   c. Older adults should receive a one-time revaccination for pneumonia if they were initially vaccinated more than 5 years previously and were less than 65 years of age at the time of the initial vaccination.
   d. All of the above

2. Health care providers should recommend that older adults engage in:
   a. 20 minutes of moderate-level physical activity 3 days a week.
   b. 20 minutes of moderate-level physical activity 3 days per week with 1 day per week for resistance exercise.
   c. 30 minutes of physical activity most days of the week, and this activity should incorporate aerobic activity, resistance training, and flexibility.
   d. 30 minutes of physical activity 3 days per week, and this activity should incorporate aerobic activity, resistance training, and flexibility.

3. Teriparatide is recommended as an alternative to traditional therapies for osteoporosis as long as there is scheduled monitoring for adverse effects, such as:
   a. Hypernatremia and hypercalcemia
   b. Hypercalcemia and urinary calcium excretion.
   c. Hypokalemia and hypercalcemia
   d. Hypophosphatemia and hypercalcemia

PRETEST ANSWERS

1. a
2. b
3. a

POSTTEST ANSWERS

1. d
2. c
3. b

Clinical Pharmacology

Mark A. Stratton and Robert C. Salinas

Upon completion of this chapter, the reader will be able to:

● Discuss four reasons why older people experience more morbidity and mortality from medication-related problems than younger people.

● Identify four pharmacokinetic and three pharmacodynamic changes that occur with aging that make older people more likely to experience problems with medications.

● Provide six practical solutions to minimize the risk associated with medication use in older people.

PRETEST

1. People age 65 and over account for 13% of the population in the United States and account for
   a. Less than 10% of all prescriptions that are written
   b. More than 90% of all prescriptions that are written
   c. More than 30% of all prescriptions that are written
   d. Less than 2% of all prescriptions that are written

2. Which of the following statements regarding adverse drug reactions in the elderly are correct?
   I. Elders are admitted to the hospital at three times the rate of younger people as a consequence of an adverse drug reaction (ADR).
   II. The elderly are more likely to suffer greater morbidity and mortality from ADRs because of a decrease in physiologic reserve.
   III. Over one-fourth of hospital admissions through the emergency room by older people are due to poor outcomes from drug therapy.

   a. I only
   b. II only
   c. I and III only
   d. II and III only
   e. I, II, and III

3. Which of the following pharmacokinetic changes that occur in the elderly is least clinically important?
   a. Distribution
   b. Elimination
   c. Absorption
   d. Metabolism

People over the age of 65 currently represent approximately 13% of the population in the United States, yet they account for more than 34% of all health care utilization and expenditures. Because of the continued need to treat chronic medical conditions and provide symptom relief of disabling diseases, the elderly receive a disproportionately large number of medications compared with younger individuals.

The elderly are particularly impacted because it is estimated that they use more than 30% of all prescriptions written and 40% of all over-the-counter medications that are sold in the United States (ASCP Update 2000). Along with the use of medications, there exists potential harm. In 1986, of all deaths caused by adverse reactions to medications, 51% occurred in persons more than 60 years of age, and of all hospitalizations resulting from adverse reactions to medications, 39% occurred in those over 60.[1] These alarming statistics led to the coining of the phrase "America's other drug problem" in 1988 by former Secretary of Health and Human Services Lewis Sullivan.

The estimated cost to the health care system of inappropriate drugs and their consequences approaches $200 billion per year, with half of that attributed to the elderly.[2,3] The following are among the many reasons for this problem.

Mr. Jones

Mr. Jones is a 74-year old widowed white gentleman who lives in an assisted living facility and is brought to clinic today by his daughter. According to his daughter, Mr. Jones had contacted her and informed her that his legs were swelling and that he was experiencing difficulty with breathing for the past 6 days. Mr. Jones' weight today is recorded at 168, approximately 10 pounds over his previous weight from 1 month ago. You ask Mr. Jones if he has been taking his medications, and he informs you that, in fact, he has not. He tells you that because of the holidays, he has omitted taking his diuretic for the past 10 days. In addition, he tells you that he has been taking Motrin for pain in his knees, which one of buddies at the dance hall recommended.

A review of Mr. Jones[1] medical problems includes a past medical history of hypertension, heart failure (HF) syndrome with an ejection fraction of 30%, hypercholesterolemia, depression, and osteoarthritis of the knees. A review of his medications include the following: lisinopril 40 mg once day, carvedilol (Coreg) 6.25 mg twice a day, furosemide (Lasix) 40 mg once a day, citalopram (Celexa) 20 mg once a day, and acetaminophen (Tylenol) 500 mg three times a day. In addition, he takes an over-the-counter multivitamin.

STUDY QUESTIONS

1. What factors might have been playing a role in this elderly patient's noncompliance?
2. What factors may affect his ability to respond to pharmacologic interventions to improve his heart failure?
3. Are there any over-the-counter medications that may have contributed to the exacerbation of his heart failure?

⬤ The estimated cost to the health care system of inappropriate drugs and their consequences approaches $200 billion per year, with half of that attributed to the elderly.

Mrs. Smith

Mrs. Smith is an 82-year-old woman who presents to the emergency department via ambulance because of acute confusion. According to Mrs. Smith's family, she had been doing well up until a few days ago when she began calling out the name of her deceased husband, insisting that he come home from work. Mrs. Smith was also recently discharged from another hospital where she was admitted following a fall at home 1 week ago. After it was determined that she did not suffer a hip fracture, she was discharged with new pain medication, Darvocet-N, and over-the-counter Benadryl to help her sleep. According to the family, Mrs. Smith takes medications for high blood pressure, diabetes, memory, and maybe for her heart.

On examining Mrs. Smith, you find an elderly woman who is trying to climb out of the gurney and is struggling to sit up. She is not orientated to person, place, and time. When asked her name, Mrs. Smith replies that she needs to see her son and wonders when the train will come by to get them.

STUDY QUESTION

1. Are there any medications that could contribute to Mrs. Smith's acute change in mental status?

PHARMACOKINETIC CHANGES

Pharmacokinetics is the science of the mathematics associated with the processes of drug absorption, distribution, metabolism, and elimination. Increasing age, in and of itself, is associated with significant changes in these four parameters. However, issues that include the dynamics of aging, frailty, comorbidities, heterogeneity, and inherent flaws associated with aging research impact the application of knowledge to practice. The current knowledge concerning aging and changes in kinetics has largely been derived from data in older patients between the ages of 65 and 74 years. There exist far less kinetic data for patients between the ages of 75 and 85 years and little or no information for those over the age of 85 years. The kinetic changes that have been identified for the young-old in all likelihood continue to change throughout the remainder of the age spectrum and become more clinically relevant in the drug decision-making process as the patient continues to age. The concept of frailty and its impact on kinetics has recently been introduced, and it is thought that the more frail a patient becomes, the greater this impacts kinetic changes in drug therapy. Various comorbidities associated with aging, such as heart failure syndrome, also impact the kinetics of many drugs. The heterogeneity of the aging population makes generalizations of kinetic changes in the elderly more challenging. A summary of the kinetic changes associated with age and disease is depicted in Table 6-1.

Absorption

Of the four areas traditionally included in the area of pharmacokinetics, absorption changes in the elderly are probably the least clinically important. First-pass metabolism decreases with age, which may increase systemic absorption of some medications such as oral nitrates, beta-blockers, estrogens, and calcium channel blockers. This is especially relevant when considering the dose of the oral nitrate, isosorbide dinitrate (Isordil).[4] For example, in this case the dose of isosorbide dinitrate needed to exert the desired pharmacologic effect in an 85-year-old patient is likely to be much less than that required in a 55-year-old patient because more drug is absorbed into the systemic circulation with advancing age owing to decreased first-pass

Table 6–1	Pharmacokinetic Changes of Aging and Disease	
Changes of Age and Disease	**Pharmacokinetic Effect**	**Examples of Some Drugs Affected**
↓ First-pass metabolism	↑ Drug serum concentration	Oral nitrates, beta-blockers, calcium channel blockers, estrogens
↓ Rate of absorption	↓ Clinical effect	Furosemide
↓ Lean mass and total body water	↓ Volume of distribution	Digoxin, lithium
↑ Fat content	↑ Volume of distribution	Diazepam, chlordiazepoxide. flurazepam, alprazolam
↓ Food intake/catabolic disease states	↓ Serum protein concentration with ↓ binding	Warfarin, phenytoin
↓ Approximately one-half of CYP 450 metabolic pathways (Phase I reactions)	↓ Reduction, oxidation, hydroxylation, demethylation →↑ half-life	Diazepam, chlordiazepoxide, flurazepam, alprazolam
↓ Renal elimination	↓Clearance →↑ half-life	Aminoglycosides, vancomycin, digoxin, salicylates

From Stratton MA, Gutierres S, Salinas R. Drug therapy in the elderly: tips for avoiding adverse effects and interactions. *Consultant* 2004;44:461-467.

effect. The clinical relevance is that if the older patient were to be given a larger dose, as is typically used in the younger patient, one would likely see an extension of the desired effect into undesirable effects such as significant orthostatic changes in blood pressure with a subsequent increased risk of falls and fractures. This effect is not seen with isosorbide mononitrate (Imdur).

Pathology- and age-related physiological changes can also combine to alter oral absorption of medications. For example, in older patients with worsening congestive HF syndrome and fluid retention, bowel wall edema may interfere with the absorption of many medications. With furosemide (Lasix), for example, the extent of absorption is not affected, but the rate of absorption is slowed, which can lead to a diminished clinical efficacy.[5] Recognition of this physiologic blockade to the desired effect is critical as it will avoid needless delays in obtaining the desired effect by giving furosemide via a parenteral route. The oral absorption of the loop diuretic, torsemide (Demedex), in HF syndrome patients with worsening left ventricular failure has been shown to be more predictably absorbed with improved clinical outcome when compared to furosemide.[6]

Distribution

With increasing age, the lean-to-fat ratio of the body mass decreases, as does total body water.[7] These changes significantly reduce the volume of distribution for water-soluble compounds or for those compounds that are distributed only in lean tissues. This is important to keep in mind for medications that may be commonly used such as digoxin and lithium; with decreased volume of distribution, dosage must be

decreased. The "therapeutic range" of lithium for the older population is approximately half what is now considered "normal."[8]

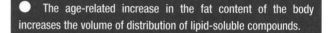

The age-related increase in the fat content of the body increases the volume of distribution of lipid-soluble compounds.

The age-related increase in the fat content of the body increases the volume of distribution of lipid-soluble compounds. For example, the volume of distribution of the benzodiazepine diazepam (Valium) increases two- to threefold from the age of 20 to 80 years.[9,10] As a result, the clearance of this and other similar lipid-soluble psychoactive compounds is markedly prolonged, increasing the likelihood of an adverse drug event with the potential for catastrophic consequences.

Although plasma protein concentrations do not normally decline with age to an extent sufficient to alter pharmacokinetics, reduced food intake or catabolic disease states may lead to decreases that become clinically relevant.[11] This becomes especially important with compounds that are normally highly protein-bound, such as the anticoagulant warfarin and the anticonvulsant phenytoin. When using either of these agents in patients with hypoalbuminemia, one can anticipate that the amount required to exert the desired pharmacologic effect will be lower. For patients with hypoalbuminemia on warfarin therapy, the initial doses required will be lower and the response quicker, and when dosage changes are required, they should be made in small increments. In the case of phenytoin (Dilantin), the therapeutic range will need to be redefined if the total plasma concentration is the method of measurement. The "therapeutic" range for phenytoin may well be 5 to 10 mcg/ml rather than 10 to 20 mcg/ml if the patient's albumin is below 3.5 g/dl.

Metabolism

Liver mass decreases by 25% to 35% and liver blood flow decreases by as much as 40% by the age of 90.[12] In addition, certain hepatic metabolic pathways diminish with age. This is the case with many phase I reactions, which include reduction, oxidation, hydroxylation, and demethylation. Many of these pathways are performed through the multiple cytochrome P450 mixed-function oxidase systems. The impact of age on these systems is mixed, with approximately one-half of these pathways being reduced in the elderly.[13] Agents that follow pathways that slow down with age include the benzodiazepines, diazepam (Valium), chlordiazepoxide (Librium), flurazepam (Dalmane), and alprazolam (Xanax). Studies have demonstrated that the half-life of diazepam and its metabolites increases two- to threefold in the elderly population.[9,10] Studies have demonstrated that the clinical effect of this metabolic change is an increased incidence of falls, fractures, and automobile accidents, with a resultant increase in morbidity and mortality.[14,15] Based on this information, these particular compounds (and others that follow this metabolic pathway) would seem to have no role in treating the elderly patient.

Phase II reactions—which include conjugation, acetylation, glucuronidation, and sulfation—do not diminish with age. Thus, if benzodiazepine therapy is necessary in the elderly, three acceptable alternatives are oxazepam (Serax), lorazepam (Ativan), and triazolam (Halcion). Sensitivity to all benzodiazepines in the elderly is enhanced; therefore, the lowest possible dose for the shortest period of time possible should be the goal. Risk of falls is increased with all benzodiazepines, especially during the first few weeks of therapy.

Elimination

It was once thought that renal function declined by approximately 10% per decade after the age of 50 in all people. However, it is now known that, in the absence of hypertension and diabetes, 35% of the elderly retain normal renal function until late in life, which still leaves the majority of elderly patients with reduced renal function.[16] The dosage of many compounds that depend solely on the kidneys for elimination will require downward adjustment in the elderly.

> ● It is now known that, in the absence of hypertension and diabetes, 35% of the elderly retain normal renal function until late in life, which still leaves the majority of elderly patients with reduced renal function.

Pharmacodynamic Changes

Pharmacodynamics relate to the observed clinical response that can also be interpreted as sensitivity. With age, sensitivity to the therapeutic as well as the toxic effects of many medications, especially those acting centrally, increases. This is further compounded by pathology and frailty. The effect of aging on receptors is thought to lead to decreased density and affinity, while the post receptor effect is mixed.[17] The effects summarized in Table 6-2 are more common and of greater intensity with frailty and advanced old age.

Table 6–2   Pharmacodynamic Changes of Aging and Disease

System	Dynamic Changes	Clinical Effect	Examples
Central nervous system	↑ Postsynaptic receptor effect mediated by GABA[18]	↑ Psychomotor impairment and delirium	Benzodiazepines
	↓ Opioid peptide content and receptors	↑ Behavioral changes	Opioids
	Changes in receptor sensitivity	↑ Behavioral changes	Alcohol and barbiturates
	↓ Choline acetyltransferase and cholinergic cell numbers[19]	↑ Delirium	Drugs with anticholinergic activity (diphenhydramine, clonidine, etc.)
	↓ D1 and D2 receptors[20]	↑ Extrapyramidal side-effects	Antipsychotics and metoclopramide
Beta-adrenergic receptor function	↓ Adenylate cyclase and cyclic AMP (no change in G-protein function)[21,22]	↑ Amounts of certain medications may be needed	Isoproterenol, beta-blockers
Baroreceptor function	↓ Baroreceptor function[21,22]	↓ Ability to ↑ vascular tone or increase heart rate in response to volume depletion or vasoactive substances	Antihypertensives (check all older patients on antihypertensives for orthostatic changes in blood pressure)
	Impaired glucose counter-regulation[17]	↑ Risk of hypoglycemia	Antidiabetics (be aware of altered presentation of hypoglycemia in the frail elder—somnolence or confusion)

From Stratton MA, Gutierres S, Salinas R. Drug therapy in the elderly: tips for avoiding adverse effects and interactions. *Consultant* 2004;44:461-467.

Polypharmacy and Inappropriate Medications

Of all prescription drugs sold in the United States, 31% are consumed by persons over 65, and more than 40% of the nonprescription drugs are estimated to be purchased by people in that age group.[23,24] In 2000 more than 2.5 billion prescriptions were sold in the United States, and by the year 2006, this is estimated to grow to more than 6 billion prescriptions annually. Recent studies have shown that elderly who live independently in a community-based setting use, on average, six different medications per day, while those living in a long-term care facility average eight different medications per day.[25,26]

In the early 1990s, the issue of inappropriate medications for the elderly became a prevalent concern. This led to the introduction of the Beer's criteria, which categorized medications according to their risk to the elderly.[27-29] Based on these criteria, it has been estimated that 20% to 25% of the elderly are taking at least one inappropriate drug and, as such, are exposing themselves to unnecessary risk of adverse drug events, which owing to frailty and decreased physiologic reserve results in unacceptable morbidity and mortality.[30] The CD ROM includes the complete Beers list of potentially inappropriate drugs.

Compliance

Compliance or adherence to a medication regimen becomes problematic for the elderly when the number of medications or the frequency of medication administration is increased. More importantly, however, the one consideration that probably plays the largest role in failure to comply to medication regimens for the elderly is the issue of cost. The result of escalating drug costs for the elderly is skipping doses to make a prescription last longer, not filling the prescription, or not getting refills. The cost of prescription drugs has increased more than two and one-half times since 1993. A recent study reported that 18% of older Californians either did not fill a prescription or skipped doses owing to the high cost of medications.[31] For those with no prescription drug coverage, the percentage increased to 29%. In Texas, the percentage of seniors failing to comply owing to cost was 31%.[31] It is yet to be determined what impact the Medicare Modernization Act will have on this picture with Medicare providing prescription benefits for its recipients effective January 2006.

Agents Requiring Special Consideration in the Elderly

ANALGESICS

Managing chronic pain in the elderly should follow the World Health Organization step care approach with the foundation consisting of a non-narcotic analgesic. However, the elderly are more likely to suffer gastritis and gastrointestinal bleeding from the use of any of the traditional nonsteroidal anti-inflammatory agents compared with younger people. The newer cyclooxygenase (COX)-2 inhibitor (celexocib [Celebrex]) has a lower incidence of gastrointestinal bleeding and would be preferred for patients with a history of peptic ulcer disease or previous gastrointestinal problems from nonsteroidal anti-inflammatory drug (NSAID) therapy.[32,33] However, the cost differences between traditional NSAIDs and COX-2 inhibitors is significant. Also, concerns regarding the increased risk of cardiovascular or cerebrovascular events with COX-2 inhibitors and possibly other NSAIDS have emerged. Therefore, acetaminophen (Tylenol) has become preferred by numerous advising bodies, including the American Geriatrics Society, as the non-narcotic agent of choice for the management of mild to moderate pain.[34] Doses should not exceed 4 g per day, and in patients who have liver enzyme abnormalities or drink alcohol on a regular basis, the dose should be lower.

Pain perception diminishes with age, and the elderly tend to be quite sensitive to the analgesic effects of narcotics. When a narcotic is necessary, it is best to begin with a relatively low-potency agent, such as codeine. However, codeine is associated with a high incidence of nausea, vomiting, and constipation. Meperidine is not an acceptable alternative, not only because of its poor oral bioavailability but also because of the accumulation of the active metabolite, normeperidine, which may produce psychosis, especially in older patients.[35] Propoxyphene is also best avoided in the elderly as it too can lead to the accumulation of the toxic metabolite norpropoxyphene. For severe chronic pain, an oxycodone-containing agent can be tried. An alternative narcotic-like agent is tramadol (Ultram), but its half-life can be prolonged in the elderly.

ANESTHETICS

Older people, especially those with multiple comorbidities, frailty, or cognitive impairment have increased sensitivity to general anesthesia and may show prolonged residual effects postoperatively.

ANTI-ANXIETY AND SEDATIVE AGENTS

It is prudent to select an antianxiety or a sedative agent that is short-acting, is metabolized in a manner unaffected by age, and has a good safety record. Among the preferred agents are oxazepam (Serax), lorazepam (Ativan), or triazolam (Halcion). As usual, the lowest possible dosage should be selected, the need for therapy should be evaluated frequently, and the quality of life and mental status should be monitored closely. Trazadone (Desyrel), an antidepressant, has also been approved for the treatment of insomnia. Some of the newer antidepressants have also been approved for anxiety disorders. It is important to consider nondrug alternatives for the older patient.

ANTIARRHYTHMICS

The pharmacokinetics of numerous antiarrhythmics are altered in geriatric patients, either as a result of age alone or of age and pathology combined.[7,36] The important aspect is that the pharmacologic effect of the antiarrhythmic agent should be judged by its electrocardiographic consequences and not necessarily by the serum levels. As stated earlier, "therapeutic range" in geriatric patients may need to be redefined.

ANTIBIOTICS

Older people, especially those with reduced renal function, will require smaller amounts of those fluoroquinolones that depend on the kidney for elimination as well as aminoglycosides, vancomycin, and many cephalosporins owing to reduced clearance. Special care should be used when using those agents with a narrow therapeutic index such as aminoglycosides and vancomycin. Risk of toxicity (confusion, weakness, QT interval prolongation) from fluoroquinolones such as ofloxacin, levofloxacin, and gatifloxacin may be increased in the presence of renal dysfunction.

Older people experience a decline in immunocompetence with advanced age, and as such, the dose and duration of antibiotics should be optimized in this age group to ensure the best likelihood of resolution of the infectious process.

ANTICANCER AGENTS

Although the pharmacokinetics of numerous anticancer drugs have shown no difference in the elderly compared with younger people, there may be pharmacodynamic differences. Some agents show a greater degree of bone marrow toxicity (docetaxel, temozolomide), and recovery of the hematopoietic system after chemotherapy can be delayed in the elderly.

ANTICOAGULANTS

Patients over the age of 65 are most likely to bleed as a result of anticoagulants and to suffer catastrophic consequences from that bleeding.[22,36] When considering the use of warfarin (Coumadin) in the older population, three important principles should be kept in mind: (1) if the total protein or albumin concentration is low, initiate warfarin at a lower dosage; (2) use the most current guidelines for anticoagulant use; and, (3) evaluate the need for therapy frequently and use warfarin for the shortest possible time.

Patients should be informed about warfarin to lessen the likelihood of bleeding, and they should be educated about the potential for drug-drug interactions with other prescription and nonprescription medications.

> ● Patients over the age of 65 are most likely to bleed as a result of anticoagulants and to suffer catastrophic consequences from that bleeding.

ANTICHOLINERGICS

Numerous medications commonly used in the elderly possess variable degrees of anticholinergic effects (Table 6-3). Common anticholinergic physiological systemic effects with these medications include dry mouth, dry skin, dry eyes, urinary retention, and constipation. The problems of urinary retention or constipation are more problematic in the elderly. Central nervous system anticholinergic effects include sedation, confusion, and psychosis with both auditory and visual hallucinations. These central nervous system effects can increase the risk of falls and fractures in this population. If the patient has any degree of cognitive impairment, these centrally mediated effects are more likely. The anticholinergic effects are thought to be cumulative, so if an elderly patient is on more than one of these medications, the anticholinergic effect is increased or more likely. This has been referred to as "anticholinergic load."

ANTIDEPRESSANTS

An antidepressant agent for a geriatric patient should be the least sedating, have minimal cardiotoxicity and minimal anticholinergic effects, and produce minimal orthostatic changes in blood pressure. On the basis of these requirements, the antidepressants of choice are the selective serotonin reuptake inhibitors (SSRIs) such as sertraline (Zoloft), paroxetine (Paxil), citalopram (Celexa), escitalopram (Lexapro), and the mixed agents venlafaxine (Effexor) and bupropion (Wellbutrin). The SSRI fluoxetine (Prozac) is probably poorly suited for

Table 6–3	Commonly Used Medications That Possess Anticholinergic Effects

• Antihistamines	• Antipsychotics
• Chlorpheniramine	• Chlorpromazine
• Hydroxyzine	• Clozapine
• Diphenhydramine	• Haloperidol
	• Thioridazine
• Antidepressants	• Anti-ulcerants
• Amitriptyline	• Cimetidine
• Nortriptyline	• Ranitidine
• Imipramine	
• Doxepin	
• Protriptyline	
• Antiemetics	• Antispasmodics
• Dimenhydrinate	• Belladonna alkaloids
• Meclizine	• Dicyclomine
• Prochlorperazine	• Hyoscyamine
• Promethazine	• Oxybutynin
• Trimethobenzamide	• Propantheline
	• Tolterodine
• Anti-parkinsonians	• Antidiarrheals
• Amantadine	• Diphenoxylate/atropine
• Benztropine	
• Miscellaneous	
• Clonidine	
• Codeine	

the older patient owing to its propensity to produce anorexia, anxiety, and insomnia, as well as its prolonged half-life in the elderly.[37] Trazodone (Desyrel) and mirtazapine (Remeron) may also be acceptable alternatives but owing to their sedating properties are best reserved for bedtime administration.

The dosages of antidepressants effective in the elderly are typically one-sixth to one-third those necessary in younger persons.

> ● The dosages of antidepressants effective in the elderly are typically one-sixth to one-third those necessary in younger persons.

ANTI-DIABETIC AGENTS

Regardless of which oral anti-diabetic agent is used in the elderly, it is suggested that they be initiated at one-half the usual dose owing to impaired glucose counter-regulation and altered presentation of hypoglycemia. It is probably best to avoid the first gener-

ation sulfonylureas owing to impaired elimination and higher incidence of hypoglycemia, especially with chlorpropamide. Glyburide (Diabeta) has a longer elimination half-life and also a higher incidence of hypoglycemic episodes in older patients compared with glipizide (Glucotrol).[38]

Insulin glargine (Lantus) is emerging as an alternative insulin preparation, with a smooth dose response curve, and, as such, may have a lower incidence of hypoglycemia.

ANTIHYPERTENSIVES

In the management of hypertension for the elderly, it is wise to remember that the studies that substantiated the benefits of treating the older hypertensive often used a low dose of diuretic as sole therapy. The benefits of diuretic therapy compared with angiotensin-converting enzyme (ACE) inhibitors and calcium channel blockers were recently reaffirmed in the Antihypertensive and Lipid-Lowering Treatment to Prevent Heart Attack Trial (ALLHAT) study, which substantiated that diuretics were superior to ACE inhibitors or calcium channel blockers in preventing major forms of cardiovascular disease, including heart attack.[39] In the elderly the dose of hydrochlorothiazide should be 12.5 mg daily, with a maximum of 25 mg daily. Doses higher than these produce no further reductions in blood pressure but certainly do result in greater electrolyte disturbances. The cost of hydrochlorothiazide ranges from $4 to $6 per month compared with $60 to $80 per month for ACE inhibitors or calcium channel blockers.

Based on the likelihood of centrally mediated side effects and the sensitivity of the elderly to these side effects, peripherally acting antihypertensives would seem to be the agents of choice to use in the geriatric patient if a low dose of hydrochlorothiazide is not sufficient or contraindicated. Agents shown to be well tolerated in older patients are ACE inhibitors or angiotensin receptor blockers (ARBs). Perhaps better matched to the pathology of hypertension in the elderly are the calcium-channel blockers, with the exception of short-acting nifedipine, which should be avoided in the elderly. Another benefit of the ACE inhibitors and ARBs is that, in patients with congestive HF and hypertension, an ACE inhibitor or ARB can be used for both conditions. In patients with hypertension and angina, a calcium-channel blocker could be used for both. Such dual functions would help minimize the number of medications.

If a centrally acting agent is being considered, such as clonidine, it is best to begin with the lowest possible dosage. If a beta-blocker is being considered, it is best to use the least lipophilic agent to minimize centrally

---

Box 6-1   MASTER: Rules for Rational Drug Therapy

- **M**inimize the number of drugs used—use the fewest number of drugs possible
- **A**lternatives should be considered—alternative therapy, alternative drugs, and alternative dosage forms should be considered
- **S**tart low and go slow—start with lowest dosage and increase gradually
- **T**itrate therapy—adjust initial dosage according to individual characteristics and readjust dosage to optimize monitored plasma levels and/or clinical response
- **E**ducate patient—instruct patient or family about the need for and potential problems of therapy to increase compliance and decrease side effects
- **R**eview regularly—monitor response regularly and re-evaluate need periodically

---

mediated side effects (e.g., atenolol would be preferable to propranolol).

ANTIPSYCHOTIC AGENTS

The most appropriate antipsychotic agent for the older population would be the least sedating with minimal anticholinergic side effects. The newer atypical antipsychotics such as risperidone (Risperdal), quetiapine (Seroquel), olanzapine (Zyprexa), ziprasidone (Geodon), and aripiprazole (Abilify) fit these criteria. Among these five agents, risperidone probably has the most dose-related extrapyramidal side effects. Olanzapine has the greatest likelihood of metabolic syndrome, with risperidone and quetiapine being less likely. Ziprasidone and aripiprazole are too new to assess their likelihood of metabolic syndrome. Quetiapine and olanzapine have greater anticholinergic effects.[40,41] Therefore, in our opinion risperidone is the antipsychotic of choice in the geriatric patient when used in the suggested geriatric dose of less than 2 mg per day. The older antipsychotics such as haloperidol (Haldol) and thioridazine (Mellaril) while minimally sedating have a much higher incidence of extrapyramidal side effects and thus are no longer preferred in the elderly. Therapy should be initiated at the lowest possible dose and continued only after careful monitoring for efficacy and toxicity.

ANTI-ULCER MEDICATIONS AND GASTROESOPHAGEAL REFLUX DISEASE MEDICATIONS

The proton pump inhibitors, omeprazole (Prilosec), esomeprazole (Nexium), lansoprazole (Prevacid), or pantoprazole (Protonix), appear to be safe to use in the elderly, with no one agent emerging as being preferable. However, omeprazole (Prilosec) is now available over-the-counter and is considerably cheaper than the other agents.

Among the H_2 antagonists, cimetidine (Tagamet) depends on the kidneys for 70% of its elimination.

Thus, when the dosage of cimetidine is not decreased in older patients with diminished renal function, they may experience more central nervous system side effects. In addition, because the elderly often take a large number of medications (many of which could interact with cimetidine) ranitidine (Zantac) or famotidine (Pepcid) would be preferable H_2 antagonists at one-half the usual adult dose.

DIGITALIS GLYCOSIDES

Because of a decrease in lean mass and a reduction in renal function in the elderly, digoxin (Lanoxin) dosage should be lower than in younger patients. Also, digoxin is sometimes used inappropriately in the elderly in the absence of atrial fibrillation. Digoxin treatment has been suspended in many of these patients without ill effects.

In older patients with recent-onset congestive HF, the predominant pathology is likely to be diastolic dysfunction, which responds better to afterload reduction than to inotropic agents. Thus, therapy with agents other than digoxin should be considered whenever possible.

NONPRESCRIPTION DRUGS AND ALTERNATIVE REMEDIES

The elderly consume more than 40% of the nonprescription drugs sold in the United States and an unknown amount of alternative or herbal products. Because of changes in kinetics and dynamics, the older population is at increased risk of serious adverse reactions and significant drug-drug interactions from these products. Particular caution should be exercised with over-the-counter analgesics and antihistamines. Patient education is most important, especially now that more prescription medications are being changed to nonprescription status.

SUMMARY

The acronym MASTER developed by Garnett and Barr,[42] provides useful guidelines for rational drug therapy in the elderly (Box 6-1). By selecting medications to minimize the risk of toxicity, by increasing communication, by applying the principles of MASTER, and by having the patient use a single pharmacy so that potential drug-drug interactions can be detected, we can begin to resolve "America's other drug problem." The goal of rational pharmacotherapy should be to maximize quality of life while reducing suffering and disability.

References

1. Knapp DE, Tomita DK. Second annual adverse drug/biologic reaction report: 1986. Office of Epidemiology and Biostatistics, Center for Drugs and Biologics, Food and Drug Administration, 1987.
2. Johnson JA, Bootman JL. Drug-related morbidity and mortality. Arch Intern Med 1995;155:1949-1956.
3. Johnson JA, Bootman JL, Cox E. The health care cost of drug-related morbidity and mortality in nursing facilities. Arch Intern Med 1997;157:2089-2096.
4. Noyes MA, Lucas DS, Stratton MA. Principles of geriatric pharmacotherapy. J Geriatr Drug Ther 1996;10:5-34.
5. Vargo D, Kramer WG, Black PK, et al. Bioavailability, pharmacokinetics and pharmacodynamics of torsemide and furosemide in patients with congestive heart failure. Clin Pharmacol Ther 1995;57:601-609.
6. Murray MD, Deer MM, Ferguson JA, et al. Open-label randomized trial of torsemide compared with furosemide therapy in patients with heart failure. Am J Med 2001;111:513-520.
7. Parker BM, Cusack BJ, Vestal RE. Pharmacokinetic optimization of drug therapy in elderly patients. Drugs Aging 1995;7:10-18.
8. Sproule BA, Hardy BG, Shulman KI. Differential pharmacokinetics of lithium in elderly patients. Drugs Aging 2000;16:165-177.
9. Divoll M, Greenblatt DJ, Ochs HR, et al. Absolute bioavailability or oral and intramuscular diazepam: effects of age and sex. Anesth Analg 1983; 62:1-8.
10. Greenblatt DJ, Allen MD, Harmatz JS, et al. Diazepam disposition determinants. Clin Pharmacol Ther 1980;27:301-312.
11. Greenblatt DJ, Sellers EM, Shader RI. Drug disposition in old age. N Engl J Med 1982;306:1081-1087.
12. Dawling S, Crome P. Clinical pharmacokinetics in the elderly: an update. Clin Pharmacokinet 1989;17:236-263.
13. Kinirons JT, Crome P. Clinical pharmacokinetic considerations in the elderly: an update. Clin Pharmacokinetic 1997;33:302-312.
14. Wang PS, Bohn RL, Glynn RJ, et al. Hazardous benzodiazepine regimens in the elderly: effects of half-life, dosage, and duration on risk of hip fracture. Am J Psychiatry 2001;158:892-898.
15. Hemmelgarn B, Suissa S, Huang A, et al. Benzodiazepine use and the risk of motor vehicle crash in the elderly. JAMA 1997;278:27-31.
16. Lindeman RD, Tobin J, Shock NW. Longitudinal studies on the rate of decline in renal function with age. J Am Geriatric Soc 1985;33:278-285.
17. Feely J, Coakley D. Altered pharmacodynamics in the elderly. Clin Geriatr Med 1990;6:269-283.
18. Castleden CM, George CF, Marcer D, Hallett C. Increased sensitivity to nitrazepam in old age. BMJ 1977;1:10-12.
19. Agostini JV, Leo-Summers, LS, Inouye SK. Cognitive and other adverse effects of diphenhydramine use in hospitalized older patients. Arch Intern Med 2001;161:2091-2097.
20. Wang Y, Chan CLY, Holden JE, et al. Age-dependent decline in dopamine D1 receptors in human brain: a PET study. Synapse 1998;30:56-61.
21. Swift CG. Pharmacodynamics: changes in homeostatic mechanisms, receptor and target organ sensitivity in the elderly. Br Med Bull 1990;46:36-52.
22. Hammerlein, A, Derendorf H, Lowenthal DT. Pharmacokinetic and pharmacodynamic changes in the elderly. Clin Pharmacokinet 1998;35:49-64.
23. Lamy PP. New dimensions and opportunities. Drug Intell Clin Pharm. 1985;19:399-402.
24. Shaughnessy AF. Common drug interactions in the elderly. Emerg Med. 1992;24:21-32.
25. Honig PK, Cantilena LR. Polypharmacy: pharmacokinetic perspectives. Clin Pharmacokinet 1994;26:85-90.
26. McCrea JB, Ranelli PL, Boyce, EG et al. Preliminary study of autonomy as a factor influencing medication taking by the elderly patients. Am J Hosp Pharm 1993;50:296-298.
27. Beers MH, Ouslander JG, Rollingher I, et al. Explicit criteria for determining inappropriate medication use in nursing homes. Arch Intern Med 1991;151:1825-1832.
28. Beers MH. Explicit criteria for determining inappropriate medication use by the elderly: an update. Arch Intern Med 1997;157:1531-1536.
29. Fink DM, Cooper JW, Wade WE, et al. Updating the Beer's criteria for potentially inappropriate medication use in older people. Arch Intern Med 2003;163:2716-2724.
30. Zhan C, Sangl J, Bierman AS, et al. Potentially inappropriate medication use in the community-dwelling elderly. JAMA 2001;286:2823-2839.
31. Neuman T, Kitchman M, McMeans T, et al. California seniors and prescription drugs. The Henry J. Kaiser Family Foundation and Tuft-New England Medical Center. 2002.
32. Simon LS, Weaver AL, Graham DY, et al. Anti-inflammatory and upper gastrointestinal effects of celecoxib in rheumatoid arthritis. JAMA 1999;282:1921-1928.
33. Langman MJ, Jensen DM, Watson DJ. Adverse upper gastrointestinal effects of rofecoxib compared with NSAIDs. JAMA 1999;282:1929-1933.
34. AGS Panel on Chronic Pain in Older Persons. The management of chronic pain in older persons: AGS Panel on Chronic Pain in Older Persons. J Am Geriatr Soc 1998;46:635-651.
35. Gloth FM. Pain management in older adults: prevention and treatment. J Am Geriatr Soc 2001;49:188-199.
36. Nielson C. Pharmacological considerations in critical care of the elderly. Clin Geriatr Med 1994;10:71-89.
37. Anderson IM. Meta-analytical studies on new antidepressants. Br Med Bull 2001;57:161-178.
38. Shorr RI, Ray WA, Daugherty JR, Griffin MR. Individual sulfonylureas and serious hypoglycemia in older people. J Am Geriatr Soc 1996;44: 751-755.
39. The ALLHAT Officers and Coordinators for the ALLHAT Collaborative Research Group. Major outcomes in high-risk hypertensive patients randomized to angiotensin-converting enzyme inhibitor or calcium channel blocker vs. diuretic: the Antihypertensive and Lipid-Lowering Treatment to Prevent Heart Attack Trial (ALLHAT). JAMA 2002;288:2891-2997.
40. Richelson E. Receptor pharmacology of neuroleptics: relation to clinical effect. J Clin Psychiatry 1999;60(Suppl 10):5-14.
41. Meyer JM. Effect of atypical antipsychotics on weight and serum lipid levels. J Clin Psychiatry 2001;62(Suppl 27):27-34.
42. Garnett WR, Barr WH. Geriatric pharmacokinetics. Upjohn Monograph Series 1984;1-27.
43. Stratton MA, Gutierres S, Salinas R. Drug therapy in the elderly: tips for avoiding adverse effects and interactions. Consultant 2004;44:461-467.

Web Resources

www.ascp.com—*this is the Web site for the American Society of Consultant Pharmacists that has probably the most up to date and useful body of information regarding drug therapy issues for older people as well as policy changes that will affect older people and their medications.*

http://www.crbestbuydrugs.org/—*is a new Web site for consumers to guide them to best prices and best choices amongst agents within therapeutic categories.*

POSTTEST

1. Which of the following statements regarding geriatric pharmacotherapy are correct?
   I. First-pass metabolism decreases with age; thus less nitrates, such as isosorbide dinitrate, would be necessary to exert their desired effect.
   II. Amitriptyline (Elavil) would be an excellent antidepressant to initiate in an 85-year-old patient with depression
   III. Phase I hepatic metabolism slows down with age.
   a. I only
   b. II only
   c. I and III
   d. II and III
   e. I, II, and III

2. When considering the use of hydrochlorothiazide in an 81-year-old patient with isolated systolic hypertension, which of the following would be the most appropriate initial dose?
   a. 12.5 mg
   b. 25 mg
   c. 50 mg
   d. 100 mg
   e. 200 mg

3. When asked to recommend a dose of warfarin for an 83-year-old patient with atrial fibrillation for the purpose of stroke prophylaxis, which of the following are likely to lead you to recommend a low dose and careful monitoring for efficacy and toxicity?
   I. Old age
   II. Reduced renal function
   III. Decreased plasma protein concentration
   a. I only
   b. II only
   c. I and III
   d. II and III only
   e. I, II, and III

PRETEST ANSWERS

1. c
2. e
3. c

POSTTEST ANSWERS

1. c
2. a
3. c

Ethnic and Cultural Aspects of Geriatrics

Jerry Johnson and Mary Beth Slusar

OBJECTIVES

Upon completion of this chapter, the reader will be able to:

- Understand the importance of culture in patient care
- Identify at least three areas in which cross-cultural differences influence doctor–patient decision-making
- State at least three general questions designed to elicit information relevant to cross-cultural communication
- Employ methods to negotiate treatment preferences with patients of diverse ethnic and cultural backgrounds
- Recognize the limitations of using family members as interpreters
- Discuss cultural influences on advance directives and other ethical matters

---

PRETEST

1. Which factor is not an important element in cross-cultural care?
   a. Individual versus family decision making about health issues
   b. Causation of illness
   c. Treatment preferences
   d. Preferences for liquid rather than pill forms of medications

2. Which statement about treatment preferences is true
   a. African Americans tend to favor more aggressive therapy than do whites.
   b. Complementary alternative therapies are used mainly by persons of higher socioeconomic class.
   c. Physicians should insist that patients accept their recommended therapies.
   d. Physicians should adamantly discourage patients from contacting folk healers.

3. Which statement about cross-cultural communication is true?
   a. Family members are often effective medical interpreters.
   b. Any person who can speak the same language as the patient can be an effective medical interpreter.
   c. Miscommunications between members of different ethnic groups originate from differences in style, grammar, word use, and body language.
   d. Medical interpreters must be the same sex as the patient.

4. As monotherapy, which antihypertensive class is relatively ineffective in African Americans compared with whites?
   a. Thiazide diuretics
   b. Beta-blockers
   c. Centrally acting agents
   d. Direct vasodilators

RELEVANCE OF ETHNICITY AND CULTURE

Racial and ethnic terms disguise vast distinctions among language, culture, and health status of persons assigned to groups of people: African American or black, American Indian or Alaska Native, Asian, Hispanics, Native Hawaiian or other Pacific Islander, and white.[1] The Asian and Native Hawaiian or other Pacific Islander category includes persons from 28 Asian countries and more than 25 Pacific Island cultures, among whom one finds vast differences in beliefs. Similar complexity is seen for Hispanics or Latinos, which are divisible into eight major cultures, and American Indians, for whom there are more than 500 federally recognized tribes and entities. Even black or African American as an ethnic group is broad, encompassing many cultures of the Caribbean, Africa, and nuances within the United States. As a result of these differences, clinicians must be cautious of generalizations about members of large racial or ethnic groups.

Excess deaths and excess morbidity and disability are prevalent among racial and ethnic minority older adults.[2] Although socioeconomic factors are the most powerful determinant of health care and health status in the U.S. population, membership in a minority racial or ethnic group is an independent risk factor for less intensive and lower quality care. As a consequence of these disparities, the Surgeon General's report, Healthy People 2010, made eliminating racial and ethnic disparities one of its two overarching goals.

Culture, the shared values, beliefs, and behaviors of members of a group, influences the presentation of symptoms by patients, the decisions of clinicians, and the patient's receptivity to recommendations. Thus, culture profoundly influences diagnosis, treatment, and responsiveness. The doctor–patient relationship merges three cultures:

1. The culture of medicine as reflected in beliefs learned from the process of education, training, and acculturation of clinicians
2. The culture unique to each physician's personal background, often because of selection factors, a culture that reflects the general beliefs, attitudes, and values of the dominant society
3. The culture of the unique patient; patients may have profoundly different views, unknown to the clinician (Table 7-1)

In contrast, cultural differences lead to miscommunications and misunderstandings, which lead to misdiagnoses. More commonly, clinicians miss opportunities for optimal illness management. Thus, clinician understanding and recognition of the cultural context of the patients' illness is essential to a successful therapeutic relationship.

Some have argued that clinicians should not attempt to learn ethnic-specific cultural characteristics but instead should learn a generic approach to cross-cultural interactions.[3] True, belonging to a racial or ethnic group is not tantamount to adherence to traditional cultural beliefs of that group. Other factors intermingled with ethnicity influence health beliefs: sex, social and economic class, age, the length of time in the United States, rural or urban area, level of education, and language. Nevertheless, because many traditional health beliefs and practices originate in distinct ethnic groups, ethnicity is an important clue to common cultural beliefs. Although a generic approach is helpful, the clinician informed of cultural tendencies is better prepared to ask the right questions, understand the patient's response, avoid confusion and misunderstandings, and negotiate differences in thinking.[4]

HEALTH BELIEFS AND CROSS-CULTURAL COMMUNICATION

Juan Gomez, *Part 1*

You are visited by an 87-year-old Mexican American whose daughter arranges the visit because of her father's weakness for 2 weeks. Because Mr. Gomez speaks little English, his daughter translates. She reveals a history of diabetes. Insulin therapy was used in the past, but more recently oral medications, of unknown type, were prescribed. The daughter, who does not reside with her father, does not think he takes his medications as prescribed. He has polyuria and polydipsia, but the review of systems reveals no other remarkable findings. He is independent in all activities of daily living. Mr. Gomez admits to not taking medications in the past 5 weeks. On examination, he is afebrile but appears fully alert as he converses with his daughter. He is not orthostatic or tachycardic. The remainder of the examination is unrevealing, but a random serum glucose is 290 mg%, and the glycosylated hemoglobin is 11.4.

Table 7–1	**Cultural Attributes/Attitudes that Influence Health Behavior**	
Attribute or Issue	**Common Physician Views**	**Examples of Other Views and Attitudes**
1. Causation (explanatory model of disease)	Genes, infectious organisms, immune system, or idiopathic	Imbalance or disharmony; spiritual intervention
2. Preference and attitudes about treatment	Deference to advice of physicians; alternative medicine is harmful or dangerous	General distrust; desire for aggressive and prolonged treatment; alternative medicine is beneficial or preferred
3. Values	Individual autonomy and aspirations	Deference and respect for others; duty to family
4. Patient decision making	Individual autonomy	Collaborative decision with family or elder
5. Communicating with physicians	Direct responses	Indirect or oblique responses; nondisclosure of bad news
6. Language	Traditional English words and meanings	General unfamiliarity with health-related terms
7. Advance directives	Acceptance; preference for written documents	Suspicious of written documents; bad news inhibits health
8. Death	Discontinuity between life and death; duty to the individual patient	Continuity between death and life; duty to prolong life
9. Diet	Balanced U.S. diet; focus on the food substance	Variable preferences; eating in a social context

You order other laboratory tests, but given the relatively stable hemodynamics, your main concern is why Mr. Gomez does not take medications as prescribed. Of course, medical considerations such as cognitive impairment are considered, but you also wonder whether Mr. Gomez willfully stopped taking his medicine. Upon questioning by his daughter, who serves as interpreter, Mr. Gomez states that he is aware that the doctors call his illness diabetes. When asked what he thinks causes diabetes, he says it derives from upset in his system, an imbalance in internal forces.

STUDY QUESTIONS

1. How should physicians respond to patients' beliefs about the cause of illness if these beliefs differ from that of the physician?
2. Name two beliefs systems distinct from Western medicine.
3. What are the limitations of family members as interpreters?

Culture clearly shapes attitudes and beliefs about disease, health, and health care.[5] Quite frequently a patient's beliefs about the causation of illness, or what is sometimes referred to as the individual's explanatory model, is quite different from the beliefs of physicians, beliefs derived from the physician's understanding of the biological basis of disease. Because of limitations of medical knowledge, physicians may give detailed explanations of pathogenesis without answering a question crucial to patients: what caused the illness or, to phrase the question another way, why me?

Although many Americans believe that germs cause disease, not all cultures and ethnic groups share that belief.[5] Mexican Americans are more likely than are whites to attribute breast cancer to breast fondling and breast trauma. Of Hispanics responding to a New York survey, 58% believed that surgery causes cancer to spread. The belief that a healthy body is in a state of balance appears to have originated in China and spread to influence beliefs in Asia, India, Spain, and Latin America. In Asia, the balance is between yin and yang; all things in the universe are primarily either yin or yang, including diseases. Other causes of disease are spirit possession; conditions of the blood (too thick or too thin); emotional states such as grief, jealousy, and malice; and social transgression such as envy or gossip. It follows, in the thinking of the patient, that treatment for illnesses resulting from such etiologies must be appropriate to the cause. If patients believe the body is out of balance, inquire as to how the person proposes to restore balance. If a spirit has taken over the body, inquire how it can be exorcised.

● Culture clearly shapes attitudes and beliefs about disease, health, and health care.

Juan Gomez, *Part 2*

On a follow-up visit, Mr. Gomez has no systemic symptoms. The physician again relies on his daughter as interpreter. He notes that Mr. Gomez tends to answer yes to an inordinate number of questions.

CASE DISCUSSION

You are aware that type II diabetes mellitus has a high prevalence among older Hispanics. You also recognize that adherence to therapy could not occur unless you somehow respond to Mr. Gomez's beliefs about the cause of diabetes. You recognize the inordinate use of yes as a reflection of respeto, or deference to the doctor, rather than acceptance of your recommended treatment regimen. Therefore, you chose to acknowledge rather than to dismiss Mr. Gomez' belief and to negotiate with him as to how he can regain balance. You ask Mr. Gomez whether the medicines create imbalance. Upon receiving a negative response, you ask Mr. Gomez if he would take the prescribed medicines for diabetes. Mr. Gomez is pleased that you have acknowledged his beliefs and consents to take the prescribed medication.

Trained interpreters should have been used instead of the daughter.[5, 21] Although it seems appropriate to use a family member as interpreter because of convenience and familiarity with the patient, evidence points to the contrary. First, relationships between patient and family member may greatly influence the information that is obtained and relayed. For instance, in many Hispanic cultures, the respect for the elder dictates a deference that will influence how much information is relayed by the family interpreter. Health systems should employ professional interpreters, a practice consistent with the view of the Office of Civil Rights that federally funded health programs provide patients with limited English skills access to services equal to those provided to English-speaking patients.

Even a trained interpreter must be aware of the dynamics of communication, of which language is but one component. Doctors and patients engage in active interpretation of verbal and nonverbal cues that determine subsequent responses and that are culturally defined. Miscommunications between members of different speech communities originate from differences in style as well as differences in grammar and word use. For instance, two elements of communication style among some Hispanics, *simpatia* (the desire for positive smooth interpersonal relations) and *personalismo* (preference for providers whom they have come to know through pleasant conversation), influence the doctor–patient interaction.[6] Japanese culture emphasizes respect, politeness, and self-control. These styles may lead to avoidance of discussing symptoms and avoidance of disagreeing with health professionals, even when not accepting recommendations. Box 7-1 gives tips regarding communications in cross-cultural interactions.

According to the 2001 Health Care Quality Survey, 16% of African Americans and 18% of Hispanics felt that they had been treated with disrespect during a health care visit.[7] In addition, almost one-third (32%) of Asians and more than one-quarter (26%) of Hispanics reported that their personal beliefs prevented them from following their physician's advice; for whites and African Americans, the numbers were only 19% and 13%, respectively. Only 49% of Asians compared with 68% of whites felt that their physician listened to them during their visit. Although much of these statistics can be improved with physicians'

increased knowledge and awareness of the distinctive needs of their diverse patients, improved care will require changes in the structure and policies of health systems. Less than one-half (48%) of non-English speakers who felt they needed an interpreter during a doctor visit actually got one either always or usually.[7]

When patients perceive that they are being treated disrespectfully in the health care setting, they are less likely to pursue preventive care, follow their physician's advice, and receive needed care, all of which have a greater impact on elderly minorities with one or more chronic diseases.[8] The physician should be conversant in the person's language or have access to a trained interpreter. One strategy to improve the doctor–patient relationship for patients of all ages and races/ethnicities is participatory decision making (PDM). PDM has been operationalized as the perception of patients that their physician involves them in treatment decisions, allows them to have some control over their treatment, and asks them to take responsibility for their treatment.[9,10] Cooper-Patrick et al.[10] found that African American patients experienced less participatory visits and were less satisfied with visits than were white patients.[10] Most important, the physician must learn how to appropriately elicit information and negotiate effectively. Box 7-2 demonstrates important cross-cultural care tips relevant to information gathering and negotiation.

Box 7-1 Tips in Cross-Cultural Communication

- When choosing an interpreter, it is not enough for the person to speak the same language as the patient. Same-sex interpreters are usually best.
- Eye contact may have different meaning in different cultures. Lack of eye contact may reflect respect or concern rather than disinterest.
- Idioms should be avoided whenever possible. Also remember that all Spanish languages and, for that matter, all English languages are not the same. The same words may have different meanings in different countries and among different ethnic groups.
- A patient should be referred to as Mr., Mrs., Miss, or Ms. unless told by the patient to do otherwise. People suffer tremendous loss of dignity when they become patients; it is important not to add unnecessarily to this loss.
- Remember that "yes" may not always mean the affirmative; for an Asian, it may be a way of avoiding the embarrassment of saying "no." Or, it may be the grammatically correct but misleading answer to a negative question, as in, "Haven't you eaten yet today?" It is best to ask open-ended questions and to avoid negatives whenever possible. Also be aware that masculine and feminine pronouns do not exist in many Asian languages and interpret statements accordingly.

Box 7-2 Do's and Don'ts of Cross-Cultural Communication

1. Do not assume that patients will view the world the same way that you do.
2. Treat the patient as a whole person with psychological, spiritual, and physical needs.
3. Respect differences; respect is demonstrated by consideration of what persons request rather than your perceptions of what is best.
4. To avoid possible stereotypes, turn assumptions into questions by asking general questions such as:
   The patient's and family expectations: How can I be most helpful?
   Language: What language do you use at home?
   Help-seeking behavior: Who helps you when you are sick? Have you seen anyone else for help, not just doctors or persons in the hospital? Are you taking any treatments at home?
   Health beliefs or explanatory model: What do you think caused your problem? What do you call it? Are you involved in a religious group?
   Social support network and role: Who should make the decisions and be part of discussions about your health?

> ● When patients perceive that they are being treated disrespectfully in the health care setting, they are less likely to pursue preventive care, follow their physician's advice, and receive needed care.

HEALTH ISSUES OF HISPANIC OLDER ADULTS

It was not until 1970 that national surveys included data on specific Hispanic ethnic groups, resulting in a paucity of accurate data on Hispanic older adults before this point. As of the 2000 census, Hispanics of all races (including people whose culture or origin is Cuban, Mexican, Puerto Rican, South or Central American, or other Spanish) accounted for 12.5% of the U.S. population, which translates to about 35 million people. Mexicans are the largest subgroup, accounting for 7.3% of the total population (but 50% of the elderly Hispanics), with Puerto Ricans following at 1.2%, Cubans at 0.4%, and other Hispanics at 3.6% of the total U.S. population. The necessity of investigating each ethnic group individually is exemplified in the variation in self-reported health ratings among Hispanic ethnicities: total Hispanic self-reported health rating as fair or poor is 22% to 25% for Mexicans, 20% for Central Americans, and 16% for Puerto Ricans.[7] The rate of health insurance among Hispanics is the lowest in the United States, a factor that undoubtedly contributes significantly to disparate health status. Box 7-3 summarizes key health issues among Hispanic older adults.

Box 7-3   Health Issues of Hispanic Older Adults

- The dominant causes of death, morbidity, and disability are diabetes and heart disease, although the rates vary among Hispanic ethnic groups.
- Hispanics were 1.9 times more likely to be diagnosed with diabetes in 2000 compared with whites, a finding most frequent among Mexican Americans and Puerto Ricans.[11]
- Among Hispanics, the mortality from cardiovascular disease is less than that for whites, although the relative risk is greater.
- Although most cancer rates are not disproportionately higher than that of whites, the stage of disease at diagnosis is often advanced. Women with Hispanic surnames have a 7.3 times greater chance of developing cervical cancer than do women with non-Hispanic surnames.
- 25% of a sample of Hispanics 60 years and above who were living in Los Angeles were suffering from major depression.[12]
- Gurland[13] diagnosed dementia in Latinos at 7.5% of the 65- to 74-year-olds, 27.9% of the 75- to 84-year-olds, and 62.9% of those 85 and older.

WORLD-VIEW RELIGIOSITY AND USE OF COMPLEMENTARY ALTERNATIVE MEDICINE

Ella Jones, *Part 1*

You are visited by Ms. Jones, a 79-year-old African American woman, who developed swelling of the face and right arm, resulting in a visit to a physician. You discover a large ulcerated mass over her right breast, which Ms. Jones had not disclosed to anyone, including family or friends. Breast cancer complicated by a superior vena caval syndrome is confirmed. The patient, initially reluctant to inform any family members, eventually consents to inform her son and daughter. She is seen by an oncologist on your recommendation and is offered chemotherapy and radiation. She refuses, stating that God will take care of her problems in due time. The oncologist is concerned about the possible life-threatening nature of the illness and is frustrated that Ms. Jones appears nonchalant.

STUDY QUESTIONS

1. How can the physician incorporate the patient's spirituality in the caring process?
2. Name two modalities of complementary alternative medicine.
3. In what ways can physicians collaborate with alternative therapists?

Closely related to an individual's beliefs about the cause of illness is the person's world view, or basic assumptions about the nature of reality, assumptions that become the foundation for all actions and interpretations.[1] Religion largely defines the world view of many African Americans and persons of other cultures. During illness, religion often becomes important in accepting and understanding the illness and in facilitating the healing process. Therefore, patients' religious beliefs should be respected and incorporated into their care whenever possible. Some religions have beliefs that conflict with Western medicine, for example, Jehovah's witnesses' beliefs about blood transfusions. When confronted with such conflicts, consider the patient's perspective. Many religions and cultures have dietary taboos or prescriptions, which should be ascertained at the intake interview. For example, Muslims and Orthodox Jews are forbidden pork. Recognize that religious symbols can take many forms, from Catholic rosary beads to Mormon long underwear. These symbols should not be removed without discussion, and it is best to try to keep them in contact with the patient's body whenever possible. Also remember that patients live within a social network in which the social cost of violating religious tenets may be high.

Another aspect of world view involves patients' relationship with nature. For example, the dominant American culture posits the belief that people control nature. If the land is dry, irrigate. If a disease is caused by bacteria, destroy them. Other cultures, such as Asian and American Indian, see people as a part of nature. They strive to maintain harmony with the earth and look to the land to provide treatment for disease. Herbal remedies are important in their cultures. These views explain partly why preventive health care measures that, to the patient, are not causally connected to the illness may be ignored.

Ella Jones, *Part 2*

Unknown to her oncologist, Ms. Jones is trying alternative therapies of a variety of sorts. When at a subsequent visit, one of her children cautiously asks the oncologist about his beliefs in folk medicine techniques, the physician states, "Why would anyone waste time with that?"

CASE DISCUSSION

You, unlike the oncologist, are aware that Ms. Jones, as we now know to be the case among many ethnic groups and across socioeconomic classes, uses complementary alternative forms of medicine. Because Ms. Jones believes God confers both health and illness, she is unenthusiastic about taking medications for breast cancer. In fact, she had largely ignored the health care system in the past, firmly believing that the will of God would control her health and illnesses. She reflects other African Americans who attribute illness recovery to God's power, in contrast to whites, who tend to view religion as a tool for coping with illness.[12] You affirm Ms. Jones's belief in God while trying to achieve compromise on conventional forms of therapy. You also elicit the assistance of her pastor. After more discussion with her adult children, Ms. Jones consents to radiation and chemotherapy.

All cultures have developed their own methods for treating illness based on presumed cause-and-effect relationships. Many Caribbean and Southern African Americans believe that certain symptoms and illnesses arise from interpersonal conflict and supernatural

activity.[14] Thus they, as did Ms. Jones, perceive perfectly understandable reasons to consult traditional healers. Others use home remedies, from prayer to herbs. Conventional folk medicine wisdom treats fever by trying to sweat it out. Some techniques, such as coin rubbing and cupping, produce marks that may appear to be signs of abuse or unrelated symptoms. It is important to recognize these signs before arriving at unwarranted conclusions.

Patients may hold beliefs regarding the necessity of certain medical procedures. For example, some feel that an injection is necessary for proper treatment. Patients may lose faith quickly in physicians who recommend multiple diagnostic tests, whether appropriate or inappropriate, when they expect a therapeutic intervention. It is often helpful with new patients to ask what treatment they feel will make them better. When doctors are unable to cure a patient or to obtain consent to certain procedures, it may be beneficial to honor a patient's request to bring in a traditional healer. Such healers are occasionally successful, whether from the efficacy of their treatments or a placebo effect. When conventional therapy contradicts complementary alternative medicine, the rationale for the conventional therapy must be explained.

THE SOCIAL CONTEXT OF HEALTH CARE: TREATMENT PREFERENCES

Albert Smith

You are visited by Mr. Smith, a 76-year-old African American man, who develops generalized weakness, weight loss, a cough, and a low-grade fever. He has a history of hypertension treated with an angiotensin-converting enzyme (ACE) inhibitor. You uncover a blood pressure of 164/90 mm Hg, respiratory rate of 26, a heart rate of 96, and a temperature of 101.8°F. A chest radiograph confirms a diagnosis of pneumonia. Further testing reveals anemia, mild chronic renal insufficiency, and a prostate specific antigen of 86. Although he has seen physicians sporadically over the years, he has not maintained a relationship with a physician. On the contrary, he commonly ignored their advice about testing and medications, preferring to treat himself. After a biopsy reveals prostate cancer, he is reluctant to receive hormonal therapy or an orchiectomy.

STUDY QUESTIONS

1. What social or historical factors have influenced the attitudes of African Americans about health care systems?
2. What are the most effective forms of monotherapy for hypertension among African Americans?
3. What are some distinctive features of prostate cancer in African Americans?

CASE DISCUSSION

Even when ethnocultural treatment preferences are evident to physicians, the enormity of their impact and the social and historical basis may be unrecognized. The controlling element in Mr. Smith's care was one of distrust in the formal health care system and in doctors in general. The origin of that distrust was evidenced when Mr. Smith disclosed the unexpected and, most likely, avoidable death of his two-year-old son at the hands of an unlicensed (unknown to Mr. Smith at the time) surgeon during a minor procedure, an event that occurred more than 50 years ago. Knowledge of this event reinforces your decision to keep Mr. Smith fully informed and in control of his treatment options. As a consequence, Mr. Smith allows himself to be hospitalized, where he responds to conventional antibiotic treatment. Later, after a full discussion of hormonal injections versus orchiectomy for metastatic prostate cancer, he elects orchiectomy. You add a thiazide diuretic to Mr. Smith's ACE inhibitor for improved treatment of hypertension. Note that the Antihypertensive and Lipid-Lowering Treatment to Prevent Heart Attack Trial (ALLHAT), a randomized effectiveness hypertension treatment trial, confirmed older reports of differential responsiveness of African Americans to monotherapy for hypertension.[22] In African Americans, a diuretic type agent was more effective in reducing cardiovascular outcomes and stroke (in particular) when used as an initial therapy compared with a dihydropyridine calcium channel agent or ACE inhibitor. However, most patients with hypertension required two or three drug regimens irrespective of the initial choice. His quality of life improves greatly for 2 years, after which he expires at home with his family, at peace and still in control.

The health preferences of African Americans are greatly influenced by their historical experiences with the formal health care system, experiences marked largely by disregard, disrespect, lack of access, and abuse; slaves as medical research subjects; deception and mistreatment in the widely known Tuskegee syphilis study subjects; and sterilization initiatives. Even today, African Americans receive less intensive health care after accounting for access to care and treatment preferences. As a consequence of this neglect, African Americans are more likely to believe that hospitals and physicians are using them for experiments, particularly when students and residents are involved.[15] Although neglect has led to distrust of the health care system, African Americans may desire aggressive medical interventions, even interventions that physicians consider to have a low probability of benefit. For instance, African Americans are more likely to want every treatment available for a hypothetical condition of persistent vegetative state,[16] and African American nursing home residents are more likely to want artificial nutrition.[17]

HEALTH ISSUES OF AFRICAN AMERICAN OLDER ADULTS

African American older adults suffer generally the same disorders as the dominant culture: cardiovascular disease, cancer, and stroke. Obesity is prevalent among African American older adults, increasing the risk of cardiovascular disease. African American women suffer the greatest disparate mortality from cardiovascular disease. The distinction is not in the type of illness but in the stage of presentation, in which illnesses such as breast and prostate cancer are diagnosed at a later stage, resulting in poorer survival. See Boxes 7-4 and 7-5 for more information regarding diseases prevalent in African Americans. Of 25 primary cancer sites, African Americans had lower survival in all but three. Osteoporosis is not as common but still causes sufficient disability so that should not be ignored in African American women. These disparities demonstrate the need for more effective efforts to screen African Americans for disorders such as hypertension, diabetes, breast cancer, glaucoma, and colon cancer, illnesses for which treatment results in significant improvements in morbidity, mortality, and disability.

Fitzpatrick[20] found higher incidence rates of dementia in African Americans, particularly African American women, compared with whites. In this particular national sample of Medicare-eligible subjects, incidence of dementia was 34.7 per 1000 person-years for white women, 35.3 for white men, 58.8 for black women, and 53.0 for black men (incidence rates were

Box 7-4	Cardiovascular Disease and Risk Factors among African American Elders

- Thirty-seven percent of all African American deaths each year can be attributed to cardiovascular disease and strokes.
- Blacks ages 65 to 74 are almost two times more likely to die of a stroke death than are whites; blacks age 75 to 84 are 1.2 times more likely.
- Seventy-nine percent of blacks who have suffered a stroke reported hypertension, making them 1.65 times more likely than similar whites to report hypertension.
- Black stroke victims were 1.89 times more likely than were whites to also have diabetes, with 32.1% of blacks who suffered a stroke also reporting being a diabetic.
- Diabetes is most common among individuals age 65 to 74 and twice as likely to afflict African Americans compared with white Americans. In 2002 more than 25% of African American men and women ages 65 to 74 had been diagnosed with diabetes.

Box 7-5	African Americans and Cancer

- African American death rates for all sites of cancer for both men and women exceed those of whites by a ratio of 1.4 and 1.2, respectively.
- African American men are more likely to have cancers of the lungs, prostate, colon, and rectum than are white men.
- Prostate cancer rates are 30% higher in African American men over 65 than in same-age whites. Older African American men also face lower survival rates for prostate cancer, 64% compared with 79% for whites.[18]
- African American women are greater than two times more likely to die of cervical cancer compared with white women and more likely to die as a result of breast cancer than are women of any other racial or ethnic group.

age-adjusted and scaled to age 80). According to another study's sample, 9.1% of African Americans ages 65 to 74 were diagnosed with dementia, 19.9% of those ages 75 to 84, and 58.6% of those ages 85 and older.[13] On a positive note, African Americans with dementia are less likely to also suffer from depression (12%) compared with whites (33%) and Hispanics (39%) with dementia.[13] These differential rates may reflect an increased predisposition for vascular dementia or accelerated rates of progression of Alzheimer's disease because of the known interaction between vascular risk factors and Alzheimer's disease.

IMPACT OF FAMILY RELATIONSHIPS AND HELP-SEEKING BEHAVIOR

Kim Duong

You are visited by Mr. Duong, an 85-year-old Chinese man who presents because of decreased appetite, weight loss, and general loss of functional status. Further history from his son reveals cognitive deficits over a period of 6 years. Mr. Duong resides with his son and daughter-in-law, both of whom are employed and lead busy lives. On examination, Mr. Duong is found to have profound cognitive deficits. He cannot ambulate and requires assistance with all basic activities of daily living. Laboratory tests reveal no acute illnesses. He is thought to have advanced Alzheimer's disease. Because of marginal food intake and evidence of malnutrition, you raise the issue of artificial feeding. The son elects artificial feeding, although he realizes it probably will not improve his father's quality of life or survival and may cause harm. When placement in a nursing facility and in-home nursing care services are offered, the son firmly refuses preferring to care for his father at home. Instead, the son takes leave from his job for a year to become the major caregiver of his father.

STUDY QUESTIONS

1. How might attitudes toward family influence use of the health care system?
2. What are some of the beliefs and attitudes of some Asians about mental health issues?

CASE DISCUSSION

Mr. Duong's son's decision reflects the traditional Chinese cultural norm that proscribes foregoing treatment or assisting in suicide and an allegiance to family. In this tradition, children are rewarded for taking all measures to extend their parent's lives. However, other Asians influenced by some eastern religions, Buddhism and Confucianism, would most likely embrace death as a natural event and encourage reverence for the deceased. In contrast to the view of Mr. Duong's son, this alternative view proposes that persons who forgo life-sustaining treatments so that the family does not suffer, emotionally or financially, are performing a valued act of compassion.[24]

This case illustrates one of the common conflicts between the health care system and persons of different cultures, in which decision-making by a family member takes precedence over the primacy of the individual. You understand Mr. Duong's position, and you make yourself available and accessible but do not try to press Mr. Duong to place his father in a nursing facility or to use in-home services. Your decision is relatively easy as Mr. Duong's son is a dedicated, informed, and effective caregiver. In other instances, home care by inadequate family support may raise questions of elder abuse. In these instances, the physician must obtain as much accurate information as possible from all relevant sources before making a decision. Encouraging and facilitating family members to discuss matters among themselves is critical. A reluctance to seek mental health services seen among Asian groups was probably not a factor in this case. Nevertheless, physicians should be mindful that Asians may view depression and dementia as stigmas.

Studies have shown important differences among ethnic groups concerning attitudes about end of life care.[25,26] Autonomy and self-determination are considered to be fundamental principles of end of life care among Western biomedicine. However, not all ethnic groups share that belief.[16] In negotiating end of life care, physicians must listen carefully to the goals of patients and family and exert every effort to avoid making culture-based assumptions that do not apply.

Family involvement in health and illness varies by culture. Self-care, a general medical goal for many patients, may appear undermined by families that take over feeding and grooming the patient. Note that these actions may be an important way for family members to demonstrate their love and respect for the patient. It may also be a way for a male patient from a hierarchical culture to demonstrate continued control over his family, despite physical weakness. African Americans, compared with Hispanic Americans or whites, are more likely to perceive family as protectors against physicians, a view related to distrust.[15] Family members share some of the emotional and physical stress and personal sacrifice of the patient's illness. In many American Indian cultures, the extended family is the network of support, which contrasts with the circumscribed nuclear family of white Americans. For these cultures,

collective needs often outweigh individual interest. Thus, the focus is on accommodating the disability and the disabled to restore harmony for the patient, family, and clan. Major decisions are collaborative and involve input from the clan, or tribal members.[19]

HEALTH ISSUES OF ASIAN AMERICAN OLDER ADULTS

Since 1980, the census has used six response categories for Asians (Asian Indian, Chinese, Filipino, Japanese, Korean, and Vietnamese), to which the category "other Asian" was added in the 2000. According to this census, Asian Americans represented 4.2% of the total U.S. population and totaled 11.9 million individuals (3.6% or 10.2 million who reported only Asian). The term "Asian" includes people from the Far East, Southeast Asia, or the Indian subcontinent (Cambodia, China, India, Japan, Korea, Malaysia, Pakistan, the Philippine Islands, Thailand, and Vietnam). Projections from the Census Bureau predict that by the year 2050, Asian Americans will account for 9.3% of the total U.S. population, or 37.6 million individuals. Box 7-6 shows major health issues among Asian American older adults.

Box 7-6 Health Issues of Asian Older Adults

- The incidence and prevalence of disease is variable across Asian American groups.
- Asians are one of the highest risk groups for osteoporosis.
- Asian Americans tend to have higher death rates from liver and gastrointestinal cancers than do whites. Vietnamese have the highest cervical cancer rates in the United States.
- More than 80% of Vietnamese older adults have been exposed to the hepatitis B virus.
- Japanese have a higher prevalence of diabetes mellitus and impaired glucose tolerance than do whites. The incidence of "possible" diabetes in the Honolulu Asian Aging Study was 12.8% for Japanese American men, and the incidence of non-insulin-dependent diabetes was 1.25 times as high in men as in women. The prevalence of diabetes in Chinese men from Boston was 13.3%, lower than that in the general elderly population.
- Vascular dementias are thought to be at an increased prevalence among Japanese older adults.
- In the Honolulu Heart program sample, the incidence rate of dementia for Japanese American men was estimated to be between 9.3% and 13%.[21]

● Who participates in health care decisions and responsibilities for care of the ill older adult varies enormously from culture to culture.

SUMMARY

The first challenge for the clinician is to recognize and acknowledge his or her own beliefs and biases about the variety of issues discussed in this chapter. No clinician can or should be expected to know all the important culture-specific features of patients. Nevertheless, the clinician can and should know the prevalent diseases, the prevalent beliefs and attitudes of cultural groups, and the distinct patterns of health decision making and help seeking behavior that he will frequently encounter. Who participates in health care decisions and responsibilities for care of the ill older adult varies enormously from culture to culture. Indeed, the distinct patterns of health care decision making may be the single most important cultural factor that clinicians must recognize. Ultimately clinicians must ask patients and families about preferences.

References

1. Recommendations from the Interagency Committee for the Review of the Racial and Ethnic Standards to the Office of Management and Budget concerning changes to the standards for the classification of federal data on race and ethnicity [notice]. Federal register. 1997; 62: 36873-36946.
2. Smedley B, Stith A, Nelson A (Eds.). Committee on Understanding and Eliminating Racial and Ethnic Disparities in Health Care, Board on Health Sciences Policy, Institute of Medicine. Unequal Treatment: Confronting Racial and Ethnic Disparities in Health Care. Washington, D.C.: National Academies Press; 2003.
3. Carrillo J, Green A, Betancourt J. Cross-cultural primary care: a patient-based approach. Ann Intern Med 1999;130:829.
4. Ethnogeriatrics Committee, American Geriatrics Society, Doorway thoughts: cross cultural health care for older adults. Boston: Jones and Bartlett Publishers, 2004.
5. Berger J. Culture and ethnicity in clinical care. Arch Intern Med 1998;158:2085.
6. Caudle P. Providing culturally sensitive health care to Hispanic clients. Nurse Pract 1993;18:40.
7. Collins KC, Hughes DL, Doty MM, Ives BL, Edwards IN, Tenney K. Diverse Communities, common concerns: assessing health care quality for minority Americans: the Commonwealth Fund 2001 Health Care Quality Survey. New York: The Commonwealth Fund, 2002.
8. Blanchard J, Lurie N. R-E-S-P-E-C-T: patient reports of disrespect in the health care setting and its impact on care. J Fam Pract 2004;53:721-730.
9. Kaplan SH, Gandek B, Greenfield S, Rogers W, Ware JE. Patient and visit characteristics related to physicians' participatory decision-making style. Medical Care 1995;33:1176-1187.
10. Cooper-Patrick L, Gallo JJ, Gonzales JJ, et al. Race, gender, and partnership in the patient-physician relationship. JAMA 1999;282:583-589.
11. Espino DV, Burge SK, Moreno C. The prevalence of selected chronic diseases among Mexican-American elderly: data from the 1982-84 Hispanic Health and Nutrition Examination Survey. J Am Board Fam Pract 1991;5:319.
12. Kemp BJ, Staples F, Lopez-Acqueres W. Epidemiology of depression and dysphoria in an elderly hispanic population-prevalence and correlates. J Am Geriatr Soc 1987;35:920-926.
13. Gurland BJ, Wilder DE, Lantigua R, et al. Rates of dementia in three ethno-racial groups. Int J Geriatr Psychiatry 1999;14:481-493.
14. Hopper S. The influence of ethnicity on the health of older women. Clin Geriatr Med 1993;9:231.
15. Hauser J, Kleefield S, Brennan T, et al. Minority populations and advance directives: insights from a focus group methodology. Camb Q Health Ethics 1997;6:58.
16. Murphy S, Palmer J, Azens, et al. ethnicity and advance directives. J Law Med Ethics 1996;24:108.
17. Obrien L, Siegert E, Grisso J. Tube feeding preferences among nursing home residents. J Gen Intern Med 1997;12:364.
18. Moul J, Sesterhenn I, Connelly R, et al: Prostate-specific antigen values at the time of prostate cancer diagnosis in African-American men. JAMA 1995;274:1277.
19. McCabe M. Patient Self-Determination Act: a Native American (Navajo) perspective. Camb Q Healthc Ethics 1994;3:419.
19. Fitzpatrick AL, Kuller LH, Ives DG, et al. Incidence and prevalence of dementia in the Cardiovascular Health Study. J Am Geriatr Soc 2004;52: 195-204.
20. White L, Petrovitch H, Ross GW, et al. Prevalence of dementia in older Japanese-American men in Hawaii: the Honolulu-Asia Aging Study. JAMA 1996;276:955-960.
21. Woloshin S, Bickell N. Schwartz L, et al. Language barriers in medicine in the United States. JAMA 1995;273:724.
22. ALLHAT Officers and Coordinators. Major outcomes in high-risk hypertensive patients randomized to angiotensin-converting enzyme inhibitor or calcium channel blocker vs diuretic. The antihypertensive and lipid lowering treatment to prevent heart attack trial. JAMA 2002;288:2981-2997.
23. Klessig J. The effect of values and culture on life-support decisions. West J Med 1992;157:316.
24. Blackhall L, Murphy S, Frank G, et al. Ethnicity and attitudes toward patient autonomy. JAMA 195;274:820.
25. Hanson L, Rodgman E. The use of living wills at the end of life: a national study, Arch Intern Med 1996;56:1018.

Web Resources

1. Stanford University Ethnogeriatrics Curriculum. stanford.edu/group/ethnoger.
2. www.cultureandhealth.org—*The Office of Minority Health offers The Cultural Competency Curriculum Modules for Physicians within "A Family Physician's Guide to Culturally Competent Care." These modules carry 9 hours of CME credit with AMA/AAFP.*
3. Cultural Positivity: Cultural Competence in Healthcare. A Diversity and Cross-Cultural Teaching Module for the Internet. www.gvhc.org/cultural/pod's_online.htm—*Detailed teaching guide for family practice residents and preceptors.*

POSTTEST

1. Which statement about biomedical ethics is true?
   a. Some cultures value extended life of their loved ones as a fundamental filial obligation.
   b. Physicians can improve patient care by insisting that mentally capable adults make decisions about their health care to the exclusion of family members.
   c. Self-determination and autonomy are accepted ethical principles in all cultures.

2. Which medical disorder is especially prevalent among African Americans, Asians, Hispanics, and American Indians?
   a. Gastrointestinal cancers
   b. Arthritis
   c. Diabetes mellitus
   d. Chronic obstructive pulmonary disease

3. Which statement about health care delivery is untrue?
   a. The quality of care provided minorities is similar once one adjusts for economic factors and prevalence of disease
   b. Urban, in contrast to rural, Hispanics have health insurance rates comparable to that of whites
   c. Part of the problem in delivering effective care to minority ethnic groups and cultures is an inadequate number of minority health providers.

PRETEST ANSWERS

1. d
2. a
3. c
4. a

POSTTEST ANSWERS

1. a
2. c
3. b

Ethics

Robert A. Zorowitz and Zachary Palace

OBJECTIVES

Upon completion of this chapter, the reader will be able to:

- Discuss the most commonly cited principles of ethical decision making in medical care
- Understand how to systematically elucidate and resolve ethical dilemmas
- Discuss the requirements of informed consent and the criteria for decisional capacity
- Discuss the role and use of different types of advanced directives, including "do not resuscitate" orders
- Understand the use of the term "futility"
- Discuss ethical concerns regarding assisted suicide and the "double effect"
- Discuss the unique issues involving provision of food and fluid

---

PRETEST

1. Which of the following statements are true?
   a. A diagnosis of dementia precludes competent decision making.
   b. Decision-making capacity can only be determined in a court of law.
   c. Lack of decision-making capacity should not be presumed if the patient goes against medical advice.
   d. Expression of a choice is sufficient to indicate decision-making capacity.

2. Which of the following statements concerning advanced directives is true?
   a. The Supreme Court has established a standard advanced directive form.
   b. The living will designates an agent to make medical decisions if an individual loses decision-making capacity.
   c. A DNR order is not equivalent to a do not treat order.
   d. Periods of acute illness are the most appropriate times to begin discussions with patients about advanced directives.

3. The following are components of the open disclosure of medical error, except:
   a. An apology to the injured patient
   b. An explanation of the error in lay language
   c. A best guess as to why the error occurred
   d. An assurance that a full investigation will take place

4. Mrs. Gloth is an 84-year-old woman whom you are admitting to the nursing home. Her son takes you aside and tells you that she has metastatic ovarian cancer but has not been told the diagnosis. He asks that you not tell her, because she would "lose all hope and die." Which of the following is an appropriate response?
   a. Tell the son that you are going to immediately inform the patient of her diagnosis.
   b. Tell the son that he can count on you to respect his wishes.
   c. Suggest that you discuss this further after getting to know the patient and family a little better.
   d. Find out from the son what the family has been telling her about her health, so you will maintain a consistent story.

INTRODUCTION

The rapid advancements in medical technology, the growing population of the elderly, and the increasing awareness of the legal and moral issues confronting the elderly, their families, and their caregivers have resulted in the need for a methodology to evaluate and resolve moral conflicts that may confront clinicians who care for older patients.

Ethics is the field that systematically studies morality, which is defined as the rightness and wrongness of human acts. Medical ethics is the discipline that studies morality in health care, generally using a process that attempts to recognize and seek solutions to moral questions or dilemmas that arise in the care and treatment of patients. As a branch of moral philosophy, medical ethics is responsive to shifts in philosophical opinion and fashion. It is also a field that is a fusion of theory and practice.[1]

Moral dilemmas arise when the rights and wishes of patients conflict with the obligations of clinicians or when there are competing obligations among clinicians. These rights and obligations may be informed by philosophical, cultural, religious, or personal principles, beliefs, and values. In geriatric medicine, rights and obligations are often influenced and complicated by factors such as limited life expectancy, cognitive impairment, impaired decision-making capacity, insufficient social and economic resources, and the complexity of multiple concomitant medical problems and functional disorders.[2]

Over the past 20 years, there has been a growing awareness of the need to institute clinical ethics as a required discipline in medical training and in health care organizations. Ethics courses are becoming more common in medical schools, and ethics committees and similar venues for the resolution of ethical conflicts have become a required and expected presence in hospitals, nursing homes, and other health care organizations. The rise of medical consumerism has resulted in a population of patients and caregivers who are increasingly well-informed about their rights and choices in the health care market. As a result, it is vital that clinicians develop a shared language of ethical decision making.

This chapter will introduce the basic principles of ethical decision making and examine common ethical issues encountered in the care of older patients.

Alice Oliver *(Part I)*

Mrs. Alice Oliver is an 83-year-old woman, an active swimmer and gardener, who suffered a right-sided stroke with mild left hemiparesis and dysphagia. During hospitalization, her motor deficits were improving, but the dysphagia persisted. A swallow evaluation indicated that she was able to tolerate a chopped or pureed diet with nectar-thick liquids, but she experienced asymptomatic aspiration with thin liquids. The speech therapist recommended thickening all liquids, and you enter this order on the chart. Mrs. Oliver, however, refuses thickened liquids, insisting that she would rather take her chances with thin liquids. The nurses and the dietician tell you they do not want to provide her with thin liquids, believing that by doing so, they will be contributing to the risk they were trying to ameliorate.

CASE DISCUSSION

You are confronted with an ethical dilemma. On one hand, you think the patient should have the right to take risks and eat what she wants. On the other hand, you can sympathize with the other health care professionals' discomfort in abetting risky behavior. Medical ethics provides a means for articulating and analyzing such dilemmas.

STUDY QUESTIONS

1. What ethical principles are in conflict in this case?
2. Is there an ethical principle that takes priority over others?

PRINCIPLES OF MEDICAL ETHICS

Traditional principles of medical ethics derived largely from the works of Greek philosophers such as Hippocrates[3] and Pythagorus.[4] During the second half of the 20th century, increasing pressure on the medical establishment from technological change, cultural upheaval, and the increasing complexity of medical care and the issues it raised resulted in the need to more explicitly frame the principles of medical ethics.

Although there are a number of alternative theories of medical ethics, such as the virtue-based theories favored by the Greek philosophers, the ethics of caring,[5] and casuistry,[6] there remain four *prima facie* principles that are most often cited as the bedrock of clinical ethics. These are autonomy, beneficence, nonmaleficence, and justice.[7]

Autonomy

The principle of autonomy refers to the duty to respect a patient's right to self-determination. This has been legally enshrined in the judicial ruling of Schloendorff v. Society of New York Hospital (NY 1914), in which Justice Cardozo found that, "Every human being of adult years and of sound mind has a right to determine what shall be done with his body."[8]

Traditionally, clinicians have assumed a strongly authoritarian and paternalistic role in the medical decision-making process. With the increase in consumerism and the availability of medical information, patients have been increasingly asserting their autonomy. Health care providers have been increasingly recognizing autonomy as a fundamental ethical principle.

Integral to the principle of autonomy is the right to be provided with sufficiently adequate and truthful information to exercise self-determination. This is the basis of informed consent, established in the Nuremberg code, which states, "The voluntary consent of the human subject is absolutely essential."[9] In Nathanson v. Kline (KS 1960), a case that centered on the failure to inform a patient of potential surgical risks, the ruling found that, "It follows that each man is considered to be master of his own body, and he may, if he be of sound mind, prohibit the performance of life-saving surgery or other medical treatment."[10]

In addition to establishing the right of an autonomous patient to refuse treatment, these rulings also introduce the concept, "of sound mind," which is indicative of a patient's capacity to understand what has been explained, appreciate the situation and its consequences, rationally manipulate information, and communicate choices.[11] Decision-making capacity is a critical requirement for providing informed consent and, therefore, for exercising autonomy.

Effective clinician–patient communication is an integral part of providing informed consent throughout the process of reaching an autonomous decision. The clinician has a duty to tell the truth and provide fact-based, objective information to the patient. Such discussions must be free of personal, subjective biases. The information must be fair and lawful and must not be swayed by any financial or personal gain.

Truth-telling is an essential component of the exercise of autonomy. The recognition that there is an obligation to provide truthful information to patients about potentially life-threatening conditions is a relatively recent phenomenon. A 1961 survey of physicians in the United States reported that 90% would not reveal a diagnosis of cancer to their patients.[12] A 1979 survey reported that 97% of physicians would reveal a diagnosis of cancer to their patients.[13] A recent survey of hospitalized patients reported that a large majority would prefer to be told of a diagnosis of cancer or Alzheimer's disease. Among those that were unsure or who did not want to be told, a majority would want to be told if it was essential to treatment. Preferences did not differ by age.[14]

Age is not, by itself, an obstacle to the full exercise of autonomy. In one study, even very old hospitalized patients were able to express their health values, underscoring the need to elicit such choices directly from the patient, unless that patient lacks decision-making capacity.[15]

Beneficence

The principle of beneficence refers to the clinician's responsibility to provide benefit or help the patient, i.e. "to do good." Beneficence is the essence of the patient–doctor relationship. Promotion of good health, curing disease, and relieving pain and suffering are all key elements in the principle of beneficence. Conversely, medical interventions that provide no benefit should be avoided.

Nonmaleficence

The principle of nonmaleficence states that throughout the physician–patient relationship, the physician shall "at the least, do no harm." It is incumbent upon all clinicians to determine what are the goals of the intervention and weigh these against the potential risk of an adverse outcome. Factors such as advanced age, concurrent disease states, and comorbidities must be considered in the equation. When available, the clinician may use formal algorithms to assess risk. For instance, preoperative cardiac risk stratification can help the clinician determine the risk of an adverse cardiac event from surgery. In essence, the duty of nonmaleficence is balanced against the duty of beneficence when weighing risks and benefits.

Justice

Justice refers to the duty to treat patients fairly. Justice can be viewed along two dimensions, access and allocation.[16] Access refers to whether those who are entitled to health care can obtain them. Allocation refers to the determination of how resources are distributed. The distribution of rights and responsibilities among the members of a society in a manner governed by consistent moral norms is often referred to as *distributive justice*.

The principle of justice can apply to either the macroenvironment, such as the decisions made to ration health care within Oregon's Medicaid program[17] or the microenvironment, such as decisions made to allocate money and other resources within a hospital or practice.

In a hospital setting, conflicts involving the principle of justice may revolve around the use of scarce, expensive, or labor-intensive medical interventions in frail, elderly patients with limited life expectancies. On a national scale, justice may be the central principle in determining whether Medicare should cover a particular procedure or in determining who should have control over allocation decisions in managed care organizations.[18]

Other Principles

In addition to the principles outlined above, there are other ethical principles that are common in geriatrics, particularly in communal settings such as assisted-living facilities or nursing homes, in which elderly residents not only obtain medical care but consider their homes. The principle of *community*, which refers to the duty to balance individual need with communal need, takes on great importance in such settings. Not only is personal autonomy important, but also *individual dignity*, a closely related but distinct value, is greatly valued. Also closely related to autonomy, the principle of *authenticity* refers to the ability to choose a lifestyle consistent with one's own values, beliefs, and habits.[19] These ethical principles largely underlie the advocacy of culture change in the nursing home industry. The culture change movement has as its goals to provide residents more homelike environments and choice over their lives, and to provide staff members the authority and empowerment to facilitate those choices.[20,21]

● In Western society, the principle of autonomy has come to dominate other ethical principles, but this may not be true of all cultures.

Case Discussion

The case of Mrs. Oliver represents a classic conflict between the duty to respect the patient's autonomy and the duty to do good—beneficence—and avoid harm—nonmalfeasance. Mrs. Oliver is unable to exercise her autonomy without the cooperation of the care team in providing her food, but the team feels this would violate the duty to avoid harm. Having identified the ethical principles that are at odds with each other, you must now systematically evaluate alternatives for resolution.

STUDY QUESTIONS

1. How would you go about devising a methodology for examining the ethical dilemma(s) in this case?
2. Is there a morally right and a morally wrong decision?

STRUCTURE FOR DELIBERATING ETHICAL DILEMMAS

There are several models for systematically evaluating and analyzing dilemmas in medical ethics. One of the most commonly used models is the "four topics" model devised by Jonsen et al.[22] This is a case-based approach that allows an organized review of the facts and issues in a given case, according to four topics: medical indications, patient preferences, quality of life, and contextual features (Figure 8-1).

Each topic represents a systematic means of organizing the questions related to the corresponding ethical principles. Under the topic "medical indications" are questions that determine how the facts of the case determine what is beneficence and nonmaleficence. The topic "patient preferences" contains questions that establish the patient's autonomy and how that autonomy fits into the ethical problem at hand. "Quality of life" contains questions that further elucidate what is considered beneficence and what is considered nonmaleficence, according to the patient's own values. "Contextual features" contains grouped questions that tease out other influences on the case and incorporate principles such as loyalty and fairness.

MEDICAL INDICATIONS

The Principles of Beneficence and Nonmaleficence

1. What is the patient's medical problem? History? Diagnosis? Prognosis?
2. Is the problem acute? Chronic? Critical? Emergent? Reversible?
3. What are the goals of treatment?
4. What are the probabilities of success?
5. What are the plans in case of therapeutic failure?
6. In sum, how can this patient be benefited by medical and nursing care, and how can harm be avoided?

PATIENT PREFERENCES

The Principle of Respect for Autonomy

1. Is the patient mentally capable and legally competent? Is there evidence of incapacity?
2. If competent, what is the patient stating about preferences for treatment?
3. Has the patient been informed of benefits and risks, understood this information, and given consent?
4. If incapacitated, who is the appropriate surrogate? Is the surrogate using appropriate standards for decision making?
5. Has the patient expressed prior preferences, e.g., Advance Directives?
6. Is the patient unwilling or unable to cooperate with medical treatment? If so why?
   In sum, is the patient's right to choose being respected to the extent possible in ethics and law?

QUALITY OF LIFE

The Principles of Beneficence and Nonmaleficence and Respect for Autonomy

1. What are the prospects, with or without treatment, for a return to normal life?
2. What physical, mental and social deficits is the patient likely to experience if treatment succeeds?
3. Are there biases that might prejudice the provider's evaluation of the patient's quality of life?
4. Is the patient's present or future condition such that his or her continued life might be judged undesirable?
5. Is there any plan and rationale to forgo treatment?
6. Are there plans for comfort and palliative care?

CONTEXTUAL FEATURES

The Principles of Loyalty and Fairness

1. Are there family issues that might influence treatment decisions?
2. Are there provider (physicians and nurses) issues that might influence treatment decisions?
3. Are there financial and economic factors?
4. Are there religious or cultural factors?
5. Are there limits on confidentiality?
6. Are there problems of allocation of resources?
7. How does the law affect treatment decisions?
8. Is clinical research or teaching involved?
9. Is there any conflict of interest on the part of the providers or the institution?

FIGURE 8–1

Four Topics for Ethical Analysis. *(From Jonsen AR, Siegler M, Winslade WJ. Clinical Ethics: A Practical Approach to Ethical Decisions in Clinical Medicine, 5 ed. New York: McGraw-Hill, 2002.)*

Once the facts of the case are organized, it is important to identify the ethical dilemma(s), if any. Only when the ethical questions are framed, is it possible to formulate potential solutions. Frequently, ethical dilemmas have more than one morally permissible alternative. When asked to participate, it may be the role of the ethics consultant or ethics committee to outline these alternatives. Nonetheless, it generally falls to the health care team and patient to determine which alternative will be followed.

● An ethical conflict may have more than one morally acceptable solution.

What appears at first to be an ethical dilemma may ultimately emerge as an interpersonal dispute among family members or between staff and family members.[23] In geriatrics, patients may have several family members, usually children, who may disagree with each other or with the health care team over decisions, large and small, sometimes making medical management time-consuming and difficult. In these cases, typical ethical deliberation may not always be useful or sufficient. Alternate techniques such as mediation,[24] negotiation,[25] or a combination of these and other methods of conflict resolution may be necessary.

● It is sometimes difficult to differentiate an ethical dilemma from an interpersonal conflict, and one may accompany the other.

Case Discussion

Mrs. Oliver's nutrition may be viewed in a dual manner. Because nutrition is considered basic to life and comfort, the team has an obligation defined by the principle of beneficence to provide it. There is, however, a therapeutic component as well, because the food must be provided in a form and texture suitable to Mrs. Oliver's swallowing disorder. You tell the team that although Mrs. Oliver is refusing the recommended therapeutic form of the nutrition, they are still fulfilling the duty of beneficence and respecting her autonomy by providing her thin liquids, although the risk may be greater. In other words, the duties of autonomy and beneficence outweigh the duty of non-maleficence. So long as Mrs. Oliver understands the increased risk she is assuming, it is ethically permissible to provide her with thin liquids. It is your responsibility, in conjunction with the care team, to establish that Mrs. Oliver has adequate information to make this decision.

STUDY QUESTION

1. Is there another morally acceptable alternative to this case?

INFORMED CONSENT

Informed consent is the foundation for the exercise of autonomy. It has become increasingly central to both the ethical and legal regulation of American medicine and the clinician—patient relationship since the concept was first used in 1957.[26] Informed consent is more than simply the required signing of permission forms before surgery or other medical procedures. In representing the means by which the principles of autonomy, beneficence, and nonmaleficence are balanced and incorporated into medical decision making,[27] informed consent requires disclosure and comprehension of information as well as voluntary and competent decision making[28] (Box 8-1).

Disclosure

The requirement for disclosure is not an obligation for the clinician to impart everything about a proposed intervention to the patient. Some states measure the adequacy of disclosure according to the standard determined by what a reasonable clinician would disclose, whereas others measure adequacy by what information a reasonable patient would need to make the decision.[29] Although this may appear at first glance to be vague, "reasonable" generally means that disclosure should provide information about the goals of the procedure, the probability of success, and the most probable adverse effects. In addition, disclosure should include information about alternative options, including foregoing of any procedure.

Disclosure should allow the patient to weigh not only the risks and benefits of the proposed intervention but also the comparative risks and comparative benefits of alternatives, including the status quo or doing nothing. The information should be provided in a form the patient can understand, in terms of both the language itself and educational level.

Voluntariness

When patients are sick, they are often vulnerable as well. There may be conflicting values, not only among the patient's own values but also among the patient's, family's, and other caregivers' values. It is important, therefore, that the clinician ascertain that the decision is not coerced, that it truly represents the free will of the patient.

Box 8-1 The Elements of Informed Consent

Disclosing Information

Steps for disclosure: Before launching into a long narrative about the decision at hand, find out what the patient knows: "Can you tell me what you know about Alzheimer's disease?" The answer will reveal the patient's understandings and appreciation, as well as misunderstanding and misappreciations. This information is a useful guide for further discussion and disclosure. After disclosing information ask, "what else?" and then wait at least 10 seconds before speaking again.

> ● Doctor means teacher, and consent means to feel together. A good physician is an empathetic teacher.

Assuring Voluntariness

Steps to ensure voluntariness: An environment such as a nursing home or assisted-living facility can impact on a person's sense of freedom and choice. Most people do not recognize the subtle impact their day-to-day environment has on their voluntariness. Open-ended questions can elicit whether this is a problem: "Do you feel like you have a choice?" Give the person time to make a decision (unless it is an emergency).

> ● Remind a person that he or she is free to choose, and give time to choose.

Assessing Competency

Steps to assess competency: In situations in which a patient is refusing what a physician considers "standard of care," a competency assessment is essential, but it can be the source of discord. Reassure the patient that the final choice is his or hers: "I am not here to argue. My duty as a doctor is to be a good teacher for you about your health and the options you have. I just want to make sure I've done an adequate job teaching you." Then assess the patient's understanding, appreciation, and reasoning by using the format of the open-ended questions described in Box 8-2.

> ● Competency derives from the ability to make a decision. Evidence of impaired decision-making capacity may be the first sign of clinically significant cognitive impairment.

From Karlawish JHT. Getting Competent at Assessing Competency. Presented at the 2003 Annual Meeting of the American Geriatrics Society.

Simply asking the patient whether he feels he has a choice or asking how much time he will need to make a choice may ensure voluntariness. Sometimes family members and friends may need to be excluded from the discussion to allow the patient to freely express himself. Overt threats from family are an obvious impediment to the free expression of choice, but subtle coercion or abuse may also occur.

The clinician may also exert undue pressure on the patient, interfering with the patient's perceived ability to express his free will. A patient may be afraid of disappointing the clinician or, worse, of being abandoned by the clinician if he or she does not consent. In some instances, abandonment may not mean the complete exit of the clinician from the clinician–patient relationship but the fear that the clinician may not be fully committed to all the patient's needs should the patient choose to pursue a course contrary to the clinician's recommendation.[30] Therefore, part of the disclosure process should include information regarding the management of the patient and an assurance of support should she or he refuse the proposed intervention.

Capacity

Although disclosure of information and voluntariness are necessary for informed consent, the patient must also be able to use the information meaningfully to render an informed decision. The ability to cognitively process the provided information appropriately and render a decision is generally referred to as decision-making capacity.

Most authors tend to use the term competence as a legal term, referring to the determination by a court that a patient no longer possesses sufficient cognitive function to make most routine decisions. This is usually accompanied by the appointment of a guardian and results in limitations in the individual's exercise of basic rights. The term capacity is used clinically on a case-by-case basis to denote the capability to render a specific decision. A patient may have the capacity to make one decision but not another. In everyday practice the distinctions between these terms often break down, leading to the use of the terms capacity and competence interchangeably.

In geriatric medicine, the prevalence of cognitive impairment owing to dementia or delirium raises difficult questions about the patient's capacity to participate in the process of informed consent. It is important to distinguish between cognitive impairment and impaired decision-making capacity. The presence of cognitive impairment does not necessarily rule out the ability to render all medical decisions, nor is an abnormal Folstein mini-mental state score,[31] by itself, an indication of incapacity.[32]

The determination of capacity should ideally be made on a case-by-case basis as part of the process of obtaining informed consent. A patient, who, because of dementia, is unable to participate in rendering a decision about a lower extremity vascular procedure, may nevertheless be able to clearly express a decision about resuscitation. Thus the inability to provide informed consent for one intervention should not necessarily imply a presumption of incapacity for other interventions. Likewise, the presence of mental illness, such as depression, should not lead to the conclusion that the patient cannot participate in decision making,[33] although there is evidence that the judgment of acutely ill adults may be sufficiently impaired in many cases to interfere with decision making.[34] This underscores the importance of using a systematic assessment of decision making specific to the decision at hand.

> ● The presence of dementia does not, by itself, indicate that the patient lacks decision-making capacity.

The set of standards that has evolved for assessing decision-making capacity includes the following components: (1) *understanding* of information that is disclosed in the informed consent process, (2) *appreciation* of the information for one's own circumstances, (3) *reasoning* with the information, and (4) *expressing* a choice[35] (Box 8-2).

Understanding represents the ability to comprehend the information provided and to be able to restate it in terms that make this evident. Thus it is helpful to ask the patient to repeat, in his or her own words, the information the clinician has provided, so it is clear that the patient fully comprehends the information.

Appreciation represents the ability to recognize that the information applies to one's self. For instance, a patient may clearly articulate information about a proposed procedure, but if the patient then asserts the procedure is not needed because of an erroneous belief that he or she does not have the condition that indicates the procedure, the patient's appreciation would be questionable.

Reasoning involves the ability to use and apply logic to information. This refers to the patient's ability to infer the consequences of a choice and to weigh the respective merits of various choices. The ability to consider the risks and benefits of a procedure or to compare the risks of two or more procedures is an example of reasoning.

Expressing a choice is self-explanatory and refers to the ability of the patient to make and state a decision. The inability to express a choice renders assessment of the other criteria for competency unnecessary, but the ability to express a choice is, by itself, inadequate to judge competency. The inability to express a choice should not be confused with the refusal to make a

---

Box 8-2   Model Questions for Assessing Capacity

Ability to choose

1. Have you made a decision about the treatment options we discussed?

Ability to understand relevant information

2. Please tell me in your own words what I've told you about

- The nature of your condition
- The treatment or diagnostic test recommended
- The possible benefits from the treatment/diagnostic test
- The possible risks (or discomforts) of the treatment/diagnostic test
- Any other possible treatments that could be used, as well as their benefits and risks
- The possible benefits and risks of no treatment at all

3. We've talked about the chance that *x* might happen with this treatment? In your own words, can you tell me how likely do you think it is that *x* will happen?

4. What do you think will happen if you decide not to have treatment?

Ability to appreciate the situation and its consequences

5. What do you believe is wrong with your health now?

6. Do you believe it's possible that this treatment/diagnostic test could benefit you?

7. Do you believe it's possible that this treatment/diagnostic test could harm you?

8. We talked about other possible treatments for you—can you tell me, in your own words, what they are?

9. What do you believe would happen to you if you decided you didn't want to have this treatment/diagnostic test?

Ability to reason

10. Tell me how you reached the decision to have [not have] the treatment/diagnostic test?

11. What things were important to you in making the decision you did?

12. How would you balance those things?

Adapted from Ganzini L, Volicer L, Nelson WA, et al. Ten Myths about decision-making capacity. J Am Med Dir Assoc 2004;5:263-267. Also from Appelbaum PS, Grisso T, unpublished.

choice when understanding, appreciation, and reasoning have been demonstrated to be intact. The latter essentially represents an endorsement of the status quo. For instance, a patient who has carefully considered a discussion about do-not-resuscitate (DNR) orders but asks that the clinician return for further discussion in a week has implicitly consented to resuscitative efforts and declined to authorize a DNR order.

How rigorously one applies these criteria to the decision-making process depends on the characteristics of the proposed intervention and the concordance between the patient's decision and the clinician's advice. For instance, few would argue that these criteria should be extensively applied to the question of drawing blood to determine basic electrolytes. In contrast, high-risk procedures or interventions with complex benefit/risk equations might require a more strict application of these criteria. Moreover, when a patient disagrees with the clinician's advice, particularly when the risk/benefit ratio of treatment is clearly favorable, a higher standard may be applied.[36]

● The process of obtaining informed consent for a given procedure is the appropriate means of determining decision-making capacity.

Case Discussion

To respect Mrs. Oliver's autonomy, it is the responsibility of you and the care team to establish that she has adequate information to make this decision, that she is making the decision of her own free will, and that she is competent to make the decision. Once the criteria for informed consent are met, it is ethically permissible to provide thin liquids despite her increased risk of aspiration.

Although it is not necessary, some institutions may require the patient to sign a written "refusal to consent" form, indicating in writing that the patient is adequately informed about the risks of deviating from the team's recommendations.

STUDY QUESTIONS

1. Is it ever morally acceptable to override a patient's wishes?
2. What can be done if a health care provider continues to have personal moral objections to a patient's autonomously derived decision?

DISCLOSURE OF MEDICAL ERROR

Studies suggest that there may be 44,000 to 98,000 deaths in the United States each year as a result of medical error.[37] A medical error may be defined as a commission or omission with potentially negative consequences for the patient that would have been judged wrong by skilled and knowledgeable peers at the time it occurred, independent of whether there were any negative consequences.[38] Preventable adverse errors may be more common in elderly patients owing to the clinical complexity of their care, the number of medications prescribed, and their increased utilization of health care.[39] This may be particularly true in nursing homes.[40] The release of the Institute of Medicine's report on medical error, *To Err is Human*, focused attention on the problem of medical error and resulted in calls for increased transparency in health care.[41] In 2001, the Joint Commission on Accreditation of Health Care Organizations introduced patient safety standards that included a requirement to disclose all unanticipated outcomes of care.[42] A national survey of risk managers conducted in 2002 revealed that more than half of respondents would disclose a death or serious injury, but respondents were less likely to disclose preventable harms than nonpreventable harms.[43]

Disclosure of unanticipated outcomes of care, including medical error, is widely accepted as an ethical obligation of both physicians and nurses.[44-46] The ethical basis for disclosure involves not only respect for the patient but also support for patient autonomy and maintenance of the confidence and trust in the relationship with the clinician. There is little empirical support for the optimal means of disclosing error,[47] but there is some agreement that disclosure should be accompanied by an apology to the injured patient, emotional support of the patient,[48] an explanation of how the error occurred, and assurance that it will be fully investigated. Although it may seem counterintuitive, there is some evidence that a policy of open communication and disclosure of medical error may reduce liability payments.[49]

EXTRAORDINARY VERSUS ORDINARY CARE

When working with a patient to make medical decisions, clinicians should be cautious about the use of terms such as *extraordinary* or *heroic*. The term *extraordinary* may have originated in the writings of Roman Catholic theologians and refers to treatments that are very expensive, are possibly painful or uncomfortable, may provide an equivocal chance of success, and are not routinely used.[50] This is hardly a rigorous definition, and it is inadequately informative to allow for moral decision making. Treatments, such as dialysis, that were once considered extraordinary are now routine. Conversely, treatments that may be considered routine under usual circumstances, such as antibiotics for pneumonia, may be considered extraordinary in some terminally ill patients. Because the distinction between *extraordinary* or *heroic* versus *ordinary* is not well demarcated, it is best to avoid the terms altogether. It is better to discuss the benefits, risks, and burdens of the possible treatments and to thereby assist the patient in making rational and informed medical decisions. In such conversations, it is critical that words have precise meanings.[51]

> ● When discussing advance directives with patients, it is better to discuss specific life-sustaining treatments rather than globally referring to "heroic" or "extraordinary" measures.

Alice Oliver (Part II)

Several days later, Mrs. Oliver suffers a second stroke. This time, the hemiparesis appears to be denser. She is now confused. The dysphagia worsens, and she is unable to take food by mouth without coughing. As you try to explain possible therapeutic options to her, you realize that she may not be able to understand what you are saying. The social worker tells you that she has three children outside in the waiting room. You wonder who will now make decisions.

STUDY QUESTIONS

1. How do you determine who is the decision maker when a patient loses decision-making capacity?
2. How do you weigh competing wishes among multiple family members?

ADVANCED DIRECTIVES

When it has been determined that a patient lacks the capacity to make decisions about medical interventions, health care providers, family, and caregivers often struggle to determine who should make the decision and what is the right decision. The process of making medical decisions on behalf of a patient is known as substituted judgment. Many states have laws governing who is entitled to exercise substituted judgment when the patient no longer possesses decision-making capacity. New York is an example of a state with no such legislation, thus forcing the initiation of guardianship proceedings to secure a legally recognized decision maker or encouraging the informal, but not legally sanctioned, use of close relatives to consent to medical procedures.

The United States Supreme Court decision, Cruzan v. Director, Missouri Department of Health[52] established a federal right to withdraw or withhold life-sustaining treatment and established that a state can set a standard of evidence for the previously expressed wishes of patients that lack decision-making capacity that is "clear and convincing," a standard sitting between preponderance of the evidence and beyond a shadow of a doubt.[53] This does not have to be written, but it is far more prudent create a written record of such wishes than to rely on the memory of family members or caregivers during a time of crisis. Such documents, known as advanced directives, ensure that the voice of the patient will be heard when the patient is no longer able to participate in making critical medical decisions.

Because it is left to the states to set the standards for advanced directives, it is important to understand the laws governing such documents and how they are used. In New York State, for instance, an individual without decision-making capacity retains the right to have life-sustaining treatment withheld or withdrawn, but the evidence of such intent must be clear and convincing. In contrast, the state of Georgia and many other states have legislation allowing family members to withhold or withdraw life-sustaining treatment for incapacitated patients under less exacting standards.

There are two commonly used categories of written advanced directives. One document appoints a surrogate or agent to make medical decisions should the individual lose decision-making capacity. This may be known variously as a health care proxy, a durable power of attorney for health care, a designation of health care surrogate, or an appointment of a health care representative. The second, the living will, is a written statement of preferences for care when decision-making capacity is lost. Some advanced directives may combine features of both types of documents.

The drawback of the living will is that the patient's actionable preferences are limited to the situations delineated in the document. It is difficult, if not impossible, to anticipate the wide variety of medical situations that might confront the incapacitated patient in the future. This risks throwing doubt on whether the stipulations in the living will might be applicable to the circumstances at hand. Some have even suggested that the concept of the living will should be abandoned in favor of the durable power of attorney for health care.[54] Such documents may include language indicating future preferences, but by appointing an agent who is familiar with the patient's values, the patient allows greater flexibility for the surrogate to make medical decisions when unanticipated circumstances arise.

Although different state legislatures have adopted different variations of these forms, a statutory form or other statement of preferences completed in one state will generally be recognized in another. The Federal Patient Self Determination Act[55] requires health care organizations to ask patients whether they possess advanced directives, provide written information regarding the individual's rights under state law, and educate the staff and community about advanced directives.

Although hospital admission may be used as an opportunity to elicit health care preferences and complete advanced directives, the stressful period at the onset of an acute illness is not the optimal time to discuss potentially difficult choices. It is more advisable to complete advanced directives in a period of good or stable health. Questions about advanced directives and an offer to help the patient complete them should be incorporated into a comprehensive geriatric assessment or the periodic examination.

A more recently developed advanced directive is the physician order for life-sustaining treatment, or POLST.[56] POLST is a document summarizing the patient's wishes for life-sustaining treatment and combines preferences that may have been expressed separately on a DNR form, living will, health care proxy, or other advanced directives. It is specifically designed to be transferred from one setting to another, a transitional period when patients are often vulnerable to errors resulting from inaccurate transmittal of information about medications, therapies and advanced directives[57] (Figure 8-2).

> ● Because patients' experiences and values may change, it is advisable to periodically review advanced directives to ascertain concordance with patients' current wishes, thus allowing for revision when necessary.

Alice Oliver *(Part III)*

One of the daughters presents to you a health care proxy naming her as agent. You tell her that Mrs. Oliver is unable to swallow a regular diet and thin liquids without coughing, a sure sign that she is aspirating. The daughter, invoking her authority as health care proxy, tells you that her mother had already refused thickened liquids and would not want them now. She requests that her mother be given thin liquids because "that was what she wanted."

CASE DISCUSSION

Although Mrs. Oliver had previously refused thickened liquids, circumstances have changed. In addition to placing her at higher risk for aspiration, she appears to be experiencing frank discomfort when taking thin liquids. Her previous refusal of thickened liquids was based on the knowledge of asymptomatic

aspiration when thin liquids were swallowed and, implicitly, on the notion that this would not be uncomfortable. Autonomy is now being exercised through substituted judgment and is conflicting to a much greater degree with the duty of nonmaleficence. After explaining to the daughter that you cannot in good conscience support her wishes if it is to cause frank discomfort, the daughter agrees to the administration of thickened liquids, expressing her understanding that the avoidance of discomfort overrides whatever pleasure Mrs. Oliver might have obtained from thin liquids. There are clearly trade-offs in achieving this resolution, which was made possible by the careful consideration of the relative benefits and burdens of different nutritional options.[58]

Carl Peterson *(Part 1)*

Mr. Carl Peterson is a 79-year-old man with diabetes who was brought by ambulance to the emergency department after experiencing severe substernal chest pain. After developing congestive heart failure and respiratory failure, he required intubation and mechanical ventilation. You have diagnosed a massive anterior wall myocardial infarction. Upon being brought to the coronary care unit, Mr. Peterson's blood pressure started to drop and he became delirious. Despite mechanical ventilation and maximum dosage of pressors, his blood pressure continued to drop.

You have explained the situation to his distraught wife and suggested that she sign a DNR order, explaining that this would apply only if his heart ceased to beat. She replies, "My husband has been through much worse and will make it through this. I want everything done to save him."

The blood pressure continues to fall, and Mr. Peterson sustains a cardiac arrest. You must decide whether to initiate cardiopulmonary resuscitation (CPR).

STUDY QUESTIONS

1. Does the absence of an order not to resuscitate obligate the clinician to initiate resuscitative efforts in every case?
2. Because the process of authorizing an order not to resuscitate is governed by varying state laws, how would the clinician reconcile state laws that he or she considered to be at variance with his or her own moral beliefs?

HIPAA PERMITS DISCLOSURE OF POLST TO OTHER HEALTH CARE PROFESSIONALS AS NECESSARY

Physician Orders for Life-Sustaining Treatment (POLST) First follow these orders, then contact physician or NP. This is a Physician Order Sheet based on the person's medical condition and wishes. Any section not completed implies full treatment for that section. Everyone shall be treated with dignity and respect.	Last Name
	First Name/Middle Initial
	Date of Birth

A *Check one*	**Cardiopulmonary Resuscitation (CPR): Person has no pulse and is not breathing.** ❏ Resuscitate/CPR ❏ Do Not Attempt Resuscitation (DNR/no CPR) When not in cardiopulmonary arrest, follow orders in **B**, **C** and **D**.
B *Check one*	**Medical Interventions: Person has pulse and/or is breathing.** ❏ **Comfort Measures Only** Use medication by any route, positioning, wound care and other measures to relieve pain and suffering. Use oxygen, suction and manual treatment of airway obstruction as needed for comfort. ***Do not transfer*** to hospital for life-sustaining treatment. ***Transfer*** if comfort needs cannot be met in current location. ❏ **Limited Additional Interventions** Includes care described above. Use medical treatment, IV fluids and cardiac monitor as indicated. Do not use intubation, advanced airway interventions, or mechanical ventilation. ***Transfer*** to hospital if indicated. Avoid intensive care. ❏ **Full Treatment** Includes care described above. Use intubation, advanced airway interventions, mechanical ventilation, and cardioversion as indicated. ***Transfer*** to hospital if indicated. Includes intensive care. *Additional Orders:*_____ _____
C *Check one*	**Antibiotics** ❏ No antibiotics. Use other measures to relieve symptoms. ❏ Determine use or limitation of antibiotics when infection occurs. ❏ Use antibiotics if life can be prolonged. *Additional Orders:*_____
D *Check one*	**Artificially Administered Nutrition: Always offer food by mouth if feasible.** ❏ No artificial nutrition by tube. ❏ Defined trial period of artificial nutrition by tube. ❏ Long-term artificial nutrition by tube. *Additional Orders:*_____
E	**Summary of Medical Condition and Signatures**

Discussed with: ❏ Patient ❏ Parent of Minor ❏ Health Care Representative ❏ Court-Appointed Guardian ❏ Other: _____	**Summary of Medical Condition**	
Print Physician/Nurse Practioner Name	MD/DO/NP Phone Number	Office Use Only
Physician/NP Signature (mandatory)	Date	

SEND FORM WITH PERSON WHENEVER TRANSFERRED OR DISCHARGED

FIGURE 8–2

Physician orders for life sustaining treatment. (© *Center for Ethics in Health Care, Oregon Health & Science University, Portland, Oregon.*)

FUTILITY

Futility is often invoked when a proposed treatment is unlikely to provide benefit or is clearly pointless. Others have proposed that the uses of the term futility in clinical medicine are too varied and diverse to allow for a precise definition.[59,60] It is more useful, perhaps, to examine the origin of the term, its possible uses in geriatric medicine, and the underlying need for its use.

The *Oxford English Dictionary* provides one definition of the term "futility" as "the quality of being futile; triflingness, want of weight or importance; esp. inadequacy to produce a result or bring about a required end, ineffectiveness, uselessness." The term derives from the Latin *futtilis*, an adjective meaning "that easily pours out, leaky, hence untrustworthy, vain, useless." The imagery conjures up a picture of bailing out a leaking boat with a sieve. It is an action that not only will fail to accomplish its intended goal but also can reasonably be predicted to fail.

The principle of beneficence, the obligation to do good, infers that actions that have a reasonable likelihood of providing no good should not be initiated or even offered. Alternately expressed, an intervention that is unlikely to achieve its intended outcome should not be undertaken.

Defining the intended outcomes of interventions in geriatric medicine is not straightforward. Within the literature of comprehensive geriatric assessment are studies that demonstrate improved diagnostic accuracy, improved functional status, improved affect or cognition, reduced prescribed medications, decreased nursing home use, increased use of home health services, reduced hospital admission, reduced medical care costs, prolonged survival, or provided comfort.[61,62] The meaning of the term "futile" therefore depends on the intended outcome of a given action.

Another definition of the term futile "refers to an expectation of success that is either predictably or empirically so unlikely that its exact probability is often incalculable."[63] To accurately define futility, one must include a component of probability or chance. Similarly, to appropriately use the term "success" one must couch it in terms of the intended outcomes. Determination of futility involves two types of value judgments. The first is the judgment that the treatment will not provide positive benefit to the patient. The second is that the likelihood of benefit is too small to justify its undertaking.[64]

If a feeding tube is inserted to prolong the life of a severely demented patient who is no longer able to eat, there may be a chance, however small, of achieving that goal. If, however, a feeding tube is inserted to provide comfort or improve the quality of life of such a patient, then it is highly unlikely to succeed. The clinician must define the intended outcomes and estimate the chances of achieving these outcomes. The purpose of evidence-based medicine is to establish treatment guidelines based on the probabilities defined in well-designed medical studies. Unfortunately, such data do not always provide guidance in an individual situation. Clinicians may have difficulty assigning a statistical probability that denotes futility. One suggestion is that futility can be presumed if a treatment has not worked in the past 100 cases and will "almost certainly" not work if it is tried again.[65] There is no consensus about this definition, and there is evidence that as an expression of probability, "futility" means different things to different doctors.[66] Other studies have shown that clinicians assign a wide variety of probabilities to define "futile."[67]

Because futility may refer to a multitude of goals, sometimes perceived differently by patient, provider, and family, there is the risk that wielding the term inevitably results in the introduction of value judgments. Jecker and Schneiderman[68] suggest that even quantitative expressions of probability cannot escape value judgments, such as the worth of taking particular chances and the quality of a patient's life.

When a patient asks for "everything to be done," it is important to explore what this means. Surely, a patient with end-stage heart failure would not request an appendectomy under the rubric "everything." Rather, the clinician must explore with the patient what are realistic goals, what interventions are possible, and what interventions are unlikely to provide benefit.

There are certainly situations in which futility is obvious. Initiating resuscitative efforts on a nursing home resident found in bed in the morning, pulseless, and cold, with the beginnings of rigor mortis is clearly futile if restoring cardiac function is the goal. Repairing a fractured hip in a bed-ridden, severely demented elderly woman may also be viewed as futile if the proposed goal is ambulation. Other situations are not so clear. For instance, the literature on the efficacy of acetylcholinesterase inhibitors for treating dementia is mixed and controversial, with clinicians staking out both sides of the treat/don't treat divide.[69,70] A clinician, who is unconvinced of the efficacy of these drugs, may, indeed, consider treatment with them to be futile, whereas others may consider these drugs to be the current standard of care.

Using futility as the basis for withholding treatments or the discussion of treatments must be done with great caution. Age alone, rarely, if ever, provides a rationale for determining that an intervention is futile, although it may be factored into calculations of risk and longevity at times. Until potential goals of treatment are articulated and understood, preferably early in the course of illness, introducing futility into the conversation is unlikely to be productive.[71]

Case Analysis

Mr. Peterson had already been on mechanical ventilation and the maximum dosage of pressor agents at the time of the cardiac arrest. This is already much of what advanced cardiac life support would have provided, absent the chest compressions. Adding chest compressions when life support has otherwise failed would be highly unlikely to restore a heartbeat, let alone blood pressure. Therefore the initiation of CPR could be considered a futile intervention that the clinician is not ethically obligated to provide. You opt not to initiate CPR and inform Mrs. Peterson that her husband has died.

ATTEMPTED RESUSCITATION AND DO NOT RESUSCITATE ORDERS

The use of closed chest cardiac massage to resuscitate an individual experiencing cardiac arrest was originally described in 1960.[72] Originally restricted to acute care facilities under specific circumstances, it is now widely accepted as a method for preventing death from cardiac arrest.

In 1974, the National Conference on CPR and Emergency Cardiac Care wrote, "The purpose of CPR is the prevention of sudden, unexpected death. CPR is not indicated in certain situations, such as in cases of terminal, irreversible illness." Discussion with the patient or family was not mentioned in the document. In 1980, the conference reiterated the purpose of CPR but noted, "The patient's family should understand and agree with the decision, although the family's opinion should not be controlling." This time, despite the comments about the family, there were no comments about the patient's wishes.[73]

Much has evolved since the original description of CPR in 1960. Because of the success of the procedure in treating sudden cardiac arrest, many cities, most notably Seattle, have promoted training the general population in techniques of basic CPR. Many office buildings and airports now maintain automatic external defibrillators. Far from being reserved for only "sudden, expected death," the initiation of CPR is almost inevitable in health care institutions if specific orders to withhold CPR have not been entered. Most states have passed legislation specifying how orders to withhold CPR can be authorized. In the absence of a DNR order, it is presumed that the individual consents to CPR. Moreover, in many institutions it is presumed that in the absence of a DNR order, a resuscitative attempt will be initiated.

Studies examining the efficacy of CPR are often flawed, resulting from insufficient elderly subjects, differing endpoints, and differing reports on postresuscitation neurologic status. Nonetheless, age alone has been shown to be a poor predictor of response to attempted CPR and should not be used as the lone determinant.[74]

In one study of out-of-hospital arrests, CPR in the elderly was found to be effective only in witnessed arrests that were not associated with asystole or electromechanical dissociation (now known as pulseless electrical activity).[75] A more recent study confirmed this, demonstrating that despite a reduction in success with increasing age, survival was greater for both octogenarians and nonagenarians who presented with pulseless ventricular tachycardia or ventricular fibrillation rather than asystole.[76]

In in-hospital cardiac arrests, age has also not been shown to be a determining factor of success by itself. One study conducted in an intensive care unit (ICU) demonstrated survival to discharge in 7% of those suffering arrests, but only 5% survived more than 6 months. No patient presenting with asystole survived, but of those surviving 6 months, mental status remained unchanged. Interestingly, of the survivors, most stated they would decline future CPR.[77] Another study demonstrated that only nine out of 52 elderly patients who survived a cardiac arrest by 1 week went on to survive a full month, and only five out of 37 previously independent patients remained independent after surviving cardiac arrest. Success was correlated with proper selection, presenting rhythm, and shorter response time, rather than age alone.[78] A subsequent study revealed poor outcomes in elderly patients presenting with hypotension, pneumonia, renal failure, cancer, coma, intubation, pressors, and previous homebound status. All survivors experienced a decrease in functional status.[79]

Survival after cardiac arrest in the nursing home has been found to be rare,[80,81] leading one study to conclude, "We favor a more radical proposal: that CPR not be offered to NH residents."[82] Another study, although conceding that survival after cardiac arrest in nursing homes was unlikely, found that with appropriate selection and effective response, the survival of certain groups was comparable to that of elderly persons suffering out-of-hospital cardiac arrest. The study recommended that resuscitative efforts be withheld for unwitnessed arrests or arrests in which the presenting rhythm is asystole or electromechanical dissociation.[83]

When discussing DNR orders with the elderly patient, it is important to differentiate resuscitation from a resuscitative effort. Because most attempts at CPR are unsuccessful, it may be misleading to discuss "resuscitation," which implies that the effort will be successful.

Using the term *resuscitative effort* or *attempted resuscitation* may be more accurate. It is also important to differentiate the DNR orders from the remainder of the care plan. A DNR order applies only to a cardiac arrest and is not equivalent to "do not treat."

A DNR order is unusual in that it is a procedure that requires informed consent to preclude its use. This presents a potential ethical problem. Although consent to resuscitation is generally presumed in the absence of a DNR order, does this mean that it is also presumed that CPR will always be initiated in the absence of a DNR order? Does offering a DNR order equate to offering resuscitation? Opinions vary on this point, but it is our opinion that the decision to initiate a resuscitative effort remains a medical decision that should be undertaken only if clinically indicated. It would make little sense to attempt resuscitation on a nursing home resident with end-stage dementia who experiences an unwitnessed cardiac arrest and presents with asystole. Likewise, it would not seem logical to initiate CPR on an ICU patient who is ventilator dependent and whose blood pressure was slowly dropping despite maximum dosing of pressor agents. Such actions must be consistent with state law and institutional policies and procedures. Furthermore, clinicians in training and nurses may feel uncomfortable making such decisions and opt instead for initiating resuscitation, despite its apparent futility.

When a patient with a DNR order undergoes surgery, additional issues must be considered. In the controlled environment of an operating room, cardiac arrest is more likely to occur, but it is also more likely to be reversible, since it would be witnessed and managed by a team experienced with such events. Because the likelihood of a successful resuscitation may be higher, it may be reasonable to offer a temporary suspension of a DNR order.[84] Some surgeons and anesthesiologists may even refuse to operate unless such contingencies are made.

Carl Peterson *(Part II)*

After Mr. Peterson's death, the nurses express their discomfort to you for withholding CPR in the absence of a DNR order. They ask whether they have breached hospital policy or state law in doing so.

CASE ANALYSIS

From a purely pragmatic standpoint, it might be difficult for a nurse at the bedside or a first-year intern to make the decision to withhold CPR in the absence of a DNR order. Furthermore, state law or hospital policy might mandate the initiation of

CPR in the absence of a valid DNR order, despite its apparent futility. Consequently, although it may be ethically permissible to withhold CPR when clearly futile, the legal obligation may be otherwise.

ASSISTED SUICIDE AND THE DOUBLE EFFECT

Social attitudes toward the morality of assisted suicide remain controversial and polarizing. In January, 2006, the Supreme court blocked Federal efforts to reverse Oregon's legalization of physician-assisted suicide. The 1997 Oregon Death With Dignity Act provides legal guidelines allowing physicians to provide lethal doses of medications to terminally ill patients who request them.[85] A qualitative study of physicians in Oregon revealed that many of them felt unprepared for such requests and were uncomfortable with issues such as pain management and symptom relief, understanding patient preferences, and concern about abandoning patients.[86] This suggests that few clinicians are prepared to confront this terribly difficult issue, and certainly medical students and medical residents are inadequately trained to make such decisions. Where there is consensus, however, is that clinicians must to a better job in providing palliative care to patients experiencing physical or psychological suffering to reduce the possibility that a patient might have to consider such a difficult question.

In providing appropriate pain and symptom management to the dying patient, it is common to worry about whether dosages of narcotics that will successfully relieve pain and discomfort might also hasten death. In fact, there is little in the medical literature to support the notion that narcotics, when properly used, will hasten death in the vast majority of terminal patients suffering pain.[87] However, in a small subset of patients who experience accelerating pain just before death despite conventional dosing of narcotics, it is possible that adequate doses of narcotics to relieve pain may also hasten death, even if by only a small time interval. Under these unusual circumstances, the double effect must be approached like other circumstances requiring informed consent and should not be presumed to be ethically acceptable in the absence of consent.[88] The following questions should be considered: (1) is the patient's suffering proportionately severe to warrant the risks of intervention; (2) has the patient or legal surrogate been fully informed of all likely outcomes of the intervention, both intended and foreseen, and is he or she aware of all the alternatives; and (3) is the intervention the least harmful one available given the patient's clinical circumstances and personal values?[89]

NUTRITION AND HYDRATION

Whether nutrition and hydration are the obligatory fulfillment of basic human needs or purely medical interventions at the end of life has been debated vigorously in the ethics literature over the past 2 decades.[90,91] The matter is not settled, and the clinician must take care to understand state laws and explore the patient's values regarding these issues. Most importantly, when discussing the possibility of withdrawal or withholding of food and fluids with patients, the clinician should have some knowledge of the medical consequences of the decision. For instance, there is little evidence that tube feeding in advanced dementia improves outcomes such as aspiration pneumonia, survival, pressure sores, infections, or comfort.[92,93] There is also evidence that food and fluid beyond that requested by terminally ill cancer patients may provide only a minimal role in providing comfort.[94] Nonetheless, the quality of informed consent for placement of gastrostomy tubes has been shown to be inadequate,[95] and using terminology such as "starvation" is unjustified and unnecessarily provocative.[96] Whether interventions such as a feeding tube or intravenous fluids should be offered when the clinician believes they will provide little benefit remains a thorny issue. It may be more appropriate to focus on those palliative interventions that will provide comfort to the patient and prepare the patient and family for the end of life rather than offer false hope.

Edward Gilliam

Mr. Gilliam is an 86-year-old widower who presents to your office for a routine checkup. He apologizes for his lateness, explaining that he got lost driving to the office, a route he has driven for many years. His past medical history is significant for hypertension, diabetes, and osteoarthritis. You have received a consultation report from his ophthalmologist indicating a diagnosis of age-related macular degeneration. On mini-mental state exam, he scores 25/30, a decline of three points since the previous year's exam. A report from a neuropsychological exam is equivocal, indicating the presence of significant but mild deficits in memory and executive function. You recommend to Mr. Gilliam that he cease driving. He responds that he has been driving for almost 70 years and insists he drives safely. He mentions that driving affords the freedom to "come and go as I please."

CASE ANALYSIS

When assessing a patient's ability to drive when possibly suffering from dementia, the ethical principle of autonomy conflicts with a potentially broader obligation to ensure reasonable safety, not only of the patient but of the public. There is evidence that self-report is an unreliable indicator of driver safety owing to denial and limited insight,[97] thus throwing into question the patient's capacity to exercise his autonomy. Although the clinician may not have a direct duty of nonmaleficence to the community, it has become increasingly evident that visits such as this may provide an opportunity for the clinician to prevent injuries or fatalities to the public. There is also evidence that although clinicians may be able to identify potentially hazardous drivers, the clinical assessment may be inadequate to accurately identify such drivers.[98] Although laws may vary from state to state, it is ethically permissible and, arguably, obligatory for the clinician to take the necessary steps to establish driver safety or, by appropriate reporting, allow relevant state agencies to make such determination.

CULTURAL AND RELIGIOUS CONSIDERATIONS

Western medical ethical principles are based largely on the perceived rights of individuals, such as privacy, liberty, and self-determination. These underlie the principle of autonomy and, implicitly, its primacy among medical ethical principles. Some religious and cultural traditions may, however, present alternate social norms. Either patient or clinician may come from a non-Western cultural tradition, possibly leading to ethical conflicts stemming from different ethical principles. This may make resolution particularly challenging, given that the usual methodology for analyzing, deliberating, and resolving ethical conflicts assumes agreement on underlying principles. It must be remembered that the extent to which a patient chooses to exercise or cede autonomy is, itself, an autonomous decision. It is important that the clinician keep an open mind to alternative values stemming from unfamiliar cultural and religious traditions and incorporate these into the process of ethical deliberation.[99]

● Do not make assumptions about the patient's moral preferences based only on the religion stamped on the chart.

SUMMARY

Medical ethics provides a moral structure for assessing the propriety of clinical decisions, particularly when patients' and clinicians' values conflict. Most health care institutions now have ethics consultants or ethics committees to assist patients and clinicians in resolving difficult ethical dilemmas. By understanding basic principles of medical ethics and the structure for methodical analysis of ethical dilemmas, the clinician can resolve the majority of common dilemmas that often arise in the care of the older patient.

References

1. Pellegrino, ED. The metamorphosis of medical ethics: a 30-year retrospective. JAMA 1993;269:1158-1162.
2. Thomasma DC. Freedom, dependency, and the care of the very old. J Am Geriatr Soc 1984;32:906-914.
3. Hippocrates. Hippocrates (Jones WJL, trans.). Cambridge: Harvard University Press, 1972.
4. Carrick P. Medical Ethics in Antiquity. Dordrecht, The Netherlands: D Reidel Publishing, 1985.
5. Gilligan C. In a Different Voice: Psychological Theory and Women's Development. Cambridge: Harvard University Press, 1983.
6. Jonsen AR, Toulmin S. The Abuse of Casuistry: A History of Moral Reasoning. Berkeley: University of California Press, 1988.
7. Beauchamp TL, Childress JF. Principles of Biomedical Ethics, 5 ed. New York: Oxford University Press, 2001.
8. Schloendorff v. Society of New York Hospital, 211 N. Y. 125, 129-130, 105 N. E. 92, 93 (1914)
9. Salgo v Leland Stanford Jr University Board of Trustees, 154 Cal App2d 560, 317 P2d 170 (1957).
10. Nathanson v. Kline, 350 P.2d 1093, 1106 (KS 1960).
11. Applebaum PS, Grisso T. Assessing patients' capacities to consent to treatment. N Engl J Med 1988;319:1635-16358.
12. Oken D. What to tell cancer patients: a study of medical attitudes. JAMA 1961;175:1120-1128.
13. Novack D, Plumer R, Smith R, et al. Changes in physicians' attitudes toward telling the cancer patient. JAMA 1979;241:897-900.
14. Keating DT, Nayeem K, Gilmartin JJ, O'Keefe ST. Advance directives for truth disclosure. Chest 2005;128:1037-1039.
15. Tsevat J, Dawson NV, Wu AW, et al. Health values of hospitalized patients 80 years or older. JAMA 1998;279:371-375.
16. Dougherty CJ. American Health Care: Realities, Rights, and Reforms. New York: Oxford University Press, 1988.
17. Garland, MJ. Justice, politics and community: expanding access and rationing health services in Oregon. Law Med Health Care 1992;20:67-81.
18. Emanuel EJ. Justice and managed care: four principles for the just allocation of health care resources. Hastings Center Rep 2000;30:8-16.
19. Kane RA. Ethics and the frontline care worker: mapping the subject. Generations 1990;18:71-74.
20. Kane RA, Caplan AL, Urv-Wong EK, et al. Everyday matters in the lives of nursing home residents: wish for and perception of choice and control. J Am Geriatr Soc 1997;45:1086-1093.
21. Mitty, EL. Culture change in nursing homes: an ethical perspective. Ann Long Term Care 2005;13:47-51.
22. Jonsen AR, Siegler M, Winslade WJ. Clinical Ethics: A Practical Approach to Ethical Decisions in Clinical Medicine, 5 ed. New York: McGraw-Hill, 2002.
23. DuVal G, Sartorius L, Clarridge B. What triggers requests for ethics consultations? J Med Ethics 2001;27(Suppl I):i24-i29.
24. Dubler NN, Liebman CB. Bioethics Mediation: A Guide to Shaping Shared Solutions. New York: United Hospital Fund, 2004.
25. Fisher R, Ury WL, Patton B. Getting to Yes: Negotiating Agreement Without Giving In, 2 ed. New York: Penguin Group, 2001.
26. Salgo v Leland Stanford Jr University Board of Trustees, 154 Cal App2d, 317 P2d 170 (1957).
27. Karlawish JHT, Schmitt FA. Why physicians need to become more proficient in assessing their patients' competency and how they can achieve this. JAGS 2000;48:1014-1016.
28. Connelly JE. Informed consent: an improved perspective. Arch Intern Med 1988;148:1266-1268.
29. Meisel A, Kuczewski M. Legal and ethical myths about informed consent. Arch Intern Med 1996;156:2521-2526.
30. Quill TE, Cassel CK. Nonabandonment: a central obligation for physicians. Ann Intern Med 1995;122:368-374.
31. Folstein MF, Folstein SE, McHugh PR. "Mini-mental state": a practical method for grading the cognitive state of patients for the clinician. J Psychiatr Res 1975;12:189-198.
32. Kim SY, Karlawish JH, Caine ED. Current state of research on decision-making competence of cognitively impaired elderly persons. Am J Geriatr Psychiatry 2002;10:151-165.
33. Applebaum PS, Grisso T. The MacArthur Treatment Competence Study, I: mental illness and competence to consent to treatment. Law Hum Behav 1995;19:105-126.
34. Cassell EJ, Leon AC, Kaufman SG. Preliminary evidence of impaired thinking in sick patients. Am Intern Med 134:1120-1123.
35. Grisso T, Appelbaum PS. Assessing Competence to Consent to Treatment. A Guide for Physicians and Other Health Professionals. New York: Oxford University Press, 1998.
36. Roth LH, Meisel A, Lidz CW. Tests of competency to consent to treatment. Am J Psychiatry 1977;134:279-284.
37. Brennan TA, Leape LL, Laird NM, et al. Incidence of adverse events and negligence in hospitalized patients: results of the Harvard Medical Practice Study, I. N Engl J Med 1991;324:370-376.
38. Wu AW, Cavanaugh TA, McPhee SJ, et al. To tell the truth: ethical and practical issues in disclosing medical mistakes to patients. J Gen Intern Med 1997;12:770-775.
39. Thomas EJ, Brennan TA. Incidence and types of preventable adverse events in elderly patients: population based review of medical records. BMJ 2000;320:741-744.
40. Kapp MB. Resident safety and medical errors in nursing homes: reporting and disclosure in a culture of mutual distrust. J Leg Med 2004;24:51-76.
41. Kohn JT, Corrigan JM, Donaldson MS, eds. To Err is Human: Building a Safer Health System. Washington, DC: National Academy Press, 2000.
42. Joint Commission on Accreditation of Healthcare Organizations, Standard RI.1.2.2, 1 July 2001.
43. Lamb RM, Studdert DM, Bohmer RMJ, et al. Hospital disclosure practices: results of a national survey. Health Affairs 2003;22:73-83.
44. Snyder L, Leffler C, et al. Ethics Manual, 5th ed. American College of Physicians, 2005. http://www.acponline.org/ethics/ethicman5th.htm.
45. American Medical Association. Code of Medical Ethics: Current Opinions, E-8.121 Ethical Responsibility to Study and Prevent Error and Harm. http://www.ama-assn.org/ama/pub/category/2498.html.
46. American Nurses Association. Code of Ethics for Nurses with Interpretive Statements.http://www.nursingworld.org/ethics/code/protected_nwcoe303.htm.
47. Mazor KM, Simon SR, Gurwitz JH. Communicating with patients about medical errors: a review of the literature. Arch Intern Med 2005;164:1690-1697.
48. Berlinger N, Wu AW. Subtracting insult from injury: addressing cultural expectations in the disclosure of medical error. J Med Ethics 2005;31:106-108.
49. Kraman SS, Gamm G. Risk management: extreme honesty may be the best policy. Ann Intern Med 1999;131:963-967.
50. Kelly G. The duty to preserve life. Theol Stud 1951;12:550-556.
51. Chambers T. Having Words with Ethicists. J Med Phil 2004;29:647-650.
52. Nancy Beth Cruzan v. Director, Missouri Department of Health, 1990, Missouri.
53. Annas GJ. Nancy Cruzan and the right to die. N Engl J Med 1990;323:670-673.
54. Fagerlin A, Schneider CE. Enough: the failure of the living will. Hastings Cent Rep. 2004;34:30-42.
55. Omnibus Budget Reconciliation Act of 1990, Pub Law 101-508, ç4206, 4751
56. Tolle SW, Tilden VP, Nelson CA, Dunn PM. A prospective study of the efficacy of the physician order form for life-sustaining treatment. JAGS 1998;46:1097-1102.
57. Coleman EA, Berenson RA. Lost in transition: challenges and opportunities for improving the quality of transitional care. Ann Intern Med 2004;141:533-536.
58. Sharp HM, Bryant KN. Ethical issues in dysphagia: when patients refuse assessment or treatment. Semin Speech Lang 2003;24:285-299.
59. Youngner SJ. Who defines futility? JAMA 1988;260:2094-2095.
60. Lantos JD, Singer PA, Walker RM, et al. The illusion of futility in clinical practice. Am J Med 1989;87:81-84.
61. Rubinstein LZ, Stuck AE, Siu AL, Wieland D. Impacts of geriatric evaluation and management programs on defined outcomes: overview of the evidence. J Am Geriatr Soc 1991;39:8S-16S.
62. Stuck AE, Siu AL, Wieland GD, et al. Comprehensive geriatric assessment: a meta-analysis of clinical trials. Lancet 1993;342:1032-1036.
63. Schneiderman LJ, Jecker NS, Jonsen AR. Medical futility: its meaning and ethical implications. Ann Intern Med 1990;112:949-954.
64. Ackerman TJ. Futility judgments and therapeutic conversation. J Am Geriatr Soc 1994;42:902-903.
65. Schneiderman LJ. The futility debate: effective versus beneficial intervention. JAGS 1994;42:883-886.
66. Nakao MA, Axelrod S. Numbers are better than words: verbal specifications of frequency have no place in medicine. Am J Med 1983;74:1061-1065.
67. Wachter RM, Cooke M, Hopewell PC, Luce JM. Attitudes of medical residents regarding intensive care for patients with the acquired immunodeficiency syndrome. Arch Intern Med 1988;148:149-152.
68. Jecker NS, Schneiderman LJ. An ethical analysis of the use of 'futility' in the 1992 American Heart Association Guidelines for cardiopulmonary resuscitation and emergency cardiac care. 1993;153:2195-2198.
69. Finucane TE. Drug therapy in Alzheimer's disease. N Engl J Med 2004;351:1911-1913.
70. Finucane TE. Another advertisement for donepezil. J Am Geriatr Soc 2004;52:843.
71. Youngner SJ. Applying Futility: Saying No Is Not Enough. J Am Geriatr Soc 1994;42:887-889.
72. Kouwenhoven WB, Jude JR, Knickerbocker GG. Closed-chest cardiac massage. JAMA 1960;173:1064-1067.
73. Paraskos JA. History of CPR and the role of the national conference. Ann Emerg Med 1993;22:275-280.
74. Schiedermayer DL. The decision to forgo CPR in the elderly patient. JAMA 1988;260:2096-2097.
75. Murphy DJ, Murray AM, Robinson BE, Campion EW. Outcomes of cardiopulmonary resuscitation in the elderly. Ann Intern Med 1989;111:199-205.
76. Kim C, Becker L, Eisenberg MS. Out-of-hospital cardiac arrest in octogenarians and nonagenarians. Arch Intern Med 2000;160:3439-3443.
77. Fusgen I, Summa JD. How much sense is there in an attempt to resuscitate an aged person? Gerontology 1978;24:37-45.

78. Gulati RS, Bhan GL, Horan MA. Cardiopulmonary resuscitation of old people. Lancet 1983;30:267-269.
79. Bedell SE, Delbanco TL, Cook EF, Epstein FH. Survival after cardiopulmonary resuscitation in the hospital. N Engl J Med 1983;309:569-576.
80. Gordon M, Cheung M. Poor outcome of on-site CPR in a multi-level geriatric facility: three and a half years experience at the Baycrest Centre for Geriatric Care. JAGS 1993;41:163-166.
81. Tresch DD, Neahring JM, Duthie EH, et al. Outcomes of cardiopulmonary resuscitation in nursing homes: can we predict who will benefit? Am J Med 1993;95:123-130.
82. Applebaum GE, King JE, Finucane TE. The outcome of CPR initiated in nursing homes. JAGS 1990;38:197-200.
83. Ghusn HF, Teasdale TA, Pepe PE, Ginger VF. Older nursing home residents have a cardiac arrest survival rate similar to that of older persons living in the community. JAGS 1995;43:520-527.
84. Choudhry NK, Choudhry S, Singer PA. CPR for patients labeled DNR: the role of the limited aggressive therapy order. Ann Intern Med 2003;138:65-68.
85. http://www.oregon.gov/DHS/ph/pas/docs/statute.pdf.
86. Dobscha SK, Heintz RT, Press N, Ganzini L. Oregon physicians' responses to requests for assisted suicide: a qualitative study. J Palliat Med 2004;7:451-461.
87. Fohr SA. The double effect of pain medication: separating myth from reality. J Palliat Med 1988;1:315-328.
88. Quill TE. Principle of double effect and end-of-life pain management: additional myths and a limited role. J Palliat Med 1998;1:333-336.
89. Quill TE, Lo B, Brock D: Palliative options of last resort: a comparison of voluntarily stopping eating and drinking, terminal sedation, physician-assisted suicide and voluntary active euthanasia. JAMA 1997;278:2099-2104.
90. Lynn J, Childress JF. Must patients always be given food and water? Hastings Cent Rep 1983;13:17-21.
91. Steinbrook R, Lo B. Artificial feeding-solid ground, not a slippery slope. N Engl J Med 1988;318:286-290.
92. Finucane TE, Christmas C, Travis K. Tube feeding in patients with advanced dementia: a review of the evidence. JAMA 1999;282:1365-1370.
93. Murphy LM, Lipman TO. Percutaneous endoscopic gastrostomy does not prolong survival in patients with dementia. Arch Intern Med 2003;163:1351-1353.
94. McCann RM, Hall WJ, Groth-Juncker A. Comfort care for terminally ill patients: the appropriate use of nutrition and hydration. JAMA 1994;272:1263-1266.
95. Brett AS, Rosenberg JC. The adequacy of informed consent for placement of gastrostomy tubes. Arch Intern Med 2001;161:745-748.
96. Ahronheim JC, Gasner MR. The sloganism of starvation. Lancet 1990;335:278-279.
97. Wild K, Cotrell V. Identifying driving impairment in Alzheimer disease: a comparison of self and observer reports versus driving evaluation. Alzheimer Dis Assoc Disord 2003;17:27-34.
98. Ott BR, Anthony D, Papandonatos GD, et al. Clinician assessment of the driving competence of patients with dementia. J Am Geriatr Soc 2005;53:829-833.
99. Turner L. From the local to the global: bioethics and the concept of culture. J Med Phil 2005;30:305-320.

Web resources

1. POLST.ORG: Physician Orders for Life-Sustaining Treatment Program. http://www.ohsu.edu/ethics/polst/index.shtml.
2. Caring Connections: National Hospice and Palliative Care Organization. http://www.caringinfo.org—*Provides resources for end-of-life planning, including advanced directives from each state.*
3. Your Life, Your Choices. http://www.hsrd.research.va.gov/publications/internal/ylyc.htm—*A workbook for advanced care planning that includes a combined durable power of attorney for health care (DPAHC) and living will.*

POSTTEST

1. Dr. Smith is obtaining informed consent from Mr. Jones to perform a colonoscopy, because the patient had blood in his stool and Dr. Smith is concerned that this might indicate the presence of carcinoma of the colon. Mr. Jones is able to recite back to Dr. Smith what a colonoscopy is, how it is done, and that a colonoscopy is performed to look for cancer. He then tells Dr. Smith that he is refusing the procedure because he knows he doesn't have cancer because he hasn't experienced any bleeding. Of the following required elements for Mr. Jones' decision-making capacity, which is impaired?
   a. Understanding
   b. Appreciation
   c. Ability to express a choice

2. George Hall is a 91-year-old man visiting his physician to receive the results of a recent computed tomography scan of his abdomen. He is cognitively intact and still works 2 days a week. He is accompanied by his daughter Eleanor. She takes the doctor aside before the appointment and says, "Please do not tell my father any bad news. It would just kill him." If the physician were to agree, which ethical principles might this violate?
   a. Paternalism
   b. Autonomy
   c. Authenticity
   d. None of the above
   e. All of the above

3. Lenore White is an 80-year-old woman who smokes two packs of cigarettes per day. She is hospitalized for pneumonia after presenting with a cough and fever. On her second day of hospitalization, she asks the nurse to please wheel her outside so she can smoke a cigarette. The nurse feels uncomfortable agreeing to this and speaks to her clinical nurse manager. What two ethical principles are in conflict?
   a. Beneficence and community
   b. Nonmaleficence and justice
   c. Autonomy and justice
   d. Autonomy and nonmaleficence

4. The director of the intensive care unit (ICU) is called to consult on an 80-year-old patient with advanced metastatic disease who presented to the emergency department with hypotension and sepsis. His decision not to admit the patient to an ICU bed should be based on which of the following ethical principles:
   a. Justice
   b. Futility
   c. Nonmaleficence
   d. All of the above

PRETEST ANSWERS

1. c
2. c
3. c
4. c

PostTEST ANSWERS

1. b
2. b
3. d
4. d

CHAPTER
9

The Health Care System

Sally L. Brooks, Michael J. Anderson, and Laura Esslinger

OBJECTIVES

Upon completion of this chapter, the reader will be able to:

- Describe the major areas of federal and state funding that support health services for the older population: Medicare, Medicaid, Title XX of the Social Security Act, the Older Americans Act, and the Veterans Administration.
- Describe and define aspects of Medicare Parts A, B, C, and D and supplemental insurance.
- Describe Medicaid programs and services for the older population.
- Describe the range, limitations, and proportions of long-term care costs paid by four sources: patient and family personal funds, Medicare, Medicaid, and private insurance.
- Describe the nature and purpose of community support programs, including available home- and community-based services and the role of case and care management.
- Describe trends in the organization and payment for health care services for the elderly and apply this knowledge to typical case scenarios.

PRETEST

1. Which one of the following statements about the Medicare program is false?
   a. Medicare Part A is generally provided to persons age 65 or over who are eligible for Social Security or railroad retirement benefits.
   b. Medicare Part B funds physician and other outpatient services.
   c. The majority of Medicare beneficiaries are enrolled in Medicare Part C.
   d. Medicare and private insurance primarily pay for hospital and physician care, whereas individuals and Medicaid pay for long-term care.

2. Recent rapid growth in Medicaid expenditures is attributed to:
   a. The expanded coverage and utilization of services
   b. An increase in the number of persons requiring extensive acute and long-term care
   c. The increase in drug costs and the availability of new expensive drugs
   d. All of the above

3. Which of the following is true in regards to funding sources for nursing home care?
   a. Most patients admitted to a skilled nursing home bed do not use the full Medicare benefit of 100 skilled nursing facility days per episode of illness.
   b. Medicare payments account for approximately 20% of the average nursing facility's revenues.
   b. Medicare Part A does not include a copayment for skilled nursing facility days.
   c. Medicare Part A covers skilled nursing facility coverage without a prior qualifying hospitalization.

Clinicians must be informed about health care funding sources for older adults. Federal, state, and local programs comprise a complex maze that consumers navigate to locate funding for their care needs. Financial constraints influence older Americans' ability to comply with treatment plans. Although the vast majority of health care funding for older Americans is public, many older adults have high out-of-pocket expenses. Medicare beneficiaries age 65 and older spent an average of 20% of their 2003 personal income on health care expenses.[1]

Older Americans consume a disproportionate share of health care services even though they comprised just 13% of the population in 1999. By 2030, there will be 80 million older adults who will account for more than 50% of the nation's medical expenditures.[2] These trends compel federal and state policy makers to explore new ways to fund care and to increase the cost-effectiveness of interventions.

The federal government recently expanded consumer choices within the Medicare program in an effort to address gaps in coverage and improve service delivery. President Bush signed the Medicare Prescription Drug, Improvement and Modernization Act of 2003 (MMA) on December 8, 2003. This act is among the most significant changes in health care funding for older adults since the Social Security Amendment of 1965 first established the Medicare program. The MMA adds a Part D prescription drug benefit, additional plan choices, and new preventive care benefits.

There are five major areas of public funding for the health care costs of older Americans: Medicare, Medicaid, Veterans Health Administration (VHA), Title XX Block Grants, and the Older Americans Act (OAA). Each program has separate funding, unique eligibility requirements and a limited set of services paid through different mechanisms (Table 9-1).

> ● By 2030, there will be 80 million older adults who will account for more than 50% of the nation's medical expenditures.

ACUTE CARE

The system of care for older Americans began with and continues to have an acute care focus with individual access to benefits largely driven by episodes of illness. Medicare, Medicaid, and VHA benefits were designed to provide coverage primarily for medically necessary care. Older adults and the clinicians who care for them experience significant gaps in coverage for primary, preventive care, and proactive interventions. The result is a fragmented system that funds the most intensive and expensive settings while requiring individuals and their families to privately fund less-expensive alternatives. New trends in public programs seek to provide consumer incentives for participation in health care decisions and coordinate care in a more cost-effective manner.

Medicare

The federal Medicare program covers a range of medically necessary services for nearly all persons age 65 or over as well as some disabled individuals (Table 9-2). Medicare traditionally consisted of two parts: Part A for hospital and postacute skilled nursing services, and Part B for physician and outpatient services. A third part of Medicare, Part C, was established as the "Medicare + Choice" program by the Balanced Budget Act (BBA) of 1997 and recently renamed as Medicare Advantage (MA) in the MMA of 2003. MMA also establishes Part D, a new prescription drug benefit that begins in 2006.

When Medicare began on July 1, 1966, approximately 19 million people enrolled. By 2004, almost 42 million people were enrolled in one or both parts of A and B, and about 5 million or 11% have chosen to participate in Part C MA plans.[3] Beginning in 2006 an estimated 25 million individuals will be eligible for Part D benefits, and it is likely that as many as 90% will enroll.[4] All parts of Medicare, including A, B, C, and D, are administered for the federal government by the Centers for Medicare and Medicaid Services (CMS) in the executive branch agency, Health and Human Services (HHS).

> ● Medicare Part A provides reimbursement for hospital services, hospice care, and some skilled care provided in nursing homes or by home health agencies.

Table 9–1 | Funding Sources for Care Services Commonly Used by Older Persons

Setting	Medicare	Medicaid	Block Grants	Older Americans Act	Veterans Health Administration
Eligibility based on:	Age	Income/Assets	Income/Other	Age	Veteran Status
Institutional					
Acute care	Yes	Yes	No	No	Yes
Rehabilitation facility	Yes	Optional[a]	No	No	Yes
Skilled nursing	Limited	Optional[a]	No	No	Yes
Mental hospital	No[c]	No	No	No	No
Community-based					
Physician services	Yes	Yes	No	No	Yes
Adult day care	No	Waiver	Some[b]	Yes	Yes
Congregate meals	No	No	Some[b]	Yes	No
Respite care	No	Waiver	No	No	Yes
In-home					
Case management	No	Waiver	Some[b]	No	Yes
Information/referral	No	No	Some [b]	Yes	Yes
Chore/repair	No	Waiver	Some [b]	Yes	Yes
Homemaker	No	Waiver	Some[b]	Yes	Yes
Home meals	No	No	Some[b]	Yes	No
Transportation	No	No	Some[b]	Yes	No
Home health aide	Yes	Waiver	Some[b]	Yes	Yes
Home health	Yes	Yes	No	No	Yes
Respite care	No	Waiver	Some[‡]	No	No

[a]*Optional* means states have the choice whether to include as a covered service.

[b]*Some* means that some states cover for the service for the elderly, and others do not.

[c]190 lifetime days only.

Table 9–2 | Medicare Plan Choices

	MEDICARE OPTIONS								
	ORIGINAL MEDICARE		MEDIGAP / MEDICARE SUPPLEMENT	MEDICARE ADVANTAGE PLANS -PART C				PROGRAM FOR ALL INCLUSIVE CARE FOR THE ELDERLY	DEMONSTRATION PROGRAMS
	PART A HOSPITAL INSURANCE	PART B MEDICAL INSURANCE		MANAGED CARE	PREFERRED PROVIDER ORGANIZATION	PRIVATE FEE FOR SERVICE	SPECIALTY		
COST	Premium-free for people or spouses who paid Medicare taxes while working. Others may pay a premium to purchase Part A. Copays and coinsurance vary by service.	Must pay monthly Part B premium. Amount higher for people who do not sign up for Part B when first eligible. 20% coinsurance on most services after annual deductible.	Additional premium amount varies based on selected plan, geography, age/sex, and may be based on experience rating.	May charge monthly plan premium (same amount for all enrollees). Generally lower out of pocket expenses than original Medicare in terms of copayments, coinsurance and deductibles.				Individual may pay a monthly premium, depending on Medicare and Medicaid eligibility.	CMS authorizes demonstration programs either via federal procurement or based on a State Medicaid agency's request. Each program is designed to test a new model of care, normally for 3 to 5 years, and may be limited to a particular subset of the Medicare population
BENEFITS	Hospital stays, skilled nursing facility care, some home health care and hospice care.	Physician care, lab, outpatient care, therapies, supplies and home health care not covered by Part A. Some preventive care.	Vary by plan but are generally designed to cover coinsurance and deductibles as well as some services not covered by Medicare.	All Medicare Part A and B covered services except hospice carveout. May offer additional benefits not covered by Medicare. A number of preventive and routine care services not covered by Medicare are generally included in Medicare Advantage plans.				All Medicare and Medicaid services plus 16 additional including personal care, adult day care, meals, restorative therapy, drugs, etc.	
FEATURES	Traditional fee for service Medicare plan available nationwide. No referrals necessary. Some doctors do not accept Medicare. Beneficiaries may get care under a private contract but must pay full fee (no limiting charge).	Automatic enrollment at 65 (if receiving social security or railroad board benefits) or after receiving disability for 24 months. Enrollment is optional.	Standard Medigap plans as well as retiree supplemental insurance offered by employers and licensed insurance companies.	Must see doctors in plan's network. Primary doctor coordinates care. Referrals may be required.	Can see any doctor. Costs less to see doctors in plan's network. No referrals needed.	Can see any doctor that accepts the plan's payment. No referrals needed.	Focused to meet the needs of a special population (institutionalized, dual eligibles or specific disease)	Generally, services provided at an adult day health center setting but may also include in-home and referral services.	
CHOICES	Automatic enrollment at 65 or after receiving disability for 24 months. If not receiving social security or railroad board benefits then must apply.	Automatic enrollment at 65 (if receiving social security or railroad board benefits) or after receiving disability for 24 months. Enrollment is optional.	Enrollment is optional. Insurers vary by area. Guaranteed issue is limited. Medigap may not be an affordable or available option for sick individuals.	Enrollment is optional. Availability varies by area. Must have Parts A and B. May not have ESRD at the time of enrollment. Some plans will offer Part D prescription drug coverage beginning in 2006.		New regional PPOs offered beginning in 2006.		Enrollment is optional. Availability varies by area. Must meet State frailty standards for nursing home care.	

MEDICARE PART A

Most individuals aged 65 or over qualify for Part A benefits without paying a monthly premium because they (or their spouse) paid Medicare employment taxes. Older persons receiving Social Security or railroad retirement benefits are automatically enrolled in Part A on the first of the month they turn 65. Disabled individuals also automatically get Part A after receiving disability benefits for 24 months. Other qualified individuals may need to apply to receive benefits. In 2003, Medicare Part A covered about 41 million people, with payments totaling $152 billion.

Medicare Part A provides reimbursement for hospital services, hospice care, and skilled care provided in nursing homes or by home health agencies (Table 9-3). Most of these services require beneficiary cost-sharing in the form of a copayment, coinsurance, or deductible. Health care services covered under Part A include the following:

- *Inpatient hospital stays* include semiprivate room, meals, general nursing, blood, and other hospital services and supplies. A "benefit period" starts the day of admission to the facility and ends when there has been a break of at least 60 consecutive days in hospital or skilled nursing facility care. There is no limit to the number of benefit periods covered by Part A. However, days 91 and beyond within a benefit period are considered "lifetime reserve days" and are counted toward a 60-day lifetime limit. Inpatient mental health care in a psychiatric facility is limited to 190 lifetime days.

- *Skilled nursing facility* (SNF) care is covered by Part A if it is certified as medically necessary and occurs within 30 days of a hospital stay of three or more days. Coverage is similar to that for inpatient hospital services but focuses on rehabilitative and nursing services. The number of SNF days provided under Medicare is limited to 100 days per "benefit period" with a copayment for days 21 to 100. Part A does not fund nonskilled or custodial care provided in a nursing facility.

- *Home health agency* (HHA) care coverage is shared under both parts A and B. Part A provides coverage for the first 100 visits following a three or more day hospital or postacute skilled nursing facility stay. Physical, occupational and speech

| Table 9–3 | Services Available under Medicare Part A (2005) |

Medicare Part A	Services Included	Conditions that Must Be Met	Deductible (d), Copayment (c)	Reimbursement
Inpatient hospital care	Semiprivate room, X-ray, laboratory, medication, supplies, blood (except for first three units), meals, nursing (not private duty)	Ordered by physician, care that can only be provided in hospital for stay approved by peer review organization	d: $952 for each benefit period[a]; c: $238 days 61 to 90; $476 days 91 to 150; no coverage beyond day 150	Prospective payment per case modified by a diagnosis-related group
SNF	Semiprivate room, rehabilitation services, meals, nursing, medications, use of appliances	For skilled nursing or rehabilitative services on daily basis after a 3-day hospital stay for a related condition within 30 days before SNF admission ordered by physician	d: none; c: $119 for days 21 to 100; no coverage beyond day 100	Cost based on approved cost of each facility
Home health care	Skilled nursing, PT, ST, OT, part-time home health aide and medical equipment	For intermittent (up to 8 hours per day for up to 21 days) skilled nursing, PT, ST, ordered by physician; patient must be confined to home	d: none; c: 20% only for durable medical equipment	Cost based on but limited by maximal approved costs
Hospice	Inpatient and outpatient nursing, PT, OT, ST, drugs, physician, homemaker, counseling, inpatient respite care, medical social services	For care of a patient certified by a physician as terminally ill, patient chooses hospice over standard Medicare benefits for terminal illness	d: none; c: none except $5 copayment for drugs and 5% of inpatient respite care; limited to 210 days, but an extension is possible	Daily fixed rate per case for up to 210 days (patient may be billed for additional days but care must be provided if patient cannot pay)

SNF indicates skilled nursing facility; OT, occupational therapy; PT, physical therapy; ST, speech therapy.

[a]Benefit period begins with day of admission and ends after patient has been out of a hospital or SNF for 60 consecutive days.

therapies are included. There is no copayment, coinsurance, or deductible for Part A HHA care. Durable medical equipment (DME) is covered with a 20% coinsurance.

- *Hospice care* is a service provided to terminally ill persons who elect to forego standard medical benefits for treatment and receive hospice care (such as pain relief, supportive medical, social, and pastoral care services). If a hospice patient requires treatment for a condition unrelated to the terminal illness, Medicare will pay for all covered services necessary for that condition. Part A requires small coinsurance amounts for drugs and inpatient respite care provided by the hospice program.

CMS pays hospital, nursing home, and home care providers for Part A services using prospective payment systems that provide a lump sum payment for care based on diagnosis, procedure, and/or intensity of services required with some modifiers for case complexity and geography. Part A providers must accept

Medicare as payment in full and only charge beneficiaries specified national standard copayments, coinsurance, and deductibles.

MEDICARE PART B

Enrollment in Medicare Part B is optional, and a monthly premium payment is required. Older adults who receive Social Security or railroad retirement benefits are automatically enrolled in Part B on the first day of the month that they turn 65. Disabled individuals are also automatically enrolled in Part B after receiving disability benefits for 24 months. Although any individual can chose to dis-enroll from Part B, 98% of those who are eligible choose to participate. The Part B premium cost is a standard national rate set each year and is normally deducted from an individual's Social Security check. Premiums are increased by 10% for each 12-month period that an older adult could have Part B but elected not to enroll. Part B coverage is subject to an annual deductible, and most services have a 20% coinsurance.

Covered services under Part B are described in Table 9-4. New preventive services such as cardiovascular screening blood tests, diabetes management, and a "welcome to Medicare" physical examination were added in 2005.

Reimbursement to physicians under Medicare Part B is based on a variable fee schedule known as the resource-based relative value scale (RBRVS), which is made up of a measure of the relative work required for different services, office overhead expenses such as malpractice insurance, and geographic factors based on labor costs.

Physicians who choose to participate in the Medicare program must accept the Medicare rate as payment in full. A physician may elect not to receive any payments from Medicare, but this choice must apply to all of his or her Medicare eligible patients. If a Medicare beneficiary seeks care from a physician who has opted out of Medicare, the patient may be asked to sign a private contract with the doctor or provider. Medicare will not pay for care received under a private contract, and Medicare limiting charges do not apply to the amount the beneficiary must pay.

> ● Medicare advantage (MA) plans (Medicare Part C) are required to provide at a minimum all Medicare parts A and B benefits, and many plans offer supplemental benefits.

MEDICARE PART C

Medicare Part C (or MA) is an expanded set of options for the delivery of health care under Medicare. Although all Medicare beneficiaries can receive their benefits through the original fee-for-service program, most beneficiaries enrolled in Part A and Part B can choose to participate in a private MA plan instead. MA plans include managed care plans (which may be offered by a health maintenance organization [HMO], a provider-sponsored organization, or insurance company), preferred provider organization (PPO) plans, private fee-for-service (PFFS) plans, and specialty plans (also referred to as special needs plans or SNPs). In 2006, a new regional MA PPO program was established under the MMA.

MA plans are required to provide at a minimum, all Medicare parts A and B benefits, excluding hospice services (which are accessed outside the plan). Most MA plans offer additional benefits and/or reduced cost-sharing. Benefit designs typically focus on making preventive care more accessible to older adults and provide incentives for beneficiaries to seek care from less intensive settings. For example, hospital and emergency department copayments are normally higher than copayments for physician services or urgent care. The need for prescription drug coverage has historically been the main reason that older adults chose to enroll in a Medicare health plan. Beginning

---

Table 9–4   Services Available under Medicare Part B (2005)

Medicare Part B	Services Included	Conditions that Must Be Met	Deductible (d), Copayment (c)	Reimbursement
Physician services	Medical and surgical services, diagnostic tests, radiology, pathology, drugs and biologicals that cannot be self-administered	Medically necessary for diagnosis and management of acute or chronic illness and approved by Medicare carrier	d: $124 deductible for all Part B services; c: 20% (50% for mental health)	Medicare fee schedule; based on the relative work for different services, modified by office, malpractice, and geographic differences
Hospital outpatient services	Ambulatory surgery services incident to services of physician, diagnostic tests (laboratory/X-ray), emergency department, hospital-based supplies	Medically necessary, approved by Medicare carrier	d: same as physician services; c: same as physician services	Varies by service; outpatient surgery based on average cost, laboratory, and X-ray on fee schedule, emergency department on hospital-specific costs
Independent laboratory services	Clinical diagnostic laboratory	Ordered by physician	d: none; c: none	Approved standard fee
Durable medical equipment	Wheelchairs, oxygen equipment for use in home	Ordered by, physician	d: same as physician services; c: same as physician services	Usually an approved amount for rental fee
Preventive services	Bone mass measurements, diabetes screening and training, mammograms, prostate cancer screening, etc.	Ordered by physician Coverage restrictions outlined in "Medicare & You 2005" (www.medicare.gov)	d: same as physician services; c: 20% except for fecal occult blood test, pap laboratory, immunizations	As above based on site of delivery

in 2006, MA plans (other than PFFS plans) must include Part D drug coverage in at least one benefit plan per area.

Although many younger and working Americans receive their care from employer-sponsored or commercial managed care organizations (such as HMOs and PPOs), less than 12% of Medicare beneficiaries were enrolled in MA plans as of 2004. Medicare health plan membership peaked in 1999 and has declined ever since through 2003. During that period, government funding for the former Medicare +Choice program did not keep pace with increases in medical costs, driving private plans to reduce member benefits and/or discontinue health plans. With benefit improvements made possible by additional funding in the MMA, membership in MA plans increased in 2004, and plans re-entered service areas or expanded into new service areas. In addition, demographic trends may drive higher future MA membership, as the baby boom generation, already familiar with managed care plans, attains Medicare eligibility.

> ● Under the new Medicare Part D benefit, prescription drug coverage for people dually eligible for Medicare and Medicaid will now be offered through Medicare rather than Medicaid.

MEDICARE PART D

The MMA creates a voluntary outpatient prescription drug benefit called Medicare Part D that will become available to Medicare beneficiaries through private plans beginning in 2006. Medicare beneficiaries may obtain Part D prescription drug coverage by either remaining in original fee-for-service Medicare or enrolling in a stand-alone prescription drug plan (PDP) or by enrolling in a MA plan with prescription drug coverage (MA-PD). Prescription drug coverage for people dually eligible for Medicare and Medicaid will now be offered through Medicare rather than Medicaid.

Medicare Part D premiums and coverage will vary based on the beneficiary's income, Medicaid eligibility, and place of residence (i.e., community versus nursing home). Part D plan sponsors may choose to offer the standard benefit design (Fig. 9-1) or one that is actuarially equivalent. Plans will compete within 34 defined regions. CMS will offer a "fallback" PDP if two or more private plans (including at least one PDP) are not available in a region. Deductibles and coverage limits are indexed to rise with growth in Medicare Part D spending. Medicare Part D benefits will be financed through both premiums and general revenues. CMS will also subsidize retiree prescription drug coverage offered by employers, provided the coverage is "comparable" to standard Part D coverage.

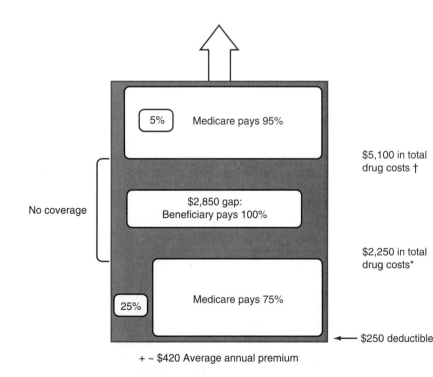

+ ~ $420 Average annual premium

* Equivalent to $750 in out of pocket spending.
†Equivalent to $3,600 in out-of-pocket spending.

FIGURE 9-1

Standard Medicare Part D Drug Benefit, 2006. (*Modified from Kaiser Family Foundation. Illustration of standard Medicare drug benefit in 2006.*)

MEDICARE SUPPLEMENTS

Older individuals enrolled in the original fee-for-service Medicare program often purchase additional private health insurance known as Medigap or Medicare supplement policies. Supplements cover copayments and deductibles for parts A and B services and help make health care costs more predictable. Medigap policies are regulated by the federal government and must conform to one of 12 standard policies that include certain specified coverage levels. Unlike MA plans, Medigap plans are available in all parts of the country and are guaranteed renewable once a person is enrolled in the plan.

As of 2001, approximately 23% of older persons have purchased Medigap policies and another 34% receive Medicare supplemental coverage from their former employers.[5] The premiums for most Medigap policies exceed $100 per month. Beneficiaries who enroll in a Part D PDP can maintain Medigap, but Medigap policies will not include coverage for prescription drugs after December 31, 2005.

HEALTH SAVINGS ACCOUNTS

The MMA authorizes tax-free health saving accounts (HSAs) to be sold in combination with qualified high-deductible health plans. Although individuals must be under age 65 when these accounts are initially opened, these accounts could enable tomorrow's older adults to save for their retirement health expenses, including premiums, deductibles, and copayments under Medicare and Medigap plans.

The intent of the accounts is to encourage individual participation in health care decision making and planning for future health needs. A qualified high-deductible health plan must meet a federally defined minimum in-network deductible and a maximum in-network out-of-pocket amount. The maximum annual contribution to the account is the lesser of the deductible, or per individual or per family amount defined by the federal government each year. Unused funds in the HSA may be rolled to the next year.

The individual, an employer, or virtually any other person may contribute money into an HSA on behalf of a beneficiary. Money in the account is owned by the individual beneficiary and, thus, can follow that person from job to job. Contributions to the account, interest or investment earnings, and distributions from the account are tax-free as long as the money is spent on qualified medical expenses (but funds can not be used to purchase Medigap coverage). This favorable tax treatment led many to suspect that HSAs would be primarily attractive for the healthy and wealthy. However, the premium savings of the underlying high-deductible health plan make HSAs attractive to lower-income employees and to some previously uninsured individuals.

> ● Medicaid provides some level of supplemental health coverage for about 6.5 million Medicare beneficiaries.

Medicaid

Title XIX of the Social Security Act, commonly known as "Medicaid," is a federal and state funded entitlement program that provides medical assistance for certain individuals and families with low income and assets. Medicaid was created in 1965. The proportion of total Medicaid costs paid for by the federal government ranges from 50% to 80%, depending on relative incomes, with the poorest states receiving a higher portion of federal funds. Each state files a Medicaid State Plan that outlines how mandatory services will be provided and additional voluntary services the state chooses to cover. Many states have reduced voluntary services (such as eyeglasses, dental care, and dentures) in an attempt to alleviate budget concerns. States also have the flexibility to expand Medicaid coverage to additional eligibility groups by raising income limits for certain populations. Finally, states can apply for a waiver of one or more federal Medicaid rules to create demonstration programs with elements such as managed care, home- and community-based alternatives to institutionalization, and/or buy-in programs with premiums and cost-sharing. No two state Medicaid programs are exactly the same.

Some Medicare beneficiaries are also eligible for assistance from the Medicaid program. These individuals are often called "dual eligibles." Medicaid is the "payer of last resort," which means that if a service is covered by both Medicare and Medicaid, then Medicare pays first and Medicaid acts as a supplemental coverage. Medicaid reimbursement levels are generally lower than those for private insurance or Medicare and must be accepted as payment in full by participating providers. Many states follow a "lesser of" methodology for dual-eligible claim payment, meaning that Medicaid pays Medicare cost-sharing amounts only up to the Medicaid allowable charge.

Medicaid currently provides some level of supplemental health coverage for about 6.5 million Medicare beneficiaries. Not all dual eligibles qualify for full Medicaid benefits based on regular state income and asset test guidelines. Special categories of Medicare beneficiaries may receive help with Medicare premium and cost-sharing payments through their state Medicaid program. Qualified Medicare beneficiaries (QMBs) are those Medicare beneficiaries with resources at or below twice the standard allowed under the Social Security Disability Insurance (SSDI) program and incomes at or below 100% of the federal poverty level (FPL). For QMBs, Medicaid offers coverage for Medicare premiums, coinsurance, and deductibles. Specified low-income Medicare beneficiaries (SLMBs) are Medicare beneficiaries with incomes less than 120% of the FPL for whom the Medicaid program pays Part B premiums. Individuals who previously qualified for Medicare because of a disability and lost entitlement when they returned to work may also receive assistance with the cost of purchasing Medicare.

Beginning in 2006, Medicare Part D will provide prescription drug coverage for dual eligibles who previously received such coverage from Medicaid. In addition, individuals eligible for both Medicare and Medicaid are eligible to receive a low-income subsidy for the Medicare drug plan premium and assistance with cost-sharing.

A significant development in Medicaid is the growth of managed care as an alternative service delivery system. HMOs or prepaid health plans (PHPs) agree to provide a specific set of services to Medicaid enrollees in return for per person per month capitation payments. These programs strive to enhance access to quality care in a cost-effective manner. Most Medicaid managed care plans offer wellness and prevention programs as well as disease management and targeted case management. The number of Medicaid beneficiaries enrolled in managed care programs has grown from 14% in 1993 to 59% in 2003.[6]

> ● Ninety percent of Veterans Administration medical centers offer long-term care services, including geriatric assessment and case management, skilled and supportive in-home services, and nursing home care.

Veterans Health Administration

Older adults who are veterans may receive benefits funded by the VHA. In 1997, VHA health care expenditures were $17 billion, most of which were spent on veterans over the age of 65. Most veterans are not guaranteed basic health care coverage, as the VHA health care system is designed to prioritize funding for services needed to treat service related injuries, conditions and disabilities. Ninety percent of Veterans Administration medical centers offer long-term care services, including geriatric assessment and case management, skilled and unskilled in-home services, and nursing home care. The limited funds available for long-term care (about 12% of the total) are directed to veterans who have service-connected disabilities or who are indigent.[7]

> ● Medicare does not fund custodial care and offers only limited skilled nursing benefits in the home or facility.

LONG-TERM CARE

The most significant coverage gaps experienced by older adults are found in the long-term care environment. Many older adults believe their Medicare benefits under parts A and B will cover long-term care services. Medicare does not fund custodial care and offers only limited skilled nursing benefits in the home or facility. Such benefits are designed to be intermittent and are triggered by hospitalization. More than a quarter of total health care out-of-pocket expenditures for persons over the age of 65 are for long-term care services. For a large majority of the elderly, the monthly cost of nursing home or assisted-living care exceeds their income.

What is statistically less obvious is the current tremendous reliance on informal caregiving by family and friends. As the baby boom generation ages and medicine continues to extend average life expectancy, our already stretched caregiving resources will not be adequate. These trends mean that many older persons will need formal sources of care in the future.

Medicaid program funds 43% of long-term care costs in the United States.[8] Many older Americans who were not originally eligible for Medicaid "spend" down to Medicaid eligibility as the cost of long-term care depletes their assets. State Medicaid programs are the primary funding source for nonskilled or custodial long-term care. The system has a strong institutional bias because all states are required to fund long-term care in a nursing home setting, while home- and community-based services are optional components of a Medicaid program. More than 43% of Medicaid individuals who are eligible for a nursing home level of care receive those services in a facility setting.[9]

Some older persons have purchased private long-term care insurance. Most policies offer nursing facility or home care coverage that is limited in duration or in total payout. Current limited benefits and high premium costs make private long-term care insurance a good choice for only a subset of older adults and an unlikely solution to our nation's overall funding crisis for long-term care.

Finally, a lack of preventive care benefits and fragmentation in service delivery make it especially difficult for chronically ill and frail elderly to access care that is critical to preventing functional decline or delaying the need for long-term care services. The latest advances in long-term care are those that seek to better integrate care and maintain the independence of older adults who want to remain in their own homes or communities.

● The Medicaid program funds 43% of long-term care costs in the United States.

NURSING HOME CARE

Mary Crane

Mrs. Crane is a 73-year-old white woman who had an uncomplicated, 5-day hospitalization for a total knee replacement and was transferred to a SNF for therapy. On SNF day 15, while demonstrating progress with all therapies, Mrs. Crane suffered a hemorrhagic stroke. She was transferred to the hospital for an additional 30 days and returned to the SNF with a feeding tube, as she was now unable to swallow and required physical, occupational, and speech therapy.

STUDY QUESTIONS

1. How many additional days will Mrs. Crane have in her Medicare SNF benefit if she continues to receive medically necessary care?
2. Has Mrs. Crane triggered another "benefit period"?
3. Given the family's joint income of $30,000 per year from Social Security retirement, what is the most likely funding source for Mrs. Crane's ongoing care in the nursing facility should she be unable to return to home?

Most states have attempted to control overall spending for Medicaid long-term care benefits by reducing nursing home expenditures. Some examples include setting lower maximum nursing home reimbursement rates, requiring higher share of cost payments from consumers, and recouping monies retroactively through estate recovery. States also constrain eligibility for care through lower maximum annual income and higher required level of frailty or disability for older adults to qualify for coverage. Adoption of case mix payment methodologies and limits on the number of certified nursing home beds also reduce access to care for less frail individuals in the hope that they will seek care in other settings.

In recent years, states have realized that short-term strategies to reduce rates paid and the numbers of individuals eligible for nursing home care are not enough to stabilize state budgets as the older adult population expands. Accordingly, many states are exploring strategies for real system change that address the broader problem of institutional bias in the long-term care system.

Case Discussion: Mary Crane

Mrs. Crane has 85 days remaining in this benefit period (100 minus 15 SNF days used in this benefit period). She has not triggered another benefit period, as she has not experienced 60 consecutive days without an inpatient hospitalization or skilled nursing facility stay. Mrs. Crane will likely spend down any savings and assets and become dependent on Medicaid to fund her long-term care bed.

HOME- AND COMMUNITY-BASED CARE

Sandra Meyer

Mrs. Meyer is an 83-year-old woman with macular degeneration, impairing her vision, and diabetes mellitus requiring insulin injections. In addition, Mrs. Meyer has an indwelling Foley catheter that requires skilled home nursing visits to assess its integrity. Mrs. Meyer resides alone and often visits the emergency department for acute problems, as she cannot drive and has difficulty accessing the public transportation system due to her eyesight.

STUDY QUESTIONS

1. Does Mrs. Meyer qualify for in-home skilled nursing and/or home aid visits and, if so, how often?
2. Where could Mrs. Meyer find transportation to her physician office visits?
3. Is an adult day program a good option for Mrs. Meyer?

A broad array of community-based long-term care alternatives are now available to older adults. Initially, home- and community-based services for older adults are often accessed after a hospitalization or SNF stay. Typically, a hospital discharge planner or case manager suggests the need for these services and obtains a physician's order.

In the home setting, a nurse and/or social worker and therapy team assess whether a patient has medically necessary skilled needs. The occupational therapist reviews the older adult's ability to perform activities of daily living such as ability to transfer, eat, and toilet independently. The team also assesses environmental barriers and adaptations required to continue independent functioning. After assessing the patient's needs, the case manager arranges for a cadre of services—within the Medicare benefit—such as home therapies, nursing visits, and home aid services and—outside of the benefit—links them to available community resources. In many cases, older adults lack sufficient private funds for the nonskilled care that is required to live independently and commonly seek volunteer, informal caregiving or other community services.

New community services have evolved, such as adult day-care programs and respite care. As with most long-term care, these services are not covered by Medicare. Adult day care centers are community settings where older adults go during the daytime hours to receive a range of social and/or health services. Most commonly, frail older persons that live with family members who work during the day require supervision that these centers provide. Most adult day care is funded by out-of-pocket payments by the older adult or their family members. However, these relatively low-cost services can offset the need for a long-term care institutional stay.

Special transportation services are often needed for the older adult to be able to use adult day care, visit senior centers, or attend required physician visits. The local area agencies of aging typically coordinate these transportation services, and it is estimated that approximately 5% of older adults use these services. Over time, a patchwork of localized services evolved in most communities, and several federal programs now contribute funding to this growing aging network. Some programs are available if the older adult is eligible for Medicaid, whereas other services are available in the community through the Older Adult Americans Act or federal block grants. Patients' access to such services depends on their geographic location. In some communities, area agencies only have contracts for delivery of services to specific high-risk individuals.

> ● The OAA funds a variety of community-based social services. These federal funds are channeled through a designated agency in each state to a local area agency on aging (AAA).

Older Americans Act

OAA funds are used to support a variety of community-based social services. These federal funds are channeled through a designated agency in each state to a local AAA. AAAs may be housed in government offices or operated through contracted private community organizations. AAAs have the authority to conduct community need assessments and to provide information and referral to community services, and they can contract for creative services to meet specific community needs. Under this provision, some local

AAAs support case management services for community-based long-term care services. In the year 2005, total OAA allocations for programs and activities totaled $1.4 billion.[10]

An example of a community program funded under the OAA provides congregate and home-delivered meals (commonly known as "meals-on-wheels"). Some of these programs are codeveloped with adult senior centers or through faith-based organizations.

Title XX Block Grants

Some case management or nonskilled services for older persons are funded via block grants the Social Security Act. Social Service block grant funds are distributed to states, each of which can determine eligibility and the services to be provided. These funds can be spent for a range of target groups. Thus, the portion of the state funds that go to elderly services tends to be limited. There is also minimal reporting required on how the Title XX funds are spent; thus, it is difficult to determine how many older persons benefit from services under this program. Examples of services are found in Table 9-1.

Medicaid Waiver Programs

Medicaid home- and community-based waiver programs have recently expanded as alternatives to institutional care. The cost of maintaining an older adult in a home- and community-based setting is roughly half that of caring for the same individual in a nursing facility. Federal 1915(c) or 1915(d) waiver programs allow states to receive Medicaid-matched funds for home- and community-based services and case management programs for high-risk populations such as frail elderly, developmentally disabled, or disease-specific populations. All 50 states have one or more of these waiver programs that are typically administered through AAAs or other local community agencies.

A smaller group of states are exploring real system change via integrated delivery models. These states recognize that the abundance of targeted waiver programs increases the complexity of finding the right care, leaves gaps in eligibility, and promotes fragmentation of medical, behavioral, and social services. Furthermore, Medicaid waiver programs each have a finite number of funded slots, and it is difficult for policy makers to see a direct correlation with reduced institutionalization. Long-term care integration pools nursing facility and community care funds to embrace a "money follows the person" concept. In these models Medicaid-eligible individuals are guaranteed equal access to community and nursing home care. In an integrated long-term care program, a care management organization receives a capitated payment to coordinate and fund acute and long-term care services. Some states fully integrate Medicaid and Medicare funding through a joint federal and state administered program. Use of an interdisciplinary care team model ensures that a full assessment of medical, behavioral, and social needs is completed and that those needs are addressed in an individual care plan. This model is also designed to put the older adult and/or their family/responsible party at the center of care decisions and facilitate consumer directed care.

Independent studies of state integrated long-term care programs demonstrate increased consumer access to and satisfaction with care versus Medicaid fee for service programs. These studies also document reductions in avoidable hospitalizations and emergency department visits, with dramatic declines in overall reliance on institutional care.

Case Discussion: Sandra Meyer

Mrs. Meyer would qualify for skilled nursing visits to load syringes with the required insulin dose and for ongoing monitoring and evaluation of her diabetes mellitus and Foley catheter. However, these visits would not typically be required daily, because with prefilled syringes, she can administer her own insulin. Blood sugars could be checked two or three times a week by the visiting nurse, and catheter integrity can be checked monthly. Mrs. Meyer should contact the social worker of her providing home health agency or the local AAA to see what transportation services are available within her geographic area. Mrs. Meyer would likely benefit from the socialization of a day care program; however, her income and transportation needs would need to be assessed.

SUMMARY

Delivery of older adult care is evolving from acute inpatient care during an "episode of illness" to preventive and long-term care services provided in the community. However, funding sources for these affordable services lags behind care delivery needs. It is imperative that clinicians update their knowledge on the financing of health care for older adults to stay abreast of funding changes.

References

1. Centers for Medicare and Medicaid Services. Proposed Regulations to Implement The New Medicare Law. http://www.cms.hhs.gov/media/press/release.asp/counter=1129.
2. Cobbs EL, Duthie Jr EH, Murphy JB, eds. Geriatric Review Syllabus, 5 ed. New York: Blackwell, 2002-2004.
3. Centers for Medicare and Medicaid Services. Medicare: A Brief Summary. http://www.cms.hhs.gov/publications/overview-Medicare-Medicaid/default3. asp.
4. The Medicare Prescription Drug Law-Fact Sheet. Henry J. Kaiser Family Foundation. http://www.kff.org.
5. Trends in Medicare Supplemental Insurance and Prescription Drug Benefits, 1996-2001. Henry J. Kaiser Family Foundation. www.kff.org.
6. Centers for Medicare and Medicaid Services. Medicaid: A Brief Summary. http://www.cms.hhs.gov/publications/overview-Medicare-Medicaid/default4. asp.
7. Department of Veterans Affairs (VA). VA Fact Sheets: VA long-term care. http://www1.va.gov/OPA/fact/ltcare.html.
8. O'Brien E, Elias R. Medicaid and Long-Term Care. Kaiser Commission on Medicaid and the Uninsured. Report no. 7089. http://www.kff.org/medicaid/loader.cfm/url=/commonspot/security/getfile.cfm&PageID=36296
9. O'Brien E, Elias R. Medicaid and Long-Term Care. Kaiser Commission on Medicaid and the Uninsured. Report no. 7089. http://www.kff.org/medicaid/loader.cfm/url=/commonspot/security/getfile.cfm&PageID=36296
10. U.S. Department of Health and Human Services, Administration on Aging, Fiscal Year 2006 President's Budget. http://www.aoa.dhhs.gov/about/legbudg/current_budg/budget-request_table.pdf.

Web Resources

Medicare site: http://www.medicare.gov
Kaiser Family Foundation: http://www.kff.org
Community Living Exchange Collaborative http://www.hcbs.org

POSTTEST

1. Which one of the following statements concerning health care funding is false?
   a. Medicare Part B is an optional program that covers excess hospital costs.
   b. Nursing home care accounts for the largest proportion of Medicaid expenditures.
   c. The Older Americans Act helps fund some home- and community-based services.
   d. Medigap is private insurance that usually includes coverage for Medicare copayments and deductibles.

2. Which one of the following statements concerning Medicaid is false?
   a. Medicaid covers Medicare deductibles and copayments.
   b. States can set a higher income limit for Medicaid eligibility than is federally required.
   c. Mandatory Medicaid benefits covered by all states include equal access to institutional and community-based long-term care services.
   d. Eligibility for Medicaid coverage is based on both low income and low assets.

3. Which one of the following statements concerning Medicare is false?
   a. Medicare Part B covers 80% of the Medicare-approved physician charge.
   b. Medicare Part B covers 70% of approved mental health services.
   c. Medicare participating physicians agree to accept Medicare as payment in full.
   d. New elements of the Medicare program include prescription drug coverage, regional PPOs, and HSAs

PRETEST ANSWERS

1. c
2. d
3. a

POSTTEST ANSWERS

1. a
2. c
3. b

Perioperative Care
Cynthia Holzer

OBJECTIVES

Upon completion of this chapter, the reader will be able to:

- Identify risk factors for cardiac complications in noncardiac surgery and approaches to managing these risk factors older patients perioperatively

- Assess perioperative pulmonary risk and its clinical implications in hospitalized older patients
- Manage the preoperative and postoperative care of the older patient
- Identify risk factors for functional deterioration during hospitalization and management strategies to minimize functional decline

---

PRETEST

1. The most important factor contributing to the increase in surgical complications among older adults is:
   a. Advanced age
   b. Underlying chronic disease
   c. Number of medications
   d. Functional status

2. Which medication reduces the risk of myocardial infarction and death in high-risk operative patients?
   a. Nitroglycerin
   b. Angiotensin-converting enzyme inhibitors
   c. Beta-blockers
   d. Calcium channel blockers

3. Alongside the cardiovascular system, which organ system is the next most important preventable source of postoperative mortality?
   a. Neurologic
   b. Hematologic
   c. Renal
   d. Respiratory

4. Which of the following is the highest predictor of perioperative cardiac risk?
   a. Advanced age
   b. Abnormal electrocardiogram
   c. Emergency surgery
   d. Compensated heart failure

5. Drugs that frequently cause adverse reactions in elderly hospitalized patients include all of the following except:
   a. Antibiotics
   b. Antidepressants
   c. Theophylline
   d. Anticoagulants

6. Which laboratory tests are routinely ordered preoperatively?
   a. Complete blood count
   b. CHEM-7
   c. Liver function tests
   d. None of the above

> ● Emergency surgery increases the risks of surgery two to four times in the elderly.

The population over age 65 has the highest rate of surgical procedures, accounting for 40% of all surgeries, 50% of emergency operations, and 75% of surgical mortality.[1] The increased rate of surgical complications in the older population correlates with the prevalence of chronic diseases and increased need for emergent surgery. Patients over the age of 65 are more than twice as likely to present for emergent surgery as are younger patients.[2,3] Emergency surgery increases the risks of surgery two to four times in the elderly. The higher rates of surgical morbidity and mortality occur with abdominal, thoracic, and aortic surgeries, which create perioperative pulmonary and myocardial infarction (MI) risks.[4,5]

The clinician is often asked to complete preoperative consultations and to manage perioperative complications. Realistic goals of preoperative evaluation include identifying patient factors that increase the risk of surgery, quantifying these risks to determine the appropriateness of and timing of the surgery, providing recommendations on how to minimize the risk, managing coexisting medical conditions, and monitoring the patient for perioperative problems.[6,7] Therefore, the aim of a preoperative assessment of an older person is to estimate, based on an individual's comorbid diseases and functional status, whether the potential benefits of the operation outweigh the potential risks.[6]

> ● The aim of a preoperative assessment of an older person is to estimate, based on an individual's comorbid diseases and functional status, whether the potential benefits of the operation outweigh the potential risks.

Mr. Miller, *Part 1*

Mr. Miller, an 80-year-old man, is in your office today for a preoperative evaluation for an upcoming elective left hip replacement surgery. He recently moved to your community to live with his daughter, and you are seeing him for the first time. Mr. Miller is alert and very talkative. According to Mr. Miller, his medical history includes "a little bit of high blood pressure." He is unsure as to why he is in your office today, stating, "I'm healthy." He denies having a history of osteoarthritis or discussing surgery with an orthopedist.

STUDY QUESTIONS

1. How will you assess the patient's perioperative cardiac risk?
2. How will you assess the patient's perioperative pulmonary risk?
3. What other factors are important in this patient's risk assessment?

> ● Limited functional capacity predicts an increased perioperative risk.

ASSESSING PERIOPERATIVE RISK

Cardiovascular

The initial history and physical examination should include documentation of coronary artery disease (CAD), prior MI, angina pectoris, heart failure (HF), symptomatic arrhythmias, presence of pacemaker or implantable cardioverter defibrillator (ICD), and a history of orthostatic intolerance. The presence of anemia may also place a patient at higher perioperative cardiac risk.[8]

It is generally accepted that the presence of CAD, HF, cerebrovascular disease, preoperative elevated creatinine greater than 2 mg/dl, insulin treatment for diabetes mellitus, and high-risk surgery (e.g., emergent operations, major vascular surgery) is associated with increased perioperative cardiac morbidity.[8] More specifically, the American College of Cardiology and the American Heart Association (ACC/AHA) updated their guidelines for perioperative cardiovascular evaluation for noncardiac surgery to include assessment of clinical markers, functional capacity, and surgery specific risk[8] (Table 10-1). Clinical predictors are based on MI history, angina, HF, and arrhythmias. Functional capacity predicts an increased perioperative risk in patients unable to meet a 4 metabolic equivalent (MET) level during most normal daily activities. Surgery-specific perioperative cardiac risk correlates to the type of surgery and the degree of hemodynamic stress associated with the procedure.[8] These factors can be integrated into a cost-efficient, step-wise approach to preoperative cardiac assessment (Fig. 10-1).

The prediction of risk in patients who are undergoing cardiac as opposed to noncardiac surgery is less of a problem for the primary care clinician, as most cardiac patients will have had sophisticated and invasive preoperative cardiac testing. Even more importantly, such patients are closely monitored postoperatively, usually in an intensive care unit.[5]

Table 10–1	Predictors of Cardiac Risk		
Markers	**High Risk**	**Intermediate Risk**	**Low Risk**
Clinical predictors	Acute MI Recent MI Unstable angina Decompensated HF Significant arrhythmia Severe valvular disease	Mild angina Remote prior MI Compensated HF Creatinine 2.0 mg/dl or more Diabetes mellitus	Advanced age Abnormal ECG Nonsinus rhythm Low functional capacity History of stroke Uncontrolled HTN
Functional capacity	Unable to meet 4 METs	Meets 4 to 10 METs	Exceeds 10 METs
Type of surgery	Major emergency surgery Aortic/vascular surgery Peripheral vascular surgery Prolonged procedures	Intrathoracic surgery Intraperitoneal surgery Carotid endarterectomy Head and neck surgery Orthopedic surgery Prostate surgery	Endoscopic procedures Superficial procedures Breast surgery Cataract surgery

MI indicates myocardial infarction; HF, heart failure; ECG, electrocardiogram; HTN, hypertension; MET, metabolic equivalent.

1 to 4 METs: Eating, dressing, walking around the house, dishwashing.

4 to 10 METs: Climbing a flight of stairs, walking on level ground at 6.4 km per hour, running a short distance, scrubbing floors, or playing a game of golf.

More than 10 METs: Strenuous sports such as swimming, singles tennis.

Adapted from Eagle KA, Berger PB, Calkins H, et al. ACC/AHA guideline update for perioperative cardiovascular evaluation for noncardiac surgery: executive summary. Circulation 2002;105:1257-1267.

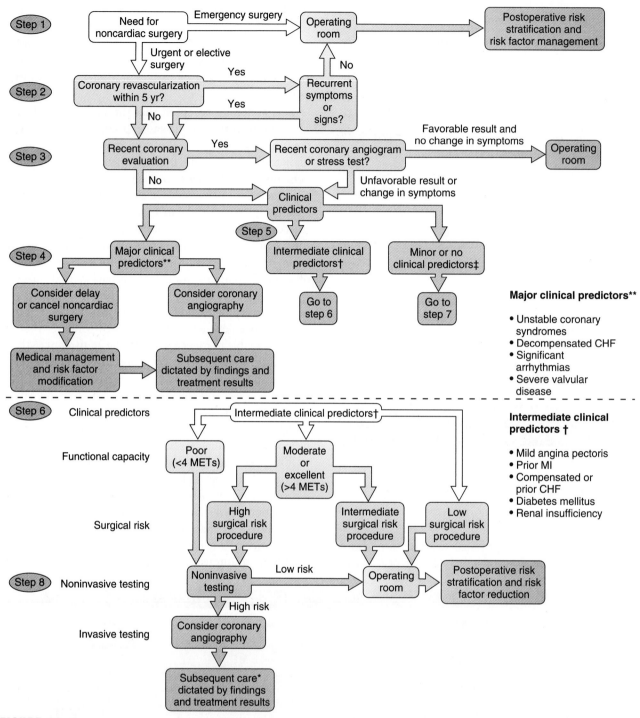

FIGURE 10–1

Step-wise approach to preoperative cardiac assessment. *(Adapted from Eagle KA, Berger PB, Calkins H, et al. ACC/AHA guideline update for perioperative cardiovascular evaluation for noncardiac surgery-executive summary. Circulation 2002;105:1257-1267.)*

(Continued)

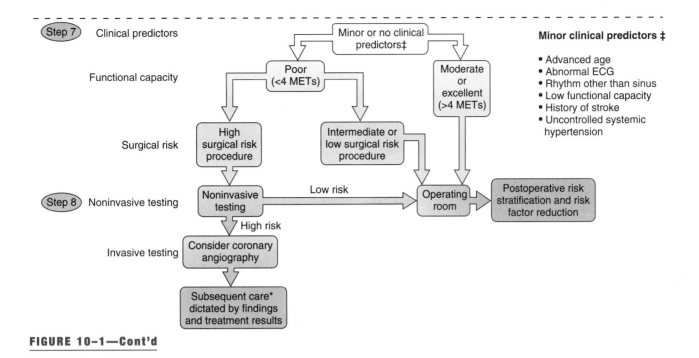

FIGURE 10-1—Cont'd

Clinicians have several options when evaluating patients judged to be at high risk for cardiac complications. The procedure can be canceled or a lower-risk surgical approach selected. If the surgery cannot be postponed, then perioperative electrocardiographic (class I) and hemodynamic monitoring (including pulmonary artery catheterization, class I) is recommended; fluids, inotropic agents, nitrates, and vasodilators can then be titrated to obtain optimal perfusion.[9]

Current studies suggest that beta-blockers reduce perioperative ischemia and may reduce the risk of MI and death in high-risk patients. Beta-blockers should be started days or weeks before elective surgery, with the dose titrated to achieve a resting heart rate between 50 and 60 beats per minute.[8] Class I recommendations exist if beta-blockers have been required in the recent past to control symptoms of angina or in patients with symptomatic arrhythmias or hypertension. Class II recommendations exist for the use of beta-blockers if the preoperative assessment identifies untreated hypertension, known CAD, or major risk factors for coronary disease.[8]

> ● Smoking represents an independent risk factor for postoperative pulmonary complications.

Pulmonary

Deaths from respiratory illness still rank alongside cardiac deaths as the major potentially preventable causes of postoperative mortality. Respiratory complications are common after surgery in older patients, increasing patient morbidity and mortality and prolonging hospital lengths of stay. These complications include pneumonia, respiratory failure, bronchospasm, atelectasis, and exacerbation of underlying obstructive and fibrotic lung disease.[1] Risk factors predisposing a patient to pulmonary complications include chronic obstructive pulmonary disease (COPD), asthma, obstructive sleep apnea, obesity, cough, dyspnea, smoking, and abdominal or thoracic surgery. The most significant risk factor is the site of surgery, with abdominal and thoracic surgery having a complication rate as high as 40%. As a rule, the closer the surgery is to the diaphragm, the higher the risk for pulmonary complications.[1,3] Surgical procedures that last more than 3 hours are also associated with a higher risk of perioperative pulmonary complications (PPCs).[3] On physical examination, prolonged exhalation, wheezing, rales, and rhonchi should prompt further investigation.[1]

Pulmonary function tests (PFTs) are not routinely indicated preoperatively. They should be reserved for risk stratification of patients with suspected lung disease who are undergoing thoracic or upper abdominal surgery. PFT abnormalities that potentially confer risk for respiratory complications and mortality include maximal breathing capacity less than 50% of predicted, forced expiratory volume in 1 second (FEV_1) less than 2 liters, and an arterial partial pressure of carbon dioxide, artery (Pco_2), greater than 45 mm Hg.[6,9] An estimated FEV_1 of 800 ml or more is required before lung resection is performed.[3]

Smoking represents an independent risk factor for postoperative pulmonary complications. Changes in respiratory epithelium and the association with chronic bronchitis are thought to be the cause. Patients with COPD have a two- to fourfold increased risk of postoperative pulmonary complications.

Anemia

Anemia is a strong predictor of death and disability in the hospital setting. The prevalence of anemia rises steadily after age 65 years. The World Health Organization defines anemia as hemoglobin less than 13 g/dl in men and less than 12 g/dl in women. If anemia is discovered on the preoperative evaluation, an investigation into and correction of the cause should be made.[7]

Renal, Fluid, and Electrolyte Problems

The assessment of pre-existing fluid and electrolyte deficits is more difficult in older patients because many of the classical signs of water and salt depletion such as reduced skin turgor and postural hypotension are neither sensitive nor specific in old age. For example, postural hypotension or lax skin tone may exist in elderly patients who are not volume-depleted, whereas a compensatory tachycardia may fail to develop in elderly people with dehydration.[5]

There are no specific guidelines formulated for fluid and electrolyte management in older patients; thus, an initial broad assessment of fluid and electrolyte needs is required and treatment is started on that basis with careful monitoring thereafter.[5]

In patients on hemodialysis, optimization of intravascular volume, correction of serum electrolyte imbalances, and the control of uremia are best accomplished by dialysis as close to the operation as possible.[1]

Diabetes Mellitus

Patients with diabetes mellitus suffer from higher rates of perioperative complications owing to increased risk of infection and delayed wound healing. Diabetic preoperative evaluation should include the type of diabetes mellitus, the type of therapy, the status of glucose control, history of ketosis, and prior surgical complications, especially cardiac or infectious.[6] The physical examination should focus on the cardiovascular findings, including peripheral pulses and checking for orthostatic hypotension and the neurologic examination.

Anesthesia Risk

Postoperative deaths occurring solely because of anesthesia are very rare at any age. The elderly have a decrease in pulmonary and cardiac reserve and a decreased response to catecholamine stimulation. Therefore, the half-lives of medications and an increased sensitivity to anesthetics are important considerations because drug pathophysiology is variable in old age, especially if polypharmacy is present. Be aware of over dosage, as the elderly tend to have a decreased metabolic rate and circulation time. The elderly also appear to have an increased sensitivity to opiates, whether given as part of anesthesia or analgesia, and these agents may also predispose the patient to late postoperative hypoxemia.[5]

Mr. Miller, *Part 2*

After reviewing Mr. Miller's records from his previous physician, you find the patient's daughter in waiting room and further discuss his history. According to the daughter, Mr. Miller's past medical history includes hypertension, congestive HF, COPD, borderline diabetes mellitus, macular degeneration, and dementia. The daughter also states that Mr. Miller has been noncompliant with his doctor appointments and medications since the death of his wife 2 years ago. She reports that her father has persistent pain in his left hip and that this is limiting his ability to ambulate.

Because of Mr. Miller's noncompliance, you perform a complete physical examination and obtain a laboratory panel in order to establish a baseline. Your laboratory studies include a complete blood count, chemistry panel, hemoglobin A_{1c}, and coagulation studies. You also perform a mini-mental status evaluation (MMSE) examination to screen for the severity of his dementia.

STUDY QUESTIONS

1. How does the updated past medical history affect your patient management?
2. Which areas of the history need to be specifically assessed?
3. How will you prevent the complications of his chronic medical problems perioperatively?

● Most preoperative laboratory tests are ordered without a clear indication, and when laboratory abnormalities are discovered, it often does not lead to changes in perioperative care.

Table 10–2 Preoperative Evaluation and Management

Evaluation	Management
Careful history and physical examination	Obtain history from caregiver if the patient has dementia Accurate BP and murmur evaluation
Laboratory evaluation	If symptoms prevail
Medication review	Avoid medications listed in Table 10-3
Cognitive, social, and functional assessment	Perform MMSE Determine decision making ability ADL assessment Emphasis on the availability of postoperative support
Nutritional assessment	Calculate body mass index Albumin level Perioperative nutritional support
Chronic obstructive lung disease	Smoking cessation Incentive spirometry Bronchodilators Antibiotics Steroids
Congestive heart failure	ACE inhibitor ARBs Diuretics Beta-blockers Digoxin
Hypertension	Blood pressure less than 200/110 mm Hg Beta-blockers
Deep venous thrombosis	Anticoagulation (see Table 10-4)
Anticoagulation management	See Table 10-5
Diabetes mellitus	Glucose less than 200 mg/dl
Endocarditis	Antibiotic prophylaxis
Anemia	Transfuse for hemoglobin less than 8 mg/dl Define and correct cause

BP indicates blood pressure; MMSE, mini-mental state examination; ADL, activity of daily living; ACE, angiotensin-converting enzyme; ARB, angiotensin receptor blocker.

PREOPERATIVE MANAGEMENT

Table 10-2 is a summary of the preoperative evaluation and management of the older patient.

History and Physical Examination

The history and physical examination should include information about the patient's current condition requiring surgery, any past surgical procedures, and the patient's experience with anesthesia. Allergies to latex should be documented. The clinician should inquire about chronic medical problems, particularly those involving the heart and lungs, and document the patient's self-reported exercise tolerance. A complete review of systems in conjunction with the medical history will help identify risk factors for perioperative complications. Informants should be sought out for further data if cognitive impairment is significant.[3]

Systolic blood pressure should be confirmed by palpation, because an auscultatory gap is often present in older patients with stiff vessels and systolic hypertension. Also, systolic ejection murmurs at the base of the heart may represent aortic valve cusp sclerosis rather than hemodynamically significant valvular obstruction. Because of the potential impact on perioperative management, the nature of a murmur should be established before elective noncardiac surgery. Echocardiography and Doppler studies may be necessary to establish a diagnosis, particularly when murmurs are long, late peaking, or transmitted to the carotids.[9, 10]

Many studies have shown that most preoperative laboratory tests are ordered without a clear indication. Moreover, when laboratory abnormalities are discovered, it often does not lead to changes in perioperative care. Thus, laboratory testing should be individualized. Most tests should be justified by a specific symptom, sign, or diagnosis identified during the patient's

Box 10–1	Drugs that Frequently Cause Adverse Reactions in Older Hospital Patients

- Antibiotics
- Theophylline preparations
- Sedative hypnotics
- Analgesics
- Digoxin
- Anticholinergics
- Antiarrhythmics
- Antiseizure medications
- Antihypertensives
- Blood products
- Anticoagulants
- Antihistamines

Adapted from Jahnigen DW. Hospital care. In Primary Care Geriatrics: A Case-Based Approach. (Ham RJ, Sloane PD, eds.). St. Louis: Mosby Yearbook, 1997.

history and physical.[11] However, a hemoglobin level is useful in identifying anemia and providing a baseline, which can be helpful postoperatively for surgeries with potential hemorrhagic complications.[3]

Medication Review

The initial preoperative encounter provides an ideal opportunity to review medications the patient is receiving and eliminate those that have no clear benefit or might contribute to complications (Box 10-1). Table 10-3 includes common perioperative medications and the appropriate timing of discontinuation.

Provisions must be made to continue essential medications throughout the perioperative period. Patients on antiepileptic, cardiovascular, and antihypertensive drugs can take their morning dose with small sips of water several hours before surgery; then appropriate parenteral alternatives should be used until oral intake is resumed. Abrupt discontinuation of beta-blockers and clonidine should be avoided; intravenous propranolol and transdermal clonidine are useful to prevent withdrawal syndromes if patients cannot ingest anything for more than 24 hours. Stable diabetics on insulin should receive one-half of their usual dose of intermediate-acting insulin subcutaneously on the morning of surgery and be provided with 5% dextrose intravenously. Patients at risk for adrenal suppression due to recent chronic corticosteroid use should receive stress coverage (e.g., hydrocortisone 100 mg intravenously every 6 hours) beginning the night before surgery, tapering to the usual maintenance dose of steroid after 3 to 5 days.[9]

Cognitive, Functional, and Social Assessment

The medical interview should also assess physical function, cognitive ability, competency, and the availability of social supports. Because impaired cognition identifies patients at risk for postoperative delirium, mortality, and prolonged hospitalization, preoperative mental status should be determined with a brief, screening mental status examination. It is important to differentiate impaired cognition from the decision-making ability to provide consent for surgery. Decision-making ability requires directly assessing the patient's ability to communicate his or her understanding of the risks, benefits, and consequences of a proposed surgical procedure and its alternatives.[9]

An important predictor of postoperative complications is preoperative functional status. The ability to perform the activities of daily living (ADLs) has been correlated with postoperative mortality and morbidity. In one study, patients identified as inactive were shown to have a higher incidence of all major surgical complications.[7] Another study targeted six conditions as markers for general functional decline in the hospitalized elderly. These conditions included pressure ulcers, poor nutrition, incontinence (urinary or fecal), confusion (delirium or dementia), evidence of falls or functional decline (e.g., impairment in mobility, ADLs), and sleep disturbances. These conditions were selected because they are common in hospitalized elderly patients and are associated with increased mortal-

Table 10–3	Common Medications and Time of Discontinuation Preoperatively	
Medication	**Potential Complication**	**Time of Discontinuation**
Aspirin	Perioperative hemorrhage	At least 7 days before surgery
Thienopyridine derivatives	Postoperative bleeding	At least 7 days before surgery
Nonsteroidal anti-inflammatories	Perioperative bleeding	At least 48 hours before surgery[a]
Anticholinergics	Postoperative delirium	Day of surgery
Benzodiazepines	Perioperative sedation, postoperative delirium	Slow taper before surgery
Diuretics	Dehydration, electrolyte imbalance	At least 48 hours before surgery
Oral hypoglycemics	Hypoglycemia	Evening before surgery

[a]Discontinuation of nonsteroidal anti-inflammatories (NSAIDs) is based on the half-life of the specific NSAID. The majority of NSAIDs are discontinued 48 hours before the procedure. However, meloxicam, nabumetone, and naproxen are discontinued 4 to 5 days prior.

ity, length of stay, need for home services, and nursing home placement.[12]

Another important aspect of history taking includes assessment of the availability of postoperative care and support. Beause patients with few family or friends are at risk for functional decline after surgery, the availability of supports should be determined. Elderly patients at risk because of poor physical function, impaired cognition, or few social supports may benefit from further evaluation by a social worker with experience in geriatrics.[9]

> ● Preoperative nutritional support should be considered in severely malnourished patients if a delay in surgery will not worsen the expected outcome.

Nutritional Assessment

A preoperative nutritional evaluation should assess any risk factors for malnutrition found during the history and physical examination (see Chapter 26). Malnutrition impairs wound healing and increases postoperative complications, thereby worsening surgical morbidity and mortality. History taking should emphasize any change in appetite, weight loss, poor dentition, vomiting, and diarrhea. Prior history of surgical procedures, particularly gastric or bowel resection, is also pertinent.

Preoperative nutritional support should be considered in severely malnourished patients if delays in surgery are not anticipated to worsen outcome. A period of 2 weeks of nutritional support is advisable before elective surgery. Oral supplementation is probably adequate as nasogastric feeding is tolerated poorly. Parenteral feeding should be used only as a last resort for patients with altered gastrointestinal tract function.[2] Avoid long periods of nothing by mouth before surgery. Fasting creates a metabolic environment that intensifies preoperative stress.[7]

> ● Patients who are identified as having chronic obstructive lung disease should begin measures to reduce PPCs *prior* to surgery.

Prevention of Perioperative Complications

CHRONIC OBSTRUCTIVE LUNG DISEASE

Patients who are identified as having chronic obstructive lung disease should begin measures to reduce PPCs before surgery. Smoking is the strongest risk factor for obstructive lung disease. Although smoking cessation leads to beneficial physiologic effects in only 48 hours, the risk for PPCs declines only after 8 weeks of preoperative cessation.[3] The use of transdermal nicotine replacement is helpful to alleviate symptoms of withdrawal.[6]

The basis of pulmonary risk reduction is lung expansion.[3] Other important measures to reduce pulmonary complications include preoperative education in the importance of deep-breathing maneuvers, coughing, and use of incentive spirometry; bronchodilators; and, where appropriate, antibiotics and steroids. It is generally accepted that incentive spirometry be performed for 15 minutes four times per day preoperatively and continued 3 to 5 days postoperatively. Bronchodilators are indicated in the presence of wheezing. Short courses of oral steroids may be required and do not increase the incidence of infection.[3] When feasible, surgery should be delayed and treatment with antibiotics instituted for 1 to 2 weeks in those patients with a new productive cough.[6] Chest physiotherapy may provoke bronchospasm in some patients, so it should be limited to patients producing more than 30 ml sputum daily or those with lobar atelectasis.[9]

CONGESTIVE HEART FAILURE

The ACC/AHA Task Force has characterized decompensated congestive HF as a major predictor of increased perioperative cardiac risk and compensated congestive HF as an intermediate predictor. Preoperative management with angiotensin-converting enzyme (ACE) inhibitors, angiotensin receptor blockers (ARBs), spironolactone, beta-blockers, and digoxin may be necessary to stabilize the patient before surgery.[13] Care must be taken to avoid diuretic-induced volume depletion, renal dysfunction, and electrolyte abnormalities, especially hypokalemia and hypomagnesemia.

HYPERTENSION

Blood pressure should be well controlled before elective surgery. Patients with elevated preoperative blood pressure appear to be more prone to experience significant fluctuations in intraoperative blood pressure and associated myocardial ischemia.[6,10] The finding of mild or moderate preoperative hypertension in the absence of associated cardiovascular or metabolic abnormalities should not necessitate delay of surgery. Surgery can be performed if the patient's diastolic blood pressure is 110 mm Hg or less and the systolic blood pressure is 200 mm Hg or less. Higher blood pressures should be controlled, preferably for 2 to 4 weeks, before proceeding with surgery. If surgery is urgent, then preoperative blood pressure control can usually be achieved in minutes or hours with the use of IV beta-blockers, calcium channel blockers, nitroglycerin, and nitroprusside.[3,10]

Table 10–4 | Deep Venous Thrombosis Prophylaxis According to Procedure

Procedure	Prophylaxis
Low- to moderate-risk general surgery	Elastic stockings plus LDUH 5000 units subcutaneously 2 hours before surgery and q12 hours after surgery
Higher-risk general surgery	LDUH every 8 hours or LMWH every 12 hours and/or IPC devices
Total hip replacement	LMWH or Warfarin (adjust INR 2.0 to 3.0) or Dose-adjusted heparin
Total knee replacement	LMWH or IPC devices
Hip fracture repair	LMWH or Warfarin plus IPC

LDUH indicates low-dose unfractionated heparin; LMWH, low-molecular-weight heparin; IPC, intermittent pneumatic compression; INR, international ratio.

DEEP VENOUS THROMBOSIS/PULMONARY EMBOLISM

Risk for deep venous thrombosis (DVT) increases with age and is high in certain procedures commonly performed in older persons. The risk of thromboembolic complications in total hip replacement has been reported to be as high as 20% to 50%.[7] The incidence of pulmonary embolism is twice as high in orthopedic procedures and five times as high for patients over age 85 years. Thus, appropriate DVT prophylaxis should always be provided (Table 10-4).

ANTICOAGULATION MANAGEMENT

For patients with prosthetic heart valves or atrial fibrillation who are on chronic anticoagulation, consideration must be given to stopping anticoagulation in the perioperative period. This must balance the risks of thrombosis versus the risks of bleeding. In almost all cases, patients must have normal to near-normal coagulation studies during the surgical procedure[1,6,11] (Table 10-5).

DIABETES

Preoperatively, glucose levels should be lower than 200 mg/dl. Elective surgery should be postponed in patients that have poor glucose control (glucose greater than 300 mg/dl). For emergency surgery, optimal control can be achieved rapidly while monitoring the patient's volume status. The primary goal of perioperative control is to avoid ketosis and maintain levels of glucose between 100 and 200 mg/dl with sliding-scale subcutaneous or constant intravenous infusion of short-acting, regular insulin. Slightly higher blood sugar levels are preferable to hypoglycemia.[9]

Type I diabetics always require insulin perioperatively to prevent ketoacidosis, even if the addition of glucose is necessary to allow the administration of insulin without hypoglycemia. Type II diabetics may require insulin perioperatively, especially if their diabetes is usually controlled with insulin and if they are undergoing major surgery.[6] Insulin can be given subcutaneously at approximately 50% of the patient's usual dose or by an intravenous infusion at approximately 1 unit per hour. Dextrose must be given along with the insulin while the patient is not allowed to take anything by mouth (NPO) to avoid hypoglycemia.

Table 10–5 | Anticoagulation Management

Risk of Thrombosis	Management
Low	Discontinue warfarin 5 days before surgery Allow INR to fall below 1.5 No preoperative heparin therapy is required Resume warfarin 12 to 24 hours postoperatively
Medium	Discontinue warfarin 4 days before surgery Allow warfarin to fall below 1.5 Use intravenous heparin if warfarin cannot be resumed within 48 hours
High	Requires concomitant heparin therapy Discontinue warfarin 4 days before surgery When INR is less than 2.0, the patient should begin heparin anticoagulation Postoperatively heparin therapy should again be reinstated 12 to 24 hours after the procedure if the bleeding risk has resolved

INR indicates international ratio. In low- and moderate-risk patients, venous thromboembolism prophylaxis should still be utilized in the perioperative period until the INR is greater than 2.0.

Adapted from Richardson JD, Cocanour CS, Kern JA. Perioperative risk assessment in elderly and high-risk patients. J Am Coll Surg 2004;199:132-146.

Serum glucose is monitored every 2 to 4 hours during surgery and while NPO.[6]

For patients who are controlled with oral agents, these drugs must be discontinued at least 1 day before surgery and 3 days preoperatively for the longer-acting chlorpropamide. Glucose can be measured every 6 hours, and regular insulin can be given for glucose levels greater than 250 mg/dl on an as-needed basis. The oral agent should then be resumed when the patient returns to a baseline diet.[6]

ENDOCARDITIS

Endocarditis is increasingly a problem of the elderly, owing to the high prevalence of degenerative valvular disease and the large numbers of older patients undergoing oral, bowel, urinary, biliary, and pulmonary procedures, which can result in bacteremia. Antibiotic prophylaxis, as recommended by the AHA, is important for patients with native valve lesions and those who have had prosthetic valve replacement.

ANEMIA

There are very few randomized trials that study when to transfuse patients in the perioperative setting. The threshold for transfusion should be based on factors such as the presence of cardiopulmonary disease, active bleeding, hypoxia, dyspnea, tachycardia, and older age. There is not an absolute hemoglobin that requires transfusion, although most patients require transfusion for a hemoglobin less than 8 mg/dl, especially in the setting of cardiac disease and/or surgery that will lead to significant blood loss. Routine postoperative iron supplementation is not recommended.[6,9]

Mr. Miller, *Part 3*

After completing your preoperative evaluation, you continue Mr. Miller on all of his previous medications. Mr. Miller's MMSE score was 25 out of 30, indicating that he is in the early stages of his dementia. His chronic medical problems are stable, and his laboratory work is within normal limits. You "medically clear" Mr. Miller for a hemi-arthroplasty of his left hip. Ten days later Mr. Miller is admitted to hospital for the hip replacement. The surgery goes smoothly, and after his procedure, he is taken to the postoperative care unit in "stable" condition. Upon arrival to the surgical floor, Mr. Miller is grimacing, agitated, and found to have a low-grade temperature.

STUDY QUESTIONS

1. What are the likely causes of Mr. Miller's postoperative symptoms and how can they be managed?
2. What other factors should be addressed during Mr. Miller's postoperative management?

● Adequate postoperative analgesia is critical as it has been shown to significantly decrease cardiovascular and pulmonary complications and mortality.

POSTOPERATIVE MANAGEMENT

Important areas to address during the postoperative period are listed in Box 10-2.

Box 10-2   Postoperative Management

- Provide effective pain management
- Encourage early mobilization
- Prevent pressure ulcers
- Remove urinary catheters
- Prevent delirium and recognize delirium if it occurs
- Encourage patient to perform activities of daily living
- Be alert for cardiac ischemia
- Manage postoperative hypertension
- Search for underlying causes of postoperative arrhythmias
- Provide adequate oxygen therapy to prevent hypoxemia
- Be suspicious for venous thromboembolism

Pain Management

Studies have documented that in hospitalized patients, older age is associated with less aggressive pain treatment and the resulting stress may worsen survival rates.[14] Pain management should be addressed early in the postoperative period. Pain is known to cause tachycardia, increase myocardial oxygen consumption, and may lead to myocardial ischemia. The anticipation that moving will worsen pain leads to splinting, resulting in poor inspiratory effort, atelectasis, pneumonia, and immobility.[7] Thus, adequate postoperative analgesia is critical, because it has been shown to significantly decrease cardiovascular and pulmonary complications and mortality (see Chapter 26).

Postoperative patients should be directly questioned about their pain at frequent intervals (not less than every 2 to 3 hours for the first 24 hours). Analgesics should be given on a regular schedule rather than "as needed."[6,9] Nonsteroidal anti-inflammatory agents may present increased hazards in the elderly because of nephrotoxicity, fluid retention, and risk for gastric irritation. Meperidine should be avoided in older persons because its metabolite, normeperidine, has considerable central nervous system toxicity and can accumulate when renal insufficiency is present. Patients with intact cognition should be considered for patient-controlled analgesia, which has been shown to provide significantly better pain relief and lower risk of postoperative confusion and pulmonary complications than intramuscular narcotic dosing.[5,9]

Mobilization

Early mobilization from bed is vital in order to reduce the risk of venous thromboembolism (VTE) and to prevent loss of the ability to walk. Bed rest leads to cardiovascular deconditioning, increased risk of orthostatic hypotension, decreased coordination and balance, loss of muscle mass (as much as 5% per day), and joint contractures, all of which threaten independent ambulation. Recumbency also contributes to urinary retention, fecal impaction, atelectasis, and pneumonia. Range of motion exercises and maintenance of upright position (e.g., sitting in chair) can reduce the severity and frequency of these complications.[9]

Pressure Ulcers

Pressure ulcers are a significant source of morbidity and mortality for postoperative patients. Age, length of surgery, nutritional status, and type of surgery are all potential risk factors.[2] Potential complications of ulcers include sepsis, cellulitis, and osteomyelitis. Frequent repositioning and early mobility will prevent against the ulcer forming properties of pressure, friction, and shear (see Chapter 28).

Urinary Catheters

Indwelling catheters are often used to manage the voiding problems that frequently accompany surgery in the elderly. However, catheters predispose to urinary tract infection and Gram-negative sepsis. In general, use of catheters beyond 48 hours should be avoided except when urinary retention cannot be practically managed by conservative measures (early mobilization, intermittent catheterization) or when wounds or pressure ulcers are being contaminated by incontinent urine (see Chapter 22).[9]

Delirium

Delirium is a common complication of surgery, with a greater incidence reported in orthopedic (40% to 55%) than in general surgery (10% to 20%) patients.[11] Type of anesthesia (general versus regional) does not appear to be an important determinant of delirium after the first postoperative day (Table 10-6).[9] The prevention of delirium is important because it places patients at risk for morbidity, higher mortality (25% to 33%), longer hospital stays, and poorer functional outcomes[9] (see Chapter 15).

Recovery of Function

Almost one-third of older adults hospitalized for acute medical or surgical illness decline in their ability to perform basic ADLs. Only half of the patients who decline in ADL function related to hospitalization recover by 3 months after discharge. It is important to identify patients at high risk for a poor functional recovery and initiate a comprehensive postoperative rehabilitation plan. Moreover, functional impairment that is slow to improve by hospital discharge may

Table 10–6	Factors that Lead to an Increase Risk of Delirium	
Surgical Procedure	**Intraoperative Factors**	**Other**
Cardiac surgery	Pre-existing dementia	Postoperative hypoxia
Hip fracture surgery (especially femoral neck fracture)	Parkinson's disease	Polypharmacy
Thoracic surgery	Low cardiac output	Preoperative alcohol abuse
Aortic aneurysm surgery	Perioperative hypotension	Advanced age
Ophthalmologic surgery	Anticholinergic medication	Male sex
Emergency surgery		Metabolic abnormalities
		Visual impairment
		Hearing impairment
		Low levels of activity

influence discharge destination, add to the patient's burden of morbidity, and increase the risk of nosocomial complications.[15,16]

> ● The incidence of postoperative cardiac complications is the highest in the first 48 hours after surgery.

Silent Ischemia

The incidence of postoperative cardiac complications is the highest in the first 48 hours after surgery. Perioperative MI is associated with a 40% to 70% mortality rate.[8] Cardiac ischemia is related to the combined effects of the changes in normal medical therapy, the underlying disease process, and stressors associated with postoperative discomfort and fluid shifts. Diagnosis of MI in the postoperative period may be difficult. Ischemia is clinically silent in up to 90% of cases.[8] The symptoms may be masked by analgesia or anesthesia. More typical symptoms in the elderly are unexplained dyspnea, hypotension, congestive HF, arrhythmia, or altered mental status.[5,10]

The ACC/AHA recommends electrocardiograms obtained at baseline, immediately after surgery, and on the first 2 days after surgery in patients with known or suspected CAD who are undergoing high-risk procedures.[8] It is important to take into consideration that the expected cardiac enzyme changes (such as rise in creatinine kinase) may be confounded by surgical trauma to muscle.[5,6]

Angioplasty should be considered in a patient with perioperative MI after the risks versus benefits have been weighed. Pharmacological therapy with aspirin should be initiated as soon as possible, and a beta-blocker and ACE inhibitor may also be beneficial.[8] At the conclusion of the perioperative period, it is important to resume the anti-ischemic medications used by the patient before surgery.

Hypertension

Postoperative hypertension has a number of causes. In the immediate postoperative period, it commonly occurs with emergence from anesthesia, which is a self-limited problem that does not cause significant morbidity. Other common causes include pain, which should be treated with analgesia; anxiety, which should be treated with anxiolytics; hypoxia, which should be treated with oxygen and therapy directed at the underlying cause; and hypothermia, which should be treated with rewarming.[6] The initial treatment of postoperative hypertension is to restart the patients' oral medications and minimize oral and intravenous sodium when possible. For patients who are unable to take oral medications and require treatment, the use of parenteral alternatives is beneficial.

Arrhythmias

Cardiac arrhythmias are common in the perioperative period, particularly in older patients, those with underlying pulmonary or cardiac disease, and those after intra-abdominal, major vascular, and intrathoracic surgery. Intraoperative arrhythmias frequently are transient and require no treatment. Postoperative rhythms may be secondary to other problems that must be looked for and treated, including hypoxia, hypotension, electrolyte imbalance, acidosis or alkalosis, myocardial ischemia, congestive HF, pulmonary embolism, drug reactions, infection, and irritation from central catheters. Therapy should be initiated for symptomatic or hemodynamically significant arrhythmias.[8] However, because of their proarrhythmic actions and potential for greater side effects in older persons, prophylactic use of antiarrhythmic agents is not recommended.[6,9]

Hypoxemia

Several factors need to be considered during the postoperative period in order to avoid respiratory complications. To minimize prolonged lobar dependence and to enhance mobilization of secretions, recumbent patients should be turned and repositioned frequently.[11] Early resumption of physical activity, adequate analgesia, incentive spirometers, breathing exercises, and intermittent positive-pressure breathing are all necessary components of postoperative care. In addition, supplemental oxygen via mask or nasal prongs should be provided to elderly patients following major thoracic and abdominal procedures.

Venous Thromboembolism

The diagnosis of VTE can be difficult, because more than half of patients with DVT are asymptomatic and the common signs and symptoms are not specific.[11] The cornerstone of VTE diagnosis is clinical suspicion. Patients with suspected VTE should be anticoagulated with heparin to prevent pulmonary embolism. Surgical patients are at increased risk for bleeding, and the individual patient risk-benefit ratio must be weighed. Initial testing of the lower extremities with duplex ultrasonography should be considered. Patients with suspected pulmonary embolism should have a lung ventilation and perfusion scan or have helical computed tomography scan of the chest.[11]

Case Discussion

Mr. Miller presents with a common scenario: multiple chronic problems in his medical history, a limited social support system, and a disorder requiring surgery. The case is further complicated by his dementia, which limits the patient's participation in his own treatment and places him at risk for perioperative delirium. It is important to gather as much information as possible on the patient and evaluate his decision-making ability. Your perioperative assessment will focus on obtaining a comprehensive history and physical, paying close attention to his cardiac and pulmonary risks; assessing his cognitive, functional, and social status; reviewing his medications carefully; assessing him nutritionally; and beginning preventive measures for his multiple medical problems.

Mr. Miller's postoperative functional outcome and long-term survival will depend on optimal medical and nursing management in the postoperative period. It would be expected that a patient with a pre-existing dementia would develop increased confusion during the hospitalization. It is the clinician's task to limit the intensity and duration of this confused episode. This requires careful attention to possible medical complications, such as hypoxia, infection, hypotension, and dehydration. In addition uncomfortable medical interventions should be withdrawn as quickly as possible (e.g., urinary catheters, intravenous lines). The patient's pain must be adequately treated. Mobility is imperative and should be instituted as soon as is feasible. Finally, the patient's confusion should be managed without the use of physical restraints or excessive sedation.

SUMMARY

A comprehensive geriatric assessment is required for older patients undergoing surgical procedures. It is imperative that the perioperative evaluation include identifying the factors that increase the risk of surgery, quantifying these risks to determine the appropriateness of and timing of the surgery, providing recommendations on how to minimize the risk, managing coexisting medical conditions, and monitoring the patient for perioperative problems.

References

1. Richardson JD, Cocanour CS, Kern JA. Perioperative risk assessment in elderly and high-risk patients. J Am Coll Surg 2004;199:132-146.
2. Beliveau MM, Multach M. Perioperative care for the elderly patient. Med Clin North Am 2003;87:273-289.
3. King MS. Preoperative evaluation, Am Fam Physician 2000;62:387-396.
4. Jahnigen DW. Hospital care. In Primary Care Geriatrics: A Case Based Approach. (Ham RJ, Sloane PD, eds.). St. Louis: Mosby Yearbook, 1997.
5. Seymour DG. Surgery and anesthesia in old age. In Brocklehurst's Textbook of Geriatric Medicine and Gerontology, 5 ed. (Tallis R, Fillit H, Brocklehurst JC, eds.). Edinburgh: Churchill Livingstone, 1998.
6. Nierman E, Zakrzewski K. Recognition and management of preoperative risk. Rheum Dis Clin North Am 1999;25:585-622.
7. Rosenthal RA, Kavic SM. Assessment and management of the geriatric patient. Crit Care Med 2004;32(Suppl):S92-S105.
8. Eagle KA, Berger PB, Calkins H, et al. ACC/AHA guideline update for perioperative cardiovascular evaluation for noncardiac surgery: executive summary. Circulation 2002;105:1257-1267.
9. Francis J. Perioperative management of the older patient. In Principles of Geriatric Medicine and Gerontology, 3 ed. (Hazzard WR, Bierman EL, Blass JP, et al. eds.). New York: McGraw-Hill, 1994.
10. Bach DS. Management of specific medical conditions in the perioperative period. Prog Cardiovasc Dis 1998;40:469-476.
11. Michota FA, Frost SD. Perioperative management of the hospitalized patient. Med Clin North Am 2002;86:731-748.
12. Inouye SK, Acampora D, Miller RL, et al. The Yale geriatric care program: a model of care to prevent functional decline in hospitalized elderly patients. J Am Geriatr Soc 1993;41:1345-1352.
13. Ahmed A. American College of Cardiology/American Heart Association chronic heart failure evaluation and management guidelines: relevance to the geriatric practice. J Am Geriatr Soc 2003;51:123-126.
14. Gloth FM. Principles of perioperative pain management in older adults. Clin Geri Med 17:553-573, 2001.
15. Hansen K, Mahoney J, Palta M. Risk factors for lack of recovery of ADL independence after hospital discharge. J Am Geriatr Soc 1999;47:360-365.
16. Hirsch CH, Summers L, Olsen A, et al. The natural history of functional morbidity in hospitalized older patients. J Am Geriatr Soc 1990;38:1296-1303.

Web Resources

1. CDC Guidelines for Preventing Health Care Associated Pneumonia. http://www.cdc.gov/mmwr/PDF/rr/rr5303.pdf.
2. ACC/AHA guideline update for perioperative cardiovascular evaluation for noncardiac surgery. http://www.acc.org/clinical/guidelines/perio/exec_summ/pdf/periop_execsumm.pdf.
3. The Seventh ACCP Conference on Antithrombotic and Thrombolytic Therapy: Evidence-Based Guidelines. http://www.chestjournal.org/content/vol126/3_suppl/.

POSTTEST

1. Factors used to assess a patient's preoperative nutritional status include
   a. Weight loss of more than 5% in 1 month or 10% over 6 months
   b. Albumin level less than 3.2 g/dl
   c. Body mass index less than 20
   d. All of the above

2. Pain assessment in the elderly should be based on
   a. Caregiver observations
   b. Anesthesia recommendation
   c. Patient perception
   d. Level of agitation

3. The most common sites of surgical infection in the elderly include all of the following except:
   a. Urinary tract
   b. Surgical site
   c. Gastrointestinal tract
   d. Respiratory tract

4. DVT prophylaxis for high-risk general surgery may include all of the following except:
   a. Aspirin
   b. Low-dose unfractionated heparin
   c. Low-molecular-weight heparin
   d. Intermittent pneumatic compression devices

5. Effective postoperative management includes:
   a. Pain management
   b. Early mobilization
   c. Removal of urinary catheters
   d. All of the above

6. Which type of surgery has the greatest incidence of postoperative delirium?
   a. General surgery
   b. Thoracic surgery
   c. Orthopedic surgery
   d. Neurologic surgery

PRETEST ANSWERS

1. b
2. c
3. d
4. c
5. b
6. d

POSTTEST ANSWERS

1. d
2. c
3. c
4. a
5. d
6. c

Long-Term Care

Deborah W. Robin

OBJECTIVES

Upon completion of this chapter, the reader will be able to:

- Explain the differences between nursing home and assisted living in terms of population served, staffing, and financing.

- Understand clinicians' roles in long-term care, including the management of family issues commonly arising in the nursing home setting, common ethical problems, and the role of a medical director.

- Outline the management of the following common medical problems in long-term care: behavioral problems in dementia, acute infections in long-term care, pressure ulcers, falls, nutrition/hydration, constipation, and terminal care.

PRETEST

1. Your patient is an 85-year-old woman who was recently widowed and has no close relatives. Because of macular degeneration, rheumatoid arthritis, and a hip fracture that was pinned 9 months ago, she is unable to drive, cook, or do housework. She requires supervision with bathing but is able to dress, ambulate, and use the toilet independently. She scores 26/30 on the mini-mental state examination. This patient is most likely appropriate for:
   a. Adult day care
   b. Assisted living
   c. A nursing home
   d. A rehabilitation hospital

2. Which one of the following is most correct about physical restraints?
   a. They reduce agitation.
   b. They result in fewer falls when used properly.
   c. Restraint reduction should begin with the hardest problem cases.
   d. Increased involvement in structured activity programs can reduce restraint use.

3. Which one of the following is most correct about nursing home patients?
   a. Injury is the most common reason for hospitalization.
   b. Empiric treatment of fever with antibiotics is rarely indicated.
   c. Vigorous prevention of falls can increase the pressure ulcer rate.
   d. Most pressure ulcers should be treated by encouraging them to dry.

Minnie Crawford

Minnie Crawford, an 86-year-old woman with hypertension and mild dementia, is hospitalized following a fall in her home for an impacted fracture of the right humeral neck. A widow, she has been your patient since moving in with her daughter and son-in-law 3 years ago. You hospitalized her briefly for a right anterior cerebral artery stroke 2 years ago, which left her with mild (4/5) weakness in the left lower extremity. She has been taking a diuretic for mild hypertension, and she complains of dizziness whenever she stands quickly. A typical blood pressure before hospitalization was 165/60 mm Hg.

In the emergency department, you note some S-T abnormalities on the electrocardiogram. You
decide to admit her for observation. Because her shoulder fracture is stable, the arm is immobilized in a sling and swathe. Acetaminophen with codeine for pain is prescribed.

By the following morning, her cardiogram has stabilized, and myocardial infarction has been ruled out. You feel that the S-T abnormalities were caused by mild hypokalemia, which you have corrected, and you plan to discharge her to home with her family to continue to assist her and home health occupation and physical therapy. Her daughter objects, however, informing you that she and her husband had planned to go out of town for 3 days next week and that she does not feel Minnie can manage on her own with the fracture. She asks if you can place her mother in a skilled nursing facility for a week or two.

After conferring with the hospital social worker, you inform Ms. Crawford's daughter that Medicare will not provide reimbursement for the nursing home stay because a shoulder fracture does not require daily rehabilitation and she has not had a 72-hour hospitalization. A long discussion ensues, during which the daughter is adamant that Minnie needs to be institutionalized for the next 10 days or so. She also expresses dismay at the idea of spending over $1000 for the stay. At last she agrees to pay for the nursing home admission, and Minnie enters as a respite patient into the nursing home where you are an attending physician.

Initially, Minnie is somewhat disgruntled, but she is befriended by the nursing home social worker who introduces her to the activities director. Two days later, when you visit to complete her admission paperwork, you find her smiling and actively participating in a reminiscence group. Your goals for care include keeping her mind active and engaged, watching for skin problems associated with the sling, having a physical therapist assess her and begin early rehabilitation (to avoid a frozen shoulder), and monitoring her for confusion or falls.

Two weeks after Minnie was admitted, you receive a call that she has been refusing food and fluids for the past 24 hours and that she seems to be limping. On examination her rectal temperature is 101°F, her pulse is 110 beats per minute, and her respiratory rate is 18 breaths per minute. She has mild muscle weakness on the left side, including a minimal facial droop. Her chest is unremarkable, but bowel sounds are diminished and a fecal impaction is noted on rectal examination. Urinalysis shows 30 to 50 white blood cells per high-power field.

You diagnose a urinary tract infection secondary to fecal impaction and a small subcortical stroke. You speak with the patient and her family; neither wants her to be hospitalized unless it is absolutely necessary. You discontinue her as-needed codeine, which she has continued receiving two or three times a day. You give her an injection of cefuroxime and then prescribe oral levofloxacin (she is allergic to sulfa drugs). She receives 1500 ml of intravenous fluid overnight. The next morning she is afebrile, eats all her breakfast, and seems less weak on the left side. You continue her daily aspirin dose and add cloprednol and ask the physical therapist to begin rehabilitation.

The need for assistance with personal care or household activities is a hallmark of aging. The proportion of individuals requiring help with activities of daily living gradually rises from around 5% at age 65 to more than 50% at age 90. With increasing disability comes the need for more assistance and more formal caregiving services. The expansion of home care has allowed a greater proportion of disabled elderly to remain at home; however, when needs are too great, residential long-term care is often required. This chapter discusses the two most common kinds of institutional long-term care—nursing homes and assisted-living facilities—with a focus on issues of relevance to medical practitioners who care for residents in these settings.

● The need for assistance with personal care or household activities is a hallmark of aging.

ORGANIZATION OF LONG-TERM CARE

Nursing Homes

Nursing homes are residential institutions that provide assistance with activities of daily living and nursing care. There are more than 18,000 nursing homes in the United States, with over 1.5 million residents.[1] Long-term care accounts for more than $110 billion dollars in health care expenditures in the United States.[2] There is a wide range of assistance required by residents in the nursing home setting—from minimal assistance with activities of daily living to total care. Nursing homes are licensed and regulated by state agencies, with considerable federal control through Medicare and Medicaid guidelines. There are two levels of care provided by nursing homes—skilled nursing care and the more traditional long-term care or intermediate level of care. These two levels differ in both the type of care provided and the payer source.

Over 50% of nursing home admissions are hospital discharges, frequently to skilled nursing units.[3] Criteria for admission are imprecise to allow individual providers to make decisions on a case-by-case basis, according to whether or not they can provide the level of care needed. Medical necessity as documented by a physician facilitates admission. Most good-quality nursing homes have waiting lists for admissions from the community.

The typical nursing home is organized into departments, which in smaller homes may consist of a single individual. Nursing home departments usually include nursing, social services, activities, administration, dietary services, housekeeping, pastoral care, and maintenance. Nursing is by far the largest department. The nursing department consists of both nurses (licensed practical nurses and registered nurses) and certified nursing assistants or nurses aides. Two of the major problems facing nursing homes are the extremely high staff turnover and the scarcity of nurses and certified nurse assistants.

● More than 50% of nursing home admissions are hospital discharges, frequently to skilled nursing units.

Carol Decker, *Part 1*

Mrs. Decker is a 79-year-old who was admitted to the nursing home where you are medical director. She spent several weeks in the hospital before transfer, during which she was treated for an acute stroke, delirium, pneumonia, and chronic renal failure. Two days before transfer, a gastrostomy tube was placed because the patient was unable to take adequate fluids and a swallowing study demonstrated aspiration. Before her hospitalization, she had lived at home with her husband but needed 24-hour supervision and assistance with dressing and bathing because of multi-infarct dementia. The family has been informed that she will require permanent nursing home care.

On admission the patient is somnolent, cachectic, and bedbound. She has a 3 × 3 cm stage II decubitus on her coccyx. She is incontinent and unable to stand without assistance. Initially she refuses to answer questions and closes her eyes, but on prompting she nods in response to simple questions and indicates that she is not in pain. Finally, she speaks, asking you to leave because she is tired. Her admission orders include haloperidol, aspirin, atenolol, and 24-hour tube feedings.

STUDY QUESTIONS

1. How would you set care priorities for Mrs. Decker?
2. What would you tell the family about her prognosis?

Assisted-Living Facilities

Assisted living is generally defined as a residential setting that provides personal care services, 24-hour supervision, and some health-related services in a homelike environment. It is estimated that there are more than 35,000 assisted-living facilities with almost 1 million residents in the United States.[4] These non-nursing home residential long-term care facilities are licensed by the states under a variety of designations, including board and care, domiciliary care, residential care, adult foster care, sheltered housing, residential care, and congregate care. These facilities are extremely diverse and include small homes caring for as few as two residents, clusters of small homes with a central administration, larger freestanding facilities that look a lot like nursing homes, and buildings or wings within a multilevel campus (continuing care retirement communities). State regulation of assisted-living facilities is variable and continues to grow owing to concerns over the quality of care provided. Most states have either created or amended regulations regarding assisted-living facilities during the past several years.[5] Most assisted-living facilities create an individualized service plan for each resident on admission, which details the services that the facility agrees to provide. Residents in assisted-living facilities tend to be somewhat less impaired than are nursing home residents; however, many facilities have a philosophy of "aging in place" and add services at increased cost or through home health agencies as resident needs increase. Therefore, it is common to encounter persons who require assistance with all activities of daily living or who are receiving terminal care in assisted-living homes. Most assisted-living facilities do not have a medical director or a routine physician presence, and the residents receive primary medical care from their own physicians.

● Most assisted-living facilities do not have a medical director or a routine physician presence, and the residents receive primary medical care from their own physicians.

Carol Decker, *Part 2*

Initial assessment identified the top care priorities to be improvement of mobility, clearing of delirium, and treatment of suspected depression. The tube-feeding regimen was changed from 24 hours a day to only 12 hours at night to allow the patient to participate better in activities and rehabilitation. Haloperidol was tapered, and the patient was begun on sertraline for depression. Rehabilitation staff was instructed to focus on getting the patient to transfer independently.

Within a few days, the patient was more alert. Within a week she was transferring with a one-person assist instead of two, and she could walk a few steps with help. By the second week, her affect was brighter and she began actively conversing with family and staff. She also showed interest in taking food by mouth, and cautious administration of thickened liquids was attempted with a speech therapist. Because this was tolerated well, over the next 2 weeks her diet was gradually advanced. By the end of a month, she was ambulating in her room with the aid of a walker, participating in activities, and eating more than 1000 calories per day by mouth. Her tube feedings were tapered and discontinued during week 5, and the family began to prepare for taking her home. Six weeks after admission, she was discharged home with follow-up monitoring by a home health nurse.

CASE DISCUSSION

Mrs. Decker had several reversible problems: depression, somnolence secondary to medication (Haldol), and a temporary swallowing disorder (owing to both the stroke and her overall debility). Without a geriatric assessment and active multidisciplinary management, however, she could well have spent the remainder of her days bedridden, tube fed, and residing in a nursing home.

PAYING FOR LONG-TERM CARE

Nursing home care is expensive, averaging between $30,000 and $50,000 per year and costing the nation more than $100 billion per year. Traditional long-term care or intermediate level of care costs per day range between $100 and $200 per day depending on the level of care and the location of the facility. Medicaid, an entitlement program for the impoverished, covers the costs of more than 50% of long term care.[6] Reimbursement of nursing facilities by Medicaid varies by state and, in 2002, ranged between $82 and $172 per day.[7] Medicaid eligibility for nursing home care is based both on lack of financial resources and on the need for care. Medicaid reimbursement is usually insufficient to cover the total cost of the resident's care. The remainder of residents pay for care privately through their own resources or those of their family's; with long-term care insurance covering less than 2%.[8] The high cost of long-term care can drain personal assets rapidly, which can be a problem for a nonresidential spouse. Of those who enter paying privately, one-third spends down their assets to Medicaid-eligible levels while there. Thus, nursing home care is a significant financial burden both on private individuals and on state Medicaid budgets.

Medicare only pays for skilled nursing care, which usually involves short-term rehabilitation stays after hospitalization. This level of care only accounts for 4% of nursing home residents.[9] This skilled level of care has strict criteria for admission, which include a 3-day hospitalization in the past 30 days and the requirement for a "skilled" service such as the need for physical, occupational, or speech therapy; intravenous antibiotics; complex wound care; or a new feeding tube. Medicare will pay for 100 days of skilled care, assuming skilled criteria continue to met. One hundred percent of the first 20 days of skilled care and then 80% of the remaining 80 days are covered by Medicare. The uncovered 20% is paid for by supplemental insurance policies (e.g., Associated for the Advancement of Retired Persons, Blue Cross/Blue Shield), Medicaid if the resident is financially eligible, or private pay. Nursing facilities were previously reimbursed for skilled care on a fee for service or cost basis. When hospitals began to be reimbursed on the basis of "diagnostic related groups" (DRGs), patients were discharged to skilled nursing facilities "quicker and sicker." However, the Balanced Budget Act of 1997 changed Medicare reimbursement of skilled nursing care to a prospective payment system (PPS) with a variable per diem rate. This rate is based on RUG (resource utilization group) categories, which are heavily weighted toward rehabilitation needs with residents requiring complex nursing care reimbursed at a lower level. The per diem rate includes all care provided in the nursing facility, including medications, blood work, X-rays, wound care supplies, ambulance transport, videofluoroscopic swallowing studies, orthotic devices, assistive devices (walkers and wheelchairs), and outside physician visits. In general, the per diem rate is insufficient to cover all patient needs. Some things are "carved out" and reimbursed separately such as chemotherapy, hemodialysis and some X-rays such as computed tomography (CT) scans and magnetic resonance imaging (MRI). There also exists a category of care called skilled Medicaid. The type of patients in this group still require skilled nursing care but have exhausted Medicare benefits and qualify financially for Medicaid

For persons concerned with paying for long-term care and preserving personal resources for a spouse or heirs, two strategies are available. Long-term care insurance, which is currently owned by only a small percentage of elderly, is slowly growing in popularity.[10] Owing to the escalating costs of nursing home care, however, purchasers (the mean age of who are 68) cannot be sure that their policy will provide adequate daily payments to meet future nursing home charges. Some older persons attempt to preserve their personal resources through artificial impoverishment by transfer of assets to heirs. This practice is unethical, and Medicaid eligibility boards look with disfavor at asset transfer and require that such transfers occur several years before application for Medicaid.

Assisted-living settings vary widely in cost but average somewhat less than does nursing home care. Neither Medicare nor Medicaid pays for most assisted living. Therefore, the vast majority of assisted-living residents pay privately or with Social Security disability payments. A recent trend is for Medicaid to pay for assisted living; this began in Oregon and has been gradually extending to other states; however, nationwide access of indigent persons to assisted living remains limited.

> ● Medicare only pays for skilled nursing care, which usually involves short-term rehabilitation stays after hospitalization; this level of care only accounts for 4% of nursing home residents.

Andrew Taylor, *Part 1*

Mr. Taylor is a large 63-year-old man with severe Alzheimer's disease who resides on the Alzheimer's unit in your nursing home. His mini-mental state examination score is less than five. He ambulates, transfers, and feeds himself without assistance, but he is incontinent and completely incapable of maintaining personal hygiene without help. A large, imposing presence in the facility, Mr. Taylor (always a wanderer) has gradually become increasingly disruptive. Nursing staff come to you because he becomes agitated every afternoon, and during the past week, he has struck at other patients twice, disrobed in the hallway, and hit himself repeatedly in the head. He is on donepezil and olanzapine; no recent change in medication has occurred.

STUDY QUESTIONS

1. How would you advise staff about assessment of Mr. Taylor's problem?
2. What medical conditions could lead to the change in behavior?

PHYSICIAN'S ROLES IN LONG-TERM CARE

Primary Care Physicians

All nursing homes are required by federal regulations to have physicians on staff to provide primary medical care to residents. Physicians treating residents in a nursing facility must be credentialed by that facility and provide 24-hour per day coverage. Physician visits are based on medical necessity; however, government regulation does require that residents be seen with some regularity. Federal guidelines for these visits are as follows:

- Initial visit after admission: none required as nursing home admission implies physician contact occurred in the period before admission
- Routine visits: every 30 days for the first 90 days after admission; then once every 60 days; timing must be less than 10 days after the date that the visit was required
- Acute visits: can be made whenever medically necessary

To some extent, long-term care residents are a medically underserved population. This does not mean that they need more medical procedures, hospitalizations, and technologic services; if anything, medicalization and dehumanization already occur too often in long-term care. Rather, many long-term care residents lack the personal relationships and individualized attention that characterize the best primary medical care. One reason for this is the logistics of traveling to a long-term care facility often reduces the number of physician visits, thus causing much decision making to be carried out over the telephone. Costs of physician care in nursing homes are primarily reimbursed through Medicare Part B and, when applicable, through Medicaid. Physician reimbursement for nursing home services by these public sources is modest. Guidelines for providing efficient care are presented in Box 11-1.

> ● To some extent, long-term care residents are a medically underserved population.

Physician visits can also be made in assisted-living facilities but are more like home visits than nursing home visits. There are fewer resources available such as nursing input and laboratory availability. In addition, visits are reimbursed at as "domiciliary" visit, which is at a lower rate than a home visit. Home health services are available to assisted-living residents but on a limited short-term basis as in the community.

Nurse Practitioners and Physician Assistants

There has been a recent trend to use both nurse practitioners and physician assistants in the long-term care setting. Nurse practitioners and physician assistants also must be credentialed by the facility and work under the supervision of a physician. Both these health professionals can make acute visits and some required medical visits (Table 11-1). Nurse practitioners and physician assistants can bill Medicare for their services and are reimbursed at rates that are approximately 80% of physician rates. Nurse practitioners and physician assistants can also be employed by the facility to provide resident care; however, in these circumstances they are no

---

Box 11-1 | **Time Management Guidelines for Physicians Working in Nursing Facilities**

1. Limit your practice to one or two facilities in which you get to know the staff well and can influence policy (e.g., by serving as medical director).
2. Employ a mid-level practitioner. A physician's assistant or nurse practitioner can manage routine patient care problems and serve as liaison between you and the nursing staff and families.
3. Work as a partner with the nursing home staff. Learn their names. Be sensitive to the challenges they face. Seek to be a supporter rather than a critic, especially in public.
4. Be consistent. Have a regular day for rounds.
5. Prioritize your time on rounds. See the sickest patients first.
6. Develop protocols for common problems such as decubitus prevention, constipation, weight loss, wound care, falls, behavioral problems, and fever.

7. Train staff to limit after-hours telephone calls to urgent medical problems. Provide mechanisms for staff to address nonurgent problems such as a daily telephone contact or regular rounds by yourself or a mid-level practitioner.
8. Speak with patients and families about advance directives soon after admission and whenever major status changes occur. Document these discussions in the medical record.
9. Communicate your expectations through discussions with staff, standing orders, and in-service programs.
10. Educate yourself about nursing home regulations, especially those that affect the provision of medical and nursing services.

Modified from Anderson EG. Nursing home practice: 10 tips to simplify patient care. Geriatrics 1993;48:61-63.

---

longer independent contractors and cannot bill Medicare for their services. Having a dedicated nurse practitioner or physician assistant who is available to see residents on a more frequent basis can provide more personalized and timely medical care.

Medical Director

By law, all skilled nursing facilities must have a medical director. Generally, this is a physician who man-

ages a significant proportion of the facility's patients and is paid on an hourly or monthly basis for the additional administrative responsibilities. The medical director is responsible for implementation of resident care policies and coordination medical care in the facility. A medical director who is committed and involved can have a tremendous impact on the health and well being of residents in a nursing facility.

The role of the medical director in a nursing home may include some or all of the following[11]:

Table 11-1 | **Authority for Nonphysician Practitioner to Perform Visits, Sign Orders, and Sign Certifications/Recertifications When Permitted by the State**

Initial Comprehensive Visit/Orders	Other Required Visits[a]	Other Medically Necessary Visits and Orders[b]	Certification/Recertification	
SNFs				
NP and CNS employed by the facility	May not perform/ may not sign	May perform	May perform and sign	May not sign
NP and CNS not employed by the facility	May not perform/ may not sign	May perform	May perform and sign	May sign subject to state requirements
PA regardless of employer	May not perform/ may not sign	May perform	May perform and sign	May not sign
NFs				
NP, CNS, and PA employed by the facility	May not perform/ may not sign	May not perform	May perform and sign	May sign subject to state requirements
NP, CNS, and PA not employed by the facility	May perform/may sign	May perform	May perform and sign	May sign subject to state requirements

This reflects clinical practice guidelines. SNF indicates skilled nursing facility; NF, nonskilled facility; PA, physician assistant.

[a]Other required visits are the required monthly visits that might be alternated between physician and nonphysician practitioner after the initial comprehensive visit is completed

[b]Medically necessary visits may be performed prior to the initial comprehensive visit

- Overseeing the medical care of the residents
- Organizing and coordinating physician services and the services of other professionals as they relate to patient care
- Organizing and supervising a quality improvement program for the facility
- Serving on required committees such as infection control, pharmacy, and quality assurance
- Reviewing incident reports
- Assisting the facility in developing and reviewing policies and procedures related to resident care
- Overseeing the health program for employees
- Conducting educational programs for employees, residents, and families
- Acting as a spokesperson for the facility in the community and with regulatory and other health care agencies

---

A n d r e w   T a y l o r, *Part 2*

During your next visit to the facility, you discuss Mr. Taylor's condition with the unit charge nurse, the social worker, and the nurse aide who knows him best. You call his daughter. You learn that his behavior is always provoked; antecedents include getting yelled at by other residents, loud noises, and being in the public area when a lot of activity is going on. His agitation builds up in the afternoon around 3 p.m., when the nursing shift changes and patients tend to get less supervision. He also becomes agitated when his clothes are being changed after an episode of incontinence, especially if staff is in a hurry.

A medical evaluation finds no new neurologic deficits, no constipation, no evidence of acute infection, and no evidence that he is in pain. You are able to exchange a few words with him, and nothing about your conversation or his reported behavior suggests that he is experiencing delusions or other psychotic manifestations. Review of his personal history reveals that Mr. Taylor was a professional musician, having contributed to a variety of musical compositions and a Broadway play. Despite being cognitively impaired by his disease, he remains a proud man who loves music.

The team develops a treatment plan for Mr. Taylor. It is decided that when he begins to get agitated, a staff member will escort him to his room, turn on an audiotape of his former band, and offer to look at an album of pictures from his career with him. His daughter agrees to visit in the late afternoons and during bath times because these

are the most difficult periods for him. In addition, his daughter helps decorate his room with personal pictures, musical instruments, and a favorite chair. Finally, staff is trained to consistently engage him in conversation about his previous career during personal care activities such as toileting and bathing.

When you visit a week later, the staff reports that Mr. Taylor's behavioral disturbances have been reduced to the point that he is now easier to manage than before the problem episodes began.

CASE DISCUSSION

Mr. Taylor's case demonstrates a number of features of dementia management. First, a patient who was stable deteriorates behaviorally for no apparent reason. This is common. Sometimes a medical cause, such as fecal impaction or an occult fracture can be identified. At other times, this is caused by progression of the disease or incidents in the life of the patient. Second, the staff took care to assess the patient's situation using the ABC framework, and they developed a multifaceted treatment plan. Finally, the problem was resolved by changes in caregiver actions and manipulation of the environment rather than with medication.

LONG-TERM CARE FACILITY RESIDENTS

The more than 1.3 million nursing home residents represent a diverse population. The largest segment of residents is over the age of 85 years. Women are more likely to use nursing homes than are men, and whites are more likely to use nursing homes than African Americans.[12] Over 90% of residents need assistance with bathing, with more than 75% needing assistance with dressing, toileting, transferring, and toileting.[13] Urinary incontinence is one of the main reasons for nursing home admission. At least 50% need assistance with feeding. Common medical diagnoses in the nursing home include Alzheimer's disease, multi-infarct dementia, stroke, atherosclerotic cardiovascular disease, diabetes, osteoarthritis, amputation (usually secondary to diabetes), or chronic obstructive pulmonary disease.

R o b e r t   J o h n s o n

Mr. Johnson is a 71-year-old white man with advanced prostate cancer and chronic pain secondary to bone metastases. Several years ago he had a radical prostatectomy with radiation therapy, and he continues to receive hormonal therapy. He is admitted to the nursing home under your care from the hospital with a 30-pound weight loss over 12 months, new-onset renal failure, and a pathologic fracture of the proximal right femur. He has been confused, restless, and agitated. The family is anxious and somewhat angry about the care they received in the hospital. His wife states that he has pulled out his intravenous line several times and that he pulled out his urinary catheter, causing bleeding from his penis. His daughter and son are worried that he might attempt to get out of bed and sustain more injury. They are requesting that a restraint be used to prevent a fall. They also express concern about how the morphine pump will be managed and who will be responsible for medication management.

On examination he is disoriented and agitated. His temperature is 101.4°F rectally, his pulse is 110 beats per minute, his respiratory rate is 38 breaths per minute, and his blood pressure is 100/60 mm Hg. He does not respond to questions or follow commands. His mouth is dry; his pupils are small but react to light. Cardiac examination reveals a tachycardia and a 2/6 systolic murmur heard loudest at the apex. His abdomen is distended and somewhat tender without rebound. Rectal examination is significant for hard stool impaction, which is heme positive.

STUDY QUESTIONS

1. What are the main issues to consider in caring for a dying patient such as Mr. Johnson?
2. How would you evaluate Mr. Johnson for causes of confusion and agitation?
3. How do you respond to the family members' concerns regarding fall risk, self-injury, and pain management?

WORKING WITH FAMILIES

Most long-term care admissions involve two parties: the resident and their family. It is often the family that constitutes the greater challenge and occupies the majority of the physician's time. This is often owing to guilt over nursing home placement and the inability to care for their family member in their own home. Recent press over the poor quality of care in nursing homes also makes families suspicious for neglect and abuse. In addition, the majority of long-term care residents are unable to communicate their needs and are poorly equipped to advocate for themselves either because of dementia or debility. Often the families are the major decision makers for the residents and take on the responsibility of looking after the interests of their loved ones.

Physicians should encourage contact with families, even though it takes extra time. Institutionalized persons who have involved families are likely to receive more staff attention and to have medical problems detected earlier.[14] The following are some general rules for working with families in the institutional setting

- The majority of physician contact is likely to be with one family member. This person is usually identified on admission as the "responsible party." If the resident is not capable of decision making on he or her own behalf, it is important to identify the individual who will be the decision maker. This should be established legally as the durable power of attorney.
- If possible, contact a family member at admission to introduce yourself and let them know how to contact you if there are problems. Let them know that most communication should occur through the nursing staff. Also let them know how often you or your PA or NP will be seeing the resident and that someone will always be available in an emergency.
- Early on, try to clarify advance directives and document patient wishes and family goals for care.
- Sometimes it is necessary for the physician to contact a family to discuss a change in resident condition. For example, when a patient with dementia is beginning to deteriorate. The physician should meet with the family before the situation reaches a crisis. Possible decision points (such as hospitalization or the use of antibiotics) should be discussed before the issue arises.
- Learn as much as possible about family dynamics and anticipate conflicts. Interpersonal discord tends to surface during a crisis. A common example of this is the son (or daughter) from out of town that materializes during a crisis and insists on reversing decisions made by the physician and responsible party.

ETHICAL ISSUES

Many long-term care residents have limited ability to make personal and medical decisions because of communication or cognitive impairment. The physician is often called upon to assess the ability of such residents to make such decisions. One general rule for decision making is to consider that the greater the risk the greater the level of understanding required for consent.[15] Surrogate decision making by next of kin is common and does not require formal legal proceedings. In all cases of surrogate decision making, the standard is substituted judgment; in other words, decisions should aim to decide in the manner that the resident would if he or she were capable.

Institution of cardiopulmonary resuscitation (CPR) in the nursing home is generally futile; less than 2% of nursing home patients survive CPR and subsequent hospitalization.[16] The exception is the patient whose arrest is witnessed and who, at the time resuscitation is attempted, demonstrates ventricular fibrillation.[17] In addition, many nursing home residents have end-stage diseases and are near the end of their lives. Consequently, it is probably most humane for the majority of nursing home residents to have do not resuscitate (DNR) status. Other issues involving withholding treatment arise frequently (e.g., whether or not to institute antibiotics for fever, whether or not to hospitalize, whether or not to initiate tube feeding). The resident's and family's preferences regarding CPR and other life-sustaining treatments should be determined on admission and reevaluated whenever there is a change in the resident's condition.

The expression of sexuality by a resident is in the nursing home is another ethical dilemma that often presents itself to long-term care staff and families.[18,19] This is particularly true if the resident has dementia and especially if a cognitively intact spouse or other relative visits the facility. In general, sexuality should be considered normal, but nursing home staff may intervene if participants are incompetent or threat of physical or psychological injury is present.

STAFFING IN LONG-TERM CARE

There is a strong relationship between staffing levels in the nursing and both quality of care and the costs of care. As expected, higher staffing levels result in better quality of care with higher costs. Nursing home staffing levels are required by federal regulations to meet minimum nursing standards defined as having enough nursing staff and related services to attain or maintain the highest practical physical, mental, and psychosocial well being of the residents.[20] The Institute of Medicine has suggested minimum staffing levels of 4.55 hours per patient per day. which includes both nursing and certified nursing assistant hours.[21]

Certified Nursing Assistants

As much as 90% of the direct patient care in nursing homes and assisted-living settings is provided by certified nursing assistants. Federal law mandates 75 hours of training for certified nursing assistants, followed by an exam for certification. The pay averages little more than minimum wage, and advancement opportunities are minimal. However, the work certified nursing

assistants do requires considerable awareness of and sensitivity to the unique and individual needs of complex geriatric patients. It is often the certified nursing assistant who identifies a change in resident condition that warrants further nursing or medical intervention.

The certified nursing assistant's work is primarily to assist residents with personal care. It is physically demanding, consisting of getting patients out of bed, washing them, brushing their teeth, grooming them, making their beds, changing their soiled linen, cleaning up after bladder and bowel accidents, monitoring them for falls, toileting them, and feeding them. Some certified nursing assistants may be responsible for restorative care, which consists of assisting patient with ambulation, range of motion to prevent contractures, and the use of splinting.

> As much as 90% of the direct patient care in nursing homes and assisted-living settings is provided by certified nursing assistants.

Licensed Nurses

Nurses are the cornerstone of care in the nursing home. Most of the hands-on nursing care is provided by licensed practical nurses. Registered nurses frequently hold administrative or supervisory positions within the nursing home such as director of nursing or unit supervisor. A registered nurse is usually available to oversee the care provided by the licensed practical nurses. Nurses must comply with the standard of care as outlined in the facility's policies and procedures. Nursing responsibilities include the following:

- Conduct resident assessments on a routine basis and for change in condition
- Administer medications
- Supervise certified nursing assistants
- Communicate with physicians
- Communicate with families
- Administer treatments such as performing wound care
- Participate in the care planning process

Staffing Crisis in Long-Term Care

The nationwide nursing shortage is also expected to affect the quality of care in nursing homes. The nursing shortage currently is at 6% but is expected to continue to increase over the next 10 years owing to the aging of current nurses, fewer persons entering the nursing profession, and developing trends to limit overtime.[20]

The certified nursing assistant field has been plagued for over a decade by turnover rates of approximately 100% per year and by low job satisfaction.[22] By the year 2000, inability of long-term care settings to recruit and retain quality nurse aides had reached an all-time high and was beginning to be considered a national crisis. Major improvement in this staffing crisis will require elevation of the certified nursing assistant position to paraprofessional status through a combination of increased educational requirements, higher wages, and improvements in the work setting (e.g., fewer patients per nursing assistant). Such a drastic change would require a significant increase in long-term care financing. In the absence of major improvements in the financing and structure of long-term care, facilities can take a number of steps to improve the recruitment and retention of quality nurse aides[23] (Box 11-2).

FUNCTION-ORIENTED CARE

Because all patients in long-term care facilities have disabilities, care providers should attempt to maximize what each patient can do independently. Such an approach requires individualization of goals and coordination of care by an interdisciplinary team. A series of federal regulations in the early 1990s introduced several procedures aimed at fostering individualized care. These include a comprehensive, standardized assessment for all patients using an instrument called the minimum data set. The minimum data set is completed by an interdisciplinary team at admission, on a quarterly basis, and with a significant change in condition. The minimum data set is computer based and can be downloaded to Medicare intermediaries for billing purposes or to the Center for Medicare and Medicaid for use in generating quality data. In addition, the information in the minimum data set is used to generate resident assessment protocols (RAPS), which in turn are used to create an individualized care plan for the resident. This care plan is reviewed with the family in a for-mal meeting attended by the interdisciplinary care team. The plan outlines the care needs of the resident, the goals of care, and who is responsible for implementation. An example of a care plan for decubitus prevention is shown in Table 11-2.

Some patients in the nursing home benefit from formal rehabilitation care aimed at restoring function after illness or injury. For some patients rehabilitative approaches such as vigorous physical therapy may increase mobility but only provide limited gains for others.[24,25] Most long-term patients, however, benefit from restorative care that focuses on maintenance of the highest maximal functional status for as long as possible. This could consist of daily ambulation with assistance or range of motion to prevent contractures in a bed-bound resident.

Within days of admission, each resident should be evaluated by the physician and nursing staff for rehabilitation potential. When appropriate, the assessment and care plan should include other health professionals such as a physical therapist, a speech therapist, and an occupational therapist. This assessment should evaluate functional status, establish a prognosis, identify specific functional objectives and a time frame to accomplish them, monitor the progress in the functional status improvement preventing iatrogenic consequences, and plan a discharge date if possible. When a resident does not have potential for improvement and discharge from the nursing home, strategies to maintain functional status should be developed. Some of these strategies are to modify the environment to enable maximal self-care (e.g., install handrails between the bed and bathroom), to eliminate any disability through medical management and the use of assistive devices, to provide a daily routine of physical and social activities that matches the resident's functional capability, and to provide a means of mobility (for immobile residents), comfortable positioning, frequent repositioning, and exercise.

Box 11-2   Steps to Improve Recruitment and Retention of Certified Nursing Assistants

1. Provide regular wage increases based on longevity or skill acquisition
2. Provide greater autonomy and decision-making opportunities
3. Involve in care planning
4. Encourage positive feedback from supervisors and especially families and patients
5. Individualize orientation
6. Be consistent in patient assignment if desired by the aide
7. Create a career ladder (e.g., restorative nurse aide or physical therapy assistant)
8. Partner with community colleges to offer short courses in care skills, the completion of which is coupled with salary increases
9. Pay greater attention to selection, orientation, and training of newly hired nurse aides (because the greatest turnover is during the first few months of employment).

Table 11–2 Example of Care Plan for Decubitus Ulcer Prevention

Problem	Goal	Approach Frequency	Discipline
6 _____ is at risk for skin breakdown due to incontinence of bowel and bladder, use of trunk restraint.	1 _____ skin will remain intact without signs of breakdown thru next review.	1 Keep resident's skin as clean and dry as possible minimizing skin exposure to moisture.	CNA
Start Date:	**Start Date:**	Check every 2 hours and at night for incontinence and provide pericare and adult incontinent briefs as needed.	CNA RN LPN
		Keep linen dry, clean, and wrinkle free.	CNA
		Conduct a systematic skin inspection weekly. Pay particular attention to the bony prominences.	CNA
		Encourage fluids up to 1500 cc per day unless clinically contradicted.	CNA
		Report any signs of skin breakdown (sore, tender, red, or broken areas) to charge nurse.	LPN
		Perform skin breakdown risk assessments per facility protocol	CNA
		Podus boots when in bed to protect heels from irritation or redness.	CNA
		Reposition while in wheelchair with restraint to possibly preserve skin.	CNA

CNA = Certified Nursing Assistant; RN = Registered Nurse; LPN = Licensed Practical Nurse.

COMMON MEDICAL PROBLEMS IN LONG-TERM CARE SETTINGS

Long-term care facilities contain a population in which the medical problems of old age are concentrated. Thus, they are settings in which expertise in geriatric medicine is particularly crucial. Professionals such as physicians, nurses, and physical therapists who work with long-term care residents should be vigilant for remediable health problems of which there are many. The practice of medical care in the nursing home and assisted-living settings is challenging and highly complex but can be very rewarding.

Many acute medical problems can be evaluated and treated on site at the nursing home. The first step is nursing recognition of a problem or acute change in medical condition. This is often noticed by the certified nursing assistant. The nurse then assesses the patient, including vital signs, oxygen saturation, pertinent physical findings, and overall patient condition. The physician, PA or NP is contacted with ordering of appropriate tests and treatment. Nursing homes have access to laboratory evaluation, X-rays, electrocardiograms, and even portable ultrasound. Stat laboratories may also be available. In addition, if the physician, PA or NP is on site, he or she can evaluate the patient. If the patient is acutely ill and cannot be managed in the nursing home or the family requests hospitalization, the patient should be sent to the emergency department.

Infections

Infections cause the majority of deaths in the nursing home and are a major reason for hospitalization.[26] The urinary tract is the most common site of serious infections followed by the respiratory tract. Common non-life-threatening infections include conjunctivitis, skin and soft-tissue infections, herpes zoster, gastroenteritis, and fungal infections of the skin.

Symptomatic urinary tract infections are the most common infection in the nursing home.[27] Asymptomatic bacteruria is also common but rarely causes problems. Indwelling urinary catheters, which are common in the nursing home, markedly increase the risk of urinary tract infections. Pneumonia is the second most common infection in the nursing home but has the highest mortality. The presentation may be atypical with fever and altered mental status. Most episodes of pneumonia are treated in the nursing home.[28] Management of these infections is discussed in relevant chapters of this text.

Management of fever in the nursing home is empirical. In contrast to the community, where viral infections predominate, as many as one-third of nursing home fevers and the majority of fevers over 102°F are caused by bacterial infection. The etiology of the fever can be assessed by getting a chest X-ray and urinalysis with urine culture. Empiric antibiotics can be initiated either by the oral or by the intramuscular route if the resident is unable to swallow. In some cases a decision must be made concerning whether or not to hospitalize the patient or to even treat with antibiotics. Pneumonia and sepsis remain the "old man's friends"—relatively rapid and comfortable ways to die. Practice guidelines for clinical evaluation of fever and infection in the nursing home have been developed.[29]

> ● Infections cause the majority of deaths in the nursing home and are a major reason for hospitalization.

Falls

Falls and fall-related injuries are extremely common in nursing homes. The mean fall incidence is about three times that of community-dwelling elderly.[24] Of these falls, 10% to 20% result in hospital admission and/or fractures, which is also higher than in the community. Common risk factors include debility from medical illnesses, decreased mobility, medications, incontinence, and dementia with poor safety awareness. On admission all residents should be evaluated for fall risk and a care plan initiated to prevent falls. Multifactoral interventions that involve environmental modifications, physical therapy, and medication adjustments have shown promising results in decreasing fall risk.

Physical Restraints

Research during the past decade and a half has demonstrated that physical restraints, although appearing to reduce fall risk, can be associated with significant morbidity and even mortality.[30,31] In addition, physical restraints in long-term care can constitute an unjustified infringement of resident autonomy. Physical restraints include vest restraints (Posey type), chairs with locking lap trays; waist restraints or roll belts; and safety belts that cannot be opened by the patient. Bed rails are considered restraints when used to keep a patient from getting out of bed. All restraints require a physician's order and family consent. Restraints are not a substitute for good care. The decision to restrain a resident must take into consideration both the benefits and the risks. In a patient who demonstrates a repetitive pattern of unsafe behavior and poor safety awareness, such as repeated attempts to ambulate without assistance, the risk of a fall with injury may outweigh the risk of restraints. A general rule would be to try the least restrictive restraint first. An initial approach might be to use a motion alarm; however, this intervention may be only minimally successful as the resident may already have fallen by the time a care person arrives to help.

Restraints have side effects, which are listed in Box 11-3. In addition, restraints do not reduce the need for close monitoring because all restrained residents

---

> **Box 11-3   Risks of Physical Restraints**
>
> 1. Increased debility and weakness from immobilization
> 2. Decubiti
> 3. Pneumonia
> 4. Injury (fall, strangulation)
> 5. Increased agitation, confusion, combativeness
> 6. Cardiac stress
> 7. Dehydration (inability to access fluids)
> 8. Physiologic sequelae of immobilization
> 9. Violation of resident rights

must be checked every 15 minutes and the restraints released every 2 hours. Restraint reduction programs are implemented in a manner that involves all staff, requires strong administrative support, and proceeds case-by-case, beginning with "easier" cases first. Programs aimed at reducing physical restraints must offer alternatives. The components of a comprehensive restraint reduction program are listed in Box 11-4.

> ● Physical restraints in long-term can constitute an unjustified infringement on resident autonomy.

Pressure Sores

A pressure ulcer is a localized area of soft-tissue injury resulting from compression between a bony prominence and an external surface. The involved tissue suffers ischemia caused by arteriolar obstruction during the period of compression. A full-thickness ischemic pressure ulcer can develop in as little as 2 or 3 hours if the patient is immobile and resting on a hard surface. Other causes of skin ulceration, which may contribute to pressure sores, include friction (e.g., by sliding a

---

> **Box 11-4   Interventions for Restraint Reduction**
>
> 1. Increased involvement for residents in structured activities
> 2. Psychosocial alternatives such as active listening, therapeutic touch, and behavior modification
> 3. Use of positioning devices such as wedge cushions and recliner chairs
> 4. Environmental modifications such as carpeted floors and lowered beds
> 5. Use of motion sensors and position monitors to alert staff when high-risk patients are attempting to get up
> 6. Alterations in nursing care such as additional observation, assisted daily ambulation, and regular toileting
> 7. Search for and treatment of physiologic causes of agitation such as pain, constipation, and infection

patient on a mattress), moisture (e.g., from incontinence), and trauma. Risk factors for pressure ulcers include increased age, immobility, malnutrition, peripheral neuropathy with decreased sensation, altered consciousness, hypotension, fever, and fecal incontinence. Many pressure ulcers treated in nursing homes arise during hospitalization for acute illnesses. All residents should have a complete skin assessment with careful documentation on admission and readmission. However, pressure ulcer development is not rare in long-term care facilities. Because most pressure ulcers are preventable, the incidence of new ulcers is considered a measure of quality of care.

Pressure ulcers are usually located on the sacrum or coccyx but can occur in any location that is unrelieved pressure. Other common locations include the ischial tuberosities (owing to sitting in a wheelchair), greater trochanteric area of the hip, heels, knees, elbows, and the back of the head. In addition, it is important to distinguish pressure ulcers from other types of ulcers such as venous insufficiency ulcers, arterial insufficiency ulcers, and diabetic foot ulcers. Pressure ulcers are described by stage (I through IV), size, and other descriptive characteristics such as type of tissue present, drainage, and presence of an odor. The staging of pressure ulcers is shown in Table 11-3.[32]

The management of pressure ulcers requires two types of interventions: the preventive one and the therapeutic one. Prevention emphasizes risk assessment, skin care, and pressure relief. Early recognition and treatment are important as most early-stage pressure ulcers can be healed within several days to several weeks. Treatment also uses relief of pressure through frequent turning and the use of positioning devices. The use of specialized beds and mattresses may augment frequent turning and repositioning, but cost usually limits accessibility. General goals of pressure sore treatment include protection of the injured area from further pressure, shear, and friction; debridement of necrotic tissue; maintenance of a moist wound environment; prevention and treatment of secondary infection; elimination of dead space; and provision of adequate nutrition. Table 11-4 describes available treatment modalities.

Pressure sores need to be identified early. Certified nursing assistants who bath residents daily should be the first line of defense in identifying early stage pressure sores. The size, stage, location, and appearance of all pressure sores should be documented weekly. A pressure sore that worsens during this period requires reevaluation of the treatment modality. Some nursing homes have designated treatment nurses, whereas others use certified ostomy and wound care nurses as consultants. Referral to a wound care specialist or plastic surgeon may be necessary for pressure sores that are not responding to treatment or require debridement.

> ● All residents should have a complete skin assessment with careful documentation upon admission and readmission.

Constipation

Long-term care residents are extremely susceptible to constipation. Half have constipation as a significant management problem, and three-quarters use at least one stool softener, laxative, or enema daily.[33] Risk factors for constipation include multiple medical problems, polypharmacy, immobility, decreased physical activity, decreased total oral intake, low dietary fiber, dehydration, and loss of functional status. Some of the most common constipating medications in the elderly are antacids, anticholinergics, tricyclic antidepressants, calcium channel blockers, nonsteroidal antiinflammatory drugs, benzodiazepines, and neuroleptics. A variety of adverse complications can arise as a result of constipation such as abdominal pain, anorexia, dehydration, urinary retention and subsequent urinary tract infection, volvulus, and megacolon. It is important to note that fecal impaction can present as

Table 11–3	Staging of Pressure Ulcers	
Stage	**Description**	**Appearance**
I	Observable pressure related alteration of intact skin	Alteration in skin temperature (warm or cold) Alteration in tissue consistency (firm or boggy) Sensation (pain or itchy) Defined area of persistent redness or purplish hue
II	Partial-thickness skin loss involving the epidermis and/or dermis	Superficial Abrasion blister shallow crater
III	Full-thickness skin loss involving damage or necrosis of subcutaneous tissue. Can extend down to fascia but not through underlying fascia	Deep crater, with or without undermining
IV	Full-thickness skin loss with extensive destruction	Tissue necrosis or damage to muscle, bone, or supporting structures

Table 11–4	Treatment Modalities for Pressure Ulcers		
Type of Dressing	**Indication**	**Uses**	**Disadvantages**
Skin sealants	Stage 1 ulcers, skin around open ulcers	Creating a protective coating on the skin, acting as a barrier between healthy skin and topical product	None
Hydrogels	Ulcers with little or no exudate	Maintaining a moist environment, promoting the wound-healing process, promoting autolytic debridement, reducing pain	May cause tissue maceration around the ulcer, a secondary dressing is necessary, may adhere to the ulcer bed if dries, may promote growth of organisms
Hydrocolloids	Stage 2 ulcers	Maintaining a moist environment, allowing clean ulcers to heal naturally, promoting autolytic debridement	Cannot be used in the presence of heavy exudate, sinus tracts, ulcers with eschar formation, exposed bones or tendons, third-degree burns, or infections
Alginates	Exudating stage 2 ulcers; stage 3 or 4 ulcers that are deep, tracking, or undermined or have moderate drainage	Maintaining a moist environment	Should be avoided in third-degree burns, heavily bleeding ulcers, and dry ulcers; may require hydration before removal; a secondary dressing is necessary
Foams	Partial-thickness or full-thickness ulcers with moderate to heavy drainage	Repelling water, bacteria, and other contaminants; maintaining a moist environment; acting as insulation; reducing odor	Some patients require a secondary dressing; maceration may occur on surrounding skin; should not be used for dry ulcers, partial-thickness ulcers, ulcers with a small amount of drainage, arterial ischemic lesions, or ulcers with exposed muscle, tendon, or bone
Sodium chloride solution–impregnated gauze	Stage 2, 3, and 4 ulcers	Maintaining a moist environment	Absorbs minimal amounts of exudate, dressing must be removed while still moist, multiple dressing changes per day

diarrhea owing to leakage of liquid stool around the impaction.

Treatment of constipation in the nursing home involves a multifaceted approach, including monitoring, prevention, and treatment. The certified nursing assistants and nursing staff need to monitor bowel function and treat appropriately before it becomes a problem. Daily documentation of bowel movements should be maintained by the certified nursing assistants. A combination of bowel training, a toileting program, adequate hydration, dietary management, and regular exercise are important aspects of prevention of constipation. Stool softeners and laxatives can be used on a daily or as needed basis.

Nutrition, Hydration, and Maintenance of Weight

Malnutrition, dehydration, and weight loss are extremely common in nursing homes. Significant weight loss is defined reduction of 5% of body weight or more in a person who is not overweight. Common treatable causes of malnutrition include the following: depression, medications that decrease appetite or cause nausea, and swallowing disorders.[34] Other causes that need to be considered are poor-fitting or absent dentures, needing assistance with feeding, restrictive diets, constipation, and failure to thrive owing to end-stage medical diseases or advanced dementia. In addition, an acute medical illness can result in temporary decreased oral intake and can contribute to malnutrition and result in dehydration.

Long-term care facilities should monitor food and fluid intake daily and should weigh patients at least once a month. When intake is reduced or weight loss is documented, the patient should be assessed for reversible causes of poor intake. Often, reduced intake can be ameliorated by changing the diet to a simpler form, such as changing a regular diet to a mechanical soft diet or changing a mechanical soft diet to a pureed diet. Finger foods may also be helpful. Between-meal snacks and liquid nutritional supplements should be ordered and their intake documented. For persons who are unable to feed themselves, the most important factor in effective nutrition is adequate staff time to assist the patient. A registered dietician should be involved in the evaluation for weight loss. Also a speech therapist can assist in determining the appropriate diet consistency. In the late stages of dementia and other terminal illnesses, weight loss is considered unavoidable.

The use of feeding tubes in long-term care is controversial. A feeding tube can supply 100% of nutrition and hydration in a patient who is unable to swallow. Short-term use of feeding tubes in the setting of an acute medical illness such as a stroke can help maintain nutrition as the patient's swallowing improves with speech therapy during recovery. However, evidence suggests that, at least in the context of end-stage dementia, feeding tubes do not prolong life.[35,36] This is probably because of the unresolved risk of aspiration. It is an important for the physician to discuss patient and family preferences regarding the use of feeding tube and to council them regarding the risks and benefits.

DEMENTIA

Dementia is one of the most common diagnoses in long-term care facilities, with almost 50% of residents having a diagnosis of either Alzheimer's disease or multi-infarct dementia.[37] The field of dementia care is changing rapidly, with new knowledge accumulating about behavioral and pharmacologic treatments that reduce disability and improve function. Therefore, physicians who manage patients in assisted-living facilities and nursing homes need to be aware of developments in dementia care and provide appropriate medical and psychiatric management of these patients. It is also important for the physician to assist in educating families about the course and prognosis of a patient with dementia, as well as assist with end-of-life decision making. Most nursing homes have psychiatric consultants who can assist in the management of dementia and associated behavioral disorders.

Recent advances in the treatment of dementia include medications that have been shown to slow the progression of dementia (cholinesterase inhibitors, e.g. donepezil). These medications do not "cure" but postpone or relatively reduce symptoms in patients with early to moderate dementia. It has been found that when these medications are discontinued, the patient's level of cognitive function will decline to what it would have been had the medication not been used. In addition, there are some data to suggest that this group of medications may also be helpful in the stabilization of behavioral disorders.

Behavioral problems are observed in up to 90% of patients with dementia and can significantly complicate the care of a resident with dementia. Examples of such behaviors include agitation, combativeness during care, repetitive yelling, and hitting other residents

or staff. In addition, these residents may also suffer from depression, anxiety, and psychosis. Interventions via nonpharmacologic or pharmacologic methods are needed if these behaviors threaten the patient or other residents' safety or decrease functional status.

Evaluating a patient with dementia-related behavioral problems requires an interdisciplinary team approach. Typically, the certified nursing assistant reports the behavior to the nurse, who then assesses the resident for potential medical causes of the behavior such as pain or an urinary tract infection. The assessment is then communicated to the physician, who helps staff members develop a plan for intervention. The plan is then implemented across all staff shifts, and the response of specific target behaviors is monitored by using behavior tracking.

Nonpharmacologic Interventions

Nonpharmacologic approaches are an important first step when managing most dementia-related behavioral problems. The goal is to identify and remove precipitating factors and diminish the aggravating consequences of the behavioral disturbances. A summary of nonpharmacologic interventions is provided in Box 11-5.

Pharmacologic Interventions

Federal regulations instituted in the early 1990s require that a behavioral management strategy be the first line of treatment for agitated residents. However, if the resident has overt psychosis, severe depression, or behavior likely to cause injury to the resident or other residents and staff, drug therapy is warranted. In addition, dangerous behaviors that constitute an immediate threat to the patient, other resident, or staff safety require psychiatric hospitalization.

For other less acute behaviors, drug therapy should be considered only after possible underlying causes such as acute medical illness, adverse drug effects, and

---

Box 11–5 Nonpharmacologic Interventions for Behavior Disorders in Dementia

1. Increase personal space (private room)
2. Reduction in noxious stimuli (noise and interactions)
3. Selection of able and willing staff
4. Pet therapy
5. Identification and modification of antecedents
6. Reminiscence
7. Validation therapy
8. Positive reinforcement
9. Special care units (dementia units)
10. Eden-ization (provide a more homelike environment)

environmental stressors have been ruled out and a behavioral approach has failed. When drug therapy is indicated, the nursing staff must identify the targeted behavioral problems and plan a timetable and objective scale to assess the response to pharmacologic therapy. After a period of behavioral stabilization, dose reduction should be attempted. If the behavior recurs, the drug dose can be reevaluated.

The following concepts should be kept in mind in the use of drug treatment for behavioral problems:

- The side effect profile should guide agent selection.
- Generally, administer medications as standing doses, not as as-needed doses. An exception is premedication before a procedure such as bathing.
- When psychotic symptoms are present, use neuroleptics as first-line treatment, keeping in mind the fluctuating nature of psychosis, the significant side effects profile, and the cost of the neuroleptic agent.
- If depression is evident, use an antidepressant agent alone, such as a serotonin selective reuptake inhibitor (SSRI).
- Trazodone has both sedative and antidepressant effects. It is especially useful if a sleep problem is present (give the majority of the dose at bedtime).
- If anxiety is evident, SSRIs, along with buspirone and benzodiazepines, have been shown to be an effective treatment for anxiety.
- If benzodiazepine has to be used, use one with a short half-life for short period.
- Recalcitrant behaviors, even in advanced dementia, may respond to a cholinesterase inhibitor.
- If the patient has a mood disorder or has had a seizure, consider an anticonvulsant such as valproic acid.

HEALTH MAINTENANCE

Screening and health maintenance in the nursing home must be individualized and based on the patient's medical status and prognosis. All new and prospective residents need to be screened for tuberculosis. The first tuberculin screen must involve booster testing and the use of controls owing to the high prevalence of delayed immunologic responses in older persons.[38] Flu vaccinations are also essential for all nonallergic residents because group immunity is important to preventing epidemics. Studies have also shown that vaccinating staff is at least as important as vaccinating residents.[39] Routine preventive care such as mammograms and colonoscopy can be considered on a case-by-case basis. Beyond these measures the medical evaluation should include a yearly history, physical examination, and appropriate laboratory testing based on these evaluations.

END-OF-LIFE CARE IN THE NURSING HOME

Many nursing home residents live out their lives in the nursing home. These older persons frequently have significant debility associated with advanced cancers, late-stage Alzheimer's disease, multiple strokes with dysphagia, and end-stage pulmonary, cardiac, and renal disease. Thus, routine care in the nursing home commonly includes end-of-life care. Although the usual course of illness is a slow decline over months to years, an acute illness can occur, causing a precipitous decline in condition. It is important for the physician and the nursing staff to understand the patient's and his or her family's goals for care. Treatment plans should be discussed with the patient early in the terminal care process and before mental status alterations, if possible. Often, however, it is the responsible party who must make the decisions during terminal care.

Although hospitalization is an option, many residents have spent years in the nursing home and wish to die in their "home" surrounded by family, friends, and caregivers. The management of terminally ill residents focuses on providing comfort measures. Comfort measures include aggressive pain management, treatment of agitation, and management of respiratory distress. This can readily be done in the nursing home setting. When oral intake is compromised, alternative routes of medication administration can be used, such topical patches (fentanyl and scopolamine), liquid medications (oral morphine solution), or orally dissolving tablets (olanzapine). Empathetic communication with family members and involvement of pastoral care are also helpful.

Some nursing homes have contractual agreements with agencies providing hospice care. This service should be reserved for residents with difficult pain management issues and families needing more support than can be readily provided in the nursing home. Some patients are admitted to the nursing home from home or after hospitalization with the goal of providing end-of-life care in conjunction with hospice.

DEFINING AND ACHIEVING QUALITY CARE

The quality of care that is provided in nursing homes has been a pressing concern for consumers, physicians, nurses, and policy makers. In 1986 the Institute of Medicine Report described widespread abuse and neglect in nursing homes.[40] Recommendations were made to strengthen federal governmental regulation of nursing homes and improve the quality of care. These nursing home reform provisions were contained in the Nursing Home Quality Reform Act of the Omnibus Reconciliation Act of 1987 and required that nursing homes that receive funds from Medicare or Medicaid must meet minimum standards of care. In addition, the states were authorized to conduct surveys to determine facility compliance with federal standards. Surveyor guidelines to assist surveyors and facilities in interpreting the regulations are published in *The State Operations Manual*. States may also have their own nursing home regulations, which are in addition to those set by the federal government. The state survey process has the following requirements:

- Every facility must have an initial survey to verify compliance with all federal regulatory requirements in order to be certified.
- Certified facilities are recertified annually.
- Follow-up surveys may be conducted to correct identified deficiencies.
- A survey can be conducted to follow-up on a complaint that alleges substandard cares.

In 2002 the Centers for Medicare and Medicaid launched the Nursing Home Quality Initiative. This initiative focuses on outcome-based quality improvement using key quality indicators. The data from individual facilities are gathered from the minimum data set. These data are published on the CMS Nursing Home Compare Web site. The quality indicators are listed in Box 11-6. During the survey process, state surveyors review the facility's quality indicator reports to identify problem areas that may require further investigation.

The federal government and state surveying agencies collect comprehensive data on many aspects of long-term care facilities. The information is collected in a data network and published as the OSCAR (Online Survey Certification and Reporting) Report. This database includes the nursing home characteristics and health deficiencies issued during the three most recent state inspections and recent complaint investigations.

As noted previously, goals of care depend on the problems and prognosis of the individual patient. Even death is not a bad outcome for many nursing home residents. However, certain outcome goals are reasonable for most residents. These include maximizing independence, autonomy, and physical function; providing safety, security, and privacy; supplying adequate nutrition, personal comfort, continuity with one's past, and a sense of home; and maintaining dignity, pride, and a sense of self-worth.

> ● The quality of care that is provided in nursing homes has been a pressing concern for consumers, physicians, nurses, and policy makers.

Box 11-6	**Nursing Home Quality Indicators**

1. Percentage of residents whose need for help with daily activities has increased
2. Percentage of residents who have moderate to severe pain
3. Percentage of high-risk residents who have pressure sores
4. Percentage of low-risk residents who have pressure sores
5. Percentage of residents who were physically restrained
6. Percentage of residents who are more depressed or anxious
7. Percentage of low-risk residents who lose control of their bowels or bladder
8. Percentage of residents who have/had a catheter inserted and left in their bladder
9. Percentage of residents who spent most of their time in bed or in a chair
10. Percentage of residents whose ability to move about in and around their room got worse
11. Percentage of residents with a urinary tract infection
12. Percentage of residents who lose too much weight
13. Percentage of short-stay residents with delirium
14. Percentage of short-stay residents who had moderate to severe pain
15. Percentage of short-stay residents with pressure sores

References

1. Harrington C, Carillo H, Wellin V, Burdin A. Nursing Facilities, Staffing, Residents and Facility deficiencies, 1996 though 2002. August 2003.
2. Knowledge Source, Inc. BusIntell Report. August 2000.
3. U.S. Department of Health and Human Services. Vital and Health Statistics. The National Nursing Home Survey, Table 11. June 2002. http://www.cdc.gov.
4. National Center for Assisted Living Policy. National Academy for Health Policy, 2002. http://www.nashp.org.
5. Mollica R. State Assisted Living Policy. National Academy for State Health Policy, 2002. http://www.nashp.org.
6. Gabrel, CS. Characteristics of elderly nursing home current residents and discharges: data from the 1997 National Nursing Home Survey. http://www.cdc.gov/nchs
7. Grabowski DC, Feng Z, Intrator O, et al. Recent trends in state nursing home payment policies. Health Affairs 2004;W4:363-373.
8. Spillman BC, Kemper P. Lifetime patterns of payments for nursing home care. Med Care 1995;33:280.
9. Department of Health and Human Services, Office of Inspector General. Trends in the Assignment of resource Groups by skilled Nursing facilities, 2001. http://www.oig.hhs.gov.
10. Butler RN, Brame JB, Kahn C, et al. Health care for all: long-term care, the missing piece. Geriatrics 1992;47:53.
11. Leveinson SA, ed. Medical Direction in Long-Term Care: A Guidebook for the Future. Durham, NC: Carolina Academic Press, 1993.
12. Murtaugh CM, Kemper P, Spillman BC, et al. The amount, distribution, and timing of lifetime nursing home use. Medical Care 1997;35:204-218.
13. Department of Health and Human Services. Vital and Heath Statistics Series 13, no. 152. The National Nursing Home Survey, 1999. http://www.cdc.gov/nchs
14. Sloane PD, Ives T. Monitoring medications in the nursing home (editorial). J Am Board Fam Pract 1995;8:249.
15. Hayley DC, Cassel CK, Snyder L, Rudberg MA. Ethical and legal issues in nursing home care, Arch Intern Med 1996;156:249-256.
16. Murphy DJ, Murray AM, Robinson BE, Campion EW. Outcomes of cardiopulmonary resuscitation in the elderly. Ann Intern Med 1989; 11:199-205.
17. Tresch DD, Neahring JM, Duthie EH, Mark DH, Kartes SK, Aufderheide TP. Outcomes of cardiopulmonary resuscitation in nursing homes: can we predict who will benefit? Am J Med 1993;95:123-130.
18. Hajjar RR, Kamel HK. Sexuality in the nursing home, part 1: attitudes and barriers to sexual expression. J Am Med Dir 2004;5:543-547.
19. Kamel HK , Hajjar RR. Sexuality in the nursing home, part 2: managing abnormal behavior: legal and ethical issue. J Am Med Dir 2004;5:549-552.

20. U.S. Department of Health and Human Services, Health Resources and Services Administration. Projected Supply, Demand and Shortages of Registered Nurses: 2000-2020, 2002. http://www.bhpr.hrsa.gov.
21. Harrington C, Kovner C, Mezey M, et al. Experts recommend minimum nurse staffing standards for nursing facilities in the United States. The Gerontologist 2000;40:5-16.
22. Caudill M, Patrick M. Nursing assistant turnover in nursing homes and needs satisfaction. J Gerontol Nurs 1989;15:24.
23. Remsburg RE, Armacost KA, Bennett RG. Improving nursing assistant turnover and stability rates in long-term care facility. Geriatr Nurs 1999;20:203.
24. Rubenstein LZ, Josephson KR, Robbins AS. Falls in nursing homes. Ann Int Med 1994;121:442-451.
25. Mulrow CD, Gerety MB, Kanten D, et al. A randomized trial of physical rehabilitation for very frail nursing home residents. JAMA 1994;271:519-524.
26. Irvine PW, Van Buren N, Crossley K. Causes for hospitalization of nursing home residents: the role of infection. J Am Geriatr Soc 1984;32:103-107.
27. O'Donnell JA, Hofmann MT. Urinary tract infections: how to manage nursing home patients with or without chronic catheterization. Geriatrics 2002;57:45, 49-52, 55-56.
28. Mybolte M, Nursing home: acquired pneumonia, Clin Inf Dis 2002;35:1205-1211.
29. Bentley DW, Bradley S, High K, et al. Practice guidelines for evaluation of fever and infection in long-term care facilities J Am Geriatr Soc 2001;49:210-222.
30. Wittman R, Altman RD, Karlan MS. Report of the Council on Scientific Affairs: use of restraints for patients in nursing homes. Arch Fam Med 1999;8:101-105.
31. Dimant J. Avoiding physical restraints in long-term care facilities. J Am Med Dir Assoc 2003;4:207-215.
32. National Pressure Ulcer Advisory Panel. Staging report 2004. http://www.npuap.org.
33. Bosshard W, Dreher R, Schnegg JF, et al. The treatment of chronic constipation in elderly people: an update. Drugs Aging 2004;21:911-930.
34. Morley JE, Silver AJ. Nutritional issues in nursing home care. Ann Intern Med 1995;123:850-859.
35. Murphy LM, Hipman TO. Percutaneous endoscopic gastrostomy does not prolong survival in patients with dementia. Arch Intern Med 2003;163:1351-1353.
36. Gillick MR. Rethinking the role of tube feeding in patients with advanced dementia. New Engl J Med 2000;342:206-210.
37. Magaziner J, German P, Zimmerman SI, et al. The prevalence of dementia in a statewide sample of new nursing home admissions. The Gerontologist 2000;30:663-672.
38. Mallet L, Strozyk WR. Tuberculosis in the elderly: incidence, manifestations, PPO skin tests and preventive therapy. DICD 1991;25:650-655.
39. Potter J, Scott OJ, Roberts MA, et al. Influenza vaccination of health care workers in long-term hospitals reduces the mortality of elderly patients. J Infect Dis 1995;175:1-6.
40. Institute of Medicine. Improving Quality of Care in Nursing Homes. Washington D.C: National Academy Press, 1986.

POSTTEST

1. All but which one of the following is a major (more than 10%) payee of U.S. nursing home expenses?
   a. Medicare
   b. Medicaid
   c. Private funds

2. Which one of the following is not true about working with families of nursing home patients?
   a. Family members are often difficult owing to their suspicions of poor-quality care and guilty feelings over nursing home placement.
   b. Admission is a good time to discuss advance directives, although it is often an emotionally traumatic time.
   c. Often a relative from out of town forces physicians to change treatment plans.

3. Which one of the following statements is most correct about medical problems in long-term care facilities?
   a. Empiric treatment of acute febrile illness is not possible in the nursing home.
   b. Weight loss can often be corrected by changing the diet.
   c. Routine laboratory testing on admission often uncovers treatable medical problems.

PRETEST ANSWERS

1. b
2. d
3. c

POSTTEST ANSWERS

1. a
2. c
3. b

OBJECTIVES

Upon completion of this chapter, readers will be able to:

- Appreciate the breadth of services available in the home.
- Define who qualifies for home care.
- Describe how home care is funded and paid for.
- Detail the clinician's role in home health care.
- Incorporate home visits into their personal clinical practices.
- Outline the evidence for the use of home care services.

PRETEST

1. An 85-year-old woman visits your office. She has a history of osteoarthritis, poor vision due to glaucoma, hypertension, and psoriasis. She reports increasing difficulty with dressing herself, bathing, and preparing her meals. Her neighbor has an "aide" who comes every day and helps her with similar issues. Which one of the following factors will impact on your patient's ability to obtain a home attendant?
   a. Being Medicaid eligible
   b. Her Medicare eligibility
   c. Having an acute skilled need
   d. A prognosis of 6 months or less

2. A 65-year-old marketing executive makes an appointment to see you in your office due to worsening knee pain. She reports 6 months of left knee pain that is worse with running and walking up stairs. She has tried using topical ice, a short course of acetaminophen, and an elastic sports knee brace—all without significant relief. Upon your examination you determine that the patient has mild to moderate osteoarthritis of the knee. Which one of the following services will the patient qualify for under the Medicare benefit?
   a. Home-based occupational therapy
   b. Home-based physical therapy
   c. Office-based physical therapy
   d. Office-based occupational therapy

3. With regard to ordering durable medical equipment for a patient with Medicare, which one of the following statements is true?
   a. The medical equipment company will not deliver the equipment until they have received payment from Medicare.
   b. The medical equipment company is ultimately responsible for ordering equipment that is medically appropriate.
   c. The main requirement for ordering durable medical equipment in the home is a patient's homebound status
   d. Medicare has specific requirements for each type of durable medical equipment covered.

Alvin Farnsworth, *Part 1*

This 84-year-old man is brought in to see you by his daughter who is very worried because he has been falling at home recently. He has a history of diabetes, hypertension and severe bilateral hip arthritis. He lives with his daughter but is alone during the day when she is at work. He reports that he has "tripped" on a few occasions when walking in his house. He reports no loss of consciousness and no presyncopal symptoms. Medications include metformin, lisinopril, aspirin, and acetaminophen. Physical examination is significant for poor vision, markedly limited range of motion of the hips, atrophy of the musculature of the lower extremities with mildly decreased strength, and bilateral sensory neuropathy in a stocking distribution. Laboratory investigation reveals HbA1C = 10.9,
and creatinine = 1.2. Mr. Farnsworth has Medicare and Medicaid.

Your assessment is that his falls are due to a variety of factors including poor vision, peripheral neuropathy, and disuse atrophy of the lower extremities. You are also concerned about the patient's poorly controlled diabetes and the daughter's stress. You make a referral to a home health care agency for services.

STUDY QUESTION

1. What services would you request?

WHAT IS HOME CARE?

The broadest definition of *home care* is "the provision of diagnostic, therapeutic, or social support services to the patient in the home fore the purpose of restoring

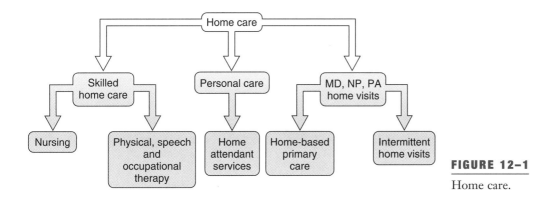

FIGURE 12–1

Home care.

and maintaining his or her maximal level of comfort, function and health."[1] In other words, the term refers to any services provided in the home to either maintain or improve a patient's well-being (Fig. 12–1).

Skilled home care, on the other hand, refers to in-home care provided by certified home health agencies. For a patient with Medicare, a physician may make a referral to a home health agency for any of the following services: nursing care, physical therapy, and speech therapy, provided that the patient qualifies for those services. Once the services are initiated, the patient may then qualify for additional services including in-home laboratory testing, social work visits, home health aide services, and occupational therapy. See Box 12–1 for examples of skilled home care services.

To obtain short-term Medicare funded home care services patients must meet three criteria: they must be homebound; they must have a qualifying skilled need; and they must have a physician willing to certify the need for home care and periodically review their treatment plan. Medicare's definition of homebound includes the following; the patient leaves the home infrequently, leaving the home requires the assistance of others, leaving the home is a taxing effort or burden for the patient, and the immobility is due to a medical or psychiatric reason.

Personal care is another important component of home care. This includes personal care aides helping patients with activities of daily living such as bathing and dressing, and instrumental activities of daily living such as meal preparation. These services are provided by Medicare-funded home health aides, Medicaid-funded home attendants, and privately paid personnel (Table 12–1). Home health aides and home attendants are not allowed to administer medications, administer enteral tube feedings, or participate in wound care. There are generally no regulations limiting the involvement of private-pay aides in these activities. However, if a private aide is hired through an agency, there may be restrictions regarding administration of controlled medications.

Home care also includes the provision of medical equipment in the home. Home medical equipment is broadly broken down into two categories: durable and nondurable. *Durable medical equipment* refers to those that are designed to hold up to repeated use such as wheelchairs, hospital beds, and walkers. *Nondurable medical equipment* refers to items that are typically used once and then disposed of, including adult incontinence pads and latex gloves.

Clinicians are responsible for ordering both types of equipment. As in the case of other home care services, insurance status will determine coverage. Medicare covers most types of durable medical equipment but does not cover nondurable equipment. Notable gaps in Medicare durable equipment coverage include canes, grab bars, and bath chairs. Medicaid typically covers durable and nondurable equipment, but there is state-by-state variability with regard to the types of items covered.

TRENDS IN SPENDING ON HOME CARE

In 2002, the last year for which such data are available, payers spent $36 billion on home care services, or

---

Box 12–1   Typical Skilled Home Care Services

- Care of a pressure or venous stasis ulcer
- Physical and occupational therapy after a stroke
- Monitoring of vital signs and other clinical parameters in a patient receiving treatment for a congestive heart failure exacerbation
- Family and patient education regarding diabetic monitoring and management
- Monitoring adherence and response to antibiotic therapy for pneumonia in a patient recently discharged from the hospital
- Pain and symptom management.
- Assessment of efficacy or side effects when introducing new medication

Table 12–1	Differences Between Home Health Aides and Home Attendants
Home Health Aide	**Home Attendant**
Medicare funded	Medicaid funded
Short duration of service	Chronic duration of service
Patient must have concurrent skilled need	No requirement for concurrent skilled need
Usually limited to 4 hours or less per day	State-by-state variability on range of hours per day

2.3% of the total national health expenditures in that year. This figure represents a substantial increase from 1988 when $8 billion were spent on home health care. In 2002, Medicare was responsible for approximately 32% of all home care expenditures, followed by Medicaid (23%), private insurers (19%), and out-of-pocket expenses (17%).[2]

Upon initial referral to the home health care agency, the clinician requests the following services:

1. Nursing care: home safety assessment, assessment of medication adherence, diabetic education, and monitoring
2. Physical therapy: strengthening, gait and balance training, assistive device selection, and assessment
3. Home health aide support: short-term help with activities of daily living
4. Social work evaluation: help with arranging long-term in-home personal care support

ARRANGING FOR HOME CARE SERVICES

The manner in which clinicians make referrals to home care agencies can have a significant impact on the success of the care plan. It is very important to provide specific information with regard to the services that the clinician believes a patient needs. If a clinician is requesting diabetic monitoring, for example, the nursing agency should receive clear instructions on what values are acceptable and what values should trigger a call to the clinician. It is equally important to provide the nursing agency with contact information for both regular work hours and evenings and weekends.

Once a referral is made and home care services are implemented, it is often useful to speak with the home care provider (nurse, physical therapist, etc.) to clarify the goals of the treatment plan, obtain and verify contact information, ask for input, and encourage open communication.

Good communication between clinicians and home care providers is critical to obtaining optimal results. When the home care nurse is comfortable contacting the clinician and feels valued as a member of the team, the nurse is more likely to provide important information in a timely manner. Critical information might include the

fact that a wound is not healing as expected, blood glucose readings are abnormal, low-salt diet recommendations have been completely misinterpreted by the patient, and there is a need for home care equipment.

Ordering home medical equipment is an important responsibility of the clinician. Therefore, it is important that clinicians are familiar with the common types of equipment and the regulations regarding the ordering of such equipment. Most durable medical equipment (DME) can be ordered by calling or faxing the appropriate information to a DME company. It is important to note that, in most cases, the DME company will deliver the equipment to the patient's home and then forward paperwork to the clinician for completion and signature. Once this paperwork is completed, the DME company will then submit it to the payer (typically Medicare) for payment. It is therefore important that equipment forms are completed and returned in a timely manner. Clinicians are ultimately responsible for equipment that they sign for and, therefore, it is important that they only authorize and sign for equipment that is medically necessary.

● When the home care nurse is comfortable contacting the clinician and feels valued as a member of the team, the nurse is more likely to provide important information in a timely manner.

Alvin Farnsworth, *Part 1*

Eight weeks later you are pleased to hear that the patient is improving. The physical therapist reports that he has participated actively in his therapy, he has adapted to his new rolling walker, and he has not fallen since services were put in place. The nurse reports that he now adheres to his medication regimen because of the introduction of a medication box, his diet has improved with counseling, and at the nurse's suggestion, his daughter has installed extra lighting so that he can see better when ambulating. A home blood draw by the nursing agency shows that the HBAIC is now down to 8.6. The nurse also reports that the patient's acute home care services will be ending soon.

STUDY QUESTION

1. With the end of Medicare-funded acute skilled services in sight, what home care options might be appropriate and available at this time?

REIMBURSEMENT FOR PARTICIPATING IN HOME CARE

When a physician authorizes acute skilled home care services, the physician will receive a "plan of care" from the nursing agency that must be reviewed for accuracy and signed. This is referred to as "home care certification." If the patient has Medicare, the physician can submit a bill to Medicare for reimbursement for this effort. Payment varies by geographic region. To bill for this service, the doctor must have seen the patient in the preceding six months. Nurse practitioners and physician assistants are not currently able to authorize and sign for home care services. Therefore, they are not permitted to bill for certification and recertification.

On the other hand, both physicians and nurse practitioners can bill Medicare for care plan oversight. *Care plan oversight* refers to activities that the clinician engages in to provide oversight to patients who are receiving Medicare-funded skilled home care. Medicare will reimburse for these activities for a given patient if they require more than 30 minutes of time in a calendar month. Covered activities include speaking with the home care nurse or physical therapist, reviewing consultant reports, and medical decision making. Time spent speaking with the patient, the patient's family members, or the clinician's medical partners do not count toward care plan oversight. Keep in mind that certification of home care services and care plan oversight reimbursement is provided through Medicare part B and patients are responsible for any co-pays not covered by a co-insurance. Clinicians may want to inform their patients of this additional charge.

> ### Alvin Farnsworth, *Part 3*
>
> *Six months later the patient suffers a severe stroke. He is hospitalized for 3 weeks and then transferred to a subacute rehabilitation facility for an additional 2 months. You receive a phone call from his daughter who reports that the rehabilitation facility is ready to discharge him. He will go home with acute nursing, physical therapy, and occupational therapy services as well as his prior personal care attendant. Because he is now wheelchair bound, he will not be able to come to the office for appointments until she is able to arrange for wheelchair ramp access to the house. You agree to see him at his home.*

STUDY QUESTION

1. With more and more of your patients needing similar care, in what ways might you incorporate house calls into your practice?

CLINICIAN (MD, NP, AND PA) HOME VISITS

Physician home visits, once the mainstay of American medicine, now constitute less than 1% of all patient–physician encounters.[3] However, a number of factors are driving a renewed interest in house calls. These include the rapid aging of the population, decreased inpatient length of stay leading to patients being discharged home when they are less clinically stable than in the past, patient preference, and recent increases in Medicare home visit reimbursement rates.[4]

Clinician house calls provide many potential benefits as compared with office-based care. For patients who are homebound and unable to get to the doctor's office, it may be the only way to receive ongoing primary care.[5] It can be an important component of post–hospital discharge assessment and management for older patients.[6] House calls can also play an important role diagnostically in assessing the environmental factors impacting on an otherwise ambulatory patient's health and well-being.[7]

There are a number of different house call models. Broadly, they break down into two categories: home-based primary care and intermittent house calls for acute problems. Some physicians make home visits full time and have no office-based practice. Others do so for a portion of their time—perhaps one session each week or each weekday afternoon after a morning of office-based care. There is a distinct set of Medicare CPT codes for home visits. This set includes five codes for new visits and four for revisits. There is a different set of codes for visits to adult homes and assisted living facilities.

Typical clinician equipment for home visits is listed in Box 12–2. With the advent of increasingly portable technology, clinicians are able to obtain better and better diagnostic information as well as provide advanced therapeutics in the home. Portable ECG machines, ultrasound bladder scanners, and bedside blood chemistry analyzers are some of the devices available to the modern home visit clinician.

Patients receiving clinician (MD, NP, PA) home visits do not need to conform to the same Medicare homebound requirement as those receiving skilled home care. However, the physician is responsible for documenting why the patient needs to be seen in the home. Most often home visits are required to provide care that cannot be provided in an office setting, such as for patients who are truly homebound (either permanently or temporarily) or to perform an assessment that can only be done in the home. Patient convenience is not considered an acceptable reason.

Box 12-2 Common Equipment for Clinician House Calls

- Stethoscope
- Blood pressure cuff
- Otoscope
- Ophthalmoscope
- Portable oximeter
- Reflex hammer
- Tuning fork
- Penlight
- Examination gloves
- Blood drawing supplies
- Wound care supplies
- Debridement kit
- Urinary catheters
- Toenail shears
- Sharps container
- Measuring tape
- Urine collection cups
- Fecal occult blood testing cards and developer
- Lubricant

● There are a number of different house call models; broadly, they break down into two categories: home-based primary care and intermittent house calls for acute problems.

THE EVIDENCE FOR HOME CARE

In 1990, the American Medical Association's Council on Scientific Affairs wrote: "More clinically oriented research is needed on patient care in the home before we can know with any assurance what interventions are most effective and appropriate."[1] Fortunately, a number of high-quality studies have been conducted since then that have helped to shape our understanding of the impact of various home care models on patient, caregiver, and health system outcomes.

Home visits have been shown to identify problems that are overlooked in the office setting. In one study, older patients referred to an interdisciplinary assessment clinic received an office-based medical evaluation and an office-based psychiatric evaluation, and these were followed by a single 90-minute home assessment. The home assessment included patient and caregiver interviews, a mental status examination, observation of the patient's function at home, inspection of all living areas with particular attention to physical hazards, and assessment of the patient's diet and medication regimen. Problems identified during the home visits that were not identified during the office-based evaluations were ranked in four categories depending on the degree of importance of the missing information to the patient's well-being. The results showed that almost 23% of patients had a problem identified only at home that conferred an increased risk of death or serious injury. Almost all patients had problems identified on the home assessment that conferred an increased risk of morbidity or loss of function. Commonly identified problems included safety problems (e.g., the need for increased supervision, bathing hazards, and wandering), medically related problems (e.g., poor medication regimen adherence, incontinence, and alcohol abuse), and psychobehavioral problems (e.g., depressed mood and confusion).[7]

At least one in-home geriatric assessment model has been shown to be associated with a lower rate of permanent nursing home placement and need for assistance with activities of daily living.[8] In this study, 414 community-dwelling men and women aged more than 74 years were randomized to usual care and usual care plus in-home assessment. The in-home assessments were conducted by geriatric nurse practitioners who evaluated problems, looked for risk factors for disability, provided health education, and gave specific recommendations to the treating physician and others. At 3 years, 4% of patients in the intervention arm of the study had been permanently placed in nursing homes as compared with 10% of those in the control arm ($p = 0.02$). The cost for each year of disability-free life was approximately $46,000.

In a groundbreaking study, Tinetti et al. were able to demonstrate that reorganizing home health agency providers into interdisciplinary teams, with appropriate training aimed at creating a restorative care team focus, could improve outcomes for home care patients without increasing costs.[9] As compared with usual care, the restorative care team model led to a higher percentage of patients remaining at home and a lower percentage of patients visiting emergency rooms. Remarkably, these outcomes were achieved even though there was a decrease in the average number of provider home visits for each patient in the restorative care team arm of the study.

On the other hand, home-based primary care models have not been well studied to date. Most studies are limited to single practice sites, do not use control groups, and are retrospective in nature. One large-scale multisite study of such programs in Veterans Affairs (VA) hospital systems showed improvements in satisfaction with care and caregiver burden, and no difference in functional outcomes with home-based primary care as compared with standard outpatient care.[10] In the absence of similar studies, it is difficult to know if these results can be generalized to other programs—particularly those that are not in the VA system.

Other studies have shown that interventions incorporating home visits can decrease subsequent risk of falls,[11] that multidisciplinary interventions incorporating home visits can reduce emergency department visits and hospital admissions,[12] and that multidisciplinary interventions that incorporate posthospitalization discharge nursing visits can decrease readmission rates for elderly patients with congestive heart failure and other selected conditions.[13,14] Other studies have shown conflicting results with regard to the impact of such home-based interventions.[15] It is likely that many of the outcomes are related to unique patient and care model characteristics of each program and intervention. Therefore, it is difficult to draw firm conclusions with regard to applying these results to other settings. The science of home care is, in many ways, still in its infancy. With more large-scale multisite trials, improved targeting of populations, improved delineation of care models, and more rigorous meta-analyses on the horizon, the future looks bright.

> ● Reorganizing home health agency providers into interdisciplinary teams, with appropriate training aimed at creating a restorative care team focus, could improve outcomes for home care patients without increasing costs.

SUMMARY

As the population ages, home care has come to play an increasingly important role in the nation's health care system. Home care includes a broad variety of services and the types of services one qualifies for is largely dependent on insurance status. Physicians are ultimately responsible for ordering most home care services, and therefore need to have a thorough understanding of who qualifies for home care, how it is funded, and how to effectively communicate with home care providers. Clinician (MD/NP/PA) home visits can play a very important role in helping selected subsets of patients to remain in their own homes and out of nursing homes.

There are adequate reimbursement structures to promote both clinician home visits and collaborative relationships with other home care providers. Lastly, there is a growing body of literature which suggests that specific home care interventions with targeted populations can have positive impacts on health outcomes, costs, and patient and caregiver satisfaction.

References

1. Council on Scientific Affairs. Home care in the 1990s. JAMA 1990;263:1241-4.
2. Levit K, Smith C, Cowan C, Sensenig A, Catlin A, Health Accounts Team. Health spending rebound continues in 2002. Health Aff (Millwood) 2004;23:147-59.
3. Meyer GS, Gibbons RV. House calls to the elderly—a vanishing practice among physicians. N Engl J Med 1997;337:1815-20.
4. Levine SA, Boal J, Boling PA. Home care. JAMA 2003;290:1203-7.
5. Fried TR, Wachtel TJ, Tinetti ME. When the patient cannot come to the doctor: a medical housecalls program. J Am Geriatr Soc 1998;46:226-31.
6. Naylor MD. A decade of transitional care research with vulnerable elders. J Cardiovasc Nurs 2000;14:1-14, quiz 88-9.
7. Ramsdell JW, Swart JA, Jackson JE, Renvall M. The yield of a home visit in the assessment of geriatric patients. J Am Geriatr Soc 1989;37:17-24.
8. Stuck AE, Aronow HU, Steiner A, et al. A trial of annual in-home comprehensive geriatric assessments for elderly people living in the community. N Engl J Med 1995;333:1184-9.
9. Tinetti ME, Baker D, Gallo WT, Nanda A, Charpentier P, O'Leary J. Evaluation of restorative care vs usual care for older adults receiving an acute episode of home care. JAMA 2002;287:2098-105.
10. Hughes SL, Weaver FM, Giobbie-Hurder A, et al. Effectiveness of team-managed home-based primary care: a randomized multicenter trial. JAMA 2000;284:2877-85.
11. Clemson L, Cumming RG, Kendig H, Swann M, Heard R, Taylor K. The effectiveness of a community-based program for reducing the incidence of falls in the elderly: a randomized trial. J Am Geriatr Soc 2004;52:1487-94.
12. Caplan GA, Williams AJ, Daly B, Abraham K. A randomized, controlled trial of comprehensive geriatric assessment and multidisciplinary intervention after discharge of elderly from the emergency department—the DEED II study. J Am Geriatr Soc 2004;52:1417-23.
13. Rich MW, Beckham V, Wittenberg C, Leven CL, Freedland KE, Carney RM. A multidisciplinary intervention to prevent the readmission of elderly patients with congestive heart failure. N Engl J Med 1995;333:1190-5.
14. Naylor MD, Brooten D, Campbell R, et al. Comprehensive discharge planning and home follow-up of hospitalized elders: a randomized clinical trial. JAMA 1999;281:613-20.
15. Kwok T, Lum CM, Chan HS, Ma HM, Lee D, Woo J. A randomized, controlled trial of an intensive community nurse-supported discharge program in preventing hospital readmissions of older patients with chronic lung disease. J Am Geriatr Soc 2004;52:1240-6.

Web Resources

1. American Academy of Home Care Physicians: www.aahcp.org.

POSTTEST

1. A 94-year-old woman with Parkinson's disease reports increasing falls at home. She denies losing consciousness, drop attacks, and has no witnessed seizure activity. She lives alone and has a home attendant for 4 hours per day, 7 days per week. Upon examination, she has a markedly stooped gait, a resting tremor, and a festinating gait with retropulsion. In addition to adjusting her medications and applying for an increase in her home attendant hours, which one of the following is appropriate at this time?
a. Home safety evaluation
b. Home physical therapy evaluation
c. Change in type of assistive device
d. All of the above

2. Your patient, a 70-year-old man, is being sent home after a lengthy hospitalization for congestive heart failure. He is significantly deconditioned, lives with no family members, and is being discharged on a higher dose of diuretic than when he presented to the hospital. Which one of the following is appropriate?
a. Nursing visits for assessment of vital signs and other clinical parameters
b. Nursing visits for patient education regarding his medication regimen and diet
c. Home physical therapy for strengthening and gait training
d. Home blood draws for assessment of electrolytes and renal function
e. All of the above

PRETEST ANSWERS

1. a
2. c
3. c

POSTTEST ANSWERS

1. d
2. e

Rehabilitation

Neil J. Nusbaum

OBJECTIVES

Upon completion of this chapter, the reader will be able to:

- Understand the burden of functional impairment in the older individual.

- Appreciate how level of function may fluctuate over time in an individual.
- Appreciate the role of rehabilitation in common diseases of the older individual.
- Understand how to support the rehabilitative needs of the patient within the primary care setting.

PRETEST

1. Of Americans over age 65, the percentage who are unable to walk two to three blocks is about
   a. 1%
   b. 5%
   c. 20%
   d. 40%
   e. 50%

2. Your patient is a 75-year-old man with a nondominant hemisphere stroke, leg weakness, and difficulty walking. Of the following, the most effective strategy for rehabilitation is
   a. Intensive inpatient therapy for 1 week, starting 1 day after the stroke
   b. Intensive inpatient therapy for 1 week, starting 1 week after the stroke
   c. Intensive outpatient therapy for 1 week, starting when discharged home
   d. Intensive therapy begun as an inpatient, continued at home
   e. Provision of an instructional video on walking

3. Leg spasticity in a patient after a stroke
   a. Does not occur in a weak muscle
   b. Is probably due to seizure activity
   c. Suggests a hemorrhagic stroke
   d. Is always undesirable
   e. Sometimes helps the patient stay upright

Alan Baker, *Part 1*

Your patient Alan Baker is a 75-year-old man with a 20-year history of diabetes who has developed peripheral neuropathy, and in recent years has had recurrent foot ulcers. He has hypertension, but his blood pressure control varies depending on whether he remembers to take his medication. His wife had driven the family car for the past 2 years, until her death 2 months ago. The patient is brought to your office by his neighbor, with a complaint of onset of one-block dyspnea on exertion beginning a month ago. When you question the patient, he says everything is going "okay." He has a few scattered rales on pulmonary exam, and bilateral pretibial edema. His EKG today shows septal Q waves not present on his EKG a year ago.

STUDY QUESTIONS

1. What are the patient's current rehabilitative needs?
2. What additional rehabilitation issues are likely to arise in the succeeding year?

> ● Rehabilitation efforts for frail elders may be directed to avoid loss of function, to help promote return of lost function, or both.

REHABILITATION AND THE OLDER INDIVIDUAL

The goal of rehabilitative care of older individuals is the prevention or delay of the onset of disability, and there is accordingly great attraction to the idea of directing rehabilitation efforts to the frail elderly.[1] Although there is a modest role of genetic factors in the risk for functional impairment in old age, environmental factors appear to be far more important.[2]

Rehabilitative care is one strategy for improving the mix of environmental factors to promote best function. Rehabilitation efforts for frail elders may be directed to avoid loss of function, to help promote return of lost function, or both.[3]

Some patients may have a sudden obvious event, such as a stroke or a hip fracture that is expected to produce an immediate severe functional decline that would benefit from rehabilitation. Many frail older individuals however may suffer progressive limitation from a gradual decline in function, and they may have gradually reduced their habitual level of activity to compensate for their decreased functional abilities. Fear of falling may have led patients to restrict walking and other activity even more severely than functional limitations might require, so that their abilities further decline from deconditioning. Many of these patients may benefit from rehabilitative regimens to help them regain their prior level of function.

An individual's level of disability is determined not just by physical and mental function. This broader view is embodied in the International Classification of Functioning, Disability and Health: "Functioning and disability are viewed as a complex interaction between the health condition of the individual and the contextual factors of the environment as well as personal factors. The picture produced by this combination of factors and dimensions is of 'the person in his or her world.' The classification treats these dimensions as interactive and dynamic rather than linear or static."[4]

Functional impairment is common among older persons, not just the small minority (5% of those aged 65 years and older) who reside in nursing homes. Of all Medicare enrollees aged 65 and over, 14% of the men and 23% of the women are unable to walk two to three blocks. There is evidence that some measures of age-adjusted rates of disability in the United States have declined, although with the growth in the total population over age 65, the absolute number of chronically disabled older individuals has modestly increased[5] (Fig. 13–1).

In the older patient, there is often more than one condition that can contribute to disability. A 1996 survey found that, of Medicare patients aged 65 years and over, 64% had at least one potentially disabling condition (blindness or low vision, deafness or hard of hearing, difficulties walking, difficulties reaching overhead, difficulties grasping and writing), and 30% had more than one of these conditions.[6]

The two most common areas of reported difficulty are in hearing and walking, both of which can benefit from medical attention, but for which the rehabilitative strategies are substantially different. Significant

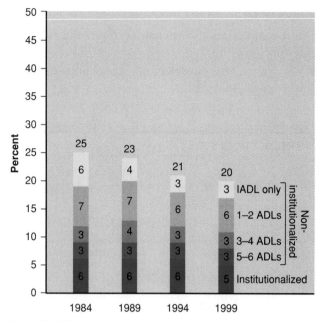

Age-adjusted percentage of medicare enrollees age 65 and over who are chronically disabled, by level and category of disability 1984, 1989, 1994, and 1999

Note: Disabilities are grouped into two categories: limitations in activities of daily living (ADLs) and limitations in instrumental activities of daily living (IADLs). The six ADLs included are bathing, dressing, getting in or out of bed, getting around inside, toileting, and eating. The eight IADLs included are light housework, laundry, meal preparation, grocery shopping, getting around outside, managing money, taking medications, and telephoning. Individuals are considered to have an ADL disability if they report receiving help or supervision, or using equipment, to perform the activity, or not performing the activity at all. Individuals are considered to have an IADL disability if they report using equipment to perform the activity or not performing the activity at all because of their health or a disability. Individuals are considered to be chronically disabled if they have at least one ADL or one IADL limitation that is expected to last 90 days or longer, or they are institutionalized. Data for 1989 do not sum to the total because of rounding. Reference population: These data refer to Medicare enrollees.

FIGURE 13–1

Age-adjusted percentage of Medicare enrollees aged 65 and over who are chronically disabled, by level and category of disability. Redrawn from National Long-Term Care Survey, with permission. Available at http://agingstats.gov/chartbook 2004/OA_2004.pdf. Accessed April 1, 2006.

hearing deficits are likely to require provision of a hearing aid, and support by the clinician to encourage the patient to obtain it and to use it once prescribed.[7] Difficulties with gait may reflect one or a combination of deficits (muscle weakness, postural instability, poor vision, peripheral neuropathy), for which the appropriate choice of management will depend in large part on the clinician's evaluation of the relevant contributory factors for the patient.

Rehabilitative strategies for older patients with weakness can be successfully linked to skills necessary to perform activities of daily living, rather than simply focused on increasing strength.[8] This may make it easier to design regimens that can directly improve functional ability, and which can be readily reinforced during physical activity while performing daily tasks.

How well or poorly an older person may be able to participate in society reflects the influence of both individual and environmental factors, and this broad view should guide rehabilitation planning. Rehabilitative measures may be directed to improve the person's own intrinsic performance. They may also involve provision of assistive devices that can compensate for the person's intrinsic impairments, as well as modifications of the wider physical environment to better fit the patient's impairments. All these approaches may fruitfully be combined; a patient with diabetic retinopathy may benefit from laser therapy of the retina, from the provision of eyeglasses for refractive correction, and from the use of large print on signs.

The evaluation of function should be tailored to the individual patient's situation, and may incorporate consideration of both objective and subjective information. It can include assessment of motor strength on the neurologic examination, as well as evaluation of the patient's ability to perform activities of daily living (e.g., getting out of bed) and instrumental activities of daily living (e.g., grocery shopping). The degree to which a patient is disabled by a loss of function depends in part on what they consider normal, as well as by their level of social supports. Even if they can still accomplish a task such as walking to go grocery shopping, they may have noted that it involves more pain from knee osteoarthritis, that they have to do it differently such as buying smaller numbers of bags at each trip, and/or that it takes more time to walk to and from the grocery store.[9] These early complaints may foreshadow the risk of being unable to accomplish the task of grocery shopping at all.

> ● Rehabilitation of older adults can take place in an acute hospital medical or rehabilitation unit, the nursing home, an outpatient area, or the patient's home.

REHABILITATION SETTINGS

Rehabilitation of older adults can take place in an acute hospital medical or rehabilitation unit, the nursing home, an outpatient area, or the patient's home. The ability to provide in-hospital rehabilitative care to Medicare beneficiaries has been influenced by changes in reimbursement formulas. Between 1994 and 2001, the median length of stay for inpatient rehabilitation fell from 20 days to 12 days.[10,11] Skilled nursing facilities may also deliver rehabilitation services to many of their residents, typically at a lower level of intensity than patients would receive in a hospital facility, and

such services may enable the resident to regain enough function to leave the nursing facility and return to the community.[12] Changes pursuant to the Balanced Budget Amendment of 1997, however, not only have affected the reimbursement structure for rehabilitation hospitals,[13] but also have made it less financially attractive for skilled nursing facilities[14] to offer their residents rehabilitation services. The ongoing changes in the Medicare program are likely to have a significant impact on the availability of rehabilitation services across a variety of care settings. The pressure of the Prospective Payment System on inpatient rehabilitation facilities for prompt discharge may have contributed to a pattern of discharges from impatient rehabilitation often being directed not to discharge home, but rather to a skilled nursing facility (SNF).[14a] The payment schema in turn places strong incentives on the skilled nursing facilities to control the intensity of the care they provide; Medicare provides reimbursement to the SNF for rehabilitative care to a certain point, but therapy beyond 720 minutes/week offers no marginal reimbursement.[14b] Yet another Prospective Payment System methodology has been adopted in the home health setting, creating a financial incentive for the home health provider to limit overall home visitors.[14c]

In the patients residing in a nursing home, the impairments are likely to be substantial and multiple[15]; they may be relatively easier to recognize but the process of rehabilitating them may be relatively more complex. Among nursing home residents, for example, those with new impairment in voluntary movement or in range of motion are at particular risk for a decrease in their ability to perform the activities of daily living.[16] The rehabilitation goals for the long-term nursing home resident are likely to be different and more modest, and a successful outcome may be to maintain level of function rather than to achieve full independence.

Rehabilitation regimens will often need tailoring to the abilities of the frail older individual. Even for those individuals in the nursing home setting, there is reason to suspect that many could benefit from an increased level of therapy, both that delivered formally by therapists and that received from the bedside nursing staff. A recent study of patients in skilled nursing facilities demonstrated that patients had a more rapid increase in their functional status, and a greater chance of leaving the nursing home to return to the community, if they were in a facility where the average resident received at least 1.5 hours of therapy per day. Likewise, both the rate of increase in functional status, and the chance of returning to the community, was higher for patients who were in skilled nursing facilities that provided higher levels of nurse staffing.[17]

REHABILITATION TEAM

Rehabilitation is an approach to care provided by a team of professionals. Although physicians specializing in physical medicine and rehabilitation, physical therapists, and occupational therapists are most closely identified with rehabilitation practice, the rehabilitation approach is applicable to older patients being cared for by geriatricians, primary care physicians, orthopedists, neurologists, nurses, psychologists, social workers, and most other health care professionals. In a given case, all rehabilitation disciplines involved will have a discipline-specific focus to their portion of the comprehensive assessment. Table 13–1 lists and briefly describes the roles of various rehabilitation professionals.

> ● An important preventive measure in primary care is to encourage physical activity to help patients achieve a higher level of baseline function, so that they will have more functional reserve during an illness.

Table 13–1	Rehabilitation Professionals
Professional	**Role**
Physiatry (physical medicine–trained MD)	Evaluates patient, integrates assessment data, determines potential, coordinates rehabilitation plan
Primary care physician	Manages acute and chronic medical care
Rehabilitation nurse	Integrates medical, nursing, rehabilitation plan
Physical therapist	Addresses mobility, strength, range of motion
Occupational therapist	Addresses activities of daily living and self-care
Speech pathologist	Addresses communication, swallowing
Psychologist and neuropsychologist	Diagnosis/treatment of mood, behavioral and cognitive conditions
Social worker	Works with family, patient, financial counseling, discharge planning
Nutritionist	Assesses nutrition status, diet plan
Pharmacist	Reviews medication use
Audiologist	Provides hearing assessment and treatment
Vocational counselor	Evaluates work potential, provides training
Recreational therapist	Assists with hobbies, leisure activities, motivation
Orthotist/prosthetist	Makes and fits orthopedic aids

Adapted from Warshaw GA. Rehabilitation and the aged. In: Gallo JJ, Busby-Whitehead J, Rabins PV, et al., eds. Care of the Elderly: Clinical Aspects of Aging. 5th ed. Philadelphia: Lippincott Williams & Wilkins, 1999:275.

PREVENTION OF FUNCTIONAL DECLINE AND ANTICIPATORY PLANNING

In planning for the primary care of an older individual, even one without current functional limitations, it is useful to consider with them the possibility that they may become frail in the future. Individuals may vary over time in their degree of disability[18] and in their needs for rehabilitation. Intermittent episodes of disability may be a marker for underlying frailty, and they may contribute to worsening frailty by leading to inactivity and deconditioning. Among the community-dwelling elderly, a commonly reported pattern is to spend occasional brief (one to several days) episodes at bed rest because of illness, injury, or other complaints. Patients with a history of episodic bed rest are at increased risk for functional decline.[19]

Advance planning for the possibility of functional decline may help ameliorate the degree of disability produced by future functional limitations. This may involve such seemingly nonmedical issues as the choice of housing in middle age, that is, an environment that will meet potential future needs. The degree of disability produced in later life by a hip fracture, and the patient's concomitant rehabilitation needs, may differ if the patient lives in a building with access only by staircase than in one with elevator or ramp accessibility. Reassessment of the patient's need for rehabilitation services, and for other services such as social services, may be particularly useful at times when their overall medical condition changes. It may also be of value at times when their system of social supports is altered, such as by the death of a spouse.

Various clinical interventions have been evaluated to test their impact on preventing disability. A detailed multispecialty evaluation of each older patient's functional status may be difficult to accomplish in routine primary care practice, and the yield may be relatively small.[20] One strategy for increasing the yield of rehabilitative care is to focus on situations of highest risk. Clinical situations that pose a particular risk for the onset of disability are hospitalizations (particularly after a fall) and episodes of restricted physical activity.[21] These clinical situations may be particularly fruitful settings for a focus on measures to decrease the risk for incident disability.

One of the important preventive measures in primary care is to encourage physical activity, to help patients achieve a higher level of baseline function, so that they will have more functional reserve. Subjects who later experience a functional decline may regain some or all of their functional loss, but are at high risk for losing function again in the near future. They are more likely to recover their independence of function, and to maintain their regained independence of function for a longer period of time, if they have a baseline pattern of habitual physical activity.[22]

Low-cost rehabilitative strategies may be most feasible for community-dwelling patients in generally stable condition.[23] These may be as straightforward as group exercise programs. In many cases, these strategies will be able to establish a higher functional status for the patient, so that if the patient has a subsequent decline in functional status it will not produce as severe a degree of functional deficit.

Alan Baker, *Part 2*

After his last visit to you, you arranged for Mr. Baker to attend a local senior center 3 days a week (Monday, Wednesday, Friday). His son has also been coming to check on him each Sunday. His son also says that he phones his father every Tuesday, Thursday, and Saturday mornings.

You receive a call Monday morning that Mr. Baker is in the emergency room. He slipped on the ice when he went to pick up his morning newspaper. The emergency room physician reports that your patient has a foul-smelling ulcer of his left heel, with bone exposed. He has no focal neurologic deficits, but he thinks he is at home. His EKG is unchanged from when you recently saw him in your office.

STUDY QUESTIONS

1. What are the patient's current rehabilitative needs?
2. What additional rehabilitation issues are likely to arise in the succeeding year?

> ● The use of an assistive device can interfere with the patient's ability to use a stairway banister or a wall for stability and actually increase the risk for a fall.

GAIT REHABILITATION, HIP REPLACEMENTS, AND FRACTURES

Patients may attempt to adjust to their gait problems by strategies such as walking more slowly. Slower walking speed by itself may prove a good compensatory strategy when walking on difficult terrain for older individuals in good health,[24] and even for those with exercise limitations from mild chronic stable angina, but is much less likely to compensate for the effects of diabetic peripheral neuropathy on proprioception.[25]

One component of therapy for patients with gait limitation is likely to be physical activity tailored to patient abilities. Frail older patients who engage in even very modest amounts of informal exercise (walking more than one block per day) are likely to preserve their residual mobility better than patients who are more sedentary.[26] Patient selection for rehabilitation should not be restricted by chronologic age, as appropriate patients even in their nineties have been shown to derive benefit from a rehabilitation program.[27,28]

Primary clinicians are in an excellent position to encourage increased physical activity by their patients. One strategy to do so is to identify particularly those patients who are already in the contemplative phase of considering an exercise program, and then to target them with motivational advice and educational materials on the benefit to them of exercise.[29] Printed patient educational materials are far less likely to be useful, however, in meeting the rehabilitation needs of patients who are more acutely ill,[30] particularly if they may suffer from delirium or dementia.

Patients with gait problems may benefit from use of a cane (used in the hand contralateral to the weak leg) or a walker, and there are a variety of each type of device available. A cane, and even more so a walker, permits the upper body muscles to support part of the person's weight. Assistive devices can also widen the patient's base of support, and can offer tactile feedback via the cane to one hand or the walker to both hands.

These mobility aids can also be associated with falls. The very reason the individual was prescribed a cane or walker may have been that their gait was unsteady and they were diagnosed as a fall risk. Use of an assistive device can interfere with the patient's ability to use a stairway banister or a wall for stability. The patient can potentially trip over the device itself. Further, use of a cane or walker requires the person to change their customary way of walking, a task that may be difficult to master, particularly in the older patient with cognitive impairment.[31]

Rehabilitation therapy can be of benefit to older individuals with a wide variety of musculoskeletal conditions,[32] including those with lower extremity fractures or following joint replacement surgery. A rehabilitation program is often an important part of the postoperative course of the older patient. The patient may often derive great benefit if the rehabilitation is begun in the early postoperative period in the hospital, rather than being delayed until the patient is discharged from the acute care setting. In one small study of unilateral hip replacement, early postoperative rehabilitation shortened the mean length of stay in hospital by 6 days.[33]

● A patient who has a hip fracture may still be ambulatory. EARLY recognition of the fracture is important for appropriate managemaent.

● Better functional outcomes for frail, older hip fracture patients may occur if (following their routine postoperative physical therapy) they undergo an additional 6 months of supervised outpatient rehabilitation.

Hip fractures are classified into three major categories according to anatomic location: femoral neck (subcapital or intracapsular), intertrochanteric, and subtrochanteric. Femoral neck fractures account for one-third of the hip fractures in the elderly and place the blood supply to the femoral head at risk, resulting in a higher incidence of avascular necrosis. Intertrochanteric fractures account for the other two-thirds of hip fractures and usually unite, but they are associated with significant blood loss and more early complications than femoral neck fractures. Subtrochanteric fractures are uncommon in the older patient, result from very significant force, and are more difficult to repair.

Hip fractures are an important cause of functional decline in the older individual. The presentation is often clear in a patient with inability to walk and with pain and limb deformity after a fall, but some patients will have much less striking findings.[33a] Early recognition of the fracture facilitates prompt management, which is usually surgical in nature, to achieve the best outcome in subsequent rehabilitation. The particular surgical approach to a fracture will vary depending according to the surgeon's technical preference, the patient's comorbidities, as well as the site of the fracture[33b] and whether it is displaced.

Efforts to avoid medical complications in the immediate postoperative period are imperative. Deep venous thrombosis is a particular risk with and after hip surgery, and it has been recommended that patients receive at least ten days of antithrombotic therapy.[34] Attention to removing bladder catheters postoperatively will help avoid urinary tract infections. Delirium is also a potential concern in the older individual with recent hip fracture, who has undergone the stresses both of a hip fracture and of the orthopedic surgical procedure for repair of the fracture.

Pressure ulcers may result from a combination of factors, all of which may be present in the patient undergoing rehabilitation (sustained high local pressures such as at the site of a bony prominence, shear forces on the underlying tissue, frictional damage to the skin, moisture of the skin).[34a] Medications that cause decreased level of consciousness, and devices and lines that restrict patient mobility, may increase the risk for pressure ulcers. Adequate skin care requires exemplary nursing care, including repeated repositioning of those patients with impaired mobility.

Even in frail older patients, prompt surgical intervention is commonly required for hip fracture to achieve the best functional result. Early mobilization postoperatively is also an important part of the patient's care, and the recent trend has been to be more liberal in allowing in patient weight-bearing postoperatively.[34b] The older patient with a preexisting cognitive deficit may be unable to participate in any therapy that involves degrees of weight bearing. As a practical matter, it is much easier for the physical therapist to administer postoperative rehabilitation if the doctor's orders allow.

A randomized controlled trial has demonstrated better functional outcomes for older hip fracture patients if (following their routine postoperative physical therapy) they undergo an additional 6 months of supervised outpatient rehabilitation, rather than the control condition of simply being discharged from postoperative therapy with advice on home exercise.[35] Attention during rehabilitation to factors that may have placed the patient at risk for their first hip fracture (osteoporosis, gait unsteadiness) is important because the older patient with a hip fracture remains at risk for a second hip fracture.[36]

Osteoarthritis of the hip or knee can produce significant limitation of function, and the primary therapy for long-term treatment of severe osteoarthritis is surgical in nature. Rehabilitation therapy[37] has a role in some patients with milder disease as a component of nonsurgical management; in other cases it helps delay the need for surgery, and in still others to assist in postoperative recovery after orthopedic surgery.[38-40]

STROKE REHABILITATION

An important setting where rehabilitation is often needed is in the older patient following a stroke. The nature of rehabilitation services required will reflect the array of neurologic deficits following the event. Patient participation in a rehabilitation program may require emotional support for the patient who is suffering from depression after a stroke. Communication difficulties between patient and therapist, such as in the patient who has a receptive aphasia following a stroke, may also require special attention in order to work effectively with the patient on rehabilitation of various neurologic deficits.

Rehabilitation efforts can begin even during the stroke hospitalization. In particular, efforts should be made to avoid or minimize deconditioning while in hospital, using measures consistent with the patient's overall condition. Even if the patient is not capable of walking, periods of standing up or even sitting in a chair can help to minimize the deconditioning from bed rest in hospital.[41] The interdisciplinary rehabilitation approach should include not only the therapy disciplines themselves, but also other caregivers including the nursing staff and family.[42]

Given the risk for episodic disability, important goals of a rehabilitative program may be to try to decrease the risk for recurrent episodes of disability, as well as to help diminish the length and severity of episodes of present and potential future episodes of disability. In a study of hospitalized ischemic stroke patients, those who achieved higher levels of physical function after their stroke were less likely to require hospital readmission in the succeeding 12 months.[43]

Rehabilitation treatment for the stroke patient derives from an ongoing team assessment. The physical therapist's focus is on strength, endurance, and mobility. Motor recovery may display a sequence of patterns. The stroke patient initially may have a flaccid paralysis, which may be followed by phase(s) where groups of muscles act in synergy, before the patient finally regains ability to move individual joints. Only some recovering stroke patients go through such a sequence, and it is often associated with limb spasticity.[43a] Although this sequence can vary from case to case, it is helpful to recognize that certain patterns can be capitalized on to assist with particular activities (e.g., extensor synergy and walking).[44] Treatment begins with bed mobility and progresses to balance training and sitting. Ambulation requires adequate strength and trunk stability. Patients with severe impairments may begin walking in parallel bars and then be advanced to walkers or canes. If weakness in the lower leg is present, an ankle-foot orthosis (short leg brace) can promote more efficient ambulation by ensuring fixed dorsiflexion at the ankle and minimizing toe dragging in the swing phase of gait.

The occupational therapist addresses upper extremity function and the ability to perform activities of daily living (ADLs), instrumental ADLs, and visual-spatial perception deficits. Maintenance of range of motion in the affected upper extremity is essential to avoid the development of a painful shoulder or contractures. When distal upper extremity spasm is present, wrist splints are prescribed. To avoid shoulder subluxation, transfers are managed without additional stress on the shoulder joint, and pillows and arm boards are used to support the affected arm.

These positioning techniques maintain the humeral head in its proper position when the muscles usually responsible for this alignment are flaccid. Dressing aids, such as clothes reachers, button hooks, sock donners, and Velcro closures may be prescribed. Feeding aids, such as rocker knives and plate guards, can be helpful.

Impairment of language function can be the most frustrating consequence of stroke. Dysarthria and aphasia require assessment by a speech pathologist. Communication boards can be provided to help patients with expressive aphasia make their wishes known. The speech pathologist can also help rehabilitation team members communicate with the patient. The patient's ability to swallow should be assessed before oral fluids and food are started.

Often the most important goal for rehabilitative efforts after stroke is to enable the patient to return home. Depending on the patient's rehabilitative needs, and on the level of support available in their home environment, the process may involve a stay in a subacute unit or a skilled nursing facility after discharge from the acute hospital setting. Many rehabilitative services can be delivered in the home (or other outpatient) setting, and rehabilitative care begun in hospital may often be continued at home after discharge. An important primary care goal in such cases is to make sure that there is continuity of the rehabilitative plan across changes in the care setting.

A home rehabilitation process can decrease overall length of stay compared to a program that delivers all the rehabilitation as an inpatient in one or a mix of facilities (e.g., acute care hospital, subacute unit, skilled nursing facility).[45] The therapist in the home setting can ensure that patients can transfer the rehabilitation skills learned in hospital and apply them in the environment where they are residing, to help them maintain their ability to live independently.[46,47] It also provides an opportunity to directly evaluate the home setting across a variety of dimensions[48] (Box 13–1). Evaluations to determine, for example, if the level of home lighting and the arrangement of furniture will help the patient to maneuver safely in the home.

The use of earlier hospital discharge, coupled with post discharge rehabilitation services at home, has been demonstrated to decrease health care costs and improve functional outcomes.[48a] A Swedish randomized study of poststroke rehabilitation suggests durable benefit for stroke patients if one supplemented their inpatient stroke unit rehabilitation, by adding the use following discharge home of a course of home rehabilitation. Although this intervention involved only a mean of 12 home visits delivered over

---

Box 13-1 **Assessment of Discharge Environment**

Functional needs

Motivation and preferences

Intensity of tolerable treatment

    Equipment

    Duration

Availability and eligibility

Transportation

Home assessment for safety

Available at VA/DoD clinical Practice guideline for the management of stroke rehabilitation in the primary care setting, http://www.oqp.med.va.gov/cpg /STR/STR_base.htm. Accessed April 2, 2006.

---

a mean of 4 months, the patients receiving the home rehabilitation showed benefit on functional outcomes assessed 5 years later.[49]

● Common poststroke medical complications include depression, shoulder pain, falls, and urinary tract infection.

Rehabilitative efforts may often be designed to meet goals of particular relevance to patient quality of life. A focus of rehabilitation may often be to increase the individual's ability to participate in society, such as to leave their home, and even modest interventions may have significant effects. An occupational therapy intervention for stroke patients, for example, significantly improved patients' outdoor mobility even though it involved a mean of only 230 minutes total contact time (spread over several visits) of the patient with the therapist.[50]

In patients recovering from a stroke, functional impairment may result not just from muscle weakness alone, but also from its combination with other neurologic deficits. The goals of rehabilitation efforts typically are designed around improving function, rather than around improving a specific neurologic parameter, such as the degree of spasticity. Spasticity after a stroke can further interfere with function. Spasticity however can also be used as part of a compensatory strategy for poststroke weakness in the same muscle group.[51]

In the ongoing care of the patient, of particular concern are the complications that may follow a stroke or other disabling event, and can potentially interfere with successful rehabilitation. In a Canadian study of a group of stroke patients admitted for inpatient stroke rehabilitation, during their rehabilitation stay (mean length of stay 40 days) two-thirds had at least one event characterized by the study author as a medical complication, and a quar-

ter of the patients had multiple such complications. The four most common complications noted were depression, shoulder pain, falls, and urinary tract infection.[52]

The propensity for falls is of special concern because many elderly stroke patients may have baseline osteoporosis, a condition that will likely worsen over time (particularly if they have poor mobility after their stroke).[53] The combination of fall risk and osteoporosis places these patients at risk for hip fracture when they walk or transfer. Interventions to preserve bone mass (bisphosphonate therapy, dietary and/or supplemental calcium and vitamin D) will commonly be useful as part of their management.

CARDIAC REHABILITATION

A common area where rehabilitation may be underutilized is across the spectrum of patients with cardiac disease,[54,55] and the patient may benefit from clinician encouragement to enter and then to remain with a rehabilitation program. A patient who has just undergone hospitalization for a cardiac event may be particularly motivated to begin a cardiac rehabilitation program.

Patient participation in rehabilitation may be compromised particularly if the patient does not drive, and lacks ready access to other transportation to the rehabilitation setting.[56] Cardiac rehabilitation may successfully be delivered in the home setting if resources to do so are available.[57]

A cardiac rehabilitation program can appropriately incorporate an individualized exercise program, as part of the effort to prevent a recurrent cardiac event, and in order to improve the patient's capability to perform daily activities. Occasional cardiac events have been reported during the exercise component of cardiac rehabilitation, and a subset of patients may benefit from more intensive monitoring of their cardiac status during exercise. The long-term benefits in general far outweigh the very small risk of engaging in a supervised cardiac exercise program.

The American Heart Association[58] has strongly endorsed the benefits of a coordinated approach to cardiac rehabilitation, including exercise training, modification of cardiac risk factors, and attention to psychological and social function. A cardiac rehabilitation program may include simultaneous attention to both increasing physical activity and to a variety of other lifestyle changes, such as smoking cessation. A regular exercise program may complement a smoking-cessation program, particularly in patients who have been advised to stop smoking and are concerned about attendant weight gain.

Both younger and older patients can benefit from cardiac rehabilitation. Cardiac patients in general, and in some studies the older cardiac patients in particular, are often either not receiving referrals to cardiac rehabilitation or are failing to participate after being referred.[59] The clinician in the primary care setting is an excellent position to reinforce at outpatient office visits the need for cardiac rehabilitation[60] and to encourage continuing adherence to rehabilitation attendance and lifestyle changes. One innovative strategy that has been suggested to increase referrals for cardiac rehabilitation is to use a system of automated referrals of eligible patients, as triggered by the electronic medical record, but still coupled with a personalized letter to the patient.[61]

> ● There is evidence for the benefit of starting a program of pulmonary rehabilitation within 10 days following hospital discharge following an exacerbation of chronic obstructive pulmonary disease (COPD).

PULMONARY REHABILITATION

Rehabilitation including exercise training may be of particular value for patients with COPD, in order to improve exercise tolerance, reduce dyspnea, and improve quality of life.[62]

There is evidence for benefit from starting a program of pulmonary rehabilitation within 10 days following hospital discharge following an exacerbation of COPD.[63] Much of the benefit of pulmonary rehabilitation by exercise training, such as lower extremity exercise (e.g., bicycle riding), comes from the improvement of peripheral muscle function rather than from an effect on the ventilatory muscles.[64,65] Home pulmonary rehabilitation has also been delivered in a program using telephone follow-up by the therapist,[66] but such minimally supervised exercise strategies requires a cognitively intact, motivated patient.

REHABILITATION IN CANCER PATIENTS

Older patients with incurable malignancy may derive significant benefit from a brief and focused rehabilitation program.[67] Rehabilitation may help the patient cope with functional deficits related to the effects of the cancer itself or the therapy received for the cancer. A cancer patient, for example, may have gait difficulty and associated rehabilitative needs for a wide variety of reasons, ranging from pathologic lower extremity fracture from metastatic cancer, to stroke from brain metastases, to postoperative deficits following surgical excision of a lower extremity sar-

coma. Therapy in the cancer setting may also often appropriately consider strategies to help the patient cope with potential future deficits if the cancer progresses.

A particular challenge may be how to integrate a rehabilitation program with a program of cancer treatment, particularly in a patient who may be experiencing fatigue and cachexia related to cancer. However, a variety of studies have been done of exercise programs for cancer, with some evidence that exercise in the setting of cancer can promote a decrease rather than an increase in patient fatigue.[68]

AGING WITH A LONGSTANDING DISABILITY

One of the most challenging areas in geriatric rehabilitative care is the treatment of older patients who have longstanding disabilities from early in life. They may lose some of the physical strength and other reserves they had drawn upon earlier to cope with their baseline disability. The ongoing challenge of coping with their disability may lead to complaints including sleep disorders, pain, or fatigue even in late middle age. Patients may perceive this as aging more rapidly and/or with more complications. In the patient with spinal cord injury,[69] for example, even young patients may have issues of skin breakdown from immobility, and these issues may become even more pressing as the patient ages and becomes less mobile. Individuals with spinal cord injury are at high risk for functional decline if they suffer medical complications such as pressure ulcers.[70]

The care of aging adults with disability may be especially complicated when their parents provide the patient's care, and then the parents themselves become disabled or die. The patients and their families in the past may have given more consideration to their medical needs in the short to medium term, and less to the issues of aging that have become important as patients have prolonged survival despite their disability.[71] Rehabilitation efforts should consider how to address the patient's long-term disability, and how those efforts may need to be reshaped as the patient ages and as their network of social supports may change.

Declines in functional reserve may impact on the patient's use of compensatory strategies. A person with baseline paraplegia, for example, may achieve mobility by wheelchair. If the patient later loses upper extremity strength, for example, the patient may lose some of the ability to accomplish wheelchair ambulation. In some cases, these functional declines can be addressed by a change in the rehabilitative regimen, such as from a manually operated wheelchair to an electrically powered wheelchair.

REHABILITATION IN SETTING OF MULTIPLE COMORBIDITIES

Older individuals with a functional limitation may have a combination of other acute and chronic illnesses, many of which can also influence their rehabilitation. Meeting the rehabilitative needs of these complex patients is likely to require a high degree of communication and individualized planning of care. Care planning requires a thorough understanding of the full range of the patient's medical problems, and this task may be particularly complex in the oldest old. Rehabilitative needs should be addressed in the context of other medical issues; rehabilitation following a stroke is important, but even more valuable is stroke reduction by more effective treatment of hypertension.

REHABILITATION AND COGNITIVE PROBLEMS

An issue that commonly arises in rehabilitative geriatric care is the role of rehabilitation in the patient with cognitive impairment.[72,73] Cognitive impairment may tend to lessen the benefit an individual may derive from a rehabilitation program.[74] This may be particularly the case if the rehabilitative program calls on the patient to perform cognitive tasks that are beyond his or her ability. Even mild degrees of cognitive impairment have been demonstrated to predict for a lesser degree of functional recovery among hospitalized elders.

Rehabilitative efforts in patients with traumatic brain injury, stroke, or other neurologic insults may be particularly difficult if the insult itself has impaired the patient's self-awareness of a deficit. This lack of self-awareness may manifest itself as a marked difference in how the patient sees the severity of their condition compared to how the family members view it.[75] There is evidence from a study of postmenopausal women with stroke that patients' own assessment of their level of function frequently differs from that shown on standardized tests, and this disparity was particularly common in women in certain subgroups such as those with multiple comorbidities and those with cognitive impairment. For those women for whom self-assessment of function and objective assessment of function were discordant, it was overwhelmingly the case that the patients overestimated their level of function compared to that seen on objective testing. In the setting of reduced self-awareness of one's own deficits, it may be particularly challenging to simultaneously promote patient independence while managing the risk to the patient from injudicious choices.[76]

Learning strategies may work better if tailored to meet the cognitive abilities and learning style of the patient.[77,78] Appropriate rehabilitative exercise interventions can benefit patients with cognitive impairment, not only in terms of physical endpoints such as strength and flexibility, but also in terms of cognition and behavior.[79]

> ● Even minor depression may be associated with a poorer degree of short-term functional improvement during a course of subacute rehabilitation.

REHABILITATION AND DEPRESSION

Depression is common in the rehabilitation setting, and can be exacerbated by the patient having experienced the functional loss that precipitated the need for rehabilitation. Depression is commonly seen in the older stroke patient, but can also be present in the patient with disabilities arising from a variety of causes. There is evidence that even minor depression may be associated with a poorer degree of short-term functional improvement by the patient from a course of subacute rehabilitation.[80] Depression also is a risk factor for early re-hospitalization following a course of inpatient medical rehabilitation.[81]

REHABILITATION AND NUTRITION

One factor that may complicate the patient's hospital course[82] and make rehabilitation more difficult is inadequate nutrition. An older patient after a stroke may have difficulty consuming adequate calories because of dysphagia, inability to handle eating utensils, or even depression.[83,84] Malnutrition may limit the patient's ability to cooperate in a poststroke rehabilitation program or to gain muscle mass. In the patient with malnutrition, rigid restrictions on the dietary content (e.g., salt, saturated fats) may often be counterproductive, since increasing caloric intake and protein intake may be the overriding nutritional goals.

Dietary modifications may include changes in the consistency or the caloric density of the food. The patient may benefit from assistance during meals, including reminders to eat, and may need an extended time for meals. Clinical monitoring of the patient's hydration status is also important to avoid dehydration, particularly in older patients who may have a decreased sense of thirst and/or a decreased ability to communicate to caregivers that they are thirsty (see Chapter 27).

ASSISTIVE DEVICES

Assistive devices are used to relieve pain and maintain or restore function. Patients with functional losses who perceive a need for an assistive device need help choosing appropriate equipment. Assistive devices that address problems with hearing, vision, mobility, and most ADLs and instrumental ADLs are available. Most require patient education and training for proper use. Physical and occupational therapists can assist the physician, patient, and family in the selection and proper use of available products. Table 13–2 is a summary of selected assistive devices.

Deciding which is the most appropriate device and teaching the patient its appropriate use are probably beyond the scope of the average primary care physician. However, many older persons use canes for which they were never appropriately evaluated, and as many as 75% may be using the wrong type of cane, using a cane in ill repair, using the device improperly, or have an improperly sized device. Thus, the primary care physician who sees a patient with a cane should ascertain that it is in good repair (rubber tip, no cracks, etc.), that it is the right size (height of greater trochanter) and that the patient uses it properly (e.g., for patient with osteoarthritis, advances cane at the same time as the affected hip but holds the cane on the contralateral side).

A common fate of rehabilitative equipment is for it to go unused by the patient. This may result if the equipment is not a good fit for the patient's cognitive abilities. It may occur if use of the equipment requires more physical strength or coordination than the patient possesses. It may also occur if the patient has unrealistic expectations of what the equipment will accomplish, and is disappointed when these expectations are not fulfilled. Or it may be that the patient does not wish to display in public that they have a need for adaptive equipment.

Fig. 13–2[85] displays a checklist that can be helpful in planning with patient and caregivers whether to issue a particular device to them. As part of the primary care follow-up of a patient who has recently been issued a device such as a wheelchair, it is helpful to ask them about their experience using it, and also to note whether they in fact use it when they come to their follow-up primary care appointment.

Case Discussion, *Part 1*

Mr. Baker is a man with two chronic illnesses, both poorly controlled. His history of erratic compliance with his antihypertensive regimen suggests that noncompliance may also be a factor in his diabetes management. His history suggests that this patient with diabetes suffered a silent myocardial infarction a month ago, with resultant congestive heart failure.

He is a candidate for cardiac rehabilitation, but is also likely to have additional rehabilitative needs now or in the future. He has recently lost his wife, who was important in meeting his transportation needs. The fact that he was brought in by a neighbor rather than a family member may suggest that his other family supports are limited. Further history is necessary to determine whether he has functional limitations that impair his ability to care for himself in other ways as well, and which would require rehabilitation.

An assessment for cognitive impairment is indicated, this may have contributed to his giving up driving and to his forgetfulness about taking his medicines. He is also at risk for depression in the wake of the death of his wife. His cardiac event may be related to the stress of that loss.

Case Discussion, *Part 2*

Mr. Baker had been managing at home with a social support system consisting of both family and institutional supports. He had developed a lower extremity ulcer, which he either did not notice or ignored, and his physical findings suggest that it has likely progressed to osteomyelitis.

His neurologic findings are more consistent with delirium rather than a stroke. Control of his foot infection may help with his confusion, but he clearly cannot manage for now living alone at home.

An immediate rehabilitation goal is to avoid deconditioning while he begins therapy (debridement, systemic antibiotic treatment) for his infection. Preserving his muscle strength is important to preserve his ability to walk, whether or not he ultimately requires surgery. If he responds to conservative measures, he will benefit from shoes designed to avoid pressure on the healing area. He is at high risk for needing an amputation if he does not quickly respond to more conservative measures. If he does undergo amputation, he will need rehabilitation to walk with a prosthesis, a process that may be complicated by his cardiac disease and resultant impaired exercise tolerance.

Table 13–2	Selected Assistive Devices	
Functional Problem	**Device**	**Comments**
Bathing	"Soap on a rope" Long-handle back sponge	Will help when reaching is impaired. These aids will require adequate grip strength and range of motion.
	Tub seat or bench Grab bars Hand-held shower hose	Allows for safe sitting in the bathtub. Reducing the risk of falls during transfers is crucial. Tub transfer bench bridges the tub side with two legs in the tub and two legs beside the tub.
Toileting	Raised toilet seat Versa frames Bedside commode	Handrails can be attached to the wall or a free-standing frame can be used.
Oral care	Toothbrush grip	
Dressing	Reaching devices Button hooks Sock donners Velcro closures Elastic shoe laces Clothes hook Long shoe horns	Aids in picking things off the floor. Helps with hand weakness or loss of agility. Sock aid helps if hip flexion is limited. Velcro substitutes for buttons or shoelaces. Aids in dressing.
Grooming	Electric razor Tilt mirror Built-up grips on handles	
Eating	Built-up grips High-edged plates and non-skid pads Rocker knives Cups with lids	Grips help with arthritis or decreased strength. Keeps food on plate and plate on table. Allows one-handed food cutting. Useful to prevent spilling that occurs with intention tremor.
Mobility		
Orthoses	Foot Ankle-foot (AFO) Knee-ankle-foot (KAFO)	Modified shoes and lifts. Plastic shell or metal brace used for mild limb weakness (foot drop) after stroke. Aids weight bearing or alignment.
Canes	Hemi-cane or hemi-walker Tri- or quad-cane Standard cane	Aids knee support. With or without hinge. A four-point frame that provides considerable support to the hemiplegic patient. All canes held on the side opposite involved leg. More support than single-point cane. Comes with wide or narrow base. Pistol grip is best. With tip positioned on ground, elbow is flexed 25 degrees.
Walkers	Standard Roller	Rubber tips. Need to lift when moving. Helps with weakness or imbalance if grip strength is poor, but can be fitted with platform grip attached to forearm, if proximal strength is adequate. Front, three- or four-wheel models. Can have brakes and cargo baskets. Provides help with balance, but less support than standard walker. Can help patients with Parkinson's disease, unstable gait, or person with limited cardiorespiratory reserve for whom lifting would intolerably increase work (e.g., COPD, CHF).
Wheelchairs	Standard	Provided if limited endurance or inability to walk. Need to be carefully fitted: seat width, arm height, seat cushion, foot rests. Folding models available.
Scooter	Powered	A three-wheeled, electric scooter can help with mobility over long distances.

Adapted from Brummel-Smith K. Rehabilitation. In: Ham R, Sloane P, eds. Primary Care Geriatrics. 2nd ed. St. Louis: Mosby Yearbook, 1992:137–161; Friedmann LW, Capulong ES. Specific assistive aids. In: Williams TF, ed. Rehabilitation in the Aging. New York: Raven Press, 1984:315–44; Wasson JH, Gall V, MacDonald R, Liang MH. The prescription of assistive devices for the elderly: practical considerations. J Gen Intern Med 1990;5:46–54; and Wilson GB. Progressive mobilization. In: Sine RD, Liss SE, Roush RE, Holcomb JD, Wilson G, eds. Basic Rehabilitation Techniques. 3rd ed. Rockville, MD: Aspen Publishers, 1988:132–6.

**Make sure the medical device you choose
is designed for you**

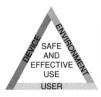

This checklist is designed for health care professionals and patients to use when choosing a medical device that is best for the patient. It is intended to be modified by health professionals to focus on particular devices for certain target populations (e.g., arthritics, diabetics, heart patients).

FIGURE 13-2

Checklist to use when choosing a medical device for a patient. Data from Medical Device Use Safety: Incorporating Human Factors Engineering into Risk Management, Available at http://www.fda.gov/cdch/humfac/you_choose_checklist.pdf. Accessed April 1, 2006.

1. Do you have limitations that can affect your use of the device?
- ☐ Could your health (stress, tired, medication effects, disease) affect the way you use the device?
- ☐ Do you have the physical size and strength (hand strength, lifting ability, and endurance) to use the device?
- ☐ Will you be able to see the display, hear the alarm, and feel the controls (knobs, buttons, switches, and keypads)?
- ☐ Do you have the coordination (manual dexterity, balance) to adjust the controls?
- ☐ Will you be able to understand and use the device?
- ☐ Do you need to remember complex instructions to use the device?

2. Is the device right for the environment where you plan to use it?
- ☐ Does the device have safety features to prevent it from harming your children or pets, and to prevent them from harming the device?
- ☐ Will you be able to hear the device's alarm in a noisy environment?
- ☐ Will the light levels (low or bright) in your environment affect your ability to use the device?
- ☐ Are you using other devices at the same time?
- ☐ Will sources of electromagnetic interference (e.g., Ham radio, AM FM TV broadcast antenna, electrical machinery, hand-held transmitters) affect the device?
- ☐ What things about your home will affect your use of the device (e.g., high heat and humidity, very dry air in the winter, too few electrical outlets, narrow doorways, wood stove heating)?
- ☐ What happens if you put the device in an inappropriate environment?

3. Are there device characteristics that can affect its use?
- ☐ Is the device simple to set up, operate, clean, maintain, and dispose of, and what happens if you don't do these things properly?
- ☐ What replacement parts or batteries are required, how frequently are they needed, how expensive are they, and are there special instructions for safely disposing of the device or its parts?
- ☐ What reading or training is required of you?
- ☐ Are there things about this device that are different from other similar devices you have operated?

SUMMARY

Many older individuals have difficulty with gait or other areas of function that interfere with their ability to accomplish the activities of daily living. The level of function can fluctuate over time, and rehabilitation efforts can be directed to preserve current function and to seek to recover lost function. Many older individuals have a variety of comorbidities rather than just an isolated functional deficit. An important goal of primary care is to ensure that these multiple medical and rehabilitative needs are addressed in a coordinated and comprehensive fashion.

ACKNOWLEDGMENT

The author is an investigator on Project EXPORT (grant 5 P20 MD 524-2), National Center of Minority Health and Health Disparities, National Institutes of Health. The contents are solely the responsibility of the author and do not necessarily represent the official view of the National Institutes of Health.

References

1. Wells JL, Seabrook JA, Stolee P, .et al. State of the art in geriatric rehabilitation. Part I. Review of frailty and comprehensive geriatric assessment. Arch Phys Med Rehabil 84:890, 2003.
2. Gurland BJ, Page WF, Plassman BL. A twin study of the genetic contribution to age-related functional impairment. J Gerontol Med Sci 59A:859, 2004.
3. Gill TM, Baker DI, Gottschalk M, et al. A prehabilitation program for the prevention of functional decline: effect on higher-level physical function. Arch Phys Med Rehabil 85:1043, 2004.
4. National Center for Health Statistics. Classification of diseases and functioning & disability. Available at: www.cdc.gov/nchs/about/otheract/icd9/icfhome.htm. Accessed February 23, 2005.
5. Federal Interagency Forum on Aging-Related Statistics. Older Americans 2004: key indicators of well-being. Washington DC: Government Printing Office, 2004.
6. Iezzoni LI, Davis RB, Soukup J, O'Day B. Quality dimensions that most concern people with physical and sensory disabilities. Arch Intern Med 163:2085, 2003.
7. Nusbaum N. Aging and sensory senescence. South Med J 92:267, 1999.
8. de Vreede PL, Samson MM, van Meeteren NLU, Duursma SA, Verhaar HJJ. Functional-task exercise versus resistance strength exercise to improve daily function in older women: a randomized, controlled, trial. J Am Geriatr Soc 53:2, 2005.
9. Gregory PC, Fried LP. Why do older adults decide they are having difficulty with a task? Am J Phys Med Rehabil 82:9, 2003.
10. Ottenbacher KJ, et al. Trends in length of stay, living setting, functional outcome, and mortality following medical rehabilitation. JAMA 292:1687, 2004.
11. Disler PB, Wade DT. Should all stroke rehabilitation be home based? Am J Phys Med Rehabil 82:733, 2003.
12. Likourezos A, Si M, Kim W-O, et al. Health status and functional status in relationship to nursing home subacute rehabilitation program outcomes. Am J Phys Med Rehabil 81:372, 2002.

13. Dobrez DG, Lo Sasso AT, Heinemann AW. The effect of prospective payment on rehabilitative care. Arch Phys Med Rehabil 85:1909, 2004.
14. Murray PK, Singer M, Dawson NV, et al. Outcomes of rehabilitation services for nursing home residents. Arch Phys Med Rehabil 84:1129, 2004.
14a. Rao P, Boradia P, Ennis J, Shift happens. Top Stroke Rehab 12:1, 2005.
14b. White C. Rehabilitation therapy in skilled nursing facilities. Health Affairs 22:214, 2003.
14c. Schlenkar RE, Powel MC, Goodrich GK. Initial home health outcomes under prospective payment. Health Services Research 40:1, 2005.
15. National Nursing Home Survey. Selected characteristics of homes, beds, and residents. Available at http://www.cdc.gov/nchs/nnhs.htm. Accessed April 1, 2006.
16. Bean J, Kiely DK, Leveille SG, Morris J. Associating the onset of motor impairments with disability progression in nursing home residents. Am J Phys Med Rehabil 81:696, 2003.
17. Jette DU, Warren RL, Wirtalla C. Rehabilitation in skilled nursing facilities: effect of nursing staff level and therapy intensity on outcomes. Am J Phys Med Rehabil 83:704, 2004.
18. Gill TM, Kurland B. The burden and patterns of disability in activities of daily living among community-living older persons. J Gerontol Med Sci 58A:70, 2003.
19. Gill TM, Heather A, Guo Z. The deleterious effects of bed rest among community-living older persons. J Gerontol Med Sci 59A:755, 2004.
20. Fletcher AE, Price GM, Ng ESW, et al. Population-based multidimensional assessment of older people in UK general practice: a cluster-randomised factorial trial. Lancet 364:1667, 2004.
21. Gill TM, Allore HG, Holford TR, Guo Z. Hospitalization, restricted activity, and the development of disability among older persons. JAMA 292:2115, 2004.
22. Hardy SE, Gill TM. Factors associated with recovery of independence among newly disabled older persons. Arch Intern Med 165:106, 2005.
23. Phelan EA, Williams B, Penninx WJH, LoGerfo JP, Leveille SG. Activities of daily living function and disability in older adults in a randomized trial of the health enhancement program. J Gerontol Med Sci 59A:838, 2004.
24. Shkuratova N, Morris ME, Huxham F. Effects of age on balance control during walking. Arch Phys Med Rehabil 85:582, 2004.
25. Menz HB, Lord SR, St George R, Fitzpatrick RC. Walking stability and sensorimotor function in older people with diabetic peripheral neuropathy. Arch Phys Med Rehabil 85:245, 2004.
26. Simonsick EM, Guralnick JM, Volpato S, et al. Just get out the door! Importance of walking outside the home for maintaining mobility: findings from the women's health and aging study. J Am Geriatr Soc 53:198, 2005.
27. Ergeletzis D, Kevorkian CG, Rintala D. Rehabilitation of the older stroke patient: functional outcome and comparison with younger patients. Am J Phys Med Rehabil 81:881, 2001.
28. Kevorkian CG, Ergeletzis D, Rintala D. Nonagenarians on a rehabilitation unit: Characteristics, progress and outcomes. Am J Phys Med Rehabil 83:266, 2003.
29. Ackermann RT, Deyo RA, LoGerfo JP. Prompting primary providers to increase community exercise referrals for older adults: a randomized trial. J Am Geriatr Soc 53:283, 2005.
30. Jones C, Skirrow P, Griffiths M, et al. Rehabilitation after acute illness: a randomized, controlled trial. Crit Care Med 31:2456, 2003.
31. Bateni H, Maki BE. Assistive devices for balance and mobility: benefits, demands, and adverse consequences. Arch Phys Med Rehabil 86:134, 2005.
32. Hebela N, Smith DG, Keenan MA. Specialty update: what's new in orthopaedic rehabilitation. J Bone Joint Surg 86A:2577, 2004.
33. Suetta C, Magnusson SP, Rosted A, Aagaard P, Jakobsen AK, Larsen LH, Duus B, Kjaer M. Resistance training in the early postoperative phase reduces hospitalization and leads to muscle hypertrophy in elderly hip surgery patients—a controlled, randomized study. J Am Geriatr Soc 52:2016, 2004.
33a. Brunner LC, Eshilani-Oates L. Hip fractures in adults. Am Fam Physician 67:537, 2003.
33b. Bedi A, Toan Le T. Subtrochanteric femur fractures. Orthop Clin N Am 35:473, 2004.
33c. Cameron ID. Coordinated multidisciplinary rehabilitation after hip fracture. Diability and Rehabilitation 27:1081, 2005.
34. Geerts WH, Pineo GF, Heit JA, Bergqvist D, Lassen MR, Colwell CW, Ray JG. Prevention of venous thromboembolism: the Seventh ACCP Conference on Antithrombotic and Thrombolytic Therapy. Chest 126(Suppl 3): 338S–400S, 2004.
34a. Grey JE, Enoch S, Harding KG. ABC of wound healing: pressure ulcers. BMJ 332:472, 2006.
34b. Parker MJ, Gurusamy K. Modern methods of treating hip fractures. Disability and Rehabilitation 27:1045, 2005.
35. Binder EF, Brwon M, Sinacore Dr, et al. Effects of extended outpatient rehabilitation after hip fracture: a randomized controlled trial. JAMA 292:837, 2004.
36. Shabat S, Gepstein R, Mann G, et al. The second hip fracture—an analysis of 84 elderly patients. J Orthop Trauma 17:613, 2003.
37. Weigl M, Angst F, Stucki G, Lehmannn, Aeschlimann A. Inpatient rehabilitation for hip or knee osteoarthritis: 2 year follow-up study. Ann Rheum Dis 63:360, 2004.
38. Gidwani S, Fairbank A. The orthopaedic approach to managing osteoarthritis of the knee. BMJ 329:1220, 2004.
39. American Academy of Orthopedic Surgeons. Osteoarthritis of the Knee: Treatment Options. Available at: www3.aaos.org/research/imca/OAknee Contents/OA_knee_m5_3.htm. Accessed February 20, 2005.
40. American Academy of Orthopedic Surgeons. Osteoarthritis of the Hip: Treatment Options. Available at: www3.aaos.org/research/imca/OAhip Contents/OAHip_treatment.pdf. Accessed February 20, 2005.
41. Gordon NF, Gulanick M, Costa F, Fletcher G, Franklin BA, Roth EJ, Shephard T. American Heart Association scientific statement: physical activity and exercise recommendations for stroke survivors. Circulation 109:2031, 2004.
42. Nir Z, Zolotogorsky Z, Sugarman H. Structured nursing intervention versus routine rehabilitation after stroke. Am J Phys Med Rehabil 83:522, 2004.
43. Bohannon RW, Lee N. Association of physical functioning with same-hospital readmission after stroke. Am J Phys Med Rehabil 83:434, 2004.
43a. Welmer A-K, Holmqvist LW, Sommerfeld DK. Hemiplegic limb synergies in stroke patients. Am J Phys Med Rehabil 85:112, 2005.
44. Mosqueda L, Brummel-Smith K. Rehabilitation. In: Ham R, Sloane P, Warshaw GA, eds. Primary Care Geriatrics. 4th Ed. St. Louis: Mosby, 2002: 149-163.
45. Weiss Z, Snir D, Klein B, et al. Effectiveness of home rehabilitation after stroke in Israel. Int J Rehabil Res 27:119, 2004.
46. Meijer R, van Limbeek J. Early supported discharge: a valuable alternative for some stroke patients. Lancet 365:455, 2005.
47. Pardessus V, Puisieux F, Di Pompeo C et al. Benefits of home visits for falls and autonomy in the elderly: a randomized trial study. Am J Phys Med Rehabil 81:247, 2002.
48. VA/DoD Clinical Practice Guideline for the Management of Stroke Rehabilitation in the Primary Care Setting, version 1.1, October 2003. Available at: www.oqp.med.va.gov/cpg/STR/STR_base.htm, module CAccessed February 10, 2005.
48a. Langhorne P, Taylor G, Murray G, et al. Early supported discharge services for stroke patients: a meta-analysis of individual patients' data, Lancet 365: 501, 2005.
49. Thorsén A-M, Holmqvist LW, de Pedro-Cuesta J, von Koch L. A randomized controlled trial of early supported discharge and continued rehabilitation at home after stroke: five-year follow-up of patient outcome. Stroke 36:295, 2005.
50. Logan PA, Gladman JRF, Avery A, Walker MF, Dyas J, Groom L. Randomized controlled trial of an occupational therapy intervention to increase outdoor mobility after stroke. BMJ 329:1372, 2004.
51. Satkunam LE. Rehabilitation medicine. 3. Management of adult spasticity. CMAJ 169:1173, 2003.
52. McLean DE. Medical complications experienced by a cohort of stroke survivors during inpatient, tertiary-level stroke rehabilitation. Arch Phys Med Rehabil 85:466, 2004.
53. Watanabe Y: an assessment of osteoporosis in stroke patients on rehabilitation admission. Int J Rehab Res 27:163, 2004.
54. Stewart KJ, Badenhop D, Brubaker PH, Keteyian SJ, King M. Cardiac rehabilitation following percutaneous revascularization, heart transplant, heart valve surgery, and for chronic heart failure. Chest 123:2104, 2003.
55. Dolansky MA, Moore SM. Effects of cardiac rehabilitation on the recovery outcomes of older adults after coronary artery bypass surgery. J Cardiopulmon Rehabil 24:236, 2004.
56. Worcester MUC, Murphy BM, Mee VK, Roberts SB, Goble AJ. Cardiac rehabilitation programmes: predictors of non-attendance and drop-out. Eur J Cardiovasc Prev Rehabil 11:328, 2004.
57. Smith KM, Arthur HM, McKelvie RS, Kodis J. Differences in sustainability of exercise and health-related quality of life outcomes following home or hospital-based cardiac rehabilitation. Eur J Cardiovasc Prev Rehabil 11:313, 2004.
58. Leon AS, Franklin BA, Costa F, et al. AHA scientific statement: cardiac rehabilitation and secondary prevention of coronary heart disease: an American Heart Association statement from the Council on Clinical Cardiology (Subcommittee on Exercise, Cardiac Rehabilitation and Prevention) and the Council on Nutrition, Physical Activity and Metabolism (Subcommittee on Physical Activity), in collaboration with the American Association of Cardiovascular and Pulmonary Rehabilitation. Circulation 111:369, 2005.
59. Johnson N, Fisher J, Nagle A, et al. Factors associated with referral to outpatient cardiac rehabilitation services. J Cardiopulmon Rehabil 24:165, 2004.
60. Jackson L, Leclerc J, Erskine Y, Linden W. Getting the most out of cardiac rehabilitation: a review of referral and adherence predictors. Heart 91:10, 2005.
61. Grace SL, Evindar A, Kung TN, Scholey PE, Stewart DE. Automatic referral to cardiac rehabilitation. Med Care 42:661, 2004.
62. Rossi G, Florini F, Romagnoli M, Bellantone T, Lucic S, Lugli D, Clini E. Length and clinical effectiveness of pulmonary rehabilitation in outpatients with chronic airway obstruction. Chest 127:105, 2005.
63. Man WD-C, Polkey MI, Donaldson N, Gray BJ, Moxham J. Community pulmonary rehabilitation after hospitalization for acute exacerbations of chronic obstructive pulmonary disease: randomized controlled study. BMJ 329:1209, 2004.
64. Rochester CL. Exercise training in chronic obstructive pulmonary disease. J Rehabil Res Dev 40:59, 2003.
65. Plankeel JF, McMullen B, MacIntyre NR. Exercise outcomes after pulmonary rehabilitation depend on the initial mechanism of exercise limitation among non-oxygen-dependent COPD patients. Chest 127:110, 2005.
66. Ferrari M, Vangelista A, Vedovi E, .et al. Minimally supervised home rehabilitation improves exercise capacity and health status in patients with COPD. Am J Phys Med Rehabil 83:337, 2004.

67. Nusbaum N. Rehabilitation and the older cancer patient. Am J Med Sci 327:86, 2004.

68. Galvão DA, Newton RU. Review of exercise intervention studies in cancer patients. J Clin Oncol 23:899, 2005.

69. McColl MA, Charlifue S, Glass C, Lawson N, Savic G. Aging, gender, and spinal cord injury. Arch Phys Med Rehabil 85:363, 2004.

70. Liem NR, McColl MA, King W, Smith KM. Aging with a spinal cord injury: factors associated with need for more help with activities of daily living. Arch Phys Med Rehabil 85:1567, 2004.

71. McColl MA, Arnold R, Charliuffe S, et al. Aging, spinal cord injury, and quality of life: structural relationships. Arch Phys Med Rehabil 84:1137, 2003.

72. Center for Medicare & Medicaid Services: Statement of Tom Scully, administrator Centers for Medicare & Medicaid Services on therapy coverage of Alzheimer's disease patients, April 1, 2002. Available at: www.cms.hhs.gov.

73. Nas K, Gür A, Çevik R, Saraç AJ The relationship between physical impairment and disability during stroke rehabilitation: effect of cognitive status. Int J Rehab Res 27:181, 2004.

74. Landi F, Bernabei R, Russo A, .et al. Predictors of rehabilitation outcomes in frail patients treated in a geriatric hospital. J Am Geriatr Soc 50:679, 2002.

75. Prigatano GP. Disturbances of self-awareness and rehabilitation of patients with traumatic brain injury: a 20-year perspective. J Head Trauma Rehabil 20:19, 2005.

76. Nusbaum N. Safety versus autonomy: dilemmas and strategies in protection of vulnerable community-dwelling elderly. Ann Long-Term Care 12:50, 2004.

77. Fenter PC. Understanding the role of practice in learning for geriatric individuals. Top Geriatr Rehabil 17:11, 2002.

78. Dewing J. Rehabilitation for older people with dementia. Nurs Standard 18:42, 2003.

79. Heyn P, Abreu BC, Ottenbacher KJ. The effects of exercise training on elderly persons with cognitive impairment and dementia: a meta-analysis. Arch Phys Med Rehabil 85:1694, 2004.

80. Allen BP, Agha Z, Duthie EH, Layde PM. Minor depression and rehabilitation outcome for older adults in subacute care. J Behav Health Serv Res 31:189, 2004.

81. Mast BT, Azar AR, MacNeill SE, Lichtenberg PA. Depression and activitites of daily living predict rehospitalization within 6 months of discharge from geriatric rehabilitation. Rehabil Psychol 49:219, 2004.

82. Sullivan DH, Bopp MM, Roberson PK. Protein-energy undernutrition and life-threatening complications among the hospitalized elderly. J Gen Intern Med 17:923, 2002.

83. Asai JL. Nutrition and the geriatric rehabilitation patient: challenges and solutions. Top Geriatr Rehabil 20:34, 2004.

84. Finestone HM, Greene-Finestone LS. Rehabilitation medicine: diagnosis of dysphagia and its nutritional management for stroke patients. CMAJ 169:1041, 2003.

85. U.S. Food and Drug Administration Center for Devices and Radiological Health. Make Sure the Medical Device You Choose Is Designed for You. Available at: www.fda.gov/cdrh/humfac/ you_choose_checklist.pdf. Accessed February 20, 2005.

Web Resources

1. American Academy of Physical Medicine and Rehabilitation, Geriartic Rehabilitation, http://www.aapmr.org/condtreat/rehab/geriatric.htm

2. Journal of Rehabilitation Research and Development, http://www.vard.org/jour/about_us.htm

3. University of Oklahoma, Geriatric Rehabilitation Resource for Oklahoma, Using walkers http://www.ah.ouhsc.edu/geriatric_resources/walkers.htm, Using canes http://www.ah.ouhsc.edu/geriatric_resources/canes.htm

POSTTEST

1. In the weeks after having a right-sided (nondominant) stroke, patients are most likely to
a. Overestimate their functional ability
b. Underestimate their functional ability
c. Develop myoclonus
d. Develop mania
e. Experience phantom limb pain in their left leg

2. Your patient is a 70-year-old woman with knee osteoarthritis, who is awakened five times a night with knee pain, and who has achieved only partial relief from a variety of analgesics. The strategy most likely to bring her long-term relief is
a. Radiation therapy to her knee
b. Monthly intra-articular steroids
c. Intra-articular hyaluronic acid
d. Oral hyaluronic acid
e. Orthopedic surgery

3. Your patient is a 70-year-old man with chronic obstructive pulmonary disease and one flight dyspnea on exertion. He asks about a rehabilitation program. Of the following, you are most likely to advise him that
a. Exercise rehabilitation may increase his exercise tolerance
b. Exercise rehabilitation is contraindicated
c. He should only exercise his upper extremities
d. Exercise rehabilitation should emphasize lifting weights
e. Exercise rehabilitation should be limited to improving his balance and coordination

PRETEST ANSWERS

1. c
2. d
3. e

POSTTEST ANSWERS

1. a
2. e
3. a

OBJECTIVES

Upon completion of this chapter, the reader will be able to:

● Understand the difference between palliative care and hospice.

● Be familiar with the basics of pain management, including pain assessment and treatment.

● Be familiar with the most common non-pain symptoms encountered in palliative care.

● Create a basic framework for structuring conversations with patients and families for both breaking bad news and negotiating goals of care.

PRETEST

1. A 71-year-old man with a history of metastatic prostate cancer, hypertension, and chronic renal failure is admitted for a pathologic fracture of the right humerus. Which of the following is the most appropriate pain regimen for him?
   a. Meperidine 50 mg po q4 hours
   b. Ibuprofen 400 mg po every 4 hours as needed
   c. Morphine 5 mg po every 4 hours as needed
   d. Morphine 5 mg po every 4 hours with morphine 3 mg po every 1 hour as needed
   e. Hydromorphone 5 mg po every 4 hours with hydromorphone 3 mg po every 1 hour as needed

2. A 68-year-old man with a history of congestive heart failure, osteoarthritis, and hypertension is hospitalized for worsening of his heart disease. Getting out of bed he falls and injures his knee. He is currently written for codeine 30 mg by mouth every 6 hours as needed for pain. The patient's nurse comes to you because he is yelling in pain before the next dose is due, and this disturbs the other patients on the ward. Many of the floor staff are concerned that he is drug seeking. What behavior is he exhibiting?
   a. Tolerance
   b. Dependence
   c. Addiction
   d. Pseudoaddiction

3. A 75-year-old woman who has been your primary care patient for 10 years comes to your office complaining of fatigue and weight loss. On further testing, she is found to have a colonic mass, which is biopsied. The results return as adenocarcinoma, and she returns to your office today. After bringing her into your exam room and explaining to your office manager that you are not to be disturbed for the next 20 minutes, what is the next step in the process of informing her that she has cancer?
   a. Ask her what she wants to know
   b. Tell her the diagnosis
   c. Explain that she needs imaging of her liver so that you can have more information
   d. Ask her what she understands up to this point

Holly Johnson, *Part 1*

Holly Johnson is a 70-year-old woman who was diagnosed with stage III ovarian cancer 3 years ago. At that time, she received a total abdominal hysterectomy and bilateral salpingo-oophorectomy along with adjuvant chemotherapy. Six months ago on a routine follow-up appointment with her gynecologic oncologist, her lab results showed a rise in her CEA-125 level, and she was diagnosed with a recurrence. Despite chemotherapy, her disease showed continued progression on a follow-up imaging study. She currently lives with her husband who is in good health. While she was independent 8 months ago, her functional status has now deteriorated and she currently needs assistance with her activities of daily living. Her physicians no longer believe that she would benefit from further chemotherapy.

Pam Rodriguez, *Part 1*

Pam Rodriguez is a 70-year-old woman with a medical history significant for osteoarthritis, advanced heart failure, mild cognitive impairment, and diabetes, who has been hospitalized for 6 days with pneumonia. This is her third hospitalization in the past year; the other two were for exacerbations of her heart failure. She is currently debilitated and cannot return to her home. Prior to this hospitalization, she was living in the community with her partner (who is also in failing health). She requires assistance with shopping, cleaning, and cooking. They have two adult sons who live in neighboring towns.

STUDY QUESTIONS

1. As a member of your hospital's inpatient palliative care consult service, how would you approach the care of each patient?
2. How does palliative care for Ms. Johnson differ from that for Ms. Rodriguez?

WHAT IS PALLIATIVE CARE?

At the turn of the 20th century, the average life expectancy was 47,[1] and people usually died suddenly as the result of trauma or infection. Over the last 100 years, however, advances in medicine such as antibiotics, improvements in nutrition, and developments in public heath and safety have led to a greatly increased longevity such that the average life expectancy in 2001 was 77 years.[1] As a consequence, the typical death is no longer a sudden or unexpected event. Rather, death today usually follows a lengthy period of chronic illness and functional dependency, such that chronic disease has become the leading cause of death. Evidence across all health care settings and disease categories demonstrates a high prevalence of physical, psychosocial, and financial suffering associated with serious illness and chronic disease.

Partly in response to these changes, the field of palliative care has arisen to address the needs of patients and families that have not been well met by traditional medical care. Erroneously, the phrase "palliative care" is sometimes conceived as care that should be provided at the end of life when treatments directed at life prolongation are no longer effective and death is imminent. In actuality, palliative care is interdisciplinary care focused on the relief of suffering and achieving the best possible quality of life for patients with serious illness and their family caregivers.[2] It involves formal symptom assessment and treatment, aid with decision making regarding the benefits and burdens of various therapies, help in establishing goals of care, and collaborative and seamless transitions between models of care (hospital, home, nursing homes, and hospice). It should be offered *simultaneously* with life-prolonging and curative therapies for persons living with serious, complex, and advanced illness (Fig. 14–1). Palliative care is not simply care that should be offered at the end of life or when nothing else can be done.[3]

In this sense, the field of palliative care attempts to overcome the artificial dichotomy of cure versus com-

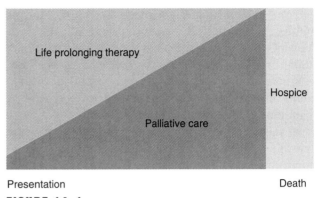

Presentation · Death

FIGURE 14–1

Palliative care is offered simultaneously with life-prolonging and curative therapies for persons living with serious, complex, and advanced illness.

fort that has been established. A key contributor to this division of health care is the Medicare hospice benefit, which requires that patients forgo life-sustaining care to be able to receive hospice and must have a predictable prognosis of 6 months or less. This ignores the fact that the overwhelming majority of older adults living with advanced illness require both life-prolonging and palliative treatments at the same time.

With this distinction in mind, it becomes clear that both patients presented in the opening of this chapter can benefit from palliative care, but in different ways. Palliative care for Holly Johnson, with her advanced ovarian cancer and poor functional status, involves treating her symptoms (e.g., nausea, pain, depression), addressing her psychological and spiritual concerns, supporting her partner, and helping to arrange for her increasing care needs. The majority of this patient's care occurs at home (with or without hospice) or in the hospital, and the period of functional debility is relatively brief (months). This differs from the care that Pam Rodriguez needs. Palliative care for this patient involves treating the primary disease process (her advanced heart failure), managing her multiple chronic medical conditions and comorbidities (diabetes, arthritis) and geriatric syndromes (cognitive impairment), assessing and treating the physical and psychological symptom distress associated with all of these medical issues; and establishing goals of care and treatment plans in the setting of an unpredictable prognosis. Additionally, the needs of her caregiver(s) are also different from that of Holly Johnson. While Ms. Johnson may only have a few months to live, the individuals caring for Ms. Rodriguez will most likely be her adult children who have their own families, work responsibilities, and medical conditions; these roles must be balanced with the months to years of personal care that they must provide to their aging parent. Like most elderly patients, both Ms. Johnson and Ms. Rodriguez can be expected to make multiple transitions across care settings (home, hospital, rehabilitation, long-term care),[4] especially in the last months of life, and palliative care programs for older adults must ensure that care plans and patient goals are maintained from one setting to another.

In this sense, palliative care in the elderly is most appropriately centered on the identification and amelioration of functional and cognitive impairment, intervening to lessen caregiver burnout, and reducing the burden of symptoms. This is in contrast to typical care for patients in a hospice setting, for example, where management is focused on advanced terminal illness and its immediate manifestations. In response to the unique needs of older adults, palliative care is an integral part of geriatric medicine.

> ● Palliative care is interdisciplinary care focused on the relief of suffering and achieving the best possible quality of life for patients with serious illness and their family caregivers. It is offered simultaneously with other treatments, as opposed to hospice, where patients must agree to forgo life-sustaining treatments.

Holly Johnson, *Part 2*

On your initial visit with Holly Johnson, she describes pain that is not well controlled. You are able to elicit that her pain is a dull ache throughout her abdomen, which is occasionally punctuated by periods of sharp pain when she turns in bed or tries to transfer from the bed to chair. She rates her pain as a 7 out of 10, and the nurse on your interdisciplinary team informs you that she is no longer getting out of bed because of the pain. She is currently on a regimen of Tylenol #3 (acetaminophen 300 mg/codeine 30 mg) by mouth every 6 hours as needed. On review of her medication records, you note that she has consistently asked for it every 6 hours since admission. When you ask if she finds the current regimen acceptable, she states that she does not want anything stronger because she wants to save the "stronger medications for when I will really need them later."

STUDY QUESTIONS

1. How would you change Holly Johnson's pain medications?
2. How would you address her concern about waiting to take pain medications until she "really" needs them?

Pam Rodriguez, *Part 2*

On your initial visit with Pam Rodriguez, you ask if she has pain. She states that while she doesn't actually have pain, she does have an intermittent diffuse ache throughout her body. When you ask her to further characterize this discomfort, she can't further elaborate on it but is able to rate it as mild-moderate. In addition, she complains of an electric, tingling sensation in both of her feet that she has had for several years. On review of her hospital medications, she currently has an order for ibuprofen 400 mg by mouth every 4 hours as needed.

STUDY QUESTIONS

1. What types of pain is Pam Rodriguez describing?
2. What changes would you suggest to her pain regimen?

ASSESSING AND TREATING PAIN IN OLDER ADULTS

Pain is an unpleasant sensory and emotional experience associated with actual or potential tissue damage.[5] Nearly 50% of severely ill hospitalized patients report that they have pain.[6,7] Pain in older patients may be poorly controlled because they may underreport pain or may have difficulty communicating, and physicians may undertreat pain due to concerns about side effects in older patients.[8]

The mechanisms underlying pain can be conceptually divided into two broad categories: nociceptive and neuropathic.[9-11] Nociceptive pain results from direct stimulation of intact pain receptors and travels along intact neurons. This type of pain may arise from tissue injury, inflammation, or mechanical deformity. Nociceptive pain can be further divided into somatic and visceral pain. Somatic pain refers to the activation or stimulation of peripheral nociceptors in cutaneous and deep tissues. Patients can localize this pain, and it is typically described as aching or gnawing. Examples of somatic pain include acute pain due to surgical procedures and chronic pain that may result from bone metastases of an underlying malignancy. Visceral pain results from infiltration, compression, or distension of abdominal or thoracic viscera. Patients often find it difficult to localize visceral pain, and they may describe it as pressure or squeezing. Examples of visceral pain include biliary colic with or without pain referred to the shoulder and back pain resulting from pancreatic cancer.

Neuropathic pain results from injury to actual nerve fibers as a result of compression, infiltration, or degeneration of neurons in either the peripheral or central nervous system.[11] Patients often describe this pain as burning, tingling, stabbing, or electrical, and they tend to experience it as severe and constant. Examples of neuropathic pain include diabetic neuropathy, pain due to spinal stenosis, and pain resulting from trigeminal neuralgia.

It is important to distinguish between the various types of pain because each is treated differently. Nociceptive pain is treated with, and often responds well to, traditional medications such as acetaminophen, non-steroidal anti-inflammatory drugs (NSAIDs), and opioids. While neuropathic pain may respond to traditional analgesic agents, it is often necessary to use adjuvant agents such as tricyclic antidepressants, anticonvulsants, corticosteroids, or local anesthetic agents.[12-15]

Pain Assessment

The treatment of pain begins with a thorough and complete assessment. The guiding principle of pain assessment is to ask patients about their pain and then believe their complaints. Several studies have shown that providers' estimate of a patient's pain severity are often lower than the patient's self-report.[16,17] Assessment of pain involves multiple components, and practitioners must consider each in order to best understand the nature and character of a patient's symptoms.

The first step of assessment is to inquire about the location of the pain as well as whether it radiates to any other part of the patient's body. A description of the pain to determine if its origin is nociceptive, neuropathic, or some combination of both should be obtained as well as questions as to when the patient's pain began, as chronic pain is often treated differently than acute pain. Additionally, it is important to ask what treatments (pharmacologic or otherwise) the patient has tried to relieve the pain as well as any factors that may exacerbate it. Temporal patterns of the patient's pain should be understood. For example, joint pain that is relieved shortly after awakening is more likely to be from osteoarthritis than from rheumatoid arthritis. If patients do not freely offer information about these characteristics, then it is important to continue probing until the physician has a complete understanding of the nature of the patient's pain and its associated factors. For a useful mnemonic device, see Box 14-1.

Patients should be asked to rate their pain both to better understand its severity as well as to give a baseline assessment to determine changes in the level of pain after treatment.[8] The same scale should be used over time in each patient, so as to best be able to reliably track changes in pain over time. Patients can be

---

Box 14-1	**Mnemonic Device for Assessing Pain**

O = Onset—When did the pain begin?

P = Provokes/Palliates—What makes the pain worse or better?

Q = Quality—What is the nature of the pain?

R = Radiation—Does the pain go to any other portion of the body?

S = Severity—How bad is the pain? (0 to 10 scale; mild, moderate, severe)

T = Temporal—Is there a certain time of day when the pain is better or worse?

---

asked to rate their pain in either words (none, mild, moderate, severe) or using a numeric scale (0 to 10 where 0 is no pain and 10 is the worst pain experienced). They can also be shown a visual analog scale, where patients place a mark indicating their level of discomfort on a horizontal line representing a spectrum of pain (the leftmost portion of the line represents no pain, the rightmost, severe pain). Another visual scale often used includes a series of faces representing various states of emotion relating to the patient's current level of pain.

In addition to the assessment principles outlined above, a crucial component of pain in older adults relates to its impact on function. The presence of symptoms that limit patients' activities of daily living (ADLs)[18] should trigger physicians to focus on the home environment and may signal the need for additional home care services. In cases where the patient cannot provide a thorough history due to conditions such as dementia or aphasia, this information can be obtained from nursing staff and the patient's family.[8] The clinician's physical exam should be used to confirm any suspicion generated during the history taking. Conditions to note include muscle spasm, gait impairment, abnormal joint alignments, and changes in skin color or integrity-to name just a few.[9]

Physicians may have particular difficulty in assessing pain in older individuals for several reasons. Patients may have physiologic barriers to reporting pain such as difficulties with hearing or vision as well as cognitive impairment. These difficulties are not insurmountable, however. Assistive listening devices or visual scales can be used to facilitate pain assessment in patients with hearing loss. Patients with poor vision should be encouraged to express their pain using either a numerical or verbal scale. For patients with both visual and hearing impairments, techniques such as pointing and gesturing are often effective.

Clinicians may assume that they cannot assess pain in individuals with cognitive impairment, but this is often not the case.[19] Patients with cognitive impairment or aphasia are often able to give basic information if questions are asked in a "yes/no" format. In addition, physicians can use signs such as elevated pulse rate, facial expressions (grimacing or frowning), diaphoresis, and changes in vocal patterns (e.g., increased moaning or changes in pitch) as signs that a patient may be in distress. Clinicians can also ask family members and paid caregivers to report their impressions of the patient's pain as well. Unfortunately, clinical studies have shown that patients' and family members' ratings of pain are not always well correlated, with family members often underestimating the patient's pain intensity.[20–22] With this in mind, however, clinicians may be able to begin with the family's assessment of the cognitively impaired patient and add to this the other visual and diagnostic clues discussed above to better estimate a patient's level of pain.

Older patients' fear of addiction has also been shown to be one of many barriers to effective pain management.[9,23] One way to counteract this barrier is to educate patients and their families about addiction and how it differs from tolerance and dependence.

Tolerance is a pharmacologic phenomenon that refers to diminished analgesic effect of a constant dose of a medication after exposure over time.[9] Tolerance routinely develops after patients receive opioid medications, and relates to both the analgesic properties of the medication (i.e., patients may need more of a medication over time to obtain the same analgesic effect) as well as to its side effects (e.g., patients will develop tolerance to the sedative effect after a short period of time). Typically when patients with cancer or other systemic diseases begin to need increasing doses of a medication, it is a result of progression of the underlying disease rather than the development of tolerance.

Dependence refers to a biological phenomenon whereupon patients may develop withdrawal symptoms once the medication is discontinued.[8] For example, patients who have been on chronic opioid therapy may experience diarrhea and a dramatic increase in their level of pain if the medication is abruptly halted. *Addiction* refers to continued use and seeking of a medication despite harm to self and others. This phenomenon is rarely seen in patients who are treated for chronic pain, and is seen no more often in patients with cancer than in the general population.[24] One way to avoid this confusion is to avoid the use of terms such as *narcotics* and *drugs* as these words may be associated with societal stigmas. Clinicians must differentiate addiction from *pseudoaddiction*, a phenomenon in which patients exhibit drug-seeking behavior due to undertreatment of their pain. This is an iatrogenic phenomenon, and will improve when patients are given an adequate medication regimen with appropriate dosing intervals.[25]

Treatment of Pain

The basic and most widely used approach to management of pain is illustrated by the World Health Organization's "pain ladder"[26] (Fig. 14–2). While originally developed to assist clinicians with assessing and managing pain in patients with cancer, the model can be extended to nonmalignant painful conditions in elderly individuals such as osteoarthritis or pathologic fractures due to osteoporosis. The first step, for patients with mild pain, encourages the use of nonopioid medications such as acetaminophen or NSAIDs with or without an adjuvant agent (see below).[27] If a patient's pain increases to a moderate level or remains poorly controlled, the next step involves adding a weak opioid medication alone or in combination with the nonopioid (e.g., acetaminophen with oxycodone) with or without the use of an adjuvant agent. The third step, for patients with severe pain, advises the use of a strong opioid (e.g., morphine, hydromorphone) with or without an adjuvant. Recent evidence suggests that patients with moderate or severe pain, especially that related to cancer, may receive faster pain relief by being started on a strong opioid regimen immediately rather than progressing in such a stepwise fashion or employing weak opioids (e.g., codeine) or combination products.[28,29]

Adjuvant agents are medications that can be combined with opioid therapies to either decrease the dose of medication needed or to avoid dose-related side

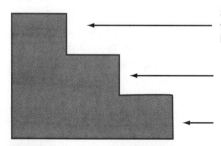

Step 3: Patients with severe pain should be treated with opioid medications (e.g., morphine or hypromorphone) ± adjuvant agents.

Step 2: Patients with moderate pain should be treated with a combination of opioid and non-opioid medications (e.g., acetaminophen + codeine) ± adjuvant agents.

Step 1: Patients with mild pain should be treated with non-opioid medications (e.g., acetaminophen or non-steroidal anti-inflamatory drugs) ± adjuvant agents.

FIGURE 14–2

Schematic of levels of pain and appropriate medications to use at each step. (*Adapted from World Health Organization (WHO). Cancer Pain Relief. Geneva: WHO, 1986, with permission.*)

effects. The term "adjuvant" refers to the fact that these medications are drugs with a primary indication other than pain, but they have analgesic properties in some painful conditions.[15] Adjuvant analgesics include antidepressants, corticosteroids, local anesthetics, anticonvulsants, muscle relaxants, osteoclast inhibitors, N-methyl-D-aspartate (NMDA) receptor blockers, alpha-$_2$ adrenergic agents, and radiopharmaceuticals, to name only a few.[30] Some experience is helpful in the use of these medications, however. For example, some of the tricyclic antidepressants (e.g., nortriptyline), SSRIs (e.g., paroxetine, citalopram), and anticonvulsants (e.g., gabapentin) are used routinely by primary care physicians as adjuvants, but at doses far below the threshold of being effective for pain management.[15] Recent evidence suggests that combination treatment with an opioid and gabapentin is superior to either agent alone.[3]

When prescribing medications for older patients, the issue of cost and accessibility must be taken into account. Analgesic medications can be expensive, particularly for patients on fixed incomes. Clinicians should inquire how patients pay for their prescriptions to ensure that they have the means to obtain the necessary medications. In addition, certain medications may be difficult to obtain due to local concerns about stocking controlled substances.[31]

While a thorough discussion of individual pain medications is beyond the scope of this discussion, what follows is a general discussion of the various classes of analgesics and some important points that clinicians should consider when prescribing these agents.

Nonopioid Medications

This category primarily consists of acetaminophen and NSAIDs. Acetaminophen is primarily metabolized by the liver, so patients should not take doses greater than 4 g/day due to hepatotoxicity. NSAIDs are limited due to the potential side effects of gastric irritation and bleeding, inhibition of platelet function, and worsening of renal function. Of note, the analgesic ceiling dose for NSAIDs is often below that of the manufacturer's recommended dose, so approaching or exceeding the maximum dose often does not result in an increase in analgesic effect.[32] The use of cyclooxygenase (COX)-2 selective agents, while once thought of as an alternative to traditional NSAIDs in older patients due to the lower incidence of gastrointestinal and antiplatelet effects, has come under considerable scrutiny recently due to cardiovascular complications, and as such these medications should be reserved for patients with clear indications after a discussion of the risks and benefits of these medications.[10]

Opioid Medications

Medications in this class mimic the action of naturally occurring opioid peptides and bind to receptors in both the brain and spinal cord. Unlike acetaminophen and NSAIDs, these medications exhibit no ceiling effect and can produce profound analgesia by gradual dose escalation. In addition, opioids have no long-term toxicity and can be used for years without concerns about organ damage. In the case of Holly Johnson, simply explaining this to her may help to assuage her fears about taking these medications before she "really" needs them.

Opioids can be administered through both enteral and parenteral routes. Morphine, for example, comes in pill, liquid, and suppository form, and can be swallowed or absorbed through the rectal mucosa. In addition, there are both short-acting (i.e., immediate release) and long-acting (i.e., sustained) preparations. Opioids can also be given intravenously, subcutaneously, intramuscularly (although this form is not preferred due to both the pain associated with the injection and erratic absorption), and absorbed transcutaneously. Rates of onset of analgesic effect differ among these various routes, however. Opioids given intravenously often have an onset within minutes; when taken orally these medications have a longer time to onset, atapproximately 1 hour. Subcutaneous injections have a time to onset of approximately 30 minutes. The transdermal fentanyl patch may take from 12 to 24 hours after first application before maximum effect is achieved.

In addition to choosing the route of medication administration, it is important to pay special attention to the dosing interval. Analgesic medications may be given either episodically (i.e., *prn* or on an "as needed" basis) or at regular intervals (i.e., around the clock).[11] Pain that occurs intermittently is best treated with episodic dosing, but pain that is expected to last for an extended period (e.g., postsurgical pain that is expected to last several days or patients with chronic pain) should be treated with both a regular dosing schedule and a backup additional medication given as needed to relieve breakthrough pain. In these cases, all patients should receive a standing dose of medication with a rescue dose that is approximately 10% of the total daily dose. For example, a regimen of sustained-release morphine 30 mg by mouth every 12 hours would be a total daily dose of 60 mg, so an appropriate dosing regimen would be written as sustained release morphine 30 mg by mouth every 12 hours along with immediate-release morphine 6 mg by mouth every 1 hour as needed for breakthrough pain.

In prescribing medications on an as needed basis, one must be sure that the dosing interval is shorter than the duration that the medication is expected to last. For example, dosing acetaminophen with codeine every 6 hours is inappropriate given that the analgesic effect of codeine lasts for approximately 4 hours. In this regimen, Holly Johnson may be in pain for 2 hours before she receives the next dose. In addition, it is important to pay attention to the maximum dose of combination medications. If a patient takes the combination above (specifically acetaminophen 300 mg combined with 30 mg of codeine, also known as Tylenol #3) as one tablet every 4 hours, the patient will receive a total of 1800 mg of acetaminophen—two tablets dosed in this manner will have a patient receive nearly the maximum daily dose of 4 g.

A complete explanation of starting dosages and titration of medications is beyond the scope of this discussion, but there are certain important points that should be stressed. Dosing of opioid medications is based on the half-life of the particular medication and its formulation. As noted above, morphine and its related compounds come in short-, intermediate-, and long-acting forms. These medications should be dosed according to manufacturer instructions, but clinicians should remember that metabolism in older individuals is affected not only by age but also the simultaneous ingestion of other medications (both prescription and nonprescription). Methadone is particularly difficult to dose due to its extremely long half-life, and its use should be reserved only for those individuals familiar with its pharmacokinetics that change over a range of doses.

No discussion of opioid medications would be complete without a discussion of common side effects. The most common side effect of this class of medications is constipation. This is so common that clinicians should start a prophylactic bowel regimen at the same time as beginning opioids,[10] unless contraindicated, especially given that many elderly patients suffer from chronic constipation. Bowel regimens should include a stool softener in addition to either one or a combination of the following laxatives: fiber/bulk-forming, stimulant, and osmotic agents. Nausea and vomiting can also be seen in patients started on opioid medications, but before starting an antiemetic, one must rule out fecal impaction. Diarrhea in the setting of opioid use should alert the clinician to the possibility of overflow incontinence, where a patient may be so obstructed by fecal material that the only matter allowed to pass around the obstruction is of a liquid nature. Other common side effects of opioids include sweating, dry mouth, and urinary retention. Physicians are often most concerned about respiratory depression, but if patients are started on appropriate doses with a gradual escalation over time, this phenomenon is rare. In addition, respiratory depression rarely occurs without a forewarning change in the patient's mental status. The other worrisome but rare side effect of opioid medications is clonus and, in rare cases, seizures. This class of medications is metabolized in the liver and then excreted by the kidney, so caution must be used in giving patients with renal failure certain opioids. For example, the metabolite of meperidine, normeperidine, can accumulate and lead to seizures in patients with decreased glomerular filtration, such as is the case in older adults. For this and other reasons, it is recommended that meperidine not be used.

In the cases discussed earlier, Holly Johnson's pain regimen is currently inappropriate. Codeine is a weak opioid agonist, and the dosing interval of 6 hours is longer than the analgesic half-life of 4 hours. An "as needed" dosing schedule is inappropriate given her level of pain. A better regimen would be to start morphine elixir 5 mg via mouth every 4 hours, with a rescue dose of 3 mg (5 mg/dose × 6 doses/day = 30 mg total daily dose; 10% or 3 mg is the as needed dose) every 1 hour as needed. Even without a history of constipation, she should be started on a bowel regimen at the same time. In terms of Pam Rodriguez's pain, ibuprofen is an inappropriate medication given her underlying cardiac disease and concerns with potentially worsening her renal failure. Given that her pain is mild and intermittent, a more appropriate starting medication for her would be acetaminophen 650 mg every 4 hours as needed for pain. She also is complaining of neuropathic pain in her feet, most likely from her underlying diabetes, and should be started on a medication such as gabapentin for this pain.

Holly Johnson, *Part 3*

The next day, you go to see Holly Johnson. She now states that her pain is well controlled, and she has only needed one of the rescue doses of morphine. However, she does note that she has vomited twice in the last 12 hours. This morning she is tearful and does not make eye contact when you speak with her.

STUDY QUESTIONS

1. What medications would you consider using for Holly Johnson's nausea?
2. Is she depressed, and if so how would you treat her given her life expectancy?

Pam Rodriguez, *Part 3*

When you go to see Pam Rodriguez the next day, she states that she had a "rough night." She was feeling extremely short of breath for most of the evening, and it took several doses of parenteral furosemide to relieve her dyspnea. While she is now comfortable, she is anxious that her shortness of breath may return. On further questioning, she admits that she has occasional problems with anxiety, and has a prescription for lorazepam at home that she takes on an as needed basis.

STUDY QUESTIONS

1. What recommendations would you have for the team to help treat Pam Rodriguez's dyspnea?
2. How would you treat her anxiety?

MANAGEMENT OF NON-PAIN SYMPTOMS

While patients with chronic illness may have multiple non-pain symptoms over the course of their illness, some of the more common ones are nausea, dyspnea, depression, anxiety, anorexia/cachexia, fatigue, and pruritis. Discussion of all of these topics is beyond the scope of this chapter, so instead we will focus on the first four.

Multiple physiologic processes underlie the sensation of nausea, so therapy is best directed at the mechanism behind the symptom. The three main areas related to the sensation of nausea are the chemoreceptor trigger zone (located in the area postrema at the base of the fourth ventricle, where the fenestrated capillary walls allow a breakdown of the blood–brain barrier, thus exposing the dopamine, serotonin, acetycholine, and opioid receptors in this area to the levels of these substances in the bloodstream), the vomiting center (located in the medulla, this area integrates information from the cortex, limbic and vestibular systems, chemoreceptor trigger zone, and vagal input, and it is rich in dopamine, acetycholine, serotonin, opioid, and histamine receptors), and the gastrointestinal (GI) tract (abdominal organs are rich in serotonin receptors as well as substance P).[33,34] The main classes of medications used for nausea and vomiting are the dopaminergic antagonists, anticholinergics, antihistamines, and serotonin antagonists. The dopaminergic agents such as prochloperazine, chlorpromazine, and metoclopramide antagonize dopamine receptors in the chemoreceptor trigger zone, but metoclopramide also increases GI motility by binding to cholinergic receptors in the GI tract, so it is contraindicated

in patients with bowel obstruction. Anticholinergic agents such as scopolamine work in the vestibular system and in the vomiting center, but these agents should be used with caution in older patients due to their numerous side effects. Serotonin agents such as ondasteron and granisteron are particularly good for patients with chemotherapy-induced nausea. Other agents used in the treatment of nausea are steroids (which act by reducing edema in the bowel wall and brain), aprepitant (which inhibits substance P in the GI tract), octreotide (which reduces GI secretions by reducing blood flow), and benzodiazepines (especially useful in anticipatory vomiting from chemotherapy). Holly Johnson should be started on prochlorperazine, and then other agents can be added that work via alternate pathways as necessary.

While depression in patients near the end of life may be difficult to diagnose, it is never normal and should always be treated to enable patients to have the highest quality of life in their remaining time. Characteristics of depression such as insomnia, weight loss, and anorexia may not be reliable in patients near the end of life, as they may be symptoms of the underlying disease. Two more reliable questions may be, "Do you feel sad or depressed?" and "Have you recently dropped many of your interests and activities?" If patients answer yes to both of these questions, then there is a high likelihood that they are depressed.[35] While a prevailing fallacy among clinical staff is often that "the patient has cancer, of course they are depressed and do not need to be treated," there are effective medications which should be tried. While the selective serotonin reuptake inhibitors (SSRIs) are usually a good place to begin therapy for depression, some of these medications may take 3 to 6 weeks before an effect is seen. If a patient has a shorter life expectancy, it may be advisable to begin a stimulant, such as methylphenidate, which should improve patients' mood and increase their energy level within days. Of note, this medication may cause anorexia, so it should be used with caution in patients who may already have this symptom. In general, anorexia can be effectively treated; numerous studies have shown that patients with cancer treated with steroids or megestrol exhibit an increased appetite, which improves their quality of life, but these medications have not been shown to have an effect on survival.[36]

One of the most distressing symptoms for patients and their families is that of dyspnea. The pathophysiology of dyspnea is complex, and it involves sensory input from the chest wall muscles, lung parenchyma receptors, and carotid bodies, as well as output from the brain respiratory center and higher input from the cerebral cortex.[34] The sensation of dyspnea is subjective. It is not correlated with oxygen saturation or partial pressures of oxygen or carbon dioxide in the blood, and thus treating it with oxygen may not always ameliorate the symptom. The most effective way to improve dyspnea is to determine its underlying cause and then treat it. The differential diagnosis for breathlessness is broad, and includes heart failure/pulmonary edema, anemia, bronchospasm, bronchial obstruction, anxiety, pulmonary embolism, pneumonia, and inability to clear/increased thickness of airway secretions. While this process is ongoing, treating dyspnea with small doses of morphine (2 to 4 mg by mouth in an opioid-naive patient) can be very effective. There is a large body of evidence to show that morphine is effective in treating dyspnea,[37–39] and mechanisms for this action include its ability to decreases respiratory drive in the brainstem, its binding to opioid receptors in the lung itself,[8] and its central ability to decrease the sensation of breathlessness.[40] While there is not as much evidence supporting the use of benzodiazepenes in the treatment of dyspnea, this class of medications may certainly relieve the anxiety associated with breathlessness, and they may decrease central respiratory drive as well. Opioids and benzodiazepines should be used with caution, however, to ensure that they are used to decrease the sensation of dyspnea but not at doses to inhibit the respiratory drive completely so as to cause oversedation and apnea. Finally, nonpharmacologic therapies such as reducing room temperature, repositioning the patient, introducing humidity, and educating patients and families may also help to reduce the sensation of dyspnea. A fan blowing air across the face of a patient is thought to stimulate the V_2 branch of the trigeminal nerve, thus inhibiting respiratory drive and decreasing the sensation of breathlessness.

Anxiety in patients with chronic disease can be distressing to patients and families, and it can interfere with care. While anxiety itself causes patients to suffer, it can also lead to insomnia, depression, fatigue, and withdrawal from social supports.[34] Patients should be asked routinely about anxiety, as too often it is ignored, trivialized, or accepted as inevitable. Like dyspnea, it is important to determine other factors that may be adding to the patient's anxiety. For example, pain that is not well controlled, dyspnea, and side effects of other medications (e.g., steroids, albuterol, or withdrawal from alcohol, opioids, and sedatives) may all contribute to anxiety. Anxiety that is incapacitating, induces behavioral changes, or that is continuous and ongoing should be treated pharmacologically. In the case of Pam Rodriguez, she has a longstanding history of anxiety and has been treated

for it as an outpatient, two factors that indicate that she should be treated with medications in the inpatient setting as well. While there is not a great deal of evidence comparing benzodiazepines, lorazepam is the most commonly used agent. Other benzodiazepines may have half-lives that are either too long or short (e.g., clonazepam and alprazolam, respectively) to be effective, especially at the end of life.[41] Neuroleptic medications may be useful in certain conditions. If a patient's anxiety is not treated by benzodiazepines, or if delirium or psychotic symptoms are present, haloperidol may be effective.[34] To date, there are no data to suggest that newer, more expensive, atypical antipsychotic agents (e.g., olanzapine, risperidone, quetiapine) are more effective than haloperidol for this condition, although some patients (i.e., those with Parkinson's disease) may benefit from their different side-effect profile (quetiapine in particular is thought to have a more favorable side effect profile, although the evidence for this is mostly anecdotal). Given recent data demonstrating a possible relationship between antipsychotic agents and increased mortality, these medications should be used with caution in older adults. Thioridazine may be a useful agent if sedation is desired, especially if a patient has insomnia or agitation.[34] Agents such as buspirone may be effective for patients who have anxiety associated with depression, but antidepressants can take weeks to become effective and as such are not efficacious in treating patients with acute anxiety. Education can be an important component in the treatment of anxiety. For Pam Rodriguez, education about the cause of her dyspnea and the medication that can be used to help relieve it (e.g., morphine, furosemide) may be as effective as a benzodiazepine.

> ● Patients with chronic disease, regardless of etiology, have multiple symptoms—both pain and non-pain (e.g., nausea, dyspnea, depression, anxiety). There are effective treatments for these, and no patient should be left feeling uncomfortable or with uncontrolled symptoms.

Holly Johnson, *Part 4*

Now that Holly Johnson's symptoms are well controlled, you arrange a family meeting to talk with her, her husband, and her adult children. The gynecologic oncologist is unable to attend, but has made it clear that there are no other surgical, radiologic, or chemotherapeutic options. Before you are even able to sit down in the room for the family meeting, the patient asks, "What other options are there for treating my cancer?"

STUDY QUESTION

1. How would you go about answering Holly Johnson's question about other medical interventions?

Pam Rodriguez, *Part 4*

By the end of the week, Pam Rodriguez is greatly improved, and the primary team has asked you to help arrange a safe discharge plan for the patient. All parties involved, including the patient and her partner, are in agreement that subacute rehabilitation is the next appropriate step. The patient seems to understand the plan, but she asks, "How long will I have to keep coming back and forth to the hospital?"

STUDY QUESTION

1. What more would you want to know about Pam Rodriguez before you were able to come up with a plan for her care?

Box 14–2	Six-Step Protocol for Communicating Bad News

Getting started.
    Create an environment conducive to effective communication.
What does the patient know?
    Find out what the patient and the family know about the illness and their current understanding of the medical facts.
How much does the patient want to know?
    Determine what quantity and quality of information the patient and family want to know.
Sharing the information.
    Deliver the information in a straightforward and sensitive manner.
Respond to feelings.
Plan and follow up.

Adapted from Buckman R. How to Break Bad News: A Guide for Health Care Professionals. Baltimore: Johns Hopkins University Press, 1992; and American Medical Association's Institute for Ethics. Education for Physicians on End-of-Life Care (EPEC): Trainer's Guide. Chicago: American Medical Association, 1999, with permission.

COMMUNICATING WITH PATIENTS AND FAMILIES

One of the most important components of palliative care is communication skills, particularly when it comes to breaking bad news. While there is no substitute for observing a skilled physician having these conversations or being observed while delivering bad news and then subsequently receiving feedback on one's performance, experts in patient–physician communication have developed a six-step protocol for breaking bad news[42] that can be used as a guide to communication (Box 14–2).

The first step begins with deciding who the meeting's key participants are, obtaining necessary background information, and arranging for an appropriate time and place for the meeting. In the case of Holly Johnson, as the gynecologic oncologist is unable to attend the meeting, it is critical for the meeting leader to understand from the oncologist the options and treatments that have already been explored and what information has already been communicated to the family. This step also involves finding a setting that ensures privacy and that will be free of interruptions, and determining whom the patient would like to have present for the discussion (e.g., family, clergy, durable power of attorney for health care).

The second step involves determining what the patient already knows, remembering that while information may have been presented to the patient, it may not have been well understood. This inquiry should begin with open-ended questions, such as "what do you understand about your illness" or "tell me what your doctors have told you about what has happened here in the hospital." This helps to determine the patient and family's level of understanding, and can ascertain whether they will be able to comprehend the bad news.

Next, determine how much the patient wants to know. Patients have the right to know as much—or as little—as they want about their medical illness and their prognosis. Questions such as "how much do you want to know about your illness?" or "whom should I talk to about what is going on with your health?" are open-ended question that can help the medical team determine how much detail to give patients about their illness.

The fourth step involves communicating the results. It is useful to deliver a "warning shot" so that patients will be prepared. Phrases such as "I'm afraid I have bad news" or "the results are not what we would like them to be" can alert patients and families that they are about to receive difficult information. The information itself should be delivered clearly and succinctly, without the use of jargon. In the case of Holly Johnson, an appropriate phrase might be "there are no other medical interventions left to try to cure your cancer at this point." Well-intentioned efforts to "soften the blow" may lead to vagueness and confusion. It is also important to avoid phrases such as "there is nothing else we can do" (patients may interpret as abandonment) and "I'm sorry" (may be interpreted as the medical team is responsible for the situation or as pity).

Responding to feelings is an important next step in the process of communicating unfortunate information. Patients and families have a variety of ways in which they react to bad news, from anger to denial to sorrow to acceptance. Outbursts of emotion may make the clinician uncomfortable, so it is important to anticipate these feelings so that the clinician will not be surprised when they are expressed. Allowing the patient and/or family to express these feelings is an important step in building the patient–clinician relationship.

The final step involves making a plan for follow-up. Patients and families have a basic need for education, and guiding them by explaining what the next steps to happen is important at this point. The clinician must walk a line between being too vague (e.g., "we need to do some tests") and too specific (e.g., "chemotherapy consists of taxol and vincristine"). For example, a phrase such as "we need to image your stomach before we can decide which chemotherapy is most appropriate for you" gives the patient both an idea of what is to come without providing too much information that might overwhelm the patient. Establish when the next visit will be, and begin that session by repeating the news and asking how the patient is coping with it.

While Pam Rodriguez's statement does not actually involve a need to deliver bad news, it is clearly a way of asking for more information about her medical care. Does she mean that she no longer wants life-sustaining treatment if it means having to return to the hospital? Or is she merely asking what her future holds? Responding with a more open-ended question will help clarify the motivation for her question (e.g., "What do you mean when you ask that?"). Regardless of the motivation, given her frequent re-hospitalizations, this would seem an appropriate point to renegotiate the overall goals of care.

What is meant by the phrase "goals of care"? While patients have a fundamental right to choose what forms of care they do and do not want, they may not always be well informed enough to be able to make these decisions. Physicians can help patients make decisions by understanding what is important to the patient, and then after eliciting these preferences, tailor treatments to these goals. For example, instead of asking a patient, "Do you want us to try to restart your heart?" when asking about the option of a do-not-resuscitate order, the clinician might better serve the patient to understand what factors are important in her or his overall medical care (e.g., avoidance of pain, quality of life, ability to interact with family) and then suggest which treatments are aligned with those goals.

> **Box 14–3 Seven-Step Protocol to Negotiate Goals of Care**
>
> Create the right setting.
> Determine what the patient/family know.
> Explore what the patient/family hope for or want.
> As necessary, suggest realistic goals of the patient's care.
> Respond appropriately to emotions that are expressed.
> Create a plan of care based on the goals established.
> Review the plan over time and revise it as appropriate.
>
> Adapted from American Medical Association's Institute for Ethics. Education for Physicians on End-of-Life Care (EPEC): Trainer's Guide. Chicago: American Medical Association, 1999, with permission.

While conversations about goals of care can be difficult, having a basic structure (Box 14–3) upon which to base these discussions can be quite helpful.[43] The first steps are similar to that used for breaking bad news. First, create the right setting, which includes getting all information that may be necessary from other providers in order to be able to understand the patient's illness and available treatment. Second, determine what the patient and family knows. Next, explore what they hope for and desire in terms of their overall goal. These may not always be appropriate or possible, so the next step for the physician is to suggest more realistic goals. Phrases such as "we can't cure your illness, but perhaps we can instead focus on keeping you at home, pain free, and able to meaningfully interact with your family for as long as possible" are ways to redirect conversations if patients have unrealistic goals. These two steps are often done in combination, and depending on the patient's and family's level of understanding, can be the most difficult portion of these conversations. As in breaking bad news, it is important to respond empathetically to the emotions and reactions that may arise, and then create a plan for care based on the goals that have been established. Finally, it is important that these goals be written clearly in the medical record, and that these goals must be reviewed and revised periodically as appropriate.

● When communicating bad news or having conversations to negotiate goals of care, it is important to have a method of approach for these often difficult conversations.

SUMMARY

Palliative care for older adults differs from the traditional hospice model in that it is offered simultaneously with life-sustaining treatments. It consists of managing pain and other symptoms, clarifying goals of care, and ensuring continuity across systems of care. Pain management in palliative care involves clear assessment and then establishing a regimen that meets the patient's overall pain needs. Treating non-pain symptoms such as nausea, dyspnea, depression, and anxiety is a cornerstone of palliative care, and this treatment is best served by having a clear understanding of the underlying pathology. When communicating bad news or having conversations to negotiate goals of care, it is important to have a method of approach for these often difficult conversations.

ACKNOWLEDGMENT

Portions of this chapter are adapted from Goldstein and Morrison.[44,45]

References

1. Arias E, Anderson RN, Kung HC, Murphy SL, Kochanek KD. Deaths: final data for 2001. Natl Vital Stat Rep 2003;52:1-115.
2. National Consensus Project for Quality Palliative Care. Clinical Practice Guidelines for Quality Palliative Care. Brooklyn, NY: National Consensus Project for Quality Palliative Care, May 2004.
3. Morrison RS, Meier DE. Clinical practice. Palliative care. N Engl J Med 2004;350:2582-90.
4. Coleman EA, Boult C. Improving the quality of transitional care for persons with complex care needs. Position statement of the American Geriatrics Society Health Care Systems Committee. J Am Geriatr Soc 2003;51(4):556-7.
5. World Health Organization (WHO). Cancer Pain Relief. Geneva: WHO, 1986.
6. Desbiens NA, Wu AW, Broste SK, et al. Pain and satisfaction with pain control in seriously ill hospitalized adults: findings from the SUPPORT research investigations. For the SUPPORT investigators. Study to Understand Prognoses and Preferences for Outcomes and Risks of Treatment. Crit Care Med 1996;24(12):1953-61.
7. Goodlin SJ, Winzelberg GS, Teno JM, Whedon M, Lynn J. Death in the hospital. Arch Intern Med 1998;158(14):1570-2.
8. Morrison RS, Meier DE, eds. Geriatric Palliative Care. New York: Oxford University Press, 2003.
9. Ferrell BA, Whiteman JE. Pain. In: Morrison RS, Meier DE, eds. Geriatric Palliative Care. Oxford: Oxford University Press, 2003:205-29.
10. American Geriatrics Society. The management of persistent pain in older persons. J Am Geriatr Soc 2002;50(Suppl 6):S205-24.
11. Doyle D, Hanks GW, Cherny N, Calman K. Oxford Textbook of Palliative Medicine. 3rd ed. Oxford: Oxford University Press, 2004.
12. Wolfe GI, Trivedi JR. Painful peripheral neuropathy and its nonsurgical treatment. Muscle Nerve 2004;30(1):3-19.
13. Beydoun A. Neuropathic pain: from mechanisms to treatment strategies. J Pain Symptom Manage 2003;25(Suppl 5):S1-3.
14. Guay DR. Adjunctive agents in the management of chronic pain. Pharmacotherapy 2001;21(9):1070-1081.
15. Lussier D, Huskey AG, Portenoy RK. Adjuvant analgesics in cancer pain management. Oncologist 2004;9(5):571-91.
16. Teske K, Daut R, Cleeland C. Relationships between nurses' observations and patients' self-reports of pain. Pain 1983;16:289-96.
17. Camp L. A comparison of nurses' record assessment of pain with perception of pain as described by cancer patients. Cancer Nurs 1988;11:237-43.
18. Katz S, Downs T, Cash H, Grotz R. Progress in development of the index of ADL. Gerontologist 1970;10(1):20-30.
19. Ferrell BA, Ferrell BR, Rivera L. Pain in cognitively impaired nursing home patients. J Pain Symptom Manag 1995;10(8):591-8.
20. Madison JL, Wilkie DJ. Family members' perceptions of cancer pain. Comparisons with patient sensory report and by patient psychologic status. Nurs Clin North Am 1995;30(4):625-45.
21. Lobchuk MM, Kristjanson L, Degner L, Blood P, Sloan JA. Perceptions of symptom distress in lung cancer patients: I. Congruence between patients and primary family caregivers. J Pain Symptom Manag 1997;14(3):136-46.
22. Weiner D, Peterson B, Keefe F. Chronic pain-associated behaviors in the nursing home: resident versus caregiver perceptions. Pain 1999;80(3):577-88.
23. Thomason TE, McCune JS, Bernard SA, Winer EP, Tremont S, Lindley CM. Cancer pain survey: patient-centered issues in control. J Pain Symptom Manag 1998;15(5):275-84.
24. Stein WM. Cancer pain in the elderly. In: Ferrell BR, Ferrell BA, eds. Pain in the Elderly. Seattle, WA: Task Force on Pain in the Elderly of the International Association for the Study of Pain, 1996.
25. Weissman D, Haddox J. Opioid pseudoaddiction—an iatrogenic syndrome. Pain 1989;36:363-6.
26. World Health Organization (WHO). Cancer Pain Relief. Geneva: WHO, 1986.
27. Nikolaus T, Zeyfang A. Pharmacological treatments for persistent non-malignant pain in older persons. Drugs Aging 2004;21(1):19-41.
28. National Comprehensive Cancer Network. Clinical Practice Guidelines in Oncology: Cancer Pain. Available at: www.nccn.org/professionals/physician_gls/PDF/pain Accessed April 22, 2005.
29. Marinangeli F, Ciccozzi A, Leonardis M, et al. Use of strong opioids in advanced cancer pain: a randomized trial. J Pain Symptom Manag 2004;27(5):409-16.
30. Lussier D, Portenoy RK. Adjuvant analgesics in pain management. In: Doyle D, Hanks GW, Cherny N, Calman K, eds. Oxford Textbook of Palliative Medicine. 3rd ed. Oxford: Oxford University Press, 2004:349-78.
31. Morrison RS, Wallenstein S, Natale DK, Senzel RS, Huang LL. "We don't carry that"—failure of pharmacies in predominantly nonwhite neighborhoods to stock opioid analgesics. N Engl J Med 2000;342(14):1023-6.
32. Popp B, Portenoy RK. Management of chronic pain in the elderly: pharmacology of opioids and other analgesic drugs. In: Ferrell BR, Ferrell BA, eds. Pain in the Elderly. Seattle, WA: International Association for the Study of Pain, 1996:21-34.
33. Lipman HI, Meier D. Treatment of nausea and vomiting in the older palliative care patient. Geriatr Aging 2004;7(10):62-7.
34. Waller A, Caroline NL. Handbook of Palliative Care. 2nd ed. Boston: Butterworth Heinemann, 2000.
35. Whooley MA, Avins AL, Miranda J, Browner WS. Case-finding instruments for depression. Two questions are as good as many. J Gen Intern Med 1997;12(7):439-45.
36. Jatoi A, Loprinzi CL. An update: cancer-associated anorexia as a treatment target. Curr Opin Clin Nutr Metab Care 2001;4(3):179-82.
37. American Thoracic Society. Dyspnea. Mechanisms, assessment, and management: a consensus statement. Am J Respir Crit Care Med 1999;159(1):321-40.
38. Jennings AL, Davies AN, Higgins JP, Gibbs JS, Broadley KE. A systematic review of the use of opioids in the management of dyspnoea. Thorax 2002;57(11):939-44.
39. Jennings AL, Davies AN, Higgins JP, Broadley K. Opioids for the palliation of breathlessness in terminal illness. Cochrane Database Syst Rev 2001;(4):CD002066.
40. Bruera E, Macmillan K, Pither J, Macdonald R. Effects of morphine on the dyspnea of terminal cancer patients. J Pain Symptom Manag 1990;5(6):341-4.
41. Bailey FA. The Palliative Response. Birmingham, AL: Menasha Ridge Press, 2003.
42. Buckman R. How to Break Bad News: A Guide for Health Care Professionals. Baltimore: Johns Hopkins University Press, 1992.
43. American Medical Association's Institute for Ethics. Education for Physicians on End-of-Life Care (EPEC): Trainer's Guide. Chicago: American Medical Association, 1999.
44. Goldstein NE, Morrison RS. Treatment of pain in older patients. Crit Rev Oncol Hematol 2005;54:157-64.
45. Goldstein NE, Morrison RS. The intersection between geriatrics and palliative care: a call for a new research agenda. J Am Geriatr Soc 2005;53:1593-8.

Web Resources

1. Website of the American Association of Hospice and Palliative Medicine, one of the largest groups representing and providing educational resources for clinicians who practice palliative medicine: www.aahpm.org.
2. Websites for the Education on Palliative and End-of-Life Care (EPEC) and End-of-Life Nursing Education Consortium (ELNEC), two national education projects dedicated to educating clinicians on improving end of life care: www.epec.net and www.aacn.nche.edu/elnec.
3. Website providing information on the medications most commonly used in palliative care: www.palliativedrugs.com.
4. The Center to Advance Palliative Care is a project funded by the Robert Wood Johnson Foundation, which is dedicated to increasing the availability of quality palliative care services in hospitals and other health care settings: www.capc.org.
5. The End of Life/Palliative Education Resource Center is dedicated to sharing educational resource materials amongst clinicians involved in palliative care education: www.eperc.net.

POSTTEST

1. A 92-year-old woman with severe dementia and frailty is a resident of a long-term care facility. She has been admitted three times in the last six months for aspiration pneumonia. She is not enrolled in hospice. As a member of the palliative care team, what of the following services can you *not* offer her and her family?
   a. Emotional support
   b. Help with decision making
   c. Insurance coverage of medications related to her underlying disease
   d. Coordination of care across settings of care

2. A 68-year-old female with a history of end-stage emphysema is referred to you for control of her dyspnea. On physical exam she is thin and frail appearing, with a large barrel shaped chest. You note that during your interview with her, she answers only in one or two word answers and rarely makes eye contact. You ask her if she is depressed and she admits that she is. Which of the following symptoms would best confirm your diagnosis of depression?
   a. Anorexia
   b. Anhedonia
   c. Insomnia
   d. Weight loss
   e. Increasing agoraphobia

3. An 87-year-old man with diabetes, hypertension, and osteoarthritis comes to your office complaining of pain in his feet. Which of the following characteristics of the pain is NOT helpful in diagnosing his pain?
   a. That he describes the pain as burning
   b. That the pain has lasted for three years
   c. That the pain began when he completed a course of antibiotics for a urinary tract infection
   d. That the pain interferes with his ability to walk at times
   e. That he rates the pain as moderate-severe

PRETEST ANSWERS

1. d. Meperidine has toxic metabolites even at normal doses, so this drug would be contraindicated given the patient's renal failure. Likewise, a nonsteroidal anti-inflammatory drug is also relatively contraindicated given his pre-existing kidney disease. This patient has pain that is expected to last for a period of time, so only providing as needed dosing is inappropriate. The hydromorphone order is written correctly, but 5 mg is a very large starting dose—equivalent to approximately 20 mg of oral morphine.

2. d. Pseudoaddiction. The patient is on an inappropriate pain regimen because the dosing interval is too long. In addition, codeine is a weak opioid. Changing him to a more potent opioid and dosing at the proper interval will adequately treat his pain and most likely will end his disruptive behavior.

3. d. While all of these are important steps in delivering bad news to patients, after setting the scene for the discussion, the next step routinely is to ask patients what they know or what they are expecting.

POSTTEST ANSWERS

1. c. The Medicare hospice benefit will pay for medications related to the patient's diagnosis for which they are enrolled. While palliative care may sometime refer patients to hospice, the two are not synonymous.

2. b. In patients with terminal illness, many of the vegetative symptoms of depression can be a result of the underlying disease process. In this case, anorexia, insomnia, and weight loss can be a part of her underlying lung disease. Her agoraphobia may simply be related to the fact that as she becomes more frail it is difficult to leave her house. Loss of interest in activities that used to give her pleasure, however, is abnormal and helps to confirm the diagnosis of depression. Referral to a psychotherapist and treatment with medications is warranted.

3. c. This patient clearly has neuropathic pain in his feet, most likely related to his diabetes. While certain medications (e.g., antineoplastic agents) are associated with peripheral neuropathy, antibiotics in general are not associated with this phenomenon.

Geriatric Syndromes and Common Special Problems

Be near me when my light is low,
When the blood creeps, and the nerves prick
And tingle; and the heart is sick,
And all the wheels of Being slow.

— ALFRED, LORD TENNYSON (1809–1892), *from In Memoriam*

What does it matter if he can't remember them, as long as they remember him?

— *Wife of Alzheimer's patient, about the grandchildren's visits, 1995*

Perhaps being old is having lighted rooms,
Inside your head, and people in them, acting.
People you know, yet can't quite name.

— PHILIP LARKIN (1922–1985), *in The Old Fools*

Cast me not off in the time of old age;
When my strength faileth, forsake me not.

— *Psalms 71:9*

He that conceals his grief finds no remedy for it.

— Turkish proverb

Body and mind, like man and wife, do not always agree to die together.

— CHARLES C COLTON (1780–1832), British churchman

The quality of a life is determined by its activities.

— ARISTOTLE (382–322 BC), Nichomachean ethics

Wine is only sweet to happy men

— JOHN KEATS "To____ (Fanny Brawne)"

As soon as people are old enough to know better, they don't know anything at all

— OSCAR WILDE (1854–1900), in Lady Windermereís Fan

Delirium
Malaz A. Boustani and Amna Buttar

OBJECTIVES

Upon completion of this chapter, the reader will be able to:

- Discuss the definition, burden, and pathophysiology of delirium among hospitalized older adults.
- Understand the delirium vulnerability–trigger interaction model, and then use this model to characterize the vulnerability of hospitalized older adults for developing delirium and identify the precipitant factors that trigger delirium among these vulnerable individuals.
- Recognize the importance of using primary prevention to decrease the burden of delirium in hospitalized older adults, and thus the value of implementing a proactive screening to identify at-risk population.
- Discuss the management of delirium in general and delirium-induced agitation in particular.
- Describe a multicomponent hospital system to decrease the burden of delirium, and discuss the process of implementing such a program at the reader's local acute setting.

PRETEST

1. Which of the following distinguishes patients with delirium from those with depression or dementia?
   a. Presence of lethargy
   b. Experience of hallucinations
   c. Aggressiveness
   d. Symptom fluctuation

2. Which of the following describes the main stress-induced modification of brain neurotransmission in delirium?
   a. Cholinergic deficiency and dopaminergic excess
   b. Cholinergic excess and dopaminergic deficiency
   c. Cholinergic deficiency and dopaminergic deficiency
   d. Cholinergic excess and dopaminergic excess

3. All of the following are common *predisposing* factors for delirium among older adults hospitalized for a medical or a surgical illness *except*:
   a. Alzheimer's disease
   b. Dehydration
   c. Hemoglobin of 11 mg/dl
   d. Current use of anticholinergic medication

Elaine Fischer, *Part 1*

Elaine Fischer is an 83-year-old woman with mild Alzheimer's disease. She lives at home with her daughter. She is independent in all of her basic actitivies of daily living (ADLs), and dependent on her daughter for shopping, finance management, and transportation. Today, Ms. Fischer comes to your office with her daughter. She is having paranoid delusions and has stopped eating as she is convinced that her daughter is poisoning her. She has been losing weight and feels weak. She also complains of shortness of breath on exertion. The remainder of her physical examination is normal.

STUDY QUESTION

1. What is the differential diagnosis for Ms. Fischer's paranoid delusion?

DEFINITION AND PATHOGENESIS

Delirium or acute confusional state is a syndrome of a disturbance in consciousness with reduced ability to focus, sustain, or shift attention that occurs over a short period of time and tends to fluctuate over the course of the day.[1] This disturbance affects numerous domains of brain function that makes the term "acute brain failure" an accurate descriptive term of delirium.

Delirium induces various neuropsychiatric symptoms such as lethargy, aggression, and hallucinations. These symptoms can be used to divide delirium into hypoactive, hyperactive, or mixed types. Delirium's neuropsychiatric symptoms are shared across various brain disorders such as dementia, depression, and psychosis. However, the specific acute and fluctuating evolving nature of these symptoms in delirium is the main differentiating feature of delirium from depression, dementia, and other brain conditions. Box 15–1 summarizes the various categories of delirium neuropsychiatric symptomatology.

Box 15-1 Delirium Symptoms

- Acute change in mental status
- Fluctuating course
- Attention disturbance
- Memory disturbance
- Orientation disturbance
- Perceptual disturbance
- Thought disturbance
- Sleep disturbance
- Consciousness disturbance
- Speech disturbance
- Psychomotor activity disturbance

The wide spectrum of delirium-related neuropsychiatric symptoms, the generalized EEG slowing that accompanies delirium, absence of primary motor or sensory dysfunction among most delirious patients, and data from neuroimaging studies of patients with delirium suggest that prefrontal cortex, anterior thalamus, nondominant parietal and fusiform cortex are involved in inducing delirium symptoms.[2,3] On the other hand, stress is considered the cornerstone of delirium pathogenesis. It leads to various metabolic changes that alter the availability of valuable amino acids from plasma to the brain, modify the cerebral neurotransmission, and lead to the secretion of cytokines.[4-6] Such a stress state is usually triggered by multiple etiologies such as infection, hypoxia, hypoperfusion, trauma, and surgeries.[3,7,8] The main stress-induced modification of brain neurotransmission in delirium is the presence of a neurotransmission state of cholinergic deficiency and dopaminergic excess.[8] In a general and practical sense, delirium is considered a brain maladaptive reaction to acute stress.[7,8]

> ● Delirium is associated with increased mortality, poorer functional status, limited rehabilitation, increased hospital-acquired complications, prolonged length of hospital stay, increased risk of institutionalization, and higher health care expenditures.

Mary Johnson, *Part 1*

Your patient, Mary Johnson, an 82-year-old woman, is in the emergency room after having fallen and broken her hip. She is very healthy except for a history of hypertension. She is a widow who has been living in her house in a rural area. She has children who live elsewhere and only see her once or twice per year, and they report she has no problems with her ADLs, but they cannot assess

her instrumental ADLs. She is taking no routine medications. Her labs on hospital admission show evidence of dehydration with sodium of 152 mmol/l and a BUN/Creatinine ratio of >20:1. The nurses administer the Mini-Mental Status Examination (MMSE) and the Geriatric Depression Scale (GDS). The patient scored 21/30 on the MMSE and 7/15 on the GDS. She had no evidence of attention deficit nor fluctuating mental status.

STUDY QUESTION

1. What is Ms. Johnson's probability of developing postoperative delirium?

PREVALENCE AND IMPACT

In 2002, there were 12.7 million hospital discharges (38% of all hospital discharges in the United States) for patients aged 65 and older with an average length of hosptial stay of 5.8 days.[9] As demonstrated in Table 15–1 and depending on the reasons for hospitalization (medical illness, urgent surgical repair of hip fracture, elective noncardiac surgery, or cardiac surgery), the prevalence rates for delirium among hospitalized older adults vary from 10% to 52%,[10-33] These rates increase dramatically among hospitalized older adults with dementia, where delirium occurred in 32% to 86% of this vulnerable population.[34] Delirium occurs in the home, assisted living, and nursing home settings in association with acute illness. The prevalence and incidence of delirium in settings outside the hospital is not known. Delirium is associated with increased mortality, poorer functional status, limited rehabilitation, increased hospital acquired complications, prolonged length of hospital stay, increased risk of institutionalization, and higher health care expenditures.[35] Among patients aged 50 and older who had undergone elective noncardiac surgery, delirium increased major complications (15% in delirious patients vs. 2% among those with no delirium), death (4% vs. 0.2%), length of hospital stay (15 day vs. 7 days), and being discharged to an institution (36% vs. 11%).[24]

Elaine Fischer, *Part 2*

In your office you obtain laboratory tests including a urine analysis, metabolic profile, and chest x-ray. The results of these tests are normal. You prescribe haloperidol 0.5 mg a day and send Ms. Fischer home with her daughter after providing reassurance and family education. However, Ms. Fischer continues to complain of shortness of

Table 15–1   Delirium Prevalence Among Hospitalized Older Adults

Setting and Population	Delirium Prevalence Range	References
Older adults hospitalized for medical illness	11%–26%	Thomas et al.,[10] Rockwood,[11] Chisholm et al.,[12] Francis et al.,[13] Johnson et al.,[14] Jitapunkul et al.,[15] Kolbeinsson and Jonsson,[16] Levkoff et al.,[17] Inouye et al.[18]
Postoperative: Older adults undergoing surgical repair of hip fracture	40%–52%	Galanakis et al.,[19] Berggren et al.,[20] Gustafson et al.,[21] Williams et al.[22]
Postoperative: Older adults undergoing elective major noncardiac surgery	10%–39%	Bohner et al.,[23] Marcantonio et al.,[24] Gustafson et al.,[25] Williams-Russo et al.,[26] Fisher and Flowerdew,[27] Rogers et al.[28]
Postoperative: Older adults undergoing cardiac surgery	13%–30%	Bucerius et al.,[29] Van der Mast et al.,[30] Roach et al.,[31] Newman et al.,[32] Smith and Dimsdale[33]

breath and the delusions persist. The next day she "runs away" from home, and the police find her wandering in the neighborhood. She is brought to the emergency room for assessment and a CT scan of her head and chest radiograph are negative. Pulse oximetry shows mild hypoxia, which is corrected by oxygen. Her haloperidol dose is increased to 0.5 mg BID. She is also started on trazodone 50 mg qd by the emergency department physician, and given codeine for off-and-on cough complaints. She is sent home with her daughter for follow-up in your office.

STUDY QUESTION

1. If Ms. Fischer does not currently have delirium, what is her current risk for developing delirium in association with an acute illness?

RISK FACTORS AND PRECIPITATING FACTORS

It has been demonstrated that the occurrence of delirium among hospitalized older adults is the result of a complex interaction among various degrees of insult severity and different levels of patient's vulnerability.[36] This vulnerability–trigger interaction is responsible for the wide range of delirium prevalence rates (10% to 86%) reported among hospitalized older adults. For example, a simple urine infection can trigger delirium among a nursing home resident with a moderate level of dementia. In contrast, severe perioperative hypotension accompanied by a postoperative sepsis and exposure to numerous anticholinergic medications might not lead to delirium among a syoung adult following a surgical repair of a gunshot injury.

Finding a single factor that is responsible for the onset of delirium is rare and thus by using the vulnerability–trigger interaction model, clinicians can categorize the contributing factors of delirium into two groups. First is the cluster of predisposing or vulnerability factors (Table 15–2). Second, is the cluster of precipitating or trigger factors (Table 15–3). However, some factors can have a precipitating or predisposing role. A common example of such a dual factor is a drug with anticholinergic properties. The delirium vulnerability of a female older adult who is taking an anticholinergic drug such as oxybutinin for urine incontinence is already high. Prescribing a sleeping pill with anticholinergic properties such as diphenhydramine to manage her postoperative sleep problem might be the only insult that leads to the development of delirium during her hospital admission for elective knee replacement.

Due to the important role that anticholinergic medications play in the development of delirium as predisposing and precipitating factors, we have summarized the most common anticholinergic medications that are used in older adults. In recent years, the concept of total anticholinergic burden has been used to reflect the cumulative anticholinergic activities of all medications taken by an individual patient.[37] Thus, both a single drug with strong antimuscarinic properties and a combination of multiple drugs, each with a relatively small antimuscarinic effect, might lead to the development of delirium in older adults.[37-40]

Various methods are used to determine the anticholinergic activities of a given drug, and thus the anticholinergic burden faced by a particular patient. One method uses the drug's in-vitro affinity to the muscarinic receptor,[41] another method uses the opinion of clinical experts regarding the drug's clinical

Table 15–2 | Predisposing Factors for Delirium Among Older Adults Hospitalized for Medical or Surgical Illness

Risk Factor	Odds Ratio Range[a]	Delirium Vulnerability Scale
Cognitive impairment		Choose one score only
Chart diagnosis of dementia	3.5–5	3 points
MMSE <24	2–4	2 points
Prior history of delirium	4	1 point
Current history of depression	2–4	1 point
Current history of alcohol abuse	3–6.5	2 points
Current and untreated hearing loss	2	1 point
Current and untreated vision loss	2–3.5	1 point
Need assistance in two basic activities of daily living	2.5	1 point
Current use of anticholinergic	1.5–2.7	2 points
Dehydration defined by BUN/creatinine >21:1	1.8–2	1 point
Sodium abnormality (Na <130 or Na >150)	2–4	1 point
Vascular risk factors: history of		Choose a score of 1 point if at least one risk factors was present (maximum score is also 1 point)
HTN	2.3	
CHF	1.3–2.9	
DM	1.3	
CVA	2.2	
Atrial fibrillation	1.4	
Admitted for		Choose one score only
Urgent surgical repair of hip fracture	3	2 points
Elective aortic aneurysm repair	6	3 points
Total score range	—	0–17
Score range	**Risk category**	**Probability of developing delirium[b]**
0–1 point	Low	<5%
2–3 points	Mild	5%–20%
4–7 points	Moderate	21%–40%
>7 points	Severe	>40%

[a]Odds ratio estimates were based on review of the literature.

[b]Delirium probability estimates for each risk category were based on a literature review[13,17-19,23,24,27,29-32,34,37,39,44,48-54] and the authors' clinical and research experiences. The delirium vulnerability scale has not been validated in a prospective cohort study.

anticholinergic adverse effects,[39,41] and a third method measures the serum anticholinergic activities (SAA) secondary to the intake of a single drug or multiple drugs.[42,43] Table 15–4 integrates the results of several studies to categorize the anticholinergic activities of medications into drugs with a definite central anticholinergic activity and those with a possible central anticholinergic property.

> ● Delirium is diagnosed if a patient has an acute change in mental status with attention deficit accompanied by disorganized thinking or a change in alertness status.

Elaine Fischer, *Part 3*

A week later you receive a call from the patient's daughter who reports that her mother is now very lethargic. You instruct the daughter to take her mother back to the emergency room to be evaluated. She again is hypoxic and has a rapid pulse, and is found to be somnolent and obtunded. In consultation with the emergency room physician you obtain a ventilation perfusion (VQ) scan, which shows a large right-sided pulmonary embolism with several small chronic emboli in the left lung.

Table 15–3	Precipitating Factors for Development of Delirium During Hospitalization for Medical or Surgical Illness[a]	
Precipitating Factor		**Odds Ratio**
Use of physical restraints		4.4
Malnutrition		4
Using more than three new medications during hospitalization		2.9
Use of bladder catheterization		2.4
Exposed to any iatrogenic event		1.9
Intraoperative hypotension (at least 31% drop in mean perioperative BP or a SBP <80 mmHg		1.4
Postoperative Hct <30%		1.7
Untreated postoperative pain		5.4–9
Use of anticholinergic drug		1.5–2.7

[a]Summary of Bucerius et al.,[29] Inouye and Charpentier,[36] Tune et al.,[43] Litaker et al.,[51] and Morrison et al.[52]

STUDY QUESTION

1. What is the most urgent next therapeutic intervention?

DIAGNOSIS AND ASSESSMENT

Delirium diagnosis is one of the most difficult tasks faced by a clinician caring for a hospitalized older adult who is suffering from a neuropsychiatric symptom such as hallucinations, delusion, or agitation in medical or surgical units. In order to differentiate among dementia, delirium, and other psychiatric illnesses with similar neuropsychiatric symptom profile, a clinician needs to be familiar with the core diagnostic features of delirium and understand that having a diagnosis of dementia does not rule out delirium. As a matter of fact, a systematic review of the literature reported that delirium occurs in up to 86% of hospitalized dementia patients.[34]

Table 15–5 provides a structured method to obtain the necessary information to diagnose delirium. Delirium is diagnosed if a patient has an acute change in mental status with attention deficit accompanied by disorganized thinking or a change in alertness status.[1] This diagnostic approach has acceptable feasibility, reliability, sensitivity (94% to 100%), and specificity (90% to 95%).[1]

After making the diagnosis of delirium, a clinician can use the vulnerability–trigger interaction model to identify the underlying modifiable and nonmodifiable triggers for delirium. Nevertheless, identifying such triggers is a difficult task. In a study of delirium among hospitalized older adults with a medical illness, fluid

Table 15–4	Medications with Central Anticholinergic Activity[a]
Definite Central Anticholinergics	**Possible Central Anticholinergics**
Desmethylimipramine	Haloperidol
Doxepin	Olanzepine
Imipramine	Alprazolam
Loxapine	Clorazepate
Nortiptyline	Diazepam
Amitriptyline	Brompheniramine maleate
Amoxapine	Bupropion hydrochloride
Chlorpromazine	Codeine
Clozapine	Colchicines
Perphenazine	Coumadin
Promazine	Dipyridamole
Quetiapine	Disopyramide phosphate
Thioridazine	Hydralazine
Trifluoperazine	Captopril
Chlorpheniramine	Isosorbide
Promethazine	Nifedipine
Diphenhydramine	Chlorthalidone
Hydroxyzine	Triamterene
Hyoscyamine	Furosemide
Benztropine	Digoxin
Ipratropium bromide inhaler	Prednisone, prednisolone, hydrocortisone
Meclizine	Quinidine
Oxybutinin	Theophylline
Meperidine	Cimetidine, Ranitidine
Paroxetine	

[a]Based on the following methods: (1) drug in-vitro affinity to muscarinic receptor,[41] (2) opinion of clinical experts regarding the drug clinical anticholinergic adverse effects,[39,41] and (3) patient's serum anticholinergic activities (SAA) secondary to the intake of a single or multiple drugs.[42,43]

and electrolyte abnormalities were the possible triggers in 40% of cases, infection in 40%, drug toxicity in 30%, metabolic disorders in 26%, sensory and environmental problems in 24%, and low perfusion in 14%.[13] Among hospitalized older adults undergoing surgical repair of their hip fracture, 62% of the delirium cases had several triggers contributing to delirium development, and the most frequent comorbid causes were environmental, infection, drug use, and fluid and electrolyte disturbances.[44]

● Brain imaging or more invasive diagnostic tests for delirium assessment are not indicated without the presence of positive findings during the history, physical examination, or chart review.

Table 15–5   Delirium Diagnosis

Acute and Fluctuating Changes in Mental Status	Attention Deficit	Disorganized Thinking	Hypoalert or Hyperalert Status
As demonstrated by one of the following: 1. Family member interview 2. Nurse interview 3. Chart review 4. ≥2 points acute drops in MMSE score during the hospitalization 5. Discrepancy between different examiners regarding patient's mental status	As demonstrated by one of the following: 1. Nurse interview 2. Patient inability to spell first name backward 3. Patient inability to repeat a phone number 4. Patient inability to count backward from 20 to 1	As demonstrated by one of the following: 1. Nurse interview 2. Patient incoherent speech 3. Patient illogical speech	As demonstrated by one of the following: 1. Nurse interview 2. Chart review 3. Patient sleepiness 4. Patient restlessness
Yes or No	Yes or No	Yes or No	Yes or No

Note: Delirium = (Acute fluctuating changes *and* attention deficit) + (Disorganized thinking *or* hypo-/hyper-alert status).

Table 15–6 provides a simple approach for delirium assessment. This approach is based on our clinical experiences and reviews of the literature. However, the suggested assessment for delirium requires (1) a face-to-face interview with patients to identify the presence of emergent situation such as hypoxia, hypotension, or sepsis; and (2) subsequent comprehensive history and chart review to identify one or more of the possible reasons that led to delirium development such as dehydration, electrolyte abnormality, heart failure, infection process, or simply a new order for an anticholinergic drug. As noted in the proposed delirium assessment, there is no routine recommendation for brain imaging or more invasive diagnostic tests without the presence of positive findings during the physical examination or chart review.

● The clinician's primary objective should be the prevention of delirium; since once delirium symptoms have developed, the older patient is at risk for a poor clinical outcome.

Mary Johnson, *Part 2*

Ms. Johnson undergoes hip replacement surgery. She becomes confused on postoperative day 2. She is rambling and incoherent, but also able to recognize the individuals caring for her. She has an oxygen mask and she keeps trying to take it off and also tries to get up out of bed and pulls at her Foley catheter. She is administered lorazepam 1 mg IV to control her symptoms.

Table 15–6   Assessment and Management of Delirium

Assessment	Symptons	Intervention
Vital signs (pulse, BP, T, RR, and pulse-oximetry). Physical examination to diagnose and treat infectious process or other acute medical conditions (pneumonia, pressure ulcers, MI, CVA, etc.). Urinalysis. Cr, Na, K, Ca, glucose. CBC with differential. Review old and new anticholinergic medication (discontinue if benefit does not outweigh harms). Review old and new benzodiazepines (discontinue if benefit does not outweigh harms). Review the need for Foley catheter, IV lines, and other tethers (discontinue if benefit does not outweigh harms).	*Agitation*	Consider professional sitter. Assess the impact of agitation on patient safety and d/c Foley and other tethers if possible. Consider trazodone 25 mg po q 6 hr PRN. If h/o ETOH, consider Lorazepam 0.25–0.5 mg PO/IM/IV q 4–6 hr PRN. If safety became an issue, sitter failed to ameliorate agitation, and reversing underlying medical condition is in process, then consider using haloperidol 0.25 mg PO/IM/IV q 4 hr PRN for maximum dose of 2 mg per day, and then re-evaluate every 24 hrs and make sure to discontinue haloperidol prior to discharge.
	Lethargy	Check skin for pressure ulcer. Decrease dose of hypnotics. Decrease dose of other psychotropics.

From Boustani M, Heck D, Farlow M, et al. Managing delirium in hospitalized elderly. J Am Geriatr Soc 52(Suppl S):S199, 2004, with permission.

STUDY QUESTION

1. What are the safest and most effective strategies to manage the patient's delirium-induced agitation?

MANAGEMENT

There are limited data to guide the management of delirium among hospitalized older adults. However, recent systematic reviews of the literatures[34,45,46] indicate that prevention-, interdisciplinary-, and system-based delirium interventions constitute an effective and promising program to reduce the burden of delirium. Such preventive interventions can be categorized into nurse-target and physician-focused recommendations (Tables 15–7 and 15–8). These recommendations are based on the delirium vulnerability–trigger interaction model. They concentrate on modifying specific vulnerability or trigger factors such as the management of cognitive impairment, sleep deprivation, anticholinergic burden, pain, constipation, and restraints. The efficacy of using a preventive interdisciplinary program that includes the above interventions ranged from an absolute risk reduction of 5% to 31%, with

the total number of patients requiring treatment in order to prevent one delirium case ranging from 3 to 20 patients.[46]

The systematic reviews also found that managing delirium after its onset is a very difficult task. Once delirium develops, its successful management depends on the accurate delivery of two types of interactive therapies. First is the treatment of underlying causes such as dehydration, infection, and or exposure to one or more anticholinergic medications; and second is providing a safe and appropriate supportive pharmacological and nonpharmacological care.

Supportive care targets the two types of delirium: hyperactive (agitation) and hypoactive (lethargy). Both of these symptoms lead to higher complication rates and longer hospital stays. Table 15-6 provides a structured assessment for delirium-induced agitation and lethargy followed by specific recommendations for each category. The cornerstone for the management of delirium-induced agitation is to provide safe and supportive care that allows management of the underlying causes of delirium. Such supportive care includes access to a trained professional sitter and administration of a low dose of trazodone. The data for this recommendation are limited and are based on the

Table 15–7	Nursing-Based Interventions to Prevent Delirium
Factor	**Interventions**
Sleep	Maintain 4–6 hours of uninterrupted sleep each night. If patient complains of insomnia consider the following: 1. Decrease environmental noise at night. 2. Provide drink of hot milk. 3. Provide back rub for 15 minutes. 4. If the above failed, then consider using a hypnotic drug.
Orientation	Orient patient about the date, place, and reason for hospitalization. Keep a clock and calendar inside the patient's room. Keep light on from 7 AM (sunrise) to 7 PM (sundown).
Environment	Encourage patient's family to bring personal items. Encourage patient's family to bring hearing aid and glasses. Encourage low-stimulation family visits.
Activity	Evaluate appropriateness of restrictive activity order.
Tethers	Evaluate necessity of using Foley catheter, restraint, IV line, and monitors.
Pain	Identify and manage adequately.
Constipation	Identify and manage adequately.

From Fisher BW, Flowerdew G. A simple model for predicting postoperative delirium in older patients undergoing elective orthopedic surgery. J Am Geriatr Soc 43:175–78, 1995, with permission.

Table 15–8	Physician-Based Interventions to Prevent Delirium
Factor	**Intervention**
Cognitive impairment	Continue or start cholinesterase inhibitors if patient has possible or probable Alzheimer disease. Avoid, discontinue, or substitute all anticholinergic medications.
Anticholinergics	Avoid, discontinue, or substitute all anticholinergic medications.
Benzodiazepines	Avoid or assess need for these drugs, and then taper off.
Pain	Maintain pain level of ≤3/10: 1. Scheduled acetaminophen, and then scheduled narcotic if necessary. 2. Avoid meperidine or codeine.
Constipation	Scheduled sorbitol or stimulant (if narcotics are used for pain control).
Insomnia	Low-dose trazodone or mitrazepine.
Mobility	Eliminate Foley catheter and physical restraints and order early mobilization if appropriate.
High risk for alcohol withdrawal	Consider scheduled short-acting benzodiazepine.
Dehydration	Maintain BUN/Crt <20/1. Maintain normal level Na.

From Boustani M, Heck D, Farlow M, et al. Managing delirium in hospitalized elderly. J Am Geriatr Soc 52(Suppl S):S199, 2004, with permission.

similar effect of trazodone or haloperidol in dementia patients with behavioral symptoms in less adverse events[47] (the low dose of haloperidol at 0.25 mg every 4 hours via oral, muscular, or venous routes of administration).

Elaine Fischer, *Discussion*

Ms. Fischer's presentation is a typical example of delirium being the only manifestation of a life-threatening emergency. She is treated for the pulmonary embolism, her delusions disappear, and her psychotropic medications are reduced and eventually stopped.

Mary Johnson, *Discussion*

Ms. Johnson appears to have pre-existing, undetected, mild dementia, which places her at higher risk for a postoperative delirium. Evaluation of her delirium symptoms reveals that she has a urinary tract infection. After starting an antibiotic, you arrange for a professional sitter to stay with Ms. Johnson in her hospital room, and prescribe haloperidol 0.25 mg q 6 hours as needed to manage her agitation.

SUMMARY

Decreasing the burden of delirium in older adults requires the implementation of a specialized delirium program that includes three crucial components: (1) implementing active screening to identify patients with high vulnerability for the development of delirium (using the delirium vulnerability scale); (2) educating clinicians, including nurses and physicians, on recognizing and diagnosing delirium and identifying its triggers; and (3) structuring consultation services that provide in-depth recommendations to prevent and manage delirium. The members of such a delirium program would include at least a physician (geriatrician, geriatric psychiatrist, or a specialized hospitalist), a nurse, and an administrative assistant.

References

1. Inouye SK, VanDyck CH, Alessi CA, et al. Clarifying confusion: the confusion assessment method, a new method for detection of delirium. Ann Intern Med 113:941-8, 1990.
2. Trzepacz PT, Sclabassi RJ, Van Thiel DH. Delirium: a subcortical phenomenon. J Neuropsychiatry Clin Neurosci 1:283-90, 1989.
3. Trzepacz PT. The neuropathogenesis of delirium. A need to focus our research. Psychosomatics 35:374-91, 1994.
4. Van der Mast RC. Delirium: the underlying pathophysiological mechanisms and the need for clinical research. J Psychosomatic Res 41:109-13, 1996.
5. Flacker JM. Lipsitz LA. Neural mechanisms of delirium: current hypotheses and evolving concepts. Erratum appears in J Gerontol A Biol Sci Med Sci 54(7):B275, 1999.
6. van der Mast RC. Fekkes D. Serotonin and amino acids: partners in delirium pathophysiology? Clin Neuropsychiatry 5(2):125-31, 2000.
7. Trzepacz PT. Update on the neuropathogenesis of delirium. Dement Geriatr Cogn Disord 10(5):330-41, 1999.
8. Trzepacz PT. Is there a final common neural pathway in delirium? Focus on acetylcholine and dopamine. Semin Clin Neuropsychiatry 5(2):132-48, 2000.
9. DeFrances CJ, Hall MJ 2002 National Hospital Discharge Survey. Advance Data from Vital and Health Statistics, 342. Hyattsville, MD: National Center for Health Statistics 2004.
10. Thomas RI, Cameron DJ, Fahs MC. A prospective study of delirium and prolonged hospital stay. Arch Gen Psychiatry 45:937-40, 1988.
11. Rockwood K. The occurrence and duration of symptoms in elderly patients with delirium. J Gerontol 48:M162-6, 1993.
12. Chisholm SE, Deniston LO, Igrisan RM, et al. Prevalence of confusion in elderly hospitalized patients. J Gerontol Nurs 8:87-96, 1982.
13. Francis J, Martin D, Kapoor W. A prospective study of delirium in hospitalized elderly. JAMA 263:1097-101, 1990.
14. Johnson JC, Gottlieb GL, Sullivan E, et al. Using DSM-III criteria to diagnose delirium in elderly general medical patients. J Gerontol 45:M113-9, 1990.
15. Jitapunkul S, Pillay I, Ebrahim S. Delirium in newly admitted elderly patients: a prospective study. J Med 83(300):307-14, 1992.
16. Kolbeinsson H, Jonsson A. Delirium and dementia in acute medical admissions of elderly patients in Iceland. Acta Psychiatr Scand 87:123-7, 1993.
17. Levkoff SE, Evans DA, Liptzin B, et al. Delirium. The occurrence and persistence of symptoms among elderly hospitalized patients. Arch Intern Med 152:334-40, 1992.
18. Inouye SK, Viscoli CM, Horwitz RI, et al. A predictive model for delirium in hospitalized elderly medical patients based on admission characteristics. Ann Intern Med 119:474-81, 1993.
19. Galanakis P, Bickel H, Gradinger R, et al. Acute confusional state in the elderly following hip surgery: incidence, risk factors and complications. Int J Geriatr Psychiatry 16(4):349-55, 2001.
20. Berggren D, Gustafson Y, Eriksson B, et al. Postoperative confusion after anesthesia in elderly patients with femoral neck fractures. Anesth Analgesia 66:497-504, 1987.
21. Gustafson Y, Brannstrom B, Berggren D, et al. A geriatric-anesthesiologic program to reduce acute confusional states in elderly patients treated for femoral neck fractures. J Am Geriatr Soc 39:655-62, 1991.
22. Williams MA, Campbell EB, Raynor VJ, et al. Reducing acute confusional states in elderly patients with hip fractures. Res Nurs Health 8:329-37, 1985.
23. Bohner H, Hummel TC, Habel U, et al. Predicting delirium after vascular surgery: a model based on pre- and intraoperative data. Ann Surg 238(1):149-56, 2003.
24. Marcantonio ER, Goldman L, Mangione CM, et al. A clinical prediction rule for delirium after elective noncardiac surgery. JAMA 271:134-9, 1994.
25. Gustafson Y, Berggren D, Brannstron B, et al. Acute confusional states in elderly patients treated for femoral neck fracture. J Am Geriatr Soc 36:525-30, 1988.
26. Williams-Russo P, Urquhart BL, Sharrock NE, et al. Post-operative delirium: predictors and prognosis in elderly orthopedic patients. J Am Geriatr Soc 40(8):759-67, 1992.
27. Fisher BW, Flowerdew G. A simple model for predicting postoperative delirium in older patients undergoing elective orthopedic surgery. J Am Geriatr Soc 43:175-8, 1995.
28. Rogers MP, Liang MH, Daltroy LH et al. Delirium after elective orthopedic surgery: risk factors and natural history. Int J Psychiatry Med 19:109-21, 1989.
29. Bucerius J, Gummert JF, Borger MA, et al. Predictors of delirium after cardiac surgery delirium: effect of beating-heart (off-pump) surgery. J Thorac Cardiovasc Surg 127(1):57-64, 2004.
30. Van der Mast RC, Van den Broek WW, Fekkes D, et al. Incidence and preoperative predictors for delirium after cardiac surgery. J Psychosom Res 46:479-83, 1999.
31. Roach GW, Kanchuger M, Mangano CM, et al. Adverse cerebral outcomes after coronary bypass surgery. Multicenter Study of Perioperative Ischemia Research Group and the Ischemia Research and Education Foundation Investigators. N Eng J Med 335(25):1857-63, 1996.
32. Newman MF, Kirchner JL, Phillips-Bute B, et al. Longitudinal assessment of neurocognitive function after cardiac surgery: perioperative decline predicts long-term (5-year) neurocognitive deterioration. N Engl J Med 344:395-402, 2001.
33. Smith LW, Dimsdale JE. Postcardiotomy delirium: conclusion after 25 years? Am J Psychiatry 146:452-8, 1989.
34. Fick DM, Agostini JV, Inouye SK. Delirium superimposed on dementia: a systematic review. J Am Geriatr Soc 50:1723-32, 2002.
35. Balas MC, Richmond TS, Sullivan-Marx EM. Outcomes of delirious hospitalized older adults: a systematic review. J Am Geriatr Soc 52(Suppl S):S56-6, 2004.
36. Inouye SK, Charpentier PA. Precipitating factors for delirium in hospitalized elderly persons. Predictive model and interrelationship with baseline vulnerability. JAMA 275(11):852-7, 1996.
37. Tune LE. Anticholinergic effects of medication in elderly patients. J Clin Psychiatry 62(Suppl 21):11-4, 2001.
38. Aizenberg D, Sigler M, Weizman A, et al. Anticholinergic burden and the risk of falls among elderly psychiatric inpatients: a 4-year case-control study. Int Psychogeriatrics 14(3):307-10, 2002.

39. Han L, McCusker J, Cole M, et al. Use of medications with anticholinergic effect predicts clinical severity of delirium symptoms in older medical inpatients. Arch Intern Med 161(8):1099-105, 2001.

40. Knight EL, Avorn J. Quality indicators for appropriate medication use in vulnerable elders. Ann Intern Med 135:703-10, 2001.

41. Minzenberg MJ, Poole JH, Benton C, et al. Association of anticholinergic load with impairment of complex attention and memory in schizophrenia. Am J Psychiatry 161(1):116-24, 2004.

42. Mulsant BH, Pollock BG, Kirshner M, et al. Serum Anticholinergic activity in a community-based sample of older adults. Arch Gen Psychiatry 60:198-203, 2003.

43. Tune L, Carr S, Hoag E, et al. Anticholinergic effects of drugs commonly prescribed for the elderly: potential means for assessing risk of delirium. Am J Psychiatry 149:1393-4, 1992

44. Brauer C, Morrison RS, Silberzweig SB, et al. The cause of delirium in patients with hip fracture. Arch Intern Med 160:1856-60, 2000.

45. Weber JB. Coverdale JH. Kunik ME. Delirium: current trends in prevention and treatment. Intern Med J 34(3):115-21, 2004.

46. Boustani M, Heck D, Farlow M, et al. Managing delirium in hospitalized elderly. J Am Geriatr Soc 52(Suppl S):S199, 2004.

47. Teri L, Logsdon RG, Peskind E, et al. Alzheimer's Disease Cooperative Study. Treatment of agitation in AD. a randomized, placebo-controlled clinical trial. [See comment.] [Erratum appears in Neurology ;56(3):426, 2001.] Neurology 55(9):1271-8, 2000.

48. Elie M, Cole M, Primeau FJ, et al. Delirium risk factors in elderly hospitalized patients. J Gen Intern Med 13:204-12, 1998.

49. Marcantonio ER, Goldman L, Orav EJ, et al. The association of intraoperative factors with the development of postoperative delirium. Am J Med 105:380-4, 1998.

50. Edlund A, Lundstrom M, Brannstrom B, et al. Delirium before and after operation for femoral neck fracture. J Am Geriatr Soc 49(10):1335-40, 2001.

51. Litaker D, Locala J, Franco K, et al. Preoperative risk factors for postoperative delirium. Gen Hosp Psychiatry 23(2):84-9, 2001.

52. Morrison RS, Magaziner J, Gilbert M, et al. Relationship between pain and opioid analgesics on the development of delirium following hip fracture. J Gerontol A-Bio Sci Med Sci 58(1):76-81, 2003.

Web Resources

1. ICU Delirium and Cognitive Impairment Group at Vanderbilt University Medical Center: www.icudelirium.org/delirium/index.html.

2. Geriatric Web, Division of Geriatrics at Palmetto Health Richland Hospital, University of South Carolina, School of Medicine Library: http://geriatricweb.sc.edu/.

3. The Hospital Elder Life Program: http://elderlife.med.yale.edu/public/public-main.php.

POSTTEST

1. All of the following are common *precipitating* factors for the development of delirium during hospitalization for medical or surgical illness *except*:
   a. Physical restraints
   b. Bladder catheter
   c. Early referral to physical therapy
   d. Untreated postoperative pain

2. All of the following medications may precipitate or contribute to delirium in older adults *except*:
   a. Atorvastatin
   b. Amitriptyline
   c. Oxybutinin
   d. Diphenhydramine

3. Interventions that may prevent the onset of delirium among older adults hospitalized for a medical or surgical illness include all below *except*:
   a. Professional or family sitter
   b. Encourage 6 hours of uninterrupted sleep per night
   c. Use of lorazepam for excessive anxiety
   d. If needed, ensure that patient wears hearing aid/eyeglasses

---

PRETEST ANSWERS

1. d
2. a
3. c

POSTTEST ANSWERS

1. c
2. a
3. c

Alzheimer's Disease and Other Dementias

Malaz A. Boustani and Richard J. Ham

OBJECTIVES

Upon completion of this chapter, the reader will be able to:

- Implement a risk assessment model for the future development of dementia in primary care.
- Differentiate among dementia, delirium, and mild cognitive impairment.
- Understand the balance between the benefits and the harms of dementia screening in primary care.
- Implement a comprehensive dementia management program in primary care.

PRETEST

1. D.S., a 76-year-old widow, presents for follow-up of her hypertension, diabetes, and chronic heart failure. She is taking six prescribed medications in addition to aspirin and a multivitamin. She reports a family history of dementia and heart disease and was involved in motor vehicle accident 10 years ago. What approach to dementia screening is recommended for this patient?
   a. No dementia screening is necessary.
   b. Include the patient in the decision of screening for dementia.
   c. Use the Mini-Mental Status Examination (MMSE), Mini-Cog, or the Clock-Drawing Test (CDT) to screen for dementia.
   d. Refer the patient to memory clinic to conduct a formal dementia evaluation.

2. On taking a clinical history of an 82-year-old patient, his wife tells you that he has had trouble remembering to take his medications. Furthermore, last week he got lost while driving alone and had to be escorted home by strangers. What would be the most appropriate next step?
   a. Refer the patient to the local memory clinic for formal evaluation.
   b. Conduct simple cognitive screening using the MMSE, Mini-Cog, or CDT.
   c. Order a brain imaging to detect any cortical infarct.
   d. Assure the patient that her symptoms are normal part of the aging process.

3. A.J., a patient with moderate dementia, was admitted last summer to a nursing home. Today, her daughter brings her in for her annual follow-up. The daughter tells you that over the past 2 months her mother has become increasingly irritable. She now spends most of the time in her room, no longer playing cards and bingo. Last week she declined her daughter's invitation to join a family picnic, something that she always used to enjoy. In addition, staff tell the daughter that A.J. has been resisting taking her medication and is sleeping poorly at night. What is the most likely diagnosis?
   a. An episode of acute delirium
   b. Primary insomnia
   c. Depression superimposed on dementia
   d. An evolving serious medical problem, such as cancer or severe anemia

---

Harold Franklin, *Part 1*

You have been Thelma Franklin's personal physician for many years. During a routine pelvic examination, she breaks down and weeps uncontrollably when asked about sexual activity. She describes a traumatic period of nearly a year during which her husband Harold, 68, who runs his own small business, has been much more sexually demanding. This was acceptable to her at first but now is getting embarrassing. For example, when *they are out to eat, he makes loud remarks about her sexual responsiveness. Several times he has gone out alone in the car in the evening, which is quite unlike him, and has sometimes returned showing evidence of drinking. She thinks he may be having an affair and blames her involvement in voluntary activities and neglect of her husband and herself (she is somewhat overweight and has type 2 diabetes). She asks if you know a good marriage counselor. She doubts that Harold would see one or see you.*

One afternoon Harold drives his car off the road and hits a tree. He is not injured, but a police breathalyzer test leads to a court case, and he is banned from driving for a year. Humbled into coming for a checkup, he finally sees you, and you are frank regarding Thelma's concerns. He declares that he feels he has been "going crazy," and finds it increasingly difficult to remember what he has done and whom he should call. As a result, his business is failing. Now he has so much trouble remembering things that he has had to delegate much of the day-to-day running of his business to others.

Mr. Franklin is not taking medication, and a physical examination reveals him to be in good shape. His MMSE score is 22/30, with poor short-term memory, inability to subtract 7s (serial 7s), and uncertainty regarding which year it is. (He jokes about this, but is clearly embarrassed.) He denies that sexuality is a problem, saying that their sex life has been poor for years. He says his drinking is not a problem; he feels that he was unlucky to have been booked. He does agree to submit to brain imaging and blood tests.

STUDY QUESTIONS

1. What tests should be done at this stage?
2. What diagnostic possibilities exist?
3. What, if anything, should you tell the family?

PREVALENCE AND IMPACT

Dementia is a growing global public health problem. In the United States, there were an estimated 7 million cases of dementia in 2000, and this number may grow to 19 million by 2050.[1] It is projected that every 7 seconds there will be one additional patient diagnosed with dementia across the globe.[2] In a primary care setting, 6.0% of patients aged 65 and older have dementia: 2% of those aged 65 to 69 years, 7% of those aged 70 to 79 years, and 17% of patients aged 80 and older.[3] Among primary care patients with dementia, 70% suffer from Alzheimer's disease (AD), 5% have vascular dementia (VaD), and 22% have mixed AD and VaD.[3]

According to the Global Burden of Disease estimates for the 2003 World Health report, dementia contributed 11% of all years lived with disability by people aged 60 years and older.[2] This disability translates to a high burden of suffering for patients, families, and society, with an annual estimated cost of $100 billion in the United States alone.[4,5] Most of this high burden falls on the patients' informal caregivers. The average family care-giver spends 6 hours per week caring for patients who are independent in their basic activities of daily living and 35 hours caring for those with significant functional dependency.[6] However, the discovery of research breakthroughs that would slow the onset and progression of Alzheimer's might reduce the projected future burden of AD,[1] such as that 3 million fewer Americans would suffer from AD by 2025 and that Medicare could achieve an annual saving of $444 billion by 2050.[1,7] Figure 16–1 illustrates that projected prevalence of Alzheimer's disease in the United States in 2050, based on four scenarios of treatment advances. As can be seen from this figure, Alzheimer's disease will be very common under all scenarios; however, the projected distribution of mild and moderate/severe cases varies depends on treatment advances.

PATHOPHYSIOLOGY AND RISK FACTORS

Pathophysiology

The precise etiology of AD is not fully understood; however, it appears to involve several pathways in the central nervous system that result in neuronal death. One pathway involves alteration in one or more aspects of beta amyloid, leading to proliferation of extracellular amyloid plaques. Another possibly related pathway involves alteration in one or more aspects of tau protein metabolism, leading to intracellular neurofibrillary tangles. As part of these processes, an inflammatory cascade appears to be catalyzed, leading to oxidative neuronal injuries and, finally, depletion of several neurotransmitters (for example, the cholinergic system).[8] The interac-

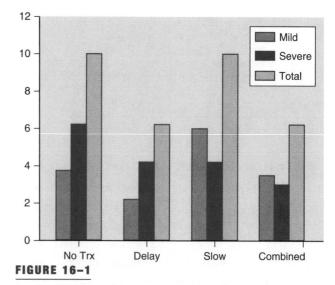

FIGURE 16–1

Projections of prevalent cases of AD (in millions) in 2050, based on three models of the effects of significant therapy advances introduced in 2010: medications that delay onset, that slow progression, and that both delay onset and slow progression.

tions among these numerous processes over decades lead to neuronal dysfunction and eventually to neuronal death. Early on, the brain compensates for these disturbances without manifesting clinically significant cognitive or behavioral symptoms. However, the continuous loss of neurons eventually overwhelms the brain's reserve capacity, and symptoms start to surface. This relatively long process offers a good opportunity for early presymptomatic interventions toward slowing or stopping the neuronal damage.

The two well-recognized pathophysiological features of AD are the presence of the intracellular neurofibrillary tangles (NFT) and the extracellular amyloid plaques within selected brain regions. NFTs are composed of an abnormally aggregated, hyperphosphorylated form of the protein tau, which is a microtubule-binding protein that stabilizes the neuronal cytoskeleton and participates in vesicular transport and axonal polarity of the neuron.[9] Amyloid plaques consist primarily of extra-cellular accumulation of a 40- to 42-amino acid amyloid-beta peptide derived from the amyloid precursor protein (APP). In the absence of AD pathology, an enzyme called alpha secretase breaks the APP and produces a soluble alpha fragment that gets excreted. In the presence of AD, two different enzymes, beta secretase and gamma secretase, cleave the APP, leading to the formation of an insoluble fragment that aggregates to form the pathological plaques.[8,9] Over the years, experts have debated about the individual and separate contribution of the amyloid plaques and the NFT to the underlying AD pathogenesis. However, recent evidence suggests that both proteins are interconnected and lead synergistically to the progressive neuronal death in AD.[8,9]

Risk Factors

The current conceptual model for the development of dementia takes into account the interaction among individuals' genetic susceptibility, their exposure to various known and unknown environmental insults, and the time available for such interactions (Fig. 16–2). Numerous epidemiological studies have demonstrated that age is the best studied and strongest risk factor for AD. The incidence rate among people aged 65 to 69 years is about 2.4 cases per 1,000 person-years, and it doubles in each subsequent 5-year period.[10] In addition to age, family history of AD is considered a strong risk factor; individuals with both parents suffering from AD have a 54% cumulative risk of developing this condition by age 80. This risk is about 1.5 times greater than the risk faced by those with one parent with AD and nearly five times greater than for those with neither parent affected. First-degree relatives of patients with AD have a cumulative

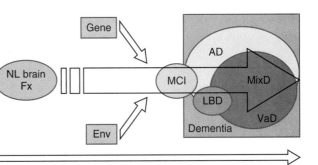

NI: normal; Fx: function; Env: environment; MCI: mild cognitive impairment; AD: Alzheimer's disease; LBD: Lewy body dementia; VaD: vascular dementia; MixD: mixed dementia.

FIGURE 16–2

Current conceptual model for development of AD and other dementias. Nl, normal; Fx, function; Env, environment; MCI, mild cognitive impairment; AD, Alzheimer's disease; LBD, Lewy body dementia; VaD, vascular dementia; MixD, mixed dementia.

lifetime risk of 39%, approximately twice the risk of AD in the general population.[11]

Some genetic mutations have been associated with AD. It is estimated that 20% to 30% of the general population and 45% to 60% of people with late-onset AD have the apolipoprotein E-4 gene.[12] Down's syndrome conveys a markedly increased risk; 55% of individuals between 50 and 59 years and 75% of those 60 years of age and older have AD.[13] Head trauma is also a risk factor for AD; a case–control study found the odds ratio of AD to be 3.5 among persons with a history of significant head trauma compared to controls.[14]

Cardiovascular risk factors such as hypertension, hyperlipidemia, and diabetes mellitus are associated with vascular dementia. A cross-sectional study found all indicators of atherosclerosis (vessel wall thickness, plaques of the carotid arteries, and the ratio of ankle-to-brachial systolic blood pressure) to be associated with all dementias, with odds ratios ranging from 1.3 to 1.9.[15]

Although meta-analysis of observational studies in the late 1990s suggested that hormone replacement therapy (HRT) might reduce the risk of AD; the Women's Health Initiative Memory randomized clinical trial indicated the contrary. This trial found that in comparison to women receiving placebo, those who used HRT had double the risk of developing AD (95% confidence interval [CI], 1.21–3.48).[16]

Protective Factors

Targeting various factors that decrease the individual's vulnerability for the development of AD has received serious attention from national and international organizations. The National Institute on Aging (NIA) initiated the Cognitive and Emotional Health Project that aims to optimize the emotional and cognitive reserve of aging persons by conducting various critical analyses of the literature to identify the factors that contribute to such reserve.[17] Similar to the NIA project, the National Alzheimer Association has launched the Maintain your Brain campaign that provides various steps for the general public to decrease the risk of developing AD (http://www.alz.org/maintainyourbrain).

A recent comprehensive review of the literature has identified several protective factors or strategies that are associated with AD, included educational attainment, cognitive and leisure activities, exercise, statins, a cholesterol lowering diet, and protection from head trauma.[18] In comparison to patients aged 75 and older who had at least 8 years of education, those with less than 8 years of education have 2.6 times the odds of developing AD (95% CI, 1.5–4.4).[18] Multiple observational and experimental studies showed a protective benefit for leisure activities such as playing board games, musical instruments, and reading. For example, the 7-year Observational Religious Orders study of 733 individuals aged 65 and older found that a 1-point increase in a cognitive activity score resulted in 33% lower risk of developing AD.[18] Based on a meta-analysis of 18 studies, being involved in aerobic and strength training exercises have preventive effects against AD.[18] Although no randomized clinical trials have investigated the role of statins or other cholesterol-lowering methods in preventing AD, a review of observational studies suggests the presence of a relationship between cholesterol or statins and the risk of cognitive decline, AD, or dementia.[18]

Despite the involvement of oxidative stress and inflammation in the pathophysiology of AD, the current evidence does not support the use of antioxidants, such as vitamin E or C, or anti-inflammatory agents, such as prednisone or nonsteroidal anti-inflammatory drugs (NSAIDs), in the prevention of AD. On the contrary, recent studies identified significant harms associated with the general use of these agents.[18]

In summary, a number of risk factors and preventive strategies for AD have been identified (see Table 16–1). An elderly patient with hypertension, diabetes, hyperlipidemia, and family history of AD, for example, would be at high risk for the development of both cardiovascular disease and dementia. Therefore, the patient's primary care physician should provide counseling about the benefits of brain exercise, heart exercise, a cholesterol-lowering diet, and head trauma protection. In addition, the physician should maintain the patient's blood pressure within recommended range of 140/80 without causing orthostatic hypotension, keep the LDL below 130 mg/ml, and aim for HbA1c level below 7%.

Table 16–1 Risk Factors and Protective Factors in Alzheimer's Disease

Risk Factors	Protective Factors
Age	Involvement in leisure activities
Family history of Alzheimer's disease	Involvement in aerobic and strength training
Head trauma	Cholesterol-lowering strategies
Low education level	Optimized management of hypertension, diabetes mellitus, hyperlipidemia
Hypertension	
Diabetes mellitus	
Hyperlipidemia	
Cerebrovascular events	

Harold Franklin, *Part 2*

All tests for contributory factors are negative, including a CT scan of the brain. Mr. Franklin's daughter, aware of her mother's concerns about her stepfather's drinking, driving, and sexuality, calls to say she is appalled that the possibility of AD is being considered. She had thought he was suffering from male menopause.

STUDY QUESTIONS

1. What are the other diagnostic possibilities?
2. Can anything further be done to confirm the diagnosis at this stage?
3. If this is AD, how would you explain the implications of the diagnosis to the family members?
4. How should you address the daughter's doubts?

DIFFERENTIAL DIAGNOSIS

The differential diagnosis of cognitive impairment is fairly extensive and needs to be approached in a systematic manner. The following sections discuss the main diagnostic considerations.

Mild Cognitive Impairment

Over the past 4 decades a variety of terms have been used to describe heterogeneous conditions of cognitive deficits that reflect intermediate and possibly transit states between normal aging and dementia. Previously used terms included malignant senescent forgetfulness, age-associated memory impairment, aging-associated cognitive decline, and questionable dementia. Over the past decade, however, clinicians and researchers have been widely using the term mild

| Box 16-1 | Diagnostic Criteria for Mild Cognitive Impairment |

- Presence of one or more subjective cognitive complaints such as memory or executive problems
- Presence of objective deficit in one or more cognitive domains
- Absence of impairment in activities of daily living
- Absence of dementia
- Absence of delirium

cognitive impairment (MCI). The interest of the research community in this concept reflects their efforts to identify a group of patients with a high probability for the future development of AD that could be the target for secondary prevention.

Box 16–1 describes features commonly seen in MCI. They include memory complaints, normal activities of daily living, normal general cognitive functioning, abnormal memory function on objective testing, and absence of dementia.[19] In 1999, a consensus conference on MCI expanded the definition to include three subtypes: amnestic MCI (memory impairment only); nonmemory, single-domain MCI; and multiple domain MCI.[20] In primary care, 33% of older patients with positive cognitive screening had MCI on a subsequent diagnostic workup.[3] Conversion rates from MCI to dementia range from 3% to 30% annually, 20% to 66% over 3 to 4 years, and 51% to 100% in 5 to 10 years, with the amnestic type having the highest rates of conversion to AD.[19-21]

> ● 33% of older patients with positive cognitive screening in primary care have mild cognitive impairment, and between 20% and 66% of these will have dementia in 3-4 years.

Delirium and "Reversible Dementia"

Early in 1980s, clinicians and researchers estimated that up to 25% of dementia cases could be reversible. Their optimistic estimates were not based on adequate prospective trials and did not tease out the interaction between delirium and dementia. Although dementia could be considered a chronic brain failure and delirium as an acute brain failure, the two syndromes occur together in approximately 20% to 60% of hospitalized older patients with cognitive deficits.[23,24] Demented patients have five times the odds of developing delirium compared to those with no dementia.[25] In comparison to those with no delirium, delirious hospitalized older adults have three to six times the odds of developing dementia in subsequent years.[26,27]

Beside the interaction between delirium and dementia, the issue of dementia reversibility is based on the clinical observation that hypothyroidism, vitamin B_{12} deficiency, neurosyphilis, and subdural hematoma have cognitive symptoms, and that treating these conditions might lead to reversing the dementia process. However, a systematic review of the literature showed that, in specialty clinical settings such as memory clinics, the probability of discovering a truly reversible cause is less than 1.5%, and that this rate is most likely even lower in primary care settings.[4] Therefore, the typical workup of a patient with a cognitive deficit might include investigating for the presence of delirium and the above comorbid conditions, but the expectation of finding a fully reversible condition should be very low. Such low expectations might need to be communicated clearly with the patients and their family.

Dementia

Dementia is an acquired syndrome of decline in memory and at least one other cognitive domain (for example, language, visuospatial, or executive function), leading to impairment sufficient enough to interfere with social or occupational functioning in an alert person (see Box 16–2).[22] The majority of patients with dementia have Alzheimer's disease or vascular disease as the underlying cause.

ALZHEIMER'S DISEASE

AD is the most common etiology of dementia, with estimated rates approaching 75% to 80%.[3,4] The diagnosis of AD can be categorized based on its certainty

| Box 16-2 | DSM-IV Diagnostic Criteria for Dementia |

- Multiple cognitive deficits, including memory impairment and at least one of the following: aphasia, apraxia,[a] agnosia,[b] or disturbed executive functioning (planning, organizing, sequencing, abstracting)
- Cognitive deficits severe enough to impair occupational or social functioning
- Cognitive deficits representing a decline from previously higher function
- These deficits not occurring exclusively during the course of delirium

Modified from American Psychiatric Association. *Diagnostic and Statistical Manual of Mental Disorders.* 4th ed. Washington, DC: The Association, 1994.

[a] *Apraxia* is the inability to carry out purposeful movements even though there is no motor or sensory impairment, including the inability to use objects, such as constructional apraxia (cannot copy simple drawings), motor apraxia (cannot use an object even though its nature is recognized), sensory apraxia (cannot use an object because its nature and purpose are not recognized).

[b] *Agnosia* is a failure to recognize sensory stimuli: for example, visual agnosia (cannot recognize objects by sight), tactile agnosia (cannot recognize objects by feel), ideational agnosia (cannot make up the idea of an object from its components).

into definite AD (requires tissue sampling such as a brain biopsy), probable AD, or possible AD. In general, a probable AD diagnosis requires the presence of dementia for more than 6 months with a slow and gradual onset, predominant deficits in memory, and absence of other comorbid conditions contributing to the cognitive impairment.[22]

VASCULAR DEMENTIA

In the primary care setting, pure VaD or mixed with AD is considered the second most common cause of dementia, with a prevalence rate reaching 30%.[3,4] Four subtypes of VaD have been described:

Cortical or multi-infarct VaD, characterized by stepwise deterioration

Subcortical VaD, characterized by progressive cognitive decline and prominent executive dysfunction

VaD due to single strategic vascular insults (such as one involving the thalamic or parietal areas), which tend to have a sudden onset and then a plateau of stability

VaD due to generalized severe cerebral hypoperfusion (for example, from anoxic encephalopathy due to a cardiac arrest and resuscitation)[28]

> ● In practice, *recognizing* dementia, especially when social skills are preserved, is challenging; ask direct questions—believe the family!

Vascular risk factors or insults, such as cerebrovascular events, diabetes, hypertension, atrial fibrillation, and hyperlipidemia, are common in both AD and VaD. Nevertheless, in comparison to patients with AD, those with VaD have better performance in verbal memory and worse performance in executive function.[29] The presence of vascular insults on brain imaging is consistent with the diagnosis of VaD. Such insults might include cortical or subcortical infarcts, abnormalities in white matter lucency, ventricular enlargement, and cortical atrophy.[28]

DEMENTIA OF LEWY BODY TYPE

Dementia of Lewy body type (DLB) may be a common type of dementia in some memory clinics, but it is considered a rare syndrome in community and primary care settings. This discrepancy could be due to lack of recognition in community settings or higher rates of referral to subspecialty settings. DLB is characterized by the presence of fluctuating cognitive deficits, Parkinsonian signs, oversensitivity to adverse effects of antipsychotic therapy, delirium-like attention deficits, and predominant visual hallucinations.

PARKINSON'S DISEASE DEMENTIA

Dementia occurs in 25% to 30% of patients with Parkinson's disease, but it usually occurs late in the disease course.[30,31] Separating Parkinson's disease dementia (PDD) from DLB is challenging. The pathology and symptomatology of the two diagnoses are similar, making the differential diagnosis particularly difficult. For a diagnosis of DLB to be appropriate, Parkinsonian symptoms must not pre-date the symptoms of dementia by more than 12 months.[32]

Treatment options in PDD are limited. Dopaminergic agents have been shown to produce only limited improvements in cognitive function. Antipsychotics can aggravate any movement disorder. The observation that cholinergic functioning decreases in PDD has led to suggestions that cholinesterase inhibitors may have utility in PDD. However, cholinergic enhancers may, theoretically, worsen Parkinsonian symptoms. A systematic evidence review found that such agents might have clinically relevant benefit in treating patients with PDD with somewhat tolerable adverse events.[31]

Rare diagnoses that should be kept in the differential include:

Frontotemporal dementia: Very rare neurodegenerative dementia disorders with a predominant frontal lobe involvement. Consequently, personality changes, disinhibition, apathy, and executive dysfunction are prominent presenting symptoms and signs. These "frontal" signs and symptoms may be benign and eccentric, but often they are unpleasant, resulting in an unattractive or belligerent personality and often leading to assumptions that the patient has a psychiatric illness.

Primary progressive aphasia: Dementing disorders characterized by a progressive expressive aphasia and hand/motor abnormalities that mimic a cerebrovascular event located in the frontal or prefrontal area.

Normal-pressure hydrocephalus (NPH): A rare but well-recognized syndrome, with a triad of concurrently developing progressive dementia, urinary incontinence, and apraxic gait. The significance of recognizing NPH is due to its possible response to surgical interventions. The excess fluid is drained through an internally placed shunt and, if caught early, the brain changes might be reversible. Assessment would generally involve a neurologist and neurosurgeon assessing the patient, often including a videotape of the gait, and demonstrating that reduction of the spinal fluid pressure by spinal tap leads to improvement in the gait.

Huntington's disease (HD): HD is a rare primary neurodegenerative dementing disorder with an autosomal dominant inheritance. It is characterized by chorea, a jerking uncontrollable movement of the limbs, trunk, and face; progressive cognitive decline; and a cluster of behavioral and psychological symptoms. Genetic counseling would certainly be indicated if the patient had a positive family history.

Creutzfeldt-Jakob disease (CJD): CJD is a rapidly progressive fatal dementia disorder. It is caused by an infectious condition that is transmitted by a prion, and therefore is transmitted at autopsy and surgery from infected patients. Tending to be seen in younger patients, the disease generally develops with a more erratic and progressive course. Neurological, EKG, and EEG findings may confirm the diagnosis. Mad cow disease (a variant of CJD) is also very rare, although it caused a large number of deaths in the United Kingdom. Such infection causes a progressive dementia associated with depression that starts at an early age and inevitably and uniformly leads to death.

Acquired Immunodeficiency Syndrome (AIDS): This disease is an important cause of progressive dementia among patients who are generally younger than most dementia patients seen in primary care practice. It is not clear whether the natural history of this syndrome is changing with current antiviral therapy for HIV.

In summary, an elderly patient who presents to a primary care clinician with cognitive problems that affect his or her functional performance, in the absence of delirium, is usually suffering from dementia. Diagnosis of the specific type of dementia relies on the overall dominant pattern of cognitive deficit. The predominant symptom early on (see Table 16–2) offers important clues: AD first affects memory, VaD executive function, LBD attention and mood, and FTD language, personality, and social function. However, all severe and late-stage cases of dementia are similar.

Harold Franklin (Part 3)

You see Harold and Thelma together to review the results of your tests. Harold is able to be frank with his wife about the progressive memory problems, his anxiety concerning them, and his difficulty coping at work. She tells you that she has noted a change in him, with loss of appetite, diminished sexual interest, sad feelings, and disturbed sleep since about 2 months ago. You point out that the symptoms suggest an existing memory problem that is getting worse plus an illness you would describe as depression, with symptoms that might response to antidepressant medication. You tell them frankly that Harold's continued drinking is making the memory loss, the emotional disturbance, and the sexual performance worse. Harold declines sexual or marriage counseling and says he will try to reduce his alcohol consumption, but he does not wish to go to a support group. Ms. Franklin is interested in the latter, and you give her the contact numbers for Al-Anon. You tell them that you want to prescribe an antidepressant and that you may later prescribe other medication specifically for the memory. In the few minutes that you are alone with Thelma, she says that although challenged by the news and fearful of the future, she is at least relieved to know that there is an explanation for Harold's behavior. She had been blaming herself and felt that their marriage was at an end.

You tell the Franklins that their daughter is concerned about Harold, and ask if you may see her to talk about the diagnosis. They agree. You subsequently discuss the situation with her, clarify the likelihood of the diagnosis, and have her contact the Alzheimer's Association for literature about the illness and about depression so that she can better understand what's going on.

Two months after starting a selective seratonin reuptake inhibitor (SSRI) (sertraline), and with his drinking moderated, Harold feels somewhat better, especially in the morning. His sleeping is better, and he is not so sad. However, he still lacks energy and drive. Your nurse repeats his cognitive testing, with results virtually identical to those at presentation. You explain to him and Thelma that you believe he is in the mildest stages of AD and that medication to slow down worsening of his memory function should be started and can be given concurrently with the

---

Table 16–2	Characteristic Patterns for Dementia Subtypes						
Dementia Type	Memory Deficit	Visuospatial Deficit	Executive Deficit	Attention Deficit	Frontal Lobe Deficit	Parkinsonian Signs	Asymmetrical Neurological Findings per Exam or Brain Imaging
Alzheimer's disease	+++	++	+	–	–	–	–
Vascular dementia	+	–/+	+++	–	–	+	+++
Lewy body dementia	+	+++	+	+++	–	+++	–
Parkinson's disease–associated dementia	+	+	+	–	–	+++	–
Frontotemporal dementia	++	–	++	–	+++	–	–

+++, significant positive effect; +/–, possible positive effect; –, negative effect.

antidepressant. You encourage Thelma, like her daughter, to contact the Alzheimer's Association and join a support group.

Treatment with a cholinergic agent is initiated, and by 4 weeks Harold is taking 10 mg of donepezil daily. Despite some transient nausea both at the 5-mg dose and when the dose is increased to 10 mg, the effect wears off in a few days and there are no other problems. Two months later, at a scheduled follow-up visit, Harold says he feels about the same and is taking his medications regularly. The family has been advised by the Alzheimer's Association to address the issues of advance directives, name a health care proxy, and to be sure that he has a will.

STUDY QUESTIONS

1. What problems can be anticipated in the short and long term, and how will you help the family to be prepared for them?
2. What else could be done at this stage to ease the situation and reduce Mr. Franklin's impairment?

ASSESSMENT OF SUSPECTED DEMENTIA

Patients with dementia can be divided into two major groups in primary care: those with unrecognized dementia (approximately 66% to 80% of all dementia cases) and those with documented dementia.[3,4] Nevertheless, both groups present to their physicians with various cognitive, functional, and behavioral complaints.

In order to diagnose dementia (see Box 16–2), a clinician needs to establish the presence of two deficits. First, an impairment in the patient's memory and at least one other cognitive domain, such as visuospatial or executive function; and second, functional disability that is caused by the cognitive impairment and has affected the patient's occupational and social performance in comparison to patient baseline.[22] Determining the presence of cognitive impairment requires the use of various neuropsychological tests; and evaluating the patient's functional status requires obtaining information from a valid informant such as the patient's spouse.

● See family members separately, so they can be frank about their concerns.

Assessing Cognitive Status

As a first step in assessing cognitive status, the clinician must review the patient's attention and alertness. The presence of any deficit in attention suggests the need to evaluate for delirium (acute brain failure). In the primary care setting, cognitive status can be assessed using a combination of short neuropsychological tests that accommodate the time constraints faced by primary care providers. The most feasible combined tests are the MMSE combined with the CDT and the Animal Fluency Test (AFT). However, these tests have significant limitations, such as low specificity, and need to be interpreted with caution. The companion CD-ROM contains files explaining the process of conducting the MMSE, the CDT, and the AFT. Following the implementation of the MMSE and CDT, the clinician needs to interpret their results. The MMSE requires 5 to 10 minutes to complete and consists of five subtests in the domains of orientation, memory, attention, language, and praxis; total scores range from 0 to 30 correct, with 30 the optimal score. The CDT can evaluate executive function and has various scoring methods; the most feasible one is to simply evaluate the CDT performance on a scale from 1 to 5 with 5 indicating a normal score. A patient aged 65 and older with 12 years of education can generate 12 to 16 animals within 1 minute on the AFT (see Fig. 16–3).

Assessing Functional Status

In addition to cognitive decline, a dementia diagnosis requires the presence of functional disability caused by the cognitive impairment. This assessment is difficult in primary care because it requires access to an informant who can provide information on the patient's baseline and current functional performance. Figure 4-5 (see chapter 4) provides an example of a scale that can help in assessing the patient's functional status.

Neurological Physical Examination

The goal of the physical examination in a patient with suspected dementia is to look for the presence of localized neurological signs that might indicate VaD; gait abnormality that might suggest LBD, PDD, or NPH; and Parkinsonian signs such as rigidity, which triggers the possibility of LBD or PDD diagnosis. Table 16–2 provides a summary of some of the relevant neurological examination findings in patients with a suspected dementia diagnosis.

Medication History

Obtaining a list of medications that are taken by the patient with a suspected dementia diagnosis is very important for two reasons: (1) medications with sedative or other CNS effects can contribute to or cause a superimposed delirium, and (2) medications with anticholinergic side effects can accumulate, impairing cognitive function and interfering with treatments for AD.

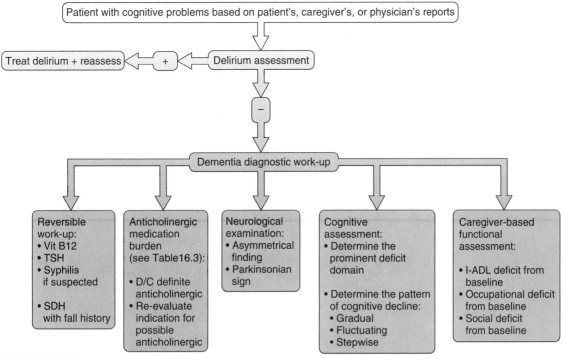

FIGURE 16-3

Overview of evaluation of patient with cognitive impairment.

The concept of cholinergic burden has gained considerable attention. The idea is that, although often the effect of a single medication is low, the combination of half a dozen or more medications with mild anticholinergic side effects can equal a strong overall effect. In a primary care setting, it is estimated that approximately 50% of patients with dementia receive at least one medication with anticholinergic effects.[33] Table 16–3 provides a list of such medications that should be at least considered for possible discontinuation in patients with a dementia diagnosis.

Laboratory Testing and Brain Imaging

The American Academy of Neurology recommends the following laboratory tests for reversible or comorbid conditions in patients with a suspected dementia diagnosis: screening for hypothyroidism, and vitamin B_{12} deficiency, and for syphilis when clinical suspicion is high.

The current guidelines for the diagnosis of VaD recommend brain imaging to determine the presence of a cortical or subcortical cerebrovascular event. In addition, brain imaging might be necessary to determine the presence of subdural hematoma or NPH. However, in the absence of symptoms during history taking or of physical signs suggesting VaD, NPH, or subdural hematoma, brain imaging is not required. Selecting the type of brain imaging for a patient with a suspected

dementia diagnosis depends on the rationale for such imaging. Computerized tomography is appropriate to detect a subdural hematoma (i.e., if this is suspected due to a history of falls); brain MRI might be more sensitive to detect cortical or subcortical vascular lesions; and positron emission tomography (PET) scans may have a place in differentiating between AD and FTD.

Staging the Patient with Dementia

It is valuable and fits current Food and Drug Administration (FDA) terminology for approved medications to divide dementia into three simple stages: mild, moderate, and severe. The MMSE can be used to define such a categorization. Patients with mild dementia have an MMSE score above 17 points; those with moderate dementia have an MMSE score between 11 and 17 points, and finally patients with severe dementia have a MMSE score below 10 points. In primary care settings, the mean MMSE score in patients with dementia is approximately 18 points.

Harold Franklin, *Part 4*

Six months after starting the donepezil, Harold and his wife and daughter return for a follow-up visit. Soon after the last visit, the decision had been made to sell the business. Harold describes himself as relieved, and selling the business to his partner has

Table 16–3 Anticholinergic Burden Scale

Definite Central Anticholinergics	Score	Possible Central Anticholinergics	Score
Amitriptyline	3	Alprazolam	1
Amoxapine	3	Brompheniramine maleate	1
Benztropine	3	Bupropion hydrochloride	1
Chlorpromazine	3	Captopril	1
Chlorpheniramine	3	Chlorthalidone	1
Clozapine	3	Cimetidine	1
Desmethylimipramine	3	Clorazepate	1
Diphenhydramine	3	Codeine	1
Doxepin	3	Colchicine	1
Hydroxyzine	3	Coumadin	1
Hyoscyamine	3	Diazepam	1
Imipramine	2	Digoxin	1
Ipratropium bromide inhaler	2	Dipyridamole	1
Loxapine	2	Disopyramide phosphate	1
Meclizine	3	Furosemide	1
Meperidine	3	Haloperidol	1
Nortiptyline	2	Hydralazine	1
Oxybutinin	3	Hydrocortisone	1
Paroxetine	3	Isosorbide	1
Perphenazine	3	Nifedipine	1
Promazine	3	Olanzepine	1
Promethazine	3	Prednisone	1
Quetiapine	2	Quinidine	1
Thioridazine	3	Ranitidine	1
Trifluoperazine	3	Theophylline	1
Tolterodine	3	Triamterene	1
Total score (range from 0 to 96)			

From Schubert CC, Boustani M, Callahan CM, Perkins AJ, Carney CP, Fox C, et al. Comorbidity profile of dementia patients in primary care: are they sicker? J Am Geriatr Soc 54(1):104–9, 2006, with permission.

been financially quite successful. He is still frustrated on a daily basis by his memory loss, and you urge his wife to remind him to carry a notepad and write down things he has forgotten and things he must remember to do. Harold has been enjoying his grandchildren and, with continual encouragement from his family, has done a little painting, a passion of his that he had long ago given up. Your nurse administers the MMSE, and his score and performance remain approximately the same as before, at 22/30, with the same calculation and short-term memory difficulties.

Then, 3-1/2 years after his initial presentation, despite some backsliding, when he has finally given

up alcohol altogether, completion of an MMSE at the office by the nurse produces a score of just 16/30. His cognitive clock is also quite a bit more disorganized than the relatively good clock he drew in the early days. He does not appear overtly depressed, and in fact his social skills seem well preserved during the interview. He is still living at home and is on his own for much of the day, since Mrs. Franklin has taken a full-time job to maintain the family's finances.

A few weeks later, she calls you because, although Harold has seemed to do all right in the day, in the evening he has been increasingly agitated. By around 11 pm he becomes unreasonable, will not *get ready for bed, and rambles on loudly about many topics. Mrs. Franklin believes he spends most of his afternoon asleep in the chair. The interrupted nights are exhausting her.*

STUDY QUESTIONS

1. How do you evaluate this situation?
2. What do you tell Mrs. Franklin over the phone?

MANAGEMENT

Dementia is characterized by complex interacting clusters of cognitive, functional, behavioral, and psychological symptoms that decrease the quality of life for both the patient and the caregiver (see Box 16–3). Thus, successful management needs to be composed of interventions for both the patient and the caregiver. The scope of such integrated management includes medications and psychosocial interventions that target the entire spectrum of dementia syndrome symptomatology. An efficacious management would most likely stabilize or slow the cognitive decline, stabilize or prevent additional functional disability and decrease the frequency or the severity of behavioral and psychological symptoms of dementia (BPSD) or delay their emergence. Current FDA standards for testing drugs in AD and other dementing illness trials require demonstration of "dual efficacy"; that is, trials must show improvement on a performance-based neuropsychological measure and demonstrate clinically meaningful change.[4] Table 16–4 provides an overview of current data on drug effectiveness; specific management recommendations are included in the following sections.

Managing Cognitive Symptoms

Currently the FDA has approved two classes of medications for the treatment of AD: cholinesterase inhibitors (ChEIs) for patients with mild to moderate AD, and memantine, an NMDA (N-methyl-D-aspartic acid) receptor antagonist, for patients with moderate to severe AD. Recently, the European Union drug evaluation agency has approved the use of rivastigmine, a ChEI, in patients with PDD.

ChEIs are generally considered the first-line treatment, especially in mild dementia. In comparison to a placebo, 6-month therapy with a ChEI, such as donepezil, rivastigmine, or galantamine, has demonstrated statistically significant positive effects on cognition.[4] The level of improvement shown was approximately equivalent to a 5- to 10-month delay in the progression of the disease.

Memantine was approved recently for the treatment of patients with moderate to severe AD (MMSE <18). In comparison to a placebo, memantine produces a similar effect to ChEIs on patients' cognition with a mean difference of 4 points on the Severe Impairment Battery (SIB, with a range of 0 to 100 points).[34] Moreover, memantine has been evaluated also as an add-on (combined) therapy to ChEIs among patients with moderate to severe dementia, and has led to a significance additional cognitive difference of 3 points on the SIB.[34]

Treatment may, however, lead to adverse effects such as nausea, vomiting, and diarrhea. The number-needed-to-harm (NNH), that is, to cause one patient to stop the treatment due to an adverse effect, is in the range of 5 for rivastigmine, 7 for galantamine, and 13 for donepezil (a high NNH means better tolerability).[4] Memantine, however, has a better tolerability profile, with NNH of 50 with headache, confusion, and constipation as the main side effects.[34]

In addition to pharmacologic interventions to manage the cognitive deficits of patients with dementia, investigators have been evaluating the efficacy of using cognitive training. Such training might involve a "guided practice on a set of standard tasks designed to reflect particular cognitive functions, such as memory, attention, or problem-solving."[35] However, cognitive training has not been adequately studied, and a recent Cochrane review failed to demonstrate its efficacy.[35]

Managing Functional Disability

There is a lack of universally accepted measures to evaluate the impact of ChEIs and memantine on the functional performance of patients with AD and other

---

Box 16–3   Domains of Dementia Symptomatology

Cognitive Impairment
Memory deficit
Language deficit
Executive deficit
Visuospatial deficit
Stimulation recognition
   deficit (agnosia)

Behavioral and Psychological Symptoms
Apathy
Depression/dysphoria/irritability
Anxiety
Agitation/aggression
Delusions/hallucinations
Elation/euphoria
Disinhibition
Aberrant motor behavior
Sleep
Appetite/eating disorders

Functional disability
Basic activities of daily living
   disability
Instrumental activities of
   daily living disability

Caregiver Burden
Sleep problem
Mood problem
Coping problem

Table 16–4	Effects of Various Pharmacological Treatments on Alzheimer's Disease				
	Target Symptoms				
Drug or Drug Class	**Cognition**	**ADL Decline**	**Aggression/Agitation**	**Depression/Apathy**	**Psychosis**
Cholinesterase inhibitors	+++	+	+/–	+	NE
Memantine	+++	+	+	+/–	NE
Neuroleptics	–	–	++	NE	+
Antidepressants	NE	NE	+	+++	NE
Anticonvulsants	–	–	+/–	NE	NE

Note: None of the neuroleptics have been evaluated by the Food and Drug Administration for use in Alzheimer's disease.

+++, significant positive effect; +/–, possible positive effect; –, negative effect; ADL, activities of daily life; NE, no effect.

dementias. Thus, it is hard to appreciate the clinical relevance of these medications' efficacy in functional disability. In general, the effect of ChEI and memantine on daily function appears minimal.[4] However, using time to functional decline as an outcome measure and in comparison to placebo, donepezil demonstrated a 5-month delay in reaching such a decline.[4] Furthermore, 34% of patients with moderate to severe AD were at least functionally stable after 6 months of treatment with memantine versus 20% of those receiving a placebo, with an NNT of 7.[36]

Managing Behavioral and Psychological Symptoms of Dementia

The noncognitive BPSD can be defined as verbal, vocal, or motor behavior that is inappropriate for the setting or the incident, and that reflects inadequate ability to cope with internal and/or environmental stressors. BPSD includes a heterogeneous range of psychological reactions, psychiatric symptoms, and behaviors. A variety of both external and internal stressors can be involved (Box 16–4). More than 90% of patients with dementia will experience BPSD at some point during the course of their illness.[37] Among BPSD, aggression is the most

serious symptom; it is seen in 30% of patients with dementia attending primary care clinics.[38]

The current management of aggression is, at best, moderately successful, even in controlled trials. One reason for the limited effectiveness of aggression management is the current focus on pharmacologic interventions used in the setting of an acute crisis. This approach fails to incorporate primary prevention strategies that would target modifiable vulnerability factors. It also fails to recognize the potential benefit of an individualized care plan built on the interaction among the patient, caregiver, and environment (Fig.16–4). The traditional pharmacologic management of BPSD in general and aggression in particular includes the use of typical and atypical neuroleptics, antidepressants, anticonvulsants, hypnotics, and ChEIs. However, these pharmacologic interventions have not been approved by the FDA for such therapy, their efficacy is limited, and they produce numerous side effects. Neuroleptics in particular lead to the development of extrapyramidal signs, gait abnormalities and potential fractures, sedation, increased incidence of cerebrovascular events, and higher mortality rates.[39] The NNT to relieve agitation

Box 16–4 Triggers of Agitation in Dementia

Internal Stressors	External Stressors
Delirium	Unaccommodating physical environment
Depression	Unaccommodating social environment
Mania	Caregiver burden
Anxiety	Unskilled caregiver
Psychosis	
Activities of daily living difficulties	
Pain	

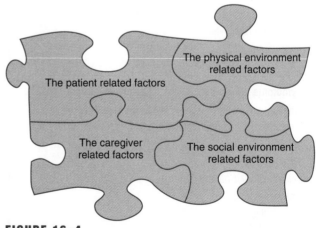

FIGURE 16–4

Theoretical framework for the assessment and management of agitation in dementia.

in a patient is between 4 to 8; in contrast, the NNH in terms of a patient needing to stop the medication due to an adverse event ranges from 8 to 13.[40] Moreover, the NNH for the development of stroke ranges from 45 to 111.[39] Thus, the therapeutic margin for the use of neuroleptics is narrow.

Over the past three decades, various nonpharmacologic interventions have been suggested to manage agitation and aggression related to dementia. Overall, the most effective approach is a multicomponent program that targets both the patient and the caregiver. Such a program has been able to delay the need to institutionalize dementia patients by 11 to 19 months without increasing the burden on their caregivers.[42] Such a program includes:

- Enhancing the caregiver's skills in problem solving
- Providing the caregiver with counseling, emphasizing the need for the caregiver to use respite care for their loved one (e.g., enrolling them in a day care setting or collaborating with other family members in providing care)
- Encouraging the caregiver to belong to a local support group
- Using environmental and nonpharmacologic interventions to compensate for the patient's disability
- Collaborating with the primary care physician to enhance the cholinergic system of patients with dementia by using ChEIs and discontinue the use of anticholinergic medications
- Screening and treating depression superimposed on dementia

- Detecting and treating delirium superimposed on dementia
- Facilitating medication adherence

Overall, the management of BPSD in dementia should be systematic, beginning with assessment, and aimed at a comprehensive approach to prevention and management (Box 16–5). One such program, the PREVENT program, has been tested in primary care clinics and demonstrated good efficacy, with an NNT for reaching a clinical improvement in BPSD of 4.[38,41] For this program to be delivered, it requires the enhancement of the current primary care system by integrating a nurse practitioner trained in dementia management and support for such a clinician, with access to a geriatrician, geriatric psychiatrist, and geriatric psychologist. Figure 16–5 provides a graphic representation of the PREVENT program.

Box 16–5   Overview of Management of Agitation in Dementia

Define target agitated behavior
Assess impact of agitation on patient's and others' safety
Identify triggers
- Caregiver related
- Environment related
- Patient related
Institute nonpharmacologic interventions
Institute pharmacologic interventions
Provide intermittent follow-up

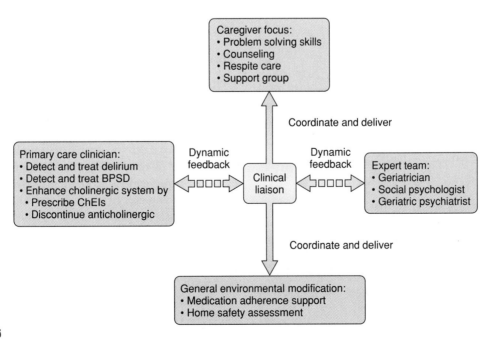

FIGURE 16–5

Outline for PREVENT program in primary care.

Harold Franklin, *Part 5*

Management of insomnia includes an increase in companionship and activity in the day and environmental changes (night light, radio), but it also requires risperidone (Risperdal) in low doses. After 2 months of taking the medication, Mr. Franklin lets himself out of the house one day. The police bring him home after a supermarket manager has intercepted him attempting to walk out with bread and eggs for which he has not paid. On being challenged, he had become hostile and agitated. According to his wife, Harold has been going out for walks during the daytime and has so far not become lost. Reassessing him, you find that his mental status remains at 15/30 on the MMSE. The Franklins' daughter calls, saying that this is an unsafe situation and her father must be institutionalized soon in view of the danger he is in.

STUDY QUESTIONS

1. Does this incident mean that Mr. Franklin should be in a nursing home?
2. Can anything be done to control wandering behaviors?

Additional Care Issues

As dementia progresses and the person needs regular supervision and monitoring, a number of issues become prominent. These include maintenance of safety, concerns about driving, relocation, managing the caregiver's burden, and preparing for the future.

Safety

Where the person lives and who they live with becomes of great importance when dementia is suspected and confirmed. The familiarity and security of home may be important; home can also be dangerous, with dark corners, bad lighting, and complicated arrangements for safety and bathing. A home visit can be very revealing, especially about fire hazards, fall risk, alcohol use, and medication adherence. In addition to assessing home safety, patients with mild to moderate dementia might have significant disorientation and thus are at high risk of getting lost. Enrolling them in the Alzheimer's Association's Safe Return program, which provides a bracelet or necklace with a toll-free number and PIN, can reduce risk.

Driving

As dementia progresses, the risk of driving accidents increases; so when to advise about driving is impor-

tant. In mild dementia, driving may be fairly safe, provided that visuospatial skills are good (e.g., the patient can copy intersecting pentagons and a formal driving assessment reveals adequate function). In addition, restrictions may allow the patient to continue longer; these can include driving during daylight only, on familiar routes, at quiet traffic times, off freeways, and avoiding inclement weather and days when the patient feels physically unwell.

It is advisable to recommend that a family member drive with the person from time to time (even if there is a spouse who usually accompanies) and make judgments as to the person's ability to handle such emergencies as a child running out into the street or some other sudden occurrence. Driving is more fully handled in Chapter 25.

Relocation

Relocating a patient with dementia can be very disruptive. There are some basic rules:

- Transfer from one place to another, even if it is short term, should be done in the day time. Even acute hospitalization should occur early in the day if possible.
- In any transfer, it is important that familiar people accompany the patient and that familiar objects from home go with them.
- It often takes weeks for a person with dementia to "settle down" in a new location (6 to 8 weeks of relatively disruptive behavior is quite common).
- The clinician must be prepared to counsel staff and family that the person may be frightened and may develop transient depressive symptoms.

Managing the Caregiver's Burden

Dementia is a chronic, debilitating disease, which is not only devastating to the patients but tremendously burdensome to those who care for them. Besides the significant amount of time spent on caregiving, there are monetary costs in terms of time lost from work, remodeling of the home, payment for respite or day care, and other expenses. Dementia caregivers are usually elderly spouses or their adult children, who may also be physically limited due to disease or age, and who may have difficulty meeting the financial, medical, and emotional needs of the demented patient. The detrimental health consequences for these caregivers are significant and sobering. Caregiving spouses have a 63% increased mortality within 4 years as compared to non-caregiving controls.[4] Negative psychological effects of caregiving are demonstrated by an increase in clinical depression, anxiety, and use of psychotropic medications.[4] The consequences of caregiver burden are not limited to the caregivers but also are an important factor in early institutionalization of dementia patients.[4]

In an attempt to lessen the burden of caregiving and/or improve or stabilize the condition of the demented patient, many different services and interventions targeting the caregiver have been developed. A sympathetic, informed, available primary care provider can be very helpful. Simple advice, such as that provided in Box 16–6, can often go a long way in aiding family caregivers. However, as has been shown by a systematic review of the literature, the best results are obtained by comprehensive, multicomponent caregiver interventions, including a support group, skills training, counseling, and education.[4]

Preparing for the Future

Most families now realize that a living will, or some other form of advance directive, should ideally be worked out while the patient can still provide meaningful input. At the very least, there should be a discussion and a written statement of the patient's desires about intensity of any future medical treatment, specifically institutionalization, tube feeding, surgical interventions, and resuscitation. This has some legal binding, but of course, naming of a health care proxy, or the formal implementation of a "durable power of attorney for health care" is also important.

Box 16–6	**Advice to Family Caregivers of Persons with Dementia**

1. Be realistic about the nature of the illness and plan accordingly.
2. Recognize your personal need for help and respite. Seek respite, accept it, and pay for it if necessary.
3. Seek a support group, usually through the Alzheimer's Association, for specific advice and psychological support.
4. Encourage communication within the family so that the caregiving burden is shared among family members.
5. Ensure optimal caregiver health: enough sleep, exercise, and social contacts.
6. Remember that there will be life after the patient is gone.
7. Become informed about the illness to anticipate problems and to plan strategies.
8. Plan financial and legal aspects early, including the will, placement, and intensity of treatment issues.
9. Be aware of the most positive and important work of the caregiver: to continually look for and maintain the preserved function of the patient. This not only reduces the burden, but also increases the quality of life of the patient and the caregiver and improves the quality of their relationship with each other.

Harold Franklin, *Part 6*

A year later the family has become organized around Mr. Franklin's disabilities, and he remains at home most of the time, attending a day program three times a week. He can still be left safely alone in the house for short periods of time. His wandering phase has come to an end assisted by attention to perimeter control in the house, which was accomplished with complex locks and some disguising of the doors. The family has been careful to provide a fenced and gated place where he can walk in his own yard.

SCREENING FOR AND EARLY DETECTION OF DEMENTIA

It is estimated that 66% to 80% of patients with early dementia are not recognized by the current primary care system.[3-5] As the prevalence of dementia increases with age, the prevalence of missed dementia cases is likely to increase. A systematic evidence review by the U.S. Preventive Services Task Force (USPSTF) found that (1) pharmacologic and psychosocial interventions are available to decrease dementia burden, (2) various brief cognitive screening questionnaires are available to identify unrecognized dementia cases, and (3) screening tests have good sensitivity but only fair specificity in detecting dementia. However, the USPSTF found insufficient evidence to determine whether the benefits observed in drug trials are generalizable to patients whose disease would be detected earlier by screening in primary care settings. Furthermore, although the systematic review established the existence of potential benefit for screening, it found no consensus regarding the patient's acceptance of, perceived harms associated with, or benefits of dementia screening.

> ● Screening for dementia is controversial, in part because of potential psychological morbidity associated with a false positive screen, and in part because there is controversy about the effectiveness of treatment in early disease.

Since that review, evidence has begun to emerge suggesting that dementia screening might lead to psychological morbidity such as depressed mood, suicidal thoughts and attempts, anxiety, societal stigmatization, and possible discrimination due to adverse decisions from insurers or employers.[41,42] Moreover, a recent study conducted in primary care identified various barriers for the implementation of feasible dementia screening and diagnosis such as the necessity of confirming the results of any screening instrument, a high patient refusal rate for post-screening follow-up, and an estimated cost of $4,000 for each dementia case recognized by the screening and diagnosis program.[3]

Despite the lack of support for dementia screening by the USPSTF, various organizations have advocated such screening. For example, some groups have suggested including a memory screening in the "welcome to Medicare" examination, several major pharmaceutical companies have promoted regional and national screening efforts, and the Alzheimer's Association (AA) declared November 16 the National Alzheimer's Screening Day. These groups argue that early screening and diagnosis of dementia would allow patients and families to make decisions regarding transportation, living arrangements, and other aspects of care when the patient is functioning at the highest possible level. Thus, screening for dementia needs to be individualized based on patients' risk profile and their acceptance for the screening process. Figure 16–6 provides a suggested algorithm. Other factors to consider are symptoms associated with early dementia but often not recognized as such: i.e. consider screening after delirium, during or after depression, or if a catastrophic reaction occurs in a patient not known to suffer dementia.

Harold Franklin, *Part 7 — the rest of the journey*

The family's long journey into Alzheimer's is well into its middle, "moderate" stage. With better knowledge about sleep and how to achieve it, the nocturnal symptoms become managable without medication. A year later, an episode of abrupt change in personality, with aggressive episodes and confusion leads to an ER visit, where the workup reveals bilateral pneumonia and dehydration. His hospitalization is behaviorally stormy, with restraints used in order to keep his IV in place. The option of tube feeding is discussed, as his swallowing is impaired and "the pneumonia was possibly from aspiration". His Advance Directive is however clear about not wishing to be maintained by tube feeding, and the family decide against. He survives, and returns home slightly more dependent, needing spoon feeding, and assistance for transfers, after a two-week hospitalization. He never returns to his prior baseline. Two years later, despite efforts to keep him mobile, his mobility has declined. He loses urinary continence, and is losing weight. His speech gradually declines until he speaks little – although he appears to mostly understand. The Alzheimer's Association group that has supported Mrs Franklin in her care of him suggests Hospice, which is locally available. At first she feels he is

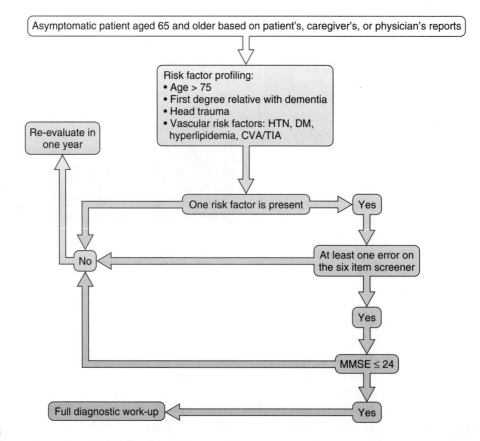

FIGURE 16–6

Recommended approach to screening for dementia.

"not ready", but remembering the trauma of the prior hospitalization and his statements earlier in the illness about dying at home, she asks for an assessment. Supported by Hospice, he declines over the next seven months and, a palliative approach having been decided upon in advance of the event, he dies quietly at home of a further episode of pneumonia, with his family present. Mrs Franklin makes a good recovery, and uses her experiences as a volunteer for both organizations, and returns to work for a further ten years before her retirement.

Case Discussion

The case of Harold Franklin illustrates how long and circuitous the primary care management of dementia can be. While the presentation and course of cognitive impairment are extremely variable, in all cases a primary care physician who knows the patient and family, and approaches the issues from a biopsychosocial perspective, providing compassionate, evidence-based care over time can be invaluable to the patient and family. Without the guidance and case management provided by his physician, Mr. Franklin would quite possibly have been institutionalized far sooner, his wife distressed to a much greater extent and his care inappropriate during his final years. Although the indication for considering tube feeding was incorrect (aspiration risk is not reduced by tube feeding!) his Advance Directive lead to a much more realistic, patient-centered approach, with his family and clinicians certain that he would have approved their approach. Further hospitalization was avoided, and the family were truly well-prepared for his death.

SUMMARY

Even though Alzheimer's disease cannot be cured, there is much that can be done to reduce disability, relieve suffering, prevent complications, and improve quality of life. When earlier recognition and diagnosis than is often achieved occurs, with prompt education of the caregiving family (if available), and using resources outside the primary care practice setting, many patients and families suffering from progressive dementia such as Alzheimer's disease can have a far less stressful, less harsh experience of this generally prolonged illness, with more appropriate treatment than our acute care oriented system often provides. There is considerable experience and advice available, especially through the Alzheimer's Association, about when and how to act to reduce the burden of care, and to manage or prevent behavioral and other disturbances. In the many situations where there is not an identifiable caregiver, or where the carer is also compromised, or in rural areas where "hands on" support and care are much less accessible, the challenge to the primary clinician is to bring as much as possible of such an ideal approach to these situations, and to be pro-active, recognizing that the most needy patients and families will not know how to seek or request the help they need.

References

1. Sloane PD, Zimmerman S, Suchindran C, Reed P, Wang L, Boustani M, Sudha S. The public health impact of Alzheimer's disease, 2000-2050: potential implication of treatment advances. Annu Rev Public Health 23:213-31, 2002.
2. Ferri CP, Prince M, Brayne C, Brodaty H, Fratiglioni L, Ganguli M, et al. Alzheimer's Disease International. Global prevalence of dementia: a Delphi consensus study. Lancet 366(9503):2112-7, 2005.
3. Boustani M, Callahan CM, Unverzagt FW, Austrom MG, Perkins AJ, Fultz BA, et al. Implementing a screening and diagnosis program for dementia in primary care. J Gen Intern Med 20(7):572-7, 2005.
4. Boustani M, Peterson B, Hanson L, Harris R, Krasnov C. Screening for Dementia. Systematic Evidence Review. Rockville, MD: Agency for Healthcare Research and Quality, 2003. Available at: www.ahrq.gov/clinic/uspstfix.htm.
5. Boustani M, Peterson B, Hanson L, Harris R, Lohr KN. U.S. Preventive Services Task Force. Screening for dementia in primary care: a summary of the evidence for the U.S. Preventive Services Task Force. Ann Intern Med 138(11):927-37, 2003.
6. Moore MJ, Zhu CW, Clipp EC. Informal costs of dementia care: estimates from the National Longitudinal Caregiver Study. J Gerontol B Psychol Sci Soc Sci 56(4):S219-28, 2001.
7. The Lewin Group. Saving Lives. Saving Money: Dividends for Americans Investing in Alzheimer Research. Report of the Lewin Group to the Alzheimer's Association, 2004 http://www.alz.org/Resources/Factsheets/Lewin_FullReport1.pdf.
8. DeKosky ST. Pathology and pathways of Alzheimer's disease with an update on new developments in treatment. J Am Geriatr Soc 51(5 Suppl):S314-20, 2003.
9. Cotman CW, Poon WW, Rissman RA, Blurton-Jones M. The role of caspase cleavage of tau in Alzheimer disease neuropathology. J Neuropathol Exp Neurol 64(2):104-12, 2005 (review).
10. Jorm A, Jolley D. The incidence of dementia: a meta-analysis. Neurology 51:728-33, 1998.
11. Lautenschlager N, Cupples L, Rao V, et al. Risk of dementia among relatives of Alzheimer's disease patients in the MIRAGE study: what is in store for the oldest old? Neurology 46:641-50, 1996.
12. Blacker D, Tanzi R. The genetics of Alzheimer disease: current status and future prospects. Arch Neurol 55:294-6, 1998.
13. Lai F, Williams R. A prospective study of Alzheimer disease in Down syndrome. Arch Neurol 46:849-53, 1989.
14. Skoog I, Nilsson L, Palmertz B, Andreasson LA, Svanborg A. A population-based study of dementia in 85-year-olds. N Engl J Med 328:153-8, 1993.
15. Hofman A, Ott A, Breteler M, et al. Atherosclerosis, apolipoprotein E, and prevalence of dementia and Alzheimer's disease in the Rotterdam Study. Lancet 349:151-4, 1997.
16. Shumaker SA, Legault C, Rapp SR, Thal L, Wallace RB, Ockene JK, et al. Estrogen plus progestin and the incidence of dementia and mild cognitive impairment in postmenopausal women. The Women's Health Initiative Memory Study: a randomized controlled trial. JAMA 289(20):2651-62, 2003.
17. Hendrie HC, Albert MS, Butters MA, Gao S, Knopman DS, Launer LJ, et al. The NIH Cognitive and Emotional Health Project Report of the Critical Evaluation Study Committee. Alzheimer Dementia 2:12-32, 2006.
18. Jedrziewski MK, Lee VM-Y, Trojanowski JQ. Lowering the risk of Alzheimer's disease: Evidence-based practices emerge from new research. Alzheimer Dementia 1(2):152-60, 2005.
19. Petersen RC. Mild cognitive impairment as a diagnostic entity. J Intern Med 256(3):183-94, 2004.

20. Petersen RC, Doody R, Kurz A, Mohs RC, Morris JC, Rabins PV, et al. Current concepts in mild cognitive impairment. Arch Neurol 58(12): 1985-92, 2001.
21. Unverzagt FW, Gao S, Baiyewu O, Ogunniyi AO, Gureje O, Perkins A, et al. Prevalence of cognitive impairment: data from the Indianapolis Study of Health and Aging. Neurology 57(9):1655-62, 2001.
22. American Psychiatric Association. Diagnostic and Statistical Manual of Mental Disorders. 4th ed. Washington, DC: American Psychiatric Association, 1994.
23. Schor JD, Levkoff SE, Lipsitz LA, et al. Risk factors for delirium in hospitalized elderly. JAMA 267:827-31, 1992.
24. Webster R, Holroyd S. Prevalence of psychotic symptoms in delirium. Psychosomatics 41:519-22, 2000.
25. Elie M, Cole MG, Primeau FJ, Bellavance F. Delirium risk factors in elderly hospitalized patients. J Gen Intern Med 13:204-12, 1998.
26. Rockwood K, Cosway S, Carver D, Jarrett P, Stadnyk K, Fisk J. The risk of dementia and death after delirium. Age Ageing 28:551-6, 1999.
27. Lundstrom M, Edlund A, Bucht G, Karlsson S, Gustafson Y. Dementia after delirium in patients with femoral neck fractures. J Am Geriatr Soc 51:1002-6, 2003.
28. Garrett KD, Paul RH, Libon DJ, Cohen RA. Defining the diagnosis of vascular dementia. Appl Neuropsychol 11(4):204-9, 2004.
29. Misciagna S, Masullo C, Giordano A, Silveri MC. Vascular dementia and Alzheimer's disease: the unsolved problem of clinical and neuropsychological differential diagnosis. Int J Neurosci 115(12):1657-67, 2005.
30. Maidment ID, Fox C, Boustani M. A review of studies describing the use of acetyl cholinesterase inhibitors in Parkinson's disease dementia. Acta Psychiatr Scand 111(6):403-9, 2005.
31. Maidment I, Fox C, Boustani M. Cholinesterase inhibitors for Parkinson's disease dementia. Cochrane Database Syst Rev (1):CD004747, 2006.
32. Samuel M, Maidment I, Boustani M, Fox C. Clinical management of Parkinson's disease dementia: pitfalls and progress. Adv Psychiatr Treatment. 2006; 12:121–129.
33. Schubert CC, Boustani M, Callahan CM, Perkins AJ, Carney CP, Fox C, et al. Comorbidity profile of dementia patients in primary care: are they sicker? J Am Geriatr Soc 54(1):104-9, 2006.
34. Areosa Sastre A, Sherriff F, McShane R. Memantine for dementia. Cochrane Dementia and Cognitive Improvement Group. Cochrane Database Syst Rev (1), 2006.
35. Clare L, Woods RT, Moniz Cook ED, Orrell M, Spector A. Cognitive rehabilitation and cognitive training for early-stage Alzheimer's disease and vascular dementia. Cochrane Database Syst Rev (4):CD003260, 2003.
36. Livingston G, Katona C. The place of memantine in the treatment of Alzheimer's disease: a number needed to treat analysis. Int J Geriatr Psychiatry 19(10):919-25, 2004.
37. Finkel SI, Burns A, Cohen GD. Overview. Int Psychogeriatr 12(Suppl): 13-18, 2000.
38. Callahan CM, Boustani M, Unverzagt FW, Austrom MG, Damush TM, Perkins AJ, et al. Effectiveness of guideline-level care for older adults with Alzheimer's disease in primary care: a clinical trial. JAMA 2006;295:2148–2157.
39. Schneider LS, Dagerman KS, Insel P. Risk of death with atypical antipsychotic drug treatment for dementia: meta-analysis of randomized placebo-controlled trials. JAMA 294(15):1934-43, 2005.
40. Sink KM, Holden KF, Yaffe K. Pharmacological treatment of neuropsychiatric symptoms of dementia: a review of the evidence. JAMA 293(5):596-608, 2005.
41. Austrom MG, Hartwell C, Moore PS, Boustani M, Hendrie HC, Callahan CM. A care management model for enhancing physician practice for Alzheimer disease in primary care. Clin Gerontol 29:35-43, 2005.
42. Boustani M, Watson L, Fultz B, Perkins AJ, Druckenbrod R. Acceptance of dementia screening in continuous care retirement communities: a mailed survey. Int J Geriatr Psychiatry 18(9):780-6, 2003.
43. Boustani M, Perkins A, Fox C, Unverzagt F, Hendrie H, Siu Hui, et al. Who refuses dementia assessment in primary care? Int J Geriatr Psychiatry. (In press).

POSTTEST

1. G.K. comes to your office with his wife. She takes you aside before the visit and tells you that over the past year she has had to take over the driving, the checkbook, and managing his medications. Your examination reveals an MMSE of 28 and an otherwise normal neurological exam. The cardiovascular exam is unremarkable, and your blood work rules out vitamin B_{12} deficiency and hypothyroidism. Which one of the following would be most appropriate for this patient?
   a. Review the medications for side-effects.
   b. Counsel the patient and spouse about Alzheimer's disease.
   c. Ask for a follow-up appointment in 6 months and repeat the MMSE.
   d. Start treatment with donepezil.

2. Which one of the following is approved by the FDA for the treatment of mild Alzheimer's disease?
   a. Vitamin E
   b. Memantine
   c. Donepezil
   d. Risperidone

3. L.W. is an 87-year-old woman with Alzheimer's disease who is managed at home on donepezil 10 mg per day. One afternoon her daughter, with whom she lives, calls to say that L.W. has become more confused lately and has been seeing the devil for the past 3 days. What is the most appropriate next management step?
   a. Start a low dose of olanzapine.
   b. Assure the daughter that these symptoms are part of the natural progression of the disease and arrange for a follow-up visit in 2 weeks.
   c. Stop her ChEIs.
   d. Ask the daughter to bring her mother to your office immediately.

PRETEST ANSWERS

1. b
2. b
3. c

POSTTEST ANSWERS

1. a
2. c
3. d

<table><tr><td>CHAPTER</td><td>**Depression**</td></tr><tr><td>**17**</td><td>J. Eugene Lammers</td></tr></table>

OBJECTIVES

Upon completion of this chapter, the reader will be able to:

- Distinguish between major depression, adjustment disorder with depressed mood, bereavement, and dysthymia.
- Describe differences in presentation of depression in the elderly compared with younger persons.
- List common medications and physical illnesses associated with depressed mood.
- Understand the use of screening tools and diagnostic testing in the diagnosis of depression.
- Discuss treatment options for depression, including both pharmacological and nonpharmacological therapy.
- Recognize urgent cases that need hospitalization or referral to a psychiatrist.
- Explain the role of electroconvulsive therapy (ECT) to a patient and family and be able to assist a psychiatrist in its medical management.

PRETEST

1. Which one of the following statements regarding depression is false?
   a. Treatment of depression in the elderly is difficult because the elderly do not respond well to antidepressant medications.
   b. Many depressed elderly patients do not report feelings of dysphoria.
   c. Despite concerns about anorexia and weight loss, selective serotonin reuptake inhibitors (SSRIs) are the current antidepressant drugs of choice in the elderly.
   d. Depressed elderly patients respond better to counseling plus antidepressant medication than to medication alone.

2. Which of the following antidepressants should always be initiated as an evening dose in elderly patients?
   a. Nortriptyline
   b. Fluoxetine
   c. Paroxetine
   d. Escitalopram

3. Depressed patients who are to receive ECT should have, as part of a pre-ECT medical screen, all of the following except:
   a. CT brain scan
   b. Cardiac history
   c. ECG
   d. Spinal film series

4. Symptoms of depression are associated with all of the following medications *except*:
   a. Benzodiazepines
   b. Digoxin
   c. Codeine
   d. Methylphenidate

Thomas Xing, *Part 1*

Mr. Xing is brought to your office with the history that he has not been doing well since the death of his wife 18 months ago. He had cared for her during a long illness, and after her death, shortly before their 52nd anniversary, he became withdrawn from his family, lost weight, slept poorly, and seemed to have increasing problems with his memory.

Clara Knighton, *Part 1*

Clara Knighton is a 78-year-old retired nurse who was brought to live in your area by her niece. While visiting her aunt, the niece discovered Ms. Knighton's home to be unkempt and with little food in the house. The niece found that her aunt had lost over 50 pounds. Neighbors confirmed that she had been having a significant decline in her physical and mental status for the previous 6 months.

Martha Jenkins, *Part 1*

Martha Jenkins is a 77-year-old woman who has been your patient for over 20 years. She has resided in the assisted living section of a retirement community for 5 years. She comes to you for help with her osteoporosis and compression fractures, which have limited her mobility and cause significant pain.

STUDY QUESTIONS

1. One diagnosis is a possibility in all three of these cases, but what is the differential diagnosis in each case?
2. What information would you seek to confirm or exclude the possibility of depression?

PREVALENCE AND IMPACT

Depression is the most common of the affective disorders seen by primary care physicians.[1] Depending on the diagnostic criteria used, major depression and related disorders affect between 5% and 20% of persons over age 65 living in the community.[2] Depression is even more common in acutely ill, hospitalized elderly patients, with a prevalence of 25% noted in some studies. Nursing home residents also have a very high prevalence at 25% to 40%.[3]

Suicide is associated with depression in the elderly, as it is with other age groups. Elderly white men have the highest rate of suicide of the entire adult population.[4-6] Atypical presentation, concomitant acute and chronic diseases, and widely held myths regarding the demeanor and personality of older persons are among the reasons that depression is often overlooked.[7,8] DSM-IV criteria are useful in distinguishing major depression from other depressive syndromes, such as adjustment reactions, dysthymia, and bereavement.[9] Although the stresses found in the life histories of many older adults can lead to sadness and depressed mood, true clinical depression is not a part of the normal aging process. Depression is associated with functional decline and excess mortality. Health professionals' clinical suspicion for depression must remain high so that it is diagnosed and treated whenever possible.

> ● Atypical presentation, concomitant acute and chronic diseases, and widely held myths regarding the demeanor and personality of older persons are among the reasons that depression is often overlooked.

DIFFERENTIAL DIAGNOSIS AND ASSESSMENT

Diagnosis

Diagnosing depression in the elderly is often difficult. Rather than having symptoms of depressed mood or crying spells, older persons are likely to have nonspecific somatic complaints, such as fatigue, abdominal pain, or headache. Family members may bring the patient to the physician with a presentation of "just not doing well." Somatic complaints may be even more prominent in persons with limited education and no previous psychiatric history. Another common presentation of depression in old age is the so-called "pseudodementia" ("the dementia syndrome of depression") in which the patient has memory loss and functional decline but of a generally more recent and abrupt onset than the more common progressive dementias, such as Alzheimer's disease. Making the clinical evaluation even more confusing is the strong association of depression with dementia. Caregivers of persons with dementia or depression are frequently depressed themselves and may be unreliable reporters of symptoms.

The diagnosis of depression should be considered in all older persons who report somatic symptoms, particularly those having chronic symptoms that appear to have no definite organic basis. However, because of the association of depressive symptoms with many medical illnesses, a full medical workup should be performed to avoid missing a concomitant or causative illness.[10] Patients with nonspecific symptoms, such as weight loss, malaise, low energy, and fatigue, should be evaluated for untreated medical causes before the diagnosis of depression is made. Many elders have several concurrent illnesses, some of which may first be discovered during the "depression workup."

Major depression and other less specific depressive symptoms are associated with many medical illnesses, including stroke, thyroid disorders, Parkinson's disease, heart disease, and dementia. Chronic pain syndromes such as diabetic neuropathy and trigeminal neuralgia are also associated with an increased risk of depression. Stroke is a particularly important factor, with 60% of patients suffering major depression in their first year after a stroke; those with a left-sided cerebrovascular accident are particularly predisposed to depression. It is also recognized that major depression occurring in the first 6 months after myocardial infarction actually increases mortality. Screening for underlying malignancy, endocrine problems, and other metabolic disorders is warranted. A careful history and physical examination should be performed to detect other medical problems such as clinically silent ischemia or stroke, both of which can lead to depression. Concomitant medical problems not only contribute to depression but also influence the choice of therapy.[11,12,13]

In addition to medical illnesses, certain medications, including digitalis, propranolol, benzodiazepines, and alcohol, are associated with causing depressive symptoms. Unfortunately, some clinicians persist in using benzodiazepines in patients who are depressed, despite evidence that shows the inappropriateness of this strategy.[13] An in-depth review of potential side effects of all the patient's prescriptions and over-the-counter medications must be done because the list of medications potentially implicated in causing depression is long (Box 17–1).[14,15]

Box 17-1   Drugs That Commonly Cause Symptoms of Depression

Antihypertensives
- Reserpine
- Methyldopa
- Propranolol
- Clonidine
- Hydralazine
- Guanethidine

Analgesics
- Narcotic: morphine, codeine, meperidine, pentazocine, propoxyphene
- Non-narcotic: indomethacin

Antiparkinsonian Drugs
- Levodopa

Antimicrobials
- Sulfonamides
- Isoniazid

Cardiovascular Preparations
- Digitalis
- Diuretics
- Lidocaine

Hypoglycemic Agents
- Psychotropic Agents
- Sedatives: barbiturates, benzodiazepines, meprobamate
- Antipsychotics: chlorpromazine, haloperidol, thiothixene
- Hypnotics: chloral hydrate, flurazepam

Steroids
- Corticosteroids
- Estrogens

Other
- Cimetidine
- Cancer chemotherapeutic agents
- Alcohol

Data from Kane RI, Ouslander JG, Abrass IB. Essentials of Clinical Geriatrics. 4th ed. New York: McGraw-Hill, 1999; Levenson AJ, Hall RCW, eds. Neuropsychiatric Manifestations of Physical Disorders in the Elderly. New York: Raven Press, 1981, with permission.

● Rather than having symptoms of depressed mood or crying spells, older persons are likely to have nonspecific somatic complaints, such as fatigue, abdominal pain, or headache.

Thomas Xing, *Part 2*

Assessment of Thomas Xing in your office reveals a frail man who is tearful at times. The physical examination shows apparent weight loss and a slow, slightly wide-based gait, with slight pitting edema of the lower legs. The Geriatric Depression Scale (GDS) and a Mini-Mental Status Examination (MMSE) are administered; the GDS score is 7/15, and the MMSE score is 22/30. Screening laboratory work reveals a normochromic normocytic anemia, a T_4 level of 1.9, and TSH level of 98. Because of the patient's history of coronary artery disease, T_4 replacement therapy is instituted cautiously; you anticipate that it may take 2 or 3 months to reach an appropriate replacement dose.

CASE DISCUSSION

The death of a spouse often leads to depressive symptoms. However, Mr. Xing's symptoms are clearly beyond normal bereavement. The GDS score in combination with the history of the present illness is consistent with major depression. The MMSE score is consistent with the pseudodementia of depression, although mild dementia is possible. Medical screening for other illnesses is needed before a diagnosis of depression is made. In this case, the profound hypothyroidism could account for most or all of the features seen.

Clara Knighton, *Part 2*

Examination of Clara Knighton in your office reveals a very thin, frail woman who is slow to answer questions and who sits passively, holding her head in her hands. Blood pressure supine is 120/75 mm Hg, standing 100/70 mm Hg. She has cataracts, dry skin, tobacco-stained fingers, and a 2/6 systolic ejection murmur. Her MMSE score is 24/30, and her GDS score is 11/15. In response to direct questioning, she admits feelings of hopelessness and worthlessness, loss of appetite, and difficulty sleeping. She feels that life is not worth living, but she denies suicidal ideation. Laboratory test results include a blood urea nitrogen (BUN) level of 55, creatinine of 1.8, and albumin of 2.9. The ECG and chest x-ray examination are normal. A diagnosis of MDE and dehydration is made, and you admit her to the local community hospital.

CASE DISCUSSION

Weight loss, functional decline, and mental decline can be associated with many medical illnesses, medication complications, and disorders of mood such as depression and dementia. A full medical evaluation is needed. However, Clara meets the criteria for a major depressive episode (MDE). Initiation of treatment on an inpatient basis is prudent when there have been significant metabolic disturbances, such as dehydration or serious weight loss. Suicidal patients should also be admitted. In addition, the social situation in this case is unstable, and an inpatient stay allows the treatment team the opportunity to address these issues.

STUDY QUESTIONS

1. Does hypothyroidism fully explain Mr. Xing's symptoms?
2. Is specific treatment for depression indicated?
3. Ms. Knighton is deeply depressed as well as dehydrated; what will the roles of the psychiatrist and family be?

Assessment

Assessment of the patient with symptoms suggestive of depression includes a complete history and physical examination, with particular emphasis on the history of the present illness, past history of similar symptoms, and a review of systems. Screening laboratory work should be performed, with more specialized testing performed depending on the clinical presentation. Patients should be screened for malignancy, renal and liver disease, and electrolyte abnormalities; a complete blood count, chemistry panel, and chest x-ray examination are generally sufficient. In addition, T_4 and thyroid-stimulating hormone (TSH) measurements should be ordered for all patients to address the possibility of hypothyroidism or hyperthyroidism. Vitamin B_{12} and folate levels should be evaluated, as they would be in patients with cognitive changes, because abnormalities are also seen in association with depression. If a rheumatologic disease such as polymyalgia rheumatica or rheumatoid arthritis is suspected, an erythrocyte sedimentation rate may be a useful test. A CT scan or an MRI of the brain is indicated only if there are neurologic abnormalities or unusual behavioral manifestations suggestive of, for example, frontal lobe problems. An electrocardiogram is useful as a baseline and may reveal cardiac disease; it is specifically indicated before initiation of any antidepressants that influence cardiac conduction, such as the tricyclic antidepressants.

It is always a clinical challenge to know how far to go with the workup of an older patient. The differential diagnosis of nonspecific symptoms such as weight loss or fatigue is long, and in many cases depression is the most precise medical diagnosis that can be made. Fortunately, the history and physical, combined with screening tests, usually uncover serious occult disease appearing as depressive symptoms. If occult disease is not quickly found to precisely explain symptoms, a trial of antidepressant therapy should be initiated while further medical evaluation is pursued or while the patient's physical symptoms are carefully observed over time, with strict attention to compliance with follow-up.

The DSM-IV criteria for MDE,[9] as well as the related disorders of dysthymia and adjustment disorder, would appear to be straightforward and easy to apply to the diagnosis of older persons with depression (Boxes 17–2 to 17–4). The patient and, if appropriate, the family are asked direct questions derived from these criteria. It is usually necessary to ask direct questions because many of the symptoms are nonspecific or are misattributed by the patient or family. The history of previous depression, as well as any history of mania or hypomania (Box 17–5), should be explored thoroughly. Unfortunately, as with many common illnesses, "atypical" presentations seem to be the rule in the elderly population (Box 17–6). Because of these difficulties, especially when associated with other chronic diseases, a number of screening instruments have been developed and validated for use in elderly patients. These include the GDS (Fig. 17–1)[16] for outpatients, the Center for Epidemiologic Studies-Depression instrument (CES-D) (Fig. 17–2),[17] and a scale (Fig. 17–3) for medically ill elderly inpatients.[18] These screening tools can be administered to such patients quickly, are easily reproducible, and correlate well with more traditional diagnostic evaluations such as structured psychiatric interviews. A "positive" score on one of these screening tools can increase or confirm a clinical suspicion of major depression. However, a "false negative" score can be seen in a patient who is denying the symptoms. These questionnaires do not replace specific questions directed toward uncovering vegetative symptoms of the type implied in the DSM-IV description of an MDE. In spite of these limitations, the use of such structured questionnaires is strongly considered in primary care practices because they can help keep the diagnosis of depression in the forefront as a patient is being evaluated for nonspecific signs or symptoms. As many older adults are reluctant to admit to any type of depressive symptoms, reports from family and friends are often critical in obtaining accurate information.

Box 17-2   Criteria for Major Depressive Episode

Five (or more) of the following symptoms have been present during the same 2-week period and represent a change from previous functioning; at least one of the symptoms is either (1) depressed mood or (2) loss of interest or pleasure. *NOTE: Do not include symptoms that are clearly the result of a general medical condition, mood-incongruent delusions, or hallucinations.*

- Depressed mood most of the day, nearly every day, as indicated by either subjective report (e.g., feels sad or empty) or observation made by others (e.g., appears tearful).
- Markedly diminished interest or pleasure in all, or almost all, activities most of the day, nearly every day (as indicated by either subjective account or observation made by others).
- Significant weight loss when not dieting or weight gain (e.g., a change of more than 5% of body weight in a month), or decrease or increase in appetite nearly every day.
- Insomnia or hypersomnia nearly every day.
- Psychomotor agitation or retardation nearly every day (observable by others, not merely subjective feelings of restlessness or being slowed down).
- Fatigue or loss of energy nearly every day.
- Feelings of worthlessness or excessive or inappropriate guilt

(which may be delusional) nearly every day (not merely self-reproach or guilt about being sick).

- Diminished ability to think or concentrate, or indecisiveness, nearly every day (either by subjective account or as observed by others).
- Recurrent thoughts of death (not just fear of dying); recurrent suicidal ideation without a specific plan; suicide attempt or specific plan for committing suicide.
- *The symptoms do not meet criteria for a mixed episode (see Box 17–5).*
- *The symptoms cause clinically significant distress or impairment in social, occupational, or other important areas of functioning.*
- *The symptoms are not a result of the direct physiologic effects of a substance (e.g., drug abuse, medication) or a general medical condition (e.g., hypothyroidism).*
- *The symptoms are not better accounted for by bereavement. After the loss of a loved one, the symptoms persist for longer than 2 months or are characterized by marked functional impairment, morbid preoccupation with worthlessness, suicidal ideation, psychotic symptoms, or psychomotor retardation.*

From American Psychiatric Association. Diagnostic and Statistical Manual of Mental Disorders (DSM-IV). 4th ed. Washington, DC: Association, 1994, with permission.

Most clinicians use a combination of screening questions and directed questions, asking them intuitively at the appropriate points in the interview, physical examination, or review of systems. The important thing is to ensure that specific questions are asked, with the physician directly inquiring as to the presence or absence of the specific symptoms as described in DSM-IV in the definition of an MDE. Clinicians

Box 17-3   Abbreviated Criteria for Adjustment Disorder with Depressed Mood

- Emotional or behavioral symptoms in response to an identifiable stressor within 3 months
- Either excessive distress or significant impairment of social or occupational functioning
- Do not meet the criteria for another clinical psychiatric disorder
- Do not represent bereavement
- Do not persist for more than an additional 6 months after the stressor is terminated

From American Psychiatric Association. Diagnostic and Statistical Manual of Mental Disorders (DSM-IV). 4th ed. Washington, DC: Association, 1994, with permission.

Box 17-4   Abbreviated Criteria for Dysthymia

- Depressed mood for most of the day, for more days than not, for at least 2 years
- While depressed, has two or more of the following:
  - Poor appetite or overeating
  - Insomnia or hypersomnia
  - Low energy or fatigue
  - Low self-esteem
  - Poor concentration or decision-making capability
  - Feeling of hopelessness
- Never without the symptoms for more than 2 months at a time
- No major depressive episode present
- No manic, mixed, or hypomanic episodes present
- Does not occur exclusively during a psychotic disorder
- Not caused by a medication or other drug or medical condition
- Causes functional deficit

Modified from American Psychiatric Association. Diagnostic and Statistical Manual of Mental Disorders (DSM-IV). 4th ed. Washington, DC: Association, 1994, with permission.

Box 17-5 Abbreviated Criteria for Manic and Hypomanic Episodes

- A distinct period of elevated, expansive, or irritable mood, lasting 4 days (hypomanic) or 1 week (manic).
- Three or more of the following (four if the mood is irritable only):
  - Inflated self-esteem or grandiosity
  - Decreased need for sleep
  - More talkative than usual or pressure to keep talking
  - Flight of ideas or subjective experience of racing thoughts
  - Distractibility
  - Increased goal-directed activity (may be social, sexual, or work related) or psychomotor agitation
  - Excessive pleasurable activities with potentially painful consequences (e.g., buying sprees, sexual indiscretion, foolish business activities)
- An unequivocal change in functioning.

- Clearly observable by others (hypomanic) or causing marked impairment in functioning or relationships, or requiring hospitalization, or with psychotic features (manic).
- Not caused by substance abuse or a general medical condition nor clearly caused by antidepressant treatment.

Mixed Episode
- The criteria for both a manic episode and major depressive episode are met nearly every day for a week.
- There is marked impairment, or psychotic features, or a need for hospitalization.
- It is not caused by a medication (including an antidepressant or other drug) or a medical condition.

From American Psychiatric Association. Diagnostic and Statistical Manual of Mental Disorders (DSM-IV). 4th ed. Washington, DC: Association, 1994, with permission.

working with the elderly should be thoroughly familiar with the DSM-IV criteria for dysthymia, bereavement, and adjustment disorders, as well as with the features of mania or hypomania that would make bipolar illness (manic-depressive disorder) a consideration. These criteria are summarized in Boxes 17-2 to 17-5.

Even if MDE is confidently diagnosed, contributory factors and concurrent illnesses must be sought and addressed if the treatment is to succeed.

In the treatment of depression in the elderly by primary care physicians, biologic tests such as dexamethasone suppression tests and platelet monoamine oxidase have no value. They have not been found to have sufficient sensitivity or specificity to be useful in clinical management of depression in the elderly.

Box 17-6 How Depression Symptoms Differ in the Older Patient

- Sadness of mood is usually present but is often masked by other symptoms.
- Impairment in cognition may be marked and may dominate the clinical picture; it may even mimic dementia.
- A psychosomatic tendency often dominates, and the patient complains of aches and pains or other physical symptoms. (Older patients with depression are more likely to have exaggerated and ruminative fears about their physical well-being than do younger patients).

Modified from From American Psychiatric Association. Diagnostic and Statistical Manual of Mental Disorders (DSM-IV). 4th ed. Washington, DC: Association, 1994, with permission. From Ham RJ, Meyers BS. Late Life Depression and Suicide Potential. Washington, DC: American Association of Retired Persons, 1993, with permission.

● The differential diagnosis of nonspecific symptoms such as weight loss or fatigue is long, and in many cases depression is the most precise medical diagnosis that can be made.

SUICIDE POTENTIAL

The risk of suicide must be assessed in every elderly depressed patient by direct questioning (Box 17–7).[6] Clinicians should inquire directly about suicidal ideation and plans, the availability of family or other social support, and the ability to access the means of suicide, including guns and medications. It is important to note that possibly 80% of those who commit suicide have visited their primary care physician within a month of their death, with 20% doing so within 24 hours.[6,10] Whereas major depression is not necessarily the cause of all suicides, it is likely to be a factor in more than half of the cases, and therefore will often be found if it is sought. Those with active suicidal ideation should be considered for referral to a psychiatric unit or an acute care hospital. Even those at relatively low risk should be monitored closely by family or friends and need frequent scheduled follow-up in the physician's office, particularly during the early phases of treatment.

Always ask direct questions of the patient and family about suicide risk. Some clinicians feel uneasy broaching this topic, for fear that it will suggest the idea of suicide, but there is no evidence to support this concern.[19] Insist that the family dispose of guns and pills, and not leave the patient alone if suicide risk exists.

● Always ask direct questions of the patient and family about suicide risk.

Geriatric Depression Scale (short form)		
Choose the best answer for how you felt the past week		
Are you basically satisfied with your life?	Yes	No*
Have you dropped many of your activities and interests?	Yes*	No
Do you feel that your life is empty?	Yes*	No
Do you often get bored?	Yes*	No
Are you in good spirits most of the time?	Yes	No*
Are you afraid that something bad is going to happen to you?	Yes*	No
Do you feel happy most of the time?	Yes	No*
Do you often feel helpless?	Yes*	No
Do you prefer to stay at home rather than going out and doing new things?	Yes*	No
Do you feel you have more problems with memory than most?	Yes*	No
Do you think it is wonderful to be alive now?	Yes	No*
Do you feel pretty worthless the way you are now?	Yes*	No
Do you feel full of energy?	Yes	No*
Do you feel that your situation is hopeless?	Yes*	No
Do you think that most people are better off than you are?	Yes*	No
Each answer indicated by an asterisk counts as one point. Scores between 5 and 9 suggest depression; scores above 9 generally indicate depression.		

FIGURE 17-1

Geriatric Depression Scale (Short Form). *From Sheikh JL, Yesavage JA. Clin Gerontol 1986;5:165, with permission.*

UNDERNUTRITION

Change in weight is one of the criteria for MDE, but it must be recognized that weight loss also indicates unmet nutritional needs.[20] A significant degree of weight loss (e.g., more than 10% in 6 months, more than 7.5% in 3 months, or more than 5% in 1 month) requires a specific nutritional investigation and approach.[21] Depression must always be considered in the differential diagnosis of significant weight loss.[22]

DECONDITIONING

The interrelationship between physical deconditioning and depression is of interest. After several months of depressive illness, an elderly person is likely to be physically as well as emotionally deconditioned; the combination of undernutrition, poor muscle strength relative to mobility, increased dependency for physical functioning, and, especially in the more frail, development of difficult symptoms such as incontinence, loss of confidence for mobility, or even falling can mean that full recovery from a depressive episode requires extensive rehabilitative techniques. Because of the Medicare program's emphasis on steady progress in its reimbursement of outpatient physical therapy, it may be necessary to initiate the treatment of depression of depression several weeks prior to starting a physical therapy program, so that the patient can have enough energy or interest to participate.

Undernutrition and physical deconditioning with all of their consequences are frequently the permanent sequelae of unrecognized depression, continuing as long-term disabilities after the depression resolves. Prevention is superior to rehabilitation, hence the importance of early detection of depression.

> ● Undernutrition and physical deconditioning with all of their consequences are frequently the permanent sequelae of unrecognized depression, continuing as long-term disabilities after the depression resolves.

Center for Epidemiological Studies Depression (CES-D)				

Responses: **A**   Rarely or none of the time (less than 1 day)
              B   Some or a little of the time (1–2 days)
              C   Occasionally or a moderate amount of time (3–4 days)
              D Most of the time (5–7 days)				

"During the past week:..."	**A**	**B**	**C**	**D**
1. I was bothered by things that usually don't bother me.				
2. I did not feel like eating, or my appetite was poor.				
3. I felt that I could not shake off the blues even with the help of my family or friends.				
4. I felt that I was just as good as other people.				
5. I had trouble keeping my mind on what I was doing.				
6. I felt depressed.				
7. I felt that everything I did was an effort.				
8. I felt hopeful about the future.				
9. I thought my life had been a failure.				
10. I felt fearful.				
11. My sleep was restless.				
12. I was happy.				
13. I talked less than usual.				
14. I felt lonely.				
15. People were unfriendly.				
16. I enjoyed life.				
17. I had crying spells.				
18. I felt sad.				
19. I felt that people disliked me.				
20. I could not "get going."				
Total score ranges from 0–60. Patients with scores over 15 are likely to be depressed. Score A = 0, B = 1, C = 2, D = 3 for all questions except **4, 8, 12, and 16 which are scored:** A = 3, B = 2, C = 1, D = 0.				

FIGURE 17–2

Center for Epidemiologic Studies-Depression (CES-D). *From Radloff L, Center for Epidemiologic Studies, National Institute of Mental Health, 1977, with permission.*

Thomas Xing, *Part 3*

Mr. Xing has characteristic symptoms of depression; to address this while slowly initiating the thyroid treatment, you decide to start sertraline (Zoloft) 25 mg per day. The patient and family are apprised of potential side effects, the time course for the medication to be effective, and the long-term treatment plan. Mr. Xing is reevaluated in 1 week to reassess suicide potential and to look for medication side effects. Because he has no side effects, the dose is increased to 50 mg per day. At the next scheduled visit, 3 weeks later, he is showing improvement in his mood, affect, and energy level. His symptoms are virtually resolved within 2 months. The patient and family receive counseling from a social worker who helps them deal with the many changes in Mr. Xing's living situation. Three months after his initial visit, Mr. Xing's GDS score is 1/15, his MMSE examination

Scale for detecting major depression in hospitalized patients		
Choose the best answer for how you have felt over the past week.		
1 Do you often get bored?	Yes	No
2 Do you often get restless and fidgety?	Yes	No
3 Do you feel in good spirits?	Yes	No
4 Do you feel you have more problems with memory than most?	Yes	No
5 Can you concentrate easily when reading the papers?	Yes	No
6 Do you prefer to avoid social gatherings?	Yes	No
7 Do you often feel downhearted and blue?	Yes	No
8 Do you feel happy most of the time?	Yes	No
9 Do you often feel helpless?	Yes	No
10 Do you feel worthless and ashamed about yourself?	Yes	No
11 Do you often wish you were dead?	Yes	No
Scoring: Assign 1 point for each "yes" response except 3, 5 and 8 score 1 for each "no". A score of 3 or more generally indicates depression.		

FIGURE 17–3

Scale for detecting major depression in hospitalized patients. *From Koenig HG, Blazer DG. Clin Geriatr Med 1992;8:235, with permission.*

score is 26/30, and he is euthyroid. The sertraline is continued for a total of 9 months, at which time Mr. Xing is slowly weaned. Some feelings of low energy and sleep disturbance begin to return within 1 month of stopping the sertraline, and it is restarted, with plans to continue it for a total of 2 years before weaning him again.

CASE DISCUSSION

Simultaneous treatment of depression and intercurrent medical problems is often needed in elderly patients. It was appropriate to initiate sertraline while his hypothyroidism was being addressed. Counseling and family support are helpful as adjunctive therapy, especially when clear social stressors or lifestyle changes are present.

MANAGEMENT

Overall Approach

Many family members or even physicians may see a case of depression as a normal response to life changes and stressors. Although depression may seem

reasonable in the circumstances, depression is disabling and dangerous and, because it may respond to treatment, should be treated (Fig. 17–4).

Box 17-7   Assessing the Potential for Suicide

- Does the patient volunteer suicidal thoughts?
- Has the patient thought through plans for suicide?
- Does the patient have access to the means of suicide?
- Does the patient have an exaggerated concern about a real or imagined physical illness?
- Is there evidence of a sense of hopelessness?
- Is the patient extremely depressed and withdrawn?
- Is this an elderly white male?
- Is there alcohol involved?
- Are there social contacts with whom to share emotional thoughts?
- Does the patient's cognitive status vary from day to day?
- Do you have reason to suspect that the patient might not be taking the prescribed medications?
- Is someone available at home for companionship until the depressed mood is controlled or resolved?

From Ham RJ, Meyers BS. Late Life Depression and Suicide Potential. Washington, DC: American Association of Retired Persons, 1993, with permission.

As with the other major syndromes of the elderly, effective treatment of depression generally requires a *multidisciplinary approach*. It is possible that ongoing stressors contribute to the persistence or relapse of depressive illness. The efficacy of pharmacologic therapy appears to be enhanced by simultaneously addressing the social support structure of the patient. This can be as simple as encouraging mildly symptomatic patients to return to previously enjoyable social activities or to take up new ones and facilitating such participation. It may be useful to minimize home stressors by organizing appropriate community services, such as case management or Meals on Wheels. Many patients with major depression respond better to psychotherapy in combination with antidepressant medications than with medication alone.[23] This can often be arranged through the local mental health association or clinic. However, many patients and families resist such treatment because of the stigma of mental illness.

Close follow-up by the primary care physician is imperative in the treatment of depression. Patients need to be seen in the office frequently during the early part of treatment to assess side effects, observe for signs of functional decline or suicidal ideation, and evaluate efficacy of the medical regimen. Asking patients to return "as needed" is not enough.[24]

Early treatment of depression with pharmacologic agents is highly recommended in the elderly, particularly for patients with major depression or depressive symptoms associated with functional decline. The primary physician's knowledge and enthusiasm for the use of these medications are vital; many families and patients associate antidepressants with the stigma of mental illness or are concerned of the possibility of harm from them. Advances in the development of antidepressants make it even more reasonable now to mount an enthusiastic "therapeutic trial" in a patient in whom depression (i.e., MDE) is present or even highly likely. The factors increasing the likelihood of antidepressant response are summarized in Box 17–8. A therapeutic trial should be started on the basis of clinical suspicion, given the prevalence and treatability of these illnesses and their potential for producing both morbidity and mortality.[7,25,26]

Medications

The broad classes of available medications for the treatment of depression include selective serotonin reuptake inhibitors (SSRIs), tricyclic antidepressants, monoamine oxidase inhibitors (MAOIs), and atypical agents (Table 17–1). Because of the serious side effects associated with many of these medications and the sensitivity of older patients to such effects, primary care physicians must focus on the safest regimens and reserve the more risky modalities for refractory situations. Some regimens should be handled only by practitioners with special skill in dealing with the elderly, such as psychiatrists or geriatricians.[24,26]

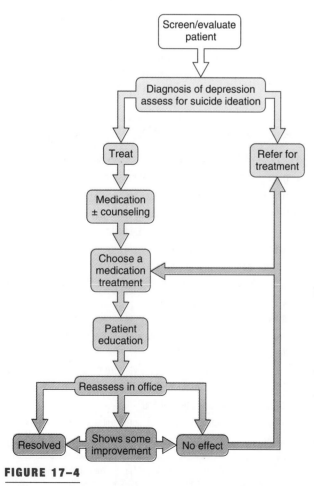

FIGURE 17–4

Depression management.

From Ham RJ, unpublished educational materials.

> **Box 17–8 Factors Increasing Likelihood of Response to an Antidepressant**
>
> - Presence of clear-cut DSM-IV criteria for major depressive episode
> - Somewhat abrupt onset of symptoms (may be over weeks, often over days, sometimes overnight)
> - History of depression or depressive episodes (especially if responsive to antidepressants)
> - Convincing biologic or vegetative symptoms of depression (diurnal variation in mood, sleep disturbance, appetite change, constipation, weight loss)
> - Family history of affective illness

Table 17–1	Antidepressants Used in Primary Care Treatment of the Elderly

Name	Sedation	Excitation	Anticholinergic Effects	Gastrointestinal Upset	Orthostasis	Range (mg)	Half-life
Nortriptyline	X		X		X	25–50	Long
Fluoxetine		XX		X		10–30	Very long
Sertraline		X		X		25–150	Very long
Paroxetine		X	X (mild)	X		10–40	Very long
Duloxetine				X		40–60	Long
Venlafaxine				X		37.5–150	Moderate
Bupropion		X	X	X		150–300	Moderate

Many family members of older patients, the patients themselves, and a surprising proportion of practicing physicians are filled with doubts and uncertainties about the reasonableness of using a psychoactive medication in an older individual (Box 17–9). Extensive press coverage of the harm caused to elders by drugs and the overuse of antipsychotics in the past can combine with old-fashioned, prejudicial thinking about the nature of "mental illness" to create a high degree of resistance to the use of psychoactive medications. Patients and families willing to undergo all kinds of other therapies may hesitate to use these medications. The primary care physician has a central leadership role in clarifying the issues so that the opportunity for useful treatment is not missed. Evidence-based guidelines exist and may be useful educational tools for reluctant families and colleagues[27] (Table 17–2).

Families and patients must understand that depression is a physical illness of the brain and that physical treatments are thus a reasonable and basic approach; this physical view of depression as a "chemical imbalance" overcomes the fear of giving medications that act on the mind. In speaking with patients and families, it is helpful to stress that, although circumstances may have precipitated the depression, the final effect is a biochemical one, which is why a pharmacologic approach is logical. Patients and families must be reassured about improvements in antidepressant medications and the relative lack of side effects compared with medications widely used in the past.[13] Patients and families need to know that the medications are not addictive, that stopping them is easy, and that each person's response is unique so that it may be reasonable to try other pharmacologic alternatives if a first trial does not work or causes a systemic upset. Lastly, the family in particular must understand exactly what the "target symptoms" are, that is, which of the range

Box 17–9	Why Patients and Families Resist the Use of Psychoactive Drugs

- Nonrecognition of the essentially chemical nature of mood disorders
- Assumption that if an event or an environment has caused the problem, the passing of the event or modification in the environment will reverse it
- Opinion that the depressed mood is reasonable, given the patient's circumstances (e.g., seeing an elderly, frail, dependent patient in a nursing home and thinking, "I don't want to live like that when I am old.")
- Belief that the individual should be strong enough to control his or her own mood without resorting to medications
- Nonrecognition that this is a physical illness of the brain and likely to respond to the physical treatment of medication
- Fear of addiction or habituation
- Fear of confusion or being "drugged"
- Fear of other side effects
- Fear of suicide induction, personality change, and other well-publicized but rare effects

From Ham RJ, unpublished educational material.

Table 17–2	Evidence-Based Treatment Recommendations for Depression

Primary care clinicians need access to providers trained in psychological interventions such as cognitive-behavioral therapy (CBT) (A).

Antidepressants are effective in moderate to severe nonpsychotic depression (A).

Referral to a specialist is indicated in psychotic depression (B).

SSRIs are better tolerated and safer in patients with medical comorbidity (C).

"Low-dose" antidepressant treatment is not recommended for older adults (A).

Adapted from Baldwin RC, et al. Guideline for the management of late-life depression in primary care. Int J Geriatr Psychiatry 2003;18(9):829–38, with permission.

of symptoms the physician believes may respond to the drug. Either the family or the patient will be reporting back to the physician, and they need to know for what they are supposed to be looking. Happily, very few physicians still exclusively use amitriptyline (Elavil), once the most popular tricyclic. Because of its dangerously sedative and anticholinergic effects, it is the least desirable of all antidepressants to use in older individuals. Recent studies confirm that some physicians tend to use benzodiazepines rather than antidepressants, which can make the depression worse. Such treatments demonstrate both a lack of knowledge about and a lack of confidence in appropriate treatment for this common illness.[28]

> ● In speaking with patients and families, it is helpful to stress that, although circumstances may have precipitated the depression, the final effect is a biochemical one, which is why a pharmacologic approach is logical.

SSRIs are the medication class of first choice according to most experts. The SSRIs (fluoxetine [Prozac], citalopram [Celexa], escitalopram [Lexapro], paroxetine [Paxil]) and sertraline [Zoloft]), share a well-tolerated side effect profile in the elderly. The most common side effect is gastrointestinal distress, but this rarely leads to discontinuation of the medication. Insomnia is a side effect related to the tendency of these agents to cause activation. They should therefore be given initially in the morning. The single daily dose is convenient and aids with compliance. Occasionally they cause sedation; should this occur, the dose is switched to bedtime. There are differences in plasma half-life and the sites of metabolism as well as the degree of "activation" or stimulation seen with each of these medications; this profile should be considered in choosing a particular agent for a given patient. Some patients respond to one SSRI and not to others. Practitioners should start with a low dose for a week or so, but an adequate trial is not complete until the patient has taken the medication at the usual recommended adult dose for at least 6 weeks.

Tricyclics (TCAs) are the most well-studied therapeutic agents. They have an established and well-understood side effect profile. For many agents in this class, blood levels are routinely available and help ensure that the patient is not receiving too much or too little. Unfortunately, the side effects of TCAs can be difficult for older patients to tolerate. Of particular concern are the anticholinergic effects such as drowsiness, constipation, blurred vision, urinary hesitancy, and dry mouth. Orthostatic hypotension can also be a problem. Nortriptyline is the least sedating of the TCAs and has a lower anticholinergic effect than most other tricyclics; therefore it should be the TCA of choice in the elderly. Other TCAs should be considered in primary care only in the case of recurrent depression that has previously responded to one such specific medication. Nortriptyline seems to be especially effective in helping depression associated with or manifested by chronic pain, insomnia, and psychomotor agitation. Usually it can be taken as a single bedtime dose and should always be initiated as such.

Martha Jenkins, *Part 2*

Evaluation of Martha Jenkins in the office reveals lethargy, a depressed mood, and feelings of hopelessness and helplessness. She experienced an episode of depression 4 years ago that responded well to nortriptyline, so nortriptyline is restarted. Over the next 6 weeks she begins to sleep better and seemingly has an improved mood, but within 3 months she begins to feel ill again, with increasing pain, weakness, fatigue, and worsening mood. Laboratory evaluation reveals an Hct of 28, mean corpuscular volume of 91, BUN of 66, creatinine of 3.2, total protein of 8.2, albumin of 2.2, and alkaline phosphatase of 303. Serum protein electrophoresis, x-ray examination, and bone marrow biopsy confirm the diagnosis of multiple myeloma. The patient is referred to an oncologist, and after beginning treatment with oral chemotherapeutic agents, she begins to feel much better.

CASE DISCUSSION

Martha Jenkins has typical features of, and a history of, depression. Because of her prior response and the usefulness of tricyclic antidepressants in chronic pain, nortriptyline is a good choice for initial therapy. However, although depression is common in older patients, so are cancer and other chronic illnesses. A complete history, physical, and appropriate screening laboratory work might have discovered this hidden malignancy earlier. The patient still needed treatment for depression, but therapy for the multiple myeloma was also required.

MAOIs (monoamine oxidase inhibitors) have been found to be effective in the treatment of depression in the elderly and have little cardiotoxic or cholinergic effect. However, the required dietary restrictions to prevent hypertensive crises and orthostatic hypotension from these drugs make them problematic. Many clinicians, including many psychiatrists, have little experience in the use of them. Therefore, this class of medications probably has little place in primary care clinicians' care of elderly patients.

Trazodone has low anticholinergic side effects, but it is highly sedating and is associated with orthostatic hypotension. In addition, the rare but serious complication of priapism has caused some practitioners to avoid its use in men. These side effects can make it difficult to titrate up to the dosage level needed to achieve reliable antidepressant results. It can be helpful as a second medication for SSRI-associated sleep disturbances.[29]

Bupropion (Wellbutrin) has many features that favor its use in the elderly population. Although its mechanism of action is unclear, it is effective for major depression and perhaps for bipolar depression (manic depression). It has energizing properties, and therefore rarely causes sedation, although it can cause nervousness. It has minimal anticholinergic side effects and no significant cardiac effects. It does reduce the seizure threshold in patients who are predisposed to them.

Duloxetine (Cymbalta) and *Venlafaxine* (Effexor) are agents with a side effect profile similar to that for SSRIs, but with the potential advantage of working at the sites of both serotonin activity and norepinephrine activity. Although this may be of theoretic benefit only, there is some evidence that this mechanism leads to a faster onset of action. They are available in a once daily formulation, and the safety profile appears satisfactory for elderly patients. Because of concerns about exacerbation of hypertension, these agents are often reserved for patients who fail to respond to an SSRI.

Mirtazipine (Remeron), can be a highly sedating agent, but in some patients may have the beneficial side effect of appetite stimulation. It is a unique drug in that its side effect of sedation seems to improve as the dose increases, so moving to a higher dose more quickly may be prudent.

TITRATION

With most antidepressants, an *initial low dose is slowly titrated upward* until the individual is on a dose that is likely to be therapeutic (Box 17–10). Most experienced clinicians recommend that a *trial of therapy* with an antidepressant last *for at least 6 weeks at the dose that is likely to be therapeutic.*[30] Establishing this dose for an individual can be difficult. It may be necessary to leave an individual on what may be the therapeutic dose for

4 weeks after which, lacking a definite response, a further increase with a further period of observation might be justified; then if there is no response after the further 4-week trial (ensure that there is compliance with the medicine), then a change of medication is necessary.[30]

DURATION

After the patient achieves a remission of the symptoms of depression, it is vital to persist with the medication, continuing the dose that has been effective. The dose should not be reduced once the patient has responded. Rather, that dose should be continued for at least 6 months, and most physicians would recommend 1 year. This is based on the assumption that the natural history of an episode of major depression is often as long as 1 year, and therefore the episode needs to be "covered" until its natural resolution. The high relapse rate of individuals responding successfully to these medications is leading some physicians to recommend more persistent therapy.[28] It is possible that as many as 20% of individuals require continuing, potentially lifelong, treatment to avoid relapse. Many authorities currently recommend that a patient whose depression relapses on withdrawal of the antidepressant be treated again for a period of at least 1 further year before another attempt at reduction, and many would consider that even one such relapse justifies continuing the medication for life. Others go further, recommending that a severe antidepressant-responsive depression in old age, especially if there

---

> **Box 17–10 Titrating Antidepressant Dosage**
>
> - Define the target symptoms and ensure that the family (and patient if cognizant) understands them.
> - Titrate carefully (slowly if possible, quickly if urgent) to the dose that is likely to be effective.
> - Persist at the "likely-to-be-effective" dose for at least 6 weeks.
> - Consider increasing after only 4 weeks at the "likely-to-be-effective" dose if there is no response, there is urgency, and the patient is tolerating the medication well.
> - When the target symptoms respond, you are at the effective dose.
> - Persist at the effective dose for at least 6 months but generally 1 year (some authorities now recommend 2 years) or longer (possibly lifelong) if this is a recurrent or relapsing depression.

has been a prior episode of depression, suicide attempt, or depression with psychosis, should lead to lifelong treatment with antidepressants at the full effective dose.[30,31]

Clara Knighton, *Part 3*

In the hospital you begin treating Clara Knighton with 10 mg of fluoxetine every morning, along with IV hydration. After several days, her BUN level is normal and with the addition of trazedone 25 mg every night, she is sleeping well at night, but she refuses to eat and sits in her chair all day. A psychiatric consultation is obtained and ECT is recommended. A normal CT scan completes the medical clearance for the ECT. You initiate detailed discussion with the family, involving the psychiatrist in the discussion, and the family agrees to ECT. However, the patient refuses, and she also refuses transfer to an inpatient psychiatric unit. The fluoxetine is increased to 20 mg per day, causing some mild nervousness.

Five days later she is more alert in the daytime but still refuses to eat. The patient refuses a temporary feeding tube, so central hyperalimentation is started. The treatment team thinks that Ms. Knighton lacks the capacity to accept or refuse potentially life-saving treatment and that a guardian is needed. Social Service assists her niece in arranging to become Ms. Knighton's temporary guardian. After the legal matters are completed, the niece signs for the transfer to the psychiatric unit and for the ECT. The psychiatrist assumes primary responsibility, with you as personal physician managing Ms. Knighton's medical problems and assisting in maintaining the family's support and the patient's compliance.

After four treatments, the patient's affect begins to brighten and she starts eating. After ten unilateral treatments she is greatly improved, walking well, eating well, and participating in group therapy sessions. She is discharged to the care of her niece with plans to continue nortriptyline for at least 2 years; if any sign of recurrent depression is noted, outpatient "maintenance" ECT will be a consideration.

CASE DISCUSSION

Fluoxetine was a good choice because of Ms. Knighton's marked vegetative symptoms, as it is the most stimulating of the SSRIs. However, ECT needs to be considered early in elderly patients who are in medical danger from their depression. Such dangers include weight loss, recurrent dehydration, and suicide. Legal hurdles can be great in cases in which the patient will not agree, and there is no guardian to make decisions. Families can be resistant to the idea of ECT, and it is important for the primary physician to be involved in these discussions. Appointing a guardian can be problematic: respect for patients' rights can lead to uncertainty as to what is in the best interest of the patient. Nonresponders to medical therapy often respond to ECT. This type of depressive episode needs long-term follow-up and treatment. The medication, if tolerated, should probably be continued for life.

ECT is an effective treatment for major depression in the elderly, with success rates approaching 90%. Although some experts call ECT the treatment of choice in the elderly, most clinicians reserve ECT for refractory cases or for cases in which a high risk of morbidity or mortality would be associated with waiting as much as 4 to 6 weeks for a significant response to medications. Such high-risk patients include those who are actively suicidal or are unwilling to take adequate nutrition and hydration. Psychotic or delusional depression is highly responsive to ECT and much less responsive to pharmacotherapy; ECT should thus be considered as primary treatment in those cases.

Medicolegal concerns, as well as the social stigma attached to ECT, can interfere with the willingness of patients and families to accept ECT as a treatment. In addition, in some parts of the country few psychiatrists perform this procedure because of a lack of training or the cost of medical liability insurance. Reassurance by the personal physician regarding the appropriateness of ECT can be helpful in getting patients and families to have an open mind regarding this treatment. Physicians should be aware of the nearest center available for referral of potential ECT patients because ECT therapy can be life saving in major depression that is refractory to pharmacologic therapy.

The main side effect of ECT, other than the transient tachycardia and elevation in blood pressure seen in the immediate postictal stage, is transient confusion. This seems to be a more serious problem in persons who have both dementia and depression. The use of unilateral electrode placement may minimize any cognitive change associated with ECT.

Referral to a psychiatrist is generally necessary for ECT, but the primary care physician is in the best position to know whether the person is a medical candidate for it. ECT is performed under brief general anesthesia, so the usual guidelines for preoperative clearance apply. In particular, patients considered for ECT should not have unstable angina, active CHF, or unstable dysrhythmias. Severe hypertension should be controlled. In addition, persons considered for ECT should have a CT brain scan or MRI to rule out the presence of a significant tumor. A small, benign tumor such as a meningioma is not an absolute contraindication to ECT; it should be discussed with a neurosurgeon if there are any doubts. The previous practice of doing complete spine films before performing ECT, to assess for the presence of fractures, is no longer necessary because the concurrent use of paralytic anesthesia minimizes the possibility of skeletal injuries. However, this practice persists in some areas of the country because of medicolegal concerns. To disallow ECT for all older persons with osteoporosis and compression fractures would be excessively cautious.

A course of ECT often ranges from 6 to 20 treatments, given two to three times per week. Response is often noticed within the first week or two.

There are roles for *combination therapy* with more than one antidepressant and for use of *augmentation agents* such as lithium, thyroid hormone,[32] methylphenidate, and dextroamphetamine.[33] Because of the risk of unfavorable side effects in the elderly population, these therapies, as well as MAO inhibitors, should be reserved for refractory cases or patients with intolerable side effects on therapeutic doses of an effective agent, and in consultation with an experienced clinician such as a gero-psychiatrist.

> ● Psychotic or delusional depression is highly responsive to ECT and much less responsive to pharmacotherapy; ECT should thus be considered as primary treatment in those cases.

Phototherapy

In phototherapy, depressed patients are exposed to extra quantities of light; this is a further consideration in patients not responding to traditional approaches.[34] Data suggest that some patients respond to light therapy of 2000 to 3000 lux for 2 hours or more, particularly those who are depressed in the winter or do not go outdoors. This is probably related to seasonal affective disorder, one element of which is thought to be light deprivation.[35,36] More research is needed, but for now it seems reasonable to at least address the gloomy environment in which many dependent elders live, and to increase the quantity and duration of lighting as an adjunctive, inexpensive, and rarely iatrogenic method for helping resolve this prevalent problem.

SUMMARY

Although a debilitating and sometimes fatal illness, depression is treatable and responds to antidepressant and other modes of therapy in the vast majority of cases. All members of the team must take part both in finding the cases and ensuring the patient's adequate treatment. All involved professionals must respond to the great need that exists for better education about depression, using widely available professional and lay resources.[37] Family involvement is crucial, not only in identifying the illness and assisting in compliance, but also in reporting back to the physician on whether the target symptoms of depression are resolving. Depression is often comingled with many other medical and social problems, so clinicians in primary care must become expert at initial treatment with antidepressants and knowledgeable about the indications for psychiatric consultation and hospitalization when necessary.

ACKNOWLEDGMENT

The author is indebted to Richard Ham, MD, for provision of material used in this chapter, including tables without citations.

References

1. Koenig HG, Blazer DG. Epidemiology of geriatric affective disorders. Clin Geriatr Med 8(2):235, 1992.
2. Prestidge BR, Lake CR. Prevalence and recognition of depression among primary care outpatients. J Fam Pract 25(1):67, 1987.
3. Parmelee PA, Katz IR, Lawton MP. Incidence of depression in long-term care settings. J Gerontol 47:M189, 1992.
4. Rousseau P. Suicide in later life and its risk factors.. Clin Geriatr 3(7):41, 1995.
5. Blazer D. Depression in the elderly. N Engl J Med 320(3): 164, 1989.
6. Ham RJ, Myers B. Late Life Depression and Suicide Potential. Washington, DC: American Association of Retired Persons, 1993.
7. McCullough PK. Geriatric depression: atypical presentations, hidden meanings. Geriatrics 46(10):72, 1991.
8. Feightner JW, Worrall G. Early detection of depression by primary care physicians. CMAJ 142(11):1215, 1990.
9. American Psychiatric Association. Diagnostic and Statistical Manual of Mental Disorders (DSM-IV). 4th ed. Washington, DC: American Psychiatric Association, 1994.
10. NIH Consensus Conference. Diagnosis and treatment of depression in late life. JAMA 268(8):1018, 1992.
11. Drugs for psychiatric disorders. Med Lett 36(933): 89, 1994.
12. Yesavage J. Depression in the elderly. Postgrad Med 91(1):255, 1992.
13. Sewitch MJ, Blais R, Rahme E, Galarneau S, Bexton B. Pharmacotherapy for late-life depression: a population study in Quebec. American Psychosomatic Society 64th Annual Scientific Meeting, Vancouver, Canada. Psychosomatic Med 2005;67(1):A-52.

14. Kane RL, Ouslander JG, Abrass IB, eds. Essentials of Clinical Geriatrics. 4th ed. New York: McGraw-Hill, 1999.
15. Levenson AJ, Hall RCW, eds. Neuropsychiatric Manifestations of Physical Disorders in the Elderly. New York: Raven Press, 1981.
16. Sheikh JL, Yesavage JA. Geriatric Depression Scale (GDS): recent evidence and development of a shorter version. Clin Gerontol 5:165, 1986.
17. Radloff L. Depression Test. Center for Epidemiologic Studies, National Institute of Mental Health, 1977.
18. Koenig HG, et al. A brief depression scale for use in the medically ill. Int J Psychiatry Med 22(2):183, 1992.
19. Hirschfeld R, Russell JM. Assessment and treatment of suicidal patients. N Engl J Med 1997;337:910-5.
20. Morley JE, Kraenzle D. Causes of weight loss in a community nursing home. Am Geriatr Soc 42(6):583, 1994.
21. Ham RJ. Indicators of poor nutritional status in older Americans. Am Fam Physician 45(1):219, 1992.
22. Cohen D. Dementia, depression and nutritional status. In Ham RJ, ed. Nutrition in old age: primary care clinics in office practice. Vol. 21. Philadelphia: WB Saunders: 1994.
23. Shearer SI, Adams GK. Nonpharmacologic aids in the treatment of depression. Am Fam Physician 47(2):435, 1993.
24. Reynolds CF III. Treatment of depression in late life. Am J Med 97(suppl 6A):39S, 1994.
25. Rovner BW. Depression and increased risk of mortality in the nursing home patient. Am J Med 95(suppl 5A):19S, 1993.
26. Stewart JT. Diagnosing and treating the hospitalized elderly. Geriatrics 46(1):64, 71, 1991.
27. Baldwin, RC,, et al.Guideline for the management of late-life depression in primary care. Int J Geriatr Psychiatry 2003;18(9):829-38.
28. Wells KB, et al. Use of minor tranquilizers and antidepressant medications by depressed outpatients: results from the medical outcomes study. Am J Psychiatry 151(5):694, 1994.
29. Nierenberg AA, et al. Trazodone for antidepressant-associated insomnia. Am J Psychiatry 151(7):1069, 1994.
30. Old Age Depression Interest Group. How long should the elderly take antidepressants? A double-blind placebo-controlled study of continuation/prophylaxis therapy with dothiepin. Br J Psychiatry 162:175, 1993.
31. Cadieux RJ. Geriatric psychopharmacology: a primary care challenge. Postgrad Med 93(4):281, 1993.
32. Joffe RT, et al. A placebo-controlled comparison of lithium and triiodothyronine augmentation of tricyclic antidepressants in unipolar refractory depression. Arch Gen Psychiatry 50(5):387, 1993.
33. Nelson JC. Combined treatment strategies in psychiatry. J Clin Psychiatry 54(suppl):42, 55, 1993.
34. Genhart MJ, et al. Effects of bright light on mood in normal elderly women. Psychiatry Res 47:87, 1993.
35. Kripke DF, et al. Controlled trial of bright light for nonseasonal major depressive disorders. Biol Psychiatry 31:119, 1992.
36. Chung YS, Dhaghestani AN. Seasonal affective disorder: shedding light on a dark subject. Postgrad Med 86(5):309, 1989.
37. National Institute of Mental Health: If You're Over 65 and Feeling Depressed . . . Treatment Brings New Hope. – Washington, DC: U.S. Department of Health and Human Services, 1990.

Web Resources

National Mental Health Association: www.nmha.org.
National Institute of Mental Health: www.nimh.nih.gov/.
National Mental Health Information Center: www.mentalhealth.samhsa.gov/.

POSTTEST

1. Referral to a psychiatrist or geriatric medicine specialist should be considered in all of the following situations except for:
a. A depressed patient develops increased nervousness after 3 weeks of fluoxetine therapy.
b. A depressed elderly white man expresses suicidal thoughts.
c. A depressed patient continues to have inadequate oral intake despite antidepressant therapy.
d. A depressed patient fails to respond to an adequate trial of two different classes of antidepressants.

2. Diagnostic evaluation to rule out medical causes of depressive symptoms should include all of the following except for:
a. Thyroid-stimulating hormone
b. Complete blood count
c. CT brain scan
d. Electrolytes

3. Which one of the following statements regarding depression is false?
a. ECT is one of the safest and most effective treatments for depression in the elderly.
b. Although safer than the tricyclics, SSRIs are slower to cause a treatment response.
c. Depression in the elderly often shows as chronic pain.
d. Persons who have a good response to an antidepressant should receive continued therapy for 9 to 12 months.

4. Orthostatic hypotension may be a serious side effect of all of the following antidepressants except:
a. Amitriptyline
b. Trazodone
c. Nortriptyline
d. Bupropion

PRETEST ANSWERS
1. a
2. a
3. d
4. d

POSTTEST ANSWERS
1. a
2. c
3. b
4. d

CHAPTER 18

Gait and Mobility

Allon Goldberg and Neil B. Alexander

OBJECTIVES

Upon completion of this chapter, the reader will be able to:

- Discuss the prevalence of gait/mobility deficits in older adults.
- List some of the deleterious impacts of gait disorders on the health of older adults.
- Discuss risk factors for mobility/gait deficits in older adults.
- Describe common diagnoses and impairments contributing to gait disorders in older adults.
- Formulate a differential diagnosis to determine the cause of a gait disorder in older adults.
- Describe and discuss some of the low-tech performance-based measures used to evaluate gait and mobility in the older adult.
- Describe and discuss some of the management options, including treatment outcomes, for gait and mobility deficits in the older adult.

PRETEST

1. Mr. Jones, a 67-year-old man, arrives at your clinic complaining of difficulty walking. He reports no pain in the hip. Among other things, your clinical examination reveals that he has marked weakness of the right hip abductors. The most likely gait pattern he exhibits is:
   a. Antalgic gait
   b. Steppage gait
   c. Trendelenburg gait

2. As part of your clinical examination of Mr. Jones, you wish to determine whether he has a leg length discrepancy. With the patient in the supine position, the accepted method of determining leg length is to measure the distance between the following anatomical landmarks:
   a. Anterior inferior iliac spine and the medial malleolus
   b. Anterior superior iliac spine and the medial malleolus
   c. Anterior superior iliac spine and the lateral malleolus

3. Mr. Jones tells you that although he did not fall this time, he has fallen in the past. A useful and easy-to-administer test of functional mobility and falls risk in the older adult is the Timed Up and Go (TUG) test. You administer the test on Mr. Jones. A TUG that may be predictive of a fall is:
   a. ≥14 seconds
   b. 12 to 13 seconds
   c. 10 to 11 seconds

Ms. Henderson, *Part 1*

Ms. Henderson is a 78-year-old patient in your practice. She has had depression, backache, and neck pain for years, has a 1-year history of left hip pain on ambulation, and reports a recent onset of intermittent confusion. You have managed her depression and arthritic pain with an SSRI antidepressant and anti-inflammatory medications. At your suggestion she has been ambulating with a quad-cane for the past year as needed. Six months ago you referred her to an orthopedic surgeon, who concurred with your diagnosis of moderately severe osteoarthritis of the hip and recommended a trial of physical therapy. She attended outpatient physical therapy three times a week for a month, and had some relief with range of motion and strengthening exercises, although some residual pain remained. She now reports that the pain has become severe over the past 3 months, and that the exacerbation coincided with a fall at home 3 months ago. She went to the emergency room after the fall, but radiographs revealed no fractures. She reports no loss of consciousness after the fall. She is currently on multiple medications for pain, including acetaminophen with codeine and a PRN muscle relaxant. Her chief complaints today are pain in the hip during ambulation, and headache and neck pain.

Your examination reveals a score of 22 on the Mini-Mental State Examination, with decreased attention and disorientation, suggestive of delirium. Her score on the Geriatric Depression Scale is 8, suggesting mild residual depression. Range of motion of the left hip is decreased when compared to the right hip, and all hip motions elicit pain. Her TUG score is 14 seconds, indicating increased risk for a fall. She is tender on palpation of the neck musculature, with reduced range of motion and pain on neck flexion and rotation. You order radiographs of the neck, which show signs of degenerative joint disease.

STUDY QUESTIONS

1. What diagnoses would you place on her problem list?
2. What would you do next?

PREVALENCE AND IMPACT

The term *mobility* may encompass a variety of functional activities including transfers to and from a bed and chair, walking, stair climbing, getting in and out of vehicles, and others.[1] Difficulty ambulating and problems with general mobility are frequent complaints of older adults. Each year about 1 in every 100 older adults develops new severe mobility disability, defined as the inability to walk across a small room or the need for help from another person to do so.[2] Approximately 20% of noninstitutionalized older adults admit to having trouble walking or require assistance from another person or equipment to ambulate,[3] and the prevalence of limitations in walking in noninstitutionalized adults 85 years and older can exceed 54%.[3]

The impact of gait and mobility deficits can be devastating for the older adult. Impairments in gait and mobility are associated with depressive symptoms,[4] falls,[5] functional dependence,[6,7] and death.[1,6]

> ● Approximately 20% of noninstitutionalized older adults admit to having trouble walking or require assistance from another person or equipment to ambulate, and the prevalence of limitations in walking in noninstitutionalized adults 85 years and older can exceed 54%.

RISK FACTORS AND PATHOPHYSIOLOGY

Many adults maintain normal or near normal gait and mobility well into old age. Thus, gait and mobility dysfunctions are not an inevitable consequence of aging, as is often thought, but in many cases are a reflection of chronic diseases[8] or of recent or remote trauma. Age-related declines in gait speed are well documented, and are due to decreases in stride length, rather than decrease in cadence (steps per minute).[9] Shorter, broader strides, longer stance, and shorter swing durations are some of the gait characteristics apparent after age 75 or 80.[10,11]

Often the cause of a gait disorder is multifactorial. Among the common contributing factors are:

- Chronic diseases, such as osteoarthritis, sensory impairment, Parkinsonism, and a variety of vascular disorders (Table 18–1).[12]
- Fear of falling, often with consequent deconditioning.
- Brain changes, such as ventricular enlargement, white matter hyperintensities, and subcortical and basal ganglia infarcts—frequent findings on magnetic resonance imaging (MRI) studies of the brain of older adults, each of which as been associated with declines in gait speed.[13,14]
- Reduced lower extremity power and strength. Loss of muscle mass (sarcopenia) is common in old age and is primarily due to decreases in size and number of type II (fast-twitch) muscle fibers.[15-17] As fast-twitch fibers are functionally associated with strength and power activities, the loss of these fibers explains at least partially, both the decreases in strength and velocity of muscle contractions in older adults.
- Coimpairments, such as when leg weakness is found in the patient with balance deficits, may have a greater effect on deficits in mobility than the sum of the single impairments.[18]

Table 18–1	Diagnoses Contributing to Gait Abnormalities in Primary Care Geriatrics	
Primary Diagnosis Contributing to Gait Disorder		**Percentage**
Degenerative joint disease/gouty arthritis		43
Sensory imbalances (e.g., peripheral neuropathy)		9
Parkinsonism		9
Orthostatic hypertension		9
Intermittent claudication		6
Postcerebrovascular accident		6
Congenital deformity		6
Postorthopedic surgery		3
Vertebrobasilar insufficiency		3
Heart disease		3
Idiopathic gait disorder: fear of falling		3
Total		100

Adapted from Hough JC, McHenry MP, Kammer LM. Gait disorders in the elderly. Am Fam Physician 1987;35(6):191–6, with permission.

DIFFERENTIAL DIAGNOSIS AND ASSESSMENT

One way of organizing a differential diagnosis for a gait disorder is to consider three levels of sensorimotor function: peripheral, subcortical, and cortical. Table 18–2 outlines for each of the three sensorimotor levels the most common conditions and the gait char-

acteristics presenting for each condition.[19] To this must be added consideration of diseases of other organ systems that commonly affect gait. Finally, one must consider whether medication-related effects are a contributor.

Peripheral sensorimotor deficits are divided into sensory and motor dysfunction, and include musculoskeletal

Table 18-2	Classification of Gait Disorders by Sensorimotor Level		
Sensorimotor Level	**Within-Level Classification**	**Condition (Pathology, Symptoms, Signs)**	**Typical Gait Characteristics**
Peripheral	Peripheral sensory	Sensory ataxia (posterior column, peripheral nerves)	Unsteady, uncoordinated, especially without visual input
		Vestibular ataxia	Unsteady, weaving ("drunken")
		Visual ataxia	Tentative, uncertain
	Peripheral motor	Arthritic (antalgic, joint deformity)	Avoids weight bearing on affected side, shorten stance phase
			Painful hip may produce "Trendelenburg" (trunk shift over affected side)
			Painful knee is flexed
			Painful spine produces short, slow steps and decreased lumbar lordosis
			Other nonantalgic features: contractures, deformity-limited motion, buckling with weight bearing
			Kyphosis and ankylosing spondylosis produce stooped posture
			Unequal leg length can produce trunk and pelvic motion abnormalities (including "Trendelenburg")
		Myopathic and neuropathic (weakness)	Pelvic girdle weakness produces exaggerated lumbar lordosis and lateral trunk flexion ("Trendelenburg" and "waddling" gait)
			Proximal motor neuropathy produces "waddling" and "foot slap"
			Distal motor neuropathy produces distal weakness (especially ankle dorsiflexion, "foot drop"), which may lead to exaggerated hip flexion, knee flexion and foot lifting ("steppage gait") and "foot slap"
Subcortical	Spasticity	Hemiplegia/paresis	Leg swings outward and in semicircle from hip ("circumduction"). Knee may hyperextend ("genu recurvatum"), and ankle may excessively plantar flex and invert ("equinovarus"). With less paresis, some may only lose arm swing and only drag or scrape the foot
		Paraplegia/paresis	Both legs circumduct, steps are short shuffling and scraping, and when severe, hip adducts so that knees cross in front of each other ("scissoring")
	Parkinsonism		Small shuffling steps, hesitation, acceleration ("festination"), falling forward ("propulsion"), falling backward ("retropulsion"), moving the whole body while turning ("turning en bloc"), absent arm swing
	Cerebellar ataxia		Wide-based with increased trunk sway, irregular stepping, staggering, especially on turns
Cortical	Cautious gait		Fear of falling with appropriate postural responses, normal to widened base, shortened stride, decreased velocity, and en bloc turns
	Frontal-related gait disorders, other white matter lesions	Cerebrovascular, normal pressure hydrocephalus	Frontal gait disorder: difficulty initiating gait and short shuffling gait similar to Parkinson's but wider base, upright posture, preservation of arm swing, leg apraxia, may freeze with diversion of attention or turning
			May also have cognitive, pyramidal, and urinary disturbances

Adapted from Alexander NB. Differential diagnosis of gait disorders in older adults. Clin Geriatr Med 1996;12(4):689–703, with permission.

(arthritic) and myopathic/neuropathic disorders (i.e., disorders distal to the central nervous system). With peripheral sensory impairment, unsteady and tentative gait is common; causes include vestibular disorders, peripheral neuropathy, posterior column (proprioceptive) deficits, and visual impairment. With peripheral motor impairment, a number of classical gait patterns emerge, including obvious compensatory strategies. Examples of these strategies include: Trendelenburg gait (hip abductor weakness causing weight shift over the weak hip); antalgic gait (avoidance of excessive weight bearing and shortening of stance on one side due to pain); and steppage gait (excessive hip flexion facilitating foot clearance of the ground in patients with foot drop due to ankle dorsiflexor weakness). These conditions involve extremity (both body segment and joint) deformities, painful weight bearing, and focal myopathic and neuropathic weakness. Note that if the gait disorder is limited to this low sensorimotor level (i.e., the central nervous system is intact), the person can adapt well to the gait disorder, compensating with an assistive device or learning to negotiate the environment safely.

Subcortical sensorimotor deficits result from lesions of the midbrain, brainstem, cerebellum, and spinal cord. At the middle level, the execution of centrally selected postural and locomotor responses is faulty, and the sensory and motor modulation of gait is disrupted. Gait may be initiated normally, but stepping patterns are abnormal. Examples include diseases causing spasticity (such as related to myelopathy, B_{12} deficiency, and stroke), Parkinsonism (idiopathic as well as drug induced), and cerebellar disease (such as alcohol induced). Classical gait patterns appear when the spasticity is sufficient to cause leg circumduction and fixed deformities (such as equinovarus), when Parkinsonism produces shuffling steps and reduced arm swing, and when cerebellar ataxia increases trunk sway sufficiently to require a broad base of gait support.

Cortical sensorimotor deficits often involve cognitive dysfunction and slowed cognitive processing. Gait characteristics tend to be nonspecific. Behavioral factors such as fear of falling are also important, particularly in cautious gait. The presence of dementia and depression are often major contributors. Frontal-related gait disorders tend to have a cerebrovascular component but may also result from dementia, normal pressure hydrocephalus, or a frontal mass. The severity of the frontal-related disorders run a spectrum from gait ignition failure, that is, difficulty with initiation, to frontal dysequilibrium, where unsupported stance is not possible. Cerebrovascular insults to the cortex and/or basal ganglia and their inter-connections may relate to gait ignition failure and apraxia.[20,21] Cognitive, pyramidal, and urinary disturbances may also accompany the gait disorder. Gait disorders that might fall in this category have been given a number of overlapping descriptions, including gait apraxia, *marché a petits pas*, and arteriosclerotic (vascular) Parkinsonism.

Other diseases and impairments may contribute to decreases in gait speed. They are frequently associated with cardiopulmonary or musculoskeletal disease, and include reductions in leg strength, vision, aerobic function, standing balance, and physical activity, as well as joint impairments, previous falls, and fear of falling.[18,22-27] Other less common diagnoses and factors contributing to gait disorders include metabolic disorders related to renal or hepatic disease, tumors of the central nervous system, subdural hematoma, depression, and psychotropic medications. Hypo- and hyper-thyroidism and B_{12} and folate deficiency may also be associated with reversible gait disorders (reviewed in Alexander[9]).

Approach to Patient Assessment

Patients consider pain, stiffness, dizziness, numbness, weakness, and sensations of abnormal movement to be the most common impairments contributing to walking difficulty.[12] In many cases, the older adult presents with a gait disorder as a manifestation of acute or chronic disease (or in some cases, diseases). Thus, the aim of the primary care practitioner should be to diagnose the underlying disease state to determine whether the gait disorder is cardiovascular, musculoskeletal, or neurological in etiology, or due to some other pathology. Components of the clinical assessment can include the traditional history and physical examination, performance-based assessments, and laboratory and imaging tests. All of these will assist the primary care practitioner in formulating a clinical and/or impairment-based diagnosis as it relates to the gait dysfunction.

> ● Thus, the aim of the primary care practitioner should be to diagnose the underlying disease state to determine whether the gait disorder is cardiovascular, musculoskeletal, or neurological in etiology, or due to some other pathology.

History and Physical Examination

The evaluation should begin with a careful medical history (Box 18–1). Inquire as to past medical history including history of injuries, accidents, and falls, as these may predispose the older adult to a mobility disorder. Determine if the patient uses an assistive device and if their level of physical activity is as expected in comparison to age-matched individuals. Enquire if they are fearful of falling, as this may cause the older adult to limit activity levels. Review medications including adherence to the prescribed regimen. A systems review is conducted to elucidate the multiple factors

---

Box 18-1   History Checklist for Patients Presenting with Falls or Mobility Problems

The in-depth history should include the following elements:

- Past medical history including:
  - History of injuries, accidents
  - Falls (recently and past 12 months)
  - History of diseases and surgeries (recent and longer term)
  - Hospitalizations
- Social/functional history including:
  - Home: levels and steps to enter, modifications
  - Lives alone, or with someone
  - Uses of assistive device
  - Usual level of activity (times leaves home per week)

- Review of systems including:
  - Acute illness (infection/sepsis)
  - Auditory: difficulty hearing, vertigo/dizziness, Meniere's disease
  - Visual: visual impairments, cataracts, glaucoma
  - Cardiopulmonary: shortness of breath, chest pain
  - Neurological: lower extremity sensory changes, numbness/tingling, muscle weakness, poor balance/unsteadiness during standing and walking
  - Musculoskeletal: joint/muscle pain, stiffness, feeling of joint instability "giving way", difficulty walking

---

potentially contributing to the gait disorder. Systemic evaluation should include evaluation for acute cardiopulmonary disorders such as myocardial infarction, and other acute illness such as sepsis, because an acute gait disorder may be the presenting feature of acute illness in the older adult. Review auditory and visual systems, inquiring as to hearing and visual impairments, including Meniere's disease, vertigo, cataracts, and glaucoma. For the neurological and musculoskeletal systems, inquire as to lower extremity sensory changes including numbness and tingling, joint and muscle pain, stiffness, joint instability, or muscle weakness limiting the patient's mobility during performance of daily activites such as ambulation, poor balance, and unsteadiness, including dizziness during upright posture and gait. Evidence of subacute metabolic disease (such as thyroid disorders) also warrants evaluation.

The physical examination (Box 18–2) should entail a thorough evaluation of the patient's gait pattern, and should begin when the patient enters the room.[28] The

---

Box 18-2   Physical Examination Checklist for Patients Presenting with Falls or Mobility Problems

Gait Examination

- Observe the patient's gait pattern beginning as she or he enters the room
- Initially observe generally to gain an overall impression and to determine if there are problems with:
  - Gait initiation; unsteadiness, short shuffling steps
  - Asymmetric weight distribution and poor toe clearance
- Then observe patient's gait in detail from behind, in front, and the sides. Observe from proximal to distal motions at lumbar spine and pelvis down to the foot. The following should be noted:
  - Sideways swaying of trunk
  - Bowing of femur or tibia
  - Medial/lateral hip rotations
  - Abduction or circumduction of lower extremity
  - Width of base of support
  - Foot position (toe and heel in or out)
  - Step and stride length deficiencies
- Check for classical gait abnormalities (see text):
  Trendelenburg gait
  Gluteus maximus lurch

- Steppage gait
- Ataxic gait

Physical Examination Procedures

- Identify motion-related deficits:
  - Vestibular
  - Orthostatic
- Musculoskeletal: evaluate neck, spine, extremities for:
  - Pain
  - Deformities
  - Range of motion (including contractures at hip and knee)
  - Leg length discrepancies
- Neurological: include evaluation of:
  - Strength
  - Muscle tone
  - Reflexes
  - Sensation including proprioception
  - Coordination
  - Balance
  - Ambulation
- Evaluation of other systems as necessary (e.g., cardiovascular, visual)

examiner should first get an overall impression of the gait; does it seem abnormal? In this initial impression, one should consider global gait problems such as difficulty with initiation, unsteadiness, short or shuffling steps, asymmetric weight distribution, and poor toe clearance. Then a closer inspection is warranted, observing the patient's gait pattern from the front, behind, and sides, in each instance from proximal to distal the motions at the pelvis and lumbar spine down to the ankle and foot.[29] Observation from the front and behind enables the examiner to observe sideways swaying of the trunk, bowing of the femur or tibia, medial or lateral hip rotations, abduction or circumduction actions of the lower extremity during swing phase, width of the base of support, and foot position (toe and heel in or out). The classical Trendelenburg gait, in which there is weakness of the hip abductors (gluteus medius muscle), is characterized by trunk shift over the affected hip and is best visualized from behind or in front of the patient.[28,29] Observation of the patient's gait from the side enables the examiner to detect stride and step length deficiencies as well as motions of the trunk and lower extremity in the sagittal plane, including the extensor or gluteus maximus lurch in which the patient thrusts the trunk posteriorly to compensate for weak hip extensors (gluteus maximus muscle).[28,29] Observation from the side also enables detection of ankle dorsiflexor weakness and footdrop leading to inability of the foot to clear the ground, which is compensated for by excessive lower extremity flexion to facilitate foot clearance of the ground (steppage gait).[28,29]

The physical examination should include an attempt to identify motion-related factors, such as by provoking both vestibular and orthostatic responses. Visual screening should be performed. Musculoskeletal examination should include evaluation of the neck, spine, extremities, and feet for pain, deformities, and limitations in active and passive range of motion, particularly regarding subtle hip and/or knee contractures. Leg length discrepancies may occur post–hip prosthesis,[30] and can be measured with the patient in supine as the distance from the anterior superior iliac spine to the medial malleolus. The neurological assessment should include assessment of strength, tone, reflexes, sensation (including proprioception), coordination (including cerebellar function), balance, and station and gait. Balance assessment should include determination of unipedal stance time, as a time of less than 5 seconds is an indicator of increased risk for an injurious fall.[31] The Romberg test screens for simple postural control and whether the proprioceptive and vestibular systems are functional when the eyes are closed. Screening for mental status is also indicated.

> ● The physical examination should entail a thorough evaluation of the patient's gait pattern, and should begin when the patient enters the room.

Performance-Based Assessments

Timed or scored functional gait and mobility tests are used in clinical settings to detect deficits in gait and mobility. These measures are valid and low tech, making them easy to use by virtually all levels of appropriately trained personnel. They are usually quick to administer, and generally require little to no equipment other than a stopwatch. They are useful in that not only can they detect deficits in mobility, but they also can be used to track progress and response to pharmacological or physical therapy interventions. Selection of the measure will depend on the level of participant ambulation impairment (e.g., community ambulator versus homebound) and the need for simple (e.g., busy clinic or hospital setting) versus more time-consuming but informative multiple task assessments (e.g., rehabilitation setting). Table 18–3 summarizes known characteristics of these tests. A few tests that are particularly useful in the primary care setting are described below.

USUAL AND MAXIMAL GAIT SPEED

Usual walking speed over distances as short as 5 m has been shown to predict functional disability in people aged 75 and older.[7] Determination of slow (<0.6 meters/second) versus fast (>1.0 meter/second) walking status is useful in predicting hospitalization and functional decline.[32] Comfortable gait speed over a 5-m distance is thought to be particularly capable of detecting clinically relevant change (e.g., post-stroke).[33]

PERFORMANCE-ORIENTED MOBILITY ASSESSMENT (POMA)

Also known as the Tinetti Balance and Gait Scale, the POMA is one of the earliest and most widely used batteries designed to assess balance, gait, and fall risk in older adults. It includes an evaluation of balance under perturbed conditions (such as while rising from a chair, after a nudge, with eyes closed, and while turning), as well as an evaluation of gait characteristics (including gait initiation, step height, length, continuity and symmetry, trunk sway, and path deviation).[34] A score less than 19 out of 28 has a sensitivity of 68% and a specificity of 88% for predicting an individual who will have two or more falls.[34] There may be a ceiling effect associated with the POMA, even in moderately disabled Parkinson's patients, while gait speed will continue to differentiate subtle changes in functional ability.[35]

Table 18–3	Characteristics of Physical Performance Tests in Older Adults				
Test	**Domain Predicted**	**Sensitivity (%)**	**Specificity (%)**	**Cox Proportional Hazard Ratio[a]**	**Reference Number**
Gait Speed					
Usual gait speed	Functional dependence[b]	—	—	6.18	7
Maximum gait speed	Functional dependence[b]	—	—	5.15	7
Multiple Tasks Tests					
POMA	Falls	68	88	—	34
TUG	Falls	80	100	—	38

[a]Cox proportional hazard ratio is a measure of risk. Lowest performance levels on the "usual gait speed" test are associated with a 6.18-fold increased risk for functional dependence compared with highest performance levels on the test. The higher the ratio, the greater the risk for functional dependence.

[b]Functional dependence is defined as a new disability in one or more of the five basic activities of daily living, or death.

POMA, Performance-Oriented Mobility Assessment, used to assess balance, gait, and fall risk in older adults; TUG, Timed Up and Go, an indicator of functional mobility and dynamic stability, including falls risk in older adults.

TIMED UP AND GO

An indicator of functional mobility and dynamic stability, the TUG test measures the time taken to stand up from a chair with armrests, walk 3 m, turn, walk back to the chair, and sit down.[36] Difficulty and/or unsteadiness in TUG performance is recognized as an important part of fall risk assessment.[37] A cut-off score of 14 seconds or greater has been proposed as predictive for falls.[38] With its simplicity in administration and scoring, the TUG is particularly relevant to primary care.

Laboratory and Imaging Tests

Laboratory and radiological testing may be warranted, depending on the findings of the history and physical examination. Complete blood count, blood chemistries, and other metabolic studies may be useful when systemic disease is suspected. If neurologic symptoms or signs were identified in the history and physical examination, head and spine x-rays, computed tomography, or magnetic resonance imaging may be needed, and additional tests such as electromyography and nerve conduction studies considered. Brain neuroimaging helps rule out ventricular enlargement, white matter hyperintensities, and subcortical and basal ganglia infarcts, each of which has been associated with gait abnormalities.[13,39] Age-specific guidelines, sensitivity, specificity, and cost-effectiveness of these workups remain to be determined.

MANAGEMENT

Treatable medical problems, such as medication side effects, B_{12} deficiency, folate deficiency, hypothyroidism, hyperthyroidism, knee osteoarthritis, Parkinson's disease, and inflammatory polyneuropathy, show improvement as a result of medical therapy.[9] However, many conditions predisposing the older adult to a gait disorder are only partially treatable, and the patient is often left with some degree of disability. In these patients, functional outcomes, such as reduction in weight-bearing pain, improvement in walking distance, or reductions in overall walking limitation, are the most relevant outcomes to seek (and evaluate) in treating patients with gait disorders.

Exercise and Gait Training

A variety of modes of physical therapy for diseases such as knee osteoarthritis and stroke result in modest improvement. In patients with knee osteoarthritis, a combined aerobic, strength, and functionally based group exercise program caused a 5% increase in gait speed.[40] The focus of exercise programs is on strengthening the extensor groups (especially knee and hip extensors) and stretching commonly shortened muscles (such as the hip flexors[41]). Using a body weight support and a treadmill to provide-task specific gait training post–total hip arthroplasty,[42] in Parkinson's disease[43] and particularly in hemiparetics post-stroke,[44] can lead to incremental reductions of gait impairment. Parkinson's gait disorders are often minimally responsive to physical therapy,[45] but audio and visual cueing can improve gait speed.[46]

Participation in exercise groups can provide motivation for patients. A number of studies have demonstrated improvements in gait parameters such as gait speed, with the most consistent effects occurring when varied types of exercise are provided in the same program.[47-49] A 12-week combined program of leg resistance, standing balance, and flexibility exercises increased usual gait speed 8% in minimally impaired community residents.[47] A similar varied 16-week format with more intensive individual support and prompting in select demented older adults (mean MMSE 15) resulted in a 23% improvement in gait speed.[48]

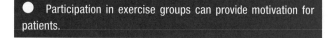

● Participation in exercise groups can provide motivation for patients.

Behavioral and Environmental Modifications

Improved lighting (particularly for those with vestibular or sensory impairment) and avoidance of pathway hazards (such as clutter, wires, and slippery floors) are some behavioral and environmental modifications that can be used to make the environment safer for the older adult with a mobility disorder. Light touch of any firm surface such as walls or furniture provides proprioceptive feedback that can often enhance balance.[50,51]

Shoes, Orthoses, and Assistive Devices

In general, to maximize balance and improve gait, well-fitting walking shoes with low heels, relatively thin firm soles, and if feasible, high, fixed heel collar support are recommended.[52] Assistive devices such as canes and walkers reduce load on a painful joint and improve stability.[53]

Use of orthoses and assistive devices may help ameliorate the effects of many gait disorders. While there are few data supporting their use, lifts (either internal or external) to correct for limb length inequality may be helpful; they should be provided in a conservative, gradually progressive manner.[54] Ankle braces, shoe inserts, shoe body and sole modifications, and their subsequent adjustments are part of standard care for foot and ankle weakness, deformities, and pain.[55]

Surgical Management

The role of surgery in the management of gait disorders is unclear. Improvement with some residual disability is commonly reported after surgical treatment for compressive cervical myelopathy, lumbar stenosis, and normal-pressure hydrocephalus. However, few controlled prospective studies and virtually no randomized studies address the outcome of surgical versus nonsurgical treatment for these disorders.

There are generally better outcomes for hip and knee replacement surgery for osteoarthritis than for surgery of the above conditions, although these studies have some of the same methodological problems. Pain relief and sizable gains in gait speed and joint motion occur, although residual walking disability may continue for a number of reasons, including residual pathology on the operated side and symptoms on the nonoperated side. For total knee replacements, despite rehabilitation postoperatively, some residual weakness, stiffness, and slowed/altered gait may remain.[56,57] Simple function may be maintained post–knee replacement, such as maintaining the ability to clear an obstacle safely, but this is usually at the expense of additional compensation by the ipsilateral hip and foot.[58]

Ms. Henderson, *Part 2*

Your initial diagnoses are depression, delirium (possibly medication induced), difficulty walking due to pain from hip osteoarthritis, and chronic headache, possibly associated with cervical spine arthritis. Your initial management is as follows: referral to the orthopedic surgeon for left hip arthroplasty, antidepressant medication, and reassessment and removal of some pain medications (especially the codeine and the muscle relaxant). To reduce the likelihood of gastrointestinal side effects, you reserve anti-inflammatory medications for exacerbations of neck symptoms, and prescribe around-the-clock acetaminophen for routine pain. Also, you document in your note that, if these do not provide relief, you plan on referring her to a physical therapist specializing in manual therapy for further management of her neck/headache symptoms.

Your patient undergoes a left hip arthroplasty and, after discharge from the acute care hospital, 12 days of inpatient rehabilitation. She is educated in the precautions necessary to avoid hip dislocation, and engages in ambulation as tolerated with a walker, isometric and range of motion exercises, and transfer training. After discharge from inpatient rehabilitation, she receives 6 weeks of outpatient physical therapy for gait and lower extremity training.

She progresses satisfactorily in outpatient physical therapy showing significant improvements in lower extremity strength, range of motion, and ambulation on level ground and up and down stairs. Her pain level has decreased significantly, but she elects to continue ambulation with the quad-cane for safety. At the surgeon's instructions, she adheres to the hip dislocation precautions for at least 12 weeks. Six weeks postsurgery she sees you for follow-up. At that visit she displays no confusion and reports minimal headache/neck pain. She reports no loss of balance since the fall nearly 6 months ago.

POSTTEST

1. Ms. Smith is a 75-year-old patient with a history of falls. She consults you today after falling approximately 1 week ago while walking in her apartment. She did not injure herself as a result of that fall, but you are concerned that she may incur an injurious fall at some time in the future. The test result that is most likely to be predictive of an injurious fall is:
   a. TUG of 10 seconds
   b. Unipedal stance time of 4 seconds
   c. Gait speed of 0.7 msec

2. After total hip replacement, it is important that the patient avoid certain motions and positions of the operated extremity in order to avoid dislocation of the prosthesis. The length of time for which these precautions should be adhered to varies according to different orthopedic surgeon's preferences, but is usually:
   a. At least 12 weeks
   b. At least 4 to 6 weeks
   c. At least 2 to 3 weeks

3. Gait speed has been shown to be a strong predictor of disability, hospitalization, and functional decline in older adults. The speed considered to indicate gait impairment and which is predictive of functional decline is:
   a. 0.9 to 1.0 m/sec
   b. 0.6 to 0.8 m/sec
   c. <0.6 m/sec

References

1. Khokhar SR, Stern Y, Bell K, et al. Persistent mobility deficit in the absence of deficits in activities of daily living: a risk factor for mortality. J Am Geriatr Soc 2001;49(11):1539-43.
2. Guralnik JM, Ferrucci L, Balfour JL, Volpato S, Di Iorio A. Progressive versus catastrophic loss of the ability to walk: implications for the prevention of mobility loss. J Am Geriatr Soc 2001;49(11):1463-70.
3. Ostchega Y, Harris TB, Hirsch R, Parsons VL, Kington R. The prevalence of functional limitations and disability in older persons in the US: data from the National Health and Nutrition Examination Survey III. J Am Geriatr Soc 2000;48(9):1132-5.
4. Lampinen P, Heikkinen E. Reduced mobility and physical activity as predictors of depressive symptoms among community-dwelling older adults: an eight-year follow-up study. Aging Clin Exp Res 2003;15(3):205-11.
5. Menz HB, Lord SR. The contribution of foot problems to mobility impairment and falls in community-dwelling older people. J Am Geriatr Soc 2001;49(12):1651-6.
6. Hirvensalo M, Rantanen T, Heikkinen E. Mobility difficulties and physical activity as predictors of mortality and loss of independence in the community-living older population. J Am Geriatr Soc 2000;48(5):493-8.
7. Shinkai S, Watanabe S, Kumagai S, et al. Walking speed as a good predictor for the onset of functional dependence in a Japanese rural community population. Age Ageing 2000;29(5):441-6.
8. Bloem BR, Haan J, Lagaay AM, van Beek W, Wintzen AR, Roos RA. Investigation of gait in elderly subjects over 88 years of age. J Geriatr Psychiatry Neurol 1992;5(2):78-84.
9. Alexander NB. Gait disorders in older adults. J Am Geriatr Soc 1996;44(4):434-51.
10. Murray MP, Kory RC, Clarkson BH. Walking patterns in healthy old men. J Gerontol 1969;24(2):169-78.
11. Kaneko M, Morimoto Y, Kimura M, Fuchimoto K, Fuchimoto T. A kinematic analysis of walking and physical fitness testing in elderly women. Can J Sport Sci 1991;16(3):223-8.
12. Hough JC, McHenry MP, Kammer LM. Gait disorders in the elderly. Am Fam Physician 1987;35(6):191-6.
13. Rosano C, Kuller LH, Chung H, Arnold AM, Longstreth WT, Jr. Newman AB. Subclinical brain magnetic resonance imaging abnormalities predict physical functional decline in high-functioning older adults. J Am Geriatr Soc 2005;53(4):649-54.
14. Camicioli R, Moore MM, Sexton G, Howieson DB, Kaye JA. Age-related brain changes associated with motor function in healthy older people. J Am Geriatr Soc 1999;47(3):330-4.
15. Frontera WR, Hughes VA, Lutz KJ, Evans WJ. A cross-sectional study of muscle strength and mass in 45- to 78-yr-old men and women. J Appl Physiol 1991;71(2):644-50.
16. Evans WJ. What is sarcopenia? J Gerontol A Biol Sci Med Sci 1995;50:5-8.
17. Candow DG, Chilibeck PD. Differences in size, strength, and power of upper and lower body muscle groups in young and older men. J Gerontol A Biol Sci Med Sci 2005;60(2):148-56.
18. Rantanen T, Guralnik JM, Ferrucci L, Leveille S, Fried LP. Coimpairments: strength and balance as predictors of severe walking disability. J Gerontol A Biol Sci Med Sci 1999;54(4):M172-6.
19. Alexander NB. Differential diagnosis of gait disorders in older adults. Clin Geriatr Med 1996;12(4):689-703.
20. Liston R, Mickelborough J, Bene J, Tallis R. A new classification of higher level gait disorders in patients with cerebral multi-infarct states. Age Ageing 2003;32(2):252-8.
21. Jankovic J, Nutt JG, Sudarsky L. Classification, diagnosis, and etiology of gait disorders. Adv Neurol 2001;87:119-33.
22. Bendall MJ, Bassey EJ, Pearson MB. Factors affecting walking speed of elderly people. Age Ageing 1989;18(5):327-32.
23. Tinetti ME, Mendes de Leon CF, Doucette JT, Baker DI. Fear of falling and fall-related efficacy in relationship to functioning among community-living elders. J Gerontol 1994;49(3):M140-7.
24. Woo J, Ho SC, Lau J, Chan SG, Yuen YK. Age-associated gait changes in the elderly: pathological or physiological? Neuroepidemiology 1995;14(2):65-71.
25. Buchner DM, Cress ME, Esselman PC, et al. Factors associated with changes in gait speed in older adults. J Gerontol A Biol Sci Med Sci 1996;51(6):M297-302.
26. Gibbs J, Hughes S, Dunlop D, Singer R, Chang RW. Predictors of change in walking velocity in older adults. J Am Geriatr Soc 1996;44(2):126-32.
27. de Rekeneire N, Visser M, Peila R, et al. Is a fall just a fall: correlates of falling in healthy older persons. The Health, Aging and Body Composition Study. J Am Geriatr Soc 2003;51(6):841-6.
28. Hoppenfeld S. Physical Examination of the Spine and Extremities. New York: Appleton-Century-Crofts, 1976.
29. Magee DJ. Orthopedic Physical Assessment. 2nd ed. Philadelphia: WB Saunders Company, 1992.
30. Gurney B. Leg length discrepancy. Gait Posture 2002;15(2):195-206.
31. Vellas BJ, Wayne SJ, Romero L, Baumgartner RN, Rubenstein LZ, Garry PJ. One-leg balance is an important predictor of injurious falls in older persons. J Am Geriatr Soc 1997;45(6):735-8.
32. Studenski S, Perera S, Wallace D, et al. Physical performance measures in the clinical setting. J Am Geriatr Soc 2003;51(3):314-22.
33. Salbach NM, Mayo NE, Higgins J, Ahmed S, Finch LE, Richards CL. Responsiveness and predictability of gait speed and other disability measures in acute stroke. Arch Phys Med Rehabil 2001;82(9):1204-12.
34. Tinetti ME, Williams TF, Mayewski R. Fall risk index for elderly patients based on number of chronic disabilities. Am J Med 1986;80(3):429-34.
35. Behrman AL, Light KE, Miller GM. Sensitivity of the Tinetti Gait Assessment for detecting change in individuals with Parkinson's disease. Clin Rehabil 2002;16(4):399-405.
36. Podsiadlo D, Richardson S. The timed "Up & Go": a test of basic functional mobility for frail elderly persons. J Am Geriatr Soc 1991;39(2):142-8.
37. Guideline for the prevention of falls in older persons. American Geriatrics Society, British Geriatrics Society, and American Academy of Orthopaedic Surgeons Panel on Falls Prevention. J Am Geriatr Soc 2001;49(5):664-72.

38. Shumway-Cook A, Brauer S, Woollacott M. Predicting the probability for falls in community-dwelling older adults using the Timed Up & Go Test. Phys Ther 2000;80(9):896-903.

39. Baloh RW, Ying SH, Jacobson KM. A longitudinal study of gait and balance dysfunction in normal older people. Arch Neurol 2003;60(6):835-9.

40. Fransen M, Crosbie J, Edmonds J. Physical therapy is effective for patients with osteoarthritis of the knee: a randomized controlled clinical trial. J Rheumatol 2001;28(1):156-64.

41. Kerrigan DC, Xenopoulos-Oddsson A, Sullivan MJ, Lelas JJ, Riley PO. Effect of a hip flexor-stretching program on gait in the elderly. Arch Phys Med Rehabil 2003;84(1):1-6.

42. Hesse S, Werner C, Seibel H, et al. Treadmill training with partial body-weight support after total hip arthroplasty: a randomized controlled trial. Arch Phys Med Rehabil 2003;84(12):1767-73.

43. Miyai I, Fujimoto Y, Yamamoto H, et al. Long-term effect of body weight-supported treadmill training in Parkinson's disease: a randomized controlled trial. Arch Phys Med Rehabil 2002;83(10):1370-3.

44. Hesse S, Werner C, von Frankenberg S, Bardeleben A. Treadmill training with partial body weight support after stroke. Phys Med Rehabil Clin N Am 2003;14(Suppl 1):S111-23.

45. Deane KHO, Jones D, Playford ED. Physiotherapy versus placebo or no intervention in Parkinson's disease. In: Cochrane Library, Issue 1. Chichester, UK: John Wiley and Sons, 2004.

46. Rubinstein TC, Giladi N, Hausdorff JM. The power of cueing to circumvent dopamine deficits: a review of physical therapy treatment of gait disturbances in Parkinson's disease. Mov Disord 2002;17(6):1148-60.

47. Judge JO, Underwood M, Gennosa T. Exercise to improve gait velocity in older persons. Arch Phys Med Rehabil 1993;74(4):400-6.

48. Toulotte C, Fabre C, Dangremont B, Lensel G, Thevenon A. Effects of physical training on the physical capacity of frail, demented patients with a history of falling: a randomised controlled trial. Age Ageing 2003; 32(1):67-73.

49. Ettinger WH, Jr. Burns R, Messier SP, et al. A randomized trial comparing aerobic exercise and resistance exercise with a health education program in older adults with knee osteoarthritis. The Fitness Arthritis and Seniors Trial (FAST). JAMA 1997;277(1):25-31.

50. Iezzoni LI. A 44-year-old woman with difficulty walking. JAMA 2000; 284(20):2632-9.

51. Jeka JJ. Light touch contact as a balance aid. Phys Ther 1997;77(5):476-87.

52. Menz HB, Lord SR. Footwear and postural stability in older people. J Am Podiatr Med Assoc 1999;89(7):346-57.

53. Van Hook FW, Demonbreun D, Weiss BD. Ambulatory devices for chronic gait disorders in the elderly. Am Fam Physician 15 2003;67(8):1717-24.

54. Brady RJ, Dean JB, Skinner TM, Gross MT. Limb length inequality: clinical implications for assessment and intervention. J Orthop Sports Phys Ther 2003;33(5):221-34.

55. Shrader JA, Siegel KL. Nonoperative management of functional hallux limitus in a patient with rheumatoid arthritis. Phys Ther 2003;83(9): 831-43.

56. Ouellet D, Moffet H. Locomotor deficits before and two months after knee arthroplasty. Arthritis Rheum 2002;47(5):484-93.

57. Benedetti MG, Catani F, Bilotta TW, Marcacci M, Mariani E, Giannini S. Muscle activation pattern and gait biomechanics after total knee replacement. Clin Biomech (Bristol, Avon) 2003;18(9):871-6.

58. Byrne JM, Prentice SD. Swing phase kinetics and kinematics of knee replacement patients during obstacle avoidance. Gait Posture 2003;18(1):95-104.

PRETEST ANSWERS

1. c
2. b
3. a

POSTTEST ANSWERS

1. b
2. a
3. c

OBJECTIVES

Upon completion of this chapter, the reader will be able to:

● Describe the physiological mechanisms that give rise to a complaint of dizziness, and discuss how these mechanisms relate to specific dizziness symptoms and to the creation of a differential diagnosis.

● Explain how the epidemiological and clinical features of dizziness in the elderly population differ in comparison to younger adults.

● Use key history and physical examination data to create a differential diagnosis, given a patient who reports dizziness on initial examination.

● Identify and describe the presentation, prognosis, and treatment of the common causes of dizziness in the elderly.

PRETEST

1. Which of the following type of dizziness is most commonly reported by older persons?
   a. Vertigo
   b. Feeling of about to pass out
   c. Disequilibrium
   d. Combination of two or more types of dizziness

2. Which of the following is the least common cause of dizziness in primary care geriatrics?
   a. Anxiety
   b. Vertebrobasilar transient ischemic attacks
   c. An acoustic nerve tumor
   d. Cervical spine disease
   e. Cerumen against the tympanic membrane

3. Which of the following historical or physical examination details would most effectively argue against benign paroxysmal positional vertigo as a cause of dizziness?
   a. Brief episodes of dizziness accompanied by nausea
   b. A negative result on Romberg's test
   c. Failure to reproduce the dizziness with Dix-Hallpike's maneuver
   d. Episodes lasting 4 to 6 hours, with progressive unilateral hearing loss
   e. Multiple similar episodes over many years

4. Ms. Smith is a 60-year-old woman who presented to your office with complaints of sudden onset dizziness, and a feeling of spinning and wooziness for last 1 to 2 weeks. She also complains of feeling of ear fullness, tinnitus in her left ear, and fluctuating hearing loss. Dizziness spells usually last for few hours. On examination, her vitals signs are within normal limits. She has horizontal nystagmus. Her cardiac, respiratory, and neurological examination is normal except she is not able to do a tandem walk and one leg stand. Which of the following tests should be ordered next?
   a. Magnetic resonance imaging of the head
   b. Audiometery
   c. Computerized tomography of the head
   d. Electroencephalogram

Thelma Franklin, *Part 1*

Ms. Franklin, 82, complains of dizziness on and off for the last 4 to 5 months. She also gives a history of having fallen thrice in the last 6 months while walking in the house. She lives with her daughter who witnessed the falls. Falls did not result in any serious injury. Ms. Franklin denies any history of head trauma, nausea, or vomiting. The daughter also noticed that her mother has had mild memory problems for the past 8 to 10 months. She has a past medical history of mild bilateral cataracts, coronary artery disease, hypertension, chronic backache, and diabetes mellitus. She has been using a cane for the past 6 to 7 months. Medications are metformin 500 mg twice a day, baby aspirin, metoprolol 12.5 mg twice a day, nifedipine XL 60 mg qd, ranitidine 150 mg twice a day, acetaminophen prn, and a multivitamin tablet.

STUDY QUESTIONS

1. What is the prevalence of dizziness in older persons?
2. What anatomic structures generally give rise to the type of dizziness reported by Ms. Franklin?
3. What factors related to Ms. Franklin's medical history could contribute to her dizziness?

4. What questions should you ask to identify the type of dizziness?
5. What are the precipitating or provoking factors?
6. What is the differential diagnosis based on the clinical history?

PREVALENCE AND IMPACT

Dizziness is one of the most common presenting complaints in older persons. Like other classic geriatric syndromes, dizziness is both a diagnostic and a management challenge. The complaint of "dizziness" is subjective, cannot be measured, and can be produced by several different mechanisms. In older persons, multiple causal or contributing factors are often involved.

> ● The complaint of "dizziness" is subjective, cannot be measured, and can be produced by several different mechanisms.

Dizziness is reported more commonly by women than men age 65 years or older; the overall prevalence ranges from 4% to 30%.[1-3] The likelihood of reporting dizziness increases by 10% for every 5 years of increasing age. Dizziness has been associated with increased fear of falling, and with worsening of depressive symptoms and of self-rated health.[4] Chronic dizziness has a negative effect on quality of life among older persons,[5] and it has been associated with increased risk for falls, orthostatic hypotension, syncope, stroke, and disability. In one study, after 2 years of follow-up in older persons, dizzy older persons were more likely to become disabled than those who were not.

> ● Chronic dizziness has a negative effect on quality of life among older persons, and it has been associated with increased risk for falls, orthostatic hypotension, syncope, stroke, and disability.

RISK FACTORS AND PATHOPHYSIOLOGY

Dizziness refers to a variety of abnormal or disturbing sensations related to the body's position, movement, or stability. Multiple body systems are normally involved in the maintenance of postural stability; disturbance of any of these systems can lead to dizziness. These postural control systems (Fig. 19–1) include the cerebral cortex, brainstem, cerebellum, eyes and visual pathways, labyrinth and the vestibular pathways, and the proprioceptive fibers in peripheral joints and their associated pathways.

Since so many different body systems can give rise to dizziness, it is not surprising that the differential diagnosis is immense. In evaluating a person with

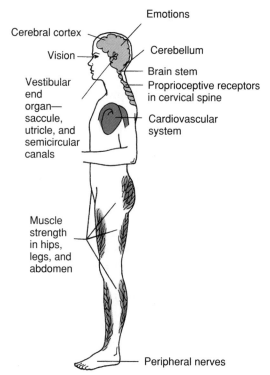

FIGURE 19–1

Components of the balance system.

dizziness, you can narrow the differential diagnosis by systematic history taking, as will be described in the next sections. You also will want to keep in mind the most common conditions, and to rule out treatable causes (Table 19–1). In addition, one should keep in mind that two or more conditions may be contributing to dizziness in your patient, and that you do not want to miss identifying contributing factors that you can treat effectively in the older person.

Chronic Dizziness as a Geriatric Syndrome

In the past clinicians have assumed that dizziness is a symptom of one or more discrete diseases. Chronic dizziness in elderly persons differs, in that multiple conditions usually contribute to the complaint. Thus, chronic dizziness is best considered as a *geriatric syndrome*, that is, a combination of symptoms and signs that often reflects impairment or disease in multiple systems.[6,7] For example, 51% of elderly reported dizziness if they have four or more of the following problems: depressive symptoms, cataracts, abnormal gait, postural hypotension, diabetes, past myocardial infarction, and/or use of three or more medications.

> ● Chronic dizziness is best considered as a *geriatric syndrome*, that is, a combination of symptoms and signs that often reflects impairment or disease in multiple systems.

Table 19–1	Key Points in Taking a Dizziness History

1. Try to Classify Dizziness Sensation

Sensation	Description	Mechanism
Vertigo	Spinning, sense of rotation	Impairment of vestibular system
Presyncopal lightheadedness	Feeling that one is about to pass out	Cerebral ischemia
Imbalance (dysequilibrium)	Loss of balance	Multiple mechanisms; abnormal proprioception, cerebellar, motor or vestibulospinal function
Lightheadedness, floating, tingling, giddiness	Difficult to describe; vague	Anxiety, depression, or other psychosomatic disorders

Caution: About half of dizziness in older persons cannot be clearly assigned to one type. (Many have imbalance plus some other sensation.)

2. Determine If Dizziness Is Episodic or Continuous

Temporal Nature	Common Causes
Episodic	Recurrent vestibulopathy, BPPV, TIA, Meniere's disease
Continuous	Medications, psychological

3. Ask What Other Symptoms Accompany the Dizziness

Symptom	Possible Diagnosis
Ear fullness	Meniere's disease, otitis media
Unilateral hearing loss	Labyrinthitis, Meniere's disease, acoustic neuroma
Weakness or diplopia, dysarthria	Vertebrobasilar insufficiency, TIA
Stiff, sore neck	Cervical osteoarthritis
Tinnitus	Meniere's disease, acoustic neuroma

4. Search for Factors That Bring on or Worsen the Dizziness

Factor	Suggested Cause
Nervousness, worry, or emotional stress	Psychological dizziness
Looking up (e.g., to a high shelf)	Cervical osteoarthritis
Rolling over in bed, bending over	BPPV, vestibulopathy
After meals	Postprandial hypotension
Standing from supine position	Postural hypotension, postural dizziness

Catherine Arnold, *Part 1*

Ms. Arnold, an 84-year-old woman, presented to your office with complaints of episodes of severe dizziness for the last 3 to 4 days. She reports that when she woke up one morning everything began to spin around. She felt nauseated and was not able to stand secondary to significant dizziness. The symptoms subsided after 10 to 15 seconds. After some time she got up and felt lightheaded. She sat on the bed for awhile and the dizziness subsided. Yesterday while cooking she suddenly noticed that the room was spinning; she sat on a chair for a time and symptoms subsided, but she still felt a little lightheaded. She noticed similar episodes while turning her head or changing position. She had similar episodes 3 to 4 years ago lasting for about 5 to 6 days. She has no history of head trauma, severe exertion, coughing or sneezing, loud noises, flu-like symptoms, new medications, twisting or turning activities, or emotional stress.

STUDY QUESTIONS

1. What other questions would you ask?
2. What is the likely diagnosis?
3. What will you do next?

DIFFERENTIAL DIAGNOSIS AND ASSESSMENT

Clinical History

Diagnosis is often difficult when dizziness first presents. Some diseases require observation of a pattern over time to make the diagnosis. Nevertheless, the initial evaluation should create a differential diagnosis from which a plan for further evaluation, treatment, or observation can be developed.[8]

Often, especially in chronic dizziness, the goal of assessment should be to identify factors that can be modified, some of which may not be the most immediate cause of dizziness. Associated symptoms should be sought (see Table 19–1). Certain factors about the onset, duration, and course of dizziness will, during the initial evaluation, help differentiate between the causes of dizziness (Tables 19–2 and 19–3). Among the most common treatable factors that contribute to dizziness-related impairment in older persons are physical deconditioning, visual problems, lack of use of proprioceptive aids (e.g., handrails or a cane), medications, and psychological problems.

In taking a clinical history and developing a differential diagnosis, the first steps involve reviewing the medications, identifying the dizziness subtype, establishing the duration of the symptoms (acute or chronic) and determining whether or not the dizziness occurs in episodes. Taking time to learn about these key characteristics will markedly narrow your differential diagnosis and will guide the remainder of your evaluation.

> ● In taking a clinical history and developing a differential diagnosis, the first steps involve reviewing the medications, identifying the dizziness subtype, establishing the duration of the symptoms (acute or chronic) and determining whether or not the dizziness occurs in episodes.

Medications

In most dizzy patients, an early step in the differential diagnosis should be a medication history, because medications so often contribute to and cause dizziness in this population.[7-9] Common classes of medications contributing to or exacerbating dizziness are aminoglycosides, anxiolytics, antihistaminics, antidepressants, antipsychotics, antihypertensives, antiepileptics, chemotherapeutic agents, and nonsteroidal anti-inflammatory drugs. Different classes of medications can provoke dizziness through different mechanisms. Aminoglycosides, loop diuretics, and NSAIDs can cause ototoxicity when used in higher dosages or for longer durations, especially when renal function is impaired. Antihistamines, tricyclic antidepressants, some cold remedies, and antihypertensives typically cause dizziness by contributing to orthostatic hypotension. Studies have also reported an independent association between the use of multiple medications and dizziness.[6,7]

Specifying the Type of Dizziness

Patients describe dizziness by various names such as giddiness, vertigo, wooziness, and lightheadedness. Classically, dizziness is divided into four types: vertigo, presyncopal lightheadedness, disequilibrium, and other.[10] A fifth category, which is common in the elderly, is "mixed dizziness."

> ● Classically, dizziness is divided into four types: vertigo, presyncopal lightheadedness, disequilibrium, and other — a fifth category, which is common in the elderly, is "mixed dizziness."

Vertigo

Vertigo is an illusion of movement, usually of rotation. Occasionally, vertigo is described as linear displacement or tilt, but usually the patient talks about the environment spinning or whirling about. Vertigo arises from disturbance of the vestibular system or its connecting pathways. The most common causes of vertigo in older persons are acute neurolabyrinthitis, recurrent vestibular syndromes, and benign paroxysmal positional vertigo. Each is described briefly below.

ACUTE (NEURO) LABYRINTHITIS

Caused by viral or vascular injury of all or part of one vestibular labyrinth, neurolabyrinthitis is characterized by rapid onset of vertigo accompanied by nausea, vomiting, sweating, and horizontal nystagmus. In young persons, the vertigo fades within a week; in older persons it resolves more slowly and often leaves a residual disequilibrium. If the auditory portion of the labyrinth is also affected, hearing loss and tinnitus are also reported. Treatment is supportive. Meclizine or promethazine may help during the acute phase; low-dose benzodiazepines may provide some relief of the more protracted disequilibrium and lightheadedness, but must be used with caution because of sedation. It is important to consider acute cerebellar hemorrhage or infarct in an older person with cardiovascular risk factors that present with acute vertigo. The initial presentation can look like vestibular vertigo. Look for gaze-evoked nystagmus, cerebellar coordination signs, or ataxia. If present, the patient must be imaged immediately.

Table 19–2 Common and/or Curable Causes of Dizziness in Older Patients

Diagnosis	Types of Dizziness	Characteristics Episodic vs. Continuous	Frequency in Primary Care	Life Threatening?	Response to Treatment
Anemia and/or hypovolemia	Presyncopal lightheadedness	Continuous	M	Y	H
Anxiety (including panic disorder)	Lightheadedness, often vague	Continuous	H	N	M
Benign paroxysmal positional vertigo	Vertigo	Episodes of <1 minute	H	N	M
Cardiac dysrhythmia	Presyncopal lightheadedness	Episodic	M	Y	H
Cerebellar atrophy	Dysequilibrium	Continuous	L	N	L
Cervical vertigo	Vertigo, often with occipital headache	Episodic	M	N	H
Cerumen against tympanic membrane	Variable, usually vertigo	Variable	M	N	H
Drug adverse effect	Variable, often postural lightheadedness	Variable	H	Y	H
Depression	Lightheadedness, often vague	Continuous	M	Y	M
Infection, systemic (viral or bacterial)	Presyncopal lightheadedness	Continuous	H	Y	H
Meniere's disease	Vertigo (with hearing loss)	Episodes of 2 to 12 hours	M	N	M
Middle ear disease (e.g., serous otitis)	Vertigo or lightheadedness	Continuous	M	N	H
Migraine	Vertigo	Episodic	L	N	H
Multiple neurosensory impairments	Dysequilibrium	Continuous	H	N	M
Myocardial infarction (acute)	Presyncopal lightheadedness	Continuous	L	Y	M
Neurolabyrinthitis	Vertigo; later disequilibrium	Continuous, abrupt onset	H	N	M
Ocular	Lightheadedness and/or imbalance	Continuous	L	N	M
Neurosyphilis	Vertigo (with hearing loss)	Episodic	L	Y	H
Perilymphatic fistula	Vertigo	Episodes associated with Valsalva	L	N	H
Recurrent vestibulopathy	Vertigo	Episodes of hours to days	M	N	L
Transient vertebrobasilar ischemia	Vertigo	Episodes of 5 to 120 minutes	H	Y	L
Stroke, vertebrobasilar system	Vertigo, later dysequilibrium	Continuous	L	Y	L
Tumor, acoustic nerve sheath	Unilateral hearing loss, occasionally with lightheadedness or vertigo	Continuous	L	N	M
Vasovagal	Presyncopal lightheadedness	Brief episodes	H	N	M

H, high; M, moderate; L, low; Y, yes, at times; N, no.

Table 19–3   Evaluation and Management of Common Causes/Contributors of Dizziness

Possible Causes/Contributors	History	Examination/Laboratory Tests	Therapy
Vestibular System			
Benign paroxysmal positional vertigo	Sudden episodes of intense vertigo often associated with nausea or vomiting; provoked by changes in head positions (e.g., looking upward; rolling over in bed into lateral position; bending forward); episodes are recurrent, often last days to months.	Rotational nystagmus; definitive diagnosis by Dix Hallpike maneuver.	Epley maneuver or Brandt and Daroff's exercises are helpful in treatment.
Vestibular neuronitis/ labyrinthitis/recurrent vestibulopathy; mostly viral or idiopathic	Can be associated with upper respiratory infection; sudden onset of severe vertigo with nausea or vomiting; hearing is normal in vestibular neuronitis while impaired in labyrinthitis.	Spontaneous nystagmus with absence of auditory or neurologic signs; head thrust test; fukuda stepping test. Unilateral reduced or absent caloric response.	Spontaneous recovery in few days; may need a short course of vestibular suppressants; vestibular rehabilitation.
Meniere's disease	Episodic vertigo lasts for a few hours; associated with tinnitus, fluctuating hearing loss, and sensation of fullness in ears.	Head thrust test and fukuda stepping test are abnormal on the ipsilateral side. Tests: An audiogram will reveal a sensorineural hearing loss (low more than high frequencies).	During acute attacks, vestibular suppressants may be helpful. Salt restriction and diuretics are the mainstay. In severe cases, may need surgical interventions, including intratympanic gentamicin ablation or transmastoid labyrinthectomy.
Vision			
Cataract; glaucoma; macular degeneration; presbyopia	Abnormality in near or distant vision; use of bifocals.	Tests: Vision screening (Rosenbaum card). Referral to ophthalmologist.	Appropriate refraction. Avoid bifocals. Cataract surgery. Medical or surgical management for glaucoma.
Hearing			
Presbycusis; otosclerosis; cerumen	Difficulty in hearing on phone, in social situations; unilateral or bilateral deafness.	Otoscopy, cerumen, abnormal findings with whisper test, Rinne's test, Weber's test. Tests: audioscopic examination; audiometery.	Ear wax drops. Wax removal/irrigation of ears. Hearing aids.
Hypotension			
Orthostatic—volume/salt depletion; medications; vasovagal episodes; autonomic dysfunction—Parkinson's disease, diabetes mellitus; Shy Drager syndrome	Near fainting/presyncope—most commonly when getting up from supine position, walking, exercising; medication history; complaints consistent with predisposing diseases.	Orthostatic changes in blood pressure and heart rate; signs of predisposing diseases. Tests: investigations relevant to predisposing diseases.	Proper hydration; dosage adjustment or removal of the offending drugs; treatment of relevant diseases; slow rising; graduated stocking; reconditioning exercises; drug therapy—fludrocortisone, etc., if needed.
Postprandial	Lightheadedness or dizziness within 1 hour of eating.	Postprandial orthostatic blood pressure changes.	Small frequent meals (five or six times a day); have caffeine with meals; slow rising after meals.
Peripheral Nerves			
Vitamin B12, folate deficiency; diabetes mellitus; idiopathic	Wooziness, dysequilibrium; worse in dark or on uneven surfaces.	Abnormal vibration or position sense; gait and balance examination. Tests: serum glucose, B12, RBC folate levels.	Good lighting; appropriate walking aids; gait and balance training and exercises. Avoid high heels in footwear. Treatment of specific disease.

Table 19–3	Evaluation and Management of Common Causes/Contributors of Dizziness—Cont'd		
Possible Causes/Contributors	**History**	**Examination/Laboratory Tests**	**Therapy**
Cervical Spine			
Cervical spondylosis, degenerative or inflammatory arthritis	Pain in neck on movement, episode of dizziness secondary to change in position of the neck, history of arthritis.	Limitation of range of motion of neck; abnormal vibratory or joint position sense; signs of radiculopathy or mylopathy. Tests: Cervical spine series.	Cervical collar; cervical or balance exercises.
Central Nervous System			
Vertebrobasilar insufficiency—transient ischemic attacks	Transient episodes of dizziness; usually associated with diplopia, dysarthria, visual disturbances, etc.	Detailed neurological examination can be normal or abnormal findings can be transient. Tests: Doppler ultrasound, arteriography is diagnostic for TIA.	Depends on cause and site of lesion; low-dose aspirin and/or clopidegel may be indicated.
Brain stem (vertebrobasilar insufficiency) and or cerebellar infarct/hemorrhage	History of dizziness (e.g., vertigo, near fainting) usually associated with slurred speech; visual changes; ipsilateral hemiparesis and/or gait ataxia.	Neurological examination to localize lesion. Tests: CT or MRI scan. MRI is preferred.	Low-dose aspirin and/or clopidigel; rehabilitation therapy.
Cerebellopontine angle tumor: acoustic neuroma	History of vertigo or imbalance or disequilibrium; unilateral hearing loss; tinnitus; may complain of parasthesias in trigeminal nerve distribution.	Detailed neurological examination. Tests: audiometery reveals sensorineural hearing loss (more with higher frequencies) in case of acoustic neuroma; brain stem auditory evoked potentials: MRI.	Surgical excision.
Psychiatric Disorders			
Anxiety, depression	Usually continuous nonspecific dizziness; poor appetite; fatigue; sleep problems; somatic complaints.	Positive results on anxiety or depression screening (e.g., anxiety rating scales, Geriatric Depression Scale).	Psychotherapy; antidepressant therapy after considering risks and benefits.

RECURRENT VESTIBULAR SYNDROMES

Recurrent attacks of vertigo, generally lasting hours to days, are common. When accompanied by hearing loss and tinnitus, they are referred to as Meniere's disease; when consisting purely of dizziness the syndrome is called recurrent vestibulopathy. Meniere's disease leads to progressive low-frequency hearing loss over time[11]; recurrent vestibulopathy generally resolves over time.[12] Meniere's generally responds to salt restriction and diuretics, but recalcitrant cases may require specialist care. Recurrent vestibulopathy tends to be milder and to respond to symptomatic treatment using antihistamines such as meclizine. A common cause of recurrent vestibulopathy is migraine related. Treat migraine with control of triggers and possibly prophylactic medications. Consider sudden hearing loss with vertigo in the differential of vertigo and hearing loss. This is important since prompt treatment of sudden hearing loss with prednisone is associated with improved hearing outcomes.

BENIGN PAROXYSMAL POSITIONAL VERTIGO (BPPV)

An extremely common cause of dizziness among elderly patients, BPPV presents as bouts of vertigo lasting less than a minute and brought on by position change, such as by rolling over in bed or by bending over and straightening up. Attacks tend to come in flurries, lasting a week or two, separated by months to years without symptoms. Unilateral hearing loss, tinnitus, and cranial nerve deficits are generally absent.[13] Most BPPV is caused by small dense calcific particles (otoliths) from the saccule or utricle of the inner ear that breaks loose and migrates into the posterior semicircular canal, where they amplify rotational movements in the plane of the canal. With time, particles are absorbed, scarred down, or otherwise dealt with so that symptoms abate. A definitive diagnosis of BPPV can be made by Dix-Hallpike test (discussed later).[14]

Presyncope

Presyncope is the sensation that one is about to pass out. It usually is described as a severe lightheaded feeling, often associated with unsteadiness or falling. The sensation arises because the cerebral cortex is temporarily not receiving adequate oxygen, usually because of diminished blood flow. Most adults have experienced transient presyncope after rapidly standing from the lying or sitting position. Usually some aggravating factor, such as lying in the hot sun, using medication, or excess alcohol intake, can be implicated in these benign episodes. Common causes in the elderly are orthostatic hypotension (OH), vasovagal episodes, carotid sinus syndrome (CSS), medications, anemia, viral infections and cardiac arrhythmias. OH, vasovagal disorders, postprandial hypotension, and CSS are described below; see Chapter 20 for a detailed discussion of syncope and its differential diagnosis.

ORTHOSTATIC HYPOTENSION (OH)

The classical definition of OH is a reduction of at least 20 mm Hg in systolic or of at least 10 mm Hg in diastolic blood pressure, measured 3 minutes after changing from a lying to standing position. However, some older patients have dizziness due to impaired cerebral blood flow when standing, even though they do not meet these criteria. Some take longer than 3 minutes to drop their blood pressure, and that in others cerebral blood flow is impaired in spite of minimal reduction in peripheral blood pressure.[15-17] The first step is elimination of medications that impair venous tone; the next step is use of fitted elastic stockings. If these do not work, then treatment with beta-blockers, disopyramide, transdermal scopolamine, and fludrocortisone can be considered.[18]

> ● There are several reasons why some patients with true orthostatic dizziness fail to meet the classical definition of orthostatic hypotension.

VASOVAGAL DISORDERS

Vasovagal disorders results from either excessive vagal tone or impaired reflex control from of the peripheral circulation. Episodes are characterized by a sudden hypotension, bradycardia, nausea, pallor, and diaphoresis. Most common causes or precipitating factors are severe pain, emotional stress, extreme fatigue, and during micturition or defecation. The prognosis is usually favorable as it is not associated with cardiac disease. Excessive sympathetic activity causes cardiac hyperactivity and excessive stimulation of cardiac mechanoreceptors (afferent vagal C fibers) leading to a sympathetic withdrawal and activation of parasympathetic activity resulting in hypotension and bradycardia. Low-dose beta-blockers treatment are often effective.

POSTPRANDIAL HYPOTENSION

Postprandial hypotension, defined as a decrease in systolic blood pressure of 20 mm Hg or more in a sitting or standing posture within 1 to 2 hours of eating a meal, may also cause dizziness.[19,20] One study has shown that the effects of postprandial hypotension and orthostatic hypotension are additive but not synergistic, suggesting that the two entities may have different pathophysiologic mechanisms.[21]

CAROTID SINUS SYNDROME (CSS)

CSS is a controversial diagnosis, but one that probably causes considerable presyncope in older persons. There are two types—cardioinhibitory (caused by bradycardia or temporary asystole) and vasodepressor (caused by a marked reduction in systolic blood pressure). Studies indicate that between 36% and 48% of dizzy patients have CSS,[22,23] but the extent to which CSS is incidental, contributory, or causal is uncertain.[24] Probably the most reasonable clinical conclusion to draw from this controversy is that older persons, in general, are more susceptible to vasovagal and other stimuli that reduce cerebral blood flow and that certain patients (i.e., those with demonstrable CSS) appear particularly susceptible.

Disequilibrium

Disequilibrium is a sense of imbalance. Patients with this type of dizziness can usually recognize that they are experiencing a body sensation rather than a head sensation. Disequilibrium is a multisensory disorder, which can arise from combinations of disorders of the musculoskeletal system interfering with gait, such as arthritis, proprioceptive system abnormalities, diabetic peripheral neuropathy, cervical spondylosis, or cerebellar disorders. Vision problems or hearing disorders or neurodegenerative disorders such as Parkinson's disease are other important causes or contributing factors. Peripheral vestibulopathy is a common contributing factor to chronic unsteadiness.

CERVICAL CAUSES

Cervical vertigo arises from irritation of proprioceptive receptors in the facet joints of the cervical spine. Osteoarthritis or muscle spasm is usually responsible. Clinically, vertigo or a more vague lightheadedness is reported, accompanied by an occipital headache and neck stiffness or pain. Management involves treating the underlying arthritis or acute neck problem. Two mechanisms have been proposed to explain cervical dizziness: proprioceptive deficits and vascular abnormalities.[25,26] *Proprioceptive* deficits in the cervical spine can cause dizziness secondary to stimulation or proprioceptive receptors in the facet joints of the cervical spine. In older persons, cervical osteoarthritis most likely causes dizziness via this mechanism. The patient usually complains of pain in the neck upon movement, along with a worsening of dizziness. There is often a history of arthritis or whiplash injury. Further examination may reveal a decreased range of motion of the neck or signs of radiculopathy or mylopathy and/or spastic gait.

A *vascular mechanism* causing cervical dizziness is thought to result from obstruction of the vertebral arteries. One theory is that when there is extensive blockage of one vertebral artery, rotation of the head can cause sufficient obstruction of the other vertebral artery to cause brainstem ischemia. Another theory is that when a person turns his/her head or neck, an osteoarthritic spur may press on the nearby vertebral artery, causing a transient disruption of the blood flow.

VISION AND HEARING PROBLEMS

Visual and auditory systems also help in spatial orientation by interpreting the respective stimuli. Common ocular diseases include cataracts, macular degeneration, and glaucoma. Age-related visual changes include a decrease in visual acuity, dark adaptation, contrast sensitivity, and accommodation.[27,28] Hearing is especially helpful when other sensations are impaired. Impairment in hearing, common in older persons, may be secondary to aging, to disease processes, or to the presence of excess cerumen.

Causes of Dizziness That Often Do Not Fit Neatly into a Subtype

The "other" category of dizziness includes vague, difficult to categorize dizziness. Patients may describe feeling of dissociation, floating, swimming or giddiness. In such situations the physician should not exclude vertigo, presyncopal lightheadedness, or disequilibrium merely because the patient was not able to articulate the problem adequately. On the other hand, dizziness that is difficult to describe often accompanies a psychological condition such as anxiety and depression.

A feature of dizziness in the elderly, in contrast to younger adults, is greater difficulty in assigning patients to one dizziness subtype. Between 42% and 56% of older patients are unable to identify their dizziness as exclusively vertigo, presyncope, disequilibrium, or other; instead, they describe multiple dizziness sensations.[6] Persons with these multiple sensations can be categorized as having *mixed dizziness*.

ANXIETY AND DEPRESSION

In various studies in older persons with dizziness, psychological diagnoses have been reported to occur in as many as a third. The most common conditions in older persons are depressive symptoms and anxiety disorders. These patients tend to report a vague lightheaded or floating sensation or continuous dizziness. Accompanying signs and symptoms may include headache, fatigue, neck soreness, and abdominal pain. Psychologic symptoms are more often secondary to the dizziness rather than a cause of it; however, treating the psychological disorder may often reduce the disability when the dizziness itself cannot be cured. Peripheral vestibulopathy is a common contributing factor in patients with "nonspecific" dizziness symptoms and anxiety. This is particularly true for patient with a history of panic disorder and/or migraine.

Finally, there are several diagnoses whose symptoms do not fit neatly into one classical dizziness subtype. These include cerebrovascular disease and acoustic neuroma. Each is described briefly below.

CEREBROVASCULAR DISEASE

Acute posterior circulation cerebrovascular disease (TIA, stroke, or migraine[29]) usually presents as vertigo; however, lacunar infarcts and small strokes in the same area often present with a sudden or insidious onset of imbalance. In severe acute disease, associated neurologic symptoms, such as diplopia, ataxia, dysarthria, unilateral weakness or numbness of one side of the body, and perioral numbness, occur frequently. However, their absence does not rule out a cerebrovascular event—up to a quarter of posterior circulation strokes begin as vertigo.

Dizziness due to cerebrovascular disease is almost always a posterior circulation problem; TIAs involving the anterior circulation rarely produce vertigo. In fact, patients with vertigo who have carotid endarterectomies frequently fail to improve because the carotid disease is incidental. The course of TIAs is variable. Less than half progress to a completed stroke, and symptoms frequently resolve completely.[30] Therefore, although therapy is largely limited to antiplatelet agents and control of risk factors, the prognosis is by no means hopeless.

ACOUSTIC NEUROMA

A benign tumor of the eighth cranial nerve, acoustic neuroma typically presents with progressive unilateral high frequency sensorineural hearing loss, and occasionally with mild vertigo or disequilibrium.[31]

Acute or Chronic Nature

Dizziness can be divided into acute or chronic, depending on its duration. *Acute dizziness* is defined by having been present for less than 2 months; chronic dizziness is defined by having been present for more than 2 months. Acute dizziness usually results from a disorder of one of system (e.g., acute labyrynthitis), and approach to its management is as in younger patients. *Chronic dizziness* in older persons, on the other hand, is most often secondary to the combined effects of disorders or impairments in the multiple systems responsible for maintaining equilibrium. The management approach is to intervene at multiple levels in chronic dizziness.

Episodic or Continuous Nature

If the patient has vertigo, it should be determined whether the dizziness is episodic or continuous. If dizziness is episodic, the duration and frequency of the episodes should be identified, along with any associated symptoms such as hearing loss, tinnitus, ear fullness, diplopia, dysarthria, and syncopal episodes.

- Episodes of vertigo lasting less than 1 minute suggest benign paroxysmal positional vertigo (BPPV).
- Episodes of vertigo lasting between 15 minutes and several hours suggest a transient ischemic attack (TIA) or migraine.
- Episodes of vertigo lasting between several hours and a couple of days suggest recurrent vestibulopathy or, if accompanied by tinnitus and hearing loss, Meniere's disease.

Continuous dizziness has a broad differential diagnosis. If dizziness begins abruptly and improves or remains the same, common causes include stroke, neurolabyrinthitis, cerebellar degeneration, peripheral neuropathy, physical deconditioning, drugs, anxiety, and depression. If onset is insidious, then psychological causes are particularly common, but acoustic neuroma should be ruled out.

Provocative or Precipitating Factors

Determining whether rolling over in bed or changing the position of the head or neck brings on the dizziness is useful; such patients usually have cervical or vestibular etiology. Dizziness on standing from the supine position is seen in postural hypotension. One should ask whether dizziness occurs after eating meals as is seen in postprandial hypotension. Dizziness developing after a change in medication needs careful review of side effects of that medication. Depressive

disorders should be sought, using a standardized instrument, such as the Geriatric Depression Scale (GDS).[32]

> ● Dizziness on standing from the supine position is seen in postural hypotension.

Thelma Franklin, *Part 2*

On further questioning about the type of dizziness, Ms. Franklin says sometimes she feels woozy, sometimes spinning or lightheadedness. The episodes usually occur when she tries to stand up from sitting or lying down. Sometimes she complains of dizziness on change in head and neck position. She denies any nausea or vomiting. Her daughter reports that she has seen no loss of consciousness during the falls. The patient denies any sensation of fullness in the ears, which is usually seen in Meniere's disease.

One of the frustrations a clinician faces in managing dizziness in the elderly is that most of the time patients are not able to specify the type of dizziness. If she would have complained of only vertiginous or spinning sensation, a vestibular lesion could be implicated. Sudden onset can suggests a vascular or traumatic process. Head stuffiness reported several weeks beforehand could indicate a viral process (neurolabyrinthitis) or the first episode of Meniere's disease. Other features of the history that may be important include use of nifedipine, a calcium channel blocker (raising suspicion for postural hypotension), her living situation (potential stress), and bilateral cataracts (raising concern about the adequacy of compensation for a vestibular problem). Based on the initial history, Ms. Franklin's physician could construct the following list of most likely diagnoses: postural hypotension, cervical arthritis, vestibular causes, anxiety, and depression.

Catherine Arnold, *Part 2*

The remainder of Ms. Arnold's history is noncontributory. An 84-year-old grandmother, Ms. Arnold shares her home with another elderly woman for whom she serves as a part-time caregiver. She is generally healthy, does her own shopping, needs some help with housework, has hypertension, and left hip arthritis. She takes enalapril 10 mg po qd and acetaminophen prn.

Based on her initial history the differential diagnosis includes BPPV, acute neurolabyrhinthitis, TIAs or brainstem infarction, or cervical vertigo.

STUDY QUESTIONS

1. What should be kept in mind during physical examination?
2. What are the bedside tests that can provoke dizziness?
3. What laboratory tests are helpful in the diagnosis?

Physical Examination

The physical examination should be individualized based on patient symptoms. However, most examinations of a patient with dizziness should include evaluation for pathologic nystagmus; fundoscopy; hearing screening; otoscopic evaluation of both ears; testing for restricted cervical spine motion and tenderness; screening for a peripheral neuropathy, and examination of the cranial nerves, peripheral arteries (especially the carotid arteries), and heart. Postural blood pressure measurement is used to diagnose postural hypotension, defined as a drop in systolic blood pressure of 20 or more mmHg, a diastolic drop of 10 or more mmHg, or both, noted 3 minutes after the patient goes from lying down to standing. Gait and balance examination should be performed. Positive Romberg's sign suggests vestibular or proprioceptive etiology. Depressive disorders should be sought, using a standardized instrument—usually the GDS.

Several bedside tests and maneuvers are helpful in certain patients. These include evaluation for forced hyperventilation, head-thrust test, marching in place with the eyes closed (Fukuda stepping test), and Dix-Hallpike's maneuver.

> ● Several bedside tests and maneuvers are helpful in certain patients: evaluation for forced hyperventilation, head-thrust test, marching in place with the eyes closed (Fukuda stepping test), and Dix-Hallpike's maneuver.

Forced hyperventilation is useful when anxiety is a possible diagnosis. Anxiety and, in some cases, depression can cause a lightheadedness that probably arises from hyperventilation. Having such patients hyperventilate in the examining room may elicit the same dizziness they are concerned about, thus making the diagnosis. Deep breathing at a rate of 20 to 30 breaths per minute for 2 or 3 minutes usually provokes dizziness, often accompanied by finger and perioral numbness. Once dizziness develops, the patient should be asked if his or her dizziness symptoms are similar. In interpreting this maneuver, be aware that it may aggravate symptoms in certain vestibular disorders, and therefore is not specific for anxiety; so other historical and examination data should be considered in interpreting the result of forced hyperventilation.

The *head thrust test* can help in determining if the vestibuloocular reflex (VOR) is intact. The VOR helps in maintaining visual stability during head movement and is impaired in patients with reduced peripheral vestibular function and some central nervous system diseases (e.g., stroke). This reflex depends on information relayed by the vestibular nucleus to the sixth cranial nerve nucleus in the pons and, via the median longitudinal fasciculus, to the third and fourth cranial nerve nuclei in the midbrain.

In this test, the patient is asked to fixate on the examiner's nose, and the head is rotated rapidly by the examiner about 10 degrees to the left or right. If the VOR is functioning normally, the eyes will remain fixed on the target; in patients with a vestibular deficit, the eyes move away from the target along with the head, followed by a corrective saccade back to the target. For example, in a patient with a left-sided vestibular lesion, head thrusts to the left will produce a movement of the pupils from the target to the left, along with the head, followed by a corrective movement back to the target, whereas head thrusts to the right will produce the normal response of continued fixation on the target.[33]

The *Fukuda stepping test* (marching in place with the eyes closed) is a sensitive test for unilateral vestibular hypofunction (e.g., from a prior neurolabyrinthitis or from Meniere's disease). To conduct the test, the patient is asked to march in place for 30 seconds with his or her eyes closed and arms extended in front. Care must be taken not to orient the patient with sound, such as the examiner's voice, a radio, or a ticking clock. Patients with absent or reduced vestibular function rotate more than 30 degrees.

The *Dix-Hallpike maneuver* attempts to induce symptoms of BPPV by provoking rotation in the posterior semicircular canals. In this maneuver, the patient is seated on the examining table so that he or she can be comfortably and rapidly eased backward to a recumbent position. Standing to the patient's right, the physician cradles the patient's head and neck in both hands turning the head about 30 degrees to the right, advising the patient to hold the physician's upper arm for stability. At the count of three, the patient relaxes and the physician quickly lays the patient backward. This places the patient's right posterior semicircular canal in the vertical plane, causing that single canal to experience a rotatory stimulus-angular acceleration. The examiner maintains the patient in this head hanging right position for at least 10 to 20 seconds or until vertigo subsides. Then the patient is returned to the initial position, again holding the position for at least 10 seconds. Next, the procedure is repeated with the physician on the patient's left side to test the left posterior semicircular canal.

A classic positive response to Dix-Hallpike maneuver includes four components: dizziness (vertigo), rotatory (torsional) nystagmus, latency (i.e., the dizziness and nystagmus do not begin immediately, but rather after a few seconds), and, fatigue such that repeating the same maneuver should result in reduced symptoms (i.e., if three or four repetitions are made, no more symptoms should be noted). A positive response to the Dix-Hallpike maneuver is diagnostic of BPPV. Because BPPV is generally unilateral, response is generally either limited to one side or unequal in intensity between sides. Negative Hallpike testing in BPPV is most common when an episode is mild or when the patient is already recovering.[34]

Laboratory Testing

The causes of dizziness are so diverse that no laboratory test should be considered routine or mandatory in the primary care setting. Test selection should be guided by the presentation, duration, and severity of the problem and by the clinician's concern about possible progressive or life-threatening conditions. Among the laboratory tests useful in certain patients are the following:

> ● No laboratory test should be considered routine or mandatory in primary care patients with dizziness.

1. Hematologic and biochemical studies to screen for systemic and metabolic causes of dizziness, such as anemia, hyperthyroidism, and syphilis.
2. Audiometry with speech discrimination is the best screening test for acoustic neuroma. It can also identify the progressive low-frequency hearing loss of Meniere's disease.
3. Electrocardiography (ECG) identifies rhythm disturbances such as atrial fibrillation, ventricular tachycardia, or complete heart block. In episodic dizziness, capturing an episode of the dysrhythmia is often difficult, and prolonged ambulatory cardiac monitoring may be necessary; however, the vast majority of cardiac monitoring for dizziness fails to identify a cardiac etiology.
4. Brainstem auditory evoked potentials can isolate the anatomic site of a vestibular or auditory nerve deficit; they are useful in further evaluation of patients with unilateral hearing loss (to rule out eighth nerve tumor).
5. Doppler examination of the cranial blood vessels and cerebral angiography can be used to diagnose vertebrobasilar disease. The usefulness of such information when the clinical picture already suggests posterior circulation TIA is questionable, however, because treatment is nonspecific. The greatest use of these tests is in differentiating migraine from vertebrobasilar insufficiency and in identifying subclavian steal, a surgically treatable cause of vertebrobasilar TIAs.
6. Brain imaging is used to rule out a mass lesion, such as an acoustic neuroma, and to identify stroke. Magnetic resonance imaging (MRI) is preferable to computed tomography in most cases because clinically significant lesions (i.e., tumor or infarction) may be small. Demonstration of increased periventricular white matter signal in MRI presents a diagnostic challenge; how much is normal in older people and how much indicates lacunar infarct disease is unclear.
7. Electronystagmography (ENG) is used to evaluate vestibular function by measuring the effect of selected stimuli on eye movements, using recordings from electrodes placed over the eye muscles. The test is based on the vestibulo-ocular reflex, which, in many pathologic states, generates subtle oculomotor abnormalities that can be appreciated only with the eyes closed. The routine ENG can often differentiate between central and peripheral causes of vertigo; however, abnormal responses are so common in older persons that the test is highly nonspecific in this population.

Consultation with an appropriate specialist is often more fruitful than performing multiple laboratory examinations, particularly in patients with chronic dizziness. This is especially true if the physician suspects a diagnosis within the province of a specific medical subspecialty, such as neurology, otolaryngology, or cardiology. Be aware, however, that consultants tend to arrive at diagnoses within their specialty and to miss diagnoses outside their field. Therefore, the importance of the generalist's role in integrating consultant opinions with the entire clinical picture cannot be overemphasized.

> ● Consultants can be helpful, but tend to miss diagnoses outside their field.

Thelma Franklin, *Part 3*

On examination, Ms. Franklin's pulse is 82 beats per minute, supine blood pressure is 116/70 (standing 100/64), and temperature is 98.4 degrees F. She complains of dizziness on standing. Cardiac and respiratory system are unremarkable.

Neurological examination reveals difficulty in getting up from chair without using arms of the chair. Romberg sign is negative, but she is not able to do a one-leg stand secondary to pain in the back. There is no nystagmus at rest or on head thrust test. She scores 27/30 on Mini-Mental Status Examination. Dix-Hallpike test is negative. She scores 3/15 on the GDS.

CASE DISCUSSION, THELMA FRANKLIN

Ms. Franklin most likely suffers from postural hypotension as the cause of her dizziness. Her gait abnormality secondary to backache and bilateral cataracts may be contributing factors. Her postural hypotension is most likely secondary to nifedipine XL. Her blood pressure measured in the office suggests she may not need nifedipine at all; it should be discontinued. Her blood pressure should be monitored and if needed, the dose of metoprolol can be increased. In addition, her backache should be adequately controlled with scheduled dosage of acetaminophen instead of using it prn. She should also have her vision tested.

MANAGEMENT

Treatment of dizziness depends on making the correct diagnosis. Many causes of dizziness are curable: examples include adverse drug effects, cerumen in the ear, anemia, cardiac dysrhythmias, depression, and perilymphatic fistula. Other causes of dizziness, such as BPPV and many vasovagal phenomena, are benign and self-limited. When dizziness cannot be cured, treatment should strive to reduce disability and minimize symptoms. Box 19–1 identifies a general approach to treatment of the patient with dizziness.

Because multiple neurosensory problems contribute to dizziness in many elderly persons, physicians should search for such problems and seek to ameliorate them. Vision is the key adaptive mechanism for vestibular and proprioceptive deficits; cataract surgery and use of a night light are two examples of ways vision can be enhanced. If loss of proprioception in the ankles and feet contributes to dizziness, the patient can get additional sensory input by touching the wall or another person; a cane can serve a similar function.

The extent to which anxiety and depression contribute to dizziness should not be overlooked. Dizziness is a common symptom of panic disorder, and vertigo is not an unusual description of the symptom. Admittedly, dizziness of purely psychiatric origin is relatively rare

Box 19–1	Treatment of Dizziness in Old Age: General Principles

1. Identify the primary diagnosis and use a specific therapeutic agent, if available.
2. Provide symptomatic relief when needed, but be wary of medications; they can worsen dizziness and increase the risk of falls. Peripheral vestibular problems respond well to antihistamines or benzodiazepines; central problems often do not. Small doses of promethazine may relieve nausea during acute problems. Low-dose haloperidol or ginger root may help in refractory cases.
3. Identify contributing sensory deficits and manage them. Vision is a key factor in compensating for vestibular and proprioceptive deficits. Visually dependent individuals benefit from using a night light. Individuals with proprioceptive problems in the legs can gather compensatory information by touching walls or using a cane. Cataract surgery, when indicated, is essential for visual compensation.
4. Exercise (physical therapy) can treat benign paroxysmal positional vertigo, reduce balance problems, help adapt to vestibular deficits, and lower the risk of falls by improving strength in deconditioned muscle groups. If possible, consult a physical therapist with special expertise in balance and vestibular problems.
5. If anxiety or depression is present and appears to impair function, treat it.
6. If the patient is at risk for falls, consider use of walking aid and home assessment to reduce hazards.
7. Work with the patient over time, providing small adjustments and always seeking to improve function.

among older patients compared to younger adults; in fact, physicians often hesitate to make a psychiatric diagnosis without a long history of similar symptoms. However, secondary psychiatric problems such as anxiety and depression are common in older persons who are dizzy. One study of 56 elderly patients with chronic dizziness identified a psychologic diagnosis meeting DSM-III criteria in more than one-third of patients. In most cases, the diagnosis was a contributing factor to rather than the primary cause of the dizziness; anxiety disorders, depression, and adjustment reactions predominated.[35]

Pharmacological Treatment

Antihistamines and sedatives are probably overused in the treatment of dizziness among elderly patients. Sedation, imbalance, and postural hypotension are common side effects, and may be more dangerous than the dizziness itself. Small doses of medication can, however, help in certain circumstances. Meclizine, dimenhydrinate, and other antihistamines provide relief for acute peripheral vestibular problems, such as labyrinthitis or attacks of Meniere's disease. Benzodiazepines reduce central sensitivity to some dizziness symptoms, but should be used with extreme caution because they cause sedation and increase the risk of falls; oxazepam and temazepam have short half-lives and are preferable to longer-acting agents. Antiemetics or antinausea medications are also sometimes useful.

Vestibular Rehabilitation

A growing body of literature indicates that physical therapy can result in significant functional gains in older persons with dizziness and imbalance.[36,37] Vestibular rehabilitation includes combinations of exercises involving head, neck, and eye movements designed to provoke dizziness and imbalance. Initially these exercises may worsen dizziness, but over a period of weeks to months dizziness improves, most likely because of central adaptation or desensitization. Desensitization exercises seek to reduce the brain's responsiveness to the stimuli from the affected labyrinth, making use of a normal compensatory mechanism by provoking vertigo spells in a safe environment. Specific dynamic balance exercises can help strengthen muscle groups that stabilize the patient, thereby reducing falls and fear of falling. A recent randomized trial of vestibular rehabilitation (a specific group of exercises consisting of eye, head, and body movements designed to stimulate the vestibular system) resulted in a significant improvement in patients with chronic dizziness.[38] Another randomized trial found that physiotherapy aimed at reducing neck discomfort resulted in both improved symptoms and better postural performance among patients with suspected cervical dizziness.[39]

Physical exercises do appear to help many patients with BPPV and should be recommended. Two forms of exercise are particularly suitable for primary care older patients:

Modified Epley's canalith repositioning maneuver represents a specific treatment for BPPV[40] (Box 19–2). The purpose of this maneuver is to move free-floating debris by the effect of gravity from the posterior semicircular canal into the utriculus, where it will no longer affect the dynamics of the semicircular canals. For a videotaped demonstration of the Epley maneover, see the CD–Rom that accompanies this text.

If Modified Epley's maneuver is not helpful, the patient can do Brandt and Daroff's exercises.[41] These exercises involve sitting on the bed and falling or rolling, in a controlled manner, toward the side of the injury,

---

Box 19-2	Modified Epley's Canalith Repositioning Maneuver

1. Start by sitting on a bed. Turn your head 45 degrees to the right. Place a pillow behind you so that on lying back it will be under your shoulders.
2. Lie back quickly with shoulders on the pillow, neck extended, and head resting on the bed. In this position, the affected (right) ear will be on the pillow. Wait for 30 seconds.
3. Turn your head 90 degrees to the left (without raising it) and wait again for 30 seconds.
4. Turn your body and head another 90 degrees to the left and wait another 30 seconds. You should now be lying on your left side with your head turned 45 degrees into the mattress.
5. Sit up slowly by elevating yourself from your side. Perform this maneuver three times a day until you have been free from positional vertigo for 24 hours.

---

precipitating the dizziness, and doing this three or four times in a row. Typically, this causes relief of symptoms, although relief may only last a few hours. The exercises likely work either by habituation or by dislodging debris from the posterior semicircular canals.[42]

Surgical Therapy

Surgery is almost never indicated for dizziness. It is reserved for (1) persons with cerebellopontine angle tumors, (2) patients with severe Meniere's disease or refractory BPPV whose dizziness is so severe and chronic that an ablative (e.g., intratympanic gentamicin ablation, a common ablative procedure used in the geriatric population, or transmastoid labyrinthectomy) or nonablative (e.g., endolymphatic sac decompression and posterior canal occlusion) procedure is considered.[43,44]

● Surgery is almost never indicated for dizziness.

Patient Education

Fearing that a dizziness attack will come on or that they will fall, many older persons with dizziness give up activities crucial to their independence and self-image, such as going to church, shopping, visiting friends, and driving. For these reasons, the effective management of dizziness requires counseling the patient and family about these issues. Patients should be given basic education regarding the pathophysiology of dizziness and its provocation to help the patient understand, and therefore be more realistic and less anxious about dizziness. At times, modifying activities is indicated; for example, in case of postural dizziness, patients should be instructed to rise slowly from the sitting or supine position. Deconditioning plays an important role in the persistence of symptoms; accordingly, activities are to be encouraged. Finally, dizzy patients should avoid over-the-counter sleeping pills or cold medicines, and their prescription medications should be carefully reviewed.

Case Discussion, Catherine Arnold

Examination reveals that vital signs are within normal limits. No orthostatic hypotension is noted. Respiratory, cardiovascular, and neurologic exam-

ination findings are normal. Rapid positional testing using Hallpike's maneuver reproduces her dizziness in the right head-hanging position. On further questioning, she admits to having greater difficulty rolling over to the right than to the left when in bed. She is given instructions for positional exercises. These consist of reproducing her vertigo by rolling over rapidly to the right.

After doing so, she is instructed to wait for her dizziness to resolve and then to roll over rapidly again in the same direction. She is instructed that, within five repetitions, the dizziness response should be fatigued temporarily and she can go about her day. As instructed, she performs the exercises every 3 hours while awake. Within 2 weeks she reports no more dizziness.

POSTTEST

1. You are asked to evaluate to see an 80-year-old man, a nursing home resident with past medical history of mild Alzheimer's disease, hypertension, and reflux oesophagitis, who complained of feeling dizzy, a sensation of about to pass out on the dining table after eating his breakfast. He had similar episodes in the past after finishing his meals. He denies any chest pain or shortness of breath. On examination, he is alert, awake, oriented to person and place. Vital signs show heart rate of 74 per minute and blood pressure of 110/70. His vital signs in the morning at 7 AM were heart rate 70 per minute and blood pressure 130/80. Other system examination was unremarkable. No recent medication changes were made. What is the most likely diagnosis?
   a. Cerebrovascular stroke
   b. Recurrent vestibulopathy
   c. Postprandial hypotension
   d. Benign paroxysmal positional vertigo

2. Mr. K.G. is a 68-year-old retired insurance salesman with a 2-day history of dizziness. He describes a lightheaded sensation as though he is about to pass out, that occurs whenever he is standing or walking. He has a milder sensation in the sitting position and is completely relieved when he lies down. There is no sense of spinning accompanying this sensation. What is the likely physiologic mechanism underlying Mr. K.G.'s dizziness?
   a. Depression or anxiety
   b. Diminished oxygenation of the cerebral cortex
   c. Cardiac dysrhythmia
   d. Stimulation of the vestibular system when he stands
   e. Irritation of neck proprioceptive fibers

3. What laboratory test provides the best method of screening for an acoustic neuroma?
   a. Magnetic resonance imaging of the head
   b. Computerized tomography of the head
   c. Brainstem-evoked potentials
   d. Electroencephalography
   e. Audiometry with speech discrimination

4. A 74-year-old man is brought to your office by his concerned wife. At about 2:30 this morning he got up to go to the bathroom, feeling a little lightheaded. He sat on the toilet, but even as he did so he could feel himself blacking out. His wife heard a thud and found him unconscious. He became conscious in about 10 to 15 seconds. He did not feel chest pain or palpitations before or after the episode, and he was not incontinent. On further questioning, he states that he has had a cold for the past 4 days, for which he has taken a combination medication containing pseudoephedrine and chlorpheniramine. Rarely an alcohol drinker, he admits to having few beers last evening while watching Monday night football with his son, who is visiting. He does not have a history of seizures. Four months ago, he had a normal cardiac treadmill test performed by his cardiologist as part of a routine evaluation. Other than the cold preparation and one aspirin a day, he is not taking medication. Which of the following conditions contributed to this episode of vasovagal dizziness and syncope?
   a. History of alcohol intake last night
   b. Common cold for 4 days, probably viral illness
   c. Use of medications containing pseudoephedrine and chlorpheniramine
   d. Postural hypotension secondary to rapidly getting up from lying-down position
   e. All of the above

References

1. Hale WE, Perkins LL, May FE, Marks RG, Stewart RB. Symptoms prevalence in the elderly. An evaluation of age, sex, disease, and medication use. J Am Geriatr Soc 1986:34;333-40.
2. Sloane P, Blazer D, George LK. Dizziness in a community elderly population. J Am Geriatr Soc 1989:37;101-8.
3. Colledge NR, Wilson JA, Macintyre CCA, MacLennan WJ. The prevalence and characteristics of dizziness in an elderly community. Age Aging 1994:23;117-20.
4. Tinetti ME, Mendes de Leon CF, Doucette JT, Baker DI. Fear of falling and fall related efficacy in relationship to functioning among community-living elders. J Gerontol 1994:49;M140-7.
5. Grimby A, Rosenthall U. Health related quality of life and dizziness in old age. Gerontology 1995:41;286-98.
6. Tinetti ME, Williams CS, Gill TM. Dizziness among older adults: a possible geriatric syndrome. Ann Intern Med 2000;132:337-44.
7. Kao AC, Nanda A, Williams CS, Tinetti ME. Validation of dizziness as a possible geriatric syndrome. J Am Geriatr Soc 2001;49:72-5.
8. Baloh RW. Dizziness in older people. J Am Geriatr Soc 1992;40:713.
9. Davis LE. Dizziness in elderly men. J Am Geriatr Soc 1994;42:1184-8.
10. Drachman DA, Hart CW. An approach to the dizzy patient. Neurology 1972;22:323-34.
11. Green DJ, BLUM DJ, Harner SG. Longitudinal follow-up of patients with Meniere's disease. Otolaryngol Head Neck Surg 1991;104;783-8.
12. Rutka JA, Barber HO. Recurrent vestibulopathy: third review. J Otolaryngol 1986;15:105.
13. Baloh RW, Honrubia V, Jacobson K. Benign positional vertigo: clinical and oculographic features in 240 cases. Neurology 1987;37:371.
14. Dix MR, Hallpike CS. The pathology, symptomatology and diagnosis of certain common disorders of the vestibular system. Proc R Soc Med 1952;45;341-54.
15. Hackel A, et al. Cardiovascular and catecholamine responses to head-up tilt in the diagnosis of recurrent unexplained syncope in elderly patients. J Am Geriatr Soc 1991;39:639.
16. Hargreaves AD, Muir AL. Lack of variation in venous tone potentiates vasovagal syncope. Br Heart J 1992;67:486.
17. Streeten DHP, Anderson GH. Delayed orthostatic intolerance. Arch Intern Med 1992;152:1066.
18. Grubb BP, et al. Utility of upright tilt-table testing in the evaluation and management of syncope of unknown origin. Am J Med 1991;90:6.
19. Jansen RWMM, Lipsitz LA. Postprandial hypotension: Epidemiology, pathophysiology, and clinical management. Ann Intern Med 1995;122:286-95.
20. Lipsitz LA, Fullerton KJ. Postprandial blood pressure reduction in healthy elderly. J Am Geriatr Soc 1986;34:267-70.
21. Maurer MS, Karmally W, Rivdeneira H, Parides MK, Bloomfield DM. Upright posture and postprandial hypotension in elderly persons. Ann Intern Med 2000;133:533.
22. McIntosh SJ, Lawson J, Kenny RA. Clinical characteristics of vasodepressor, cardioinhibitory, and mixed carotid sinus syndrome in the elderly. Am J Med 1993;95:203.
23. Lawson J, et al. Diagnosis of geriatric patients with severe dizziness. J Am Geriatr Soc 1999;47:12.
24. Sloane PD, Dallara J. Clinical research and geriatric dizziness: the blind men and the elephant. J Am Geriatr Soc 1999;47:113.
25. Sloane PD. Evaluation and management of dizziness in the older patient. Clin Geriatr Med 1996;12(4):785-801.
26. McClure JA. Vertigo and imbalance in the elderly. J Otolaryngol 1986;15:248-52.
27. Sekuler R, Hutman LP. Spatial vision and aging. 1: Contrast sensitivity. J Gerontol 1980;35:692-9.
28. Hutman LP, Sekuler R. Spatial vision and aging. 2: Criterion effects. J Gerontol 1980;35:700-6.
29. Fisher CM. Late-life migraine accompaniments as a cause of unexplained transient ischemic attacks. Can J Neurol Sci 1980;7:9.
30. Fisher CM. Vertigo in cerebrovascular disease. Arch Otolaryngol 1967;85:529.
31. Selesnick SH, Jackler RK, Pitts LW. The changing clinical presentation of acoustic tumors in the MRI era. Laryngoscope 1993;103:431-6.
32. Yasavage JA, Brink TL. Development and validation of a geriatric depression screening scale: a preliminary report. J Psychiatry Res 1983;17:37-49.
33. Walker MF, Zee DS. Bedside vestibular examination. Otolayngol Cli North Am 2000;33(3):495-506.
34. Dix MR, Hallpike CS. The pathology, symptomatolgy and diagnosis of certain common disorders of the vestibular system. Proc R Soc Med 1952;45:341-5.
35. Sloane PD, Hartman M, Mitchell CM. Psychological factors associated with chronic dizziness in patients aged 60 and older. J Am Geriatr Soc 1994;42:847.
36. Shepard NT, Smith-Wheelock M, Telian SA, Raj A. Vestibular and balance rehabilitation therapy. Ann Otol Rhino Laryngol 1993;102:198-205.
37. Cowand JL, Wrisley DM, Walker M, Strasnik B, Jacobson JT. Efficacy of vestibular rehabilitation. Otolarngol Head Neck Surg 1998;118:49-54.
38. Yardley L, et al. A randomized controlled trial of exercise therapy for dizziness and vertigo in primary care. Br J Gen Pract 1998;48:1136.
39. Karlberg M, et al. Postural and symptomatic improvement after physiotherapy in patients with dizziness of suspected cervical origin. Arch Phys Med Rehabil 1996;77:874.
40. Radtke A, et al. A modified Epley's procedure for self- treatment of benign paroxysmal positional vertigo. Neurology 1999;53:1358.
41. Brandt T, Daroff RB. Physical therapy for benign paroxysmal positional vertigo. Arch Otolaryngol 1980;106:484-5.
42. Tusa RJ. Episodic vertigo. In: Conn HF, et al., eds. Conn's Current Therapy, 2000. Philadelphia: Saunders, 2000:884-92.
43. Gacek RR. Technique and results of singular neurectomy for the management of benign paroxysmal positional vertigo. Acta Otolaryngol (Stoch) 1995;115:154-7.
44. Parnes LS, McClure JA. Posterior semicircular canal occlusion for intractable benign paroxysmal positional vertigo. Ann Otol Rhinol Laryngol 1990;99:330-4.

PRETEST ANSWERS

1. d
2. c
3. d
4. b

POSTTEST ANSWERS

1. c
2. b
3. e
4. e

Syncope

Lorraine M. Stone and Philip D. Sloane

OBJECTIVES

Upon completion of this chapter, the reader will be able to:

- Describe the physiological mechanisms that give rise to a complaint of syncope.

- Use key history and physical examination data to create a differential diagnosis for the patient experiencing syncope.

- Identify and describe the presentation, prognosis, and treatment of the common causes of syncope in the elderly.

PRETEST

1. A 71-year-old woman with hypertension, diabetes mellitus, and ischemic cardiomyopathy presents after a witnessed episode of syncope at a church gathering. She does not remember the event, but her daughter describes her suddenly appearing pale while sitting and then slumping over and hitting her head on the side of a table. After about 30 seconds she came to on her own. She has a normal physical exam except for an abrasion on her forehead, and her only electrocardiogram abnormalities are the changes from her previous myocardial infarction. What type of syncope is most likely in your differential diagnosis?
   a. Neurologic
   b. Neurally mediated
   c. Cardiac
   d. Orthostatic
   e. Psychiatric

2. Which of the following evaluation methods is *not* considered part of the routine workup for a first episode of syncope?
   a. Electrocardiogram
   b. Complete history and physical exam
   c. CT scan of the brain
   d. Review of medication use

3. A 65-year-old man presents to you after an episode of feeling lightheaded and nauseous, and then passing out briefly. A friend was with him at the time and caught him as he was sliding against a wall to the floor. He has a history only of longstanding hypertension. His comprehensive physical exam and electrocardiogram are normal. Are carotid Dopplers indicated as part of the evaluation to determine the etiology of his syncope?
   a. Yes
   b. No

Lucia Alvarez, *Part 1*

You are called to the emergency department to see Lucia Alvarez, a 67-year-old who passed out at her granddaughter's wedding reception. Upon questioning, she tells you that the reception was held outdoors, in 85° heat. After standing for a long time in the sun, she felt flushed and a little nauseous. The next thing she knew she was lying on the ground.

Lucia's past medical history is significant for obesity and hypothyroidism. Her only medication is levothyroxine, at a stable dose for several years. Three months ago she was hospitalized overnight after an episode of chest pain. During that hospitalization she had a normal electrocardiogram and a negative cardiac stress echocardiogram.

STUDY QUESTIONS

1. Based on the history alone, what is in your differential diagnosis regarding the possible cause of Lucia's syncope?
2. Is Lucia at high risk for cardiac syncope?

George Fallon, *Part 1*

George Fallon, age 75, "fell out" while eating lunch with a friend. He was talking normally and feeling well when, according to his friend, George suddenly slumped over at the table, plopping his head into his pasta salad. His friend called for the waiter, but by the time he arrived, about 10 or 15 seconds later, George had awakened and lifted his head, looking very pale. His speech and actions were sluggish for another minute or two, but soon he was feeling back to normal. George adamantly rejected the idea of calling EMS, so his friend agreed to drive him to your office for a same-day appointment.

You have been George's physician for the past 15 years and know that he is an active retiree with longstanding but controlled hypertension, elevated cholesterol, and benign prostatic hyperplasia. His medications include hydrochlorothiazide, metoprolol, lovastatin, aspirin, tamsulosin and trazodone occasionally for sleep. His last electrocardiogram was 5 years ago and was normal. George has never had an echocardiogram or cardiac stress test. This is his first episode of syncope.

STUDY QUESTIONS

1. Which aspects of George's history put him at increased risk of syncope?
2. Based on the brief description of the syncopal event, what causes of syncope do you suspect?
3. Could any of George's medications have contributed to the event?

PREVALENCE AND IMPACT

Syncope is defined as the sudden loss of consciousness and postural tone with spontaneous recovery. It is distinct from dizziness, vertigo, seizures, prolonged decreased mental status, drop attacks without loss of consciousness, and cardiac arrest. During a 10-year period, approximately 6% of adults have syncope. The prevalence rises steeply, however, after age 70.[1] A recent cross-sectional survey of over 7 million hospital discharges found that 1.3% of all U.S. hospitalizations had the discharge diagnosis of syncope. This translates to an estimated annual cost for syncope-related hospitalizations of $2.4 billion.[2] In spite of the high frequency and economic impact of this condition, diagnostic testing is applied inconsistently, specific therapies are often not begun, and a large number of syncopal events remain undiagnosed at the time of hospital discharge. These facts emphasize a need for more stringent use of algorithms and evidence-based guidelines in the evaluation and management of patients with syncope.[2]

RISK FACTORS AND PATHOPHYSIOLOGY

The underlying pathophysiology leading to syncope is inadequate oxygenation of the cerebral cortex and reticular activating system, resulting in loss of consciousness. A variety of mechanisms lead to this outcome, but the final common pathways involve reduced blood flow or reduced oxygen-carrying capacity. Fig. 20–1 is a graphic identifying the main physiological factors that can lead to inadequate brain oxygenation. The differential diagnosis is extensive, as many diseases and conditions can lead to this outcome. They fall into these general categories: neurally mediated (reflex) causes, orthostatic hypotension, cardiac causes, central nervous system diseases, and psychiatric disorders.

In a study of 655 cases of syncope among community elderly, a history of stroke or transient ischemic attack (TIA) was, by far, the greatest potential risk factor for syncope (odds ratio [OR] = 2.96).[3] Use of cardiac medication (OR = 1.70) and a diagnosis of high blood pressure (OR = 1.50) were also significant predictors of a syncopal event.[3] The cause of these associations is probably multifactorial, with side effects from medications and autonomic insufficiency as possible contributing factors.

In addition to having more underlying chronic conditions and being on more medications than younger adults, older persons also tend to have several age-related physiological changes that increase their syncope risk. These include[4]:

- Atherosclerosis (impairing dilation of cerebral blood vessels in the face of reduced blood flow)
- Increased endothelin production (increasing vasoconstriction of cerebral arterioles)
- Left ventricular dysfunction, due to longstanding hypertension and/or heart disease (causing decreased cardiac output)
- Cardiac valvular disease (increasing the likelihood of arrhythmias and heart block)
- Blunting of autonomic responses (predisposing the person to orthostatic hypotension)

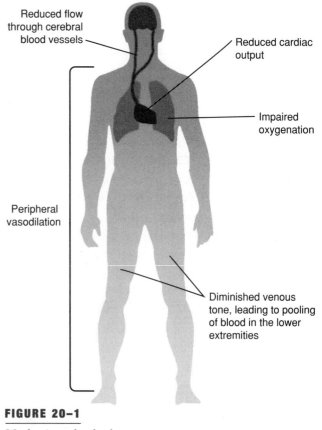

Reduced flow through cerebral blood vessels

Reduced cardiac output

Impaired oxygenation

Peripheral vasodilation

Diminished venous tone, leading to pooling of blood in the lower extremities

FIGURE 20–1

Mechanisms that lead to syncope.

Lucia Alvarez, *Part 2*

In the emergency department, Lucia is sitting on a gurney in the hallway. She looks comfortable, but tired, and is sipping a large cup of ice water. She tells you that she "just got too emotional." The triage vital signs show that she had a pulse of 105 and a blood pressure of 122/76, with no significant difference between the supine and upright positions. The other vital signs were normal. You recheck her pulse and notice that it is down to the 80s and regular. The EMS technician has already placed a peripheral IV, and Lucia is on her second liter of normal saline.

You can find no abnormalities on Lucia's exam, including a comprehensive cardiac and neurological exam. She is alert and well oriented. There are no signs of trauma from her fall. Her electrocardiogram shows normal sinus rhythm at 90 beats per minute, no conduction delays, and no signs of ischemia.

STUDY QUESTIONS

1. Based on the history, physical exam, and ECG, what other testing is warranted?
2. Are there any new findings that make you think Lucia is at high risk for cardiac syncope?
3. Can you diagnose the cause of Lucia's syncope?
4. Will you hospitalize Lucia or her follow-up in clinic?

George Fallon, *Part 2*

On entering the examining room, you find George sitting in a chair chatting with his wife and looking comfortable. He is alert and fully oriented. His vital signs are normal, including blood pressure in the supine and upright positions. There are no signs of trauma, and his head, neck, and pulmonary exams are normal. The cardiovascular exam is reassuring, with normal heart sounds, no murmur, and a regular rhythm. Carotid arteries are without bruits, and a comprehensive neurological exam is negative.

The ECG reveals a heart rate of 72 beats per minutes with a regular rhythm. Changes from his previous ECG include signs of left ventricular hypertrophy and a new right bundle branch block.

STUDY QUESTIONS

1. What is the differential diagnosis for the etiology of George's syncope?
2. Based on the history and examination, what further testing is warranted?
3. What findings indicate that George is at increased risk of syncope due to cardiac arrhythmia?
4. Does George need any additional neurological workup, such as computed tomography or magnetic resonance imaging of the brain, or electroencephalography?
5. Should George be hospitalized or worked up as an outpatient?

DIFFERENTIAL DIAGNOSIS AND ASSESSMENT

Differential Diagnosis

The differential diagnosis of syncope is long, and traditionally many cases have gone undiagnosed. Causes can be categorized as neurally mediated, orthostatic, cardiac, cerebrovascular, psychiatric, or multifactorial (Box 20–1). In geriatric practice, a high proportion (perhaps half) of cases are multifactorial.

Neurally mediated syncope involves the initiation of reflexes that lower blood pressure (through venous pooling in the legs) or slow the heart rate, usually through stimulation of the vagus nerve.[5,6] A variety of physiological stimuli can trigger this reflex; they include urination, defecation, cough, gastrointestinal stimulation (especially pain), and stimulation of the carotid sinus (e.g., by a tight collar), and intense emotions. Neurally mediated syncope is often considered a benign etiology, but it has a high prevalence and can therefore cause a large burden. It can be difficult to diagnosis accurately because of multiple contributing factors.

Vasovagal or neurocardiogenic syncope is the most common type of neurally mediated syncope; it includes the common faint. Typically, a situation involving prolonged standing, emotional distress, or exertion in a warm environment causes peripheral venous pooling and a drop in blood return to the heart. As the heart recognizes a sudden decrease in preload, it tries to compensate by contracting harder. The quick increase in contraction activates mechanoreceptors in the ventricles that start a reflex mechanism causing the central nervous system to stimulate vasodilation and bradycardia. As the drop in cardiac output becomes more profound, syncope may occur.[7] When suspecting a neurally mediated syncope, look for associated symptoms of nausea and/or vomiting,

---

Box 20-1 Differential Diagnosis of Syncope

Neurally Mediated (Vasovagal or Reflex) Syncope
- Common faint
- Situational syncope
  - Postmicturition
  - Cough induced
  - Associated with stimulation of the gastrointestinal tract (pain, swallowing, defecation)
  - Postprandial
- Carotid sinus syncope

Orthostatic Hypotension
- Medications (e.g., diuretics, antihypertensives)
- Alcohol
- Volume depletion (hemorrhage, dehydration)
- Associated with viral illness

Reduced Cardiac Function
- Arrhythmia (sinus bradycardia, sinus pause, atrioventricular block, supraventricular tachycardia, torsades de pointes, pacemaker malfunction)
- Valvular disease (especially aortic stenosis)

- Angina pectoris or myocardial infarction
- Obstructive (hypertrophic) cardiomyopathy
- Other (aortic dissection, atrial myxoma, pericardial tamponade, pulmonary embolism, severe pulmonary hypertension)

Cerebrovascular Disease
- Transient ischemic attack
- Stroke
- Subclavian steal
- Seizure (not technically considered syncope because of different mechanism, but important to consider)

Psychiatric Disorders
- Depression
- Anxiety disorders (especially panic disorder, with hyperventilation)
- Phobias
- Somatization

Multifactorial

---

prolonged standing, hot environments, and unpleasant situations. You should be cautious to not assume this diagnosis in patients with known heart disease or repetitive episodes of syncope.

Carotid sinus syndrome is often listed as a cause of syncope.[8] This is because manual stimulation of the carotid sinus can, in susceptible individuals, stimulate neurally mediated syncope. A few individuals (e.g., wearing tight collars) have true carotid sinus syncope; however, in most cases the provocation of syncope with carotid sinus massage indicates a susceptibility to neurally mediated syncope rather than a diagnosis.

Orthostatic hypotension is a drop in arterial pressure that occurs when an individual moves to an upright position. Typically, the autonomic nervous system rapidly compensates for this by increasing the venous tone in the legs; when this system fails, syncope may occur. When the circulating blood volume is depleted, as in dehydration, orthostatic hypotension, and syncope may occur even with appropriate autonomic compensation.[9] This diagnosis should be considered in individuals who are on medications that can predispose to hypotension, who have reason due to illness or blood loss to be dehydrated, or have autonomic insufficiency from a neurological disorder such as Parkinsonism. A typical case occurs soon after standing up or after prolonged standing in a hot, crowded environment.

The traditional definition of orthostatic hypotension is a drop in systolic blood pressure of ≥20 mm of mercury, or a drop in the diastolic pressure of ≥10 mmHg, 3 minutes after assuming the upright position. While this definition remains in use, numerous studies have demonstrated that syncope due to orthostatic cerebral hypoperfusion can occur when the standard criteria for orthostasis are not met. Three general mechanisms can lead to this orthostatic syncope (or near-syncope) that does not meet the definition of orthostatic hypotension:

- Early orthostatic hypotension (i.e., a drop in blood pressure immediately upon standing that becomes normalized within 3 minutes)
- Late orthostatic hypotension (i.e., a drop in blood pressure that occurs after prolonged standing)
- Impaired cerebral perfusion and syncope with mild decreases in systemic blood pressure (often due to atherosclerotic narrowing of the carotid and/or vertebral arteries)

Cardiac syncope occurs when reduction in cardiac functioning by arrhythmia, death of myocardium, or outflow obstruction leads to decreased blood flow to the brain. Several studies have shown an increase in overall mortality and sudden death among patients with cardiac syncope compared to patients with syncope from other causes.[1,10] A cardiac cause should be considered when syncope is preceded by palpitations or chest pain, or when it occurs during exertion. Patients with known severe structural heart disease should be considered to have cardiac syncope until proven otherwise.

Cerebrovascular disease is a rare but plausible cause of syncope. Most transient ischemic attacks or strokes do not cause loss of consciousness, but occasionally this can occur. There is a low yield to use of neurological testing in the evaluation of individuals with syncope unless it is directed at those with neurological findings on initial evaluation.[5,11]

Psychiatric causes should be considered in patients with repetitive syncope of unknown origin after cardiac causes have been effectively ruled out.[12,13] They are more common in younger patients. Prodromal symptoms, such as dizziness, are common. Several hypotheses exist regarding the connection between psychiatric disorders and syncope. Hyperventilation can increase susceptibility to neurally mediated syncope. There is also a term called pseudosyncope, which has been used to describe patients with syncope of unknown but presumed psychiatric origin, who have no pathological findings on exam and documented syncope without any change in blood pressure or pulse.[14]

Evaluation of the Patient with Syncope

The most common cause of syncope in older persons is one of the neurally mediated syndromes (Table 20–1). However, cardiac syncope is also quite common and, if untreated, is associated with a higher risk of sudden death. Therefore, evaluation of the patient with syncope involves the parallel process of seeking a specific diagnosis and ruling out cardiac causes. The initial history, examination, and electrocardiogram are sufficient in most cases to rule in or out cardiac disease. However patients without a diagnosis, but with a high likelihood of cardiac disease, should have additional studies.

> ● Because cardiac causes of syncope are associated with a higher risk of sudden death, evaluation of the patient with syncope must include ruling out a cardiac cause. In most cases, a history, examination, and electrocardiogram are sufficient.

In recent years, considerable evidence has accumulated that diagnostic yield and cost-effectiveness are greatest if an initial history, a standardized physical examination battery, and an electrocardiogram are applied to all older patients with syncope (strength of evidence = B).[5,9,10,15] The history can identify symptoms and situations surrounding syncope that can help diagnose three common etiologies, neurally mediated (vasovagal), orthostasis, and drug related. The physical

Table 20–1	Causes of Syncope in Older Adults: A Summary of 1516 Hospitalizations (Median Age 75 Years)
Unknown	41.6%
Vasovagal	11.5%
Orthostasis or dehydration	10.9%
Other noncardiovascular (infections, vertigo, hypoglycemia, subclavian steal, and miscellaneous noncardiac causes)	5.7%
Drug induced	3.6%
Bradycardia	3.4%
Complete heart block	2.4%
Ventricular tachycardia	2.3%
Atrial fibrillation or flutter	2.2%
Bleeding or anemia	2.2%
Seizures	1.9%
Other cardiovascular (unspecified arrhythmias, carotid sinus syncope, ruptured aorta, and miscellaneous cardiac causes)	1.8%
Supraventricular tachycardia	1.6%
Sick sinus syndrome	1.5%
Transient ischemic attack	1.2%
Micturition or tussive	1.2%
Myocardial ischemia	1.1%
Aortic stenosis	0.9%
Cerebrovascular accident	0.9%
Pulmonary embolus	0.7%
Mobitz 2 heart block	0.6%
Psychiatric	0.6%
Pacemaker dysfunction	0.2%

From Getchell WS, Larsen GC, Morris CD, McAnulty JH. Epidemiology of syncope in hospitalized patients. J Gen Intern Med 1999;14:677–87, with permission.

exam may uncover signs of a cardiovascular or neurologic process, as well as orthostasis. History and physical exam alone may be diagnostic in almost a third of syncope cases.[5] The electrocardiogram alone has little yield, due to the intermittent nature of arrhythmias; however, it is important to use along with the history and physical to risk stratify patients and direct further testing. Fig. 20–2 is an algorithm that guides the clinician through the syncope evaluation.

RULING OUT CARDIAC CAUSES

Structural heart disease, defined as coronary heart disease, congestive heart failure, valvular disease, or congenital heart disease, is the only independent risk factor for a cardiac cause of syncope. Electrocardiograms and echocardiograms may not be diagnostic in many cases,

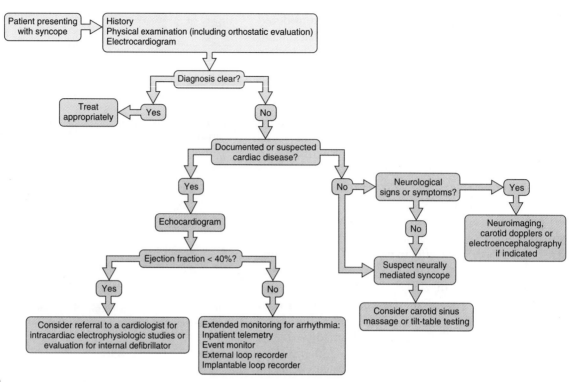

FIGURE 20-2

Syncope evaluation algorithm.

but they can stratify patients' risk by identifying who has structural heart disease. The intensity of the cardiac "rule out" evaluation depends on the patient's risk status and the history of the event.

The electrocardiogram (ECG) is an inexpensive and noninvasive test that can diagnose some cases of syncope and guide further testing in others. In a review of six inpatient and outpatient studies involving 1110 people with syncope, electrocardiography diagnosed only 5% of the cases, mostly arrythmias.[5] More importantly, it is excellent at identifying who has structural heart disease. Abnormal findings include previous myocardial infarction, bundle branch block, evidence of ventricular hypertrophy, atrioventricular blocks, brady- or tachycardias, premature ventricular contractions, pacemaker, or significant ST abnormalities.[4,10,16] These are the patients who should receive cardiac testing, as there is very poor diagnostic yield in further cardiac testing of patients with a normal ECG and no cardiac history.[4]

Patients with a cardiac history or abnormal ECG should have an echocardiogram if the etiology of syncope is still unknown after the initial history and physical exam. Similar to the ECG, it can diagnose a few rare causes of syncope such as critical aortic stenosis, myxoma, or tamponade. Otherwise, the systolic function can be used as a marker of risk for arrhythmia. An ejection fraction of 40% or less places a patient at significantly higher risk of arrhythmia.[16]

The continued search for arrhythmia in patients with undiagnosed syncope may include 24-hour Holter monitoring, external loop recorders, and implantable loop recorders. These should be reserved for the select group of patients with unexplained syncope who are at increased risk for arrhythmia based on history and initial workup. The generalized use of these studies is inefficient and expensive.[4,15,16] The finding of arrhythmia correlating with syncope or syncopal events without arrhythmia is both prognostically important and should be considered a successful test. The implantable loop recorder deserves special mention because it can be used for 18 months after implantation, increasing the likelihood of identifying another syncopal event. It can store data for 20 minutes prior to activation, allowing patients or their companions a longer time window to activate the device.[17]

Cardiac stress testing is rarely diagnostic in the evaluation of syncope. It should be considered in patients who have syncope during exertion or experience chest pain associated with syncope.[4,9,15] These select patients may show cardiac ischemia or arrhythmias associated with exercise.

Intracardiac electrophysiologic studies are invasive and very expensive. They should be reserved for patients with known structural heart disease who have very high risk for arrhythmias due to depressed ventricular function. This will most likely include patients with previous myocardial infarction. In this procedure catheters are inserted from the femoral vein into the heart near the electrical conduction system. Atrial and ventricular pacing along with electrical stimulation are used to assess sinus node recovery time, sinoatrial conduction time, and AV node function. This allows detection of conduction abnormalities that can predispose to arrhythmia.[4,15,16]

NEUROLOGIC EVALUATION

Neuroimaging and electroencephalography (EEG) have been used frequently in the routine workup of patients with unexplained syncope. Retrospective reviews have shown them to have a poor yield and high cost when used on unselected patients. In a review of 649 cases of syncope, 253 patients received electroencephalography testing, and only six had abnormal results that explained the cause of syncope (i.e., a yield of 2%). All six of those patients had a history and physical examination that was consistent with seizure. In the same group, 283 patients had brain CT scanning, also with a yield of 2%; all had a history and examination consistent with acute stroke. Carotid Dopplers were done in 185 patients, with a 0% yield.[18] In summary, consistent with published recommendations for syncope evaluation, neuroimaging and EEG can be limited to patients with symptoms or signs of acute stroke or seizure.[5]

EVALUATION FOR NEURALLY MEDIATED SYNCOPE

Many cases of neurally mediated syncope will be diagnosed by the initial evaluation alone, usually with a classic history. When the etiology of syncope is unknown and the syncopal events have become repetitive or dangerous, tilt table testing and carotid massage can be useful as confirmatory tests. It is important that cardiac syncope be effectively ruled out by prolonged cardiac monitoring if there is known or suspected cardiac disease.

Tilt table testing evaluates whether a patient is susceptible to neurally mediated syncope.[4,9] There are multiple protocols for tilt table testing, some including the use of drugs such as isoproterenol or nitroglycerin to increase susceptibility to syncope and improve the sensitivity of the test. The procedure involves baseline measurement of blood pressure and heart rate while supine, then quickly bringing the patient to an upright position by tilting to approximately 60 degrees. A foot board is in place for support. The patient is then kept in the tilted position for 45 minutes to observe for syncope or presyncopal symptoms while continuing to monitor heart rate and blood pressure. Some protocols include giving isoproterenol or nitroglycerin after the patient has been asymptomatic in the tilted position for 10 to 15 minutes, followed by further monitoring. If syncope symptoms occur during testing and correlate with a quick drop in blood pressure or pulse rate, it is considered a positive test. Likewise, if syncope occurs without a change in vital signs, a neurally mediated syncope is less likely and other etiologies should be reconsidered.

Standardized carotid sinus massage (CSM) in the supine and upright positions can help differentiate carotid sinus syndrome, or carotid sinus hypersensitivity, another risk factor for neurally mediated syncope. The carotid sinus is located in the common carotid artery at the branching point of the internal and external branches. There are baroreceptors in the carotid sinuses that respond to changes in pressure. These, via nerve centers in the brain stem, stimulate the vagus nerve, causing inhibition of the sinus node of the heart or a reduction in blood pressure.[19] A positive cardioinhibitory result is present if a cardiac pause (asystole) of 3 seconds or longer occurs during or immediately after CSM; a positive vasopressor result is present if the systolic blood pressure drops 50 mmHg or more, and is accompanied by symptoms.[20]

CSM is performed as follows[4,19]:

1. Confirm that no carotid bruits are present and that there is no known significant cerebral vascular disease. If bruits are present, or the patient is at high risk for atherosclerotic disease, consider carotid Doppler ultrasound to evaluate for significant plaque.
2. Have the patient supine, on continuous ECG monitoring and beat-to-beat blood pressure monitoring. An IV line should be in place, and atropine and transcutaneous pacing available.
3. Turn the patient's head to the left in the supine position and find the maximum impulse in the right carotid artery at the level of the thyroid cartilage. Use two fingers, firmly press down, and massage longitudinally for 5 to 10 seconds. Wait a few minutes and repeat on the left carotid sinus. Repeat in the head-up tilt position if symptoms do not occur in the supine position.

DIAGNOSING ORTHOSTATIC HYPOTENSION

To test for orthostatic hypotension, have the patient lie supine for 3 minutes, after which you check the blood pressure and pulse. Then have the patient stand for 3 minutes, during which you monitor the pulse and blood pressure. Orthostatic hypotension is said to be present if the patient experiences a drop of at least 20 mm Hg in systolic blood pressure or at least 10 mm HG in diastolic blood pressure within 3 minutes after standing from the recumbent position. This can also be demonstrated using the tilt table in the head-up position at a minimum 60-degree angle.

Multiple variables can affect the blood pressure readings, including the time of day, ambient temperature, postural deconditioning, and medications. Also, it is known that some patients may not show the diagnostic drop in blood pressure until they have been standing for at least 10 minutes. For these reasons, it is important to repeatedly check for a significant orthostatic blood pressure reduction while keeping in mind when medications are taken, time of meals, and any other factors that may have contributed to the syncopal episode under evaluation. Many patients who demonstrate a significant drop in blood pressure after standing will also have an increase in pulse rate, but it is not necessary for the diagnosis of orthostasis.

PSYCHIATRIC EVALUATION

Clues to a psychiatric origin include a history of anxiety or depression, repetitive syncope of unknown origin, a repeatedly negative cardiac workup, and multiple episodes of syncope without injury. In patients with suspected psychiatric disease, consulting with a psychiatrist is important both to identify or rule out a psychiatric diagnosis and to review the potential psychotropic effects of medications. Tilt table testing can also be helpful, because, if syncope is provoked, the physician can readily differentiate psychogenic (i.e., with no blood pressure or pulse changes) from neurally mediated syncope.[10,21]

George Fallon, *Part 3*

Concerned about a cardiac arrhythmia as the cause of George's syncope, you admit him to the hospital for cardiac monitoring and further risk stratification. The LVH and bundle branch block on the EKG, combined with his history of multiple cardiac risk factors, place him at high risk for having coronary heart disease, and therefore of arrhythmia. His medication list is also worrisome, because it contains drugs that have been implicated in hypotension, electrolyte imbalances, and dizziness. A reflex-mediated situational syncope from swallowing is unlikely, since George had no prodromal symptoms. The reassuring neurological exam and lack of postictal symptoms eliminate the need for further neurological testing at this time.

An echocardiogram shows an ejection fraction of approximately 40% with mild hypokinesis of the left ventricle and trace mitral valve regurgitation. You have George do a stress treadmill test along with the echo to make sure there is no

reversible ischemia. George is able to exercise to about 80% of his maximum heart rate, but has to stop before goal due to fatigue. However, there are no signs of ischemia on the ECG or echocardiogram. George's blood chemistries including sodium, potassium, chloride, blood urea nitrogen, creatinine and magnesium, are all within normal limits. His cardiac enzymes are also normal.

By this time, George has been in the hospital for almost 24 hours with telemetry cardiac monitoring. You received one call about a 2.5-second sinus pause, and another call about three consecutive beats of ventricular tachycardia. During both events George was talking to his wife and felt nothing unusual.

You explain to George that his ECG and echocardiogram make you think that he probably had a myocardial infarction at some point in the past couple years, and you are worried that he passed out from a cardiac arrhythmia. You decide to discharge him home with a 30-day event monitor and arrange for an appointment with the cardiologist. He is not to drive in the interim. You also start him on an ACE inhibitor to try to improve his cardiac function.

STUDY QUESTIONS

1. What evidence do you have to make you more concerned about a cardiac arrhythmia?
2. What are your options to further investigate for a cardiac arrhythmia?
3. How do you defend your decision to hospitalize George? Could all of this been done as an outpatient?

MANAGEMENT

The aggressiveness of evaluation and treatment of syncope will largely depend on the presence of cardiac disease and other comorbidities. First-time syncope in patients without known or suspected heart disease usually warrants the reduction of risk factors for further syncope. This includes reducing polypharmacy and medication misuse, treating underlying illness, and education regarding avoidance of triggers. Individuals with cardiac disease deserve a more aggressive effort in establishing an etiology of syncope and treatment of cardiac causes. Identifying and treating structural heart disease will help reduce the risk of recurrent syncope.

Lucia Alvarez, *Part 3*

The history of Lucia's syncopal event is confirmed by her husband and daughter. They explain that Lucia had been standing in the sun for over an hour even though they tried encouraging her to take a rest in the shade. It had been a long day, full of excitement and emotion, in the hot sun, and possibly with a glass or two of champagne. The bride and groom were just getting ready to leave the reception when Lucia passed out. This confirms your theory that Lucia most likely experienced a situational neurally mediated syncope. You have her get up and walk around, making sure that she feels steady on her feet. Then you send her home with her family with instructions to drink plenty of fluids and follow up with her primary physician within a week.

George Fallon, *Part 4*

Two days later, George's wife calls you after he passed out again briefly while working in the yard. You are able to get the report from the event monitor and it shows that George had 30 seconds of ventricular tachycardia. You have George readmitted to the hospital immediately where an implantable cardioverter-defibrillator is inserted the following day.

● Not everyone with syncope needs to be admitted to the hospital.

When to Hospitalize

Not everyone with syncope needs to be admitted to the hospital. Individuals for whom cardiac syncope is not suspected can usually be safely managed as an outpatient. While many hospitalizations for monitoring fail to identify a reoccurrence of symptoms, hospitalization gives rapid access to evaluation tools that can quickly assess the risk of cardiac syncope. The hospital is also a good place to change a patient's medications in a monitored environment.[22] The following are general principles about hospitalization in patients with syncope:

- Consider hospitalization of older patients with multiple comorbidities when the etiology seems multifactorial and a monitored environment is needed to sort it out.
- Hospitalize patients with known or suspected potentially fatal arrhythmias.
- Hospitalize patients with unknown etiology of syncope when cardiac disease is known or suspected by initial evaluation.

- Hospitalize when the cause is identified and requires admission (e.g., myocardial infarction or pulmonary embolism).

Permanent Cardiac Pacemakers

When syncope is a sign of symptomatic bradycardia, not caused by medications, a pacemaker will be the treatment of choice. The cardioinhibitory form of neurally mediated syncope may also be an indication for permanent cardiac pacing, especially if it is repetitive and dangerous for the patient.[22] However, evidence to support this approach has been mixed.[23,24]

Implantable Defibrillators

Patients with unexplained syncope, documented structural heart disease, and left ventricular ejection fractions of less than 30% are at high risk of sudden death due to arrhythmia. These patients warrant referral to cardiac specialists to evaluate for implantable cardiac defibrillators. When ventricular tachycardia or fibrillation is documented, the defibrillator may be clearly indicated. However, some patients with a low ejection fraction may be considered for empiric treatment with the device.

Treatment of Orthostatic Hypotension and Neurally Mediated Syncope Without Cardiac Abnormalities

For patients with orthostatic hypotension or neurally mediated syncope that does not require a pacemaker, the treatment approach is similar. The first step is elimination of medications that may contribute to orthostasis (see Box 20-1), and an admonition to refrain from alcohol. The next step is to focus on lifestyle changes to reduce recurrence, including (1) instruction to stay adequately hydrated by drinking at least 8 glasses of water a day; (2) prescription of compression stockings to reduce venous pooling in the legs (the drawback is that many patients find them uncomfortable and difficult to use); and (3) education on safer ways of assuming an upright position by rising (i.e., doing so in two stages—sitting and then standing—and using counterpressure maneuvers to avoid a drop in blood pressure.[22,25] If these measures fail to relieve symptoms, then pharmacological treatment should be considered. Drugs that have provided relief in some cases have included sympathomimetics (e.g., midodrine), beta blockers (e.g., atenolol), and mineralocorticoids (e.g., fludrocortisone). As always, any new medication should be monitored carefully for adverse effects and interactions.

Lucia Alvarez:
Case Discussion

Lucia Alvarez's case was fairly straightforward because of her uncomplicated past medical history. After hearing her initial medical history, you do not think the syncope is related to medications and you are fairly certain that she is at low risk for cardiac syncope. You believe that she was probably dehydrated from standing in the sun, and that her venous tone may have been impaired by a glass or two of champagne. As she became overheated and overcome by emotion, she was at risk for neurally mediated syncope. The nausea she experienced prior to passing out is consistent with this explanation.

The lack of cardiac or neurologic findings on examination was reassuring. She had no signs or symptoms of trauma that would necessitate radiographic evaluation. Her slower pulse rate after receiving some fluids again suggest she was dehydrated. The normal electrocardiogram along with no history of heart disease and a recently normal echocardiogram convince you that she does not have structural heart disease that would put her at increased risk for cardiac syncope. Therefore, you feel confident diagnosing Lucia with situational syncope and sending her home with her family.

If similar syncopal events become a reoccurring problem for Lucia, you could consider tilt table testing to confirm your suspicion of her susceptibility to neurally mediated syncope. It would also be helpful to have her wear a cardiac event monitor to see if it captures bradycardia or another arrhythmia that would be an indication for a pacemaker or implantable defibrillator. Also, educating her on prodromal symptoms and situations associated with neurally mediated syncope may help avoid injury.

GEORGE FALLON: *Case Discussion*

George Fallon's case presents an example of syncope that cannot be diagnosed by history, exam, and electrocardiography alone. You should be concerned about cardiac syncope from the beginning after hearing about the sudden nature of his syncope and the lack of prodromal symptoms. Even more convincing is the fact that he was actually witnessed falling into his plate of pasta salad. Other red flags from George's history include his longstanding hypertension and cholesterol, and the multiple cardiac medications that he takes daily. While the history alone should make you suspect possible cardiac disease and the need for further workup, the abnormal electrocardiogram provides additional evidence. The echocardiogram helps to risk stratify George since his low ejection fraction is an additional risk factor for arrhythmia.

In this case, the cardiac stress testing is not done as part of the syncope workup, but to further investigate the new diagnosis of cardiac disease. If you already knew about George's cardiac disease and the abnormalities on the electrocardiogram, the echocardiogram and cardiac monitoring would have been sufficient.

Hospitalization was warranted for George because of the high suspicion of cardiac syncope and the need to further evaluate his cardiac disease. The sinus pause and several beats of ventricular tachycardia that occurred in the hospital were not diagnostic because George experienced no symptoms. On discharge, George had a support system in place and would always have someone around who could call for help and activate the event monitor if he became symptomatic again. Finally, do not forget to think of safety issues such as driving, flying, operating heavy machinery, and risk of injury from falls.

SUMMARY

The multifactorial nature of syncope in older individuals makes it a very challenging problem to diagnose and treat. For many patients, the etiology of syncope will never be clear. A directed approach to evaluating syncope after an initial history, physical exam and electrocardiogram is well described. The future may bring increased use of algorithms and dedicated syncope units that will more efficiently risk stratify patients with syncope and guide appropriate testing. This will reduce excessive use of resources, prevent hospitalizations, and help to more quickly diagnose a frustrating problem.

POSTTEST

1. An 87-year-old man gets up at night to urinate, something he has done for years. However, this time, after urinating, he feels nauseated and "woozy," and passes out as he tries to return to his bed. Given this brief history, what is the most likely cause of this syncopal episode?
   a. Micturition
   b. Cerebrovascular disease
   c. Medication-induced postural hypotension
   d. Multiple factors
   e. Cardiac arrhythmia

2. A positive response to carotid sinus massage indicates a high likelihood of which one of the following types of syncope?
   a. Neurally mediated
   b. Cardiac
   c. Neurological
   d. Orthostatic
   e. Psychiatric

3. A 74-year-old patient comes to see you because she is frustrated with her previous physician, who was unable to diagnose her recurrent syncope. She describes multiple episodes of passing out and near passing out, which have occurred over several years. She often feels dizzy before the syncope. She lives at home, golfs regularly, and is active in her church. Medications include hydrochlorothiazide, a multivitamin, and PRN loratadine. She has no history of cardiac disease, and previous evaluations have included several normal electrocardiograms, a normal Holter monitor, and a normal echocardiogram. Your neurological examination is normal. Which of the following would be a logical next step in evaluating this patient?
   a. Event monitor
   b. Tilt table testing
   c. CT scan
   d. Orthostatic blood pressure evaluation
   e. Referral to a neurologist

4. A 65-year-old female patient who is new to your practice presents after one episode of syncope that was sudden and without prodromal symptoms. She has hypertension, hypothyroidism, and depression, all controlled on medication per her report. Her physical exam reveals an obese woman with 2+ pretibial edema and a normal cardiovascular and neurological exam. Her electrocardiogram shows left ventricular hypertrophy. Which of the following would be reasonable as the next step in determining the etiology of her syncope?
   a. Carotid Dopplers
   b. Transthoracic echocardiogram
   c. CT scan of head
   d. Tilt table testing
   e. Referral to a psychiatrist

5. A 67-year-old man with no significant medical problems passes out at a cookout soon after standing up. He had recently finished his barbeque dinner and admits to having consumed three beers. He denies any previous syncopal episodes. His complete physical exam reveals a very healthy-appearing man with no abnormal findings. His electrocardiogram is normal. What should you do?
   a. Admit him to the hospital for telemetry monitoring.
   b. Refer him to a cardiologist for intracardiac electrophysiologic studies.
   c. Schedule an exercise treadmill cardiac stress test.
   d. Reassure him and follow up with him in clinic again later in the week.

References

1. Soteriades ES, Evans JC, Larson MG, et al. Incidence and prognosis of syncope. N Engl J Med 2002;347:878-85.
2. Sun BC, Emond JA, Camargo CA. Direct medical costs of sycope-related hospitalizations in the United States. Am J Cardiol 2005;95:668-71.
3. Chen L, Chen MH, Larson MG,, et al. Risk factors for syncope in a community-based sample (the Framingham Heart Study). Am J Cardiol 2000;85:1189-93.
4. Sim V, Pascual J, Woo J. Evaluating elderly patients with syncope. Arch Gerontol Geriatr 2002;35:121-35.
5. Linzer M, Yang EH, Estes NAM, et al. Clinical guideline: diagnosing syncope. Part 1: value of history, physical examination, and electrocardiography. Ann Intern Med 1997;126:989-96.
6. Abboud FM. Neurocardiogenic syncope. N Engl J Med 1993;15:1117-20.
7. Grubb BP. Neurocardiogenic syncope. N Engl J Med 2005;352:1004-10.
8. Kenny RA, Richardson DA, Steen N, Bexton RS, Shaw FE, Bond J. Carotid sinus syndrome: a modifiable risk factor for nonaccidental falls in older adults. J Am Coll Cardiol 2001;38:1491-6.
9. Brignole M, Alboni P, Benditt DG, et al. Guidelines on management (diagnosis and treatment) of syncope—update 2004, executive summary. Eur Heart J 2004;25:2054-72.
10. Sarasin FP, Louis-Simonet M, Carballo D, et al. Prospective evaluation of patients with syncope: a population-based study. Am J Med 2001;111:177-84.
11. Getchell WS, Larsen GC, Morris CD, et al. Epidemiology of syncope in hospitalized patients. J Gen Intern Med 1999;14:677-87.
12. Kapoor WN, Fortunato M, Hanusa BH, et al. Psychiatric illnesses in patients with syncope. Am J Med 1995;99:505-12.
13. Luzza F, Di Rosa S, Pugliatti P, et al. Syncope of psychiatric origin. Clin Auton Res 2004;14:26-9.
14. Lombardi F, Calosso E, Mascioli G, et al. Utility of implantable loop recorder (Reveal Plus) in the diagnosis of unexplained syncope. Europace 2004;7:19-24.
15. Linzer M, Yang EH, Estes NAM, et al. Clinical guideline: diagnosing syncope. Part 2: unexplained syncope. Ann Intern Med 1997;127:76-86.

16. Sarasin FP, Junod A, Carballo D, et al. Role of echocardiography in the evaluation of syncope: a prospective study. Heart 2002;88:363-7.
17. Armstrong VL, Lawson J, Kamper AM, et al. The usage of an implantable loop recorder in the investigation of unexplained syncope in older people. Age Ageing 2003;32:185-8.
18. Pires LA, Ganji JR, Jarandila R, et al. Diagnostic patterns and temporal trends in the evaluation of adult patients hospitalized with syncope. Arch Intern Med 2001;161:1889-95.
19. Cummins RO, ed. ACLS Provider Manual. Dallas, TX: American Heart Association, 2001.
20. Kumar NP, Thomas A, Mudd P, et al. The usefulness of carotid sinus massage in different patient groups. Age Ageing 2003;32:666-9.
21. Parry SW, Kenny RA. Tilt table testing in the diagnosis of unexplained syncope. Q J Med 1999;92:623-9.
22. Morillo CA, Baranchuk A. Current management of syncope: treatment alternatives. Curr Treat Options Cardiovasc Med 2004;6:371-83.
23. Connolly SJ, Sheldon R, Roberts RS, et al. The North American Vasovagal Pacemaker Study (VPS): a randomized trial of permanent cardiac pacing for the prevention of vasovagal syncope. J Am Coll Cardiol 1999;33:16-20.
24. Connolly SJ, Sheldon R, Thorpe KR, et al. Pacemaker therapy for prevention of syncope in patients with recurrent severe vasovagal syncope: second Vasovagal Pacemaker Study (VPS II). JAMA 2003;289:2224-9.
25. Wieling W, Colman N, Krediet CTP, et al. Nonpharmacological treatment of reflex syncope. Clin Auton Res 2004;14(Suppl 1):I/62-70.

PRETEST ANSWERS

1. c
2. c
3. b

POSTTEST ANSWERS

1. d
2. a
3. b
4. b
5. d

Falls

Diana C. Schneider and Scott L. Mader

OBJECTIVES

Upon completion of this chapter, the reader will be able to:

- Describe the incidence and consequences of a fall in older individuals residing in the community or long-term care setting, or in acute care.

- List the major medical, physical, psychological, and environmental risk factors for falls in older individuals.

- Develop a plan for evaluating an older individual who falls, including an appropriate history, physical examination, and laboratory assessment.

- Identify useful strategies for the management and rehabilitation of patients who fall.

- Recognize the interventions that are effective in preventing falls and preventing injury from falls.

PRETEST

1. Which of the following is a true statement regarding falls in elderly persons?
   a. Most falls in elderly persons are associated with significant injury.
   b. Falls are the leading cause of accidental death in the elderly.
   c. Approximately 5% of elders residing in a nursing home fall each year.
   d. Survivors of hip fractures secondary to falls are rarely institutionalized.

2. A 76-year-old man who is a resident of an Alzheimer's unit of a long-term care facility has had three falls since admission 1 month ago. Which of the following medications is least likely to contribute to his falls?
   a. Diazepam, 5 mg twice daily
   b. Sertraline, 50 mg daily
   c. Metformin, 500 mg daily
   d. Risperidone, 2 mg at bedtime

3. An 83-year-old female patient with a history of Parkinson's disease and macular degeneration is brought to your clinic after a fall. She was discharged from the hospital 2 days ago with a diagnosis of pneumonia. Which of the following statements is true regarding her risk for falls?
   a. Since she has been discharged from the hospital, this patient is no longer at risk for falls.
   b. This patient is only at risk for falls until her pneumonia has completely resolved.
   c. This fall proves that this patient should not have been discharged from the hospital.
   d. This patient's Parkinson's disease and macular degeneration as well as recent hospitalization all place her at higher risk for falls.

4. An 86-year-old woman has had two recent falls in her home. She fractured her humerus 3 months ago and presents today with some bruising on her right cheek from a fall yesterday. She has a history of hypertension and osteoporosis. Which of the following should be the first step in evaluating the falls?
   a. Carotid sinus massage
   b. History, medication review, and observation of gait
   c. Electrocardiogram
   d. Computed tomography of the head
   e. Chest x-ray

PREVALENCE AND IMPACT

Falls and fall-related injuries are common in older adults and can be associated with significant morbidity and mortality. Each year, approximately 30% of community-dwelling persons over age 65 years and 50% of those over 80 years will fall.[1,2] Among older adults residing in institutions, more than 50% will fall each year.[3] Fortunately, most falls result in minor or no physical injury. An estimated 5% of falls result in a fracture, but many other injuries can occur, including lacerations, sprains, dislocations, subdural hematomas, and hemarthroses.[4] However, falls can also result in serious injury and even death. Unintentional injuries are the fifth leading cause of death for persons aged 65 to 84,[5] and falls are the leading cause of accidental death in older adults, accounting for 9600 deaths in the United States in 1998.[6] Of all fall-related fractures, hip fractures cause the greatest number of deaths and lead to the most severe health problems and reduced quality of life.[7,8] The risk of dying from a fall increases with increasing age. Table 21-1 demonstrates the rate of falls and injuries from falls in older adult populations.

Table 21–1	Prevalence and Complications of Falls			
Setting	**Rates of Falls (per Year)**	**Injury (per Fall)**	**Death (per Fall)**
Community-dwelling adults >65 years	30%	5% fractures 10% serious injury 30%–50% minor injury	Men 32.7/100,000 Women 27.3/100,000
Community-dwelling adults >85 years	50%		
Nursing home residents	50% or 1.5 fall/bed/year	1%–10% fractures 1%–36% injuries	1800 fatal falls per year
Acute hospital adults	2.3–7 per 1000 patient days	30% injury 4%–6% serious injury	

Major sources include Blake et al.,[1] Tinetti et al.,[2] Rubenstein et al.,[3] Centers for Disease Control and Prevention,[9] and Hitcho et al.[10]

For those older adults who survive a fall, there may be significant consequences. Approximately 8% of older adults visit an emergency room because of a fall-related injury each year and almost half of these are admitted to the hospital.[6] Of the elders admitted to a hospital after a fall, only 50% will be alive 1 year later.[11] A fall can result in a long lie on the floor due to the faller being unable to rise from the floor. It is estimated that close to 50% of noninjured fallers are unable to rise from the floor after a fall.[12] This can place an older adult at risk for pneumonia, pressure sores, dehydration, and rhabdomyolysis (muscle breakdown). Falls and recurrent falls can be associated with many psychological consequences. Older individuals who have fallen may develop a fear of falling and avoid activities in order to avoid falling. One in four older adults reported avoiding activities because of fear.[2] This self-induced restriction in activity can lead to loss of function and loss of independence. Compared to older adults who do not fall, those who fall experience more functional decline in activities of daily living and in physical and social activities.[13] Falls have also been shown to be a strong predictor of nursing home placement.[14] A survey found that 80% of older women would rather be dead than experience the loss of independence and quality of life that results from a hip fracture followed by nursing home placement.[15] There is also significant cost associated with falls. In 1991, Medicare costs for hip fractures were estimated to be $2.9 billion.[16] Hip fractures are the most costly fall-related injuries, often resulting in hospitalization. In 1996, over 250,000 older Americans suffered a hip fracture, at a cost in excess of $10 billion.[17]

> ● Of the elders admitted to a hospital after a fall, only 50% will be alive 1 year later.

RISK FACTORS AND PATHOPHYSIOLOGY

Falls in older adults result from the inability to maintain postural stability in the face of the demands of the environment.[18] There are many risk factors for falls, and it is the interaction of these factors that predisposes an individual to a fall. These risk factors are commonly divided into intrinsic and extrinsic factors. The risk of falling increases with the number of risk factors.[19] Intrinsic risk factors include age-related physiologic changes, acute or chronic medical conditions, mobility disorders, and medications. Extrinsic risk factors include risks in the environment, activity performed and restraints. Some common risk factors are listed in Box 21–1. A recent review of fall risk factor studies found the most predictive risk factors to be lower extremity weakness, history of previous falls, and gait and balance disorders.[20]

Box 21–1 Common Risk Factors to Inquire About During Falls Assessment

Intrinsic
- Age and age-related physiologic changes
- Acute illness
- Chronic illness
- Mobility factors

Medications
- Polypharmacy
- Diuretics (electrolyte imbalance, orthostasis)
- Hypnotics and sedatives (sedation)
- Antidepressants (sedation, central nervous system activity)
- Psychotropics (sedation, central nervous system ativity)
- Antihypertensives (orthostasis, hypotension)

Extrinsic
- Environmental factors
- Footwear
- Use of ambulatory assistive devices
- Mechanical restraints

George Binson, *Part 1*

George Binson is an 82-year-old male who is initiating outpatient care with you. He was recently widowed and is now living alone. His daughter, who lives nearby but works full-time, has urged him to make an appointment to begin taking better care of himself. He has a history of hypertension, diabetes mellitus, intermittent nausea with possible gastroparesis, benign prostatic hypertrophy, and osteoarthritis of the knees. He takes multiple medications to manage his medical conditions, but did not bring these with him today. His only complaints are increased urinary frequency and feeling bored. You note bent glasses frames, a small abrasion on his forehead, and another on his right arm. When you ask him about these, he reluctantly admits that he fell 2 days ago in his house and that this was not the first time. He does not want his daughter to know about the falls because he would like to continue to live on his own and does not wish to be dependent on her.

STUDY QUESTION

1. What are Mr. Binson's intrinsic and extrinsic risk factors for falls?

Intrinsic Factors

Falls increase with increasing age, and the risk triples from age 70 to age 90.[21] It is likely that this is partially explained by physiologic changes associated with aging. Visual changes that occur with aging include decreased depth perception, decreased dark adaptation, and greater sensitivity to glare. Muscular strength in the legs and ankles declines, and joint flexibility also becomes impaired with aging. Proprioceptive feedback declines with age, leading to more postural sway. The vestibular righting response diminishes with age, thus decreasing the chance of recovering once balance is lost. Gait changes that occur with aging include slower speed, decreased stride length, and decreased heel lift. Reaction time is prolonged with aging. Although orthostatic hypotension is not more common in healthy elderly, susceptibility to orthostatic hypotension increases with age. All of the above changes may increase the propensity to fall.

Nonspecific presentation of disease is more common in older patients. Acute illness, such as pneumonia or myocardial infarction, may present as a fall in an older individual. It is important to consider this when evaluating an older patient for a fall, especially in the acute environment, such as an emergency room. Older adults are also vulnerable to falls after treatment in the emergency room or hospital. The risk of a fall in older persons recently discharged from the hospital and receiving home care is four-fold higher than well elders for 2 weeks after discharge.[22] This increased risk may be due to the illness itself, deconditioning, or possibly medication effect.[6]

Many studies have revealed that older adults who fall tend to have more medical diagnoses than those who do not fall.[2,23] Thus, the risk of falling increases with increased numbers of simultaneously occurring diseases. However, many chronic illnesses, especially those that affect the visual and neuromuscular systems, are also independent risk factors for falls. Visual impairment from any cause, Parkinsonism, stroke, and arthritis have been found to be correlated with falls in multiple studies.[1,2,23-25] Older women with circulatory disease, chronic obstructive pulmonary disease, depression, and arthritis are at higher risk of falling.[26] Depression has been found to be an independent risk factor for falls.[2,27,28] Dementia can increase the risk of falling, possibly through impairment of judgment, motor function, or visual spatial perception.[28-30] Other conditions that have more recently been found to increase risk for falls include peripheral neuropathy and urge urinary incontinence.[31,32] Any condition that causes impairment in muscle strength, gait, hearing, cognition, or blood pressure regulation should be considered a fall risk factor. Some investigators believe there are subsets of fallers who actually have syncopal disorders. Studies have shown that carotid sinus hypersensitivity with bradycardia and hypotension may be present in some older patients who have falls but deny syncope, and that management focused on this can decrease subsequent falling.[33]

Patients with either very low mobility or very high mobility are at the greatest risk for falling. Impairments in mobility increase the risk for falls and patients who have low activity levels and impaired activities of daily living have been found to have more falls.[2] Lower extremity disability, arthritis of the knees, and abnormalities in gait and balance from any cause also increase fall risk.[2,34] Lower extremity weakness is an independent risk factor for falls.[35] Foot disorders, in particular calluses, hallux valgus, and lesser digital deformity are common in older individuals and may contribute to functional impairment and falls in this age group.[36] Additionally, a history of one or more falls in the previous year, a fall occurring indoors, or the inability to get off the floor after a fall are predictive of future falls.[37]

> ● A history of one or more falls in the previous year, a fall occurring indoors, or the inability to get off the floor after a fall are predictive of future falls.

Medications

Medications play a significant role in falls among the elderly. Patients taking four or more chronic medications (polypharmacy) are at increased risk of falling.[19,23] Individual medications with the potential to cause sedation, dizziness, hypotension, or fluid or electrolyte abnormalities or arrhythmias are most often implicated as increasing risk for falls. It is clear that many psychotropic medications can cause falls and as a group, psychotropic medications may double the risk of falling.[38] Use of both tricyclic antidepressants and selective serotonin reuptake inhibitors (SSRIs) increase the fall risk.[39] Long-acting benzodiazepines, sedative hypnotics, and antipsychotics have all been found to increase the risk of falls. Topical eye medications have been associated with increased risk for falling, especially beta-adrenergic antagonists.[40] See Box 21–2 for a list of medications implicated in falls.

Extrinsic Factors

Extrinsic risk factors have been implicated in one-third to one-half of all falls. This risk appears to be highest for persons with underlying frailty or mobility disorders. Some environmental risk factors that have been implicated include low or elevated bed heights, bed rails, low toilet seats, poorly illuminated areas, upended carpet or rug edges, uneven sidewalks or cur edges, highly polished or wet floors, and icy walkways.[11] Footwear style may also be considered an extrinsic risk factor. Fall risk has been found to be increased in older adults who were barefoot or wearing only stockings.[41] Older adults who wear multifocal glasses have been found to be more than twice as likely to suffer falls when compared with those who did not wear these glasses.[42] Most falls in older adults occur during usual activities, such as walking or changing position, but a small percentage occur during more risky activities, such as climbing a ladder or sports activity.[2]

Mechanical restraints, which were once used in an effort to prevent falls and injuries, have been found to increase the risk of falls and injuries from falls.[43] Restraints have never been shown to prevent falls or control agitation, and complications resulting directly from restraints include falls, death from strangulation, stress, pressure sores, social isolation, and incontinence.[44]

> ● Extrinsic risk factors have been implicated in one-third to one-half of all falls.

Risk for Injury from Fall

Because of age-related changes and comorbid disease, older persons have a higher risk of injury from a fall than younger individuals. Any fall may result in injury, but there are certain conditions that make injury from a fall more likely. The presence of osteoporosis increases the likelihood of a fracture with a fall. Additionally, older individuals with less body fat and lower body weight appear to fracture more easily.[11] Some characteristics of the fall itself may predispose to more injury, including a fall from a greater height, landing on a hard surface, landing sideways onto a hip (hip fracture), or landing on an outstretched hand (Colles wrist fracture).[6]

Box 21-2   Medications That Increase Risk of Falling

- Polypharmacy
- Sedative hypnotics
- Antidepressants (both tricyclics and SSRIs)
- Antipsychotics
- Antihypertensive agents
- Cardiac medications
- Anticholinergic drugs
- Hypoglycemic agents
- Antiparkinsonian medications
- Topical eye medications

George Binson, *Part 2*

You have only a short clinic appointment, so your plan is to examine Mr. Binson briefly. On examination, you find a thin elderly male who is slightly disheveled and wearing glasses with bent frames. He did not bring in any gait assist device. Vital signs show him to be afebrile with BP 135/80, pulse 80 (sitting) and BP 130/85, pulse 88 (standing). The cardiovascular exam shows a regular rate and rhythm without murmurs. Pulmonary and gastrointestinal exams are noncontributory, with the exception of mild tenderness in the suprapubic area. He is unable to rise without using his hands, and casual examination of his gait is that it is slow and unsteady.

Urinalysis obtained at the end of your visit reveals too numerous to count white blood cells and many bacteria. Post-void residual as assessed by ultrasound is 77 cc. You treat his urinary tract infection, make a referral to physical therapy, and ask him to return in 1 week for a review of his medications and a thorough neurologic examination.

STUDY QUESTION

1. Is the urinary tract infection significant with regard to Mr. Binson's falls?

DIFFERENTIAL DIAGNOSIS AND ASSESSMENT

A fall may be a seminal event in an older individual's life with the possibility of a subsequent decline in function. However, sometimes a fall may be truly accidental (e.g., an active 72-year-old who falls while hiking). The clinician's role is to determine whether the fall is indicative of an underlying problem, and if so, to initiate management strategies to prevent further falls. A history of a single fall in the past year should prompt at a minimum, an observation of gait. *Recurrent falls*, defined as two or more falls in a 6-month period, should definitely prompt a thorough evaluation. The American Geriatrics Society, British Geriatrics Society, and the American Academy of Orthopedic Surgeons provided a guideline for the assessment and management of falls in older adults (Fig. 21–1).[45] This evaluation will often reveal multiple risk factors possibly contributing to the falls.

Differential Diagnosis

A fall in an older adult may be the result of an accident, environmental hazard, gait or balance disorder, dizziness, vertigo, hypotension, dementia, visual disorder, syncope, or another cause. In considering the etiology of a fall, the clinician must determine whether there was any loss of consciousness, particularly if the fall was unwitnessed. This would suggest possible syncope, and further evaluation must center on the conditions that may precipitate syncope. Falls and syncope are distinct syndromes with various differential diagnoses; however, there is some evidence that lack of history of loss of consciousness does not always rule out syncope.[46] Thus, syncope (due to vasovagal reaction, carotid sinus hypersensitivity, cardiac arrhythmias, or orthostatic or other situational hypotension) should be considered in older patients with recurrent unexplained falls. The basic approach to fall assessment should include a focused history, physical examination, balance and gait assessment, and laboratory and diagnostic studies. The assessment of the older adult who falls may consist of many components, listed in Table 21–2.[47]

> ● In considering the etiology of a fall, the clinician must determine whether there was any loss of consciousness, particularly if the fall was unwitnessed.

Screening for Falls

Because falls are a commonly under-reported problem in the elderly, clinicians should ask about falls and near-falls as part of every geriatric review of systems or at least annually. Community physicians tend to underdetect falls and gait disorders in their older patients.[48] Memory problems may impair the ability of some patients to report falls, so questioning the caregiver or family is important. Some older adults may be reluctant to disclose a fall as they want to avoid an image of frailty, preserve their autonomy, or are fearful of institutionalization.[11] Screening instruments have been

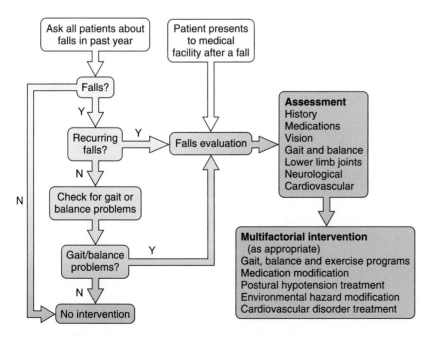

FIGURE 21–1

Algorithm summarizing assessment and management of falls. From American Geriatrics Society, British Geriatrics Society, American Academy of Orthopedic Surgeons Panel on Falls Prevention. Guideline for the prevention of falls in older persons. J Am Geriatr Soc 2001;49(5):664–72, with permission.

Table 21–2	Assessment Strategies and Diagnostic Maneuvers to Evaluate Older Persons with a History of Falling

Indication	Assessment Strategy	Level of Evidence for Recommendation	Comments
All older adults	Screening for falls	D	Yearly screening.
Older adults with one fall or no fall	Gait and balance assessment	D	If problem identified, complete the comprehensive fall evaluation below.
Older adult with recurrent falls	Comprehensive fall evaluation (includes all tests below)	A	Referral to a specialist for particular components may be required.
	Fall history Number of risk factors History of a fall Fear of falls	C	History, circumstances, symptoms associated with falls; assess fear of falling; note number of risk factors.
	Health and functional assessment Acute illness Gender Advanced age Sleep problems Sensory deficits	C	Assess ADLs, IADLs, ability to transfer safely.
	Medication and alcohol review Polypharmacy Drug side effects Alcohol	A	Review medications, check for polypharmacy, ask about alcohol.
	Postural vital signs	A	Check for orthostatic hypotension.
	Vision screening	C	Note problems with acuity, visual fields; check glasses.
	Gait/balance screening	A	Target fall prevention strategies based on deficits.
	Musculoskeletal and foot assessment Osteoarthritis Amputation Foot problems	C	Disability, osteoarthritis, range of motion, corns, calluses, bunions.
	Continence assessment	C	Note history of incontinence and medications used.
	Cardiovascular ssessment Cardiac medication review Postprandial hypotension Carotid sinus massage	B	Note any cardiac symptoms, consider carotid sinus massage.
	Neurologic assessment History of cerebrovascular accident (CVA) History of Lewy body dementia Reduced grip strength	A	Note history of CVA, transient ischemic attack, dementia, vestibular dysfunction, any neurological disease. Assess grip strength, proprioception, peripheral innervation, rigidity, Mini-Mental Status Exam.
	Depression screening Depression medication	A	Note history of depression and any medications used.
	Walking aid and protective device assessment Wheelchair, scooter Footwear	A	Note use of walking aids, wheelchairs, other devices. Note use of footwear.
	Environmental assessment	C	Identify modifiable risk factors
Older long-term care residents	Resident assessment protocol (RAP) trigger		RAP can be used to guide a comprehensive fall evaluation

See footnote at end of Table 21-3 for level of evidence scale.

developed to predict which patients in a hospital or institutional setting may be at increased risk for falls, such as the Morse or STRATIFY risk assessment tool. Use of these instruments may help to focus prevention strategies on a high-risk group of patients.[49]

Fall History

The fall evaluation and risk assessment begins with a directed history of the events surrounding the fall. An initial open-ended question such as "tell me about your fall(s)" allows patients to describe the event in their own words. It is important to identify the circumstances surrounding the fall. For some patients, a falls diary may be useful.[50] It is important to determine if acute illness or syncope is present.

Once it has been determined that acute illness or syncope is not involved, then questioning should relate to the other common risk factors for falls. Specific questions to ask include any symptoms experienced at the time or prior to the fall. Common fall-associated symptoms and their diagnostic implications include:

- Drugs (new prescriptions, polypharmacy, centrally active, hypotensive, alcohol/illicit)
- Abnormal mobility (previous cerebrovascular accident, Parkinsonism, foot disorders, neuropathy, arthritis, use of gait assist device)
- Cognitive impairment (judgment problems other signs of dementia)
- Dizziness (hypotension from orthostasis, meals, medications, Valsalva), audio/vestibular problems, dehydration, drug effect)
- Impaired vision (glasses, date of most recent eye exam, eye medications)
- Environmental hazards (clutter, poor lighting, poor vision, stair/rails in need of repair, uneven outdoor surfaces/curbs)

A history of any previous falls or near falls must be elicited. The risk of falling has been shown to be increased with the frequency of near falls.[51] Activity performed at the time of a fall can provide clues as to the etiology. Examples include a fall with standing (orthostatic hypotension), reaching (balance), carpet edge (weakness), flexion of the neck (basilar artery), and after a meal (postprandial hypotension). The location of a fall or time of day may suggest a mechanism (nocturia, poor vision). The injuries incurred from a fall (bruises on one side of the face, upper extremity fracture) may also suggest a mechanism for the fall. Psychological factors, history of depression, and fear of falling should also be assessed in the fall history. Assessment of incontinence symptoms should be obtained. It is essential to review all current medical diagnoses and medications, including any recent changes in dosing, over-the-counter medications, eye drops, and alcohol.

Baseline Functional Level

It is also important to ask about prior functional activity level to determine if there has been a recent change in functional status or usual activity level. Baseline cognitive status and any recent changes (confusion, worsening memory loss) would be significant. Family members or neighbors may supplement these data. In addition, gathering information about environmental factors including ambulatory assistive devices (and if

they were appropriately prescribed and fitted), shoes, and home structure can reveal hidden hazards within the home. The patient's social situation in terms of living environment and support will become important in implementing treatment strategies.

Physical Examination

A comprehensive physical examination should be performed with special emphasis given to skin, cardiac, neurologic, musculoskeletal, and cognitive evaluation. The clinician should review the vital signs for evidence of occult infection or cardiac or pulmonary disease. Pain should be assessed with a standardized pain assessment tool.[47] Orthostatic vital signs should be measured, as orthostatic hypotension may be present without symptoms. The patient's subcutaneous fat and temporal areas should be assessed to evaluate nutritional status. On cardiac examination, particular attention should be paid to rhythm, murmurs, bruits, and jugular venous pressure. The musculoskeletal system should be examined for arthritic deformity, impairments in range of motion, or disability. Examination of the feet should be performed to evaluate for deformities, contractures, calluses, pain, and footwear.

The neurologic examination should include mental status testing if there is evidence of dementia, delirium, or depression. Depression screening, with a tool such as the Geriatric Depression Scale, should be performed as depression may contribute to fall risk.[47] Cranial nerve examination should include tests of visual acuity, visual fields, extraocular movements, and hearing. In the upper extremities, increased muscle tone, cogwheeling, or other signs of Parkinsonism should be noted. Evaluation of upper and lower extremities should include strength, sensation, and tone. Cerebellar function, Romberg testing, and reflexes should be performed. It is essential that gait be observed as well as the use of any walking aids.

> ● The neurologic examination should include mental status testing if there is evidence of dementia, delirium, or depression.

Balance and Gait Evaluation

Balance and gait are complex tasks that are affected by age, disease, lifestyle, and impairments in sensory, neurologic, and musculoskeletal function. There is strong evidence that balance and gait assessment is the single best predictor of individuals at increased risk of falling.[2,52] A careful assessment of the older person's balance and gait is a crucial part of the fall evaluation. This allows the clinician to observe the patient perform position changes and gait maneuvers used in daily activities. A simple reliable method for evaluating balance and gait is the Timed Up and Go Test

(TUG).[53] The TUG test is quick and simple and can be performed in a clinic, emergency room, hospital ward, long-term care setting, or a home (Box 21–3). While the patient is ambulating, the clinician can observe gait initiation, step height, length, continuity, symmetry, speed, path, and deviation. When evaluating the turn, look for smoothness of movement, tempo, and foot placement. The sternal nudge test (Box 21–4) adds important information about the patient's postural stability. Patients who have difficulty on this screening test should undergo further gait assessment.[54] There are many variations of balance and gait tests that can be used (such as the Tinetti Gait and Balance Assessment). Based on this evaluation, a clinician can make medical, rehabilitative, and environmental recommendations. It is important to remember that these assessments only analyze balance and gait, and do not specifically address other risk factors for falls, such as delirium.

Laboratory and Radiologic Studies

All older persons who have experienced recurrent falls should undergo some laboratory testing, although there are no specific guidelines. This may include complete blood count, thyroid function tests, electrolytes, glucose, calcium and vitamin B_{12} level, urinalysis (for both infection and specific gravity).[18] These tests are warranted because of the high prevalence of potentially treatable conditions.[14] Further laboratory

---

> ### Box 21-3 Timed Up and Go Test
>
> **Performing the Test**
>
> Time the patient performing the following steps:
>
> 1. Rise from a standard armchair.
> 2. Walk a distance of 3 m (10 feet); may use walking aid (cane, walker).
> 3. Turn around.
> 4. Walk back to the chair.
> 5. Sit down without using arms.
>
> **Scoring the Test**
>
> - 10 seconds or less indicates low risk for falling.
> - 11 to 19 seconds indicates low to moderate risk for falling.
> - 20 to 29 seconds indicates moderate to high risk for falling.
> - 30 seconds or more indicates that the patient has impaired mobility and is at high risk of falling.

Adapted from Podsiadlo D, Richardson S. The timed "Up & Go": a test of basic functional mobility for frail elderly persons. J Am Geriatr Soc 1991;39:142–8, and National Guideline Clearinghouse (www.guideline.gov), with permission.

> ### Box 21-4 Sternal Nudge Test
>
> **Performing the Test**
>
> 1. Ask the patient to stand with both eyes open.
> 2. Ask the patient to place feet as close together as possible.
> 3. Ensure safety by having another person stand behind the patient.
> 4. Nudge the patient's sternum lightly with your fingers three times (with enough force to induce balance displacement).
>
> **Scoring the Test**
>
> Normal response is to stretch arms forward and take a step backward if needed to maintain balance.

Adapted from Tinetti ME. Performance-oriented assessment of mobility in elderly patients. J Am Geriatr Soc 1986;34:119–26, with permission.

---

and diagnostic testing may be warranted based on the history and physical examination. Drug levels or urine toxicology screening may be indicated if the patient is taking medications whose levels can be assessed, such as anticonvulsants or if there is suspicion of other substance use. Brain or other imaging and cardiac evaluation should be directed by the clinical history and examination.

Special Tests

Special tests might be helpful if any abnormalities are found on examination. If acute illness is suspected, additional tests might include urinalysis, chest x-ray, electrocardiogram, and cardiac enzymes. In cases of falls where the older adult has a significant cardiac history or symptoms suggestive of syncope or arrhythmia, an electrocardiogram, 24-hour Holter monitoring and echocardiogram may be warranted. In the older patient with recurrent falls, the clinician may consider monitoring heart rate and blood pressure responses to carotid sinus massage (in a monitored environment).[55] Tilt table testing may be appropriate in patients with recurrent falls, unclear history, and no orthostasis on repeated assessments.

> ### George Binson, *Part 3*
>
> *Mr. Binson returns feeling better and notes that his urinary symptoms are improved. When you ask him about falls, he seems hesitant to answer any questions. He has not yet seen the physical therapist. You reassure him that your goal is to prevent further falls or serious injury. You tell him that studies have shown that some treatments may*

prevent falls in older people. You obtain a complete fall history and learn that Mr. Binson has fallen more than five times. He usually falls during the day and has had such frequent near falls that he admits to limiting many activities he used to enjoy, because "I'm sure I would fall." He does not notice any premonitory symptoms and states, "I just trip over my own feet." He denies any syncope, chest pain, palpitations, or shortness of breath. He does admit to some numbness in his feet. When asked about his memory, he states, "It's fine." His answers to all questions are slow and when you ask about his mood, he admits to feeling very bored since the loss of his wife. He denies alcohol use and this is corroborated by family. He has a large bag of medications that includes metoclopramide, acetaminophen, metoprolol, hydrochlorothiazide, aspirin, glipizide, terazosin, and temazepam (which he has taken since his wife had been ill).

On examination, he has an early cataract in the right eye. Extraocular muscles are intact. Hearing is normal by whisper test and external auditory canals are clear. Cranial nerves are intact. Strength is normal. Sensory exam shows decreased sensation to light touch and vibration in both lower extremities to the knee. There is mild rigidity but no cogwheeling. Romberg exam shows slight sway and patient has difficulty maintaining balance with a sternal nudge. Musculoskeletal exam shows arthritic changes in both knees. Ankle dorsiflexion is also limited. Mini-mental status exam score is 29/30. You perform the TUG test and the patient has difficulty rising without use of his arms. He gait is slow and antalgic, steps are discontinuous, and the turn appears unsafe. It takes the patient 40 seconds to complete the test. The Geriatric Depression Scale reveals a score of 2 out of 15, which is in the nondepressed range. You order the following laboratory tests: complete blood count, electrolytes, vitamin B_{12}, thyroid stimulating hormone, glucose, and glycosylated hemoglobin.

STUDY QUESTIONS

1. Based on your complete fall evaluation, what further risk factors does Mr. Binson have for falls?
2. What interventions would you propose at this visit to decrease his risk for falls?

MANAGEMENT

Once the fall evaluation is complete, interventions should be initiated to treat acute conditions and injuries, minimize the risk of future falls, and prevent any injuries from future falls. Identification and modification of risk factors for falls have been shown to reduce the number of recurrent falls, and significantly reduce 1- and 2-year hospitalization rates.[56] Table 21–3 reviews the efficacy of fall management and prevention strategies that have been studied. Because falls usually result from the interaction of multiple risk factors, there is no standard approach to the treatment of falls. The management of an acute fall depends upon the fall history and evaluation of the individual patient and that patient's predisposing and precipitating risk factors. The goal of treatment is to minimize fall risk and maximize functional independence.

Elimination of Specific Risk Factors

All injuries from the fall should be treated with attention to the potential psychologic consequences from falls. Any acute illness or change that may have contributed to the fall should be treated. Specific medical factors that were identified through the fall evaluation as possible causes should be improved by appropriate interventions. Review of all medications should be performed, and an attempt made to reduce the number of medications and eliminate high-risk medications. The patient should be questioned and counseled about alcohol.

Exercise and Balance Training

Physical therapy is an integral part of a fall treatment program. A physical therapist can instruct the patient in muscle strengthening and balance exercises (such as Tai Chi), prescribe an appropriate ambulatory assistive device and train in its use, perform transfer and gait training, and potentially perform a home safety evaluation designed to modify and adapt the environment for fall reduction.[14] Teaching someone to get up from the floor may avoid a potentially dangerous long lie-down on the floor.[4]

Environmental Modification

In falls where the cause seems predominantly environmental, a home evaluation by an occupational or physical therapist can be helpful in preventing future injury. A home safety checklist can be given to patients at risk for falls as a preventive measure. See Table 21–4 for commonly reported environmental risk factors and

Table 21–3	Evidence-Based Management and Prevention Strategies		

Population	Strategy	Level of Evidence for Recommendation	Comment
Community-dwelling older adults	Exercise/physical therapy, individually targeted—muscle strengthening and balance retraining	A	Decreased falls and injuries from falls.
	Tai Chi group exercise (15 weeks)	A	Lower rate of falling.
	Multidisciplinary, multifactorial health/environmental risk factor screening and intervention program for older people with/without risk of falls	A	Most studies assess orthostatic BP, vision, drugs,and environmental risks. Most interventions include exercise, environmental modification, and education.
	Review and modification of medications, particularly psychotropic medication	B	Reduction in falls.
	Cardiac pacing for fallers with cardioinhibitory carotid sinus syndrome	B	Reduction in syncope and falls.
	Vitamin D	B	In meta-analysis, 22% decrease in falls in both community and long-term care; some studies show no effect.
	Home hazard assessment and modification, professionally prescribed for persons with fall history	C	Reduction in number of falls. Most effective for persons with history of falls.
Older long-term care residents	Multidisciplinary assessment and intervention program	A	
	Review and modification of medications, particularly psychotropic medication	B	Reduction in falls.
	Staff education programs	B	
	Gait training and use of assistive devices	B	
	Hip protectors for residents at high risk of falling	B	

A, evidence from well-designed meta-analysis, or well-done synthesis reports such as those for the Agency for Healthcare Policy and Research or the American Geriatrics Society; *B,* evidence from well-designed controlled trials, both randomized and nonrandomized, with results that consistently support a specific action; *C,* evidence from observational studies or controlled trials with inconsistent results; *D,* evidence from expert opinion or multiple case reports.

From National Guideline Clearinghouse. Fall prevention for older adults, 2004. Available at: *www.guideline.gov.*

A, Supported by one or more high-quality randomized clinical trials (RCTs) in an appropriate population, without contradictory evidence from other clinical trials; *B,* supported by one or more high quality nonrandomized cohort studies or low-quality RCTs; *C,* supported by one or more case series and/or poor-quality cohort and/or case–control studies; *D,* supported by expert opinion and/or extrapolation from studies in other populations and/or settings; *X,* The preponderance of evidence supports the treatment being ineffective or harmful.

Major sources include American Geriatrics Society et al.,[45] Gillespie et al.,[60] Tinetti et al.,[61] Campbell et al.,[64] Bishoff-Ferrari et al.,[65] Ray et al.,[67] and Close et al.[75] From Sackett DL, Straus SE, Richardson WS, Rosenberg W, Haynes RB. Evidence-Based Medicine. 2nd ed. Edinburgh: Churchill-Livingstone, 2000, with permission.

recommended modifications. Several studies have demonstrated a reduction in falls with home hazard reduction, especially when combined with other risk factor interventions.[57-59]

Other Methods

Appropriate aids can be ordered to assist with activities of daily living, including eyeglasses, hearing aids, and proper footwear. Follow-up of interventions and reports of further falls or near falls is important in assessing the utility of interventions. The patient can be asked to keep a fall diary to record any future falls. An alarm device (such as an emergency call system or lifeline) may help to alleviate some of the fear of falling and reassure the patient and family that help could be summoned in the event of another fall.

George Binson, *Part 4*

You recommend discontinuation of metoclopramide and a slow taper off of temazepam. No changes to hydrochlorothiazide or terazosin because there has been no orthostatic hypotension on repeated assessments. You emphasize the importance of the physical therapy evaluation and also order an evaluation by ophthalmology. The patient agrees with this plan. In a discussion with the patient's daughter, she agrees to have family members visit more frequently, help identify senior activities, and assist with the patient's medication changes.

The patient returns 6 weeks later with a rollator walker given to him by physical therapy and new eyeglasses with plans to follow up his cataract. He states that he is feeling much more confident

Table 21–4	Commonly Reported Environmental Risk Factors for Falls and Recommended Modifications	
Risk Factor	**Strength of Evidence**	**Recommended modifications**
Physical restraints	A	Avoid restraints.
Bedrails/siderails	B	Provide beds that permit safe movement.
Lack of handrails	C	Ensure stairways have secure handrails. Install grab bars in bathrooms. Install grab bars in bathtub/shower.
Slippery/shiny floor surfaces	C	Provide nonskid floors. Avoid waxing kitchen floors. Clean wet floor immediately. Cover slippery surfaces with nonskid carpeting. Place nonskid strips or mats in bathtub to avoid slipping.
Snow, ice, cold weather	C	Exercise caution in cold weather.
Inadequate lighting	C	Provide sufficient lighting, especially in high-risk areas (bedroom, bathroom, stairways). Provide illuminated light switches. Place nightlights along the pathway from bedroom to bathroom. Avoid lighting glare.
Uneven flooring	C	Avoid thick pile carpet to minimize tripping. Mark step edges with bright nonskid tape. Ensure that step surfaces are in good repair and nonskid.
Loose throw rug, cord, frayed carpet, wire	D	Replace throw rugs with nonskid rugs. Ensure that carpet edges are flat. Ensure that loose lamp and telephone cords are not in walkways.
Cracked or uneven sidewalk	D	Repair sidewalk cracks. Mark step edges with bright nonskid tape.
Toilet, tub, or furniture at inappropriate height	C	Provide seating of proper height to permit safe sitting and standing. Provide beds that permit safe movement. Use toilet risers if toilet seat too low.
Temporary environmental hazard	C	Ensure wheelchairs and ambulatory assistive devices are properly fitted. Avoid placing equipment in hallways. Avoid clutter and low-lying objects.

A, evidence from well-designed meta-analysis, or well-done synthesis reports such as those for the Agency for Healthcare Policy and Research or the American Geriatrics Society; *B*, evidence from well-designed controlled trials, both randomized and nonrandomized, with results that consistently support a specific action; *C*, evidence from observational studies or controlled trials with inconsistent results; *D*, evidence from expert opinion or multiple case reports.

From Tideiksaar R. Falls in Older People. 3rd ed. Baltimore: Health Professions Press, 2002; and Lyons SS. Fall Prevention for Older Adults. Iowa City: University of Iowa Gerontological Nursing Interventions Research Center, Research Dissemination Core, 2004. Available at: www.guideline.gov, with permission. Evidence grades from National Guideline Clearinghouse. Fall Prevention for Older Adults, 2004. Available at: *www.guideline.gov.*

with walking and is steadier on his feet. In fact, he has had no falls since the last visit. His laboratory tests return normal except for a slightly elevated glucose and HbA1c. On examination, his muscle tone is normal. No rigidity is noted. His gait is steadier, and with the use of the walker he ambulates with more speed. He is much more steady with sternal nudge. He also tells you that he has been able to perform more activities at home (because of some modifications made by physical therapy) and in the community (because he can ambulate more). He feels his mood has improved as well as his sleep. You remind him to continue doing the exercises recommended by physical therapy and ask him to return in 3 months.

PREVENTION OF FALLS

Because of the profound impact of falls on the elderly individual and the community, there has been much research in methods to prevent falls in the elderly and there are now evidence-based recommendations for prevention of falls in the elderly. A review of interventions to prevent falls was conducted with the Cochrane Database of Systematic Reviews. This review considered only randomized studies and evaluated 62 trials involving 21,668 people as of July 2003.[60] Interventions that were likely to be beneficial based on this review included multidisciplinary, multifactorial health/environmental risk factor screening/intervention programs, individually prescribed muscle strengthening and balance training, Tai Chi, home hazard assessment and modification, withdrawal of psychotropic medication, and cardiac pacing for persons with cardioinhibitory carotid sinus hypersensitivity.

There have been several studies evaluating the utility of a multidisciplinary screening and assessment of risk for falls and interventions to reduce risk. Most of the studies involve an initial assessment by a health care professional with expertise in falls and recommendations made to decrease risk for falls. These interventions are effective in reducing falls in community dwelling elders and institutionalized elders.[60,61] This suggests that clinicians should evaluate risk for falls in their older adult patients who have or have not fallen and provide interventions to reduce risk.

Exercise for strength and balance training has been suggested as a preventive measure for falls for many years. Many studies now support this recommendation, especially programs that are individually prescribed at home. These studies have found that older adults with individualized physical therapy programs directed at strength and balance have less falls and less injuries than control groups.[62] A group-based exercise program also showed benefit in fall reduction.[60] Therefore, there is now evidence that a home-based, individualized exercise program for strength and balance can prevent falls and injuries. Additionally, the Frailty and Injuries: Cooperative Study of Intervention Techniques (FICSIT) revealed that certain balance exercise programs, such as Tai Chi are associated with a significant reduction in the fall rate (at one site a 25% reduction).[63]

Home evaluation for hazard reduction (a home visit performed by an occupational therapist to reduce the number of potential hazards within the home) has also been shown to be an effective technique to prevent falls, but mainly in elders who have already had a fall.[60] This effect may be due in part to home modifications. However, it has been suggested that home visits by occupational therapists may also lead to some behavioral changes in the elderly individual that may decrease the risk of falls.[57] A separate Cochrane review regarding home modification concluded that there is not enough evidence to state that modification of home hazards definitely reduces injuries from falls.[50]

A medication withdrawal program, focused on psychotropic medications, was paired with a home-based exercise program.[64] In this study, there was a 66% fall reduction rate in the medication withdrawal group. As medications (especially psychotropic medications) are a strong risk factor for falls in the elderly, the results of this study are not surprising. Thus, it appears that a focused review of medications and withdrawal of psychotropic medications can reduce falls. Clinicians should be careful in prescribing to older adults and carefully review and withdraw unnecessary medications.

There may be at least some older patients who may fall due to carotid sinus hypersensitivity, causing bradycardia and falls. This group of older adults has been shown in one study to benefit from the insertion of a cardiac pacemaker, with a significant reduction in the number of falls after pacer insertion.[60] A recent meta-analysis of Vitamin D supplementation has shown fall risk reduction in groups of elders at high risk for vitamin D deficiency.[65]

In addition to the above interventions that have demonstrated definite benefit, there are several interventions of currently unknown efficacy. Exercise programs such as group-delivered exercise and lower limb strengthening programs may be beneficial in reducing falls for a specific subgroup of elders. Nutritional supplements are currently being evaluated in terms of their efficacy in reducing falls. Correction of visual impairment in an elderly patient may be beneficial for many reasons (improved quality of life, less depression, etc.). However, there is no evidence to date that correcting vision has any effect on falls.[60] Hormone replacement therapy, although still beneficial in treating osteoporosis, is not protective against falls. Pharmacological therapy with raubasine-dihydroergocristine (a vasoactive medication) had some efficacy in one study. A few studies have attempted a cognitive/behavioral (or educational) intervention to decrease falls and were not found to be efficacious.[60]

A second systematic review revealed conclusions similar to that in the Cochrane Review. It found that multifactorial falls risk assessment and management programs were the most effective at reducing falls (18%) and exercise was also effective (14%). However, it found no evidence for the efficacy of environmental modification or education programs.[66]

Prevention of Falls in Nursing Homes and Assisted Living

Older residents of nursing homes and assisted living tend to be more frail, and it is uncertain whether the modalities successful in preventing falls in community-dwelling older adults are effective in these residents. There are now several studies of fall prevention programs in the nursing home setting.[56,67,68] The effective components of these studies appear to be a comprehensive assessment by an interdisciplinary team, staff education, assistive devices, and the reduction of medications. Additional components include resident education, environmental adaptations (lighting, grab bars), personal safety (footwear) and progressive balance and resistance training.

Prevention of Injury from Falls

In older individuals who are at high risk for future falls, measures should be taken to attempt to prevent injury from future falls. There is now evidence that population-based interventions (such as mass media education, exercise promotion, and home visits) are effective in reducing injuries from falls.[69] It has not yet been determined that the measures proven effective in reducing falls are equally effective in reducing injuries from falls.[70] For all older adults, osteoporosis should be considered, and calcium, vitamin D, exercise and osteoporotic medication prescribed as indicated. Hip protectors have been suggested as a method to pad the greater trochanteric region of the hip from direct contact with the ground in the event of a fall. There are now several studies evaluating hip protectors, and a systematic review of these studies reveals that they may be effective in reducing hip fractures in older adults residing in institutional care settings (effect only seen for those residing in institutional care with high background incidence of falls), but not in older adults living in the community.[71] They may improve confidence in ability to perform activities of daily living.[72] One obstacle with hip protectors is compliance. Many older adults prefer not to wear them as they are bulky. Helmets are sometimes used in patients with recurrent head injury from falls. In institutionalized patients who fall from bed, using a low mattress bed frame may be beneficial.

> ● There is now evidence that population-based interventions (such as mass media education, exercise promotion, and home visits) are effective in reducing injuries from falls.

Education

The U.S. Preventive Services Task Force recommends that all persons 75 years of age and older, as well as those 70 to 74 years of age who have a known risk factor, be counseled about specific measures to prevent falls.[73] Most behavioral-educational trials to reduce falls in older adults have demonstrated little or no effect. However, a recent study of Stepping On (a small-group–based educational program) demonstrated a 31% reduction in falls.[74] Thus, teaching older adults about falls, home hazards, and safety may be effective in preventing further falls.

SUMMARY

Falls are common among older persons and result in morbidity, loss of independence, higher health care costs, and sometimes death. There are many intrinsic and extrinsic risk factors for falls and multiple factors may be present in an older individual who falls. A fall may be the presenting feature of an acute illness. Medications can increase fall risk, and the more medications used by a patient, the greater their risk. All clinicians who care for older patients should periodically ask about falls and near falls. Balance and gait assessment is the single best predictor of individuals at

---

POSTTEST

1. An 86-year-old woman on 12 medications with a history of hypertension, mild dementia, and painful bunions could potentially reduce her risk of falling with all except which one of the following?
   a. Reduction in medication number
   b. An exercise program for balance and strength
   c. A prescription for sertraline
   d. Podiatry evaluation
   e. Evaluation for orthostatic hypotension

2. A 74-year-old male patient has had three falls within the last 6 weeks. Which of the following would be reasonable studies to perform at this time?
   a. Complete blood count, urinalysis, and 24-hour urine for heavy metals
   b. Complete blood count, electrolytes, glucose, and thyroid-stimulating hormone
   c. Electrolytes and PET scan
   d. Electrolytes, antinuclear antibody, erythrocyte sedimentation rate, and follicle-stimulating hormone

3. A 69-year-old female patient asks you what sort of exercise she should do to prevent falls. You tell her:
   a. Jogging or other aerobic exercise
   b. Deep-breathing exercises daily
   c. Balance and strength exercises
   d. Bicycling and swimming (non–weight-bearing exercise)

4. A 90-year-old male patient has come to see you in clinic after a second fall at home. As part of your assessment, you ask an occupational therapist to evaluate his home. The therapist finds multiple environmental risk factors in the home. Which of the following is *not* an environmental risk factor for falls?
   a. Throw rug
   b. Freshly waxed kitchen floor
   c. Electrical cords lying on the floor
   d. Grab bars in the bathroom

increased risk of falling. All patients with an injurious fall or multiple falls should undergo a fall evaluation, including a history, physical examination, balance and gait evaluation, and diagnostic studies. There are many interventions that have been shown to prevent falls. The most efficacious interventions include a multidisciplinary risk factor assessment and intervention program, an exercise program of muscle strengthening and balance training, Tai Chi, a home hazard assessment by a professional, and the withdrawal of psychotropic medications.

References

1. Blake AJ, Morgan K, Bendall MJ, et al. Falls by elderly people at home: prevalence and associated factors. Age Ageing 1988;17:365-72.
2. Tinetti ME, Speechley M Ginter SF. Risk factors for falls among elderly persons living in the community. N Engl J Med 1988;319:1701-7.
3. Rubenstein LZ, Josephson KR, Robbins AS. Falls in the nursing home. Ann Intern Med 1994;121:442-51.
4. Sattin RW, Lambert Huber DA, DeVito CA, et al. The incidence of fall injury events among the elderly in a defined population. Am J Epidemiol 1990;131:1028-37.
5. Weigelt JA. Trauma. In: Advanced Trauma Life Support for Doctors: ATLS. 6th ed. Chicago: American College of Surgeons;, 1997:26.
6. King MB. Falls. In Hazzard WR, Blass JP, Halter JB, Ouslander JG, Tinetti ME, eds. Principles of Geriatric Medicine and Gerontology. 5th ed. New York: McGraw-Hill, 2003.
7. Wolinsky FD, Fitzgerald JF, Stump TE. The effect of hip fracture on mortality, hospitalization, and functional status: a prospective study. Am J Public Health 1997;87:398-403.
8. Hall SE, Williams JA, Senior JA, et al. Hip fracture outcomes: quality of life and functional status in older adults living in the community. Aust N Z J Med 2000;30:327-32.
9. Centers for Disease Control and Prevention. Falls and Hip Fractures Among Older Adults. September 2005. Available at: www.cdc.gov/ncipc/factsheets/falls.htm.
10. Hitcho EB, Krauss MJ, Birge S et al. Characteristics and circumstances of falls in a hospital setting: a prospective analysis. J Gen Intern Med 2004;19:732-9.
11. Tideiksaar R. Falls in Older People. 3rd ed. Baltimore: Health Professions Press, 2002.
12. Tinetti ME, Liu WL, Claus EB. Predictors and prognosis of inability to get up after falls among elderly persons. JAMA 1993;269:65-70.
13. Kiel DP, O'Sullivan P, Teno JM, et al. Health care utilization and functional status in the aged following a fall. Med Care 1991;29:221-8.
14. Tinetti ME, Williams CS. Falls, injuries due to falls, and the risk of admission to a nursing home. N Engl J Med 1997;337:1279-84.
15. Salkeld G, Cameron ID, Cumming RG, et al. Quality of life related to fear of falling and hip fracture in older women: a time trade off study. BMJ 2000;320:341-5.
16. Centers for Disease Control and Prevention. Incidence and costs to Medicare of fractures among Medicare beneficiaries aged >65 years—United States, July 1991-June 1992. MMWR Morb Mortal Wkly Rep 1996;45(41):877-83.
17. Fuller GF. Falls in the elderly. Am Fam Physician 2000;61:2159-68.
18. Thomas DC, Edelberg HK, Tinetti ME. Falls. In: Geriatric Medicine. 4th ed. New York: Springer-Verlag, 2003.
19. Tinetti ME, Williams CS, Mayewski R. Fall risk index for elderly patients based on number of chronic disabilities. Am J Med 1986;80:429-34.
20. Rubenstein LZ, Josephson KR. The epidemiology of falls and syncope. Clin Geriatr Med 2002;18:141-58.
21. Campbell AJ, Borrie MJ, Spears GF, et al. Circumstances and consequences of falls experienced by a community population 70 years and over during a prospective study. Age Ageing 1990;19:137-41.
22. Mahoney J, Sager M, Dunham NC, Johnson J. Risk of falls after hospital discharge. J Am Geriatr Soc 1994;42:269-74.
23. Robbins AS, Rubenstein LZ, Josephson KR, et al. Predictors of falls among elderly people. Results of two population-based studies. Arch Intern Med 1989;149:1628-33.
24. Campbell AJ, Borrie MJ, Spears GF. Risk factors for falls in a community-based prospective study of people 70 years and older. J Gerontol 1989;44:M112-7.
25. Lord SR, McLean D, Slathers G. Physiological factors associated with injurious falls in older people living in the community. Gerontology 1992;38:338-46.
26. Lawlor DA, Patel R, Ebrahim S. Association between falls in elderly women and chronic diseases and drug use: cross sectional study. BMJ 2003;327:712-7.
27. Turcu A, Toubin S, Mourey F, et al. Falls and depression in older people. Gerontology 2004;50:303-8.
28. Rubenstein LZ. Falls in the nursing home. Ann Intern Med 1994;121:442-51.
29. Van Doorn C, Gruber-Baldini AL, Zimmerman S, et al. Dementia as a risk factor for falls and fall injuries among nursing home residents. J Am Geriatr Soc 2003;51:1213-8.
30. Buchner D, Larson E. Falls and fractures in patients with Alzheimer-type dementia. JAMA 1987;257:1492-5.
31. Richardson JK, Hurvitz EA. Peripheral neuropathy: a true risk factor for falls. J Gerontol 1995;50A(4):M211-5.
32. Brown JS, Vittinghoff E, Wyman JF, et al. Urinary incontinence: does it increase risk for falls and fractures? J Am Geriatr Soc 2000;48:721-5.
33. Kenny RA. Neurally mediated syncope. Clin Geriatr Med 2002;18:191-210.
34. Nevitt MC, Cummings SR, Kidd S, et al. Risk factors for recurrent nonsyncopal falls: a prospective study. JAMA 1989;216:2663-8.
35. Moreland JD, Richardson JA, Goldsmith CH, Clase CM. Muscle weakness and falls in older adults: a systematic review and meta-analysis. J Am Geriatr Soc 2004;52:1121-9.
36. Menz HB, Lord SR. Foot problems, functional impairment, and falls in older people. J Am Podiat Med Assoc 1999;89:458-67.
37. Close JCT, Hooper R, Glucksman E, et al. Predictors of falls in a high risk population: results from the prevention of falls in the elderly trial (PROFET). Emerg Med J 2003;20:421-5.
38. Cumming RG. Epidemiology of medication-related falls and fractures in the elderly. Drugs Aging 1998;12(1):43-53.
39. Liu B, Anderson G, Mittmann N, et al. Use of selective serotonin-reuptake inhibitors or tricyclic antidepressants and the risk of hip fractures in elderly people. Lancet 1998;351:1303-7.
40. Glynn RJ, Seddon JM, Krug JH, et al. Falls in elderly patients with glaucoma. Arch Ophthalmol 1991;109:205-10.
41. Koepsell TD, Wolf ME, Buchner DM, et al. Footwear style and risk of falls in older adults. J Am Geriatr Soc 2004;52:1495-501.
42. Lord SR, Dayhew J, Howland A. Mulifocal glasses impair edge-contrast sensitivity and depth perception and increase the risk of falls in older people. J Am Geriatr Soc 2002;50:1760-6.
43. Tinetti ME, Liu WI, Ginter SF, et al. Mechanical restraint use and fall-related injuries among residents of skilled nursing facilities. Ann Intern Med 1992;116:369-74.
44. Marks W. Physical restraints in the practice of medicine. Current concepts. Arch Intern Med 1992;152:2203-6.
45. American Geriatrics Society, British Geriatrics Society, American Academy of Orthopedic Surgeons. Guideline for the prevention of falls in older persons. J Am Geriatr Soc 2001;49:664-72.
46. Davies AJ, Steen N, Kenny RA. Carotid sinus hypersensitivity is common in older patients presenting to an accident and emergency department with unexplained falls. Age Ageing 2001;30:289-93.
47. Lyons SS. Fall Prevention for Older Adults. Iowa City: University of Iowa Gerontological Nursing Interventions Research Center, Research Dissemination Core, 2004. Available at: www.guideline.gov.
48. Rubenstein LZ, Solomon DH, Roth CP, et al. Detection and management of falls and instability in vulnerable elders by community physicians. J Am Geriatr Soc 2004;52:1527-31.
49. Oliver D, Britton M, Seed P, et al. Development and evaluation of evidence based risk assessment tool (STRATIFY) to predict which elderly inpatients will fall: case-control and cohort studies. BMJ 1997;315:1049-53.
50. Lyons RA, Sander LV, Weightman AL, et al. Modification of the home environment for the reduction of injuries. Cochrane Database of Systematic Reviews 2004;4.
51. Teno J, Kiel DP, Mor V. Multiple stumbles: a risk factor for falls in community dwelling elderly: a prospective study. J Am Geriatr Soc 1990;38:1321-5.
52. Maki BE, Holliday PJ, Topper AK. A prospective study of postural balance and risk of falling in an ambulatory and independent elderly population. J Gerontol 1994;49:M72-84.
53. Podsiadlo D, Richardson S. The timed "Up & Go": a test of basic functional mobility for frail elderly persons. J Am Geriatr Soc 1991;39:142-8.
54. Tinetti ME. Performance-Oriented Assessment of Mobility in Elderly Patients. J Am Geriatr Soc 1986;34:119-26.
55. O'Shea D, Perry SW, Kenny RA. The Newcastle protocol for carotid sinus massage. J Am Geriatr Soc 2001;49:236-7.
56. Rubenstein LZ, Robbins AS, Josephson KR, et al. The value of assessing falls in an elderly population: a randomized clinical trial. Ann Intern Med 1990;113:308-16.
57. Cumming RG, Thomas M, Szonyi G, et al. Home visits by an occupational therapist for assessment and modification of environmental hazards: a randomized trial of falls prevention. J Am Geriatr Soc 1999;47:1397-402.
58. Day L, Fildes B, Gordon I, et al. Randomized factorial trial of falls prevention among older people living in their own homes. BMJ 2002;325:128-31.
59. Nikolaus T, Bach M. Preventing falls in community-dwelling frail older people using a home intervention team (HIT): results form the randomized falls—HIT trial. J Am Geriatr Soc 2003;51:300-5.
60. Gillespie LD, Gillespie WJ, Robertson MC, et al. Interventions for preventing falls in elderly people. Cochrane Database of Systematic Reviews 2004;4.
61. Tinetti ME, Baker DI, McAvay G, et al. A multifactorial intervention to reduce the risk of falling among elderly people living in the community. N Engl J Med 1994;331:821-7.

62. Campbell AJ, Robertson MC, Gardner MM, et al. Randomised controlled trial of a general practice programme of home based exercise to prevent falls in elderly women. BMJ 1997;315:1065-9.

63. Province MA, Hadley EC, Hornbrook MC, et al. The effects of exercise on falls in elderly patients. A preplanned meta-analysis of the FICSIT trials. JAMA 1995;278:557-62.

64. Campbell AJ, Robertson MC, Gardner MM, et al. Psychotropic medication withdrawal and a home-based exercise program to prevent falls: a randomized, controlled trial. J Am Geriatr Soc 1999;47:850-3.

65. Bishoff-Ferrari HA, Dawson-Hughes B, Willet WC, et al. Effect of vitamin D on falls. A meta-analysis. JAMA 2004;291:1999-2006.

66. Chang JT, Morton SC, Rubenstein LZ, et al. Interventions for the prevention of falls in older adults: systematic review and meta-analysis of randomized clinical trials. BMJ 2004;328:680-7.

67. Ray WA, Taylor JA, Meador KG, et al. A randomized trial of a consultation service to reduce falls in nursing homes. JAMA 1997;278:557-62.

68. Becker C, Kron M, Lindemann U, et al. Effectiveness of a multifaceted intervention on falls in nursing home residents. J Am Geriatr Soc 2003;51:306-13.

69. McClure R, Turner C, Peel N, et al. Population-based interventions for the prevention of fall-related injuries in older people. Cochrane Database of Systematic Reviews 2005;1.

70. Tinetti ME. Preventing falls in elderly persons. N Engl J Med 2003;348: 42-9.

71. Parker MJ, Gillespie LD, Gillespie WJ. Hip protectors for preventing hip fractures in the elderly. Cochrane Database of Systematic Reviews 2004;4.

72. Cameron ID, Stafford B, Cumming RG, et al. Hip protectors improve falls self-efficacy. Age Ageing 2000;29:57-62.

73. Preventive Services Task Force. Guide to Clinical Preventive Services: Report of the U.S. Preventive Services Task Force. 2nd ed. Baltimore: Williams & Wilkins, 1996–.

74. Clemson L, Cumming RG, Kendig H, et al. The effectiveness of a community-based program for reducing the incidence of falls in the elderly: a randomized trial. J Am Geriatr Soc 2004;52:1487-94.

Web Resources

1. American Geriatrics Society link to Health in Aging: www.healthinaging.org (links to public education site for falls prevention).
2. Centers for Disease Control and Prevention link to National Center for Injury Prevention: www.cdc.gov/ncipc/factsheets/falls.htm.
3. National Guideline Clearinghouse: www.guideline.gov (published guideline on exercise and fall prevention).

PRETEST ANSWERS

1. b
2. c
3. d
4. b

POSTTEST ANSWERS

1. c
2. b
3. c
4. d

CHAPTER

22

Urinary Incontinence

Charles A. Cefalu

OBJECTIVES

Upon completion of this chapter, the reader will be able to:

- Articulate the definition, prevalence, and significance of urinary incontinence in the elderly.
- Summarize the epidemiology of urinary incontinence in various clinical settings and elderly subgroups.
- Describe the various classifications, schemes, and rationales for determining the types of incontinence.
- Summarize the factors necessary for maintaining and restoring continence and the factors associated with precipitation and aggravation of urinary incontinence.

- Summarize the major types, frequency, and causes of urinary incontinence.
- Perform the primary care workup for urinary incontinence.
- Describe the various nonpharmacologic and pharmacologic treatment options for urinary incontinence in the primary care setting.
- Articulate the general and specific indications for referral of an elderly patient with urinary incontinence for urodynamic assessment.
- Summarize the indications and complications of indwelling urinary catheterization and the indications and place for diapers and other incontinence aids.

PRETEST

1. Normal aging of the lower urinary tract includes:
   a. Bladder capacity decreases with age while residual urine volume decreases.
   b. Aging leads to a decline in bladder outlet and urethral resistance pressure.
   c. Ten to twenty percent of elderly patients with no medical problems will have involuntary contractions of the bladder.
   d. As many as 75% of elderly patients with functional incontinence will have involuntary bladder contractions.
   e. All of the above.

2. An abnormal flow rate is specific for the following types of incontinence:
   a. Overflow incontinence
   b. Urge incontinence
   c. Stress incontinence
   d. Intractable incontinence
   e. Transient incontinence

3. The best way to initially assess incontinence in an older patient is by a combination of:
   a. Urinalysis, culture and sensitivity, residual volume determination, and clinical symptoms
   b. Catheterization
   c. Cystourethrography
   d. Renal ultrasound
   e. Cystoscopy

Harold Burnhart, *Part 1*

Mr. Burnhart is a 60-year-old Caucasian male who is widowed and lives with his son. He is independent with activities and instrumental activities of daily living. He has been your patient for 30 years and he is seeing you in your office today for a 3-month checkup. His problem list includes hypertension, osteoarthritis, longstanding type II diabetes controlled on oral medications, and benign prostatic hyperplasia. His medications include hydrochlorothiazide 25 mg daily, glyburide 2.5 mg daily, and atenolol 25 mg once daily. His blood pressure today is 135/75 mm Hg, and his latest

glocosylated hemoglobin is 7%, with previous readings in the 7% to 7.5% range. During the last 15 months, Mr. Burnhart has complained of frequency and urgency during the day and especially at night during which times he reports getting up to urinate four to five times per night. Today he reports he has had some dysuria for the last several weeks. His normal pattern of urination at bedtime prior to this was once or twice at night. When questioned, he admits to hesitancy, straining to urinate, and decreased caliber of his urine stream for about 2 to 3 years, all of which have been gradually getting worse.

Linda James, *Part 1*

You are seeing Ms. Linda James, an 80-year-old African-American female, who is in the hospital for a cerebrovascular accident (CVA) involving the left lower extremity. Her past history includes a history of mild dementia secondary to probable Alzheimer's disease, hypertension, and osteoarthritis. Her surgical history includes a total abdominal hysterectomy 30 years previously. She attained an 11th grade education. Her medications include aspirin 81 mg and a multivitamin daily, acetaminophen for pain as necessary, hydrochlorthiazide 12.5 mg daily, and donepezil 10 mg daily. She has 10 grown natural children. Her blood pressure on admission is noted to be 130/80 mm Hg. Her strength in the left lower extremity on admission is 2 out of 5 (best) but has improved to a 4 out of 5 with inpatient physical therapy. She initially had an indwelling urinary catheter due to urinary incontinence that was removed on day 3 of her hospitalization. Prior to this hospitalization, Ms. James was independent with activities of daily living including toileting, but has become incontinent since the catheter was removed. She describes no symptoms of urgency, frequency, dysuria, hesitancy, or loss of urination on coughing or straining. You arranged for a bedside commode. Prior to discharge on day 6 of the hospitalization, she is able to balance herself and stand and ambulate with assistance only. A brief inspection of the external genitalia on insertion and removal of the urinary catheter reveals no abnormalities. Prior to discharge from the hospital, a urinalysis is performed, which showed 2 to 5 white blood cells per high power field and no blood on a routine specimen. Serum chemistry values were also within normal limits including a blood sugar, sodium, potassium, blood urea nitrogen, and creatinine. A walker is prescribed by the physical therapist, and she is discharged to the nursing home for skilled care and rehabilitation. Her Mini-Mental Status Examination results on discharge are 26 out of 30, and she is noted to be alert and oriented to person and place with some cueing needed relative to time.

PREVALENCE AND IMPACT

Urinary incontinence, defined as the involuntary loss of urine in sufficient amounts or frequency to be a social or health problem, is one of the major geriatric syndromes. Urinary incontinence may not be addressed during a typical primary office visit for one of several reasons: its silent presentation may appear peripheral to the major presenting complaint in an acutely or chronically ill older patient; the patient seldom complains; and the confusing nature of the subject, complicated by complex chapters on the subject often written by subspecialists. However, evaluation and management of urinary incontinence deserves special consideration because it has an enormous economic, psychologic, social, and physical effect on patients.

> The onset of urinary incontinence is associated with psychologic, medical, social and financial consequences.

The evaluation and management of urinary incontinence can seem so simple that it becomes complicated. The 10 principles of the primary care approach to urinary incontinence are listed in Box 22–1.

Box 22–1 Ten Principles of Primary Care Evaluation and Management of Urinary Incontinence

1. Assessment can be achieved in two or three office visits in 66% of cases.
2. The best clinical tools are a comprehensive history and a physical examination.
3. An understanding of basic physiology and pharmacology is essential.
4. Laboratory assessment includes a complete urinalysis, urine culture, chemistry profile, and serum calcium.
5. Patients who do not fit a simple pattern of incontinence should be referred promptly for urodynamic assessment.
6. Holistic thinking is key to evaluation and management of incontinence; one must take into account the effects of aging, acute illness, chronic illnesses, medications, and the environment.
7. Communication and rapport with the patient are crucial, as are education and behavioral therapy.
8. Complicated urodynamic studies play little to no role in the primary care evaluation of incontinence. However, a simple assessment to rule out overflow incontinence is important.
9. A combination of nonpharmacologic and pharmacologic treatment approaches usually works best.
10. Diapers and incontinence pads may serve a useful purpose, but only after a base assessment has been performed and a diagnosis has been made.

Urinary incontinence is common, affecting 12% or more of the elderly population, and is more frequent in women than in men. Its frequency is 10% to 30% among the elderly who live in communities, 30% to 35% among the elderly who are in hospitals, and 50% among those living in nursing homes. It may be as mild as occasional dribbling of urine to continuous urinary and fecal incontinence. The prevalence of urinary incontinence is also related to the type of incontinence, with urge occurring more in younger women and stress occurring more in older women.[1] Urinary incontinence is a dynamic state; some women move back and forth along a continuum between continence and incontinence, with increasing age being a significant predictor.[2] Difficulty holding urine is a prevalent condition in the community-dwelling elderly, and is highly associated with a number of functional problems and health conditions.[3]

Psychologic consequences of urinary incontinence include depressive symptoms secondary to embarrassment and anxiety about appearance and the odor of urine. This may lead to restricted excursions away from home, restricted social interactions with friends and family, and avoidance of sexual activity.[4] Whereas physicians often focus on the effect of urinary incontinence on patient function, patients more often cite the effect on their emotional well-being and on the interruption of services.[5]

Urinary incontinence and sleep disturbance have been shown to be significant predictors of perceived limitations in usual role activities because of physical health problems[6,7]. Therefore, prompt evaluation and treatment of depression and mobility problems are paramount in the evaluation and management of urinary incontinence.[8] In the nursing home setting, incontinence care accounts for a significant amount of sleep disturbance.[9]

The physical consequences of urinary incontinence may include falls on slippery floors, skin rashes and dermatitis, and the development of skin infections and pressure ulcers in bedridden patients, since moisture is a risk factor.[10] Incontinent patients are also at greater risk for urinary tract infections alone or in association with urinary catheters.

> ● The occurrence of urinary incontinence is associated with the increased frequency of comorbid disease and medications.

Urinary incontinence may be a reason for institutionalization. One study showed that urinary incontinence alone was one of four independent risk factors for institutionalization. The other factors were cognitive impairment, dependence in ambulation, and being unmarried.[11] Another study showed that urinary incontinence was an independent predictor for skilled nursing home placement.[12] In homebound, cognitively intact elderly, urinary incontinence tends to be severe in terms of frequency and number of accidents. These patients perceive the problem to be a very disturbing one that further restricts their activities.[13]

RISK FACTORS AND PATHOPHYSIOLOGY

Aging of the urinary tract is associated with an increased frequency of involuntary bladder contractions in about 10% to 20% of well elderly. Post–void residual urine volume increases to 75 to 100 ml in some cases. First urge to void occurs at a lower bladder volume of 150 to 300 ml and total bladder capacity decreases to 300 to 600 ml.[10-16] Because of these changes, older patients void more frequently. Nocturnal awakenings associated with urination may average two or three times per night. Aging of the urogenital tissues associated with thinning, atrophy, and weakness, especially in women, is associated with a reduced urethral resistance and a decline in bladder outlet pressure. This leads to involuntary loss of urine associated with increased abdominal pressure.[10,16]

Normal bladder function is coordinated by the autonomic parasympathetic and sympathetic nervous systems that innervate smooth muscle in the bladder resulting in a filling or a relaxation phase and a micturition or contraction phase. Inhibition of parasympathetic tone and stimulation of sympathetic tone by the brain results in relaxation of the bladder wall and trigone smooth muscle and contraction of the sphincter, resulting in bladder dilation and filling. Inhibition of sympathetic tone and stimulation of parasympathetic tone by the brain results in contraction of the bladder wall and trigone smooth muscle and relaxation of the urethral sphincter resulting in micturition.[10,16,17]

Components of Continence

Four principal components are necessary for continence: effective functioning of the lower urinary tract, adequate cognitive and physical functioning, motivation, and an appropriate environment.[10] Impairment of any one may cause incontinence.

> ● An intact nervous system and lower urinary tract, a motivated patient, and an appropriate environment are necessary to maintain continence.

Classification of Incontinence

Three classification schemes have traditionally been recommended for classification of urinary incontinence: anatomic, chronologic, and symptomatic.

Although anatomic classification is helpful in understanding function, the other two are useful clinically and easy to remember when classifying the type of incontinence. Chronologic classification divides cases between acute and chronic. Urinary incontinence that does not resolve within 3 to 6 weeks is defined as chronic incontinence.[10,16,17]

> ● New onset incontinence is associated with delirium. Incontinence that does not resolve within 6 weeks is classified as chronic, established incontinence.

ACUTE OR TRANSIENT INCONTINENCE

Patients with acute or transient incontinence have an abrupt onset, which usually is associated with the administration of medications or onset of acute illness. Discontinuance of the offending medication or successful resolution of the acute medical illness results in resumption of a continent state (Table 22–1). The mnemonic device DRIP is often used to recall the various causes of acute incontinence:

D: Delirium, usually caused by drugs or an acute illness

R: Retention of urine caused by obstruction or to a dilated and flaccid bladder as a result of neuropathy; restraints preventing ambulation or mobility; restricted mobility as a result of musculoskeletal or neurologic problems; inability to get to the bathroom

I: Impaction of stool causing obstruction to emptying the bladder; infection of the urinary tract or other infection; inflammation caused by arthritis, infection, or other causes

P: Polyuria caused by high or low output states such as congestive heart failure, chronic venous insufficiency, diabetes mellitus, and hypercalcemic states; polypharmaceuticals such as diuretics (alcohol, caffeine, thiazides and loop diuretics, and theophylline) and other agents that affect the bladder wall or sphincter (beta-blockers, anticholinergics, alpha-blockers, hypnotics, narcotics, antidepressants, antipsychotics, and calcium channel blockers). In summary, drugs may cause incontinence by having a diuretic effect or by causing outlet obstruction with retention or flaccidity with retention.[10,16,17]

> ● The most common type of urinary incontinence is urge incontinence. The rarest but most serious form of urinary incontinence is overflow incontinence.

CHRONIC OR ESTABLISHED INCONTINENCE

A classification system clinically useful in categorizing chronic urinary incontinence is organized by symptom. Urge incontinence is characteristically associated with the sensation of urgency. Stress incontinence is usually associated with stress related to increased abdominal pressure secondary to coughing

Table 22–1	Effect of Various Medications on the Development of Urinary Incontinence	
Pharmacologic Agent	**Mechanism of Action**	**Clinical Consequences**
Alcohol	Sedation, delirium, diuresis	Frequency and urgency
Caffeine	Diuresis	Frequency and urgency
Diuretic	Diuresis	Frequency, urgency, and polyuria
Narcotics	Sedation, delirium; reduces bladder wall contractility leading to overflow	Urinary retention with resultant frequency
Antipsychotics (tricyclic antidepressants, major tranquilizers, antispasmodics)	Reduces bladder wall contractility leading to overflow	Urinary retention with resultant frequency
Calcium channel blockers	Reduces bladder wall contractility leading to overflow	Urinary retention with resultant frequency
Alpha-agonist (pseudophederine, phenolpropalamine)	Increases urethral sphincter pressure	Urinary retention with resultant frequency
Alpha-antagonist (phentolamine)	Reduces urethral sphincter pressure	Stress leakage associated with elevated intraabdominal pressure
Beta-agonist	Reduces bladder wall contractility leading to overflow	Urinary retention with resultant frequency
Minor tranquilizers (particularly long-acting benzodiazepines)	Sedation, delirium	Frequency and urgency
Antispasmodics (dicylomine)	Reduces bladder wall contractility leading to overflow	Urinary retention with resultant frequency
Anticholinergics (diphenhydramine)	Reduces bladder wall contractility leading to overflow	Urinary retention with resultant frequency

or straining. Mixed incontinence implies a combination of urge and stress incontinence. Overflow incontinence implies the overflow of urine from an over distended bladder resulting from the inability to empty because of an obstruction or loss of function. Loss of function may be caused by drugs or by denervation of the bladder (neuropathy). However, symptoms associated with any type of urinary incontinence can be misleading and are generally poorly correlated with the specific type of incontinence. For instance, frequency may be caused by overflow or urge type, as well as by other chronic clinical states such as anxiety, depression, prostatism, social circumstances, and high output states such as congestive heart failure, poorly controlled diabetes, or hypercalcemia.[10,16,17]

The most common type of urinary incontinence is *urge*. Incontinence occurs as a result of irritability of the trigone of the bladder, causing involuntary bladder contractions and the sensation or urge, urgency, and frequency. Many patients describe the "abrupt sensation that urination is imminent." Other patients describe it as "reflex" or "unconscious" incontinence or "precipitant leakage" with no warning of imminent urination. Urge incontinence can be divided further into sensory and motor urge subtypes. Sensory urge incontinence usually occurs as a result of local or surrounding infection or inflammation or irritation caused by urinary tract infection, cystitis, prostatitis, atrophic vaginitis, or radiation therapy to the pelvic area. Motor urge incontinence usually occurs as a result of cerebral disinhibition of the reflex sensory and motor arc. This results in an uninhibited trigone of the bladder and involuntary bladder contractions. Common neurologic causes of motor urge incontinence, referred to as detrusor hyperreflexia, include stroke, dementia, and Parkinson's disease. A temporary urge incontinence occurs for several weeks after transrectal resection of the prostate as a result of the irritation of the trigone by infection or inflammation.[4,10,16,17]

The second most common type of urinary incontinence is *mixed urge and stress incontinence*. The third most common type is *stress incontinence*, and is more common in women. Stress incontinence occurs as a result of one of or a combination of several of the following mechanisms. First, aging is associated with weakness of the pelvic floor musculature and thinning and atrophy of the perineal and vaginal tissues. This is to some extent related to hormonal deficiency and multiple childbirths. This may lead to the development of detrusor instability and urethral sphincter laxity and even incompetence. This can lead further to descensus of the pelvic organs (uterus, cervix, and ovaries) into the vaginal canal, which reduces the acute angle normally present between the proximal urethra

and the base of the bladder. Loss of urine then occurs when abdominal pressure increases as a result of coughing, sneezing, lifting, or straining. Stress incontinence can be further classified as mild, moderate, or severe. A rare but serious cause of stress incontinence in men is secondary to sphincter damage that occurs after prostate surgery, particularly the most invasive types of surgery, suprapubic and radical.[4,10,16,17]

Vaginal delivery is a risk factor for transient postpartum incontinence and incontinence that develops later in life. The results of several studies indicate that damage to nerve and muscle provides a physiologic basis for this association. Although studies indicate no association between the development of urinary incontinence in the first few years after hysterectomy, other studies point to an increased risk many years after hysterectomy and with advancing age. Although the consensus has been that menopause is associated with the development of urinary incontinence, epidemiologic studies have not proved this association.[18]

> ● A postvoid residual urine determination of 200 ml or greater is a sign of overflow incontinence.

The fourth and rarest but most serious form of urinary incontinence is *overflow incontinence*, which accounts for 5% of incontinence. Overflow of urine from a distended bladder can occur when the bladder is prevented from emptying because of an obstruction at the base of the bladder, sphincter, or urethra. Causes of overflow incontinence include a tumor at the base of the bladder, benign prostatic hyperplasia, urethral stricture, prostate carcinoma, uterine or cervical obstruction from a carcinoma, and an ovarian mass. Although pelvic prolapse may be associated with stress incontinence, in the case of severe prolapse, obstruction also may occur. Another type of overflow incontinence is that related to an atonic or flaccid bladder that has lost its neuronal innervation or is affected by pharmacologic agents with anticholinergic activity such as tricyclic antidepressants, phenothiazine tranquilizers, narcotics, antispasmodics, and antihistamine agents commonly present in over-the-counter cold medications. These products may cause an anatomic or chemical denervation. Any drug that inhibits detrusor function or contracts the sphincter or the bladder wall may cause overflow incontinence.[4,10,16,19] Cardinal symptoms and signs of overflow incontinence that should be inquired about include straining to urinate or decreased flow rate or size of stream, dribbling, and hesitancy. Overflow incontinence caused by obstruction is more common in older men. One study involving 100 hospital patients showed that a postvoid residual greater than 50 ml was not correlated with urinary tract infection or renal failure but was strongly associated with incontinence.[20]

Finally, *functional incontinence* is incontinence with a functional cause such as mobility problems from neurologic or musculoskeletal disease that impair mobility and prevent the patient from getting to the bathroom. It is hypothesized that functional incontinence occurs in these patients because of involuntary bladder contractions that occur in as many as 75% of patients affected. Other causes of functional incontinence include diarrhea or drugs that cause diarrhea and autonomic neuropathy or neurologic or anatomic lesions from pelvic surgery or pelvic trauma.[10,16]

Harold Burnhart, *Part 2*

During your exam of Mr. Burnhart you perform an abdominal and rectal examination. The prostate is noted to be about 75 g in size and rubbery firm. The abdominal examination is within normal limits. During this office visit, a fingerstick blood sugar (nonfasting) and a clean catch voided urine dipstick for sugar protein, white cells, nitrite, and bacteria is obtained, and you order a fasting chemistry profile, a prostatic-specific antigen (PSA), and a complete blood count.

The fingerstick blood sugar is reported at 150 mg/dl. The urine dipstick also indicates 2-plus sugar in the urine, 1-plus protein, 4-plus white blood cells, and positive nitrite. The PSA is noted to be 4 ng/ml (normal range 0 to 4). A culture of the urine is requested. The next day, results of the blood tests reveal a blood sugar 120 mg/dl (normal range 109 to 120), BUN 25 mg/dl, creatinine 1.2 mg/dl, Na 136 mEq/L, and K of 4 mEq/L. Forty-eight hours later, his urine culture reveals E. coli greater than 100,000 colonies per ml. Your office nurse calls Mr. Burnhart and requests that he go to the hospital radiology department for a scheduled postvoid bladder sonography. The results are faxed to your office and reveal a postvoid residual of 175 cc of urine.

Linda James, *Part 2*

Ms. James is admitted to the skilled nursing unit of the nursing home after discharge from the hospital, and you continue to manage her rehabilitation. She is ambulatory with a walker.

She is alert and oriented to person and place, but needs cueing relative to time. She requires assistance with activities of daily living including toileting (assistance of one). After a period of 6 weeks of rehabilitation, her mobility improves and the walker is replaced by a cane. However, Ms. James continues to experience 12 to 14 episodes of incontinence per day. She has no urinary symptoms of hesitancy, urgency, frequency, loss of urination on straining, or dysuria. She describes her incontinence as of "abrupt onset without notice." Your evaluation of the perineal area and vaginal canal reveals no abnormalities. You order a serum chemistry profile and urinalysis and culture, all of which are reported to be "within normal limits." The nursing home staff that she has a near fall while trying to get to the bathroom due to slipping on the floor wet from an incontinent episode.

● In most cases, the primary care assessment for urinary incontinence can be performed in a few office visits using simple clinical tools. Formal urodynamic testing evaluation is time consuming, expensive, and usually does not add to diagnostic accuracy.

DIFFERENTIAL DIAGNOSIS AND ASSESSMENT

The tools useful for office assessment of urinary incontinence are part of the everyday armamentarium of the primary care physician. First and foremost, a thorough history and physical examination are essential, cost efficient, and expedient.

History

A detailed description of the incontinence from the patient or caregiver focusing on its onset, frequency, severity, pattern, precipitants, alleviating features, and associated symptoms and conditions is important. Specific questions that the physician should investigate with the patient include the following: when the incontinence started; its association with some other illness or episode such as childbirth; its progression; whether it occurs during the day or night, how many times per day or night; its association with symptoms such as urge, stress, straining, or unawareness of passing urine or being wet; the status of the patient's normal environment; access to toilets; time it takes to get to the bathroom; and frequency of trips to the bathroom during the night to empty the bladder.

Vaginal wetness, dryness, or discharge and burning also should be inquired about and may be associated with atrophic vaginitis. Frequency of bowel movements, a history of constipation, immobility, and the time of the last bowel movement may be an indication of fecal impaction associated with and causing the incontinence. The presence of diarrhea or formed stool during an incontinent episode may be an indication of neurogenic combined urinary and fecal incontinence. Back, perineal, or testicular pain may be associated with prostatitis represented by a sensation of frequency and urgency. The concurrent administration of drugs that may cause incontinence or cause diarrhea should be inquired about, especially those with anticholinergic activity.

Other pertinent information gathered during an office visit includes a history of previous stroke, Parkinson's disease, or dementia. Arthritis or amputation that prevents or impairs mobility may be responsible for neurogenic or functional causes. A history of metabolic problems such as diabetes mellitus, clinical states associated with hypercalcemia, and high output states such as congestive heart failure, anemia, and chronic venous insufficiency may be responsible for incontinence associated with polyuria. Obtaining a psychological history is important because urgency, frequency, and nocturia may be associated with low output states such as chronic anxiety, depression, and insomnia.

A telltale sign of overflow incontinence whether the result of a neurogenic flaccid or obstructed bladder is a history of straining to urinate, decreased caliber of urine, hesitancy, and periods of interrupted urination during micturition. Painful urination may indicate the presence of a renal stone or malignancy. A sensation of a "bulging," uncomfortable feeling or the sensation that "my bottom is falling out" may be an indication of pelvic prolapse. Lastly, historical information about surgical or natural menopause, previous childbirths, gynecologic surgery, and the previous use of hormone replacement therapy may be associated with stress, urge, or overflow incontinence. A history of falls may be a clue to other environmental barriers. A skilled home care visit or physician home visit may help identify barriers to bathroom access such as cluttered hallways, inadequate lighting, or an upstairs bathroom (level of evidence=D).[10,16,21]

The response to key questions can differentiate urge incontinence from stress incontinence. Incontinence that occurs precipitously, while standing or sitting quietly rather than running, is of the urge type. Incontinence that occurs in the absence of stress maneuvers and several seconds after the patient first stands is of the urge type. This is not the case with stress incontinence (level of evidence=D).[10,16,17]

Voiding Record

A voiding record is one of the most valuable but overlooked aids in evaluation of urinary incontinence. The patient or caregiver notes the occurrence and volume of each void or incontinent episode for 1 to 3 days by using a measuring cup or plastic "hat" inserted beneath the toilet seat. The voiding record involves the patient, legitimizes the problem, documents the severity of the problem, and in complex cases may even provide a clue to the etiology. For example, a voiding record may help identify the source of the incontinence that occurs between 8:00 AM and noon; it may be caused by a morning diuretic. Others cases in which a voiding record would help identify the cause of incontinence include (1) incontinence that occurs at night while supine but not during a 4-hour nap in the wheelchair may be caused by the postural diuresis of congestive heart failure or chronic venous insufficiency; (2) incontinence occurring indiscriminately on the hour because of a metabolic problem such as diabetes or hypercalcemia; (3) isolated incontinence occurring at the same hour every day (e.g., at 1:00 AM as a result of the regular use of a hypnotic); and (4) incontinence occurring only on first arising in the morning in an elderly woman related to volume-dependent stress incontinence (level of evidence=D).[21,22]

> ● The diagnosis of stress incontinence is made by a history of urinary leakage associated with any maneuver that increases abdominal pressure or the direct observation of urinary loss on bearing down.

Physical Examination

Physical findings are also key to determining the cause of incontinence. The presence of neurologic findings related to cognitive status and sensory and motor deficits help establish the diagnosis of neurogenic urge incontinence. Arthritis of the hips, knees, and lumbar spine can contribute to the development of functional incontinence. Varicosities, sensory neuropathy of the lower extremities, ulcerations of the digits or feet, and the status of pulses in the extremities are helpful in making a diagnosis of acute or overflow incontinence.

A rectal and pelvic examination is helpful in determining the cause of overflow, stress, or neurogenic incontinence. Abdominal examination may reveal a suprapubic mass, possibly indicative of a pelvic mass or distended bladder. Specifically, an enlarged prostate, pelvic prolapse, or an ovarian mass may indicate obstructive overflow incontinence. An atrophic vaginal mucosa may indicate the presence of stress incontinence or sensory urge incontinence. Pelvic examination with visual inspection may also indicate the presence of laxity of the anterior or posterior vaginal wall resulting in a cystocele, cystourethrocele, or rectocele, a result of bulging of the bladder, bladder and proximal urethra, or rectum into the vaginal canal. Although the isolated findings of urethrocele or cystourethrocele are not directly correlated with stress incontinence, they may be associated with symptomatic stress incontinence. Laxity of the rectal sphincter may be an indication of neurologic or metabolic problems related to spinal cord disease or autonomic neuropathy resulting in overflow incontinence. Direct visualization of the external genitalia and urethra while asking the patient to "bear down" to detect evidence of urinary leakage may indicate the presence of stress incontinence (level of evidence=D).[10,16,17,21]

Other, more sophisticated tests that can be performed in the primary care setting include the pelvic laxity test, the Q-tip test, and the Bonney (Marshall) tests. One checks for pelvic laxity by sequentially applying the blades of the vaginal speculum to the anterior and posterior vaginal walls and asking the patient to cough. If bulging of the anterior wall occurs when the posterior wall is stabilized, a cystocele may be detected if pelvic laxity is present. The reverse is true for the detection of rectocele. The presence of pelvic laxity is a good indication to the treating surgeon of the type of surgery that will surgically correct incontinence as discussed later in surgical options. The Q-tip test involves placing a lubricated Q-tip in the urethra and asking the patient to "bear down" or apply abdominal pressure. Significant change in the angle of the Q-tip is a useful measure in indicating pelvic laxity but does little to indicate the type of incontinence. The Bonney (Marshall) test is useful in determining if surgical intervention will provide symptomatic relief of stress incontinence. This is performed by placing two fingers in the lateral vaginal fornices and asking the patient to cough. If urine leakage occurs on coughing initially but is prevented on applying finger pressure, significant pelvic laxity is present and the patient should benefit from pelvic floor exercises or surgery if the stress incontinence is severe (level of evidence=D).[21,22]

Laboratory Tests

The primary care workup of urinary incontinence includes a urinalysis, urine culture, and sensitivity test (when indicated), serum electrolytes, fasting blood sugar, and serum calcium. Although urinary catheterization usually is performed to obtain a urine sample for bacteriologic culture, microscopic and macroscopic and microbiologic analysis of the urine performed by extraction from disposable diapers has been shown to be a simple and reasonably reliable method of urine sampling. In particular, incontinent female nursing home residents do not necessarily have to be catheterized to obtain an accurate quantitative urine culture.[23] Similar results from sterile catheterization are obtained when using a careful clean catch technique from a urine-soiled diaper or from a condom catheter (level of evidence=D).[24]

An intravenous pyelogram offers little to no diagnostic value in the workup of a patient with urinary incontinence. This procedure may actually lead to morbidity secondary to allergic reactions, dehydration, or renal failure in volume-contracted elderly or those with preexisting renal disease such as nephrosclerosis or diabetic nephropathy.

A postvoid residual urine determination should be performed at some point in every primary care incontinence evaluation. This is performed by asking the patient to empty their bladder completely followed by and "in and out" catheterization performed under sterile conditions. An elevated postvoid residual urine of 200 ml is indicative of overflow incontinence and is an absolute indication for referral for urodynamic evaluation and specialty consultation. In patients with cognitive dysfunction, the post void urine collection should be performed after the last scheduled void. Newer technology now allows the noninvasive ultrasonic evaluation of the bladder for determination of postvoid urinary estimation.[24] It has a sensitivity of 55.7% and a specificity of 96.5% in detecting a postvoid residual of more than 100 ml. This method is quick and easy to use.[25,26] However, ultrasonic evaluation is expensive and impractical in the primary care office setting because the cost of the equipment ranging from $5,000 to 10,000 (level of evidence=C).

Postvoid urine volumes of between 100 and 200 ml are equivocal and should receive consideration for referral for workup depending on the results of other historical, physical, and laboratory findings, operative risk, and wishes of the patient. In other cases, close monitoring or nonpharmacologic and a pharmacologic treatment trial may be considered (level of evidence=D).[4,10,16,21,22] Indications for further urodynamic assessment and urologic referral are reviewed in Box 22–2.

Harold Burnhart, *Part 3*

Mr. Burnhart comes to your office for a follow-up appointment to discuss the results of his tests. You tell Mr. Burnhart that he has an enlarged prostate but no evidence of carcinoma, and that the enlarged prostate is "pressing" on his urethra and preventing him from fully emptying his bladder. You explain that his kidney function is normal but

---

Box 22-2 General and Specific Indications for Urologic Referral and Urodynamic Assessment of Urinary Incontinence

General

1. Diagnosis is unclear.
2. Risk of empiric drug therapy is unacceptable because of increased risk of side effects.
3. Empiric therapy has failed and other therapy is desired.

Specific

1. Recent history of urinary tract infection.
2. Previous pelvic surgery or irradiation.
3. Relapse or recurrence of urinary tract infection.

4. Marked pelvic prolapse.
5. Severe stress incontinence.
6. Marked benign prostatic hyperplasia or suspicion of carcinoma.
7. Severe hesitancy, straining, or interrupted urinary stream.
8. Difficulty passing a large-lumen catheter (e.g., no. 14 Fr).
9. Hematuria.
10. Postvoid residual urine greater than 200 ml.
11. Uncertain diagnosis.

---

that the retained urine at the end of his urination is also contributing to the development of a urinary infection since bacteria are entering the bladder due to age and reduced resistance and the blockage from the prostate. You prescribe trimethoprim sulfamethoxazole twice daily for the urinary infection, discontinue the atenolol, and begin prazosin 1 mg at bedtime to prevent bladder spasms and assist with symptoms. You schedule a repeat bladder sonography in 6 months, and a trial of medication to reduce the size of the prostate (finasteride) will be started after the infection has cleared.

Linda James, *Part 3*

You order bladder (Kegel) exercises to be administered by the nursing aide four times per day. Due to Ms. James' cognitive status, she is unable to complete the exercises. You order a continence diary and the patient is assisted to the bathroom to urinate at scheduled intervals to avoid incontinent episodes. This activity is continued for a period of 2 months. Her incontinent episodes are subsequently reduced in frequency to six to eight episodes per 24 hours. The patient subsequently develops superficial stage II pressure ulcers to both buttocks approximately 5 cm × 5 cm, which is treated with saline occlusive dressings. The patient and family request that the attending prescribe a medication to prevent the urinary incontinence or insert an indwelling urinary catheter. The attending indicates that he is concerned about prescribing medication for this purpose since its side effects could affect her cognitive function. He also indicates that a urinary catheter would promote infections and dependence and advises against both.

● Most cases of chronic urinary incontinence can be managed effectively, but complete resolution rarely occurs.

MANAGEMENT

The treatment of urinary incontinence is summarized in Table 22–2.

Functional Incontinence

Addressing the underlying functional problem is the best approach to functional incontinence. When a patient is unable to get to the bathroom because of mobility problems, physical therapy and exercise, as well as assistive devices, should provide some improvement. When suspected environmental barriers are the problem, a home visit by a skilled home nurse or physician may be beneficial. An example of a flexible approach to mobility or environmental barriers and incontinent episodes is the use of a bedside commode, especially when associated with diuretic use for a patient with chronic congestive heart failure or diarrhea-producing agents used to treat constipation.[10,16,17]

Acute or Transient Incontinence

Treatment of transient or acute incontinence depends on treatment of the suspected cause. It commonly occurs in the acute hospital setting, since any acute illness or drug interaction may cause incontinence. A study evaluating potentially remediable causes of urinary incontinence in the frail elderly population showed that impairment in activities of daily living, dementia, physical restraints, use of bed rails, and use of antianxiety/hypnotic medications were independent risk factors.[27]

Early attention to the functional needs of the patient while treating the acute illness and associated confusion is therapeutic. Use of a urinal and bedside commode and reorientation can prevent the need for

Table 22–2 Behavioral, Medical, and Surgical Treatment Options for Urinary Incontinence

Type of Incontinence	Clinical Entity	Behavioral Therapy	Medical Therapy	Surgical Therapy
Urge	Dementia	Prompted voiding initiated by caregiver	Oxybutynin, imipramine, tolterodine, darifenacin, trospium	Not applicable
Urge	Stroke, Parkinson's disease	Pelvic floor exercises, scheduled voiding by patient	Oxybutynin, imipramine, tolterodine, darifenacin, trospium	Not applicable
Urge	Atrophic vaginitis, urinary tract infection, cystitis, radiation	Not applicable	Estrogen vaginal cream or oral preparation, antibiotics	Not applicable
Mild to moderate stress	Aging, estrogen-deficient vaginal mucosa, previous childbirth	Pelvic floor exercises	Estrogen vaginal cream or oral preparation, pseudoephedrine	Anterior repair of vagina, uterine suspension, bladder suspension, bulking procedures, tension-free vaginal tape, cone insertion, electrical stimulation with biofeedback, extracorporeal magnetic intervention
Severe stress	Severe uterine prolapse, urethral sphincter damage from prostate surgery	Ineffective	Ineffective	Vaginal hysterectomy, surgical implantation of sphincter, tension-free vaginal tape
Overflow	Obstruction caused by ovarian, uterine, bladder, or urethral pathology (stricture), benign prostatic hyperplasia	Not applicable	Not applicable in most cases; pessary for nonsurgical female; alpha-blocker for mild to moderate prostatic hyperplasia	Abdominal hysterectomy and oophorectomy, dilation of stricture, transurethral resection of prostate
Overflow	Flaccid and atonic bladder caused by neuropathy anticholinergic drug administration	Not applicable except for intermittent or chronic urinary catheterization	Discontinue implicated drug therapy; chronic indwelling catheterization	Permanent urostomy

a urinary catheter in many cases. Indwelling urinary catheterization may be temporarily necessary in monitoring output in the case of dehydration, renal insufficiency, or congestive heart failure. However, removal of the urinary catheter should be encouraged as soon as the patient can tolerate oral medications and hydration. Early diagnosis of a fecal impaction as a cause of the transient incontinence can restore continence promptly (level of evidence=B).[28]

> ● Drug therapy for urge incontinence is directed at relaxing smooth muscle of the base (trigone) of the bladder wall or blocking the involuntary bladder contractions of the base of the bladder.

Urge Incontinence

The initial therapy for urge incontinence should be bladder exercises (pelvic floor), commonly referred to as Kegel exercises. This involves voluntary contraction of the bladder in a sequence of 10 contractions several times per day, in between and during micturition. When used regularly in a motivated and compliant patient, studies indicate that urge incontinence may resolve or improve significantly.[29] Bladder–sphincter biofeedback provides another nonpharmacologicl approach to therapy for urge incontinence that may be more effective than pelvic floor exercises.[30]

Nonpharmacologic therapy should be combined with pharmacologic agents when nonpharmacologic therapy alone is ineffective. Research indicates that the combination may produce better results than either pharmacotherapy or nonpharmacologic methods alone (level of evidence=A).[31]

The pathophysiology of urge incontinence involves irritability of the base or trigone of the bladder, whether initiated by local irritation or neurogenic denervation by the brain or spinal cord. Pharmacologic management is targeted at this irritability. In the case of local irritation, antibiotic treatment of a cystitis or urinary tract infection or topical estrogen vaginal cream may suffice to resolve the irritation and subsequent incontinence. Often, atrophic vaginitis may be the cause not only of the urgency and frequency but also of the incontinence and associated urinary tract infection. In the absence of incontinence, the primary care physician may be fooled into performing repeated microscopic analysis of the urine and may perform bacterial analysis by culture before a thorough vaginal inspection actually reveals the cause of the symptoms.

In the case of neurogenic urge incontinence (referred to as detrusor hyperreflexia) secondary to stroke, Parkinson's disease, or dementia syndromes, anticholinergic, antimuscarinic, or smooth muscle-relaxing pharmacologic agents may provide symptomatic and incontinence relief by relaxing the trigone of the bladder (level of evidence=A).[10,16,17]

Tricyclic agents (e.g., imipramine) that possess moderate anticholinergic properties may provide relief. Imipramine may be given before bedtime in as low a dose as possible—10 to 25 mg/day. Other agents that possess smooth muscle and anticholinergic relaxing properties that might be beneficial include oxybutynin chloride in a dose of 2.5 to 5 mg two to three times per day. Oxybutynin may cause cognitive dysfunction especially in the advanced elderly and should be used with caution due to its chemical properties of being able to cross the blood–brain barrier by virtue of its lipophilic nature.[32,33] Flavoxate hydrochloride is another agent that relaxes smooth muscle.[10,16,17,34] It is not effective. Tolterodine tartrate is a newer agent similar to oxybutynin but with muscularinic or weaker anticholinergic properties, and therefore may have the advantage of causing fewer side effects, especially those related to cognition.[17,35] This is since it is hydrophilic and has less potential for crossing the blood–brain barrier.[32] Newer formulations of oxybutynin and tolterodine, the XL (long-acting) given once per day provides a more stable blood level, and therefore have fewer side effects.[36] Additionally, a patch formulation of oxybutynin was recently released that can be given twice per week with significantly less central nervous system side effects than the XL formulations of oxybutynin or tolterodine.[37]

Darifenacin and solifenacin are antimuscarinic agents which appear to be even more specific on the various muscarinic receptor sites than tolterodine. Darifenacin was approved for use in early 2005.[38,39] Trospium is a quaternary ammonium derivative recently approved in the United States for treatment of urinary incontinence with unique properties of being minimally metabolized, not highly protein bound, and with low potential for crossing the blood–brain barrier, and therefore less risk of anticholinergic/antimuscarinic side effects, especially cognitive dysfunction.[40] Caution is advised when using anticholinergic or antimuscarinic agents in combination with cholinesterase agents since the two classes of agents may antagonize the other's effects (level of evidence=A).[41]

Temporary urge incontinence (caused by local inflammation or infection) occurring after prostate surgery should be treated with one of the above agents together with a 2-week course of antibiotics such as nitrofurantoin or trimethoprim-sulfamethoxazole.

> ● Pelvic floor (Kegel) exercises are the first line of therapy for both urge and stress incontinence and can be effective in 60% to 80% of cases.

Stress Incontinence

Mild to moderate stress incontinence is also treated most effectively with a combined nonpharmacologic and pharmacologic approach. Since stress incontinence occurs as a result of pelvic muscle weakness and atrophic changes of the vaginal tissues as a result of aging and hormonal insufficiency, pelvic floor exercises, and hormone replacement are the mainstays of treatment. As is the case for urge incontinence, pelvic floor exercises are an effective first line treatment for mild and some moderate stress incontinence, particularly if a patient is educated and compliant.[10,16,17,29] Pelvic floor exercises have also been shown to be effective in cognitively intact homebound older patients who have high levels of comorbidity and functional impairment. Exercise adherence is the most consistent predictor of responsiveness to this therapy.[42] Selected older women with mild to moderate stress urinary incontinence can achieve results within as little as a week by acquiring the skill of using a properly timed pelvic floor muscle contraction to significantly reduce urine leakage during a cough.

When the stress incontinence is associated with vaginal atrophic changes, the addition of estrogen vaginal cream or an oral dose of estrogen may also be beneficial. However, the addition of oral estrogen at menopause has little clinical benefit on urinary incontinence initially, and is associated with an increased risk of urinary incontinence in women aged 60 and older according to epidemiologic studies.[19] In addition, an alpha-stimulating agent such as pseudoephedrine, 30 mg three times a day, to tighten the bladder sphincter may prove helpful in some cases. However, these medications may aggravate cardiac arrhythmias, anxiety disorders, congestive heart failure, or hypertension, and may therefore be contraindicated in many patients. Pelvic exercises have been shown to be as beneficial as phenylpropanolamine in reducing stress incontinence.[10,16,17,43]

The dual-acting serotonin and norepinephrine reuptake inhibitor, duloxetine, recently released for the treatment of depression, also appears to reduce the frequency of stress incontinence episodes. Duloxetine does not have Food and Drug Administration approval for the pharmacologic management of stress incontinence.[44] A common side effect of duloxetine at the incontinence dose range of 40 mg twice daily is nausea. Mixed urge and stress incontinence should be treated with a combination of bladder exercises, topical or oral estrogen preparations, and either alpha stimulants such as pseudoephedrine or anticholinergic/antimuscarinic smooth muscle relaxer–type medications, depending on which of the components (stress or urge) is thought to be the major contributor to the incontinence (level of evidence=A).[10,16,17]

Severe stress incontinence usually is caused by some amount of pelvic laxity and therefore is most likely to respond only to surgical therapy or pessary insertion. In general, surgical procedures are more likely to cure severe stress urinary incontinence but are also associated with more adverse events.[45] Insertion of a pessary restores the acute angle of the bladder, preventing loss of urine associated with increased abdominal pressure. Use of a pessary may be indicated in a patient who is not a good preoperative candidate or when the patient refuses surgery.[46]

A vaginal hysterectomy should be considered if the incontinence is associated with other pelvic disease or severe prolapse. The vaginal hysterectomy may be combined with resection of the redundant portion of the anterior vaginal wall, which strengthens and lifts the pelvic floor and restores the acute angle of the bladder. This is referred to as an *anterior repair*. Anterior repair alone is useful to treat mild to moderate stress incontinence when empiric drug therapy has failed. Other procedures include bladder suspension (tacking the bladder to the symphysis pubis) procedure and the pubo-fascial or vaginal sling procedure.[47] A newer technique involves injection of the periurethral or transurethral space with collagen (bulking procedures), which are efficacious in a significant number of cases with minimal morbidity.[17,48] In older women with genitourinary prolapse with associated occult stress incontinence, transvaginal prolapse repair, and the prophylactic tension-free vaginal tape (TVT) procedure at 27 months follow-up were associated with significant improvement of the stress incontinence from baseline and were found to be safe. It also appears to be a shorter and easier procedure than the traditional Burch (retropubic urethropexy) or culposuspension procedure and is associated with a shorter learning curve. However, unlike the Burch procedure, long-term data on efficacy are pending.[49,50]

Newer nonpharmacologic procedures that may be used as an alternative to surgery include the use of a vaginal 150-g ceramic cone coupled with pelvic floor exercises and functional electrical stimulation (FES) using biofeedback and extracorporeal magnetic innervation (ExMI) for pelvic muscle strengthening.[51]

Stress incontinence caused by a damaged sphincter in older men can be treated with artificial sphincter implantation with variable results or a plastic surgery procedure involving a sling operation to the sphincter muscle (level of evidence=B).[4,10] Tissue engineering and regenerative medicine may also provide new and exciting treatment strategies for the management of urinary incontinence.[52]

> ● The initial urgent management of obstructive overflow incontinence is the use of an indwelling or suprapubic catheter to decompress the bladder.

Overflow Incontinence

The treatment of overflow incontinence depends on the underlying pathologic condition: an obstructed versus a dilated and flaccid bladder. For the *acutely obstructed* patient, prompt diagnosis should be followed by decompression using an indwelling or suprapubic catheter, for symptom relief and prevention of renal damage. This should be followed by referral, further workup to determine the cause of the obstruction, and usually by surgical intervention.

Medications that directly cause constriction of the urinary sphincter may also cause acute obstruction (see Table 22–1).[4,10,12,17] For the older male patient with symptomatic bladder outlet obstruction from benign prostatic hyperplasia and associated urge incontinence secondary to detrusor hyperreflexia, one study indicated that the combined use of doxazosin with tolterodine versus doxazosin alone resulted in a significant improvement of urinary symptoms of urgency, frequency and incontinence (level of evidence=B).[53]

Drugs with anticholinergic or antimuscarinic activity are common causes of overflow incontinence. Removal of the offending drug followed by observation usually restores continence after 24 to 48 hours. Chronic disease processes associated with neurogenic uropathy include longstanding diabetes, chronic renal failure, vitamin B_{12} deficiency, multiple sclerosis, and tertiary syphilis. Depending on the amount of neuronal function that remains, drugs with cholinergic activity such as urecholine may restore some bladder function by causing contraction of the bladder wall. These agents are best used when associated with acute overflow incontinence secondary to anticholinergic drug therapy or postoperatively. These agents are seldom used for chronic drug therapy because of the variable response and associated side effects. They are contraindicated in patients with asthma, congestive heart failure, peptic ulcer disease, and thyrotoxicosis. Another agent, phentolamine, an alpha-adrenergic receptor blocker, relaxes the sphincter. Before use in an acute situation, obstruction of the bowel and bladder should be ruled out (level of evidence=B).[4,10,16,17]

Depending on the amount of residual damage as a result of long-standing obstruction (dilated collecting ducts and calyces) or neuronal innervation remaining in the case of neuropathic bladder, residual urine volumes left at the end of urination may lead to urinary tract infection and stone formation. Further renal insufficiency may also develop as a result of sustained elevated intravesicular and renal tubular pressure. Intermittent urinary (in and out) catheterization performed under clean conditions may prevent this complication. This intervention works best in a well-educated, compliant diabetic patient. Other patients with an atonic flaccid bladder need either indwelling or suprapubic catheterization (level of evidence=B).[10]

Behaviorally Oriented Training

Behaviorally oriented training procedures include biofeedback, habit training, and scheduled toileting. These can be divided into patient-dependent and caregiver-dependent procedures. *Patient-dependent procedures* include pelvic floor exercises and biofeedback. Biofeedback involves use of bladder, rectal, or vaginal pressure or electrical activity recordings to train patients to contract the pelvic floor muscles to relax the bladder. It can be used to treat urge and stress incontinence. Limitations include the need for an extensively trained individual and equipment, as well as the invasive nature of the procedure. This makes biofeedback unacceptable in many cases. For these reasons, biofeedback remains useful as a research tool but is of limited use in the clinical setting. Scheduled or timed voiding is another patient-dependent procedure involving voiding at regularly scheduled intervals to prevent incontinent voids as a result of an uninhibited bladder contraction. This type of behavioral therapy would be indicated for a patient with precipitous urge incontinence or the type of incontinence in which the patient is "unaware." Patients may determine the frequency of the scheduled voiding by keeping an incontinence record. Initial improvement may be high, but long-term compliance tends to be low (level of evidence=A).[4,10,16,17]

A *caregiver-dependent procedure* involves habit training or prompted voiding in a patient with neurogenic incontinence related to detrusia hyperreflexia secondary to dementia, Parkinson's disease, or stroke. In such cases, cognitive or neurologic deficits prevent awareness of the need for voluntary micturition. The caregiver prompts the patient to void at scheduled intervals to prevent incontinent episodes, depending on the frequency of involuntary voids. Micturition is modified according to the patient's schedule of continent voids and incontinent episodes according to the monitoring record. After taking the patient to the bathroom and placing the patient on the toilet seat, the caregiver uses various adjunctive techniques to initiate prompted voiding such as running tap water, stroking the inner thigh, suprapubic tapping, or bending forward after completion of voiding to help empty the bladder.[10,16,17] This procedure has been shown to reduce incontinent episodes by 32% and may be useful in some dementia patients.[54] Success of this procedure is related to the motivation and knowledge of the caregiver rather than the physical, functional, and mental status of the patient. To be cost-effective in the home or nursing home, the time spent on this treatment should not exceed the time spent changing the patient. Those patients with the most severe dementia, those who are least mobile, and those with the more severe incontinence benefit the least from this procedure.[54] This procedure also works best for those patients who have less frequent voiding and large bladder capacities or voided volumes (level of evidence=C).

Incontinence in the Long-Term Care Setting

Federal regulations require that a resident who enters a long-term care facility with urinary incontinence receives appropriate treatment to prevent urinary tract infections, and services should be provided to restore normal bladder function when possible.[55] Implementing an exercise and/or incontinence management protocol may be expensive but is associated with improved "dryness," reduced pressure ulcer incidence, less urinary and fecal incontinence, better physical activity, and skin wetness outcome measures with a cost of $573 per resident per day.[56-58] A practical clinical practice guideline for urinary incontinence that addresses the key elements of diagnosis, treatment and monitoring is available from the American Medical Directors Association.[59]

> ● Indications for urinary catheterization are to relieve obstruction, monitor output, keep the patient dry, manage incontinence that cannot be treated medically or surgically, or for patient or caregiver preference.

Indications for Urinary Catheterization

Approximately 10% to 15% of nursing home residents have chronic urinary catheters. Types include transurethral, suprapubic and condom, with the transurethral being more common, but with none of these have being proven to be more effective than another.[60] Indications for indwelling urinary catheterization include obstructive pathology if the patient has a high preoperative risk or the quality of life to be gained does not justify the risk of surgery.[10] A common scenario is an older man with obstructive disease of the prostate caused by benign prostatic hyperplasia or prostate carcinoma with severe congestive heart disease or angina or a demented and bedridden nursing home or homebound elderly patient.[10] Chronic indwelling urinary catheterization also may be indicated to keep a patient in a dry environment until a buttock, sacral, or hip decubitus heals or for a terminal patient to prevent caregiver burden and physical exhaustion associated with frequent diaper changes (level of evidence=C). Complications of indwelling catheters include an increased risk of urinary tract infection and urosepsis, increased frequency of bladder stones, periurethral abscess, bladder cancer, and an increased risk of chronic bacteremia and bacteriuria (Box 22-3).[10]

CHRONIC CATHETER CARE

Within 2 to 5 weeks after continuous indwelling catheterization has been initiated, patients routinely develop chronic bacteriuria (usually polymicrobial), pyuria, and occasionally microscopic hematuria. Attempts to eradicate the bacteriuria are unsuccessful and may be followed by bacterial resistance to common antibiotics and subsequent life-threatening urosepsis. Chronic bacteriuria should be treated only in the presence of acute symptoms such as fever, low back pain, chills, or persistent gross hematuria. Systemic broad-spectrum antibiotic therapy should be instituted after a fresh urine specimen is obtained from the bladder after catheter change. Post-treatment cultures are not useful to assess results because of the chronic colonization of bacteria that is present.[10,61,62]

Catheter management and infection control measures vary widely among nursing homes, though some are supported in the medical literature.[60] From a practical standpoint, a good rule of thumb is that indwelling catheters should be changed routinely when the following end point is reached: significant sludge or catheter debris (exfoliation) has accumulated and is causing reduced urinary catheter drainage by partially obstructing the catheter lumen. In addition, several attempts at irrigation of the catheter with a sterile solution is not associated with increased urinary catheter drainage. In this scenario, further obstruction could lead to significant residual urine accumulation and urosepsis.[10] In addition, in chronic care institutions, indwelling catheters are changed regularly for convenience. Routine scheduled catheter irrigation is not recommended because it has not been found to be effective and may introduce infection.[10] Recurrent episodes of urinary tract infection or urosepsis that develop as a result of chronic indwelling catheter placement in which there is an absolute indication for continued catheter drainage are difficult to manage. Urologic consultation should be performed, and further urodynamic assessment may be necessary to rule out other causes of obstruction or nidus for infection (level of evidence=C).

Condom catheters are preferred by both male patients and nursing staff because of patient comfort and ease of administration. Dislodgment and leakage are major drawbacks of condom catheters (level of evidence=C).[63]

Box 22-3   **Indications for and Complications of Indwelling Urinary Catheters**

Indications

- Acute overflow incontinence caused by obstruction or atonic flaccid bladder.
- Obstructive incontinence in patient who is not candidate for surgical intervention.
- Temporarily to manage output (e.g., high-output states or dehydration).
- To keep the patient dry until a buttock, sacral, or hip decubitus heals.

- For caregiver preference to prevent burnout in the care of a patient who requires bed sheets to be changed more than several times per day because of incontinent episodes.

Complications

- Increased risk of urinary tract infection and urosepsis.
- Increased frequency of bladder stones.
- Periurethral abscess.
- Increased risk of bacteremia and bacteriuria.
- Increased risk of bladder carcinoma.

Diapers and Continence Aids

Diapers and continence pads and other aids are commonly used in the management of urinary incontinence in the cognitively and functionally impaired and to some extent in elderly dwelling in the community. Diapers and continence pads should be reserved for an incontinent patient in whom at least a primary care workup of urinary incontinence has been performed and urologic referral and urodynamic workup has been performed when indicated. In addition, the patient should have failed attempts at behavioral and medical therapy. This is referred to as refractory, or intractable, incontinence. Garments and pads are nonspecific and should not be used as a first line of treatment before a workup or as a substitute for workup of chronic continence (level of evidence=D).[64]

Harold Burnhart, *Part 4*

Mr. Burnhart is seen back in your office for follow-up in 2 weeks for his urinary tract infection and to determine his response to the prazosin. He indicates that his frequency and nocturia is "better." His urine dipstick is negative for nitrite and white blood cells. He still gets up to urinate two or three times at night but does not have to urinate as frequently during the day. He is scheduled for a 2-month follow-up appointment, but you are called to see the patient at 2:00 AM 2 weeks later at the hospital emergency room. Mr. Burnhart is noted to have a fever of 102 degrees and is confused to time and place. He is attended by his son. His physical examination reveals positive flank tenderness on the left. Laboratory workup reveals a white blood cell count of 17,000 with 80% neutrophils (normal range 6,000 to 10,000 and 60 to 70% neutrophils). He is also noted to have too numerous to count white blood cells and 15 to 20 red blood cells per high power field on a catheterized urinalysis. You diagnose him with pyelonephritis. You admit him to the hospital and begin intravenous antibiotics. He responds to the antibiotics after 48 hours and his confusion subsequently resolves. You consult a urologist and she indicates the need for a workup including a cystoscopy, cystourethrogram, renal ultrasound, and intravenous pyelogram. The cystoscope reveals evidence of trabeculations and the cystourethrogram shows evidence of a moderately dilated noncompliant bladder. He is subsequently scheduled for a transurethral resection of the prostate but Mr. Burnhart requests that the surgery be postponed and that a trial of medication be prescribed to "empty" the bladder. The urologist and you advise Mr. Burnhart that medical therapy is contraindicated and that surgery should be performed as soon as possible.

CASE DISCUSSION

Mr. Burnhart's urgency, frequency, and nocturia are secondary to an enlarging prostate that resulted in partial obstruction and overflow incontinence. The history of longstanding diabetes and the relatively poor blood sugar control as reflected by his elevated glycosylated hemoglobin levels probably explains his uropathy secondary to diabetes and his incomplete bladder emptying as shown on the cystourethrogram. The bladder trabeculations are characteristic of long-standing obstruction of the bladder. The urinary tract infection may also be causing urge symptoms. The symptoms of urgency, frequency, and nocturia are nonspecific for the type of incontinence. Symptoms most characteristic of overflow incontinence are straining to urinate, decreased size of the stream, and hesitancy, as Mr. Burnhart reported. The postvoid residual urine amount of 175 cc found on the bladder sonography is in the borderline range of 100 to 200 ml in which "watchful waiting" might be considered to be appropriate while administering pharmacologic therapy as indicated. Since Mr. Burnhart subsequently developed pyelonephritis within a short period of time after discontinuing the antibiotics, urological consultation and surgery is appropriate to relieve the obstruction. The suggestion by Mr. Barnhart to be prescribed a medication to empty his bladder (cholinergic agent) is not appropriate since it may be ineffective and actually detrimental due to the obstruction. Without the presence of the obstruction from the prostate, cholinergic agents may be of variable benefit in patients with uropathy depending on the degree of the uropathy and viable nerve innervation.

Linda James, *Part 4*

You order the patient to be toileted every 2 hours while awake (prompted voiding) and to be toileted before bedtime. You also discontinue the hydrochlorthiazide, and subsequent monitoring indicates that her blood pressure is in the 130/80 range without medication. After a period of 2 weeks, her pressure ulcers begin to heal. Her incontinence episodes are also reduced in frequency to two to four episodes per 24 hours and usually during the night shift. Continence pads are then prescribed for Ms. James at bedtime.

CASE DISCUSSION

Ms. James probably could be experiencing a combination of acute, functional incontinence and urge incontinence. During the hospitalization, bedrest and dysmobility secondary to the stroke (functional) could contribute to her incontinence. In such cases, it is important to provide environmental modifications such as a bedside commode and human assistance with toileting and to improve mobility. Removal of the urinary catheter is important to prevent infection and prevent dependence. Acute incontinence secondary to medical illness could also be contributing to the incontinence during the hospitalization. Appropriate management of functional incontinence would be the institution of nonpharmacologic methods such as bladder exercises and a toileting schedule around the incontinent episodes as was done. A period of 6 weeks with improved mobility but inability to complete the bladder exercises and failure of the toileting schedule to completely resolve the incontinence is sufficient time to rule out acute and functional incontinence. The introduction of an alternative nonpharmacologic approach of prompted voiding every 2 hours (caregiver-dependent procedure) and at bedtime, coupled with removal of the diuretic, is usually beneficial in reducing the frequency of urge incontinence episodes. The urge incontinence is probably secondary to the dementia and CVA (neurogenic urge). The patient has no symptoms or signs of stress incontinence despite her age and 10 childbirths. Most cases of incontinence can be managed but not cured. The use of an anticholinergic or antimuscarinic in a patient with dementia who is also prescribed a cholinesterace inhibitor can be counterproductive in worsening the dementia and negating the effects of the cholinesterace inhibitor.

SUMMARY

An intact nervous system and lower urinary tract, a motivated patient, and an appropriate environment are necessary to maintain continence. The onset of urinary incontinence is associated with psychologic, medical, social, and financial consequences.

The primary care workup of urinary incontinence includes a comprehensive history and physical examination, a complete urinalysis, urine culture, serum electrolytes and calcium, and a postvoid residual urine determination. Two-thirds of the time, the primary care workup for urinary incontinence can be performed in two or three office visits using simple clinical tools. A formal urodynamic workup is time consuming, expensive, and usually does not add to the diagnostic accuracy. Patients who do not fit a specific incontinence pattern or for whom the diagnosis is uncertain can be referred for urodynamic evaluation.

Acute or transient incontinence is common in older adults with an acute illness. Incontinence that does not resolve within 3 to 6 weeks is classified as chronic incontinence. Most cases of chronic urinary incontinence can be managed effectively, but complete resolution rarely occurs.

The most common type of chronic urinary incontinence is urge incontinence. Drug therapy for urge incontinence is directed at relaxing the smooth muscle of the base (trigone) of the bladder wall or blocking the involuntary bladder contractions of the base of the bladder. The diagnosis of stress incontinence is made by a history of urinary leakage associated with any maneuver that increases abdominal pressure or the direct observation of urinary loss on bearing down. Pelvic floor (Kegel) exercises are the first line of therapy for both urge and stress incontinence and prove effective in 60% to 80% of cases.

The rarest but most serious form of urinary incontinence is overflow incontinence. A postvoid residual urine determination of 200 ml or greater is a sign of overflow incontinence.

Indications for urinary catheterization are to relieve an acute obstruction, monitor output, keep the patient dry, manage incontinence that cannot be managed medically or surgically, or for caregiver preference. Chronic urinary catheterization is associated with the development of chronic bacteriuria and pyuria.

POSTTEST

1. The following symptoms are diagnostic for urge incontinence (detrusor hyperreflexia):
   a. Urgency, frequency, and a feeling of incomplete bladder emptying
   b. Frequency and pain or discomfort in the suprapublic area
   c. Nocturia
   d. Urgency and nocturia
   e. None of the above

2. The following drugs can cause incontinence except:
   a. Narcotics
   b. Hypnotics
   c. Antipsychotics and antidepressants
   d. Calcium channel blockers
   e. Beta blockers

3. Pelvic floor exercises (Kegel) has been shown to be effective for which type of incontinence:
   a. Urge incontinence
   b. Overflow incontinence
   c. Stress incontinence
   d. Urge and stress incontinence
   e. Acute incontinence

4. Which of the following the pharmacological agents used for urge incontinence can cross the blood–brain barrier and cause significant cognitive dysfunction in an older patient?
   a. Trospium
   b. Oxybutynin
   c. Tolterodine
   d. Darifenacin

References

1. Thom D. Variation in estimates of urinary incontinence prevalence in the community: effects of differences in definition, population characteristics, and study type. J Am Geriatr Soc 46:473, 1998.
2. Nygaard IE, Lemke JH. Urinary incontinence in rural older women: prevalence, incidence, and remission. J Am Geriatr Soc 44:1049, 1996.
3. Wetle T, Scherr P, Branch LG, et al. Difficulty with holding urine among older persons in a geographically defined community: prevalence and correlates. J Am Geriatr Soc 43:349, 1995.
4. U.S. Department of Health and Human Services. Clinical Practice Guideline: Urinary Incontinence in Adults. Rockville, MD: U.S. Department of Health and Human Services, 1992 (AHCPR 92-0038).
5. DuBeau CE, Levy B, Mangione CM, et al. The impact of urge urinary incontinence on quality of life: importance of patients' perspective and explanatory style. J Am Geriatr Soc 46:683, 1998.
6. Hunskaar S, Vinsnes A. The quality of life in women with urinary incontinence as measured by the sickness impact profile. J Am Geriatr Soc 39:378, 1991 (published erratum appears in J Am Geriatr Soc 40:967, 1992).
7. Johnson TM 2nd, Kincade JE, Bernard SL, et al. The association of urinary incontinence with poor self-rated health. J Am Geriatr Soc 46:693, 1998.
8. DuBeau CE, Kiely DK, Resnick NM. Quality of life impact of urge incontinence in older persons: a new measure and conceptual structure. J Am Geriatr Soc 47:989, 1999.
9. Cruise PA, Schnelle JF, Alessi CA, et al. The nighttime environment and incontinence care practices in nursing homes. J Am Geriatr Soc 46:181, 1998.
10. Kane R, Ouslander JG. Essentials of Clinical Geriatrics. 3rd ed. New York: McGraw-Hill, 1994.
11. Steiner JF, Kramer AM, Eilertsen TB, et al. Development and validation of a clinical prediction rule for prolonged nursing home residence after hip fracture. J Am Geriatr Soc 45:1510, 1997.
12. Osterweil D, Martin M, Syndulko K. Predictors of skilled nursing placement in a multilevel long-term care facility. J Am Geriatr Soc 43:108, 1995.
13. McDowell BJ, Engberg SJ, Rodriguez E, et al. Characteristics of urinary incontinence in homebound older adults. J Am Geriatr Soc 44:963, 1996.
14. Herzog AR, Diokno AC, Brown MB, et al. Urinary incontinence as a risk factor for mortality. J Am Geriatr Soc 42:264, 1994.
15. Shih YC, Hartzema AG, Tolleson-Rinehart S. Labor costs associated with incontinence in long-term care facilities. Urology 62:442-6, 2003.
16. Brandeis GH, et al. Urinary incontinence. In: Calkins E, Ford AB, Katz PR, eds. Practice of Geriatrics. 2nd ed. Philadelphia: WB Saunders, 1992.
17. Ouslander JG, Johnson TM. Incontinence. In: Hazzard WR, et al., eds. Principles of Geriatric Medicine and Gerontology. 4th ed. New York: McGraw-Hill, 2003.
18. Ouslander JG, Palmer MH, Rovner BW, et al. Urinary incontinence in nursing homes: incidence, remission, and associated factors. J Am Geriatr Soc 41:1083, 1993.
19. Thom DH, Brown JS. Reproductive and hormonal risk factors for urinary incontinence in later life: a review of the clinical and epidemiologic literature. J Am Geriatr Soc 46:1411, 1998.
20. Grosshans C, Passadori Y, Peter B, et al. Urinary retention in the elderly: a study of 100 hospitalized patients. J Am Geriatr Soc 41:633, 1993.
21. Brocklehurst JC. Urinary incontinence in old age: helping the general practitioner to make a diagnosis. Gerontology Suppl 36:3, 1990.
22. Resnick NM. Noninvasive diagnosis of the patient with complex incontinence, Gerontology Suppl 36:8, 1990.
23. Belmin J, Hervias Y, Avellano E, et al. Reliability of sampling urine from disposable diapers in elderly incontinent women. J Am Geriatr Soc 41:1182, 1993.
24. Ouslander JG. Urine specimen collection from incontinent female nursing home residents. J Am Geriatr Soc 43:279, 1995.
25. Ouslander JG, Simmons S, Tuico E, et al. Use of a portable ultrasound device to measure postvoid residual volume among incontinent nursing home residents. J Am Geriatr Soc 42:1189, 1994.
26. Goode PS, Locher JL, Bryant RL, et al. Measurement of postvoid residual urine with portable transabdominal bladder ultrasound scanner and urethral catheterization. Int Urogynecol J Pelvic Floor Dysfunct 11:296-300, 2000.
27. Brandeis GH, Baumann MM, Hossain M, et al. The prevalence of potentially remediable urinary incontinence in frail older people: a study using the minimum data set. J Am Geriatr Soc 45:215, 1997.
28. Cefalu CA. Hospital restraint use in the elderly: a review of the literature and practical guidelines for use. Hosp Physician 29:25, 1993.
29. Fantl JA, Wyman JF, McClish DK, et al. Efficacy of bladder training in older women with urinary incontinence. JAMA 265:609, 1991.
30. Wang AC. Bladder-sphincter biofeedback as treatment of detrusor instability in women who failed to respond to oxybutynin. Chang Gung Med J 23:590-9, 2000.
31. Burgio KL. Current perspectives on management of urgency using bladder and behavioral training. J Am Acad Nurse Pract Suppl 16:4-7, 2004.
32. Habgood MD, Begley DJ, Abbott NJ. Determinants of passive drug entry into the central nervous system. Cell Mol Neurobiol 20:231-53, 2000.
33. Katz IR, Sands LP, Bilker W, et al. Identification of medications that cause cognitive impairment in older people: The case of oxybutynin chloride. J Am Geriatr Soc 46:8-13, 1998.
34. Sourander LB. Treatment of urinary incontinence: the place of drugs. Gerontology Suppl 36:19, 1990.
35. Malone-Lee JG, Walsh JB, Maugourd MF. Tolterodine: a safe and effective treatment for older patients with overactive bladder. J Am Geriatr Soc 49:700-5, 2001.
36. Hughes DA, Dubois D. Cost-effectiveness analysis of extended-release formulations of oxybutynin and tolterodine for the management of urge incontinence. Pharmacoeconomics 22:1047-59, 2004.
37. Bang LM, Easthope SE, Perry CM. Transdermal oxybutynin: for overactive bladder. Drugs Aging 20:857-64, 2003.
38. Lipton RB, Kolodner K, Wesnes K. Assessment of cognitive function of the elderly population: Effects of darifenacin. J Urol 173:493-8, 2005.
39. Cardozo L, Lisec M, Millard R, et al. Randomized, double-blind placebo controlled trial of the once daily antimuscarinic agent solifenacin succinate in patients with overactive bladder. J Urol 172:1919-24, 2004.
40. Hofner K, Oelke M, Machtens S, et al. Trospium chloride—an effective drug in the treatment of overactive bladder and detrusor hyperreflexia. World J Urol 19:336-43, 2001.
41. Siegler EL, Reidenberg M. Treatment of urinary incontinence with anticholinergics in patients taking cholinesterase inhibitors for dementia. Clin Pharmacol Ther 75:484-8, 2004.
42. McDowell BJ, Engberg S, Sereika S, et al. Effectiveness of behavioral therapy to treat incontinence in homebound older adults. J Am Geriatr Soc 47:309, 1999.
43. Wells TJ, Brink CA, Diokno AC, et al. Pelvic muscle exercise for stress urinary incontinence in elderly women. J Am Geriatr Soc 39:785, 1991.
44. Moore K. Duloxetine: a new approach for treating stress urinary incontinence. Int J Gynaecol Obstet Suppl 86:S53-62, 2004.

45. 65. Nygaard IE, Heit M. Stress urinary incontinence. Am J Obstet Gynecol 104:607-20, 2004.

46. Zeitlin MP, Lebherz TB. Pessaries in the geriatric patient. J Am Geriatr Soc 40(6):636-9, 1992.

47. Rodrigues P, Hering F, Meler A et al. Pubo-fascial versus vaginal sling operation for the treatment of stress urinary incontinence: a prospective study. Neurourol Urodyn 23:627-31, 2004.

48. Schulz JA, Nager CW, Stanton SL, et al. Bulking agents for stress urinary incontinence: short-term results and complications in a randomized comparison of periurethral and transurethral injections. Int Urogynecol J Pelvic Floor Dysfunct 15:261-5, 2004.

49. Groutz A, Gold R, Pauzner D, et al. Tension-free tape (TVT) for the treatment of occult stress urinary incontinence in women undergoing prolapse repair: a prospective study of 100 consecutive cases. Neurourol Urodyn 23:632-5, 2004.

50. Kung RC. Laparoscopic treatment of urinary incontinence. Obstet Gynecol Clin North Am 31:539-49, viii, 2004.

51. Yokoyama T, Fujita O, Nishiguchi J, et al. Extracorporeal magnetic innervation treatment for urinary incontinence. Int J Urol 11:602-6, 2004.

52. Koh CJ, Atala A. Tissue engineering for urinary incontinence applications. Minerva Ginecol 56:371-8, 2004.

53. Lee JY, Kim HW, Lee SJ, et al. Comparison of doxazosin with or without tolterodine in men with symptomatic bladder outlet obstruction and an overactive bladder. BJU Int 94:817-20, 2004.

54. Skelly J, Flint AJ. Urinary incontinence associated with dementia. J Am Geriatr Soc 43:286, 1995.

55. American Medical Directors Association. Synopsis of Federal Regulation in the Nursing Facility—Implications for Attending Physicians and Medical Directors. Columbia, MD: American Medical Directors Association, January 2003.

56. Bates-Jensen -BM, Alessi CA, Al-Samarrai NR, et al. The effects of an exercise and incontinence intervention on skin health outcomes in nursing residents. J Am Geriatr Soc 51:348-55, 2003.

57. Frantz RA, Xakellis GC Jr. Harvey PC, et al. Implementing an incontinence management protocol in long-term care. Clinical outcomes and costs. J Gerontol Nurs 29:46-53, 2003.

58. Schnelle JF, Alessi CA, Simmons SF, et al. Translating clinical research into practice: a randomized controlled trial of exercise and incontinence care with nursing home residents. J Am Geriatr Soc 50:1476-83, 2002.

59. American Medical Directors Association. Urinary Incontinence—Clinical Practice Guideline.Columbia, MD: American Medical Directors Association, 1996.

60. Gammack JK. Use and management of chronic urinary catheters in long-term care. J Am Med Dir Assoc Suppl 4:S52-9, 2003.

61. Yoshikawa TT. Chronic urinary tract infections in elderly patients. Hosp Pract 28:103, 1993.

62. Kunin CM, Douthitt S, Dancing J, et al. The association between the use of urinary catheters and morbidity and mortality among elderly patients in nursing homes. Am J Epidemiol 135:291, 1992.

63. Saint S, Lipsky Bam Baker PD et al. Urinary catheters: what type do men and their nurses prefer? J Am Geriatr Soc 47:1453, 1999.

64. Newman DK, Lynch K, Smith DA, et al. Restoring urinary continence. Am J Nurs 91:28, 1991.

Web Resources

1. For healthcare providers: www.nlm.nh.gov/medlineplus/urinaryincontinence.html.
2. For patients: http://incontinence.org.

PRETEST ANSWERS
1. e
2. a
3. a

POSTTEST ANSWERS
1. e
2. e
3. d
4. c

CHAPTER 23 Constipation and Fecal Incontinence

Steve Bartz

OBJECTIVES

Upon completion of this chapter, the reader will be able to:

- Define constipation and understand various perceptions of the condition.
- Identify risk factors and causes of constipation.
- Recognize potential complications of constipation.
- Identify lifestyle choices used to treat constipation.
- Prescribe laxatives and know how they work.
- Define when to refer constipated individuals for specialized testing.
- Understand the etiology of, and treat, fecal incontinence.

PRETEST

1. Which diseases are implicated in constipation?
   a. Alzheimer's and anemia
   b. Hypertension and urinary incontinence
   c. Diabetes mellitus and hypothyroidism
   d. Gastroesophageal reflux disease (GERD) and depression
   e. Irritable bowel syndrome and hyperlipidemia

2. True or False. A higher level of both fluid intake and activity are well proven to improve symptoms of constipation.

3. Which of the following is the most common type of constipation in the U.S.?
   a. Diabetes mellitus
   b. Laxative abuse
   c. Low dietary fiber
   d. Normal transit
   e. Prescription medications

4. True or False: A history and focused physical exam are usually adequate in evaluating routine cases of constipation.

PREVALENCE AND IMPACT

Constipation is a common medical condition in Western societies affecting between 2% and 28% of the population.[1,2] It is particularly problematic in the elderly where it is a complaint in 25% to 30% of surveyed individuals.[3] The elderly are most affected[4] followed by children and younger adults.[5] Women tend to be more symptomatic than men. Constipation alone prompts more than 2.5 million office visits annually to physicians in the United States.[6] Sufferers spend greater than $500 million yearly seeking relieve from its symptoms.[7]

Although symptoms of constipation are generally mild and intermittent, they can be very uncomfortable and persistent in patients. Most cases can be successfully managed with simple strategies, including lifestyle modifications, dietary changes, or fiber and laxative use. A detailed workup to check for serious disease is needed only if warning signs are present.

Definition

There is no single definition of constipation. The Rome II criteria[8] (Box 23–1) is a consensus-driven set of symptom-based criteria usually used in research.

Box 23–1 Rome II Criteria for Adults with Constipation

Two or more of the following occurring during bowel movements for at least 12 weeks (need not be consecutive) in the past 12 months:

- Fewer than three bowel movements per week
- Straining during more than 25% of bowel movements
- Lumpy or hard stools for more than 25% of bowel movements
- Sensation of anorectal blockage for more than 25% of bowel movements
- Sensation of incomplete evacuation for more than 25% of bowel movements
- Manually assisted removal of more than 25% of bowel movements

Loose stools not present.
Criteria for irritable bowel syndrome not met.

Most patients define constipation as either straining during defecation (52%) or the passage of hard stools (44%). Other frequent complaints include the inability to defecate when desired (34%) and infrequent defecation (33%).[9] In contrast, physicians mainly consider the frequency of stool passages in their definition of the problem.

Most definitions of normal stooling will fit the criteria of having bowel movements from two or three times daily to three times per week. This, however, is a general rule and some individuals who have fewer than three stools per week may still be considered normal if this is not a recent change in bowel habits and is not associated with any difficulty in defecation patterns. Since constipation is such a subjective condition, a practical rule to follow is to treat constipation if a patient's stooling pattern causes discomfort or concern and to investigate when any warning signs are present.

Lydia Beulow, *(Part 1)*

Lydia Beulow is an active 85-year-old who comes to the office for a routine office visit. As a new complaint, she mentions that she is having some discomfort with her hemorrhoids and thinks it may be worsened by her infrequent bowel movements. She frequently will miss a daily bowel movement but mentions that when she was younger she would have a movement every day. She also states that her stools are harder than they used to be. Her medical history includes hypertension, urinary incontinence, GERD, and iron deficiency anemia. Surgical history reveals only a deviated septum repair.

STUDY QUESTIONS

1. Does she meet criteria for constipation?
2. Could her medical problems be contributing to her complaints?
3. What questions would you ask her next?

CAUSES AND PATHOPHYSIOLOGY

Constipation is often multifactorial and can be caused by a combination of systemic or local conditions, lifestyle issues, and/or medications. Normal colonic physiology requires the proper complex interaction of multiple organ systems including neurologic, muscular, and endocrine. Sympathetic and parasympathetic pathways from the autonomic nervous system, as well as fibers from the enteric nervous system, innervate involuntary (smooth) muscles of the bowel wall and along with voluntary (striated) muscles of the pelvic floor, coordinate transit of digested food in the small and large intestines

and rectum. Numerous neurotransmitters including acetylcholine, vasoactive intestinal peptide, nitric oxide, and substance P as well as the hormones estrogen and progesterone also participate in this process.

Stool movement is propagated by the combination of semifrequent low-amplitude contractions and infrequent high-amplitude ones. Low-amplitude waves cause small movements of colonic material and facilitate mixing of contents. High-amplitude waves occur typically after eating and early in the morning. They move larger amounts of material down the digestive tract. Nonpropagating segmental contractions also occur to facilitate mixing but tend to retard the forward movement of intestinal contents.

The defecatory process requires the coordinated activities of intestinal peristalsis, Valsalva of the intra-abdominal muscles, reflex relaxation of the internal anal sphincter, and voluntary relaxation of the external anal sphincter. Problems in any of these areas can impede successful stooling.

Normal- and Slow-Transit Constipation

The most common form of constipation in adults worldwide, although rare in the United States, is Chagas disease.[10] In the United States, the most common form is *normal-transit constipation*, also called *functional constipation*. There is no discernable secondary disorder responsible for symptoms, making the etiology idiopathic. Patients will complain of infrequent stools, hard stools, abdominal bloating, fullness, or pressure. However, when evaluated, both colonic transit time and pelvic floor function are normal. Nevertheless, patients can be very uncomfortable and desire treatment. Passage of stool through the digestive tract typically takes less than 72 hours. If stool propagation is delayed, constipation is defined as being slow transit. Besides infrequent stooling, patients often will complain of hard stools since the fecal material is more prone to water absorption due to increased contact time with the bowel lumen. There is some debate in the literature as to the frequency of this condition. The disorder may be most common in young females and present from a young age.[11] It tends to be mostly neurologic in origin resulting in fewer propagating colonic contractions and slower transit times. Treatment with dietary fiber and laxatives tends to be disappointing.

Systemic diseases can manifest in the gastrointestinal system as constipation. They generally result from disturbances of the endocrine, neurologic, or collagen-vascular systems. The most commonly implicated metabolic disturbance is diabetes mellitus, which can cause a diffuse enteroparesis.[12] Other metabolic conditions potentially resulting in constipation are hypercalcemia and hypothyroidism. Neurologic disorders associated with constipation include those causing central nervous system lesions such as Parkinson's disease, multiple sclerosis, and cerebral vascular accidents. In scleroderma, impaired colonic transit results from smooth muscle atrophy and fibrosis.

Irritable bowel syndrome (IBS) is a very common condition that can present with constipation. It typically occurs in younger adults but can persist into old age. Patients will often complain of crampy abdominal pains and either diarrhea or small, hard stools requiring excessive straining. Bloating and flatulence are also frequently present.

Historically, lifestyle issues such as diminished mobility and physical inactivity have been associated with constipation in elderly individuals. Likewise, a lack of dietary fiber can cause constipation in adults and treatment with increased fiber relieves symptoms. By increasing intake of dietary fiber, colonic transit time is enhanced resulting in stools that are bulkier and more frequent.

Colonic motility is very susceptible to various medications. Numerous medications have been implicated in constipation but those that have anticholinergic activity are most problematic. Many different classes of medications have some anticholinergic potential. Complicating the issue, the elderly are often on several different prescription and nonprescription medications with constipating potential. Commonly used classes that are frequent contributors include narcotics, urinary incontinence drugs, and antihypertensives (Table 23–1).

> ● In the United States, the most common form is *normal-transit constipation*, also called *functional constipation*.

Defecatory Disorders

Defecatory disorders encompass dysfunction of the pelvic floor or of the anal sphincter. Other names used to describe subsets in this class include recto-sigmoid outlet delay, anismus, and pelvic-floor dys-synergy.

Successful defecation requires the proper coordination of abdominal, pelvic floor, and rectoanal muscles. The individual must also be able to sense that a bolus is ready for evacuation and be willing to eliminate. Painful conditions such as external hemorrhoids or anal fissures might inhibit the desire to void contents of the rectal vault. Individuals with a history of sexual or physical abuse may also have difficulty initiating evacuation resulting in stool retention.

Anismus is a condition where the anal sphincter cannot relax during defecation impeding the elimination of feces. In pelvic floor dys-synergy, the internal anal sphincter fails to relax properly while the external anal

Table 23–1	Medications Associated with Constipation
Medications	**Examples**
Nonprescription	
Sympathominetics	Pseudoephedrine
Nonsteroidal anti-inflammatory drugs (NSAIDs)	Ibuprofen, naproxen
Antacids	Aluminum hydroxide, calcium carbonate
Calcium supplements	Calcium carbonate/citrate
Iron supplements	Ferrous sulfate/gluconate
Antidiarrheals	Loperamide, bismuth salicylate
Prescription	
Anticholinergics	Benztropine, trihexylphenidate
Antihistamines	Diphenhydramine
Antidepressants	Tricyclics, amitriptyline, paroxetine, fluoxetine, sertraline.
Anti-Parkinson agents	Levodopa
Calcium channel blockers	Verapamil, diltiazem
Antispasmodics	Dicyclomine
Antipsychotics	Chlorpromazine, haloperidol
Diuretics	Furosemide
Narcotic	Codeine, morphine, oxycodone, hydrocodone

sphincter paradoxically contracts during attempted fecal evacuation. Other disorders that can cause outlet delay include structural conditions such as rectoceles and enteroceles, colorectal tumors, and strictures.

> ● Successful defecation requires the proper coordination of abdominal, pelvic floor, and rectoanal muscles.

DIFFERENTIAL DIAGNOSIS

History and Physical Exam

A thorough patient history and physical examination is the most important step to exclude secondary causes of constipation. Often, reassurance that there is a broad range of normal frequencies of bowel movements may adequately ease concerns. Since most individuals define constipation by the frequency and consistency of stools, a good history will start with these questions. Next, collection of a dietary history will aid in determining contributing factors for constipation such as limited dietary fiber or excessive dairy product consumption. Reviewing any gynecologic/obstetric and surgical history may present clues to a pelvic outlet dysfunction. Especially in the frail elderly, realizing that physical disability may prevent easy access to a toilet may obviate unnecessary testing and laxative use. Likewise, the lack of caregiver assistance to toileting may also lead to suppression of the defecation urge. The presence of a bedside commode often is useful for individuals with a limited degree of physical mobility.

Symptoms such as persistent nausea, vomiting, and abdominal pain are important signals that should broaden the differential diagnosis, possibly signaling an intestinal obstruction. Other important questions in the history include whether the patient experiences excessive straining during defecation, has the sense of incomplete evacuation, or needs to self-disimpact, which may indicate an outlet problem.

There are several warning signs from the history that may foreshadow a colonic tumor thereby requiring a more comprehensive work-up. Constipation along with a family history of colon cancer, rectal bleeding, unexplained anemia, weight loss, or narrowed caliber stools are all important red flags. However, pain during defecation is infrequently a symptom of cancer.[7] Box 23–2 contains a guide for endoscopic referral.[16]

Although a physical exam is usually recommended by gastrointestinal experts, it is rarely helpful in detecting serious disease unless an abdominal mass is felt. Nevertheless, a rectal examination should be performed to evaluate for visible blood, painful or obstructing hemorrhoids, rectal impaction or masses, anal fissures, and to check the neurologic integrity of the perineum. Guiac testing from digital rectal examination is controversial since a positive test does not indicate the presence of a cancer and a negative test does not preclude the need for further colonic testing.

> ● Symptoms such as persistent nausea, vomiting, and abdominal pain are important signals that should broaden the differential diagnosis, possibly signaling an intestinal obstruction.

Diagnostic Testing

To rule out a secondary cause of constipation, blood tests to consider include a complete blood count, thyroid-stimulating hormone level, and calcium level. Further initial laboratory tests can include stool Guiac sampling, especially if the constipation is new onset. Abdominal radiographs are of low yield but can indicate significant colonic stool retention, a volvulus, megacolon, or mass lesion.

Patients with unrelieved or new-onset constipation should proceed with sigmoidoscopy, barium enema, or colonoscopy. Sigmoidoscopy alone is usually reserved for younger adults where constipation is the only complaint, especially if IBS is strongly suspected. By adding a barium enema to the evaluation, visualization of the extended colon lumen will highlight mass lesions, a volvulus, megacolon, or strictures. Patient cooperation is needed to perform the examination so those with moderate dementia or impaired consciousness and those with poor rectal tone are poor candidates for the procedure. A colonoscopy is preferred in most instances since, besides directly visualizing the colonic lumen, any masses can be removed or biopsied during the examination.

> ● Patients with unrelieved or new-onset constipation should proceed with sigmoidoscopy, barium enema, or colonoscopy.

Special Tests

Further testing is rarely indicated, and if performed, is usually done by a subspecialist. Four additional examinations may be performed if the constipation is refractory to treatment or the history is suggestive of an outlet disorder:

1. Colon transit testing: Radiopaque markers are ingested followed by serial radiographs as the transit of the markers through the gastrointestinal tract is timed. If, after 5 days, more than 20% of the marker is retained, colonic hypomotility is diagnosed. If markers are retained in the rectosigmoid area, an outlet delay is suspected. Patients should not use laxatives during the testing period.

2. Anorectal manometry: Pressure measurements are made at the internal and external anal sphinc-

---

Box 23–2	Indications for Endoscopic Workup in Patients with Constipation
New onset constipation with:	**Chronic constipation with:**
• Weight loss	• Anemia
• Macroscopic or microscopic blood in stool	• Weight loss
• Family history of colon cancer	• Change in stool pattern
• Anemia	• Undiagnosed abdominal pain
• Undiagnosed abdominal pain	• Chronic constipation despite trial of multiple laxatives
	• Undiagnosed cause of fecal incontinence

ters at rest and during maximal contraction. This test can be used in suspected defecatory disorders or in Hirschsprung's disease.

3. Defecography: Barium is used under fluoroscopy to record the defecatory process. Used to assess for complete rectal emptying or for distal structural abnormalities.
4. Balloon expulsion: Test using a balloon filled with 50 ml of water, which the patient is instructed to expel out.

Lydia Beulow, *(Part 2)*

Ms. Beulow states that, in general, she feels good. She admits to mild fatigue and thinks her memory is not as sharp as it used to be. No weight loss has occurred. Her cooking skills have declined recently so she is eating more prepared and fast food than in previous years. Her activities include walking about three or four times weekly at the senior center. She states that her medication compliance is good and she uses a mediset as a reminder. Her medicines include iron 325 mg three times daily, ranitidine 300 mg daily, diltiazem CD 240 mg daily, lisinopril 20 mg daily, oxybutinin 10 mg nightly, calcium carbonate 500 mg twice daily, and acetaminophen 500 mg as needed for pain. Physical exam reveals no abdominal masses, normal heart, lung, and extremity exam, and a moderate-sized external hemorrhoid. Vital signs are normal today.

STUDY QUESTIONS

1. Is her lifestyle contributing to her sense of constipation?
2. What medications could be contributing? Could any be reduced?
3. Is any further testing warranted at this time?

MANAGEMENT

The treatment of constipation is directed by information discovered during the assessment. If an identifiable cause is found (e.g., hypothyroidism), the condition should be treated. More likely, an underlying disease is not identified and an intervention is needed with lifestyle changes or medication. Ideally, lifestyle changes such as bowel retraining or dietary adjustments should be tried prior to resorting to medications. There are many classes of medication available for use alone or in combination.

Bowel Retraining

A worthwhile initial step to avoid constipation is re-establishing a regular bowel pattern. Utilizing the natural postprandial gastrocolic reflex, the patient should be encouraged to attempt defecation shortly after meals. Trying to maintain a regular schedule after the same daily meal can be effective in many individuals. In less private living environments, such as the nursing home, the nursing staff can be instructed to give residents needed privacy on a regular basis to facilitate a regular stooling schedule. Occasionally, aging brings about a diminished feeling for the need to evacuate. Over time, repeatedly ignoring this signal can lead to a distended rectum and eventual stooling delay. Attention to a regular bowel regimen should be encouraged.

> In less private living environments, such as the nursing home, the nursing staff can be instructed to give residents needed privacy on a regular basis to facilitate a regular stooling schedule.

Diet and Exercise

Despite being universally recommended, increases in fluid intake and physical activity seem to have minimal[8] to no value in relieving symptoms of chronic constipation unless patients are dehydrated.[13,14] However, since many elderly often do not hydrate adequately anyway, increasing fluid intake is a common recommendation. By using fluids with a natural cathartic effect, such as prune or pear juice, the chances of success are enhanced.

Increasing dietary or supplemental fiber, in patients with normal- or slow-transit constipation, is another frequent initial treatment. The lay public is generally aware of this recommendation, although it is easy and useful to review. An additional 6 to 15 g of bran daily in institutionalized elderly patients was noted to increase the number of observed bowel movements.[15] Wheat fiber and bran are foods with the highest fiber density. Other foodstuffs high in dietary fiber are fruits and vegetables.

> An additional 6 to 15 g of bran daily in institutionalized elderly patients was noted to increase the number of observed bowel movements.[15]

Laxatives

If lifestyle modification is unsuccessful in improving bowel function, medications are frequently taken either independently or on the advice of a physician. Unfortunately, there are few good long-term studies available comparing medical therapies in older adults.[3] Before starting new medications, review of a patient's current medication profile should be performed looking for those with constipating side effects. There are at least 700 single and multiple formulation products available without a prescription.[16] In general, their mechanisms of action are incompletely understood. Some medications, if used chronically, can paradoxically exacerbate a patient's symptoms. Avoid products that stimulate peristalsis if there is any concern for an intestinal obstruction or impaction. Any agents other than fiber products, if used on a chronic basis, should periodically be evaluated for effects on a patient's electrolyte balance (Table 23–2).

BULK-FORMING AGENTS

By adding volume and improving hydration of the stool, bulk-forming agents are the most physiologic treatment products. Both natural and synthetic forms act as hydrophilic agents that promote water retention in the bowel. Onset of action is slow (1 to 2 weeks) and side effects can be bothersome but tolerable. Slowly titrating these products while concurrently recommending increased dietary fiber will help reduce abdominal discomfort, bloating, and flatulence. Natural fiber supplements, like psyllium, tend to generate more uncomfortable side effects than synthetics such as polycarbophil and methylcellulose. Besides the traditional powder formulation that needs to be mixed into a slurry, products are now available in tablet and wafer forms that many people find more palatable. An adequate intake of fluid is needed. When increasing fiber intake, a total of at least 2 liters daily is suggested.

STOOL SOFTENERS

Stool softeners, also called surfactants, are a commonly used class of laxatives. They are poorly absorbed and have a detergent-like effect of reducing the water–oil interface in the stool. Most studies using docusate have had varying effectiveness of minimal to no difference when compared with placebo and psyllium.

SALINES

The saline class is composed of the cations sodium and magnesium. They form a hypertonic solution drawing water into the colon lumen and may also

Table 23–2	Common Laxatives			
Laxative	**Generic Name**	**Brand Name**	**Adult Dosing**	**Onset (hrs)**
Bulk forming	Bran	—	Up to 2–5 g/day	12–72
	Psyllium	Metamucil, Fiberall	1–2 tsp qd to tid	12–72
	Methylcellulose	Fiberall	16 g qd to bid	12–72
	Polycarbophil	Citrucel, FiberCon	1 g qd to qid	12–72
Surfactants (stool softeners)	Docusate sodium	Colace	100–300 mg/day	24–72
	Docusate calcium	Surfak	240 mg/day	24–72
	Docusate potassium	Dialose Plus	100 mg qd to tid	24–72
Salines	Magnesium sulfate	Epsom salt	1–2 tsp qd to bid	0.5–3
	Magnesium hydroxide	Milk of Magnesia	30–60 ml/day	0.5–3
	Magnesium citrate	Citrate of Magnesia	Up to 200 ml/day	0.5–3
	Sodium phosphate	Fleets phosphosoda	Up to 45 ml/day	0.5–3
Hyperosmotic agents	Sorbitol	—	30–60 ml/day	24–48
	Lactulose	Chronulac	15–60 ml/day	24–48
	Polyethylene glycol	Miralax	17 g/day	48–96
Stimulants	Bisacodyl	Dulcolax, Correctol	5 mg qd to tid	6–10
	Senna	Senokot, Ex-Lax	1–2 tabs qd to bid	6–10
	Cascara	—	325 mg/day	6–10
Miscellaneous	Mineral oil	—	15–45 ml/day	6–8
	Castor oil	Purge	15–60 ml/day	2–6
Chloride Channel Activator	Lubiprostone	Amitiza	24 mg bid	

Based on Drug Facts and Comparisons. 59th ed. Philadelphia: Lippincott Williams & Wilkins, 2005.

release cholecystokinin, known to promote colonic prokinesis. Magnesium products should be used with caution in patients with renal failure. Sodium products may contribute to fluid overload in vulnerable elders if used on a frequent basis.

HYPEROSMOLAR AGENTS

Like the salines, hyperosmolar laxatives also work osmotically to treat constipation. They are comprised of two main classes: semisynthetic sugars (e.g., lactulose and sorbitol) and polyethylene glycol (PEG). Humans do not possess the enzyme needed to metabolize the disaccharide sugars so they pass through the small intestines unmetabolized. In the colon, *Escherichia coli* and *Streptococcus faecalis* metabolize them to water and organic acids contributing to an osmotic gradient. Lactulose and polyethylene glycol are the only two prescription laxatives available and are significantly more expensive than other laxatives. Sorbitol works similarly but is much less expensive. These agents are generally safe for chronic use but the disaccharide sugars should be used with caution in patients with diabetes mellitus.

Polyethylene glycol is particularly effective in resistant constipation. It too is poorly absorbed and is not metabolized by colonic bacteria, causing less abdominal side effects. It is available without electrolytes as a constipation treatment and with electrolytes as a bowel evacuent. PEG is colorless, odorless, and tasteless; however, the formulation with electrolytes does have a salty taste. Although it is not approved for use longer than 2 weeks, PEG is safe and is likely a reasonable choice for longer-term use.

STIMULANTS

The stimulant class (senna, bisacodyl, cascara) is the most frequently used type of over-the-counter laxative. They promote peristalsis presumably by direct action on the colonic mucosa and by stimulating intraluminal water and electrolyte secretion. They work quicker (several hours) than most other classes of laxatives. Early data suggested that stimulants may damage the enteric nervous system or cause dependency after repeated use but this is weakly supported by the literature. Melanosis coli, a black pigmentation staining of the colon, occurs with frequent use but is a benign condition and does not have any long-term consequences.

PROKINETIC AGENTS

A number of prokinetic agents have been tried for constipation. Metoclopramide and erythromycin work mostly on the upper gastrointestinal system and cholinergic agonists (bethanechol) have not been well studied. All of these drugs have a high side effect profile in the elderly and are not recommended.

Misoprostol has also been tried but is poorly studied, especially in the elderly.

Tegaserod (Zelnorm) is a 5-HT$_4$ receptor partial agonist that has been approved for the short-term use of constipation-predominant IBS in women. It is not approved for routine constipation use and is not recommended in the geriatric population.[17]

MISCELLANEOUS

Castor oil and mineral oil are infrequently used treatments for constipation. Mineral oil softens the stool and slows water absorption in the colon. It is very lipophilic and may bind fat-soluble vitamins, inhibiting their absorption. If aspirated, it is very irritating to the lung and can cause a chemical pneumonitis. It should not be given to someone with an impaired swallowing mechanism or decreased mental alertness. Castor oil is an older agent that both inhibits glucose and sodium absorption and enhances electrolyte and water secretion in the bowel lumen. It has an unpalatable taste.

In 2006, a new product, lubiprostone (Amitiza), was approved for treatment of chronic constipation. It has a unique mechanism of action by activating chloride channels, resulting in fluid secretion into the intestinal lumen. Nausea was the main side effect (31%) in clinical trials. Like the other prescription products, it is much more expensive than OTC treatments.

The wide array of products available for constipation treatment can be confusing for patients and physicians alike. The general consensus is to try bulk laxatives first due to their long-term safety. A stool softener, saline, or osmotic laxative (some available as combinations) should be added next if the bulk laxative is ineffective. Stimulants are typically reserved for as-needed use if the other agents fail.

ENEMAS AND SUPPOSITORIES

Enemas (tap water, soapsuds, mineral oil, and phosphate) or suppositories (glycerin or bisacodyl) are commonly used after constipation persists despite trial of an oral agent. There is limited data to support their use over other therapies. They work primarily by softening and loosing the stool and by directly stimulating the rectum upon insertion. There is likely no advantage to using any medicated treatment over plain tap water.

Lydia Beulow, *(Part 3)*

All her labs were normal 3 months ago including a thyroid-stimulating hormone (TSH) test, renal panel, and complete blood count (CBC). She has tried fiber products in the past but found them too "gritty" to use. She is reluctant to try other fiber products. She would like some kind of treatment but doesn't want anything too expensive.

STUDY QUESTIONS

1. What treatment regimen would you recommend?
2. Should a different fiber product be recommended?
3. Would she be appropriate for a combination product?
4. Should she have a colonoscopy for her symptoms?

FECAL INCONTINENCE

Fecal incontinence is the involuntary passage of fecal matter. It occurs more often than is commonly recognized, and is an occasional cause for institutionalization of the elderly. The prevalence of either fecal or combined fecal and urinary incontinence is almost 50% in nursing home residents.[18] It is particularly prevalent in residents who have dementia or are immobile. In noninstitutionalized elderly, it is often under-reported due to its social stigma. Individuals quietly adapt using incontinence aids like pads and diapers. Under fear of having accidental soiling, afflicted patients often are socially isolated, not wanting to stray far from a toilet. Patients may be reluctant to discuss the issue with their physician due to embarrassment. They may use terms such as diarrhea or stooling urgency to substitute for incontinence. Some patients may be distressed with only mild soiling of undergarments while others may have frank stooling before reporting a problem.

> ● Fecal incontinence occurs more often than is commonly recognized, and is a frequent cause for institutionalization of the elderly.

Mechanisms of Continence

To maintain continence, several anatomic structures need to function in a coordinated fashion. The most important structure appears to be the puborectalis muscle, which wraps around the rectum in a horseshoe fashion between its attachments to the symphysis pubis. When it is contracted, the puborectalis muscle pulls the rectum tight, acting as a valve to shut off flow through the rectum. It does this by sharply angulating the rectum making evacuation difficult. When the puborectalis muscle is relaxed, the angle of fecal flow is straighter and evacuation can occur. This process works less well when stool contents are watery since the stool can more easily slip around this angle.

Other determinants of fecal continence include proper functioning of both the internal and external anal sphincters. Numerous diseases or disorders can affect the innervations of these muscles or can affect the muscles directly. These include systemic diseases (scleroderma, diabetes mellitus), neurologic disorders (spinal tumors, multiple sclerosis, advanced Alzheimer's disease), or local trauma (anorectal surgical procedures, rectal prolapse) (Box 23–3). One of the more common causes of fecal incontinence is, paradoxically, fecal impaction. A hard fecal bolus may become impassable allowing only liquid stool to seep around the mass. The liquid stool may overwhelm an impaired sphincter mechanism.

Diagnosis

Important components of the history should include how long the incontinence has been present, if there is associated urinary incontinence, and if the patient is able to alter the sudden defecation urge. In addition, reviewing the patient's medical history, surgical history, and medication profile can also provide insight into causative or aggravating factors.

Examining the perianal region, including a digital rectal exam, is essential in the workup. Inspection of the perineum can reveal a surgical scar, mass, rectal prolapse, or skin changes from frequent fecal soiling. Asking the patient to perform a Valsalva maneuver during the inspection can also be helpful. A digital

---

Box 23-3   Causes of Fecal Incontinence

Anatomic Problems
- Rectal prolapse
- Previous surgery
- Fistula

Muscular Dysfunction
- Fecal impaction
- Inflammatory bowel disease
- Radiation proctitis

- Myasthenia gravis
- Scleroderma

Neurologic Disorders
- Stroke
- Dementia (Alzheimer's, vascular, Lewy body)
- Multiple sclerosis
- Spinal cord lesions
- Diabetes mellitus

rectal examination will assess for rectal tone, rectal masses, or low-lying fecal impactions. Repeating the Valsalva maneuver can further quantify rectal tone. Adding a stool Guiac test is unlikely to provide useful information regarding the incontinence.

Further evaluation may include a flexible sigmoidoscopy to visualize the rectal/sigmoid lumen, anorectal manometry to assess rectal strength and distension response, and ultrasonography of the sphincter to evaluate its structural integrity.

Management

Treatment of fecal incontinence is targeted at correcting the underlying condition if possible. In many cases, this cannot be done and the treatment becomes supportive. Continence aids, like pads and adult-sized diapers, are practical solutions to allow some individuals to have more independence. Although helpful, the aids alone are frequently insufficient to deal with this difficult problem. For bed-bound or institutionalized patients, assisted defecation at timed intervals can help prevent frequent soiling. Inserting a suppository to stimulate evacuation on a routine schedule can greatly reduce sporadic episodes. Dietary factors, such as sorbitol-sweetened foodstuffs, and excessive fruit juice intake can further aggravate incontinence.

Most patients will inquire about medications that can assist in maintaining continence. Loperamide is the recommended medication choice, often given on a scheduled basis immediately after a stooling episode. Used in this manner, a dose or two daily can greatly assist in regulating an acceptable stooling pattern. Stronger opioid derivatives, like diphenoxylate (with atropine as Lomotil), should be reserved for more resistant cases.

Biofeedback has been reported to be of benefit in motivated individuals who have rectal sensation and can contract the external anal sphincter. Studies using a broad age range have reported improvement in symptoms in a majority of patients who qualify. It typically works better for individuals experiencing formed stool incontinence versus diarrhea. Surgery can be considered as a last resort for those with uncontrolled symptoms. The type of operation performed depends on the specific problem but varies from repair of the anal sphincter/perineal floor to fecal diversion via colostomy.

POSTTEST

1. Which medication class is generally *not* implicated in constipation?
   a. Calcium channel blockers
   b. Opioids
   c. Urinary incontinence aids
   d. Proton pump inhibitors
   e. Dietary supplements (calcium, iron, magnesium)

2. Which of the following is *not* a typical warning sign or symptom in patients with constipation?
   a. Weight loss
   b. Anemia
   c. Family history of colon cancer
   d. Occult blood in stool
   e. Pain with defecation

3. Options to treat fecal incontinence in elderly patients include all of the following except:
   a. Biofeedback
   b. Loperamide (Imodium)
   c. Dicyclomine (Bentyl)
   d. Adult diapers
   e. Diphenoxylate (Lomotil)

References

1. Higgins PD, Johanson JF. Epidemiology of constipation in North America: a systematic review. Am J Gastroenterol 2004;99:750-9.
2. Tally NJ. Definitions, epidemiology, and impact of chronic constipation. Rev Gastroenterol Dis 2004;4(Suppl 2):S3-10.
3. Tramante SM, Brand MB, Mulrow CD, et al. The treatment of chronic constipation in adults: a systematic review. J Gen Intern Med 1997;12:15-24.
4. Johanson JF, Sonnenberg A, Koch TR. Clinical epidemiology of chronic constipation. J Clin Gastroenterol 1989;11:525-36.
5. Nyam DC, Pemberton JH, Ilstrup DM, Rath DM. Long-term results of surgery for chronic constipation. Dis Colon Rectum 1997;40:273-9.
6. Sonnenberg A, Koch TR. Physician visits in the United States for constipation: 1958-1986. Dig Dis Sci 1989;34:606-11.
7. Cheskin LJ. Constipation and diarrhea. In: Barker LR, Burton HR, Zieve PD, eds. Principles of Ambulatory Medicine. 5th ed. Baltimore: Williams & Wilkins, 1999:498-503.
8. Whitehead WE, Chaussade S, Corazziari E, et al. Report of an international workshop on management of constipation. Gastroenterol Int 1991;4:99-113.
9. Prather CM, Ortiz-Camacho CP. Evaluation and treatment of constipation and fecal impaction in adults. Mayo Clin Proc 1998;73:881-7.
10. Gemlo BT, Wong WD. Etiology of acquired colorectal disease. In: Wexner SD, Bartolo DC, eds. Constipation Etiology Evaluation and Mangement. Oxford: Butterworth-Heinemann, 1995:3-8.
11. Preston DM, Lennard-Jones JE. Severe chronic constipation of young women: "idiopathic slow transit constipation." Gut 1986;27:41-8.
12. Casto DD, Cherry DA. Extracolonic causes of constipation. In: Wexner SD, Bartolo DC, eds. Constipation Etiology, Evaluation and Management. Oxford: Butterworth-Heinemann, 1995:23-30.
13. Young RJ, Beerman LE, Vanderhoof JA. Increasing oral fluids in chronic constipation in children. Gastroenterol Nurs 1998;21(4):156-61.
14. Meshkinpour H, Selod S, Movahedi H, et al. Effects of regular exercise in management of chronic idiopathic constipation. Dig Dis Sci 1998;43:2379-83.
15. Wrenin K. Fecal impaction. N Engl J Med 1989;321:658-62.
16. Etzkorn KP, Rodriguez L. Constipation. Rakel RE, Bope ET, eds. Conn's Current Therapy. Philadelphia: WB Saunders, 2002.
17. Zelnorm prescribing information. Monthly Prescribing Reference, October 2004:185.
18. Borrie MJ, Davidson HA. Incontinence in institutions: costs and contributing factors. CAMJ 1992;147:322-8.

PRETEST ANSWERS

1. c
2. False
3. d
4. True

POSTTEST ANSWERS

1. d
2. e
3. c

Hearing Impairment

Timothy J. Lewis

OBJECTIVES

Upon completion of this chapter, the reader will be able to:

- Identify effects of aging on the auditory system.
- Describe the psychosocial and functional consequences of hearing loss.
- Interpret common tests used to evaluate hearing impairment and disability.
- Distinguish presbycusis from other forms of hearing loss.
- Discuss the differential diagnosis for adult hearing impairment.
- List appropriate indications for audiology and otolaryngology referrals.
- Summarize effective hearing loss treatments.

PRETEST

1. A 75-year-old man presents to clinic accompanied by his wife who reports that he is having hearing difficulties. He denies hearing loss and reports that people around him "mumble too much." His ear canals are free of cerumen impaction. Which of the following is the most reliable and valid screening test for hearing loss?
   a. Whisper test
   b. Audioscopy using otoscope with built-in audiometer
   c. Tuning fork test
   d. Finger-rub test
   e. Weber and Rinné tests

2. A 67-year-old male with severe bilateral hearing loss comes to clinic to establish primary care. A nurse practitioner observes that he does not understand what is said to him during his assessment. He has no hearing aids. Which of the following actions is *least* likely to ease communication with the patient?
   a. Use a hard-wired voice amplification system such as a Pocket Talker.
   b. Ensure that the speaker's face is in full view of the listener and speak clearly at a slightly louder than normal intensity; avoid shouting.
   c. When repetition is necessary, paraphrase the message or write key words.
   d. Lean forward and speak directly into the patient's ear at a distance of 5 to 10 inches.
   e. Speak with adequate pauses between sentences and signal to the listener when the subject of conversation is changing.

3. Matching (items 1 to 4): Match each hearing aid technology item with its appropriate description:
   a. Nonprogrammable hearing aid
   b. Programmable hearing aid
   c. Compression
   d. Telecoil
   e. Channels

   (1) Circuitry that helps people talk on the telephone by converting electromagnetic signals from telephone to amplified sound.

   (2) Offers good sound quality at a reasonable price; limited flexibility in adjustments.

   (3) Circuitry that keeps loud sounds from being over-amplified while dynamically increasing the volume of soft sounds.

   (4) Refers to the number of frequency bands into which the incoming sound signal is divided; permits independent control of the intensity of low- and high-frequency sounds.

PREVALENCE AND IMPACT

Hearing loss is common in people aged over 65 and can have serious psychosocial and functional consequences. It affects one-third of individuals aged 65 years or older and ranks as the third most common chronic disease in that age category. Hearing impairment's prevalence rises with age and is about 16% at age 60, 32% at age 70, and 64% at age 80 years. The prevalence of hearing disability also rises with age, as is illustrated in Fig. 24–1. Functional deficits associated with hearing loss include diminished ability to recognize speech amid background noise and to locate and identify sounds that may have an important warning or alarm significance. The communication difficulties experienced by the hearing impaired also affect other people in their environment such as family members and coworkers. Hearing loss is associated with depression, social isolation, and poor self-esteem. Despite the importance of hearing function in everyday life, hearing loss is often an unrecognized and under-treated problem.

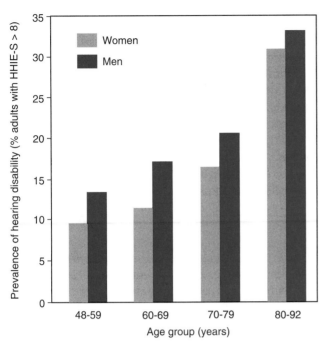

FIGURE 24–1

Prevalence of hearing disability (Hearing Handicap Inventory for the Elderly-Screening Version score >8) by age and gender. (Modified from Wiley T, et al. Self-reported hearing handicap and audiometric measures in older adults. J Am Acad Audiol 11:67–75, 2000, with permission.)

Barriers to Recognition of Hearing Loss

Several barriers exist to the recognition of hearing problems among older adults. One barrier is that individuals with hearing impairment are not always aware of their functional deficits and therefore may not know what they are missing. In contrast, some older adults are aware of their hearing loss, but view it as being so much a part of growing old that they do not consult a doctor about it. Indeed, non-consulters have been characterized by their passive acceptance of hearing problems with increasing age. Among hearing-impaired adults, however, the attitude of passive acceptance of hearing loss is in fact only slightly correlated with age, with a correlation coefficient of 0.19.[1]

> ● Hearing disability is not an inevitable aspect of aging, despite the fact that hearing ability usually decreases with age.

Not all barriers to the identification of hearing loss are patient centered. Doctors routinely fail to assess their patients for hearing loss. Primary care physicians should aid identification of individuals with untreated hearing disability by routinely asking about hearing problems and watching for potential signs or symptoms of hearing disability, such as communication difficulties, social withdrawal, or depressed mood.

> ● Timely referral for hearing health services such as hearing aid fitting can help improve the outlook for older adults with hearing disability.

Aging Changes

Usual aging changes in the auditory system contribute to diminished hearing performance among older adults (Box 24–1). The presence of noise exposure, previous middle ear disease, and vascular disease further impacts the progression of hearing loss with advancing age. Longitudinal studies demonstrate that hearing declines gradually with advancing age in the majority of the population (97%) as evidenced by diminished pure-tone threshold sensitivities with age. Individuals under 55 years of age typically lose hearing at a rate of 3 dB per decade, and those over 55 years at a rate of 9 dB per decade.[2] The ability to understand speech amid a backdrop of competing conversations begins to deteriorate slowly starting with the fourth decade of life, a decline that accelerates after the seventh decade. As adults age, it also becomes increasingly difficult for them to understand speech that is rapid, poorly transmitted, or mispronounced.

Box 24–1	**Effects of Aging on Auditory System**

Functional Effects
- Hearing loss for pure tones
- Hearing loss for speech
- Problems understanding difficult speech

Anatomic Effects
- Atrophy and disappearance of sensory cells in inner ear
- Calcification of membranes in inner ear
- Degeneration of fibers in eighth cranial nerve
- Reduced number of cells in auditory cortex

Harry Jackson, (Part 1)

Mr. Harry Jackson, a 70-year-old man comes to your office accompanied by his wife of 45 years for evaluation of gradually worsening hearing loss. His wife has noticed that he has difficulty understanding speech, especially at a distance or in noisy social gatherings. He has been gradually scaling back his work hours as a self-employed plumber in preparation for retirement. In his spare time he is an avid softball fan. He also enjoys the company of his grandchildren immensely, but is having increasing difficulty understanding them. His wife is particularly concerned about her husband's reluctance to participate in social activities. She has been encouraging him to have his hearing tested and thinks he needs a hearing aid. He denies ear pain, tinnitus, vertigo, or asymmetric hearing loss. His past medical history includes osteoarthritis, hypertension, and chronic stable angina. His only medications are 81 mg aspirin daily for heart attack prevention, metoprolol for hypertension, and Tylenol as needed for arthritis pain.

STUDY QUESTIONS

1. What factors may be contributing to hearing problems in this patient?
2. What assessments are needed to investigate this patient's hearing difficulty?

RISK FACTORS AND PATHOPHYSIOLOGY

The two major forms of hearing loss are sensorineural and conductive disorders; each form has its own risk factors and causes. Disorders of the inner ear cause sensorineural hearing loss by damaging the cochlea, eighth cranial nerve, or internal auditory canal. Presbycusis is a distinct age-related sensorineural hearing loss that is the most common cause of hearing loss in older adults. The hallmark feature of presbycusis is bilateral, symmetric, high-frequency sensorineural hearing loss. Advancing age is the predominant risk factor for its development. The cochlea appears to be the primary site of pathogenesis, although the precise cause of presbycusis remains uncertain.

Noise-induced hearing loss (NIHL) is the second most common cause of sensorineural hearing loss among older adults after presbycusis. The pathogenesis of NIHL involves direct mechanical injury to the sensory hair cells of the cochlea. Continuous noise exposure poses greater risk than intermittent exposure.

Disorders of the external ear or the middle ear can cause conductive hearing loss by interfering with the mechanical transmission of sound into the inner ear. Conductive disorders often have a mechanical cause. Occlusion of the external ear canal by cerumen is the most common cause of conductive hearing loss. Other risk factors for conductive hearing loss include perforated ear drum (i.e., due to acoustic trauma), fluid in the middle ear, and disarticulation of the ossicular chain. Specific disease entities causing conductive hearing loss are described in the discussion under differential diagnosis.

DIFFERENTIAL DIAGNOSIS AND ASSESSMENT

Hearing loss can result from diseases of the auricle, external auditory canal, middle ear, inner ear, or central auditory pathways. Diseases of the inner ear or eighth nerve cause sensorineural hearing loss, whereas diseases of the auricle, external auditory canal, or middle ear generally cause conductive hearing loss. Mixed loss refers to the combination of conductive and sensorineural hearing loss. A differential diagnosis for hearing loss is listed in Box 24–2.

Box 24-2 Differential Diagnosis of Hearing Loss

Conductive Hearing Loss	Sensorineural Hearing Loss
Outer Ear Causes	**Inner Ear Causes**
Otitis externa	Presbycusis
Trauma	Noise exposure
Cerumen	Ménière's disease
Osteoma	Ototoxic Drugs
Exostosis	Meningitis
Squamous cell carcinoma	Viral cochleitis
	Barotrauma
Middle Ear Causes	Acoustic neuroma
Otitis media	Meningioma
Tympanic membrane perforation	Multiple sclerosis
Cholesteatoma	Vascular disease
Otosclerosis	
Glomus tumors	
Temporal bone trauma	
Paget's disease	

Conductive Hearing Loss

This form of hearing loss can result from obstruction of the external auditory canal (EAC) by cerumen, debris, or foreign bodies. Otitis externa results in conductive hearing loss when inflammation leads to canal edema that blocks the EAC. Tumors of the EAC such as squamous cell carcinoma can be mistaken for otitis externa. Conductive hearing loss arises when such tumors occlude the canal. Diagnosis is made by biopsy. Additional causes of conductive hearing loss include perforations of the tympanic membrane; disruption of the ossicular chain due to trauma or infection, fluid, scarring, or tumors in the middle ear; and otosclerosis.

Cholesteatoma refers to stratified squamous epithelium in the middle ear or mastoid. This nonmalignant slowly growing lesion can cause conductive hearing loss when erosion occurs into the ossicular chain.

Suspicion for cholesteatoma should be raised in the setting of a chronically draining ear that fails to respond to antibiotic therapy. Management is surgical.

Conductive hearing loss with a normal ear canal and intact tympanic membrane should raise concern for ossicular chain disease. Otosclerosis, a bony overgrowth involving the footplate of the stapes, leads to stapes fixation and low-frequency conductive hearing loss. Systemic bone diseases such as Paget's disease and immunologic diseases such as rheumatoid arthritis can also lead to conductive hearing loss by causing ossicular pathology.

Tympanic membrane perforation causes conductive loss and usually arises from trauma, acute otitis media, or chronic otitis media. Size and location of the perforation determine the degree of hearing loss. An audiogram is indicated to determine the effect on hearing function. Small perforations tend to heal spontaneously, whereas large perforations usually require surgical repair. Otoscopy usually suffices to diagnose tympanic membrane perforation, as well as middle ear infection and cerumen impaction.

Sensorineural Hearing Loss

The most common pattern of sensorineural hearing loss in adults is presbycusis, an age-associated bilateral high-frequency hearing loss. In the early stages of presbycusis, the audiogram will usually show gentle or sharply sloping high-frequency hearing loss. Adults with presbycusis often complain of difficulty understanding speech, especially in noisy environments.

Sensorineural hearing loss may also develop from damage to the hair cells of the organ of Corti due to intense noise, ototoxic drugs, viral infections, meningitis, temporal bone fracture, or Ménière's disease. Noise is the second most common cause of sensorineural hearing loss after presbycusis. Noise-induced hearing loss is permanent but largely preventable. It begins at the higher frequencies (3000 to 6000 Hz) and develops gradually as a consequence of cumulative exposure. Hearing loss can develop following chronic exposures equal to an average decibel level of 85 dB or higher for an 8-hour period.

Older adults are at risk for ototoxicity from certain medications. Of the offending agents, aminoglycosides are the best known. Tobramycin and amikacin are more cochleotoxic, whereas gentamycin and streptomycin are more vestibulotoxic. Additional medications with known ototoxicity are listed in Box 24-3.

Ménière's disease causes sensorineural hearing loss that classically affects low frequencies and is episodic with periods of vertigo, tinnitus, and aural fullness. The associated hearing loss may become permanent over time and involve other frequencies.

Box 24-3   Ototoxic Medications

- Antibiotics: aminoglycosides, erythromycin, tetracycline, vancomycin
- Antimalarials: chloroquinine[a], quinine[a]
- Antineoplastics: cisplatin, bleomycin, 5-fluorouracil, nitrogen mustard
- Salicylates: aspirin[a]
- Diuretics: loop diuretics[a]

[a]Hearing loss and tinnitus are reversible with these agents.

Tumors of the inner ear are usually benign. Acoustic neuroma is the most common benign tumor in the inner ear and originates from the eighth cranial nerve. Acoustic neuromas are commonly either asymptomatic or cause unilateral sensorineural hearing loss, but may also be associated with other symptoms such as unilateral tinnitus, dizziness, or headaches.

Sensorineural hearing loss may also be caused by meningiomas or other neoplasms, demyelinating or degenerative disease, or infections such as HIV. Endocrine or other metabolic disorders can also cause hearing loss. For example, diabetes can cause small vessel disease inducing cochlear ischemia.

Harry Jackson, *(Part 2)*

To assess the self-perceived emotional and social impact imposed by his hearing impairment, you administer the Hearing Handicap Inventory for the Elderly–Screening Version (HHIE). Mr. Jackson obtains a total score of 10. Routine otoscopic examination reveals findings of bilateral cerumen impaction. Using a curette, you gently remove bilateral moderate cerumen plugs from the external auditory canal under direct vision of an otoscope. His tympanic membranes have normal landmarks. You proceed to perform screening audiometry using an otoscope with a built-in audiometer. He fails to hear the 2000-Hz pure tone stimulus at a screening level of 40 dB in both ears on two independent trials. After discussing your findings with the patient, he agrees to have a diagnostic hearing assessment at a local audiology center. You make his referral.

STUDY QUESTIONS

1. What is the clinical significance of the patient's score on the Hearing Handicap Inventory for the Elderly?
2. What is the traditional definition of an abnormal result on a screening audiometry test?

Office Assessment

There are three main steps in the assessment of hearing function in the primary care office: history taking, physical examination, and screening for hearing impairment and disability. Identification of hearing impairment frequently requires direct questions regarding difficulty hearing under challenging listening conditions. The patient should be asked about difficulty hearing speech in large groups, soft voices, or telephone conversation. Collateral history from a spouse or other individuals familiar with the patient's hearing performance may be useful. An important focus of the routine otologic examination is the identification of reversible causes of conductive hearing loss. These include otitis externa, cerumen impaction, foreign objects obstructing the external auditory canal, and osteoma. Assessment of the integrity and mobility of the tympanic membrane is also indicated. Tuning fork tests such as the Rinné and the Weber tests allow differentiation of conductive and sensorineural hearing loss.

RATIONALE FOR HEARING SCREENING AMONG OLDER ADULTS

The value of routine screening for hearing impairment among older adults remains to be proven in clinical trials; however, it appears advisable on epidemiologic grounds.[3] Primary care clinicians are well situated to promote early audiologic screening and hearing health education to improve recognition and rehabilitation of older adults with hearing disability.[4] One rationale for hearing screening is the belief that if such hearing-impaired individuals could be detected earlier, they, their family, and associates would suffer less from the patient's hearing impairment, and rehabilitative interventions such as hearing aids would be easier and more effective.[5]

Age-associated hearing loss meets many of the traditional epidemiologic criteria for the advisability of a screening program. Hearing impairment prevalence is high as is the associated disease burden. Hearing loss can profoundly diminish the quality of life of the aged, and is associated with a decline in functional health status and psychosocial well-being. Accurate and inexpensive screening tests for hearing impairment exist. Effective treatments for hearing impairment are also available. Furthermore, screening programs for hearing loss can likely reach the patients who could benefit, and appear feasible within the U.S. health system despite significant barriers such as lack of medical insurance coverage for expensive hearing evaluations and treatments.

Several professional organizations have advocated for greater use of audiologic screening among older adults. The American Speech-Language-Hearing Association recommends that the adult population receive both impairment and disability screening every decade after age 18 years until age 50 years with more frequent monitoring after age 50 years.[6] The U.S. Preventive Services Task Force and the Canadian Task Force on Preventive Health Care, also recommend screening older adults for hearing impairment. Ongoing clinical trials may soon help to confirm whether early detection of hearing loss among older adults via office-based screening programs will promote improved long-term health outcomes.

SCREENING TESTS

The traditional objective of a hearing screening program among older adults is to identify persons who need diagnostic hearing assessment to investigate possible untreated medical disease and/or hearing disability. There are two general screening strategies: audiometry and hearing disability self-report measures.

SCREENING AUDIOMETRY

Screening audiometry is a reliable and accurate physiologic test for identifying persons with hearing impairment. The Audioscope™ (Welch-Allyn) is a widely accepted and well-validated screening audiometry tool. This handheld otoscope with a built-in audiometer allows quick and accurate detection of hearing impairment when referenced against a conventional audiogram as the criterion standard.[7] Traditionally, older adults are considered to have failed screening audiometry testing if they fail to detect either a 1-kHz or 2-kHz pure tone signal in both ears or fail to detect both 1-kHz and 2-kHz unilaterally at a sound intensity of 40 dB. Controversy exists about the desirability of screening for more mild degrees of hearing impairment among older adults (i.e., using a 25-dB screen pure tone cutoff). Regardless of the specific screening strategy selected, the goal should be to identify persons whose hearing impairment is clinically significant because of associated hearing disability and/or medical disease. Currently available screening devices such as the Audioscope give clinicians the flexibility of screening using 25-dB and/or 40-dB pure tones. One trade-off associated with screening for milder degrees of hearing impairment is the resulting identification of a greater proportion of persons that, while failing the physiologic test, deny self-reported hearing handicaps and may therefore be less motivated to seek hearing health services. The relationship between hearing impairment and hearing disability, however, is imperfect. Some individuals do in fact experience disability and/or handicap even with a mild 25-dB-level hearing impairment. Thus, to assess the functional and social implications of hearing impairment, it is prudent to complement physiologic tests of hearing with subjective measures of hearing disability.

HEARING DISABILITY SELF-REPORT MEASURES

The Hearing Handicap Inventory for the Elderly–Screening Version (HHIE–S) is a widely accepted subjective screening tool for hearing disability (Box 24–4). The HHIE–S contains 10 questions and can be administered in less than 2 minutes. Possible scores range from 0 (no handicap) to 40 (maximum handicap). A score of 10 or more suggests a significant self-perceived hearing handicap, and should prompt referral to an audiologist. Using the 10-or-more cutoff, the HHIE–S performs with a sensitivity ranging from 63% to 80% and a specificity ranging from 67% to 77%.[8] An interactive multimedia CD-ROM version of the same questionnaire is available that incorporates informational counseling about hearing loss and treatments based on principles of the health belief model.[9]

Another efficient approach to hearing disability screening is to pose the single question: "Do you have a hearing problem now?" That single question identified older adults with unrecognized hearing impairment with both sensitivity and specificity at 71% when validated against a conventional audiogram-based criterion standard.[10]

PRACTICAL APPROACH TO HEARING SCREENING

A practical approach toward office-based hearing screening incorporates case history and pure tone audiometry combined with at least one validated hearing disability instrument (HDI). The objective of the case history is to rule out indications for otolaryngology referral (discussed below). After elicitation of the oto-

logic history, routine otoscopic examination is recommended followed by screening audiometry. Audiometry is performed in each ear using an Audioscope set at 25-dB and 40-dB screening levels. The criterion for audiology/hearing disability referral is defined as either (1) failure to hear a 25-dB tone at 1 kHz or 2 kHz in both ears or 1 kHz and 2 kHz in one ear and failure on a validated HDI, or (2) failure to hear a 40-dB tone at 1 kHz or 2 kHz in both ears or 1 kHz and 2 kHz in one ear. To screen for hearing disability, every older adult is asked if she or he has a hearing problem now, and/or completes the HHIE–S on paper. Failure on either HDI (i.e., scoring 10 or greater on the HHIE–S or answering yes to the single global assessment question) constitutes a hearing disability failure. Persons that fail the 25-dB level pure tone screen, but deny hearing disability, are designated "at risk" for hearing disability/handicap and receive recommendation for retesting in 1 year. Priority for referral is given to individuals who screen positive for both hearing impairment and disability. The above screening strategy employs the principle of only referring the most motivated persons as suggested by the HDI results, and is adapted from a model originated by the American Hearing and Speech Association.[11]

MANAGEMENT OF HEARING IMPAIRMENT

Cerumen Impaction

Cerumen impaction can usually be easily managed in the office. A small curette may be used to remove the cerumen if the clinician is familiar with the technique. Alternately, gentle warm water irrigation may be used to loosen and remove the cerumen if the tympanic membrane is visible and intact. Cerumen-dissolving drops

---

Box 24-4   Hearing Handicap Inventory for the Elderly—Screening Version

- Does a hearing problem cause you to feel embarrassed when you meet new people?
- Does a hearing problem cause you to feel frustrated when talking to a member of your family?
- Do you have difficulty hearing when someone speaks in a whisper?
- Do you feel handicapped by a hearing problem?
- Does a hearing problem cause you difficulty when visiting friends, relatives, or neighbors?
- Does a hearing problem cause you to attend religious services less often than you would like?

- Does a hearing problem cause you to have arguments with family members?
- Does a hearing problem cause you difficulty when listening to television or radio?
- Do you feel that any difficulty with your hearing limits/hampers your personal or social life?
- Does a hearing problem cause you difficulty when in a restaurant with relatives or friends?

Note: Answers scored as yes (4), sometimes (2), and no (0). Total point range, zero to 40; zero to 8 = no self-perceived handicap; 10 to 22 = mild to moderate handicap; 24 to 40 = significant handicap. Adapted from Ventry IM, Weinstein BE. Identification of elderly people with hearing problems. Am Speech Language Hearing Assoc 1983;25:37–42, with permission.

such as 10% sodium bicarbonate can also help ease cerumen removal. When severe cerumen impaction is identified, referral to an otolaryngologist may be advisable.

Counseling Patients About Benefits of Hearing Health Services

A critical aspect of managing hearing impairment in older adults is promoting health-seeking behaviors. To be effective in this regard, clinicians must understand barriers to the recognition of hearing loss, and act to help older adults become aware of hearing loss, its consequences, and the promise of rehabilitative services.

It is important to counsel patients about the benefits of hearing health services and discuss their attitudes toward treatment options such as hearing aids. Implicit in these discussions is the opportunity to dispel pessimistic views that older adults may harbor about their ability to benefit from hearing aids. The evidence supporting hearing aid effectiveness is strong, a fact that should be communicated to any patient with suspected hearing impairment. Hearing aid use can reduce the adverse impact of hearing loss on quality of life among older adults.[12] Hearing aid recipients demonstrate significant improvements in social, emotional, and communication function, as well as depression.

Enhancing Communication with the Hearing Impaired

Communication with hearing-impaired older adults can be enhanced by optimizing speaking distance, sound environment, signal clarity, and visual cues. The speaker's face should be in full view of the listener within 2 to 3 feet. Avoid excessive backlighting such as occurs when the speaker stands with their back to a bright window. Where possible, reduce background noise. Speak with adequate pauses between sentences. Avoid shouting and attempt to speak clearly at a slightly louder than normal intensity. When repetition is necessary, paraphrase the message or write key words. Speaking directly into the good ear is not advisable since the speaker's face and lips are then no longer in view.

Myths About Hearing Aids

Myths about hearing aids frequently influence decision making and may negatively impact hearing rehabilitation efforts. The common misconception that hearing aids draw increased attention to the individual and their hearing impairment merits special discussion. This misconception that hearing aids are "too conspicuous" is one of the foremost reasons that individuals reject hearing aid use. To address this misconception, clinicians should advise prospective hearing aid candidates that not hearing when spoken to and not answering correctly are more conspicuous behaviors than wearing a hearing aid.

> ● If used appropriately, a hearing aid can reduce hearing disability and thereby diminish the outward signs of hearing loss.

Harry Jackson, (Part 3)

At his hearing aid evaluation, Mr. Jackson reported to the audiologist that he is hearing somewhat better since the wax removal. His wife was amused by her husband's recent comment that "we have to get these darn floors fixed." Since the wax removal, her husband became aware of the long-standing squeak of the floor boards in their century-old home. Audiologic evaluation revealed a bilaterally symmetrical, mild to moderate, sloping high-frequency sensorineural hearing loss. On speech discrimination testing, he recognized 87% of a monosyllabic word list in his right ear and 90% in his left ear with amplification at 40 dB above his pure tone thresholds. At normal conversational level, his word recognition score dropped to 70%. Subsequently, Mr. Jackson was scheduled for a hearing aid evaluation.

At his hearing aid evaluation the audiologist obtained other audiometric measures and recommended a behind-the-ear (BTE) hearing aid with a skeleton mold to fit the left ear. The patient preferred monoaural fitting and was left-handed. Mr. Jackson experienced improved word recognition with use of the hearing aid. At a subsequent dispensing visit, the audiologist reviewed the care, use, and placement of the BTE unit and provided further instruction regarding the benefits and limitations of amplification. Mr. Jackson and his wife elected to participate in an audiologic rehabilitation course to learn about communication strategies that would aid his engagement in social activities. He received a return audiology appointment within the 30-day trial period for follow-up consultation.

STUDY QUESTIONS

1. What are appropriate indications for audiology referral? Otolaryngology referral?
2. What treatment options are there for hearing loss and are they effective?

Management of Hearing Loss by Hearing Specialists

Patients referred to an audiologist for evaluation of hearing loss often benefit from education about what to expect. Audiologic management can be summarized as a three-step process involving:

1. Comprehensive audiologic assessment
2. Hearing aid evaluation
3. Fitting and follow-up

For auditory rehabilitation to be a success, the amount of hearing loss is less critical than are patient awareness and acceptance of hearing loss, communication difficulties, and motivation to try amplification. After completing the audiologic assessment, the audiologist will help select a hearing aid or aids based on the patient's hearing needs and goals and provide training in the use of amplification and other selected rehabilitative approaches. After fitting a hearing aid for the patient, the audiologist provides supportive follow-up during the trial period and after the purchase.

Hearing Aid Selection

Hearing aid technology continues to evolve rapidly. Features include miniaturized styles, programmability, multimicrophone technology, and digital signal processing (DSP) capabilities. With symmetric hearing loss, binaural hearing aid fitting provides the most benefit. Hearing aids come in several basic types, but all are designed to increase the intensity of sound and deliver it to the ear with maximal fidelity. Body hearing aids are the largest type and are now somewhat outdated. Persons with severe profound hearing loss or those who lacked the dexterity to manipulate smaller hearing aids traditionally used these devices. Behind-the-ear (BTE) hearing aids have a case that fits behind the ear and conduct sound through a tube to an ear mold in the ear canal. Modern BTE hearing aids have greater amplification than the traditional body hearing aids.

In-the-ear (ITE) hearing aids are self-contained, fitting into the external ear, and are the preferred aids for many patients due to their cosmetic appeal and ease of insertion and adjustment. In-the-canal (ITC) hearing aids fit entirely into the outer portion of the ear canal. They provide sound amplification similar to most BTE and ITE hearing aids, but may pose a disadvantage for patients with dexterity problems because of their tiny size. Completely-in-the-canal (CIC) hearing aids are the smallest and most expensive aids and fit entirely within the ear canal. They are suitable for patients with mild to moderate hearing impairment, good manual dexterity, and a healthy ear canal.

Assistive Listening Devices

A variety of assistive listening devices (ALDs) are available to provide further benefit to hearing-impaired individuals. ALDs usually consist of a microphone placed close to the desired sound, and a means by which sound is transmitted directly to the listener. Examples of ALDs that improve signal-to-noise ratio via direct sound transmission include infrared or FM radio listening systems for televisions, stereos, concerts, and church sermons. Additional devices include amplified phones that are hearing-aid compatible, portable phone amplifiers, text telephones, signaling systems that make lamps flash on and off when the phone or doorbell rings, vibrating alarm clocks, televisions with closed captioning, and flashing smoke detectors.

Audiologic Rehabilitation Courses

In addition to assistive listening devices, audiology centers also often offer audiologic rehabilitation courses. With a focus on the development of problem-solving strategies to improve communication in everyday life situations, such courses represent an important educational opportunity for hearing-impaired individuals and their families. Referred individuals should be encouraged to attend the courses along with their communication partners since their participation helps reduce hearing handicaps for the referred individual and increases use of communication strategies.

Indications for Otolaryngology Referral

Box 24–5 lists important findings on the history or physical examination that should prompt referral for medical evaluation by an otolaryngologist. Otolaryngology referral is generally appropriate for patients who have hearing loss that deviates from the pattern characteristic for presbycusis (bilateral, symmetric, high-frequency hearing loss). Also, when visual ear inspection reveals the

---

Box 24-5   History or Exam Findings That Should Prompt Otolaryngology Referral

- Unexplained unilateral hearing loss
- Hearing loss associated with ear pain, tinnitus, or drainage
- Hearing loss associated with findings of middle ear disease such as cholesteatoma or tympanic membrane perforation
- History of fluid-filled ears or painful draining ears within the past 3 months
- History of sudden onset or rapidly progressive hearing loss within the past 3 months

presence of cerumen or a foreign body totally occluding the external auditory canal, medical evaluation by an otolaryngologist may be beneficial.

Medical-Surgical Treatments for Hearing Loss

Cochlear implants have become widely accepted as a means of hearing rehabilitation in people with advanced sensorineural hearing loss who are unable to gain effective speech recognition with hearing aids. In appropriately selected patients, cochlear implantation improves communication ability and leads to positive psychological and social benefits; furthermore, the surgery appears to be safe and well tolerated in geriatric patients.

Harry Jackson, Case Discussion

Mr. Jackson's increasing difficulty understanding his grandchildren's high-pitched voices is more likely a sign of presbycusis rather than his cerumen impaction, given that the former condition predominantly affects perception of high pitches and the latter condition mostly affects low pitches. Although he takes aspirin, a known cause of reversible hearing loss and tinnitus, hearing loss usually occurs only at higher daily doses of aspirin such as 650 mg four times a day. This case also illustrates how cerumen impaction can worsen the hearing disability imposed by other diseases such as presbycusis.

SUMMARY

Accurate and reliable hearing screening tools exist to help identify persons for whom hearing specialist referral is warranted.

Clinicians can improve the outlook for hearing-impaired persons by recognizing the serious consequences of hearing loss, assessing routinely for hearing loss, and counseling patients about the benefits of hearing health services.

Hearing aids significantly improve the quality of life of patients with sensorineural hearing loss.

POSTTEST

1. A 78-year-old woman complains of difficulty understanding conversations, especially in noisy social gatherings. Her audiogram 2 years ago showed moderately severe symmetrical bilateral sensorineural hearing loss. She declined hearing aid fitting at that time. You discover that she has some misconceptions about hearing aids. Each of the following statements reflects myths about hearing aids, *except:*
   a. Most people with hearing aids do not like how they sound.
   b. Hearing aids cannot help people with sensorineural hearing loss.
   c. All hearing aid users can achieve adequate speech recognition with hearing aids.
   d. Hearing aids restore hearing to normal.
   e. Clinical trials have demonstrated significant improvements in social, emotional, and communication function, and depressive symptoms among hearing aid recipients.

2. A 65-year-old female with type 2 diabetes and diabetic peripheral neuropathy was hospitalized 1 week ago and received piperacillin-tazobactam and gentamycin for treatment of bibasilar pneumonia. At the time of hospital discharge, she complained of dizziness and poor balance during ambulation. She now reports that her dizziness has worsened and she has been afraid to walk. Her unsteadiness is worse if she attempts to ambulate in the dark. She reports chronic bilateral hearing loss mildly worse in her left ear, but denies tinnitus. Orthostatic testing is unremarkable. Her neurological examination is remarkable only for a positive Romberg test and postural instability during ambulation. An audiogram reveals moderately severe bilateral sensorineural hearing loss (left mildly greater than right) with gently sloping high frequency hearing loss. The most likely cause of her dizziness and poor balance is:
   a. Benign positional vertigo
   b. Viral cochleitis
   c. Bilateral vestibular dysfunction induced by gentamycin
   d. Complication of diabetic peripheral neuropathy
   e. Ménière's disease

References

1. van den Brink RH, Wit HP, Kempen GI, van Heuvelen MJ. Attitude and help-seeking for hearing impairment. Br J Audiol 1996;30:313-24.
2. Jennings CR, Jones NS. Presbyacusis. J Laryngol Otol 2001;115:171-8.
3. Mulrow CD, Lichtenstein MJ. Screening for hearing impairment in the elderly: rationale and strategy. J Gen Intern Med 1991;6:249-58.
4. U.S. Department of Health and Human Services. Healthy people 2010. Washington, DC, 1999. Available at: www.healthypeople.gov/document/.
5. Stephens SD, Meredith R, Callaghan DE, Hogan S, Rayment A. Early intervention and rehabilitation: factors influencing outcome. Acta Otolaryngol Suppl 1990;476:221-5.
6. American Speech-Language-Hearing Association Audiologic Assessment Panel. Guidelines for audiologic screening. Rockville, MD: American Speech-Language-Hearing Association, 1997.
7. Lichtenstein MJ, Bess FH, Logan SA. Validation of screening tools for identifying hearing-impaired elderly in primary care. JAMA 1988;259:2875-8.
8. Yueh B. Screening and management of adult hearing loss in primary care. JAMA 2003;289:1976-85.
9. Punch JL, Weinstein BE. The hearing handicap inventory: introducing a multimedia version. Hear J 1996;49:35-49.
10. Gates GA, Murphy M, Rees TS, Fraher A. Screening for hearing loss in the elderly. J Fam Pract 2003;52:56-62.
11. Schow RL. Considerations in selecting and validating an adult/elderly hearing screening protocol. Ear Hear 1991;12:337-48.
12. Mulrow CD, Aguilar C, Endicott JE, et al. Quality-of-life changes and hearing impairment. A randomized trial. Ann Intern Med 1990;113:188-94.

Web Resources

1. National Institute on Deafness and Other Communication Disorders. National Institutes of Health. Available at: www.nidcd.nih.gov/. This site provides a wealth of information on hearing disorders, and is useful for laypersons and professionals. It also includes links to over 140 hearing-related organizations.

PRETEST ANSWERS

1. b
2. d
3. (1) d
   (2) a
   (3) c
   (4) e

POSTTEST ANSWERS

1. e
2. c

CHAPTER 25

Visual Impairment and Eye Problems

Karin Johnson and Steven Record

OBJECTIVES

Upon completion of this chapter, the reader will be able to:

● Know changes to the eye, vision, and visual function that accompany aging.

● Understand the impact of contrast sensitivity, illumination, and glare on visual acuity and visual function.

● Be familiar with the three most common age-associated ocular diseases, their diagnostic features, and treatment.

● Understand optical and nonoptical methods to enhance visual function.

PRETEST

1. A 75-year-old woman presents to your office with concerns that she may have to stop driving. You discover that she has difficulty seeing on bright, sunny days, and especially at night with oncoming automobile headlights. You suggest that she see her eye care provider for further evaluation as the most likely source of her visual difficulty is
   a. Age-related macular degeneration
   b. A cataract
   c. Glaucoma
   d. Uncorrected refractive error

2. A 70-year-old man comes into your office complaining that he just can't do what he was able to do when he was younger. He is particularly worried because he drives everywhere and now cannot see as well. He asks you what will happen to his eyes as he gets older. Which of the following ocular changes is not associated with aging?
   a. Miosis
   b. Lens yellowing
   c. Alterations in color vision
   d. Increased glare sensitivity and recovery
   e. Increased intraocular pressure

3. A 65-year-old male patient tells you that he has recently developed wet age-related macular degeneration. Which of the items listed below has not been shown to improve visual function in wet macular degeneration?
   a. Laser photocoagulation of the leaky neovascularization
   b. A hand magnifier
   c. Antioxidant vitamins
   d. Wearing a hat on bright, sunny days

VISUAL IMPAIRMENT WITH AGE

The eye is the window to the soul—and so much more. It is key to maximum functionality. With age, vision and functionality related to vision decline.[1,2] This has a major impact on quality of life and independence. Loss of vision is associated with depression, and difficulties with activities of daily living and safe driving, as well as increased risk of injury, falls, and medication errors. Surprisingly, visual acuity is not a good predictor of visual ability.[2-4] It is tested under high-contrast, ideal conditions that rarely exist outside of a doctor's office. Better predictors are contrast sensitivity, glare sensitivity, and performance under reduced illumination. Performance in these areas

declines not only for older adults with visual impairment (visual acuity worse than 20/40) but also for older adults without visual impairment. Deficits worsen when low contrast, reduced illumination, and glare co-exist. Treating refractive error and ocular disease is helpful but is not enough. Minimizing functional deficits related to the environmental conditions listed above will maximize function and independence. Success requires a team approach among the patient, family, primary care provider, eye care provider, and an occupational therapist trained in vision rehabilitation. The goal of this chapter is to provide the reader with the tools to easily deliver and coordinate such comprehensive care.

Wayne Knapp, *(Part 1)*

Wayne Knapp is a 73-year-old white male who presents to your office for a routine follow-up visit on his hypertension, hyperlipidemia, and coronary artery disease. He has been free of chest pain but is occasionally short of breath. He continues to smoke cigarettes, but says he has decided to cut down as his first grandchild has been born and he does not want to expose her to the smoke. He notes that his vision is "not as good as it used to be" and that he has "to get right under the light to see anything." He reads the paper every morning and reports that some of the words look distorted, especially with his left eye. Furthermore, he notes that he has stopped driving at night because it is even harder to see, especially with headlights coming toward him.

You have him read a distance and near Snellen chart and realize you must examine his eyes with your ophthalmoscope.

STUDY QUESTIONS

1. What is/are the most likely cause(s) of Mr. Knapp's visual complaints?
2. Which risk factors contribute to this/these conditions?

Prevalence and Impact

The Smith-Kettlewell Institute (SKI) Study evaluated vision and visual function in older adults aged 58 to 85 and older.[4] *Visual impairment* was defined as binocular acuity of 20/40 or worse. After age 60, 89% of their patients had no visual acuity impairment. Unfortunately, this percentage declined steadily with increasing age as per Table 25–1. Thus, 40% of patients 85 and older had some form of visual impairment. The statistics are even worse for the nursing home population where it is estimated that the degree of legal blindness (visual acuity worse than 20/200) is 15% in those over age 60 and up to 29% of those over age 90. This is an increase of 15

Table 25–1	Visual Decline with Aging
Age (Years)	**Percent without Visual Acuity Impairment**
58–69	99
70–74	97
75–79	91
80–84	88
≥85	60

times over community-dwelling older adults.[1] Such statistics highlight vision loss as the third leading cause of activity of daily living (ADL) impairment.[5] Over one-half of the conditions that cause visual impairment or blindness in older individuals are surgically treatable or potentially preventable.[6] Additionally, one-third of older adults with visual impairment improve vision with refraction alone. Thus, simply increasing access to eye care would significantly improve vision and function in older Americans.

Risk Factors and Pathophysiology

Vision loss and decreased vision function in older adults are related to ocular disease and age-related physiologic changes.[1-5,7] Even older patients with good visual acuity (20/40 or better) and no significant ocular disease showed deficits in visual function.[4] Visual acuity is tested under maximum contrast (i.e., black target on white background) and illumination with minimal glare. Rarely in life do people operate under these ideal conditions. "Real-life" vision occurs more commonly under decreased contrast, decreased and changing illumination, and increased glare. Contrast sensitivity is the ability to distinguish an object from its background. A visual acuity chart and most street signs provide high contrast sensitivity while camouflage demonstrates low contrast.

Measurement of visual function (rather than visual acuity) correlates highly with success in performing many common and essential daily activities.[3,8]

> ● Even older patients with good visual acuity (20/40 or better) and no significant ocular disease show deficits in visual function.

Differential Diagnosis and Assessment

Standard visual acuity can be measured with a distance and near Snellen chart. Testing the effects of decreased contrast sensitivity, decreased illumination, and increased glare is not practical for the primary care provider, as the equipment necessary for such testing is specialized, and is not widely available to primary care providers.[3,4] Rather, questioning older patients about their performance under these circumstances is easier. For contrast sensitivity, ask if a patient has much difficulty driving in the rain or seeing on a hazy day. For low illumination, ask if your patient has significantly greater difficulty seeing at dusk and at night. For glare, ask how debilitated your patient is by oncoming headlights, by walking from outside to inside on a sunny day, or by entering a tunnel from daylight.

Management

Enhancing visual function requires a team approach among the primary care provider, the eye care provider, and an occupational therapist trained in visual rehabilitation. Eye examination by an optometrist or ophthalmologist is key to providing best-corrected vision with refraction and treatment of visual deficits due to ocular disease. Despite these efforts, some patients may not be correctable to 20/20. Performance can be enhanced for patients with low vision (worse than 20/70 visual acuity) and for patients with better acuity who have difficulty in certain circumstances or settings. An ideal approach would be to have a home evaluation by a vision rehabilitation specialist. Since this is not readily available for many older adults, a more practical approach educates the primary care provider, the patient, and the patient's family about simple measures to maximize visual acuity and function.

SPECIFIC OCULAR DISEASES ASSOCIATED WITH AGING

Age-Related Macular Degeneration

PREVALENCE AND IMPACT

Age-related macular degeneration (ARMD) is the leading cause of severe vision loss in patients 75 years of age and older.[7,9] It is the most common cause of new visual impairment in patients over age 65. Over 5% of older adults beyond age 65 have some form of visual impairment due to ARMD. The National Advisory Eye Council estimates that more older adults will become blind from ARMD than from glaucoma and diabetic retinopathy combined. It targets the macula, and in particular the fovea, resulting in a loss of central vision first unilaterally and later bilaterally. This loss of central visual acuity is associated with impaired ability to perform activities of daily living, impaired mobility, increased risk of falls and fractures, increased medication errors, depression, and lower quality-of-life scores.[9] Also, visual function is adversely affected by distortion (metamorphopsia) and impaired ability to adapt to changing light levels.[4,9–11] Non-neovascular (dry) ARMD accounts for 90% of the cases and neovascular (wet) ARMD accounts for the remaining 10%.

> ● The National Advisory Eye Council estimates that more older adults will become blind from ARMD than from glaucoma and diabetic retinopathy combined.

RISK FACTORS AND PATHOPHYSIOLOGY

There is no gender predilection for the development of ARMD, but once present, neovascular disease is more prevalent in women.[9] Additionally, there is a racial predilection for disease development, with older Caucasian Americans being affected twice as often as older African Americans.[6,10] In general, risk factors for coronary artery disease and ARMD are similar. Patients with a history of hypertension, smoking, and atherosclerosis are more prone to acquire macular degeneration.[10] A supposition that oxidative damage to arterioles is causative played a role in studies examining the use of antioxidants in macular degeneration prevention and mitigation. Research also implicates phototoxicity, inflammation, and diet as other possible risk factors. A genetic link for ARMD is as yet unclear.

DIFFERENTIAL DIAGNOSIS AND ASSESSMENT

Ideally, the best way to diagnose ARMD is with a dilated fundus exam and the use of a slit lamp biomicroscope and special magnifying lenses. Florescein angiography is also helpful.[9–11] Given the specialized equipment necessary for the diagnosis, a patient with suspected ARMD is best referred to an eye care specialist for establishment of the diagnosis.

W a y n e   K n a p p, *(Part 2)*

His acuity is 20/50 in the right eye and 20/40 in the left eye. With your ophthalmoscope, you find the red reflex, and in the retroillumination, you note that there appears to be a central density in both eyes. You adjust your ophthalmoscope to focus on the retina but note that the view OU remains a little hazy despite your best efforts. You are able to detect yellowish, ground-glass–like deposits in the macula as well as patchy white and black areas indicating disruption of the retinal pigment epithelium. You suspect Mr. Knapp has nuclear sclerosis cataracts and early dry macular degeneration. You refer him to a local eye care provider who confirms your diagnosis.

STUDY QUESTIONS

1. After consultation with Mr. Knapp's eye care practitioner, what treatments do you advise?
2. What is the prognosis for his nuclear sclerosis cataracts and dry macular degeneration?

MANAGEMENT

Unfortunately, the treatment of ARMD is limited and the prognosis is poor. There is no medical management for dry or wet ARMD.[10] The Age-Related Eye Disease Study (AREDS) research group did show a reduction in the development of advanced dry ARMD in some patients with existing ARMD meeting certain specifications.[12] These patients were given an antioxidant mixture (vitamin C, vitamin E, and beta-carotene) with zinc. Pharmaceuticals to inhibit vascular endothelial growth factor are being studied to treat wet ARMD.[10] Nevertheless, standard therapy for wet ARMD remains laser photocoagulation of the leaky neovascularization.[9–11]

Cataracts

PREVALENCE AND IMPACT

A cataract is any opacity in the lens that causes it to lose transparency or scatter light.[13] Prevalence is well known to be age related, occurring in one in six patients under age 40 and 50% of patients age 80 and beyond. The Framingham Eye Study estimated the prevalence of cataracts causing acuity of 20/30 or worse to be 5% for ages 55 to 64, 18% for ages 65 to 74, and 46% for ages 75 to 80. Three main varieties of cataracts exist–nuclear sclerosis, posterior subcapsular cataracts, and cortical spoking. Cataracts reduce illumination, reduce contrast sensitivity, increase glare, and degrade blue-yellow color vision.[4,13] Any loss of visual acuity and visual function will impair activity of daily living performance, driving ability, and mobility; increase fall risk and medication errors; and reduce quality of life. Additionally, cataracts are costly. Among Medicare beneficiaries, cataracts are the most common reason for eye exams and cataract surgery is the most frequently performed surgery. Over 43% of visits by older Americans to optometrists and ophthalmologists are for cataracts. Nearly $3.5 billion each year is spent on 1.35 million cataract surgeries.

RISK FACTORS AND PATHOPHYSIOLOGY

A number of risk factors exist for cataract development. They include more hours of sunlight exposure, smoking, heavy alcohol consumption, and a low educational level. Diabetics have a higher prevalence of cortical opacities, as do women and African Americans.[6,13] Diet and vitamin use appear not to play a role in cataract development. The AREDS research group showed no link between supplementation with a combination of antioxidants (vitamin C, vitamin E, and beta carotene) and the development or progression of age-related lens opacities.[14] Pathophysiology is varied. Nuclear sclerosis results from the accumulation of high-molecular-weight protein. Subcapsular cataracts result from degenerative changes in the capsule epithelium. Cortical

cataracts develop because of damage to the lens fibers due to an increased accumulation of intracellular and extracellular water.

> ● A number of risk factors exist for cataract development. They include more hours of sunlight exposure, smoking, heavy alcohol consumption, and a low educational level.

DIFFERENTIAL DIAGNOSIS AND ASSESSMENT

Cataracts are best diagnosed with a slit lamp biomicroscope through a dilated pupil. With retroillumination off of the retina, one or more types can be detected with an ophthalmoscope but this is clearly inferior to slit lamp examination. A nuclear sclerotic cataract appears as a yellowish-brown opacity in the lens center. It is football-shaped or circular depending on your view with the slit lamp or ophthalmoscope. A posterior subcapsular cataract looks like a smudge on the back of the lens. Cortical spiking appears as whitish, triangular, or fleck-like opacities around the lens perimeter.[13–16]

MANAGEMENT

The treatment of cataracts remains surgical. Extracapsular cataract extraction with posterior chamber intraocular lens implantation continues to be the standard. No medications are known to prevent or abolish cataracts. The criterion for surgery is functional visual impairment and not a specific visual acuity. In general, visual acuity of 20/50 or worse with glare testing is considered to be a surgical level of dysfunction.

Glaucoma

PREVALENCE AND IMPACT

Primary open-angle glaucoma (POAG) affects approximately 6% of patients over the age of 65.[7] It is the second most common cause of legal blindness in the United States and the leading cause of blindness among African Americans.[17] Unlike macular degeneration, which starts with a loss of central acuity, glaucoma destroys peripheral vision first and central vision in the end stages. It limits an older adult's useful field of view, making mobility and safe driving more difficult and increasing fall risk.

> ● Primary open-angle glaucoma affects approximately 6% of patients over the age of 65; it is the second most common cause of legal blindness in the United States and the leading cause of blindness among African Americans.

RISK FACTORS AND PATHOPHYSIOLOGY

Open-angle glaucoma is characterized by progressive and initially asymptomatic optic neuropathy resulting in visual field loss in the presence of an open anterior chamber. Despite the open anterior chamber, there is resistance to aqueous outflow.[17] Intraocular pressure increases, resulting in damage to optic nerve fibers. Many risk factors exist.[18] The most well known is increased intraocular pressure (IOP). However, it is crucial to remember that the increase is relative. Some patients have low-pressure glaucoma and demonstrate optic nerve damage at pressures less than 21 mmHg, and others demonstrate ocular hypertension and have no damage at pressures greater than 21 mmHg. In general, patients with IOPs between 15 to 20 mmHG are at low risk, and patients with IOPs above 25 mmHg are at greater risk. Other contributory factors besides IOP and age are enlarged optic nerve cup (0.5 cup-to-disk ratio or larger), race (greater prevalence in African Americans), family history, and diseases affecting the vasculature such as hypertension and diabetes.

DIFFERENTIAL DIAGNOSIS AND ASSESSMENT

Intraocular pressure measurement is essential for the diagnosis of open-angle glaucoma. However, measurement of IOP with a tonometer is not practical in the primary care setting. Neither is optic nerve head evaluation through a dilated pupil with a slit lamp biomicroscope and a special magnifying lens or visual field analysis with a computer. Use of a direct ophthalmoscope to view the optic nerve head is feasible but not ideal. Glaucomatous optic atrophy results in pallor and thinning of the neural retinal rim (the donut) with secondary widening and deepening of the cup (the donut hole). The rim should be thickest inferiorly, then superiorly, nasally, and lastly temporally (ISN'T). Deviation from this, as well as a cup-to-disc ratio of greater than or equal to 0.5, should raise suspicion of glaucoma. Differential diagnosis includes ocular hypertension, a congenitally large optic nerve cup, and a myriad of other types of optic atrophy.[16,17]

MANAGEMENT

Glaucoma is amenable to medical, surgical, and laser therapy. Beta-blockers are first-line medical therapy followed by prostaglandin analogs. Second-line agents include topical carbonic anhydrase inhibitors and alpha-2 agonists. Medications that were the standard 10 years ago, such as epinephrine, pilocarpine (a cholinergic agent), and oral carbonic anhydrase inhibitors, are now infrequently used.[18] All topical ocular medications have the potential for systemic absorption and side effects. Many of these side effects have been eliminated with the less frequent use of epinephrine and pilocarpine. Selective and nonselective beta-blockers may cause the same cardiovascular and pulmonary side effects as their oral counterparts. Additionally, the alpha-2 agonists may cause hypertension. When medical management is not sufficient, other treatment options include laser trabeculoplasty and filtration surgery.[18]

Case Discussion

Mr. Knapp's age and smoking are risk factors for both his cataract and macular degeneration. His cardiovascular disease is a further risk factor for his macular degeneration. His difficulties in low light levels and with glare are consistent with cataract symptoms. The distortion he notes is typical of macular degeneration. It is not surprising that his visual acuity is reduced. When examining a patient's eyes, if the doctor has trouble seeing through the ocular media, then the patient will surely have trouble seeing out through it. If Mr. Knapp's vision is not improved with refraction, cataract surgery is a reasonable option. Unfortunately, no treatment exists for his dry macular degeneration. Mr. Knapp's best chance at mitigating progression is to quit smoking and get optimal treatment for his cardiovascular disease. In the future, he may need some of the optical and nonoptical aids discussed in the chapter.

SUMMARY

A basic principle of geriatric care is to identify functional impairment and maximize residual function. Vision care for the elderly is no exception. A difference exists between standard visual acuity and visual functional ability. Many older adults with good standard acuity will experience severe degradation due to everyday environmental factors. Thus, it is important to know how the patient functions in his or her natural setting, and not just rely on office performance. Identifying and treating refractive errors and age-related ocular disease such as macular degeneration, cataracts, and glaucoma can go a long way toward improving functionality and quality of life. However, this is not enough. Many older patients cannot be corrected to 20/40 or better despite treatment in these areas, and need to be advised of other optical and nonoptical ways to enhance visual function. This requires a team approach among the patient, the family, the primary care and eye care providers and, where available, a vision rehabilitation specialist.

POSTTEST

1. Ms. Jones is a 75-year-old female residing in a senior retirement community. She values her independence but had a mother who became blind at about age 75. Ms. Jones is concerned that the same thing may happen to her. The leading cause of severe vision loss in patients 75 years of age and older is
   a. Glaucoma
   b. Age-related macular degeneration
   c. Cataracts
   d. Diabetic retinopathy

2. You discuss the risk factors for the ocular disease mentioned in question 4 with Ms. Jones. They include
   a. Smoking
   b. Hypertension
   c. Genetics
   d. a and b
   e. All of the above

3. A 70-year-old African-American female presents to your office complaining of difficulty seeing. The most common age-associated ocular disease causing vision loss for her would be
   a. Cataracts
   b. Age-related macular degeneration
   c. Glaucoma
   d. Diabetic retinopathy

4. Your 68-year-old patient went to see her optometrist yesterday. Her best-corrected visual acuity is 20/70. She notes that this seems to get worse at times. What can you advise her to do to maximize her visual function?
   a. Improve contrast
   b. Improve illumination
   c. Reduce glare
   d. Increase stereopsis
   e. a, b, and c

References

1. Swanson M. The elderly. In Benjamin W, ed. Clinical Refraction. Philadelphia: WB Saunders, 1998.
2. Kamel HK, Guro-Razuman S, Sharceff M. The Activities of Daily Vision Scale: a useful tool to assess fall risk in older adults with vision impairment. J Am Geriatr Soc 48:11, 2000.
3. Ball K. Real-world evaluation of visual function. Ophthalmol Clin North Am 16:2, 2003.
4. Schneck ME, Haegerstrom-Portnoy G. Practical assessment of vision in the elderly. Ophthalmol Clin North Am 16:2, 2003.
5. Watson GR. Assessment and rehabilitation of older adults with low vision. In Hazzard WR, Blass JP, Halter JB, et al., eds. Principles of Geriatric Medicine and Gerontology. New York: McGraw-Hill, 2003.
6. Munoz G, West SK, Schein OD. Causes of blindness and visual impairment in a population of older Americans: the Salisbury Eye Study. Arch Ophthalmol 118:6, 2000.
7. Lighthouse International. Home page. Available at: www.lighthouse.org.
8. Rubin GS, Roche KB, Prasado-Rao P. Visual impairment and disability in older adults. Optom Vis Sci 74:12, 1994.
9. Martidis A, Tennant MTS, Age-related macular degeneration. In Yanoff M, ed. Ophthalmology. Philadelphia: Mosby, 2004.
10. Alexander LJ. Exudative and non-exudative ocular disorders. In Primary Care of the Posterior Segment. East Norwalk, CT: Appleton and Lange, 1989.
11. Age-Related Eye Disease Study Research Group. A randomized, placebo-controlled, clinical trial of high-dose supplementation with vitamins C and E, beta carotene, and zinc for age-related macular degeneration and vision loss. Arch Ophthalmol 119:10, 2001.
12. Chitkara DK, Hall AB, Rosethal AR. Pathophysiology and epidemiology of cataracts. In Yanoff M, ed. Ophthalmology. Philadelphia: Mosby, 2004.
13. Age-Related Eye Disease Study Research Group. A randomized, placebo-controlled clinical trial of high-dose supplementation with vitamins C and E and beta carotene for age-related cataract and vision loss. Arch Ophthalmol 119:10, 2001.
14. Chitkara DK. Cataract formation mechanisms. In Yanoff M, ed. Ophthalmology. Philadelphia: Mosby, 2004.
15. Grabow HB. Indications for lens surgery and different techniques. In Yanoff M, ed. Ophthalmology. Philadelphia: Mosby, 2004.
16. Distelhorst JS, Hughes GM. Open-angle glaucoma. Am Fam Phys 67:9, 2003.
17. Zimmerman R, Sakiyalak D, Krupin T, Rosenberg L. Primary open-angle glaucoma. In Yanoff M, ed. Ophthalmology. Philadelphia: Mosby, 2004.
18. Wiggington SA, Higginbotham EJ. Choosing initial and combination medical therapy for glaucoma. Ophthalmol Clin North Am 13:3, 2000.

Web Resources

www.lighthouse.org

PRETEST ANSWERS

1. b
2. e
3. c

POSTTEST ANSWERS

1. b
2. d
3. a
4. e

Persistent Pain

Jane F. Potter and Heather M. Titman

OBJECTIVES

Upon completion of this chapter, the reader will be able to:

- Define persistent pain and discuss its impact on older adults.
- Discuss the pathophysiology of persistent pain.
- Describe age-related changes that influence the presentation and treatment of persistent pain.
- Take an accurate pain history and use assessment tools to quantitate and monitor pain symptoms.
- Choose appropriate pharmacologic treatments to manage persistent pain.
- Apply nonpharmacologic interventions in the treatment of persistent pain.
- Understand the level of evidence for specific recommendations that are based on the 2002 American Geriatrics Society's "Guideline on the Management of Persistent Pain."[1]

PRETEST

1. What proportion of older people experience persistent pain?
   a. 1% to 3%
   b. 5% to 10%
   c. 15% to 20%
   d. 25% to 50%

2. Which of the following is a consequence of persistent pain?
   a. Increased pain threshold
   b. Altered self-concept
   c. Depression
   d. Mental status changes

3. Which of the following agents would be expected to have the greatest efficacy in treating persistent neuropathic pain?
   a. Acetaminophen
   b. Codeine
   c. Gabapentin
   d. Celecoxib

PREVALENCE AND IMPACT

Pain is an unpleasant sensory and emotional experience. Pain sensation is conveyed by afferent nerve fibers from the periphery to the brain. Factors such as the patient's personality, cultural background, the involved organ, individual memory, expectations, and experiences make pain a complex phenomenon.[2] An emotional response also accompanies the sensation of pain and must be addressed in assessment and treatment.

Acute pain has a well-defined temporal pattern of onset associated with physical signs and autonomic activity (e.g., elevated heart rate or blood pressure).[2] In contrast, *persistent pain* is more difficult to define and identify. Autonomic signs are usually absent. Pain becomes persistent when it continues for a prolonged period of time and may or may not be associated with a recognizable disease process. Persistent pain also occurs when healing of an underlying disease process is lacking or incomplete or when routine pain control methods are not able to adequately alleviate pain.[1] When pain becomes persistent, the patient's pain threshold is lowered. Factors such as female gender, greater pain intensity, insomnia,

and poor social network are significant predictors of the presence of persistent pain.

Persistent pain is an extremely common problem in the elderly population, but our understanding of the epidemiology remains limited. Estimates of the prevalence of persistent pain in community samples vary greatly from a low of 2% to 40% and higher depending on definition and method of detection. A Louis Harris telephone survey found that nearly one in five Americans (18%) take analgesic medications regularly (several times a week or more) and 63% of those individuals had taken prescription pain medications for more than 6 months.[3] In a general community sample, 48% of persons described having mild persistent pain, whereas 15% of the sample described severe persistent pain.[4] Certain groups within the population are more likely to experience persistent pain. Although it is fair to estimate that 25% to 50% of older community dwellers suffer from persistent pain, this problem may affect between 45% and 80% of nursing home residents.[1] Chronic conditions such as arthritis, back pain, and bone and joint disorders comprise the majority of cases of persistent pain.

Box 26–1   Consequences of Persistent Pain

- Depression
- Decreased socialization
- Sleep disturbances
- Impaired ambulation
- Increased health care cost and utilization

Persistent pain potentially affects all aspects of life, health, and safety. Persistent pain increases health care costs. Health care use depends on pain perception and intensity of pain, but is also increased by other factors such as older age, female gender, multiunit housing, and retirement or unemployment status.[4] About half of patients with persistent pain consult their primary physician, and about 7% a physiotherapist.[5] The number and type of medications prescribed for persistent pain increase the likelihood of drug side effects and interactions.

Persistent pain produces substantial morbidity in the older population. Undertreatment of pain leads to depression, social isolation, gait problems, and sleep disturbances (Box 26–1). Pain is associated with depression in the older person, and this correlation is statistically significant among nursing home residents.[6] Older patients with good coping strategies have lower pain and psychological disability. The patient's pain-related beliefs and coping strategies independently predict physical disability, whereas a patient's tendency to view pain as catastrophic predicts depression.[7] Pain problems often limit physical activity, resulting in deconditioning. Deconditioned persons are more likely to suffer injuries when they do move and are more likely to experience gait disorders and falls.

People with chronic cancer pain have increased morbidity and mortality because they suffer from symptoms such as constipation, pressure sores, urinary retention or incontinence, venous thromboses, and muscle pain.

● Undertreatment of pain leads to depression, social isolation, gait problems, and sleep disturbances.

June Morris, *(Part 1)*

June Morris is a 78-year-old white married woman who comes to your office concerned about burning and aching in the buttocks, with radiation to her thighs when she stands for more than 10 minutes or when she walks for more than one block. This problem has been present for more than 2 years and limits her ability to shop and complete household chores.

Rebecca Dixon, *(Part 1)*

Rebecca Dixon is an 80-year-old black married woman who presents to your office as a new patient. She has extremely poor vision as a result of advanced age-related macular degeneration and a history of uterine cancer treated with hysterectomy and pelvic irradiation in 1992. Seven months ago she experienced the sudden onset of severe boring pain in her right pelvis and thigh. After 4 months during which time her pain was poorly understood, she was diagnosed with a pelvic insufficiency fracture. After 6 weeks of rest and analgesics, she experienced some improvement. However, when she tries to resume household activities, the pain recurs and is severe with any level of activity.

STUDY QUESTIONS

1. What is the pathophysiology of each patient's pain?
2. How will the etiology of the pain influence therapy?
3. What would you especially seek on examination?

RISK FACTORS AND PATHOPHYSIOLOGY

Although persistent pain can take many forms, understanding its basic pathophysiology helps to target treatment. Aging could potentially play a role in the pathophysiology of pain because the perception of pain involves complex neural functions. There is altered transmission along A-delta and C-nerve fibers associated with aging; however, age-related changes in perception are not thought to be clinically significant. There is, however, reduced plasticity in the aged central nervous system (CNS) response to prolonged noxious input and a slower recovery and an increased duration of postinjury tenderness in adults of advanced age.[8] Table 26–1 lists the common causes of persistent pain according to the un... ...ory. *Nociceptive* pain arises from bon... ...l organs, and is a result of s... ...uropathic pain arises ... ...nerves or CNS. ... ...ixture of the ... ...ome pain syn- ... ...omatization disor- ... ...he approach to such pat... ...standing of the syndrome, its diag... ...he factors that are mediating it. Table 26... ...es guidelines to classifying persistent pain and predicting response to medications.

Table 26–1	Pathophysiologic Classification of Persistent Pain

Nociceptive Pain

Arthropathies (e.g., rheumatoid arthritis, osteoarthritis, gout, post-traumatic arthropathies, mechanical neck, and back syndromes)

Myalgia (e.g., myofascial pain syndromes)

Skin and mucosal ulcerations

Nonarticular Inflammatory Disorders (e.g., polymyalgia rheumatica)

Ischemic disorders

Visceral pain (pain of internal organs and viscera)

Neuropathic Pain

Post-herpetic neuralgia

Trigeminal neuralgia

Painful diabetic polyneuropathy

Post-stroke pain (central pain)

Post-amputation pain

Myelopathic or Radiculopathic Pain (e.g., spinal stenosis, arachnoiditis, root sleeve fibrosis)

Atypical facial pain

Causalgia-like syndromes (complex regional pain syndromes)

Mixed or Undetermined Pathophysiology

Chronic recurrent headaches (e.g., tension headaches, migraine headaches, mixed headaches)

Vasculopathic pain syndromes (e.g., painful vasculitis)

Psychologically Based Pain Syndromes

Somatization disorders

Hysterical reactions

Modified from Leland JY. Chronic pain: primary care treatment of the older patient. Geriatrics 54(1):26, 1999, with permission.

DIFFERENTIAL DIAGNOSIS AND ASSESSMENT

June Morris, *(Part 2)*

You suspect that Ms. Morris has spinal stenosis, which causes neuropathic pain. She also has long-standing Paget's disease and describes aching in her wrists and hands and in her left hip. Examination reveals warmth, swelling, and tenderness along both wrists. You are able to reproduce her bilateral thigh pain by having her stand, and you find the pain is greatly reduced with forward flexion. Her serum alkaline phosphatase is 1500 IU/L (range 40 to 143). On interview you learn that the patient's husband has advanced prostate cancer, and when you have the patient complete a Geriatric Depression Scale (GDS), she scores 9 out of 15 (scores higher than 5 suggest depression).

Rebecca Dixon, *(Part 2)*

You suspect that Ms. Dixon has a nonhealing pelvic fracture and classify her pain as nociceptive. She has difficulty transferring from a seated to a standing position and initiating gait, and in transferring weight from one leg to the other. She grimaces with these movements and notes that weight bearing reproduces her symptoms.

STUDY QUESTIONS

1. What diagnostic studies would confirm the diagnoses?
2. What associated conditions in each patient warrant attention and therapy?

Pain History and Examination

The patient's account of pain is considered most reliable in evaluating the presence and severity of persistent pain.[1] It is essential that the patient's complaint and perception be taken seriously. Because pain is such a common problem, all older patients presenting to a medical service should be assessed for persistent pain (level of evidence = B). In screening older patients, it is important to use a variety of terms, such as *burning, aching, soreness, heaviness,* or *tightness,* to describe the pain (Box 26–2).

When patients have cognitive or communication problems, the history should be supplemented with information from family and caregivers. The clinician should also watch for signs suggestive of pain such as groaning, agitation, crying, withdrawal of limbs, or changes in weight bearing while walking or moving (level of evidence = B). Decreased cognition complicates but does not preclude accurate pain assessment in the mild to moderate stages of dementia.

All patients with persistent pain should undergo a comprehensive pain assessment (level of evidence = D). The pain history should evaluate the presenting pain complaint, its character, location, pattern, intensity, duration, and precipitating and alleviating factors (level of evidence = D). The history of analgesic use is particularly important. Patients should be questioned on the use of prescription and over-the-counter medications, the duration of use, the effect on pain, and side effects (level of evidence = D). A detailed medical history should also be obtained.

Barriers to accurate pain assessment are often present in older persons. Patients may be reticent to report pain because they believe it is a normal part of aging or because they fear that it is a sign of serious illness or signals impending death. They may also under-report the problem out of fear of diagnostic tests or medication side effects. Others may believe that pain is sent to

Table 26–2	Guide to Classifying and Treating Chronic Pain		
Pain Type	**Localization**	**Character**	**Response to Medication**
Nociceptive (somatic)	Well localized	Aching, gnawing	Responsive to anti-inflammatory medications and opioids
Nociceptive (visceral)	Poorly localized, referred pain	Squeezing, pressure-like	Responsive to anti-inflammatory medications and opioids
Neuropathic	Referred along nerve pathway	Severe, constant with paroxysms of burning or shock-like sensations	Incomplete response to anti-inflammatory drugs and opioids; often requires adjuvant medications
Mixed type	Well localized	Throbbing, aching, constant	Variable response to medications; often requires combined approach
Psychologically based pain	Poorly localized	Burning, aching, includes autonomic symptoms like sweating, palpitations	Combined approach, psychiatric counseling

Modified from Leland JY. Chronic pain: primary care treatment of the older patient. Geriatrics 54(1):26, 1999, with permission.

them as atonement for past sins. To achieve effective management of persistent pain, the patient's pain beliefs, perspectives, expectations, and coping strategies must be understood. The cost of medications, access to health care, co-morbid disorders, attitudes of health professionals, lack of communication, and fear of losing independence all influence pain evaluation and management.[9]

Any pain that affects quality of life or the patient's ability to function in daily life must be taken seriously. To appreciate the impact that pain is having, function (see Chapter 4) should be assessed (level of evidence = B). Various instruments are used to assess function.[10,11] Essentially each of these instruments asks the patient about his or her ability to perform basic activities of daily living or self-care activities such as bathing, dressing, eating, and walking. The patient's ability to carry out more complex activities such as cooking, cleaning, and shopping (i.e., instrumental activities of daily living) may also be informative. Asking the patient how pain is affecting his or her ability to conduct each activity provides a measure of the current impact of pain on function, and serves as a baseline against which progress in pain management can be gauged.

The emotional impact of persistent pain must also be evaluated and managed (level of evidence = B). Depression and anxiety are common sequelae for such patients. Brief screening instruments, such as the GDS, may help objectively evaluate depression.[12] Anxiety symptoms are often a result of depression and will respond as the depression is treated. Symptoms of anxiety that persist after treatment of depression warrant further evaluation and treatment. Sleep disorders predict development of persistent pain, and pain disrupts sleep. Sleep disorders should be addressed first with sleep hygiene measures and medications, if necessary. If there is any indication that a psychologic-based syndrome is involved, it can be helpful to consult mental health services.

A physical examination should be completed, with special emphasis on the neuromuscular and musculoskeletal systems, including palpation for tenderness, inflammation, deformities, and trigger points. Search for neurologic impairments such as weakness, numbness, hyperalgesia, and paraesthesia (level of evidence = D). Observation of gait using a simple "Up and Go" test helps the patient and clinician see the effect of pain on movement and address gait safety as part of the treatment plan. The history and physical examination should then direct selection of appropriate laboratory and diagnostic studies.

● It is essential that the patient's complaint and perception of pain be taken seriously.

Pain Quantitation and Monitoring

Persistent pain is the personal experience of the patient and, by its nature, one that even the patient may have difficulty quantitating over time. The clinician has only a secondary and episodic involvement in the pain experience and may lack objectivity unless a standard instrument is used during each visit. Pain intensity scales bring objectivity to serial assessments and should be considered standard in managing patients with persistent pain (level of evidence = B) (Fig. 26–1).[13] Such

Box 26-2   Pain Assessment

- Ask the patient about pain (aggravating and relieving factors, quality of pain, location, severity, frequency, and duration).
- Use alternative terms (e.g., burning, aching) to elicit symptoms.
- Treat the underlying cause when possible.
- Use the mechanism of the pain syndrome to direct treatment.

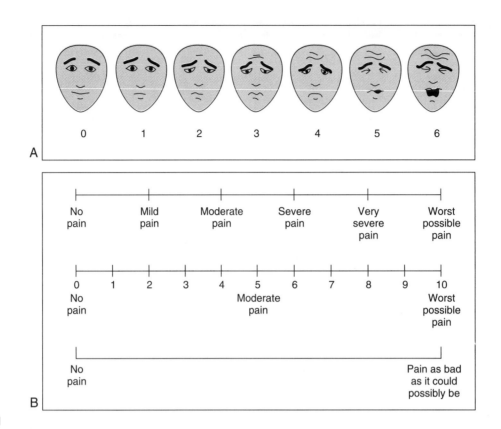

FIGURE 26–1

Pain intensity scales used in older patients. **A:** Faces scale. Ask the patient to "put an X by the face that best matches the severity of your pain right now." *(From the Pediatric Pain Sourcebook (original copyright 2001), with permission from the International Association for the Study of Pain.)* **B:** Visual analog scales. Ask the patient to "circle the number that best represents the intensity or severity of your pain right now." *(Redrawn from Carr DB, et al. Acute Pain Management: Operative or Medical Procedures and Trauma. Rockville, MD: Agency for Health Care Policy and Research, 1992 (AHCPR 92-0032), and Jacox A, et al. Management of Cancer Pain. Rockville, MD: Agency for Health Care Policy and Research, 1994 (AHCPR 94-0592), with permission.*

instruments use faces or word descriptors in a visual analog scale that asks the patient to rate the severity of pain from 0 (no pain) to 10 (the worst pain possible).[14] Repeated use of the same scale brings needed objectivity to monitoring persistent pain over time. Some scales are adapted for people with language impairment, and large-print scales are available for patients who are visually impaired. Clinicians should avoid estimates of pain based on clinical impression or surrogate report unless patients are unable to reliably report their needs (level of evidence = B).

In many cases of persistent pain, complete elimination of pain is not possible. Patients must then appreciate that the goal is pain control and be helped to set expectations for therapy. For such patients, the nonpharmacotherapies become especially important to assist them in learning to live with some element of pain and avoid the physical and psychological complications, such as physical deconditioning and depression. Patients or their caregivers should be asked to keep a daily pain log (Box 26–3) in which they record the intensity of pain, medications used and side effects, response to treatment, and activities associated with pain (level of evidence = D).

Routine health care visits can be scheduled based on the severity of pain and associated or complicating health issues. At each visit the patient should be evaluated for all relevant issues (e.g., mood, functional disability) identified during the comprehensive pain assessment. The same scales should be used to follow specific problems (e.g., pain, function, mood). Medication use should be reviewed both for efficacy and side effects and for adherence to the prescribed regimen, including any nonpharmacologic modalities.[1] It is important not to assume that a change in the patient's pain experience is simply caused by an exacerbation of the chronic problem. A change in pain should prompt a new evaluation. It is important in this context to know if this is the same pain syndrome or

---

Box 26–3 Elements of Daily Pain Log

- Date and time
- Pain intensity (use same scale daily)
- Activity, treatment, results, medication side effects

underlying disease process inadequately managed or whether this is a new symptom. A "new" pain should be classified into one of the general four categories of pain syndromes and treatment started.

June Morris, *(Part 3)*

You obtain magnetic resonance imaging (MRI) of the lumbar spine. The MRI confirms that Ms. Morris has severe spinal stenosis from L-3 to L-5. Radiographs of the wrists show bony enlargement, areas of sclerosis, and lucency and osteoarthritic changes in the joints consistent with Paget's disease. Her current therapy includes acetaminophen 1 g four times daily and hydrocodone 5 mg every 6 hours as needed for pain. She rates her pain as zero (0) at rest, and 8 to 9 out of 10 during prolonged standing or walking. She had previously been treated with bisphosphates for Paget's disease but currently receives no therapy. Back pain of moderate severity occurs with light housekeeping and meal preparation.

Rebecca Dixon, *(Part 3)*

You review a radiograph of the pelvis completed last week that confirms a fracture of the pubic ramus, at the same site as Ms. Dixon's original injury. Her current therapy includes acetaminophen 1 g four times daily; she had been offered treatment with an opioid analgesic but declined, due to fear of addiction and side effects. She also has been taking Benadryl 50 mg at night for sleep and an uncertain amount of calcium. On her current pain regimen, Ms. Dixon rates her pain as 5 to 6 on a scale of 10 while seated and 7 to 8 during any movement or activity.

STUDY QUESTIONS

1. How can each patient's pain management be improved?
2. What role should pharmacotherapy play in management?

MANAGEMENT

Analgesic medications are the most commonly used modalities for treatment of persistent pain in older people. There is no ideal drug to control pain. Usually the lowest dose of one drug is chosen and increased to therapeutic effect. "Start low, go slow" is the common adage followed. Most analgesic drugs

(even opioids) can be used safely in older people, although many older patients show increased analgesic sensitivity.[15] There is substantial heterogeneity within this population, and effective treatment may require doses similar to those used in younger persons. The least invasive route of administration (usually oral) is preferred.

In planning and prescribing the treatment regimen, patients must be educated about the expected duration and effect of the analgesic. They should also expect a period of trial and error as new treatments are introduced and titrated. Medications found to be ineffective should be tapered and discontinued. Although it is desirable to limit polypharmacy, using smaller effective doses of analgesics from different classes may provide pain relief with fewer side effects than would be associated with high doses of a single agent.[1]

In dosing analgesics, noncontinuous pain is best treated with episodic dosing, and continuous, ongoing pain with frequent continuous dosing. Additional doses may be needed to facilitate exercise and other activities that the patient has found to exacerbate pain. Efforts should be made to keep the regimen simple to fit with a lifestyle that does not focus on pain. End points to treatment should be improved functional status, sleep, gait, nutrition, and mood. If medications are not dosed or timed appropriately, patients tend to decrease physical activity to limit pain and become more deconditioned and functionally disabled. Finally, cost is a consideration with many patients in designing the regimen.[1]

Acetaminophen

Analgesia should be initiated with an effective agent that has the fewest number of side effects. Acetaminophen, salicylates, and nonsteroidal anti-inflammatory drugs (NSAIDs) are preferred over narcotics to treat mild to moderate pain, regardless of origin (Table 26–3). Acetaminophen has a much lower side-effect profile than the NSAIDs, and is as effective in the treatment of mild to moderate pain of musculoskeletal origin (level of evidence = A). The maximum dose should not exceed 4 g/day and should not exceed 3 g/day in persons with renal or liver disease and those with alcohol misuse disorders. Fixed dose combinations of acetaminophen and opioids (e.g., Percocet, Vicodin) may be useful for mild to moderate pain unrelieved by acetaminophen alone (level of evidence = A).[1]

Nonsteroidal Anti-Inflammatory Drugs

Adding NSAID drugs to acetaminophen when pain is uncontrolled by acetaminophen is rarely warranted. NSAIDs are best reserved for conditions where pain

Table 26–3	Nonopioid Analgesics and Adjuvant Agents for Persistent Pain
Drug	**Considerations**
Nonopioid Analgesics	
Acetaminophen	Hepatotoxic above 4 g/day; reduce dose to 2–3 g/day in kidney or liver disease and with harmful or hazardous drinking; >2 g/day may prolong INR in warfarin use.
Ibuprofen (Motrin, Advil, Nuprin, etc.)	Gastric, renal, platelet dysfunction may be dose dependent; constipation, confusion, headaches; avoid high doses for prolonged time.
Naproxen (Naprosyn)	Similar to ibuprofen.
Salsalate	Check levels during titration and periodically; similar to ibuprofen.
Choline magnesium	Prolonged half-life; similar toxicity to ibuprofen; check levels as for salsalate.
Trisalicylate (Trilisate)	
Celecoxib (Celebrex)	COX-2 inhibitor, GI side effects at higher doses.
Adjuvant Agents	
Desipramine, nortriptyline	Start 10 mg/day dose, titrate 1 to 2 times/week; anticholinergic side effects.
Duloxetine (Cymbalta)	Nausea, dry mouth.
Carbamazepine	Start low daily dose, monitor LFTs, CBC, BMP.
Gabapentin (Neurontin)	Monitor sedation, ataxia, edema; BID dosing usually sufficient in older patients.
Lidocaine 5% patch	Apply to affected area 12 h/day; apply only to intact skin.

has an inflammatory origin. The cyclooxegenase-2 (COX-2) inhibitors have lower gastrointestinal (GI) toxicity (ulcers, bleeding) compared to traditional NSAIDs; however, the withdrawal of refecoxib and valdecoxib from the market raises concern that any of these agents may increase the risk of adverse cardiovascular events. The nonacetylated salicylates are less expensive than COX-2 inhibitors and have somewhat lower GI toxicity than other NSAIDs.

NSAIDs should be avoided in patients with a history of renal insufficiency, peptic ulcer disease, or a bleeding diathesis, and those who are on anticoagulant, antiplatelet, or corticosteroid medications.[16] NSAID use is associated with a 3% to 4% risk of gastrointestinal bleeding among patients with a history of a previous bleeding ulcer.[17] Antacids, misoprostol, histamine-2 (H₂) blockers, and proton pump inhibitors only partially decrease the risk of gastrointestinal bleeding.[1] Short-acting NSAIDs are preferred over longer-acting agents, and all NSAIDs are best when used short-term or on an as-needed basis. Use of more than one NSAID at a time is not advisable (see Table 26–2).

All patients receiving NSAIDs, including those on COX-2 inhibitors, should be monitored closely for side effects. All NSAIDS can cause nausea, dyspepsia, and epigastric discomfort.[17] COX-2 inhibitors are similar to COX-1 inhibitors in producing renal dysfunction. Risk factors for NSAID renal toxicity include age greater than 75, congestive heart failure, dehydration, history of peptic ulcer disease, history of renal disease, hypertension, female gender, and diuretic use while on NSAIDs. Use of diuretics and NSAIDs together can lead to reduced renal blood flow, reduced glomerular filtration rate, and increased sodium retention. NSAIDs reduce renal prostaglandin and rennin secretion and may cause a sudden rise in serum potassium while patients are on ACE inhibitors or potassium-sparing diuretics. Electrolytes and creatinine should be measured before initiating treatment with an NSAID, and repeated in 1 to 4 weeks and periodically thereafter.[18]

Opioids

The use of opioids for persistent noncancer pain has gradually gained acceptance (Table 26–4). The doses used to treat persistent noncancer pain are often much lower than those used for cancer pain. Opioids may be useful for moderate to severe nociceptive pain.[19] It is safest to begin titration with a short-acting opioid given on a routine schedule for continuous pain; this allows the clinician to estimate the dose of the agent to be given as a longer-acting formulation. The long-acting agents are appropriate for continuous pain, and shorter-acting agents are then used for noncontinuous or breakthrough pain. In titrating an opioid analgesic, the number of doses needed for breakthrough pain guides further titration of the long-acting agent.

Monitoring of side effects should focus on CNS effects such as sedation, confusion, or reduced concentration, and others such as nausea and constipation (see Table 26–4). When opioids are initially started,

Table 26–4	Opioid Analgesic Drugs	
Drug	**Aging Effects**	**Precautions and Recommendations**
Short-Acting Drugs		
Tramadol (Ultram)	Older patients may require lower doses. If CrCl <30 ml/min, dose only every 12 h.	Monitor for nausea, dizziness. Use with caution in patients with history of seizure disorders.
Morphine sulfate (Roxanol, MSIR)	Older patients are more sensitive than younger patients to side effects; duration of action is longer.	Start low and titrate to comfort; anticipate and treat constipation.
Codeine (plain codeine, Tylenol with codeine, other combinations)	Reduce dose if CrCl < 50 ml/min.	Monitor for nausea, anorexia; anticipate and treat constipation.
Hydrocodone (Vicoden, Lortab, others)		Start lowest dose in liver disease and titrate; anticipate and treat constipation.
Oxycodone (Roxicodone)	Reduce initial dose by ⅓–½ in debilitated, opioid-naive patients.	Anticipate and treat constipation.
Hydromorphone (Dilaudid)	Reduce dose by 25%–50% of usual adult dose.	Anticipate and treat constipation.
Long-Acting Drugs		
Typically used after initial titration with short-acting opioids.		
Sustained-release morphine (MS Contin, Kadian, Oramorph SR)	Older patients may require lower doses.	Escalate dose slowly because of possible drug accumulation; use immediate-release opioid for breakthrough pain.
Sustained-release* oxycodone (Oxycontin)	Reduce dose if CrCl < 60 ml/min.	Start ⅓–½ usual dose in liver impairment.
Hydromorphone extended release	New agent dosed once daily; very limited experience in geriatric patients.	Consider for use only after titration with short-acting opioids.
Transdermal fentanyl (Duragesic)	Effective activity may exceed 72 h in older patient.	The lower-dose patch is recommended for patients who require 60 mg/day oral morphine equivalent.

mild sedation with minimal cognitive impairment is expected until tolerance develops.[1]

Constipation occurs very frequently with opioids, and a bowel regimen should be initiated when these drugs are used (bulking agents are not effective). Fluids, activity, and osmotic or stimulant agents are recommended. However, motility agents should not be used if there is fecal impaction. When persistent pain diminishes and opioids are no longer needed, tapering should be done by converting to an equivalent dose of a short-acting agent with very slow tapering, perhaps by as little as 10% per month in order to avoid unpleasant withdrawal effects.

> ● Constipation occurs very frequently with opioids, and a bowel regimen should be initiated when these drugs are used (bulking agents are not effective).

Adjuvant therapies

Certain medications that are not formally classified as analgesics can have important pain-relieving properties for specific types of persistent pain, especially neuro-pathic pain (see Table 26–3). These adjuvant analgesic drugs are sometimes used as the primary therapy, but are more often helpful in providing partial pain relief when combined with other strategies (level of evidence = B). Failure to respond to one agent in a class does not predict response to a different agent in that class.

It is always best to consider the safest agents first. Topical capsaicin and 5% lidocaine patches are safe and may be beneficial for local and regional pain syndromes (e.g., postherpetic neuralgia) (level of evidence = A).[1] Of the other adjuvant agents, the largest body of evidence supports the efficacy of the tricyclic antidepressants in persistent pain.[1] Although newer antidepressants are preferred to treat the affective disorders of old age, most have not shown effectiveness for persistent pain. Tricyclic antidepressants have anticholinergic side effects, and should be started at a very low dose. In fact, the effective analgesic dose of these medications is lower than that needed for antidepressant effects. The selective serotonin and norepinephrine reuptake inhibitor duloxetine (Cymbalta®) is approved as both an antidepressant and for treatment of diabetic neuropathy. Nausea is its commonest adverse effect.

Corticosteroids are also used adjunctively for inflammatory conditions (arthritis with moderate pain). Most frequently these are used in low doses of 2.5 to 5 mg of prednisone daily. Chronic use is generally avoided because of side effects such as hyperglycemia, osteopenia, and Cushing's syndrome.

The anticonvulsants may be useful for persistent neuropathic pain. Carbamazepine is used most frequently for the pain of trigeminal neuralgia, with good results. Carbamazepine is started at 100 mg daily and slowly increased. Because leukopenia, thrombocytopenia, and drug-induced hepatitis are significant side effects, complete blood counts and liver function studies must be monitored. Gabapentin may be useful for neuropathic pain syndromes such as diabetic neuropathy, spinal stenosis, postherpetic or trigeminal neuralgia, restless legs syndrome, phantom limb, stump pain, and post-stroke pain.[20] It is generally well tolerated if the dose is started low and slowly titrated. Newer anticonvulsants (oxcarbazapine, tiagabine, topiramate, lamotragine) are undergoing clinical trials for use in persistent pain.[15,20] Mexiletine and clonidine are occasionally used for neuropathic pain; effectiveness is less certain and extra care is needed because of their cardiovascular effects.[20]

Baclofen, a centrally acting muscle relaxant, is useful in the treatment of painful muscle spasms and neuropathic pain in patients with stroke. Patients need to be monitored for urinary retention and weakness.

Nonpharmacologic Therapy

Nonpharmacologic therapy (e.g., exercise, education, cognitive behavioral therapy) should play a role in the management of most patients with persistent pain (Box 26–4). Each has been shown to be effective in improving long-term pain management for older patients.[21] An exercise program tailored to the patient's condition is recommended (level of evidence = A). Moderate levels of aerobic and resistance training improve functional status and pain management in older adults. Training is usually done under supervision for 8 to 12 weeks initially, and the program should be maintained by the patient long term. Patients with specific physical impairments that are contributing to pain should be given a trial of physical or occupational therapy or both to address underlying disorders. Any of these programs should include elements to increase strength, flexibility, and endurance (level of evidence = A). Education of the patient and caregiver on the use of medications, the use of pain rating scales, what can be expected from specific analgesics, and self-help techniques (e.g., heat, cold, massage) improves management and outcomes (level of evidence = A). Cognitive therapies that aim to change thoughts, beliefs, and attitudes regarding the experience of pain are effective (level of evidence = A).[1] Behavioral therapies include relaxation, hypnotherapy, and biofeedback. Together these are known as *cognitive-behavioral therapy*. A series of sessions conducted by a trained specialist can improve coping skills and prevent relapse. The easiest way to access these services is by referral to a formal pain management program.

Chiropractic, acupuncture, and transcutaneous nerve stimulation may benefit some patients. Objective evidence to support these expensive therapies is lacking, and when used should be provided only by a trained professional. Local heat, cold, or massage therapy is inexpensive and sometimes of benefit. The major caution is to instruct patients on the correct use to avoid thermal injury.

Box 26–4	Nonpharmacologic Therapy

- Patient and family education: pain scales, medication use
- Heat, cold, and massage
- Exercise: aerobic and resistance
- Physical or occupational therapy or both
- Cognitive therapies: changing thoughts, beliefs, and attitudes about pain
- Behavioral therapies: relaxation, hypnotherapy, and biofeedback

---

June Morris, Case Discussion

Based on the diagnosis of spinal stenosis, you begin a nonopioid analgesic for Ms. Morris's neuropathic back pain. You select gabapentin (Neurontin) at 100 mg daily and plan to titrate the dose by 100 mg/week to minimize sedative side effects. You schedule a 1-month follow-up appointment, and refer her to a rheumatologist for consideration of agents to treat her symptomatic Paget's disease. When she returns 1 month later, her back pain has improved (she now rates it as mild to moderate with housekeeping activities) on a dose of 200 mg twice daily. She has experienced no significant sedation. She has been started on cyclic therapy with a bisphosphate but has yet to experience significant improvement in her wrist pain. She is obviously tearful and depressed, and a repeat depression scale score documents severe depression. She consents to a trial of an antidepressant. You also refer the patient for a physical therapy evaluation and schedule an appointment in 6 weeks for reevaluation of her mood and pain.

Rebecca Dixon, Case Discussion

Consultation with an endocrinologist confirms your impression that the cause of this patient's slowly healing pelvic fracture is radiation-induced bone injury. You elect to maximize therapy to facilitate healing. Alendronate 70 mg weekly is added, and you increase calcium to 1500 mg and vitamin D to 800 IU. You focus on pain control and patient education. Since her last visit, sequential trials of acetaminophen and celecoxib were both ineffective. After educating the patient on the safety and appropriateness of an opioid analgesic, you initiated oxycodone 5 to 10 mg orally four times daily with fair relief. Today you start oxycontin 10 mg orally twice daily. She is instructed to use oxycodone 5 to 10 mg orally as needed for breakthrough pain, and to keep a record of level of pain with activities and the frequency and dose of oxycodone used for breakthrough pain. Together you decide that improvement is sufficient to allow a referral for physical therapy. For sleep, Benadryl is discontinued, and she is given a titrating dose of trazodone and instructed on sleep hygiene measures. You schedule a return visit for 3 weeks.

SUMMARY

Persistent pain is a common problem in older people and one that is receiving increased attention. The first step that the clinician must take is to understand the cause of the pain, and then use the underlying pathophysiology to select pharmacologic therapies. The impact of persistent pain on function, the severity of the pain, and response of pain to interventions should be recorded and reevaluated systematically. Patients and caregivers benefit from education on pain management. Exercise and cognitive-behavioral training reduce morbidity and keep medications at a minimum while maximizing function. (The reader is referred to the American Geriatrics Society Clinical Practice Guidelines for extensive references and further treatment recommendations.)

References

1. American Geriatrics Society Panel on Persistent Pain in Older Persons. Clinical practice guidelines: the management of persistent pain in older persons. J Am Geriatr Soc 50:S205-224, 2002.
2. Carr DB, et al. Acute Pain Management: Operative or Medical Procedures and Trauma. Rockville, MD: Agency for Health Care Policy and Research, 1992 (AHCPR 92-0032).
3. Cooner E, Amorosi S. The Study of Pain and Older Americans. New York: Louis Harris and Associates, 1992.
4. Elliot AM, et al. The epidemiology of chronic pain in the community. Lancet 354:1248, 1999.
5. Andersson HI, et al. Impact of chronic pain on health care seeking, self care, and medication: results from a population-based Swedish study. J Epidemiol Community Health 53(8):503, 1999.
6. Parmelee PA, Katz IR, Lawton MP. The relation of pain to depression among institutionalized aged. J Gerontol 46:15, 1991.
7. Turner JA, Jensen MP, Romano JM. Do beliefs, coping and catastrophizing independently predict functioning in patients with chronic pain? Pain 85:115, 2000.
8. Zheng Z, et al. Age-related differences in the time course of capsaicin-induced hyperalgesia. Pain 85(1):51, 2000.
9. Lansbury G. Chronic pain management: a qualitative study of elderly people's preferred coping strategies and barriers to management. Disabil Rehabil 22(1-2):2, 2000.
10. Keith RA, et al. The functional independence measure: a new tool for rehabilitation. Adv Clin Rehabil 1:6, 1987.
11. Mahoney FI, Barthel DW. Functional evaluation: the Barthel Index. Md Med J 14:61, 1965.
12. Yesavage JA, et al. Development and validation of a geriatric depression screening scale: a preliminary report. J Psychiatr Res 17:37, 1983.
13. Herr KA, Mobility PR. Comparison of selected pain assessment tools for use with the elderly. Appl Nurs Res 6:39, 1993.
14. Herr K, et al. Evaluation of the faces pain scale for use with elderly. Pain 14:29, 1998.
15. Fine P. Pharmacological management of persistent pain in older patients. Clin J Pain 20:4, 2004.
16. Burris JE. Pharmacologic approaches to geriatric pain management. Arch Phys Med Rehabil 85:3, 2004.
17. Brown JA, Von Roenn JH. Symptom management in the older adult. Clin Geriatr Med 20:4, 2004.
18. Davis M, Srivastava M. Demographics, assessment and management of pain in the elderly. Drugs Aging 20:1, 2003.
19. Jacox A, et al. Management of Cancer Pain. Rockville, MD: Agency for Health Care Policy and Research, 1994 (AHCPR 94-0592).
20. Nikolaus T, Zeyfang A. Pharmacological treatments for persistent non-malignant pain in older persons. Drugs Aging 21:1, 2004.
21. Leland JY. Chronic pain: primary care treatment of the older patient. Geriatrics 54(1):26, 1999.

Web Resources

Public Education Sites

www.painfoundation.org/
www.healthinaging.org/agingintheknow/chapters_ch_trial.asp?ch=19

Professional Information Sites

http://ampainsoc.org/
www.arthritis.org
www.ascp.com/public/pr/pain
www.partnersagainstpain.com
www.geriatricsatyourfingertips.org (chapter on pain)
www.amda.com/clinical/chronicpain
www.ahcpr.gov

POSTTEST

1. Ms. Dixon is seen in follow-up for a slowly healing pelvic fracture. Current therapy is alendronate 70 mg orally weekly, calcium carbonate 500 mg orally three times daily, vitamin D 800 IU orally daily, and oxycontin 10 mg orally twice daily. A review of her pain record shows that she has well-controlled symptoms (minimal to mild pain) except during twice weekly shopping trips and when riding in a car for more than short distances. Which of the following is the most appropriate adjustment to her ongoing therapy?
   a. Oxycodone 5 to 10 mg orally every 3 to 4 hours as needed for pain
   b. Oxycontin 20 mg orally twice daily
   c. Gabapentin 100 mg orally three times daily
   d. Celecoxib 100 mg orally twice daily

2. You evaluate a 73-year-old married man for problems with leg pain. He has a 10-year history of adult-onset diabetes and currently is treated with glipizide 10 mg orally twice daily. He describes a burning sensation in his feet and ankles that causes mild to moderate pain at night but is also mildly symptomatic at other times. The most recent glycosylated hemoglobin was 8% (normal range 4.6% to 6.5%). In addition to improving his diabetes control, which of the following is the most appropriate treatment for this patient?
   a. Oxycodone 5 to 10 mg orally every 3 to 4 hours as needed for pain
   b. Oxycontin 20 mg orally twice daily
   c. Gabapentin 100 mg orally twice daily
   d. Celecoxib 100 mg orally twice daily

3. Ms. Morris returns for follow-up of painful spinal stenosis. Current therapy consists of gabapentin 200 mg orally twice daily, and sertraline 50 mg orally daily. Her mood is good, she is sleeping well, and she rates her pain as mild with household activities. However, she is concerned about ongoing pain, and is fearful about resuming her usual social and volunteer activities. Which of the following is most likely to result in the patient resuming full activities?
   a. Acupuncture
   b. Transcutaneous nerve stimulation
   c. Cognitive-behavioral therapy
   d. Chiropractic care

PRETEST ANSWERS
1. d
2. c
3. c

POSTTEST ANSWERS
1. a
2. c
3. c

Malnutrition and Feeding Problems

Migy K. Mathew and Karen Funderburg

OBJECTIVES

Upon completion of this chapter, the reader will be able to:

- Understand the impact and prevalence of malnutrition and feeding problems in older adults.
- List the risk factors for poor nutritional status in older adults.
- Describe the pathophysiology of malnutrition and feeding problems in older adults.
- List the differential diagnosis for malnutrition and feeding problems in older adults.
- Identify assessment tools and management options to address malnutrition and feeding problems in older adults.

PRETEST

1. Mr. Smith is a 75-year-old male who has been living alone, and has come to your office for a routine physical exam. During the visit you notice that Mr. Smith has lost 15 pounds since his last visit 6 months ago. You decide to get some lab work to investigate the weight loss further. Which of the following is the least useful marker for evaluating nutritional status?
   a. Serum cholesterol
   b. Total lymphocyte count
   c. Serum albumin
   d. Serial weight measurement
   e. Serum pre-albumin

2. An 83-year-old woman presents to your office with complaints of decreased appetite and weight loss. Which of the following is not responsible for reduced calorie intake in older adults?
   a. Inability to obtain food due to social factors, decreased income, social isolation and depression
   b. Illness or medication that can suppress appetite or impair absorption
   c. An increase in senses such as smell and taste that make food more palatable
   d. Increased functional problems that can make it difficult to prepare meals
   e. Improperly fitting dentures

Ms. Robinson, *(Part 1)*

Ms. Robinson is an 85-year-old white female recently widowed and living alone. She was diagnosed with macular degeneration and subsequently had to stop driving. She also has a history of osteoarthritis of the knees and uses a walker intermittently to walk. She is otherwise independent in her activities of daily living (ADLs), but has to ask neighbors for rides to the supermarket or take the bus. She often skips meals, and has lost 10 pounds within the last 4 months.

STUDY QUESTIONS

1. Which factors place Ms. Robinson at an increased nutritional risk?
2. What is Ms. Robinson's risk score and category according to the nutrition screening initiative tool?
3. How common is malnutrition in the ambulatory setting?

PREVALENCE AND IMPACT

Malnutrition, more specifically undernutrition, appears to occur frequently in older adults, and has been associated with adverse health outcomes. The outcome of chronically poor nutritional status and unrecognized or untreated malnutrition is frequently considerable dysfunction and disability,[1] reduced quality of life, premature or increased morbidity and mortality,[2–5] and increased health care cost.[4–6]

When defined as a decrease in nutrient reserve, *malnutrition* is prevalent in 1% to 15% of ambulatory outpatients, in 25% to 60% of institutionalized patients, and in 35% to 65% of hospitalized patients.[7] Review of current incidence data available suggests that unintended weight loss is a more frequent problem, especially in the older outpatient population, than previously thought. Malnutrition has been associated with increased mortality in numerous studies, with weight loss often remaining independently associated with mortality after adjustment for baseline health status, which suggests a potential causal role.[8–11]

Health outcomes other than mortality have also been associated with malnutrition in older adults. Data from National Health and Nutrition Examination Surveys (NHANES) indicated that older women (baseline age 60 to 74, mean 66 years) who lost 5% or more of their body weight over a 10-year follow-up interval had a twofold increase in risk of disability compared to weight-stable women. This risk persisted after adjustment for age, education, smoking, and multiple health conditions.[12]

RISK FACTORS AND PATHOPHYSIOLOGY

Many older adults undergo changes in their lives (e.g., physiological, social, family, environmental, economic) that could affect their nutritional intake. Identifying risk factors for malnutrition helps direct further questioning. These risk factors, listed in Fig. 27–1, are often multiple and synergistic; if left unchecked these risk factors could weaken nutrition status, increase medical complications, and result in loss of independence.[13]

Ms. Robinson, *(Part 2)*

Over the next several months Ms. Robinson notices that she has been feeling more tired and has lost her appetite, although she has well-fitting dentures and is able to eat anything she wishes. During a routine visit she tells her doctor that her favorite foods just aren't appetizing anymore and she feels full faster. On physical exam the doctor notes moderate muscle wasting and generalized weakness as well as chronic arthritic changes. Her recent lab work was significant for the following: albumin = 2.8, cholesterol = 120, and TSH = 15.

STUDY QUESTIONS

1. What are the physiologic factors that may influence her food intake?
2. What is the differential diagnosis for this patient regarding her malnutrition?

Normal Aging Changes

As one passes through the life span, we often see changes in body mass and percentage of body fat. Lean body mass declines at a rate of 0.3 kg/year beginning in the third decade. However, this decrease in lean body mass tends to be offset by an increase in body fat, which continues until at least age 65 to 70.[14,15] Body weight usually peaks at approximately the fifth to sixth decade of life and remains stable until 65 to 70, after which we see a slow decrease in body weight that continues for the remainder of life.[16]

Anorexia of Aging

Food intake is a motivated behavior between internal signals and environmental cues, and this occurs primarily through the senses of olfaction, taste, vision, and hearing. With aging we often see alterations in these hedonic qualities of food, specifically taste and smell.[14,16] The sense of smell declines dramatically with aging, with an increase in odor threshold and a decline in odor identification. Although changes in the sense of taste seem to be less important than changes in the sense of smell, many changes in taste do occur with aging. Among these changes are an increase in taste threshold, difficulty in recognizing taste mixtures, and an increased perception of irritating tastes. These chemosensory changes with aging lead to reduced appetite and subsequent weight loss.[17]

The regulation of appetite is a complex process involving feedback from a number of peripheral signals and the interactions of a variety of neurotransmitters within the central nervous system. Much of the anorexia of aging seems to be related to the changes in gastrointestinal activities that occur with aging,[17–19] with less antral distention, and thus earlier satiety.[17,20,21]

Protein Energy Malnutrition

The physiologic anorexia of aging and its associated weight loss predisposes older persons to develop protein energy malnutrition (PEM). The prevalence rate for PEM is high and has been reported in 15% of community-dwelling older persons, 5% to 12% of homebound patients, 20% to 65% of hospitalized persons, and 5% to 85% of institutionalized older persons.[14] PEM has been defined as the presence of both clinical (physical signs such as wasting, low body mass index) and biochemical (albumin, cholesterol, or other protein changes) consistent with undernutrition.[22] It is a syndrome characterized by a person's having too little lean body mass, secondary to decreased energy or protein being supplied.

Within this PEM syndrome there are two clinical patterns that need to be distinguished: marasmus and kwashiorkor (hypoalbuminemic malnutrition). Marasmus is the PEM syndrome that develops gradually over months or years when energy intake is insufficient. Skeletal muscle, rather than plasma proteins or visceral protein, is metabolized, and thus

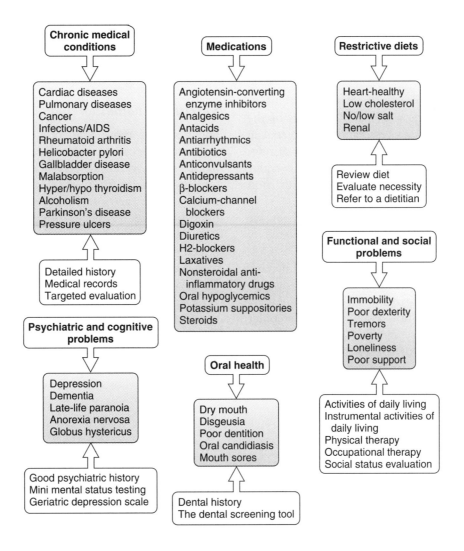

FIGURE 27–1

Risk factors for undernutrition illustrated by clinical approach. *(Redrawn from Omran ML, Salem P. Diagnosing undernutrition. Clin Geriatr Med 18:719–36, 2002, with permission.)*

there is generally a normal serum albumin level. Kwashiorkor is the more acute or subacute type of PEM and is frequently superimposed on marasmus, the precipitant being the stress of acute illness; it may develop over weeks but is often more acute. Due to elevated levels of hormones, monokines, and tumor necrosis factor, serum proteins are depleted, causing consequent edema and frequently no weight loss. Once developed, this PEM syndrome has a high mortality rate.

It must be emphasized that the symptoms and signs of PEM are nonspecific, and other conditions, such as underlying malignancy, malabsorption, hyperthyroidism, peptic ulcer, and liver disease, need to be ruled out.

> ● It must be emphasized that the symptoms and signs of protein energy malnutrition are nonspecific, and other conditions, such as underlying malignancy, malabsorption, hyperthyroidism, peptic ulcer, and liver disease, need to be ruled out.

DIFFERENTIAL DIAGNOSIS AND ASSESSMENT

Nutrition Screening and Assessment

Nutrition screening is the first step in identifying patients who are at risk for nutrition problems or who have undetected malnutrition. It allows for prevention of nutrition-related problems when risks are identified and early intervention when problems are confirmed.[23] Early detection and treatment are not only cost-effective but result in improved health and quality of life of the older patient.[23,24] An approach to the evaluation of weight loss in the elderly is illustrated in Fig. 27–2.

Several screening and assessment tools specific to the older population are available. Regardless of the tool used, the screening process can be completed in any setting. Screening includes the collection of relevant information to determine risk factors and evaluates the need for a comprehensive nutrition assessment.[24]

Nutrition assessments are more comprehensive than nutrition screens and are generally completed by a registered dietitian. The mnemonic ABCD stands for anthropometric, biochemical, clinical, and dietary, the four primary components of a nutrition assessment.[25] Box 27–1 summarizes the most common data collected during a nutrition assessment of an older patient. Assessments vary in their detail and depth depending on the level of risk identified during the screening process, and the amount of information available at the time of the evaluation.

Once the nutrition assessment is complete, it is combined with data from other disciplines to be interpreted and evaluated for the purpose of developing a patient care plan to address identified risks and problems.[24]

Nutrition Evaluation Tools

The need for more than one nutrition evaluation tool exists because the older population can be divided into several subsets, such as the healthy community-dwelling group, those that live in the community but are frail, and those that are institutionalized.[25] Three popular tools developed for older Americans as part of the Nutrition Screening Initiative (NSI) are the DETERMINE Your Nutritional Health Checklist (Table 27–1), and the Level I and Level II screens of the NSI. The NSI was a collaborative effort of the American Dietetic Association, the American Academy of Family Physicians, the National Council on Aging, and 35 other aging agencies. The Checklist tool can be self-administered or used by any member of the health care team. For those patients identified to be at high

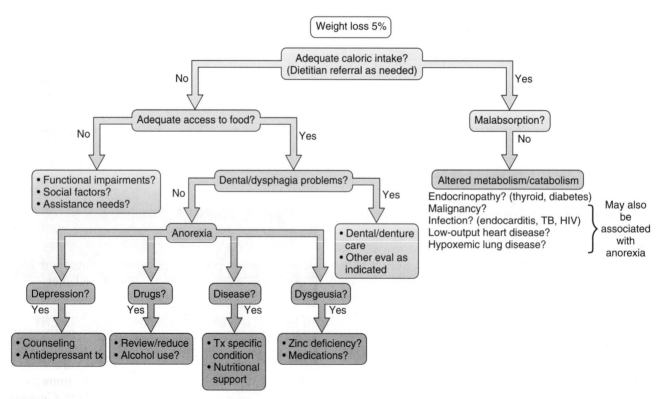

FIGURE 27–2

Weight loss algorithm. (*Redrawn from Wallace JI, Schwartz RS. Involuntary weight loss in elderly outpatients-recognition, etiologies, and treatment. Clin Geriatr Med 13:717–33, 1997, with permission.*)

Box 27-1   Components of a Nutrition Assessment

Anthropometric Measurements
- Body mass index
- Usual adult weight
- Recent weight changes
- Skinfold measurements

Biochemical Analysis
- Complete blood count
- Protein status
- Lipid profile
- Electrolytes
- BUN/creatinine

Clinical Evaluation
- Physical exam
- Chronic conditions
- Current health status

- Oral health and dentition
- Medication use and polypharmacy

Dietary History and Current Intake
- Food preferences and food habits
- Cultural or religious food habits
- Meal frequency
- Lack of control over food selection and choices
- Fluid intake
- Alcohol intake
- Special diet
- Vitamin/mineral/botanical supplement use
- Current intake compared to current nutritional needs
- Chewing and/or swallowing problems
- Functional limitations that impair independence with eating
- Cognitive changes affecting appetite and ability to feed self
- Physiological changes that affect the desire to eat

---

nutritional risk, further information should be obtained by using a more in-depth assessment tool

Table 27-1   Determine Your Nutritional Health

Questions	Yes Points
I have an illness or condition that made me change the kind and/or amount of food I eat.	2
I eat fewer than 2 meals a day.	3
I eat few fruits or vegetables or milk products.	2
I have 3 or more drinks of beer, liquor, or wine almost every day.	2
I have tooth or mouth problems that make it hard for me to eat.	2
I don't always have enough money to buy the food I need.	4
I eat alone most of the time.	1
I take 3 or more different prescribed or over-the-counter drugs a day.	1
Without wanting to, I have lost or gained 10 pounds in the last 6 months.	2
I am not always physically able to shop, cook, and/or feed myself.	2
Total score	
Interpretation of scores	
0–2: Good. Recheck nutritional score in 6 months	
3–5: You are at moderate nutrition risk. Recheck in 3 months.	
6 or more: You are at high nutritional risk. Review with a health care provider.	

such as the Level I and Level II screens, or referring to a registered dietitian.[26]

A tool that is a combination of a quick screen and a detailed assessment is the Mini Nutritional Assessment questionnaire (MNA). It is an evaluation tool using 18 items to assess the malnutrition risk of an older patient.[27] The MNA is only validated for patients over the age of 65.[28] Like the DETERMINE Checklist, the MNA provides a score on the screening section that determines the need for further assessment. Other tools include the Nutritional Risk Index, Nutritional Risk Score, Nutrition Risk Assessment Scale, Prognostic Nutritional Index, and Subjective Global Assessment. The tools vary in their length, type of data collected, and type of older patient being evaluated.

Feeding Problems

An important part of the nutrition assessment is determining barriers to eating a well-balanced diet. The loss of functional ability to eat due to acute or chronic conditions of the oral cavity has an impact on diet and nutritional status.[29] Decayed or missing teeth, ill-fitting dentures, tooth erosion, periodontal disease, gingivitis, xerostomia, taste disorders, and oral infections are factors that can have a significant impact on a patient's willingness or ability to eat.[30] Certain prescription drugs have side effects such as dry mouth, disordered taste, anorexia, nausea, and drowsiness that can also impair the ability and desire to eat.[31]

Edentulous patients are at a disadvantage when attempting to eat fresh fruits and vegetables and high-fiber foods. When a study compared the diets of denture wearers to fully dentate participants, the denture wearers had lower serum levels of beta carotene, vitamin C, and folate as well as lower dietary fiber intakes.[32]

Other problems associated with feeding include general limitations in the ability to self-feed. Conditions that cause tremors or shaking, arthritis, loss of vision, loss of memory, sedation, changes in gastrointestinal tract motility, and generalized weakness can add to the challenges of feeding the older patient a well-balanced diet.[33]

> ● An important part of the nutrition assessment is determining barriers to eating a well-balanced diet.

Swallowing Problems

The prevalence of swallowing disorders is 16% to 22% in adults over the age of 50 and up to 60% in nursing home residents.[34] Subtle changes in upper esophageal sphincter function and peristalsis can result in dysphagia.[35] Changes are associated with normal aging and with stroke, neuromuscular disorders, and central nervous system diseases.[35] Box 27–2 identifies the most common risks for swallowing problems, and Box 27–3 lists screening criteria used to evaluate swallowing problems.[36-38]

MANAGEMENT

Treatment of Common Feeding and Swallowing Problems

Once the assessment process is complete, the patient's plan of care with appropriate interventions is implemented.[24] Treatments may include environmental strategies, diet therapy, counseling, and the use of community services.

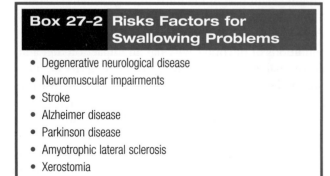

Box 27-2	**Risks Factors for Swallowing Problems**

- Degenerative neurological disease
- Neuromuscular impairments
- Stroke
- Alzheimer disease
- Parkinson disease
- Amyotrophic lateral sclerosis
- Xerostomia

Box 27-3	**Screening Criteria for Evaluating Swallowing Problems**

- Drooling
- Coughing
- Choking
- Changes in voice quality (wet, hoarse)
- Throat clearing
- Difficulty swallowing solids and liquids
- Prolonged eating time
- Pocketing food or medications
- Food or liquid leaking from the nose
- Unusual head or neck posturing while swallowing
- Pain with swallowing
- Decreased oral/pharyngeal sensation

The environment in which meals are served can have an impact on intake. Eating the majority of meals alone is a risk factor for poor nutritional intake.[39] Encouraging companionship at mealtimes for those patients routinely eating alone is a primary strategy for improving nutrient intake. Congregate meal programs established by the Older Americans Act provide a nutritious meal 5 days each week and social interaction for the adult 60 years of age or older.[40] The program is available at no cost and also provides health screens and education. Home-delivered meals are available for those who qualify. Other agencies also provide mobile meals and in-home services. The local Area Agency on Aging can provide additional information.

Problems with the oral cavity, loss of taste and smell, and poor dentition are treated with a variety of food modification strategies. Foods may be mechanically altered by chopping, grinding, or pureeing to minimize or eliminate the need for chewing. Mechanical alteration affects the appeal of foods and may not be well accepted. Every attempt should be made to serve the food in an attractive way. Offering soft, nutritious foods such as fruit and vegetable juices, cooked fruits and vegetables, milk, yogurt, custard, tender moist meats, poultry, fish, and eggs will provide a palatable diet that is familiar to the patient. Food should be well seasoned to accommodate the loss of taste and smell. The patient with xerostomia should keep a water bottle close by and avoid dry and salty foods.[31] Special dishes, drinking cups, and eating utensils are available for patients who are physically impaired.

Feeding problems associated with dementia or Alzheimer's disease consist of problems with cognition and memory along with chewing and swallowing problems. The Alzheimer's Association website has a list of feeding strategies.[41] These include providing an environment that is not distracting such as minimal noise, plain tablecloths or placemats, one food choice at a time, and one eating utensil. As the patient loses the ability to use eating utensils, finger foods are recommended. When the progression of the disease includes chewing and swallowing problems, the appropriate dietary modifications are made or aggressive nutrition support is introduced, if appropriate to the patient's condition and preferences.

The treatment of swallowing problems is an interdisciplinary approach involving the speech pathologist, the dietitian, the nurse, and the physician. Key strategies for successful eating include proper positioning and food consistency. The patient should be sitting up straight with the chin slightly down. Swallowing liquids of thin consistency require the most coordination and control.[38] The registered dietitian should be involved in making recommendations for an appropriate diet, which may range in texture from pudding-like to nearly normal-texture solids, with liquids ranging from spoon thick, to honey-like, nectar-like, and thin. It is critical that food be thickened to the recommended consistency because aspirating food or liquid into the lungs may result in life-threatening aspiration pneumonia.[38] Commercial thickeners and thickened products are available.

> ● Key strategies for successful eating include proper positioning and food consistency.

Ms. Robinson, (Part 3)

Ms. Robinson continues to have slow involuntary weight loss. She has now lost 16 pounds in 7 months. She states she tries to eat, but just doesn't have the energy to prepare meals. Her current diet consists primarily of canned soups, cold cereals, crackers, ice cream, and coffee. About once a week her neighbor will bring her a meal from a local fast food restaurant. Ms. Robinson looks forward to having her neighbor come by and enjoys the fast food meal.

STUDY QUESTIONS

1. List strategies for improving Ms. Robinson's dietary intake.
2. What suggestions can you offer to increase protein and calories in Ms. Robinson's diet?

Nutrition Interventions

When malnutrition is identified and a course of action is planned, the first strategy to consider is a diet that is as liberal as possible without endangering the patient's life. Diet orders that restrict sodium, sugar, and fat can be liberalized to improve the palatability of the diet and thus improve intake.[42]

When patients are not eating enough to maintain weight and nutritional status, the introduction of nutrient-dense foods can be incorporated into the normal diet. Calories can be added without increasing the volume of food eaten. Strategies for increasing calories include adding fat in the form of butter or margarine to hot cereals, vegetables, and breads, using whole milk or half and half in cooking and for beverages, and using full-fat salad dressings and gravies. Carbohydrate calories can be added to beverages by using extra sugar, honey, corn syrup, or a commercial glucose polymer. Dry milk powder or commercial protein powder can be added to milk, creamed soups, hot cereals, and casseroles. Small nutrient dense snacks can boost calories and protein without significantly diminishing intake at mealtime. Suggested snacks include eggnog, custard, pudding, peanut butter with bread or crackers, instant breakfast beverage, ice cream, and homemade milkshakes.

Adding calorie and protein boosters may still require some patients to eat and drink more volume than they desire or are capable of consuming. A variety of commercial supplements are available for these patients. Liquid supplements range from 1 to 2 calories per milliliter or approximately 250 to 500 calories per cup. Protein content ranges from 8 to 20 grams per cup. Supplements that provide 1.5 to 2.0 calories per milliliter help the patient who is having a problem consuming much volume. Commercial supplements also provide micronutrients and the benefits that result from their intake.[15] Disease-specific commercial formulas are also available. Other supplemental dietary products include nutrition bars, fortified cookies, baked products, and even ice cream cups. A registered dietitian can help patients identify recipes and commercial products to meet their specific needs.

Ms. Robinson, (Part 4)

Ms. Robinson is in the hospital with a stroke (CVA). Her swallowing ability is now impaired and she continues to have moderate PEM. It is likely that she will be admitted to a long-term care facility after discharge.

STUDY QUESTIONS

1. How will you meet Ms. Robinson's nutritional needs during her hospital stay?
2. What plans should be made regarding her continued nutrition support after discharge.

Nutrition Support

There comes a time for many patients when they are no longer able to meet their nutritional needs orally. At this point a decision must be made by the patient or caregiver regarding enteral or parenteral nutrition support. The position of the American Dietetic Association on ethical and legal issues in nutrition, hydration, and feeding is an excellent reference to guide the health care team when the wishes of the patient are not known.[43]

When the decision is aggressive nutritional support, enteral nutrition is the first option to consider for the patient who has a functioning gastrointestinal (GI) tract.[31] There are fewer infectious complications with enteral feedings compared to parenteral feedings (level of evidence = Grade A) and enteral feedings are more cost-effective (level of evidence = Grade B).[44] The patient's calorie, protein, fluid, vitamin, and mineral needs are all considered when selecting an enteral formula. Cost and product availability should also be considered.[45]

Parenteral nutrition support is indicated when the patient has an impaired GI tract that prevents enteral feedings.[31] Risks associated with parenteral nutrition in the older patient include impaired glucose tolerance, thin skin, and increased risk of infection.[45]

> ● The position of the American Dietetic Association on ethical and legal issues in nutrition, hydration, and feeding is an excellent reference to guide the health care team when the wishes of the patient are not known.

Case Discussion

Ms. Robinson's case illustrates the classic presentation of an older community-dwelling person with multiple comorbidities (osteoarthritis, macular degeneration, hypothyroidism, depression, etc.), along with physiological changes in aging that may be contributing to her malnutrition. Also, as we often see in this age group, a catastrophic event can often lead to a transition in living situations from independent to long-term care. Ms. Robinson incurs an adverse event that leaves her debilitated and places her at an even greater risk for malnutrition, which will need to be addressed with enteral or parenteral nutritional support, either on a short- or long-term basis.

From this case, it is evident that an interdisciplinary team care approach will be necessary to provide optimal care for Ms. Robinson. The realm of geriatric care extends well beyond the domain of the physician. The responsibility for preservation of health rests not only on the physician but also on other allied gerontologic professionals including nurses, physical therapists, pharmacists, and social workers.

SUMMARY

Age-related changes in physiology, metabolism, and function alter the older person's nutritional requirements. In order to evaluate the nutritional adequacy in older persons, clinicians must understand the general concepts of geriatric nutrition and the parameters of nutritional assessment for this age group. Nutritional care of the older person is indicated across the health care continuum and in all practice settings; therefore, clinicians need to work with other professionals from a variety of disciplines in addressing the nutritional health of older people.

References

1. Galanos AN, et al. Nutrition and function: is there a relationship between body mass index and the functional capabilities of community dwelling elderly? J Am Geriatric Soc 42:368-73, 1994.
2. Brodeur JM et al. Nutrient intake and gastrointestinal disorders related to masticatory performance in the edentuolous elderly. J Prosthet Dent 70:468-73, 1993.
3. Coe RM, et al. Nutritional risk and survival of elderly veterans: a five year follow-up. J Community Health 9:327-334, 1993.
4. Zahler LP, et al. Nutritional care of ambulatory residents in special care units for Alzheimer's patients. J Nutr Elder 12(4):5-19, 1993.
5. McEllstrum MC, Collins JC, Powers JS. Admission serum albumin level as a predictor of outcome among geriatric patients. South Med J 86:1360-2, 1993.
6. Mowe M, Bohmer T. The prevalence of undiagnosed potein-calorie undernutrtion in a population of hospitalized elderly patients. J Am Geriatr Soc 39:1089-92, 1991.
7. Silver AJ. Malnutrition. In Beck JC, ed. Geriatrics Review Syllabus. A Core Curriculum in Geriatric Medicine. Book 1/Syllabus and Questions. New York: American Geriatric Society, 1991:145-52.
8. Pamuk ER, Williamson DF, Serdula MK,, et al. Weight loss and subsequent death in a cohort of US adults. Ann Intern Med 119:744-8, 1993.
9. Satish S, Winograd CH, Chavez C,, et al. Geriatric targeting criteria as predictors of survival and health care utilization. J Am Geriatr Soc 44:914-21, 1996.
10. Sullivan DH, Walls RC, Lipschitz DA. Protein-energy undernutrition and the risk of mortality within 1 year of hospital discharge in a select population of geriatric rehabilitation patients. Am J Clin Nutr 53:599-605, 1991.
11. Wallace JI, Schwartz RS, La Croix AZ,, et al. Involuntary weight loss in older outpatients: incidence and clinical significance. J Am Geriatr Soc 43:329-37, 1995.

12. Launer LJ, Harris T, Rumpel C,, et al. Body mass index, weight change, and risk of mobility disability in middle-aged and older women: the epidemiologic follow-up study of NHANES I. J Am Med Assoc 271:1093-8, 1994.
13. American Dietetic Association. Nutrition, aging, and the continuum of care—position of American Dietetic Association. J Am Diet Assoc 100:580-95, 2000.
14. Morley JE. Anorexia of aging: physiologic and pathologic. Am J Clin Nutr 66:760-73, 1997.
15. Wallace JI, Schwartz RS. Involuntary weight loss in elderly outpatients-recognition, etiologies, and treatment. Clin Geriatr Med 13:717-33, 1997.
16. Morley JE, Thomas DR. Anorexia and aging: pathophysiology. Nutrition 15:499-503, 1999.
17. Morley JE. Pathophysiology of anorexia. Clin Geriatr Med 18:661-73, 2002.
18. Morley JE. The neuroendocrine control of appetite: the role of the endogenous opiates, cholecystokinin, TRH, gamma-amino-butyric-acid and the diazepam receptor. Life Sci 27:355-68, 1980.
19. Morley JE. Neuropeptide regulation of appetite and weight. Endocr Rev 8:256, 1987.
20. Jones KL, Doran SM, Hveem K, et al. Relation between postparandial satiation and antral area in normal subjects. Am J Clin Nutr 66:127-32, 1997.
21. Rayner CK, MacIntosh CG, Chapman IM, et al. Effects of age on proximal gastric motor and sensory function. Scand J Gastroenterol 35:1041-7, 2000.
22. Jensen GL, Powers JS. In Beck JC, ed. Geriatrics Review Syllabus. A Core Curriculum in Geriatric Medicine. Book 1/Syllabus. New York: American Geriatric Society, 2002:191-9.
23. White JV. Risk factors for poor nutritional status in older Americans. Am Fam Physician: 2087-97, 1991.
24. Council on Practice (COP) Quality Management Committee. Identifying patients at risk: ADA's definitions for nutrition screening and nutrition assessment. J Am Diet Assoc 94:838-9, 1994. (errata in J Am Diet Assoc 94:1101, 1994).
25. Dwyer JT, Gallo JJ, Reichel W. Assessing nutritional status in elderly patients. Am Fam Physician 47(3):613-620, 1993.
26. Lipschitz DA, Ham RJ, White JV. An approach to nutrition screening for older Americans. Am Fam Physician 45(2):601-608, 1992.
27. Mini Nutritional Assessment. Nestle Research Center. Nestle Clinical Nutrition 1998. Available at http:// www. nestleclinicalnutrition.com/images/MNA_Assessment.pdf.
28. User's Guide to Completing the Mini Nutritional Assessment. Nestle Clinical Nutrition. Available at http://www.mna-elderly.com/practice/user_guide.htm.
29. Mobley C, Saunders MJ. Oral health screening guidelines for nondental health care providers. J Am Diet Assoc 97:120S-2S, 1997.
30. Touger-Decker R, Mobley CC. Position of the American Dietetic Association: nutrition and oral health. J Am Diet Assoc 103:615-25, 2003.
31. Niedert K, Dorner B, eds. Nutrition Care of the Older Adult, 2nd ed. Chicago, IL: American Dietetic Association, 2004.
32. Nowjack-Raymer RE, Sheiham A. Association of edentulism and diet and nutrition in US adults. J Dent Res 82:123-6, 2003.
33. Worthington-Roberts BS, Williams SR. Nutrition throughout the life cycle. 4th ed. New York: McGraw-Hill, 2000.
34. Firth M, Prather CM. Gastrointestinal motility problems in the elderly patient. Gastroenterology 122:1688-700, 2002.
35. Orr WC, Chen CL. Aging and neural control of the GI tract IV. Clinical and physiological aspects of gastrointestinal motility and aging. Am J Physiol Gastrointest Liver Physiol 283:G1226-G31, 2002.
36. Brody RA, Touger-Decker R, VonHagen S, et al. Role of registered dietitians in dysphagia screening. J Am Diet Assoc 100:1029-37, 2000. 11th ed. Philadelphia: WB Saunders, 2004.
37. Marik PE, Kaplan D. Aspiration pneumonia and dysphagia in the elderly. Chest 124:328-36, 2003.
38. Mahan K, Escott-Stump S. Krause's Food, Nutrition, and Diet Therapy. 11th ed. Philadelphia: Saunders, 2004.
39. Wahlqvist ML, Savige GS. Intervention aimed at dietary and lifestyle changes to promote healthy aging. Eur J Clin Nutr 54:S148-56, 2000.
40. U.S. Department of Health and Human Services, Administration on Aging. Elderly Nutrition Program Fact Sheet. Available at: www.aoa.gov/press/fact/pdf/fs_nutrition/pdf.
41. Alzheimer's Association. Eating Fact Sheet. Available at: http://search.alz.org/Resources/** FactSheets/FSEating.pdf.
42. American Dietetic Association. Position paper of the American Dietetic Association. Liberalized diets for older adults in long-term care. J Am Diet Assoc 102:1316-23, 2002.
43. American Dietetic Association. Position paper of the American Dietetic Association. Ethical and legal issues in nutrition, hydration, and feeding. J Am Diet Assoc 102:715-26, 2002.
44. American Dietetic Association. Evidence Analysis Library. Available at: www.eatright.org.
45. Matarese LE, Gottschlich MM. Contemporary nutrition support practice: a clinical guide. 2nd ed. St. Louis, MO: WB Saunders, 2003.

Web Resources

www.aafp.org/x17367.xml
www.nestleclinicalnutrition.com/ solutions_content_mna.html
www.mna-elderly.com

POSTTEST

1. A recently widowed 74-year-old women presents to your office with depression and fatigue. She has a documented weight loss of 5 pounds since her last visit 3 months ago. She confesses that she has not been preparing meals and eating like she did when her husband was alive. She is not surprised that she has lost weight since her husband died last month. A nutritional assessment confirms that she is still in good nutritional health but is at risk for malnutrition due to depression, eating alone, and social isolation. What is the first nutrition strategy you recommend?
   a. She should consume a commercial high-calorie supplement once or twice a day to prevent further weight loss.
   b. Visit a senior nutrition program.
   c. Move to a retirement home.
   d. Start cooking again.
   e. Volunteer at the local food bank.

2. Your patient is hospitalized due to a CVA. He is at nutritional risk because he has dysphagia as a result of the stroke. The first step to nutrition intervention is to:
   a. Get a swallowing assessment so that the level of food texture and fluid viscosity can be determined for his diet order.
   b. Start enteral feedings via NG tube.
   c. Thicken all liquids to honey-like consistency until a complete assessment can be made.
   d. Start the patient on a liquid nutritional supplement.
   e. Order a general diet.

3. Your 86-year-old nursing home patient can no longer meet her nutritional needs orally and is losing weight. Your first consideration in addressing this situation is to:
   a. Start enteral feedings via PEG tube.
   b. Start parenteral feedings.
   c. Order a nutrition consult.
   d. Check the chart for an advanced directive.
   e. Consult with the patient's family regarding aggressive nutrition support.

PRETEST ANSWERS

1. b
2. c

POSTTEST ANSWERS

1. b
2. a
3. d

Pressure Ulcers

Banu Sezginsoy and Jonelle E. Wright

OBJECTIVES

Upon completion of this chapter, the reader will be able to:

- Describe the pathophysiology of pressure ulcer formation.
- Develop a comprehensive prevention plan addressing pressure ulcer risk factors.
- List the differential diagnostic criteria for pressure ulcer staging.
- Identify management options available for pressure ulcer care.
- Elucidate the complications that compromise pressure ulcer healing.

PRETEST

1. Mr. Lasting, a 92-year-old Caucasian male, recently discharged from the hospital where he was treated for acute cerebral vascular accident, is found supine on the bathroom floor. He is confused and has been incontinent of stool and urine. Physical evaluation reveals a stage II pressure ulcer over the sacrococcigeal area. What is the primary causative factor for his pressure ulcer formation?
   a. Chemical irritation of urine
   b. Unrelieved pressure
   c. Friction
   d. Sensory deficit
   e. Dry skin

2. Mr. Risky, a 94-year-old African-American male, with type II diabetes and its multiorgan complications, is admitted to a nursing home after suffering multiple strokes. He is severely malnourished as a result of aspiration pneumonia, but refuses alternative feeding measures other than oral. Right-sided weakness that is more pronounced in the lower extremity restricts Mr. Risky's mobility. Which of the following can be considered a pressure ulcer risk factor in this patient?
   a. Sensory perception
   b. Moisture
   c. Activity and mobility
   d. Nutrition
   e. All of the above

3. Ms. Holiheel, a 77-year-old Caucasian female with a medical history of coronary artery disease (CAD), hypertension, and restless leg syndrome, was transferred to the extended care unit (ECU) after 3 weeks of treatment for acute stroke with left-sided weakness. While in the hospital, Ms. Holiheel suffered a stage II pressure ulcer over the right heel. In the ECU, you notice that the pressure ulcer now contains necrotic tissue with foul-smelling, greenish drainage. What should you do next?
   a. Culture a swab sample.
   b. Apply topical antibiotics.
   c. Debride using sharp instruments.
   d. Cleanse the wound with antiseptics.
   e. Debride using autolytic methods.

4. Ms. Pickyrite, an only daughter, is the caregiver for a disabled 84-year-old frail lady who is bed-bound and totally dependent for activities of daily living (ADL). One day, she noticed a skin abrasion with mild erythema on both of her mother's heels. Knowing that this was a dangerous sign, Ms. Pickyrite started repositioning her mother every 2 hours and began wound cleansing with hydrogen peroxide on a daily basis to prevent infection. When she did not see any improvement, she increased the frequency of the skin care. Two weeks later, at the end of her wits, Ms. Pickyrite brought her mother to the Emergency Department after she noticed that the wound had several blisters and felt warm over an erythematous area that had significantly expanded in size. Where did Ms. Pickyrite go wrong in managing her mother's pressure ulcer?
   a. Hydrogen peroxide use
   b. Frequency of skin care
   c. Inadequate dressing changes
   d. Inappropriately positioning her mother
   e. Neglecting prophylactic antibiotic treatments

Ms. Jones, *(Part 1)*

Ms. Jones, a frail 85-year-old African American female who is 5'1", 85 pounds (having lost 10 pounds in the last 8 months), was admitted to a nursing home after a long hospitalization for congestive heart failure exacerbated by cardiac ischemia and dysrhythmia. She has hypertension and CAD with an ejection fraction of 35%; she can only sleep in her recliner (>45-degree angle). Ms. Jones suffers severe osteoarthritis, partially managed with analgesics, that limits her mobility. She now takes 15 different medications including amiodarone, and her appetite is poor. Ms. Jones is depressed and spends most of her time in her wheelchair watching TV. She frequently complains of pain, especially when walking, but her pain decreases with rest. Ms. Jones requires assistance with bathing and is incontinent of urine and feces.

STUDY QUESTIONS

1. What are the risk factors for ulcer development?
2. How common is pressure ulcer development in a nursing home setting?

PREVALENCE AND IMPACT

Pressure ulcers, defined as "lesions caused by unrelieved pressure resulting in damage to underlying tissue,"[1] are debilitating and costly complications of immobility that are considered, for the most part, preventable. However, even with the most vigilant care, seemingly insignificant areas of skin discolorations that remain under pressure can quickly develop into serious ulcerations whose complications can lead to death. As a case in point, despite the very best of care, Christopher Reeve, the famous spinal cord–injured actor who played "Superman" in several movies before a serious sporting accident, died in 2004 after a heart attack and subsequent coma suffered during treatment for an infected pressure ulcer.[2] While pressure ulcers can form in individuals of any age, most occur in the elderly; approximately 70% of all pressure ulcers occur in older individuals.[3,4]

Pressure ulcer prevention and treatment interventions cost in the billions of dollars each year in the United States,[4,5] and it is estimated that pressure ulcer–related care can increase health care costs by up to $20,000 per patient admission.[6] Reviews of various clinical databases published between 1990 and 2000 have indicated that incidence rates of pressure ulcers have approached 38% in acute care settings, 40% in critical care units, and 24% in long-term care facilities.[7] Prevalence rates reported during the same time period reached 18% in acute care settings and 28% in long-term care facilities. Certain patient populations may experience even higher risk: the Agency for Health Care Policy and Research (AHCPR) reported that almost two-thirds of quadriplegics or older persons hospitalized for hip fracture suffered pressure ulcers. The problem of pressure ulcers became so serious and widespread that national healthcare policy and funding agencies convened expert panels to develop systematic prevention and treatment strategies for public dissemination. Healthy People 2010, a set of national health objectives developed by the U.S. Department of Health and Human Services to publicize "the most significant preventable threats to health and establish national goals to reduce these threats," includes an objective that targets pressure ulcers: it seeks a 50% reduction in the proportion of nursing home residents with current diagnosis of pressure ulcers by the year 2010.[8]

> ● Even with the most vigilant care, seemingly insignificant areas of skin discolorations that remain under pressure can quickly develop into serious ulcerations whose complications can lead to death.

RISK FACTORS AND PATHOPHYSIOLOGY

Physiology

The skin, the body's largest organ, serves as the barrier between internal and external environments. As illustrated in Figure 28-1 the skin is made up of several layers dispersed throughout the epidermis and dermis.[9] The *outer*most layer of the epidermis is subjected to constant loss in the course of normal daily activities and in response to various diseases, injury, or trauma. The *inner*most layer of the epidermis is where new epithelial cells are generated to replace injured cells. The dermis is made up of important blood vessels, nerves, and lymphatic vessels. Blood vessels deliver oxygen and nutrients, sensory nerves mediate sensory pain, touch, and temperature, and motor nerves monitor arterioles and excretion production. Leukocytes, fibroblasts, mast cells, and macrophages, all cellular components of the dermis, are important in wound repair. Capillary blood flow in the dermis approaches 32 mmHg at the arterial end and 11 mmHg at the venule end. Hydrostatic capillary pressures above 32 mmHg are considered high enough to compromise blood flow to such an extent as to cause tissue ischemia (Fig. 28–1).

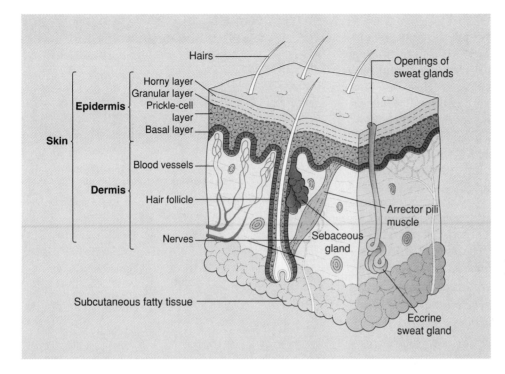

FIGURE 28-1

Basic structure of the skin.
(From Nixon J. The pathophysiology and aetiology of pressure ulcers. In Morison MJ, van Rijswijk L, eds. The Prevention and Treatment of Pressure Ulcers. Edinburgh: Mosby, 2001, with permission.) (See Fig. 3–1 on companion CD-ROM.)

Pathophysiology

Injury to various skin layers can be caused by inflammatory, mechanical, or chemical factors. Normal skin is rarely, if ever, infected by bacterial invasion, but compromised skin frequently becomes colonized with opportunistic organisms. Mechanical injury can occur either to the dermis or epidermis. Dermal damage from local impedance of capillary and lymphatic flow is considered to be associated with prolonged periods of pressurized occlusion and is the classic mechanism of pressure ulcer formation. In contrast, epidermal damage from friction, shear, or laceration caused by various factors such as quickly jerking tape from the skin is not considered an antecedent to pressure ulcer formation but can worsen tissue damage caused by pressure-related compromises in tissue perfusion. Likewise, chemical injury occurs in response to exposing the skin to caustic agents such as feces—alkaline enzymes in stool can irritate skin and cause perianal erosion if not immediately cleansed. Again, while not directly caused by pressure, such skin exacerbations complicate pressure ulcers that have erupted in the epidermis.

Pressure ulcers are the visible evidence of tissue damage caused by pressure-related compromises in dermal blood flow.[10] Pressure, the primary antecedent to impaired skin perfusion, affects individuals differently depending on nutritional status, activity level, body composition, and ability to shift weight to relieve pressure. Fundamental principles of pressure gradients, however, are in play when all pressure ulcers form. When constant force places stress on implicated tissue, resultant pressures are highest at the interface closest to the bony prominence and the soft tissue, not at the skin. Furthermore, when pressure-related anoxia ensues, fat and muscle tissues, which require greater oxygenation than skin does, are more susceptible to injury than skin. Thus, pressure ulcers originate from deep inside, at the juncture of bone and tissue rather than at the skin; such damage from pressure is most quickly manifested where nonpliable surfaces such as bone are closest to the skin. These locations are identified in Fig. 28–2.

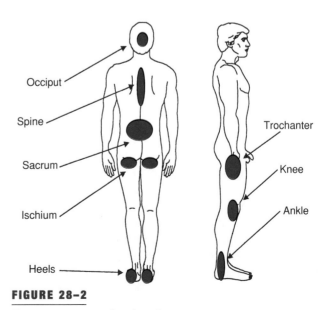

FIGURE 28-2

Common pressure ulcer locations.

Risk Factors

The primary risk factors for pressure ulcers are immobility and limited activity[11] with positioning that exerts unrelieved pressure on tissue confined between nonpliable surfaces. At greatest risk for pressure ulcers are those who are confined to bed or chair and are unable to shift weight or reposition themselves at regular intervals. Additionally, intrinsic and extrinsic etiologic factors[12] that do not actually cause pressure ulcers but do increase the probability that a pressure ulcer will emerge are described in Table 28–1.

Ms. Jones, *(Part 2)*

Two months after Ms. Jones's admission, the charge nurse notices a skin discoloration of a bluish hue on her sacral area. However, no skin tear is noted. Ms. Jones has had difficulty sleeping and now appears restless. Vital signs are stable except for a mild elevation in blood pressure (145/92); labs show mild chronic anemia, her white cell count is 7500 cells/mcl, and her urinalysis is nonsignificant. Daily skin care and appropriate positioning are routinely included in her care plan.

STUDY QUESTIONS

1. What is your differential diagnosis for this patient regarding skin status?
2. Describe the criteria that differentiate the four stages of pressure ulcers.

● At greatest risk for pressure ulcers are those who are confined to bed or chair and are unable to shift weight or reposition themselves at regular intervals.

DIFFERENTIAL DIAGNOSIS AND ASSESSMENT

In addition to a standard history and physical examination, pain assessment, and psychosocial evaluation, specific assessment strategies relative to pressure ulcers are instituted for two purposes: risk factor identification and pressure ulcer evaluation. AHCPR clinical practice guidelines recommend that all bed- or chair-bound patients be assessed upon admission to healthcare services and periodically re-evaluated for risk factors such as those identified in Table 28–1. Assessments should also be performed whenever an important change in patient status is

Table 28–1	Extrinsic and Intrinsic Risk Factors for Pressure Ulcer Occurrence	
Factor	**Example**	**Selected Consequences**
Intrinsic		
Immobility	Foot in cast	Constant pressure, poor circulation
Low body mass	Low body weight	No padding on bony prominences
Moisture	Incontinence, night sweats	Chemical irritation, skin erosion
Poor nutritional status	Protein malnourished	Decreased immunity; dehydration
Decreased consciousness	Dementia	Immobility, unable to reposition
Decreased sensory perception	Peripheral neuropathies	Unable to feel pain or tingling
Smoking[13]	Cigarettes, cigars, pipes	Poor tissue perfusion
Extrinsic		
Direct pressure	Heel of foot supported on bed foot board for 3 hours	Capillary and lymphatic occlusion when vessel lumen is compressed
Shear force	Skin of back is stuck to sheets after patient has slid down in bed when head of bed is elevated	Tissue is displaced laterally by traction on skin that bends vessels to angles that cause tissue anoxia
Friction	Pulling rather than lifting a patient up in bed	Epidermal abrasions

noted. Use of validated standardized assessment tools such as the widely available Braden Scale for Predicting Pressure Sore Risk[14] and the Norton Risk Assessment Scale[15] will assist clinicians to address these risk factors in a comprehensive and systematic manner.

Evaluation of existing pressure ulcers is also accomplished using a systematic method because information obtained during the assessment process becomes the basis for treatment and management decisions. The pressure ulcer should be assessed for location, size, depth, exudate type and amount, necrotic tissue color and amount, presence of sinus tracts, undermining, tunneling, and formation of granulation tissue and epithelialization. The quality of surrounding skin should also be examined. Published tools such as the Pressure Sore Status Tool[16] or the Pressure Ulcer Scale for Healing[17] can help clinicians conduct and document a comprehensive assessment of the pressure ulcer in an organized manner. Once important characteristics of the ulcer have been assessed, pressure ulcers are routinely classified into four categories using a widely disseminated pressure ulcer staging system that is recommended by pressure ulcer advisory panels and AHCPR clinical practice guidelines. In Table 28–2, the four pressure ulcer stages are identified and characterized, and helpful diagnostic tips are presented.

Despite clearly being useful, it should be noted that accurately "staging" pressure ulcers can be challenging. It is difficult to identify stage I pressure ulcers in darkly pigmented skin. Innocuous-appearing skin changes (e.g., localized edema or warmth) that also serve as indicators of stage II pressure ulcers can easily be missed. Third, irregularities such as undermining or sinus tracts in open pressure ulcers can make it very difficult for clinicians to accurately differentiate stage III and IV pressure ulcers.

Ms. Jones, *(Part 3)*

Ms. Jones went on pass to spend Christmas with her son's family. Days later, when she is brought back to the nursing home, her son described a fall episode in which he found his mother on the floor unable to move. She neither remembered how long she stayed on the floor nor how she fell, but refused to go to the Emergency Department despite complaining of pain on her side. Ms. Jones's physical examination now reveals an open wound on her left trochanteric area that extends through the dermis and subcutaneous tissue. Her left ankle has some abrasions but is not warm to the touch.

STUDY QUESTIONS

1. What is the stage of Ms. Jones's pressure ulcer?
2. What are the most common sites for pressure ulcer development?

MANAGEMENT

Pressure ulcer management includes strategies to prevent ulcers from deteriorating and treatments to promote healing in existing ulcers. A systematic program of careful assessment, early recognition, and comprehensive treatment can prevent nearly all stage IV pressure ulcers.[21] But when pressure ulcers do deteriorate to advanced stages, they are associated with substantial morbidity and complications, and treatment is problematic.[22] Published reports assert that the costs of a comprehensive prevention program, while seemingly substantial, prove considerably less than the costs of wound care compounded by the costs of treating the comorbidities associated with stage IV pressure ulcers.[21] Researchers also document that systematic prevention programs can decrease hospital-acquired pressure ulcers 34% to 50%.[23]

Too frequently, aggressive and expensive interventions are implemented without attention to basic care such as adequate nutrition, good hygiene, and proper positioning.[22] Skin care, nutritional support, and pressure reduction strategies should be implemented for all patients who present with or are at risk for a pressure ulcer.

Table 28–2	Pressure Ulcer Staging	
Stage	**Characteristic**	**Differential Diagnostic Tips**
I	Observable pressure-related alteration of unbroken skin that differs from adjacent or opposite area of skin in: - Temperature (warm vs. cool) - Tissue consistency (firm vs. boggy feeling) - Sensation (pain or itchiness) Induration, hardness, or edema may also be present.	Stage I pressure ulcer areas do not blanch when pressed. Convex glass lens can be used to differentiate unblanchable from blanchable skin.[18] Appearance differs with skin tone: - In lightly pigmented skin, area will appear persistently red (usually, redness should clear within 30 minutes after area is relieved of pressure; if redness persists, a pressure ulcer has begun).[19] - In darker skin tones, area will appear with persistent red, blue, or purple hues.[20]
II	Superficial ulcer with partial thickness skin loss involving epidermis, dermis, or both.	Could look like an abrasion, blister, or shallow crater.
III	Full thickness skin loss involving damage or necrosis in subcutaneous tissue that may extend down *to*, but not *through*, underlying fascia.	Looks like a deep crater with or without undermining of adjacent tissue.
IV	Full thickness skin loss with extensive destruction, necrosis, or damage in muscle, bone, or support structures such as tendons and joint capsules	Undermining and sinus tracts may also be present, making assessment more difficult.

● A systematic program of careful assessment, early recognition, and comprehensive treatment can prevent nearly all stage IV pressure ulcers.

Skin Care

Skin care includes frequent and thorough assessment, basic hygiene, and protecting at-risk areas from harmful friction and shear. Careful inspection of body sites at high risk for pressure ulcer formation should be performed daily. Skin should be kept clean, well hydrated to prevent cracking, and without excessive moisture; regularly bathing with warm water and a mild cleansing agent helps minimize skin dryness. Heat lamps are contraindicated; their use dries tissue and increases local temperature and, thus, metabolic demand of the target area. Vigorous scrubbing or friction should be avoided, and cleansing should be performed as frequently as needed to keep the skin clean and dry, especially when the patient experiences sweating or is incontinent. High temperature, humidity, and massages over bony prominences should also be avoided to prevent skin injury. Last, non–alcohol-based moisturizing agents should be used.[24] Specific strategies to reduce harmful friction and shear are summarized in Box 28–1.

Nutrition

Nutritional compromises increase pressure ulcer risk and delay healing[25]; consequently, a dietary consult should be requested for every patient at risk for pressure ulcers. Careful nutritional assessments should be performed and nutritional deficits remedied. Nutritional strategies used to prevent and treat pressure ulcers are listed in Box 28–2.

The role of specific nutrients in pressure ulcer care is detailed in Table 28–3.[26]

Pressure Reduction

Strategies for pressure reduction over bony prominences and other vulnerable skin sites are very important, especially when the patient is immobile or bed- or chair-bound. Tissue perfusion is dramatically compromised when pressure applied for extended periods of time constricts tissue between nonpliant surfaces. This is especially true in patients with diabetes, vascular disease, anemia, hyperthermia, low skin temperature, low blood pressure, poor circulation, and low serum protein.[27] Donut cushions should be avoided; their use can cause tissue ischemia. Strategies to reduce pressure on vulnerable body sites, especially bony prominences, are listed in Box 28–3.

Box 28-1 Strategies to Reduce Injury from Friction and Shear	
Strategies	**Level of Evidence for Effectiveness**
Elevate head of bed <30 degrees.	C
Transfer patient by lifting, not pulling.	C
Turn patient using lift sheets, trapezes, and so on to avoid sliding on sheets.	C
Use dry lubricants such as corn starch.	C
Use protective films (e.g., transparent film dressings, skin sealants, hydrocolloids), protective padding, or dressings.	C

From National Pressure Ulcer Advisory Panel. Statement on pressure ulcer prevention. Rockville, MD: Agency for Health Care Policy and Research, U.S. Department of Health and Human Services, Public Health Service, 1992.

Box 28-2 Nutritional Strategies in Pressure Ulcer Prevention and Treatment	
Strategies	**Level of Evidence for Effectiveness**
Nutritional assessment: weight, food and fluid intake, laboratory values	B
Dietary consultation	B
Nutritional intake of energy (30–35 kcal/kg), protein (1–1.5 g/kg), fluid (1 mL/kcal)	B
Replete vitamins and minerals if depleted	C
Supplementary support when indicated: parenteral or oral supplements, tube feeding	D

From Schols JMGA, Ende MA. Nutritional intervention in pressure ulcer guidelines: an inventory. Nutrition 2004;20:548–53, with permission.

Table 28–3 Function of Various Nutritional Elements in Wound Healing

Element	Function	Deficiency Effect
Protein	Cell proliferation, collagen metabolism	Delayed healing
Carbohydrate	Energy Source	Altered leukocyte function
Fats	Membrane function	Not known
Vitamin C	Enzyme cofactor in collagen metabolism	Scurvy, altered collagen formation, delayed healing
Vitamin A	Antagonizing effect on steroids	Not well known
Thiamine	Energy metabolism	Decreased cell proliferation and collagen metabolism
Vitamin E	Stabilization of membranes	None known
Vitamin K	Coagulation cofactor	Bleeding, hematoma, wound disruption
Water and salts (sodium, potassium, chloride)	Membrane function, hydration	Volume depletion, decreased tissue perfusion
Phosphorus	Adenosine triphosphate metabolism	Altered cell replication and protein metabolism
Calcium, magnesium, manganese	Enzyme cofactors in collagen metabolism	Altered collagen formation, delayed healing
Zinc	Ribonucleic acid metabolism	Altered cell replication, delayed healing
Iron, copper	Enzyme cofactors in collagen metabolism	Delayed healing, anemia

Box 28-3 Strategies to Reduce Pressure

Strategies	Level of Evidence for Effectiveness
Properly align patient position so as not to exert pressure on at-risk or affected sites.	C
Use appropriate physical or occupational therapy to increase activity levels.	C
Frequent reposition/turn: at least every 2 hours in those with normal circulation, and more frequently in those with circulation problems; every 15–20 minutes while sitting.	C
Elevate head of the bed <30 degrees; incline body 30 degrees laterally when positioned on side.	C
Place cushioning devices between legs and ankles.	C
Use pressure-reducing pillows or mattresses if bed-bound: foam, static or alternating air, gel, water, or low air loss.	C

From National Pressure Ulcer Advisory Panel. Statement on pressure ulcer prevention. Rockville, MD: Agency for Health Care Policy and Research, U.S. Department of Health and Human Services, Public Health Service, 1992.

Ms. Jones, *(Part 4)*

When Ms. Jones's pressure ulcer deteriorated, regular wound cleansing was instituted with dressing changes. Daily physical therapy was initiated and Ms. Jones is frequently repositioned while in bed. Unfortunately, Ms. Jones is neither motivated nor compliant with these measures; at night she still sleeps partially sitting up in her recliner. Ms. Jones's nurse has just called you about a fever of 101°. Ms. Jones's blood pressure is 84/45 and her pulse, 110–135. She is confused. Upon examination, you note that her nonhealing trochanteric pressure ulcer has increased drainage. You transfer Ms. Jones to acute care for further management and close monitoring.

STUDY QUESTIONS

1. What are the most common complications of nonhealing pressure ulcers?
2. What should you do if the ulcer does not respond to 2 weeks of topical antibiotics?

● Donut cushions should be avoided; their use can cause tissue ischemia.

ULCER TREATMENT

Ulcer treatment necessitates eliminating factors that impede healing, optimizing wound conditions for healing, and minimizing the patient's distress during treatment. Bacteria, necrosis, and imbalance in moisture, pH, and temperature are detrimental to healing and can exacerbate painful stimuli associated with wounds. Treatment modalities that minimize these factors include wound cleansing, debridement, dressings, and controlling infection.

All pressure ulcers are contaminated and most are colonized. Some experts assert that wound colonization with small amounts of bacteria can actually help improve wound healing by causing increased local blood flow, angiogenesis, and granulation.[28] However, when colonization exceeds the host's immune response, infection develops and wound healing is impaired. Risk of infection increases when wounds are not kept clean or necrotic tissue is allowed to serve as a fertile harbor for infectious organisms.

> ● All pressure ulcers are contaminated and most are colonized.

Wound Cleansing

Warm normal saline or water should be used to rid an ulcer of microorganisms and devitalized tissue because topical antiseptics, soaps, and antimicrobial solutions that are appropriate for use on intact skin can damage tissue in open wounds. For example, antiseptics that act by invading the cell wall of the target organism also invade fibroblasts and macrophages. Hydrogen peroxide produces oxygen bubbles that agitate the wound surface to loosen microorganisms and debris; while effective, it damages fibroblasts. Iodine solutions that reduce bacterial counts have been shown to be toxic to fibroblasts, neutrophils, and red blood cells.

The temperature, volume, and force of irrigation used to cleanse a pressure ulcer are also very important. Irrigation solutions should be mildly warm so as not to cause local hypothermia that is detrimental to mitogenesis and phagocyte activity and should be of sufficient volume and force to dislodge and wash away germs and debris without causing damage to healthy tissue. Experts suggest that a safe range of irrigation pressure is 4 to 15 psi, which is the median force of flushing liquid through a 19-gauge angiocatheter from a 35-ml syringe.[28]

Debridement

If a considerable quantity of nonviable or infected tissue remains in the wound after cleansing, debridement is indicated and the method used depends on the patient's physical status, the location, type, and amount of tissue to be removed, and the damage caused to surrounding tissue by the debridement method. It should be noted that the more aggressive the debridement method, the shorter the time it takes to remove tissue and vice versa. Various debridement methods are described in Table 28–4.

Wound Dressings

Broken skin exposes underlying tissue to infectious agents and allows local hypothermia and evaporation of moisture needed to maintain tissue, minimize local pain, and promote healing. Dry wound tissue can result in dehydration necrosis; conversely, an appropriately moist, warm ulcer bed optimizes epithelial cell proliferation, improves phagocyte activity, and promotes cell migration needed for healing. Decisions regarding what dressings to use are made in light of ulcer condition (e.g., presence of granulation, necrotic tissue, slough, etc.), type and amount of drainage, microbial status, and quality of surrounding skin.

Controlling Infection

Infection is the most frequent complication of pressure ulcers. Signs of infection include inflammation, increased exudate, foul odor, fever, leukocytosis, greater numbers of neutrophils, and positive cultures of biopsies (swabs frequently indicate colonization rather than

Table 28–4	Debridement Techniques Listed in Ascending Order of Invasiveness		
Type	**Means of Necrosis and Debris Removal**	**Selectivity**	**Rapidity**
Autolytic	Digested by endogenous enzymes retained on wound surface by moisture-retentive dressings	High	Slow
Chemical	Digested by proteolytic agents retained on wound surface by moisture-retentive dressings	High	Slow
Mechanical	Scrubbing with gauze, irrigating with higher pressures, whirlpool, wet-to-dry dressings	Low	Moderate
Sharp	Manual removal using scalpel or scissors (can be performed in patient room)	Moderate	Moderate
Surgical	Major surgical procedure followed by grafting	Moderate	High

infection and can result in too many false positive findings; aspirations can be low in sensitivity[29]).

Antibiotics should be used judiciously. Use of topical antibiotics is controversial; they can be toxic to healthy tissue and often prove ineffective for the mixed flora found in pressure ulcers. If a clean ulcer does not show signs of healing despite 2 to 4 weeks of treatment, however, a triple antibiotic or silver sulfadiazine can be tried for a couple of weeks.[5] Systemic antibiotics are frequently ineffective in wounds colonized by skin flora, and delivery of systemic antibiotics to infected pressure ulcers sites is impeded by the impaired tissue perfusion that originally caused the ulcer. They are, however, necessary in cases of confirmed bacteremia, sepsis, osteomyelitis, and cellulitis. An excellent algorithm used to facilitate pressure ulcer wound care decisions is presented in Fig. 28–3.

> ● Use of topical antibiotics is controversial; they can be toxic to healthy tissue and often prove ineffective for the mixed flora found in pressure ulcers.

Minimizing Pain

While ulcer debridement and dressing changes can be painful, pressure ulcer pain can also be present during periods of inactivity. Pressure ulcer-related pain has been shown not to respond well to oral analgesics, so other means including relaxation techniques, should be implemented as necessary; patients need not experience pain relative to pressure ulcers. Pain-reducing interventions should be modified according to the patient's verbalization of pain and, in the case of intractable pain, formal pain management services may be consulted.

Patient Education

Patient education facilitates adherence to treatment regimens and helps patients and families become active participants in their care. Patients' understanding of pressure ulcer care can lead to significant reductions in pressure ulcer incidence, and patients' caregivers should become knowledgeable in the prevention and treatment of pressure ulcers. Several published educational programs and guidelines are available for clinicians as well as patients. Important topics to teach are listed in Box 28–4.

Case Discussion

Ms. Jones's case is a common presentation of a nursing home admission. Any acute care admission involving an elderly individual with multiple comorbidities should be considered as an important

stress factor that often results in deconditioning and a decrease in the ability to perform ADLs. Therefore, patients should undergo comprehensive evaluation for pressure ulcer risk on each admission and with changes in medical condition. Ms. Jones's medical problem list includes congestive heart failure, peripheral vascular disease, poorly managed severe osteoarthritis, poor nutritional status, urinary incontinence, and depression. Her skin color makes it challenging to diagnose and stage her pressure ulcer. The patient's compliance with the pressure ulcer care plan is very important and requires a multidisciplinary approach involving:

> *Geropsychologist—depression management*
> *Dietary—nutrition management*
> *Physical therapy—regular exercise to reduce pressure*
> *Physician—control of chronic medical conditions*
> *Pain management—osteoarthritis management to improve mobility*
> *Wound care nurse—regular skin care for pressure ulcer*
> *Pharmacist—medication review*

Ms. Jones's lack of motivation secondary to untreated depression, poorly controlled osteoarthritic pain, and ongoing poor nutritional status needs to be addressed in her plan of care. This should be evaluated and monitored regularly by the interdisciplinary team with action plans provided.

Ms. Jones's stage I pressure ulcer is managed with pressure reduction, which prevents the progression. Her fall episode during her recovery period led this vulnerable patient to develop an advanced pressure ulcer. Ongoing poor medical status, along with poor mobility, caused a nonhealing pressure ulcer complicated with infection and sepsis.

SUMMARY

Elderly patients who experience immobility and decreased activity are at high risk for pressure ulcers and serious complications that can quickly become lethal. When pressure ulcers deteriorate to advanced stages, they are associated with substantial morbidity and treatment is problematic. While the costs of preventative measures might seem substantial, they prove considerably less than the costs of wound care compounded by the costs of treating complications

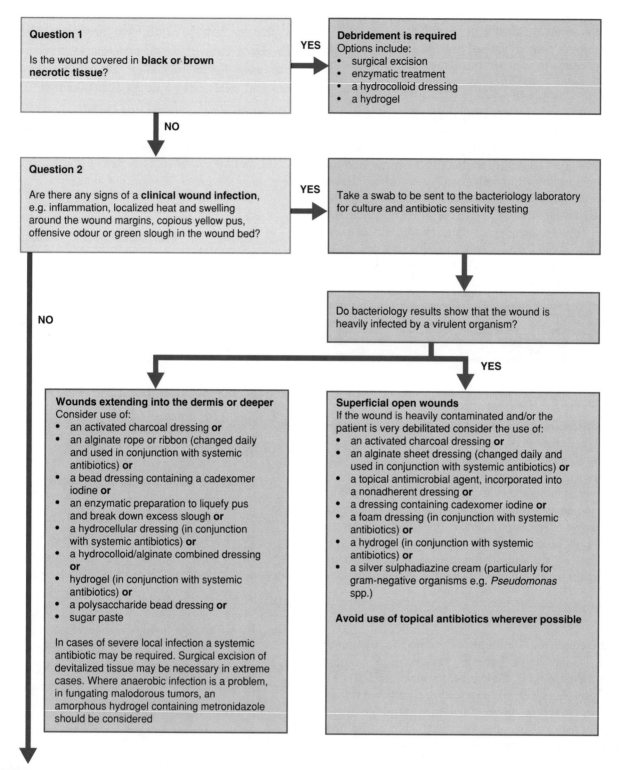

FIGURE 28–3

Selecting a wound care product. (*Modified from Ovington L. Wound management: cleansing agents and dressings. In Morison MJ, van Rijswijk L, eds. The Prevention and Treatment of Pressure Ulcers. Edinburgh: Mosby, 2001, pp. 144–146 with permission.*)

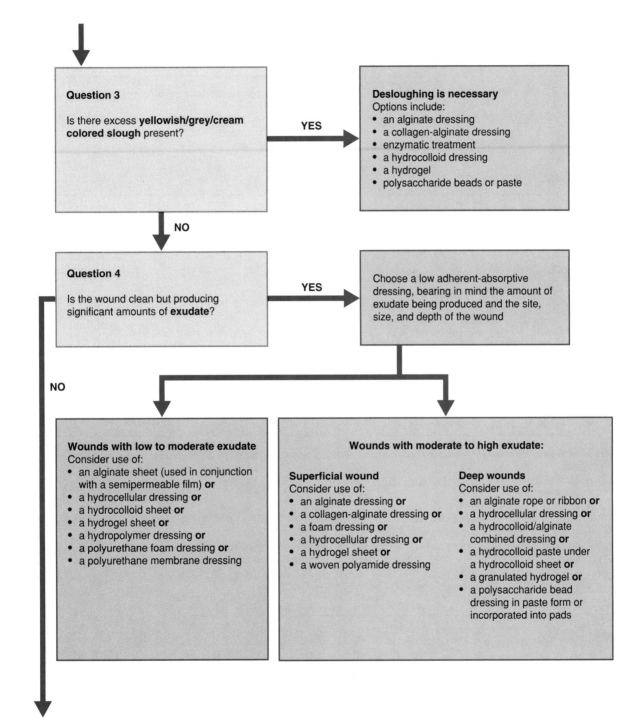

FIGURE 28-3—Cont'd

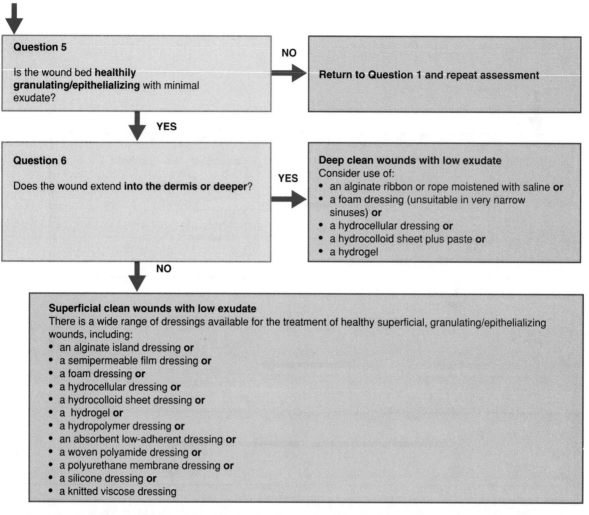

In addition to the nature of the wound bed, many other factors should be considered before a dressing is selected, including:

- the site of the wound and ease of applying the dressing
- the size of the wound
- the frequency of dressing changes required
- comfort and cosmetic considerations
- where and by whom the dressing will be changed
- the availability of the dressing, in the size required – not all dressings are available to patients whose wounds are being managed in the community, and where the dressing is available may not be available in all sizes.

Where all other considerations are equal, choose the cheapest dressing.

Before using any wound care product for the first time **ALWAYS** consult the manufacturer's recommendations, contraindications, precautions and warnings. This information can change, so it is worth re-reading the manufacturer's instructions at frequent intervals. For 'prescription only' wound care products, the relevant product data sheets **MUST** first be consulted prior to use.

If there is still any doubt about the suitability of any dressing, the patient's doctor should be consulted and further advice obtained from the local pharmacist.

FIGURE 28–3—Cont'd

Box 28-4   Patient Education Topics

- Characteristics of healthy versus damaged skin
- Pressure ulcer risk factors and prevention strategies
- Skin assessment, care, and cleansing
- Good nutrition for pressure ulcer prevention and treatment
- Techniques for relieving pressure: turning, positioning, devices, support surfaces
- Techniques to prevent injury from friction and shear
- Pain relief

From National Pressure Ulcer Advisory Panel. Statement on pressure ulcer prevention. Rockville, MD: Agency for Health Care Policy and Research, U.S. Department of Health and Human Services, Public Health Service, 1992.

associated with serious pressure ulcers. Prevention involves a systematic program of careful assessment, early recognition, and comprehensive risk reduction and treatment. Risk factors can be identified using standardized assessment tools and treatment strategies should be delegated to all members of the multidisciplinary care team. In the event of pressure ulcer formation, careful and systematic assessment can guide the clinician in providing individualized care and appropriate wound management.

References

1. Treatment of Pressure Ulcers Guideline Panel. Treatment of pressure ulcers clinical practice guideline. Rockville, MD: Agency for Health Care Policy and Research, U.S. Department of Health and Human Services, Public Health Service, 1994.
2. Holley J. Christopher Reeve, 1952-2004, a leading man for spinal cord research. Washington Post, October 12, 2004.
3. Lyder CH, Preston J, Grady JN, Scinto J, Allman R, Bergstrom N, et al. Quality of care for hospitalized Medicare patients at risk for pressure ulcers. Arch Intern Med 161(12):1549-54, 2001.
4. Langemo DK, Anderson J, Volden C. Uncovering pressure ulcer incidence. Nurs Manag 34(10):54-7, 2003.
5. Norman RA, Bock M. Wound care in geriatrics. Dermatol Ther 16:224-30, 2003.
6. Meraviglia M, Becker H, Grobe SJ, King M. Maintenance of skin integrity as a clinical indicator of nursing care. Adv Skin Wound Care 15(1):24-9, 2002.
7. National Pressure Ulcer Advisory Panel. Pressure ulcers in America: prevalence, incidence, and implications for the future. An executive summary of the National Pressure Ulcer Advisory Panel monograph. Adv Skin Wound Care 14(4):208-15, 2001.
8. U.S. Department of Health and Human Services. Healthy People 2010 Online Documents. Available at: www.healthypeople.gov/document. Accessed January 12, 2005.
9. Alterescu V, Alterescu K: Etiology and treatment of pressure ulcers. Decubitus 1(1): 28-35, 1988.
10. Thomas DR, Kamel HK. Wound management in postacute care. Clin Geriatr Med 16(4):783-804, 2000.
11. Panel for the Prediction and Prevention of Pressure Ulcers in Adults. Pressure ulcers in adults: prediction and prevention clinical practice guideline. Rockville, MD: Agency for Health Care Policy and Research, U.S. Department of Health and Human Services, Public Health Service, 1992.
12. Russell L. Physiology of the skin and prevention of pressure sores. Br J Nurs 7(18):1084, 1088-92, 1096 passim, 1998.
13. Guralnik JM, Harris TB, White LR, Cornoni-Huntley JC. Occurrence and predictors of pressure sores in the National Health and Nutrition Examination survey follow-up. J Am Geriatr Soc 36(9):807-12, 1988.
14. Braden BJ, Bergstrom N. Clinical utility of the Braden Scale for predicting pressure sore risk. Decubitus 2(3):44-51, 1989.
15. Norton D. Calculating the risk: reflection on the Norton Scale. Decubitus 2(3):24-31, 1989.
16. Bates-Jensen BM, Vredevoe DL, Brecht ML. Validity and reliability of the Pressure Sore Status Tool. Decubitus 5(6):20-8, 1992.
17. National Pressure Ulcer Advisory Panel. Push Tool 3.0. Available at: www.npuap.org/push3-0.html. Accessed January 12, 2005.
18. Halfens RJG, Bours GJJW, Van Ast W. Relevance of the diagnosis "stage 1 pressure ulcers" in acute care and long-term care hospital populations. J Clin Nurs 10:748-57, 2001.
19. Lindsey L, Klebine P, Oberheu AM. Prevention of pressure sores through skin care. Spinal Cord Injury Information Network, University of Alabama. Available at: www.spinalcord.uab.edu. Accessed January 12, 2005.
20. National Pressure Ulcer Advisory Panel. Stage I assessment in darkly pigmented skin. Available at: www.npuap.org/positn4.html. Accessed January 12, 2005.
21. Brem H, Lyder C. Protocol for the successful treatment of pressure ulcers. Am J Surg 188(1A Suppl):9-17, 2004.
22. Smith DM. Pressure ulcers in nursing homes. Ann Intern Med 123(6): 433-42, 1995.
23. Barczak CA, Barnett RI, Childs EJ, Bosley LM. Fourth National Pressure Ulcer Prevalence Survey. Adv Skin Wound Care 10(4):18-26, 1997.
24. National Pressure Ulcer Advisory Panel: Statement on pressure ulcer prevention. Rockville, MD: Agency for Health Care Policy and Research, U.S. Department of Health and Human Services, Public Health Service, 1992.
25. Horn SD, Bender SA, Bergstrom N. Description of the National Ulcer Long-Term Care Study. J Am Geriatr Soc 50(11):1816-25, 2002.
26. Schols JMGA, Ende MA. Nutritional intervention in pressure ulcer guidelines: an inventory. Nutrition 20(6):548-53, 2004.
27. Nixon J. The pathophysiology and aetiology of pressure ulcers. In Morison MJ, van Rijswijk L, eds. The Prevention and Treatment of Pressure Ulcers. Edinburgh: Mosby, 2001, pp. 17-36.
28. Ovington L. Wound management: cleansing agents and dressings. In Morison MJ, van Rijswijk L, eds. The Prevention and Treatment of Pressure Ulcers. Edinburgh: Mosby, 2001, 135-154.
29. Livesley NJ, Chow AW. Infected pressure ulcers in elderly individuals. Aging Infect Dis 33:1390-6, 2002.

Web Resources

1. National Pressure Ulcer Advisory Panel, Pressure Ulcer Prevention Points: www.npuap.org/PDF/preventionpoints.pdf.
2. National Library of Medicine, Clinical Practice Guideline: www.ncbi.nlm.nih.gov/books/bv.fcgi?rid=hstat2.section.4521.
3. National Pressure Ulcer Advisory Panel, Push Tool 3.0: www.npuap.org/push3-0.html.

POSTTEST

1. Ms. Posture is a 93-year-old Japanese, bed-bound nursing home resident with advanced Alzheimer's dementia. She is totally dependent for ADLs. What would be the appropriate measures for pressure relief with this patient?
   a. Repositioning every 2 hours
   b. Elevation of the head of the bed less than 30 degrees
   c. Placement of cushioning devices between the ankles and legs
   d. Using pressure-reducing mattresses
   e. All of the above

2. Ms. Stagefut is a frail Caucasian female with advanced dementia and type II diabetes, admitted to the nursing home because her chronically ill son is no longer able to take care of her. On admission, Ms. Stagefut is noted to have a quarter-sized erythematous skin lesion over her left heel that is mildly warm to the touch. She does not complain of pain in her heel. Her right heel has a 1-cm × 2-cm bulla, with a mildly erythematous base. What are the stages of the pressure ulcers described in this patient?
   a. Left heel, stage I; right heel, stage II
   b. Left heel, stage I; right heel, stage I
   c. Left heel, stage I; right heel, stage III
   d. Left heel, stage II; right heel, stage II
   e. Left heel, stage II; right heel, stage III

3. Mr. Cruked has been in an acute care facility for about 2 weeks for right hip fracture, status post open reduction with internal fixation. His postoperative care was complicated with a stage III pressure ulcer over the coccyx area that did not respond to topical treatment. Mr. Cruked is complaining of increased pain that is difficult to manage. What should you do next?
   a. Swab culture to determine the microorganism causing infection
   b. Use antiseptic solutions for wound cleansing
   c. Bone biopsy to rule out osteomyelitis
   d. More frequent wound cleansing
   e. Change to a different topical antibiotic

4. Mr. Jones is a frail 93-year-old who presents to the Emergency Department with a deep pressure ulcer that exposes muscle tissue and bone. The edge of the wound is erythematous with some granulation tissue, but part of it is covered with black eschar. After assessment, wound care includes pressure reduction measures, necrotic tissue debridement, and daily wound cleansing with warm saline solution followed by dressing changes. Two weeks later, the ulcer is clean and only extends to the epidermis. His dressings are changed to hydrocolloid dressings and he is sent home. What is the stage of the pressure ulcer of Mr. Jones on admission and at discharge?
   a. Stage III, healing stage III
   b. Stage IV, healing stage IV
   c. Stage III, healing stage II
   d. Stage II, healing stage II
   e. Stage IV, healing stage I

PRETEST ANSWERS
1. b
2. e
3. c
4. a

POSTTEST ANSWERS
1. e
2. a
3. c
4. b

Hypothermia and Hyperthermia

Richard Slevinski

OBJECTIVES

Upon completion of this chapter, the reader will be able to:

- Understand the risk factors and clinical features of hypothermia.
- Be able to categorize hypothermia into mild, moderate, and severe, and to outline the general princi-

ples of management of the degrees of severity, including common serious complications of severe hypothermia management.

- Comprehend the range of risk factors for hyperthermia, both environmental and endogenous.
- Define the major characteristics of the five environmental heat syndromes, and the principles of their management, including major complications of heat stroke, a medical emergency.

PRETEST

1. The effects of severe hypothermia include all except which *one* of the following?
   a. Respiratory depression
   b. Coma
   c. Metabolic alkalosis
   d. Bradycardia
   e. Ventricular fibrillation

2. Which *one* of the following is *false* regarding hypothermia?
   a. In mild hypothermia, the patient shivers.
   b. At a core temperature of 31°C or less, the patient may appear to be dead.
   c. The core temperature should be raised at least 2°C per hour.
   d. Alcohol can increase heat loss in mild hypothermia.

3. Which *one* of the following is *false* concerning hyperthermia?
   a. Heart failure is a common risk factor.
   b. Excess alcohol increases the risk.
   c. Heat cramps are principally induced by salt deficiency.
   d. In heat syncope the body temperature is normal.

4. Which one of the following is *true* regarding heat stroke and its management?
   a. Heat stroke can be fatal if untreated.
   b. The skin is hot, flushed, and sticky.
   c. Combativeness is unusual; coma is the rule.
   d. The nude patient is soaked in ice water and fanned.

HYPOTHERMIA

Fred Jones (Part 1)

You are at a nursing home seeing your patients when you hear a cry for help from the kitchen staff. Mr. Jones, your patient of 5 years, a 76-year-old Caucasian male, has been found in the walk-in freezer. He is lying on the floor, unconscious, with a respiratory rate of 6 and a pulse rate of 20. He is very cold to the touch. Before the staff drags him out, you tell them to hold on and not touch him because there was something you needed to remember about hypothermia. You whip out your trusty medically equipped personal digital assistant (PDA) and search for "hypothermia."

Prevalence and Impact

During the 1979–2002 period, an average of 689 deaths per year were attributed to exposure to excessive natural cold. Annual death rates range from 0.2 to 0.4 per 100,000 population. In 2002, a total of 646 hypothermia-related deaths were reported, with an annual death rate of 0.2 per 100,000 population. Fifty-two percent of all decedents were aged over 65 years.

Risk Factors and Pathophysiology

RISK FACTORS

Hypothermia is produced by exposure to cold temperatures (environmental) and many medical conditions (Box 29–1).[1] Hypothermia is defined as a core temperature of less than 35°C (95°F). Risk factors are many: age, health, nutrition, body size, dehydration, mental status, exposure, wind speed, temperature, humidity, medications, and alcohol all decrease heat production or increase heat loss, or interfere with the patient's ability to maintain body temperature. Body heat is lost by *conduction* (direct transfer of heat by contact with a cooler object or area); *convection* (body heat is transferred to cool air moving across the body surface, warming the air and cooling the body); *evaporation* (loss of heat through vaporization

---

Box 29-1 Differential Diagnosis of Endogenous Hyperthermia

Infections
  Bacterial, viral
Hyperactivity
  Status epilepticus, alcohol withdrawal, amphetamine use,
  psychoses
Drug reaction causing fever
  Anticholinergics (tricyclics, phenothiazines, antihistamines,
  antispasmodics), alcohol, amphetamines, cocaine, anesthetics
Immunization reactions
  Transfusion, chemotherapy
Physiologic abnormalities
  Hyperthyroidism, obesity

---

of body water); *respiration* (inspired air is heated, and then is exhaled, taking out body heat); and *radiation* (heat radiated from the body to a cooler environment).

PATHOPHYSIOLOGY

The pathophysiologic effects of severe hypothermia include severe bradycardia, respiratory depression, altered reflexes, and coma.[2] A protective mechanism during hypothermia is vasoconstriction of surface and muscle blood vessels. Rewarming reverses this vasoconstriction and cold, acidotic blood recirculates into the core of the body leading to a paradoxical drop in temperature, and creating metabolic acidosis. This is called "core temperature afterdrop." Thus, the core must be rewarmed before the periphery. Since the myocardium is severely irritable in hypothermia, rewarming can cause arrhythmias including ventricular fibrillation. Hypothermia can mimic death: a major principle of hypothermia care is that no one is dead until he or she is *warm* and dead!

Diagnosis and Assessment

The diagnosis of the *level* of hypothermia requires use of a rectal probe thermometer to measure the core temperature. Hypothermic patients must be handled gently and slowly to prevent more damage. Hypothermia can be grouped into three stages: mild, moderate, and severe.

MILD HYPOTHERMIA

The core temperature is 34 to 35°C (93 to 95°F). The patient shivers and will have muscle pains; the patient is still alert and can understand and follow commands.

MODERATE HYPOTHERMIA

The core temperature is 31 to 33°C (88 to 92°F). The patient exhibits mental status changes that may include confusion, drowsiness, and hallucinations. The muscles start to stiffen and the patient is *not* shivering. Respiratory depression is present.

SEVERE HYPOTHERMIA

The core temperature is less than 31°C (88°F). The patient's mental status changes are worse; often the patient is unconscious. The skin is waxy to cyanotic, the muscles are stiff, respiration is severely depressed, and the patient may *appear* dead.

● No patient apparently dead and at risk for hypothermia is dead until she or he is "warmed and dead"!

Laboratory tests should include a complete metabolic panel: CBC, BUN, creatinine, ABGs, clotting factors, serum and urine toxicology, ETOH, thyroid panel, cardiac isoenzymes, amylase, and lipase. An EKG and a CXR are indicated.

Management

Correctly conducted rewarming is the key good management.[3,4] There is some controversy regarding the speed of the rewarming and how to accomplish this. The guiding principle is to warm the core before the periphery in order to decrease metabolic acidosis and avoid "temperature afterdrop" (see above). The aim is to raise the core temperature 0.5°C to 2°C (0.25°F to 1°F) per hour. Clinical management depends on the severity.

MILD HYPOTHERMIA

Core temp is 34 to 35°C. Indicated treatment includes mild exercise to generate body heat; warm bath; and glucose-containing drinks to increase caloric load. *Contraindicated* actions include massage to cold limbs, and alcohol or coffee, as the vasodilatory effect of both increases heat loss.

MODERATE HYPOTHERMIA

Core temp is 31 to 33°C. Warm the core first, that is, the trunk and/or the chest. Warm humidified air at 40 to 42°C (104° to 107.5°F) by mask elevates the core temperature. Warm IV fluid boluses with dextrose give caloric supplements but do *not* provide enough heat calories to significantly raise body temperature. The trunk is wrapped in heated blankets, or specially designed heating vests are used. The trunk is heated before the limbs. Note: *no exercise, no alcohol, no caffeine, no cold air, no cold drinks,* and *no IV fluid overload.*

> ● In severe hypothermia, patient movement must be gentle to avoid the development of ventricular fibrillation.

SEVERE HYPOTHERMIA

Core temperature is less than 31°C. Such patients are very fragile and unstable. Movement of the limbs is minimized to avoid pumping the muscles, as this sends cold blood to the core. Movement must be gentle to avoid the development of ventricular fibrillation. Intubation may be needed in order to control respiration, but this can also precipitate ventricular fibrillation. Techniques for core warming include heated humidified air by mask or endotracheal tube, peritoneal lavage with warm potassium-free lavage fluids, cardiopulmonary bypass with warmed blood and fluids, and nasogastric intubation with lavage and suction of warmed fluids. Drugs, CPR, and defibrillation can be used once the hypothermic patient is properly warmed; usually, none of these is successful until the core temperature is above 32°C (90°F). The rate of ventilation must be adjusted or CO_2 added, since the hypothermic patient produces less CO_2 and therefore risks hypokapnea; the CO_2 level should be kept near 40 mmHg.

Hyperkalemia is common. Management of this complication should include administration of 1 g of calcium chloride IV, 1 ampoule of sodium bicarbonate IV, 1 ampoule of D5W plus 10 units of regular insulin IV, and a Kayexalate enema. More aggressive measures to reduce extremely high serum K include dialysis or exchange transfusion.

Hemoconcentration is common in hypothermic patients: blood viscosity increases 2% for each 1°C (2°F) drop in temperature. Physiologic vasoconstriction in the limbs may cause imprecise values on lab tests; vasoconstriction and lab test effects may shift rapidly during rewarming. IV fluids should be started with initial boluses of D5 normal saline, 250 to 500 cc, followed by re-evaluation of circulatory status. The need for more fluids may change during rewarming and is best measured by pulmonary wedge pressure monitoring and frequent reassessments of lab values. Lactated Ringer's must *not* be used as the liver is unable to metabolize it during hypothermic states.

Myoglobinuria is a common complication during resuscitation of hypothermic patients. Once the patient is warmed, treatment follows standard guidelines with the use of IV fluids: 20% mannitol (0.5 g/kg IV over 30 minutes) and furosemide (40- to 200-mg IV bolus) to maintain a urinary output of 2 ml/kg/h. Bicarbonate boluses to maintain urinary pH above 6.5 is recommended.

Acute tubular necrosis is common after prolonged hypothermia and requires referral to a nephrologist.

Clotting factor abnormalities occur as hypothermia leads to a hypercoagulable state, and the DIC (disseminated intravascular coagulation) syndrome. The prothrombin time (PT), (PTT), fibrin degradation products and platelet count direct the therapeutic approach, as in other illnesses causing such states.

HYPERTHERMIA

> ### Rosie O'Flaherty, *(Part 1)*
>
> *A 74-year-old white female is found in her home by an EMS crew in mid-July "talking out of her head." She lives in a rundown neighborhood across the street from the hospital, has burglar bars on her doors, and the home is locked tight. She has no air conditioning but does have three fans running in the house. It is stiflingly hot! The EMS crew loads her onto a stretcher and brings her into the ER; the ER physicians are occupied with handling three cardiac arrests and a major trauma victim. The nurses see you standing in the hallway and say, "We need help. I think this is your patient anyway!" You look, and indeed it is Rosie O'Flaherty. You remember her well as a mildly overweight, insulin-dependent diabetic, with poor vision, who is also bipolar and drinks alcohol to excess. You remember that you prescribed Phenergan for her last week for nausea and vomiting. The nurse gives you her vital signs: temperature is 106°F rectally, pulse is 125, and blood pressure is 80/40. Her skin is hot and dry. She is confused and mildly combative. You recognize hyperthermia and pick up your PDA:*

Prevalence and Impact

Heat-related deaths typically occur in the summer months. During the 1979–1999 period, the most recent years for which national data are available, over 8000 deaths in the United States were heat related. A total of 48% were "due to weather conditions," 5% were "of man-made origins" (e.g., heat generated in vehicles, kitchens, boiler rooms, furnace rooms, and factories), and 48% were "of unspecified origin." An average of 182 deaths per year were recorded associated with excessive heat resulting from weather conditions. Of the weather-related deaths for which age of decedent was reported, 45% of deaths occurred among persons aged over 65 years. For heat-related deaths, the mortality rate increases with age."[5] During a record-setting heat wave in Chicago in July 1995, there were at least 700 excess deaths, most of which were classified as heat related. Those at greatest risk of dying from the heat were people with medical illnesses who were socially isolated and did not have access to air conditioning.[6]

Pathophysiology and Risk Factors

PATHOPHYSIOLOGY

The regulation of temperature in the body is known as thermal homeostasis. Normal core temperature is 37°C (98.6°F). The body temperature is a balance of heat gain or loss from the environment, calories generated by metabolism, cardiac output, respiration, and sweating and diversion of the circulation to the skin to promote cooling. Alteration of the balance of any of these mechanisms can increase the core temperature and cause hyperthermia.

> ● A number of age-related factors and common comorbid conditions place older adults at greater risk for heat syndromes.

RISK FACTORS

A number of age-related factors and common comorbid conditions place older adults at greater risk for heat syndromes.[7] Heart failure, with the resulting inability to raise cardiac output to shunt more blood to the peripheral tissues in order to cool the body, is a common risk factor. Medications for hypertension, arrhythmias, and other conditions can reduce sweating and the ability to lose body heat. The aging of the skin, with the loss of subcutaneous fat, is a factor in regulation of body temperature. The social issue of the inability of the elderly to cool their homes in hot climates is a major factor. The use of alcohol to excess, leading to vasodilation in the skin and paradoxical heat gain in hot environments, is yet another.

> ● Heat stroke is a life-threatening syndrome. The mechanisms to control heat are lost and the temperature rises quickly, causing cellular and end organ damage.

Diagnosis

ENVIRONMENTAL HEAT SYNDROMES

Heat fatigue is usually caused by exposure to high outside temperatures or overexertion in a hot environment. It is the first level of heat stress and is characterized by pale and sweaty skin that is still moist and cool to touch. The heart rate is elevated and the patient feels exhausted and weak. Core temperature is normal. The important physical diagnostic point is that the patient is still able to sweat and lose heat by thermal convection.

Heat syncope is a sudden syncopal spell or dizziness after exercising in the heat. The body has lost some vascular volume and electrolytes from sweating. The skin is pale and sweaty, the pulse pressure may be weakened, and the heart rate is usually elevated. The body temperature is normal.

Heat cramps, the third stage of heat syndromes, are characterized by muscle cramping of the legs, arms, or abdominal wall. The skin is still moist and the body is able to sweat. There is a common misconception that this is caused by salt loss. It is actually caused by the *rate* of salt *and* water loss, and is not correctable with salt alone. The physiologic signs of hypovolemia (tachycardia, decreased pulse pressure, and thirst) are usually present.

Heat exhaustion, the fourth heat syndrome, signals an impending, life-threatening danger. The patient is thirsty, has altered mental status (giddy, confused, weak), skin that is cool and clammy, and there is tachycardia and possibly nausea. Core temperature is normal or mildly elevated.

Heat stroke is the most deadly of the heat syndromes. Untreated victims will die. In this stage, the mechanisms to control heat are lost, and body temperature rises quickly, causing cellular and end organ damage. The patient has an elevated temperature (>104°F), with flushed skin, and is hot and dry; there are mental status changes such as confusion, combativeness, delirium, and coma. There may be tachycardia, hypotension, and hyperventilation.

Management

Management of the five environmental heat syndromes is summarized in Table 29–1. Heat stroke is a medical emergency and requires expert management.[8]

Heat stroke treatment involves cooling the patient as rapidly as possible. There are two techniques:

1. The use of ice water soaks, covering the naked patient with ice water towels or sheets, with ice packs on the neck, and in the axillae and inguinal areas. A fan is used to circulate air over the patient, causing evaporative cooling of the cold sheets and towels.
2. Wetting the patient with tepid water spray bottles and circulating air with a fan in a low-humidity environment to cause evaporative cooling. Rapid cooling should not be allowed to cause shivering, if possible, as the latter creates unwanted metabolic heat. These patients are critically ill and will require IV hydration with normal saline.

Table 29–1 Management of Environmental Heat Syndromes

Diagnosis	Treatment
Heat fatigue and heat syncope	Oral hydration with electrolyte replacement drinks
	Cooler, less humid environment
	Rest
Heat cramps and heat exhaustion	Cool environment
	Oral hydration
	IV normal saline
	Rest
Heat stroke	Complex medical emergency!
	See text

Intubation may be necessary. A catheter is used to measure urinary output and a central monitoring line is placed. Laboratory studies include ABGs, a metabolic panel with electrolytes, BUN, creatinine, cardiac enzymes, lactate levels, and PT and PTT.

Hypotension is managed by giving a 500-cc bolus of normal saline, which is repeated depending on response. The goal is to maintain both good urinary output and a systolic pressure of 90 or above.

Shivering is managed by the administration of chlorpromazine 25- to 50-mg IV. This is often the prodrome to a seizure; the drug helps with the shivering, but lowers the seizure threshold. If *seizures do occur*, diazepam 5-to 10-mg IV or lorazepam 1- to 2-mg IV can be given. Dilantin is ineffective in the acute heat stroke patient.

Acidosis will correct itself with hydration, cooling, and proper management. Bicarbonate infusions are not indicated.

Hypoglycemia is managed via bolus therapy with D5W IV infusions, monitoring carefully every 30 minutes.

Acute renal failure can result from hyperthermia and hypotension. Initial treatment consists of IV infusions, using mannitol and furosemide to maintain urinary output. Acute dialysis is often necessary.

Clotting factor abnormalities, or a hypercoagulable state, and DIC syndrome are common results of hyperthermia. The PT, PTT, fibrin degradation products and platelet count are obtained and appropriate treatment is given.

Endogenous hyperthermia is characterized by the body itself producing too much heat, and inability to lose it to the environment. The causes are summarized in Box 29–1. Management is treatment of the underlying cause.

SUMMARY

Over 50% of all deaths from hypothermia occur in older adults. Hypothermia from cold exposure is categorized into mild, moderate, and severe depending on the core temperature, taken with a rectal probe thermometer. Management involves gentle handling of the patient, warming the core (the trunk and chest) before the limbs, and the expectation of metabolic acidosis and cardiac arrhythmias, all of which require core warming before drugs and other therapies will succeed. Other common complications are hyperkalemia, cardiac arrhythmias and acute renal failure. Initially, the patient may appear dead but he or she must be "warm and dead," before a declaration of death is made.

Hyperthermia is a syndrome with several levels of severity, ranging from common heat fatigue to life-threatening heat stroke. The most common cause is environmental exposure but the clinician should always be aware of the endogenous causes of hyperthermia. The elderly are at higher risk for the development of heat stroke due to a number of metabolic, physiologic, and social factors. The treatment of heat stroke is to identify the underlying cause, and to cool the patient as rapidly as possible. Complications during treatment include hypoglycemia, shivering, seizures, renal failure, and hypotension.

References

1. Hudson LD, Conn RD. Accidental hypothermia: associated diagnoses and prognosis in a common problem. JAMA 227:37, 1974.
2. Reuler JB. Hypothermia: pathophysiology, clinical settings and management. Ann Intern Med 89:519, 1978.
3. Danzl DF, Pozos PS. Accidental hypothermia. N Engl J Med 331:1756, 1994.
4. Medical Letter Advisory Panel. Treatment of hypothermia. Med Lett 36:116, 1994.
5. Centers for Disease Control and Prevention. Hypothermia-related deaths—United States, 2003–2004. MMWR Morb Mortal Wkly Rep 54:173, 2005.
6. Semenza JC, Rubin CH, Falter KH, et al. Heat-related deaths during the July 1995 heat wave in Chicago. N Engl J Med 329:483, 1993.
7. Kilbourne EM, et al. Risk factors for heat stroke: a case control study. JAMA 247:332, 1982.
8. Simon HB. Hyperthermia. N Engl J Med 329:483, 1993.

POSTTEST

Questions 1 through 5 are based on the Fred Jones case.

1. Your first action after you protect Mr. Jones's cervical spine is to direct the staff to:
    a. Take him by the arms and legs and carry him to a warm bed.
    b. Gently and carefully get him onto a bed or backboard.
    c. Turn him on his side so he cannot vomit and aspirate.
    d. Move him into the warm kitchen to see if he wakes up.

2. You need to know his temperature. You ask for:
    a. A rectal probe temperature
    b. An oral temperature
    c. An axillary temperature
    d. A tympanic probe temperature

3. His core temperature is 30°C. What degree of hypothermia is this?
    a. He is dead at this temperature.
    b. Mild hypothermia.
    c. Moderate hypothermia.
    d. Severe hypothermia.

4. Your first principle of treatment is to:
    a. Warm the limbs with heated blankets or warm towels.
    b. Wrap the entire body in heated blankets.
    c. Warm the chest and trunk with heated blankets.
    d. Move the arms and legs to prevent clotting.

5. You note that he has a pulse of 40, blood pressure of 80/40, and a respiratory rate of 8/min. What do you do?
    a. Provide warm humidified air and observe.
    b. Give atropine to raise the heart rate.
    c. Give lactated Ringer's IV to raise the blood pressure.
    d. Intubate him and start CPR until his core temperature is up to 34°C.

Questions 6 through 10 are based on the case of Rosie O'Flaherty.

6. Rosie has a heat-related condition known as:
    a. Heat cramps
    b. Heat syncope
    c. Heat exhaustion
    d. Heat stroke

7. You elect to cool her down with which of the following techniques:
    a. You put her in front of the air conditioning vent.
    b. You offer her cool liquids to drink and put a fan on her.
    c. You strip off her clothes, soak her in iced towels, and blow a fan across her.
    d. You pack her head in an ice soaked towel, and give chilled IV normal saline.

8. She begins to have a seizure. You give her:
    a. Dilantin 500 mg IV push
    b. Dilantin 1 g IV over 10 minutes
    c. Lorazepam 1 to 2 mg IV push
    d. Clonazepam 750 mg IV over 3 minutes

9. The nurses drew blood from the patient while she was seizing. What do you want to know first?
    a. Temperature of the blood
    b. BUN and creatinine
    c. Blood alcohol level
    d. Blood glucose level.

PRETEST ANSWERS

1. c
2. c
3. c
4. d

POSTTEST ANSWERS

1. b
2. a
3. d
4. c
5. a
6. d
7. c
8. c
9. b

OBJECTIVES

Upon completion of this chapter, the reader will be able to:

- Recognize common causes of sleep problems in older people.

- Understand diagnostic testing and appropriate treatments for common sleep disorders in older people.

- Differentiate between sleep complaints that can be managed in primary care versus those requiring referral to a sleep specialist.

PRETEST

1. Sleep disorders that increase in prevalence as people age include:
   a. Sleep disordered breathing (sleep apnea)
   b. Periodic limb movement disorder
   c. Narcolepsy
   d. a and b

2. Common age-related changes in sleep include all of the following *except:*
   a. Lower sleep efficiency
   b. A decrease in deep (stage 3 and stage 4) sleep
   c. Strengthening of endogenous circadian rhythms
   d. Increased daytime napping

3. Clues to the presence of sleep apnea include all of the following *except:*
   a. Daytime sleepiness and fatigue
   b. Large neck circumference
   c. Hypertension
   d. Anemia

4. Which of the following most accurately describes the sleep-related consequences of circadian rhythm changes commonly associated with older age?
   a. Feeling sleepy in the evening, and waking earlier than desired in the morning
   b. Feeling sleepy in the evening, and waking later than desired in the morning
   c. Inability to fall asleep at night and waking earlier than desired in the morning
   d. Inability to fall asleep at night and waking later than desired in the morning

---

PREVALENCE AND IMPACT

Jonathan Chen, *(Part 1)*

Mr. Jonathan Chen, a 66-year-old recently retired, Asian-American engineer, comes to your office for a routine visit. Near the end of his appointment, with prompting from his wife, he states that he is "up all night," and asks you for "something to help me sleep." He is concerned about his inability to sleep, and he is clearly distressed. He feels tired during the day, spending much of his time "resting," which limits the couple's social activities.

Charles Banker, *(Part 1)*

Mr. Charles Banker, a 79-year-old African-American man, arrives 1 hour late for his first appointment in your office, and apologetically explains he fell asleep at home. He admits to falling asleep during conversations and card games with friends. He is a retired security guard, and was fired several years ago for "falling asleep on the job." He sees a psychiatrist, who is treating him for depression. Mr. Banker wonders whether there is an "energy pill" that will help him stay awake during the day.

STUDY QUESTION

1. How common are sleep problems and to what extent do they affect the well-being of older people?

PREVALENCE AND IMPACT

Sleep is an essential biological process, and sleep deprivation leads to neurological, autonomic, and biochemical changes. Older people generally report more nighttime awakenings and more daytime sleeping than younger people. The primary care provider needs to understand common underlying causes of sleep problems, appropriate treatments, and indications for referral to a sleep specialist.

The reported prevalence of sleep complaints among older adults ranges from 16% to 68%.[1] There is a yearly linear increase in sleep complaints from early adulthood to old age. Also, across the life span, women report more problems with sleep than men. Insomnia is the most common sleep disturbance in the older population, with up to 40% of those over age 60 complaining of difficulty falling asleep and/or maintaining sleep, and over 20% reporting severe insomnia.[1,2] The prevalence of primary sleep disorders, such as sleep apnea, periodic limb movement disorder (PLMD), and restless leg syndrome (RLS) also increases with age, and the magnitude of sleep problems is higher in long-term care facilities than in community settings.

Sleep disruption in old age is not benign. It can have a significant impact on overall quality of life. In correlational studies, sleep disturbance and sleep disorders have been associated with cognitive impairment, poor health status, low quality of life, and increased mortality.[3,4]

RISK FACTORS AND PATHOPHYSIOLOGY

ments. Normal adults progress from NREM stages 1 to 4, then return briefly to lighter sleep (typically stage 2) before entering REM sleep, in a cycle of approximately 90 minutes, which repeats throughout the night.

The most notable change in sleep structure with aging is a decrease in deep sleep. Other common changes with age include taking longer to fall asleep, decreased sleep efficiency (time asleep over time in bed), being awake more during the night, waking earlier than desired in the morning, and more intentional and inadvertent daytime napping.[5] Age-related neuronal loss in the suprachiasmatic nucleus (SCN) of the hypothalamus and reduced melatonin production by the pineal gland weaken circadian (24-hour) rhythms, contributing to these changes. In addition, a host of other factors often cause or aggravate sleep difficulties.[6] Box 30–1 lists medical, pharmacologic, psychiatric, and psychosocial factors that commonly contribute to sleep problems in older people. Table 30–1 summarizes age-related changes in specific organ systems and the impact of these changes on sleep.

Jonathan Chen, *(Part 2)*

Mr. Chen's physical examination reveals mild arthritis in his knee, for which he takes ibuprofen as needed. He denies pain at night. He does not have hypertension or a history of heart disease. He denies a history of depression, anxiety, or other psychiatric problems. He states that his current mood is "great, except for this sleep thing."

Charles Banker, *(Part 2)*

Mr. Banker describes his mood as "tired." He is obese, with a history of hypertension, gastroesophageal reflux, high cholesterol, and type II diabetes. He takes glipizide, metformin, atenolol, rabeprazole, aspirin, and atorvastatin. On physical examination, his blood pressure is 134/76; he is 5'8" tall and weighs 190 pounds. Heart and lung examination is unremarkable.

STUDY QUESTION

1. Are the sleep complaints of Mr. Chen and Mr. Banker age-related?

Human adult sleep is comprised of two separate states: rapid eye movement (REM) sleep and non-REM (NREM) sleep. NREM sleep is further divided into four stages, which roughly parallel a "depth of sleep" continuum, from light sleep (stages 1 and 2) to deep sleep (stages 3 and 4). REM sleep is normally characterized by EEG activation, muscle atonia, and rapid eye move-

Jonathan Chen, *(Part 3)*

On further questioning, Mr. Chen reports that he has not been sleeping well for nearly a month. He drinks a glass of wine with dinner, and then later dozes while watching television. He goes to bed at 10:00 P.M. and lies awake as "the hours tick by." He awakens at 4:00 A.M. to urinate, and often has trouble falling back to sleep. He and his wife get up at 6:00 A.M., and he "rests" on the couch after breakfast. He generally exercises in the afternoon, and then rests on the couch while his wife prepares dinner. He does not drink coffee or consume other caffeine. He snores softly on some nights, and his wife has not seen him stop breathing while asleep. He denies leg discomfort at night, and his wife has not noticed that he kicks his legs during sleep.

Charles Banker, *(Part 3)*

Mr. Banker reports sleeping "off and on" throughout the day and night. He falls asleep in his recliner in the evenings, and then goes to bed around midnight. He falls asleep quickly, but awakens "too many times to count" during the night. He urinates several times during the night, but also awakens for other unknown reasons. He gets out of bed around 4:30 A.M., and then falls back asleep in his recliner until about 9 A.M. He reports being told in the past that he snored loudly.

DIFFERENTIAL DIAGNOSIS AND ASSESSMENT

Older adults seldom spontaneously report problems with sleep to their primary care providers.[7] Because of this, screening for sleep complaints is recommended. This should include asking about satisfaction with sleep, daytime fatigue and sleepiness, and unusual behaviors during sleep (especially snoring, interrupted breathing and/or leg movements). Persistent sleep problems require a detailed sleep history from the patient and the bed partner or caregiver. In addition, a "sleep diary," in which the patient tracks sleep-related behaviors for 1 to 2 weeks can be informative.

Many sleep disorders can lead to complaints of insomnia or excessive daytime sleepiness. The International Classification of Sleep Disorders, second edition (ICSD-2) Diagnostic and Coding Manual lists eight categories of sleep disorders and their diagnostic criteria.[8] They include: (1) insomnias, (2) sleep-related breathing disorders, (3) hypersomnias of central origin, (4) circadian rhythm sleep disorders, (5) parasomnias, (6) sleep-related movement disorders, (7) isolated symptoms and apparently normal variants, and (8) other sleep disorders. Sleep disorders commonly encountered by primary care providers are discussed below.

The initial evaluation of sleep should focus on medical conditions, substance abuse, mental health problems, and medications that may be contributing to sleep complaints (see Box 30–1). Patients should be queried about their usual sleep patterns and events during sleep such as limb movements, respiratory distress, panic attacks, pain, nocturia, shortness of breath, headache, or symptoms of gastroesophageal reflux. Recent stressors and symptoms of depression, anxiety, and other psychiatric disorders need to be identified, and psychosocial factors such as bereavement, loss of social supports, and lifestyle changes (e.g., retirement) should be considered. A mental status examination to identify cognitive impairment is also indicated. A full medication history, including the use of over-the-counter and herbal medications, is essential. The focused physical examination should be based on evidence from the history. For example, reports of nocturia disrupting sleep should lead to evaluation for cardiac, renal, or prostate disease. Prior treatments for sleep-related complaints should be reviewed.

Referral for an overnight sleep study (polysomnography [PSG]) is indicated when evidence suggests a primary sleep disorder, such as sleep disordered breathing or periodic limb-movement disorder (discussed below).[9] PSG is the gold standard for the evaluation of sleep and generally involves spending a night in a sleep laboratory, where physiological measures are recorded, including an electroencephalogram (EEG), electrocardiogram (ECG), electrooculogram (EOG),

---

Box 30-1   Factors That Increase Risk of Sleep Problems and Sleep Disorders in Older Adults

Medical conditions
- Chronic pain secondary to rheumatological disorders, neuropathy, or other conditions
- Dyspnea of cardiac or pulmonary origin
- Gastroesophageal reflux
- Obesity
- Nocturia, incontinence
- Neurodegenerative diseases such as Alzheimer's disease and Parkinson's disease

Psychiatric disorders
- Depression and other mood disorders
- Anxiety disorders
- Drug or alcohol abuse or dependency

Psychosocial, Psychological, and Lifestyle Factors
- Retirement
- Bereavement
- Poor sleep habits/inadequate sleep hygiene

- Daytime sleeping, extended napping
- Inaccurate, maladaptive beliefs about sleep changes with advancing age

Medications and nonprescription agents
- Benzodiazepines
- Antihistamines
- Tricyclics and other antidepressants
- Analgesics
- Clonidine
- Theophylline
- Methylphenidate
- Anticonvulsants
- Antiparkinsonian agents
- Diuretics
- Nicotine
- Caffeine
- Alcohol

Table 30–1 Impact of Specific Physiological Changes on Sleep in Older Adults

System	Changes	Consequences
Circadian rhythms	Advance (shift earlier) in normal aging	Problems maintaining sleep and with early morning awakenings
Upper airway physiology	More fatty tissue, reduced muscle tone	Obstructive sleep apnea (nightime awakenings and daytime sleepiness)
Musculoskeletal	Arthritis, other conditions causing chronic pain	Problems with falling asleep and nightime awakenings
Genitourinary		
Benign prostatic hypertrophy	Increased nightime urination	Nightime awakenings
Menopause	Hot flashes	Nightime awakenings, night sweats

electromyogram (EMG), respiratory effort and airflow, and oxygen saturation. PSGs are performed and interpreted by sleep specialists.

> ● Older adults seldom spontaneously report problems with sleep to their primary care providers; therefore, screening for sleep complaints is recommended.

Insomnia

Insomnia is a complaint of inadequate or nonrestorative sleep characterized by difficulty falling asleep, repeated awakening, inadequate total sleep time, or poor quality sleep which is reflected in poor daytime functioning. An acute stressor commonly precipitates short-term insomnia (<1 month). Long-term insomnia may be classified as a primary problem or secondary to another disorder. The diagnosis of insomnia is made based on a thorough sleep history, sometimes in conjunction with a sleep diary. The American Academy of Sleep Medicine recommends PSG in the evaluation of insomnia only when a sleep-related breathing disorder or periodic limb movement disorder is suspected as an underlying cause, the initial diagnosis is uncertain, initial treatment has failed, or precipitous arousals occur with violent or injurious behavior.[9]

True primary insomnia is quite rare among older adults, accounting for only 5% to 20% of cases. Most insomnia complaints are secondary to specific medical conditions, neurological disorders, primary sleep disorders (described below), substance abuse, prescription medications, or psychiatric conditions; multiple factors may coexist. In depression, early morning awakening is the most characteristic pattern, along with increased sleep latency (time to fall asleep) and more nighttime wakefulness. Chronic pain at night is a common medical cause, particularly in older patients with rheumatological disorders, neuropathy, or cancer.

Drug and alcohol use are thought to account for 10% to 15% of cases of insomnia. Chronic use of hypnotics can lead to fragmented sleep and rebound insomnia when stopped abruptly. Many over-the-counter medications produce side effects that are either sedating or stimulating. Older patients often take multiple medications, which may be prescribed by multiple providers, compounding the situation. Caffeine (an ingredient in many nonprescription analgesics and dietary supplements, teas, chocolate, and beverages) increases sleep latency and sleep fragmentation. Although older adults sometimes try alcohol as a sleep aid, it actually leads to fragmented sleep. The use of alcohol combined with hypnotics may further exacerbate sleep difficulties, and may worsen sleep disordered breathing.

> ● Most insomnia complaints are secondary to specific medical conditions, neurological disorders, primary sleep disorders, substance abuse, prescription medications, or psychiatric conditions; multiple factors may coexist.

Sleep Disordered Breathing (Sleep Apnea)

These conditions are characterized by repeated episodes of either a cessation or marked decrease of airflow during sleep.[10] Apneas (complete airflow cessation for 10 seconds or more) and hypopneas (partial decrease in airflow for 10 seconds or more with a drop in oxygen saturation) during sleep can result from either upper airway obstruction (obstructive apnea), loss of ventilatory efforts (central apnea), or a combination of the two.

Obstructive sleep apnea (OSA), the most common sleep disorder diagnosed in sleep laboratories, is characterized by recurrent episodes of upper airway collapse and a reduction or cessation of airflow despite persistent ventilatory efforts. When OSA is associated with symptoms such as daytime somnolence, the term obstructive sleep apnea syndrome is applied. Obesity is the strongest risk factor for OSA, which may be aggravated by alcohol (especially near bedtime), sedatives, sleep deprivation, nasal congestion, and supine sleeping posture. Consequences of OSA include hypertension, cardiac arrhythmia, heart failure, memory impairment, and increased mortality. Excessive daytime sleepiness, ranging from subtle drowsiness to falling sleep in unsafe circumstances (e.g., while driving), is the most common complaint of OSA patients.

Loud snoring, nocturnal gasping, and witnessed apneas may be reported by bed partners or caregivers and serve as an additional important clue. Apneic episodes are usually terminated by gasps, chokes, snorts, and/or brief awakenings, and patients may therefore complain of insomnia. Patients may also experience morning headaches; impaired dexterity, attention, memory, or judgment; or personality changes, such as irritability, anxiety, or depression.

Clinical examination of a suspected OSA should include an evaluation of body habitus (height, weight, and neck circumference), and a careful upper airway examination to identify structures or abnormalities that potentially narrow the airway. Thyroid disorders should be ruled out, as hypothyroidism predisposes to OSAS. Patients suspected of having sleep apnea should be referred to a sleep laboratory for overnight PSG, from which an apnea-hypopnea index (total number of apneas and hypopneas per hour of sleep) can be calculated and used to inform treatment decisions.

> ● Excessive daytime sleepiness, ranging from subtle drowsiness to falling sleep in unsafe circumstances, is the most common daytime complaint of patients with sleep disordered breathing.

Sleep-Related Movement Disorders

Among older patients, periodic limb movements during sleep (PLMS) are common.[11] PLMS involves episodes of repetitive, highly stereotyped movements (primarily of the legs) during sleep. When PLMS is associated with a complaint of insomnia and/or excessive sleepiness with no other disorder to explain the symptoms, it is referred to as periodic limb movement disorder (PLMD). Restless legs syndrome (RLS) is characterized by an irresistible urge to move the legs while awake (often when in bed trying to sleep). The restless feeling is usually associated with sensory complaints such as paresthesia (i.e., "creepy crawly" sensation), dysesthesia (i.e., "pins and needles" sensation), or "internal itching." There is usually worsening of symptoms at rest, and movement of the limbs relieves

symptoms. For many patients, symptoms are worse later in the day, making it difficult to fall asleep. RLS runs in families and, in some cases, an underlying medical disorder, such as uremia, iron deficiency, or peripheral neuropathy, may predispose a person to RLS. The diagnosis of RLS is made based on history, while diagnosis of PLMD requires both history and overnight PSG. RLS and PLMD are distinct syndromes that frequently coexist. Approximately 80% of individuals with RLS have evidence of PLMD on PSG as well.

Circadian Rhythm Sleep Disorders

These disorders result from desynchronization between patients' endogenous circadian clock and the external environment. Circadian rhythms are entrained to the 24-hour day by time cues or *zeitgebers*, the most important of which is the light–dark cycle.[12] Older adults often have an advanced sleep phase, where they go to sleep early in the evening and wake up early in the morning. On nights when they do stay up late, their biological clock still causes them to awaken in the early morning hours, making them sleepy during the day. In contrast, people with a delayed phase (which is much less common in older people) fall asleep late and wake up late in the morning. Sleep diaries and wrist activity monitoring can be used to detect these sleep patterns.

REM Sleep Behavior Disorder

The presenting symptoms of this disorder are usually vigorous sleep behaviors associated with vivid dreams. These behaviors may result in injury to the patient or bed partner, and there may be a family history of the disorder. Toxic-metabolic abnormalities, drug or alcohol withdrawal or intoxication, and certain medications (e.g., tricyclic antidepressants, monoamine oxidase inhibitors, cholinergic agents, and serotonin-specific reuptake inhibitors) can cause acute REM sleep behavior disorder. The chronic form is usually idiopathic or associated with other neurological disorders, such as dementia, Parkinson's disease, and multiple system atrophy. PSG is indicated when this disorder is suspected. Typically PSG shows a pathologic absence of the muscle atonia that should occur during REM sleep.

Jonathan Chen, *(Part 4)*

Mr. Chen's sleep problems likely result from lifestyle changes after his retirement, which led to problematic sleep patterns, poor sleep hygiene, and worry about sleep.

Charles Banker, *(Part 4)*

Mr. Banker presents with classic symptoms of sleep disordered breathing, including daytime sleepiness and snoring. PSG reveals an apnea-hypopnea index of 70 per hour, with repeated oxygen desaturations.

STUDY QUESTION

1. What treatment strategies should be initiated for each of these patients?

MANAGEMENT

Following careful assessment, primary care clinicians should be able to determine whether a sleep-related problem can be managed within the primary care setting, or whether a referral to a sleep specialist is indicated (Fig. 30–1). The following discussion will review the management of sleep problems within primary care, and will provide some detail on situations in which referrals are needed.

Insomnia

As insomnia is a symptom of a wide variety of medical, psychological, and psychiatric conditions, it is crucial to identify the underlying cause(s), which can lead to specific treatments, such as analgesics for nocturnal pain or treatment for depression. Treating insomnia with hypnotic medications without addressing the underlying cause(s) can result in treatment failure and even exacerbation of the problem. For chronic insomnia, after underlying problems have been addressed, the first-line approach should be nonpharmacologic. For short-term, stress-related transient insomnia, such as during acute hospitalization or other acute stressors, short-term use of sedative-hypnotic medications may be appropriate.

The focus of the primary care provider should be in identifying behaviors that directly contribute to sleep disruption, and providing education and instructions on the use of good "sleep hygiene" in combination with "sleep restriction" (i.e., reducing overall time in bed) (Box 30–2).[13,14] Patients should be made more aware of health practices (e.g., lack of exercise, substance abuse) and environmental factors (e.g., light, noise, temperature, mattress) that impact sleep. One or two issues of particular relevance to the patient should be identified, such as eliminating evening alcoholic beverages. The patient should be asked to institute the new practice (e.g., substituting nonalcoholic wine) for at least 2 weeks, since sleep patterns are typically slow to change. Follow-up and ongoing management should be provided.

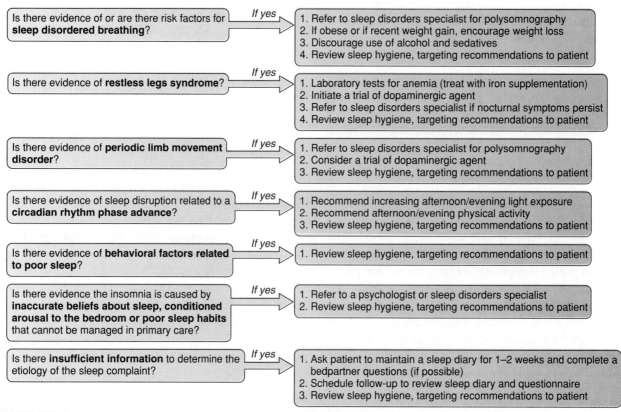

FIGURE 30–1

Evaluation and management of primary care patients with sleep complaints.[9,27]

> ### Box 30-2 "Sleep Hygiene" Measures to Improve Sleep
>
> - Maintain a regular morning rising time.
> - Avoid daytime naps, or limit napping to the early afternoon for less than 1 hour.
> - Exercise or increase activity level during the day, but not in the evening or immediately prior to bedtime.
> - Increase exposure to bright light during the day or early evening.
> - Take a hot bath about 2 hours before bedtime.
> - Avoid caffeine, nicotine, and alcohol in the evening.
> - Avoid excessive food or fluid intake at night.
> - Practice a relaxing bedtime routine.
> - Minimize light and noise exposure in the bedroom at night.

Other nonpharmacologic approaches address the behavioral and cognitive factors often underlying chronic primary insomnia, and these approaches are well supported by multiple randomized controlled trials in both younger and older adults.[15] Stimulus control therapy involves instructing the patient to reserve the bed and bedroom only for sleep and sexual activity with the goal of breaking the association between the bedroom environment and anxiety. Sleep restriction therapy involves curtailing the amount of time in bed to match the amount of time the patient actually sleeps. This method, which is often combined with stimulus control, reduces the amount of time awake at night, and leads to improved sleep over time. Relaxation techniques such as progressive muscle relaxation, yoga, and meditation can be useful for insomnia patients with high physiological arousal at night, although these methods are not universally effective. Cognitive-behavioral interventions combine the above techniques with methods to identify and address inaccurate beliefs about sleep such as "staying in bed longer will help me sleep better." Implementation of these techniques requires motivation on the patient's part and close follow-up by the clinician; involvement of a specialist can be extremely helpful.

> ● Because insomnia is a symptom of a wide variety of medical, psychological, and psychiatric conditions, it is crucial to identify the underlying causes, which can lead to specific treatments, such as analgesics for nocturnal pain or treatment for depression.

BRIGHT LIGHT THERAPY

When sleep problems are characterized by trouble maintaining sleep and early morning awakenings with-out difficulty falling asleep, and there is no evidence of another sleep disorder, evening bright light exposure can be effective.[16] Light therapy targets the underlying circadian rhythm changes that result in an advanced sleep phase. Exposure to either outdoor or artificial light via commercially available bright light boxes can be effective. As a general guide, for patients with an advanced sleep phase, at least 30 minutes of evening bright light close to bedtime for at least 2 to 3 weeks is suggested. The light intensity (brightness) used in research studies is generally between 2500 and 10,000 lux, which is comparable to daytime outdoor light levels. Potential side effects include transient headache and eye strain. Light exposure may be inappropriate for patients taking photosensitizing agents (e.g., amiodarone, hydrochlorthiazide), and a routine eye examination is recommended prior to treatment.

PHARMACOLOGIC TREATMENT

The decision to initiate drug therapy for insomnia should be based on the presence and severity of daytime symptoms and their impact on functioning and quality of life. Short-term hypnotic therapy may be appropriate in conjunction with improved sleep hygiene in cases of transient situational insomnia, particularly during bereavement or acute hospitalization.[14,17] With one exception (eszopiclone), hypnotic agents are approved by the Food and Drug Administration (FDA) only for short-term use. In patients with chronic insomnia, sedative/hypnotic agents should be considered cautiously, because of the complications associated with long-term use in older people. Altered metabolism of drugs, high rates of polypharmacy, and increased sensitivity to central nervous system depression all contribute to the high rate of adverse effects in older persons. Also, it is important to consider abuse potential on an individual basis, as some patients may be prone to psychological dependence on sleep aids. With most agents, tolerance develops over time, and dose escalation may occur as patients try to maintain therapeutic effects. When hypnotic agents are used, careful follow-up is essential, and a plan for discontinuation should be discussed when the initial prescription is provided.

Table 30-2 lists commonly used sedative-hypnotic medications. In general, agents with higher receptor selectivity and shorter half-life, and those without active metabolites have fewer adverse side effects. Benzodiazepines shorten the time to fall asleep and increase total sleep time; however, for most of these agents, sleep architecture is changed such that more time is spent in the lighter stages of sleep. Short-acting benzodiazepines may be useful for treating difficulty falling asleep; they have fewer daytime effects and are

Table 30–2 Commonly Used Sedatives/Hypnotic Medications

Generic (Trade) Name	Recommended Dose (mg)	Half-Life Range (Hours)	Chemical Class	Approval Date
Estazolam (Prosom)	0.5, 1, or 2	10–24	Benzodiazepine	1991
Temazepam (Restoril)	7.5, 15, or 30	3.5–18.4[a]	Benzodiazepine	1982
Triazolam (Halcion)	0.125 or 0.25	1.5–5.5	Benzodiazepine	1979
Lorazepam (Ativan)	0.25–2 mg	8–12	Benzodiazepine	
Eszopiclone (Lunesta)	1, 2, or 3	6.0	Non-benzodiazepine	2004
Zolpidem (Ambien)	5 or 10	1.4–4.5[b]	Non-benzodiazepine imidazopyridine	1993
Zaleplon (Sonata)	5 or 10	1.0	Non-benzodiazepine pyrazolopyrimidine	1997

[a]Up to 30 hours in older patients.
[b]Ten hours in hepatically compromised patients.

less likely to be associated with falls and hip fractures than longer-acting agents. Intermediate-acting agents are recommended for problems with sleep maintenance; using the lowest effective dose and tapering the dosage prior to discontinuation of the drug can reduce the potential for rebound insomnia. Long-acting agents (e.g., quazepam, flurazepam) should not be used in older people as these medications have active metabolites and a half-life of more than a day.

Newer nonbenzodiazepine hypnotics are gaining popularity, and may have some advantages in terms of safety and effectiveness over the older benzodiazepines. They also reduce the time to fall asleep, and some increase the duration of sleep and may be less likely to disturb sleep architecture. Because of rapid onset of action, zolpidem and zalepon should only be taken immediately prior to bedtime or after the patient has gone to bed and has been unable to fall asleep. No evidence of tolerance has been observed with either medication; however, psychological dependence may develop with continued use. Eszopiclone can be helpful for maintaining sleep during the night and has been approved for long-term use based on results of a 6-month study in younger patients (<65 years of age).

Other medications sometimes used for sleep are discussed briefly below.

Sedating antidepressants (e.g., trazodone, doxepin, and mirtazapine) are sometimes used off label to treat insomnia. They may be helpful for patients with a concomitant diagnosis of depression; however, there is no evidence to support their use in nondepressed individuals with insomnia.

Most over-the-counter sleep aids contain a sedating antihistamine, such as diphenhydramine. They should not be used in older persons, because of their potential for causing anticholinergic effects, daytime sedation, and cognitive impairment.

Melatonin, a hormone that helps control circadian rhythms, is a popular over-the-counter nutritional supplement marketed as a sleeping aid. It may be helpful for individuals suffering from circadian rhythm–related sleep disorders. To be effective, however, it must be taken at the appropriate "circadian" time, and recent studies show that very low doses (<0.5 mg) are most effective. Melatonin has not been shown to be an effective hypnotic agent for sleep problems unrelated to circadian rhythm changes, but it may be useful while discontinuing the use of sedative-hypnotic medications.[18]

Herbal agents (e.g., valerian, kava-kava) have unclear effectiveness but may potentiate the effects of prescribed sleep aids.

Obstructive Sleep Apnea

Nasally applied continuous positive airway pressure (CPAP) is the established treatment of choice for sleep apnea. It requires the patient to wear a sealed mask over the nose during sleep. Positive pressure is used as a "splint" for the airway, reducing airway collapse during sleep. CPAP is extremely effective and should be recommended as a first-line treatment for OSAS, regardless of the patient's age. Other general measures consist of weight loss (if overweight) and avoiding sedatives, hypnotics, and alcohol. Oral and dental appliances that reposition the jaw or tongue may be appropriate in mild cases or in patients who refuse CPAP. In a few severe cases, surgical treatments such as uvulopalatopharyngoplasty or hyoid suspension may be considered; however, successful resolution of OSA occurs in only about one-half of surgically treated patients.

● Nasally applied continuous positive airway pressure (CPAP) is the established treatment of choice for sleep apnea.

PLMD and RLS

Dopaminergic agents are the initial agents of choice for both PLMD and RLS. A nightime dose of carbidopa/levodopa can be used on an "as needed basis" for infrequent symptoms. Chronic symptoms are best treated with a dopamine agonist such as pramipexole or ropinorole. Benzodiazepines (e.g., clonazepam) and opioids (e.g., oxycodone) may also be effective, but have higher risks in older people and are not first-line therapy. There is limited evidence regarding the use of tegretol, gabapentin, and clonidine in the treatment of PLMD and RLS. Potentially causative or contributory factors need to be addressed. RLS in association with low ferritin levels may respond to iron replacement therapy.

Other Sleep Disorders

An advanced sleep phase may respond to evening bright light exposure, as close to bedtime as possible for 30 to 60 minutes. Clonazepam is reported to be highly effective in the treatment of REM sleep behavior disorder, with little evidence of tolerance or abuse over long periods of treatment.[19]

Jonathan Chen, *(Part 5)*

You make specific sleep hygiene recommendations to Mr. Chen, including giving up his evening alcohol and limiting daytime napping to 30 minutes in the early afternoon. After some reluctance, he agrees. Two weeks later, Mr. Chen reports that, after "a few rough days and nights" he is back on track, sleeping better most nights, and feeling better during the day.

Charles Banker, *(Part 5)*

Mr. Banker is prescribed a CPAP machine, which he uses nightly. When you see him for follow-up, he reports marked improvement in his daytime sleepiness and fatigue.

CHANGES IN SLEEP WITH DEMENTIA AND IN THE NURSING HOME

Patients with dementia have frequent sleep disruption and arousals, lower sleep efficiency, more stage 1 sleep, and less deep sleep compared to individuals without dementia.[5] Disturbances of sleep–wake cycles are common, resulting in both fragmented nighttime sleep and frequent, brief episodes of daytime sleeping. This may present a particular challenge for caregivers and can precipitate nursing home placement. Some dementia patients may "sundown," or experience an exacerbation of confusion and agitation during the evening or nighttime hours, which can be extremely difficult for caregivers.[20] Evaluation and treatment of sleep problems among patients with dementia should include input and participation from the caregiver, and should focus on improving quality of life for both. Once medical causes, such as infection, polypharmacy, and fecal impaction are excluded, sleep disturbances should be managed similarly to individuals without dementia, and recent findings suggest that, with caregiver support, dementia patients can benefit from sleep hygiene education, bright light therapy (if indicated), and even CPAP treatment for sleep apnea.[21,22]

In nursing home residents, marked disruption in sleep patterns are seen, perhaps even beyond what is found in dementia patients living at home.[23,24] In the nursing home, many of the same factors contribute to sleep problems; however, additional environmental and caregiving factors are also important to consider.[25,26] In general, the nighttime nursing home environment is noisy, lights are often left on in residents' rooms, and caregiving activities frequently interrupt sleep. In addition, daytime inactivity, excessive in-bed time, and minimal time spent outdoors exposed to bright light contribute to the commonly seen pattern of continual dozing and waking. There are, however, little data on the effectiveness of sleep medications and specific management of sleep disorders in the nursing home setting, and side effects of sedative-hypnotics can be significant in these frail older people. Behavioral factors (sleep hygiene) and environmental interventions should be the treatments of choice, and sleep medications should be used with extreme caution.[27]

> ● Evaluation and treatment of sleep problems among patients with dementia should include input and participation from the caregiver and should focus on improving quality of life for both.

SUMMARY

Most sleep disturbances in older adults are caused by specific problems, which should be properly evaluated. Obtaining a good sleep history is absolutely essential. Referral should be made when appropriate. Accurate diagnosis and appropriate therapy of sleep disorders may substantially improve sleep and quality of life in older people.

References

1. Lichstein KL, Durrence HH, Riedel BW, Taylor DJ, Bush AJ. Epidemiology of sleep. Mahwah, NJ: Lawrence Erlbaum Associates, 2004.
2. Foley DJ, Monjan AA, Brown SL, Simonsick EM, Wallace RB, Blazer DG. Sleep complaints among elderly persons: an epidemiologic study of three communities. Sleep 1995;18(6):425-32.
3. Cricco M, Simonsick EM, Foley DJ. The impact of insomnia on cognitive functioning in older adults. J Am Geriatr Soc 2001;49(9):1185-9.

4. Foley DJ, Wallace RB, Eberhard J. Risk factors for motor vehicle crashes among older drivers in a rural community. J Am Geriatr Soc 1995;43:776-81.

5. Bliwise DL. Review: sleep in normal aging and dementia. Sleep 1993;16:40-81.

6. Kryger MH, Roth T, Dement WC. Principles and Practice of Sleep Medicine. 3rd ed. Philadelphia: W.B.Saunders, 2000.

7. Shochat T, Umphress J, Israel AG, Ancoli-Israel S. Insomnia in primary care patients. Sleep 1999;22(Suppl 2):S359-65.

8. American Academy of Sleep Medicine. The International Classification of Sleep Disorders. 2nd ed. Westchester, IL: American Academy of Sleep Medicine, 2005.

9. Kushida CA, Littner MR, Morgenthaler T, Alessi CA, Bailey D, Coleman J, Friedman L, Hirshkowitz M, Kapen S, Kramer M, Lee-Chiong T, Loube DL, Owens J, Pancer JP, Wise M. Practice Parameters for the Indications for Polysomnography and Related Peocedures: An Update for 2005. Sleep 2005;28(4):499-521.

10. Ancoli-Israel S, Kripke DF, Klauber MR, Mason WJ, Fell R, Kaplan O. Sleep disordered breathing in community-dwelling elderly. Sleep 1991;14(6):486-95.

11. Ancoli-Israel S, Kripke DF, Klauber MR, Mason WJ, Fell R, Kaplan O. Periodic limb movements in sleep in community-dwelling elderly. Sleep 1991;14(6):496-500.

12. Duffy JF, Kronauer RE, Czeisler CA. Phase shifting human circadian rhythms: influence of sleep timing, social contact and light exposure. J Physiol (London) 1996;495(1):289-97.

13. Hoch CC, Reynolds CF III, Buysse DJ, Monk TH, Nowell P, Begley AE, et al. Protecting sleep quality in later life: a pilot study of bed restriction and sleep hygiene. J Gerontol B Psychol Sci Soc Sci 2001;56(1):52-9.

14. Vitiello MV. Effective treatments for age-related sleep disturbances. Geriatrics 1999;54(11):47-52.

15. Chesson AL, Jr., Anderson WM, Littner M, Davila D, Hartse K, Johnson S et al. Practice parameters for the nonpharmacologic treatment of chronic insomnia. An American Academy of Sleep Medicine report. Standards of Practice Committee of the American Academy of Sleep Medicine. Sleep 1999;22(8):1128-1133.

16. Campbell SS, Dawson D, Anderson MW. Alleviation of sleep maintenance insomnia with timed exposure to bright light. J Am Geriatr Soc 1993;41:829-36.

17. Morin CM, Colecchi C, Stone J, Sood R, Brink D. Behavioral and pharmacological therapies for late life insomnia. JAMA 1999;281(11):991-9.

18. Olde Rikkert MG, Rigaud AS. Melatonin in elderly patients with insomnia. A systematic review. Z Gerontol Geriatr 2001;34(6):491-7.

19. Schenck CH, Mahowald MW. Polysomnographic, neurologic, psychiatric, and clinical outcome report on 70 consecutive cases with the REM sleep behavior disorder (RBD): sustained clonazepam efficacy in 89.5% of 57 treated patients. Cleveland Clin J Med 1990;57:S10-24.

20. Bliwise DL, Carroll JS, Lee KA, Nekich JC, Dement WC. Sleep and "sundowning" in nursing home patients with dementia. Psychiatry Res 1993;48(3):277-92.

21. Ancoli-Israel S, Gehrman PR, Martin JL, Shochat T, Marler M, Corey-Bloom J, et al. Increased light exposure consolidates sleep and strengthens circadian rhythms in severe Alzheimer's disease patients. Behav Sleep Med 2003;1(1):22-36.

22. Ancoli-Israel S, Palmer BW, Loredo JS, Corey-Bloom J, Marler M, Greenfield D. CPAP improves cognitive function in Alzheimer's disease patients with sleep apnea: preliminary results. Sleep 28[abstract suppl.], A110-A111. 2005.

23. Ancoli-Israel S, Parker L, Sinaee R, Fell R, Kripke DF. Sleep fragmentation in patients from a nursing home. J Gerontol 1989;44(1):M18-21.

24. Ancoli-Israel S, Klauber MR, Jones DW, Kripke DF, Martin J, Mason W, et al. Variations in circadian rhythms of activity, sleep and light exposure related to dementia in nursing home patients. Sleep 1997;20(1):18-23.

25. Cruise PA, Schnelle JF, Alessi CA, Simmons SF, Ouslander JG. The nighttime environment and incontinence care practices in nursing homes? J Am Geriatr Soc 1998;??(?):463-466.

26. Schnelle JF, Ouslander JG, Simmons SF, Alessi CA, Gravel MD. The nighttime environment, incontinence care, and sleep disruption in nursing homes. J Am Geriatr Soc 1993;41(9):910-4.

27. Alessi CA, Schnelle JF. Approach to sleep disorders in the nursing home setting. Sleep Med Rev 2000;4(1):45-56.

28. Chesson AL Jr, Ferber R, Fry JM, Grigg-Damberger M, Hartse KM, Hurwitz TD, et al. The indications for polysomnography and related procedures. Sleep 1997;20(6):423-87.

Web Resources

1. American Academy of Sleep Medicine: www.aasmnet.org.
2. National Institutes of Health, National Center on Sleep Disorders Research: www.nhlbi.nih.gov/sleep.
3. National Sleep Foundation: www.sleepfoundation.org.
4. Sleep Research Society: www.sleepresearchsociety.org.

POSTTEST

1. All of the following are true about sleep of older adults, *except:*
   a. Older adults with health problems and psychiatric disorders are more likely to have sleep problems than their healthy counterparts.
   b. Older people are more likely to use medications for sleep than younger adults.
   c. Older people commonly have a delayed sleep phase, characterized by late onset of sleep and awakening later than desired in the morning.
   d. Sleep problems are associated with impaired cognitive and physical functioning in older people.

2. The treatment for sleep disordered breathing with the strongest empirical support is:
   a. Cognitive-behavioral therapy
   b. Continuous positive airway pressure (CPAP)
   c. Laser-assisted uvulopalatoplasty (LAUP)
   d. None of the above

3. When older adults complain about sleep problems, an assessment interview should include
   a. Symptoms of sleep disordered breathing, such as snoring or witnessed apneas
   b. "Hygiene"-related factors, such as caffeine, alcohol, and exercise patterns
   c. Symptoms of periodic limb movement disorder, such as leg kicking and disheveled bed coverings
   d. All of the above

4. The efficacy and safety of long-term use of sedative-hypnotic medications is supported by randomized controlled trials, in which patients have used such medications for several years.
   a. True
   b. False

PRETEST ANSWERS

1. d
2. c
3. d
4. a

POSTTEST ANSWERS

1. c
2. b
3. d
4. b

OBJECTIVES

Upon completion of this chapter, the reader will be able to:

- Understand the importance of taking a sexual history and obstacles encountered in taking it.

- List common medications that can adversely affect sexual function.

- Understand the prevalence and causes of dyspareunia as well as its identification and treatment.

- Understand the prevalence and causes of erectile dysfunction as well as its identification and treatment.

- List the advantages and disadvantages of the different types of treatments for erectile dysfunction.

P R E T E S T

1. A 71-year-old man with hypertension and diabetes mellitus continues to smoke. He also says he is able to attain an erection during sexual intercourse, but quickly becomes flaccid. Possible causes of erectile dysfunction (ED) in this man include:
   a. Vascular disease due to his hypertension
   b. Vascular disease due to his smoking
   c. An unrecognized alcohol abuse disorder
   d. Neuropathy from his diabetes mellitus
   e. Any of the above

2. A 68-year-old man notes that over the past several years his erections are becoming less firm. He has hypertension and diabetes mellitus. He has begun a new relationship and comes to your office to see if you can help. Initial treatment would be:
   a. Tell him to wait until his blood pressure and diabetes mellitus are under better control.
   b. Begin a trial of a PDE5 inhibitor.
   c. Order a testosterone and prolactin level before starting a testosterone patch.
   d. Refer the patient for a penile implant.
   e. Begin a yohimbine trial.

3. A 76-year-old woman complains of painful intercourse. On physical examination you find dry and slightly inflamed perivaginal tissue. Her past history includes a hysterectomy 20 years ago, a myocardial infarction (MI) 5 years ago, and breast cancer treated with a lumpectomy and irradiation 2 years ago. The best initial therapy for her discomfort would be:
   a. Begin oral estrogen 0.625 mg/d with a progestin.
   b. Begin oral estrogen 0.3 mg/d with a progestin.
   c. Begin oral estrogen 0.3 mg/d without a progestin.
   d. Try a vaginal lubricant prior to sexual intercourse.
   e. Begin intravaginal estrogen treatment.

Erma Watson, *Part 1*

Erma Watson is a 72-year-old woman who presents to your office for a routine visit. Her medical history includes peptic ulcer disease, osteoarthritis, and hypothyroidism. She is doing well on a proton pump inhibitor, scheduled acetaminophen, and levothyroxine. You enjoy her clinic visits as you are usually behind in your clinic, and the visits are short because she has few medical problems.

STUDY QUESTIONS

1. When should you include a sexuality history with older adults?
2. Do you believe that if patients do not bring up an uncomfortable topic (like sex), then it means they have no concerns?

PREVALENCE AND IMPACT

Sexual activity commonly, although not inevitably, declines with age.[1-4] For men, the decline is often caused by poor health or medications or both. For women, the decline is often caused by the lack of a partner or poor health. A survey of Americans age 60 or older found that nearly half (48%) of the men and women surveyed engaged in sexual activity at least once a month.[4] Among those who reported being sexually active, 79% of men and 66% of women said that maintaining an active sex life was an important aspect of their relationship with their partner. Prevalence of sexual activity varies with marital status. In a study of persons older than age 60, the prevalence was 74% for married men versus 31% for unmarried men, and 56% for married women versus 5% for unmarried women.[5]

401

RISK FACTORS AND PATHOPHYSIOLOGY

Physical and Hormonal Changes with Age

Normal aging brings about inevitable changes in anatomy and physiology that can affect sexual function, which are summarized in Box 31–1. Sexual desire wanes with age for both sexes, although low sexual desire is more commonly reported by older women. The arousal and refractory phases are longer, whereas the orgasmic phase is shorter than in younger persons. Difficulty reaching orgasms is common in women of all ages. The older man requires more prolonged, direct, and intense stimulation of the penis to attain an erection. The achieved erection is less firm, and a smaller amount of ejaculate is expelled with less force. Older women often find that it takes longer to lubricate, and that the amount of lubrication is less. In addition, vaginal tissue can be more sensitive and easily traumatized as a result of atrophy. For both men and women, although orgasms diminish in physical intensity, they can retain their psychologic or pleasurable intensity.

Psychosocial Changes That Affect Sexuality

In addition to physical changes, psychosocial changes affect the sexual lives of older persons. The loss of a sex partner through divorce, mental or physical illness, or death can affect sexual functioning. Role changes imposed by retirement or job loss can lead to boredom, low self-esteem, and lack of confidence. Depression is frequently correlated with decreases in sexual desire or function, while some antidepressants can increase sexual dysfunction. Although older persons need not be fully healthy to participate in sexual activities, the chronic illnesses that increase with age can affect desire for, enjoyment in, or performance of certain sexual activities. Should an older couple live with family, they might fear that the younger members disapprove of their continuing enjoyment of sex. Lack of privacy and suppression of all expressions of resident intimacy from staff and family members are an especially challenging problem in other communal settings such as the nursing home.

DIFFERENTIAL DIAGNOSIS AND ASSESSMENT

The Interview: Taking a Sexual History

There are many obstacles to obtaining an effective sexual history (Box 31–2). Suggestions for overcoming barriers are summarized in Box 31–3. Inhibitions, intolerance, and prejudice that both the clinician and the patient bring to the medical interview affect the discussion of sexuality. Both might assume incorrectly that sexual dysfunction is to be expected and accepted with increasing age. Becoming adept at discussing a personal, emotionally laden issue like sexuality, however, is imperative because such issues can directly affect health and may arise during any patient encounter. The topic of sexuality may be introduced in a variety of nonthreatening ways (see Box 31–3). Any time a medical or surgical procedure is considered or a new medication is prescribed, the possible effects on sexual function should be explained and the patient's concerns elicited.[6–9]

Sexually active elderly patients should be considered at risk for STDs, and discussion about STDs

---

Box 31–1 Summary of Physiologic and Anatomic Changes with Age in Women and Men

Women

- Ovaries decrease in size.
- Responsiveness of ovaries to follicle-stimulating hormone (FSH) and luteinizing hormone (LH) decreases.
- Estrogen and progesterone production are reduced.
- Testosterone and androstenedione production are reduced.
- Diminished conversion of adrenal androgens to testosterone and estrone.
- Uterus and vagina atrophy; vaginal vault shortens.
- Vaginal secretions are decreased and pH increases, which alters microbial flora.
- Glandular and ductal tissue of breast involute.
- Fat tissue increases.
- Ligamentous support of breasts relaxes.

Men

- Sperm production decreases.
- Chromosomal abnormalities in sperm increase.
- Leydig cell numbers decrease and responsiveness to LH lessens.
- Bioactive (free and bioavailable) testosterone often, but not always, decreases.
- Levels of inhibin, biofeedback for FSH, decline, resulting in a rise in FSH.
- Altered central nervous system regulation of LH and FSH occurs.
- Benign prostatic hypertrophy is present in 90% of men by age 85.
- Volume of prostate secretions decreases.

Box 31-2 Barriers to Taking a Sexual History

- Belief that topic is taboo
- Shame or embarrassment
- Anxiety or lack of confidence in asking or answering questions
- Lack of time
- Belief that older persons are not sexually active or interested
- Lack of knowledge
- Awkwardness with sexual language
- Fear of invasion of privacy, voyeurism
- Lack of understanding other than one's own experience (clinical frame of reference)
- Intolerance of certain sexual attitudes or practices

should be undertaken during the interview. Because older patients may link protection, or "safe sex," with contraception only and therefore consider themselves not at risk, clinicians need to provide education on the prevention of STDs. Age alone should not dissuade clinicians from considering the complications of human immunodeficiency virus (HIV) infection in a differential diagnosis.[10,11] Older persons with HIV experience a more rapid progression of the infection and have a shortened survival following the diagnosis of acquired immunodeficiency syndrome.

> Becoming adept at discussing a personal, emotionally laden issue like sexuality, is imperative because such issues can directly affect health and may arise during any patient encounter.

Box 31-3 How to Initiate a Sexual History

- I know it may be awkward to discuss, but I consider sexuality important to your overall health.
- Many women experience changes in sexual feelings after menopause—have you?
- Many medications and illness cause problems with sexual functioning—have you noticed any changes while on your medicines?
- I would like to ask you about diet, exercise, sexual activity, smoking, and so on.
- Are you satisfied with your sexual relationships?
- Has your illness affected your sex life?
- Some people note changes in sexual performance or desire with age—have you?

Dyspareunia

Recurrent genital pain before, during, or after intercourse is known as dyspareunia, which is truly a symptom rather than a diagnosis. Dyspareunia is common; however, the exact incidence is unknown because of under-reporting. In a study of 313 women in their thirties, more than 60% of the women studied experienced dyspareunia at some point in their lives.[12] Dyspareunia can be classified by whether the site of pain is superficial or deep. Superficial dyspareunia can be vulvar or vaginal. Patients often describe vulvar pain as "feeling inflamed" with associated burning, itching, and stinging. Some of the causes of vulvar dyspareunia are a tight hymen, urethritis, genital herpes, and topical irritants such as spermicides or feminine deodorants. Next to low sexual desire, vaginal dyspareunia is the most common sexual complaint of postmenopausal women. The urogenital atrophy accompanying hypoestrogenemia is the most common cause. Other causes of vaginal dyspareunia include vaginitis (as with a candidal infection or radiation vaginitis), chemical irritants, and physical trauma. Deep dyspareunia is pain resulting from pelvic thrusting during sexual intercourse, which can be due to positioning, postoperative or posthysterectomy adhesions, vaginal scars, piriformis syndrome, pelvic tumors, endometriosis, urinary tract infections, or ovarian cysts.

Bob Richardson

Bob Richardson is a 68-year-old man who is several years post-MI. He has hypertension, diabetes mellitus, and hyperlipidemia under fair, but not ideal, control. His medications include lisinopril, glipizide, terazosin, and simvastatin. He has not taken nitroglycerin for more than a year. He confides in a joking way that he has a "sex problem." He states that his desire for intercourse remains high, and his wife is supportive, but for many months he has been having more difficulty keeping an erection, which he loses soon after penetration.

STUDY QUESTIONS

1. What is the differential diagnosis for these symptoms, and what is the most likely cause?
2. Are any labs needed at this point?
3. Is it ever appropriate to treat nonspecifically? Or is a more detailed workup indicated, or should you refer him to a urologist?

Erectile Dysfunction

ED is the consistent inability to attain or maintain an erection sufficient for satisfactory sexual intercourse, and can have a significant impact on quality of life.[6,13-15] Vascular disease, causing poor blood inflow into the penis or increased outflow, is the most common cause of ED. In fact, ED may be the initial sign of serious vascular disease, preceding MI or stroke.[16,17] Other risk factors for ED are listed in Box 31–4. Tobacco use is a strong, independent risk factor for ED. By advising smokers of this, a clinician may give them even greater incentive to stop.

To investigate organic causes of ED, the clinician should screen for diabetes mellitus, renal insufficiency, and thyroid dysfunction. Lifestyle risk factors also play a major role in ED.[16,18-20] Based on clinical findings and the patient's lack of response to nonspecific therapy, other laboratory tests measuring levels of free or bioavailable testosterone or prolactin may then be appropriate.[21] Medications that can cause sexual dysfunction, many commonly used in elderly patients, are listed in Box 31–5. Every possible effort should be made to reduce or discontinue these medications (particularly diuretic, antipsychotic, and anticholinergic agents) when a patient has sexual dysfunction. Some medications with the side effect of inhibiting orgasm, such as serotinergic antidepressants, may actually play a therapeutic role in men with premature ejaculation.

> ● Erectile dysfunction may be the initial sign of serious vascular disease, preceding MI or stroke.

Box 31-4	Risk Factors for Erectile Dysfunction

- Atherosclerotic vascular disease
- Diabetes mellitus
- Hypertension and certain antihypertensives
- Smoking
- Hyperlipidemia
- Surgery or trauma to the pelvis or spine
- Neurologic disease
- Medications of many kinds (see Box 31–5)
- Alcohol use
- Depression and certain antidepressants
- Psychologic issues
- Relationship issues
- Obesity
- Lower urinary tract symptoms (LUTS)
- Chronic renal failure
- Physical inactivity
- Hypogonadism

MANAGEMENT

Erma Watson, *Part 2*

When you routinely inquire about Ms. Watson's sexual functioning, her demeanor changes. With encouragement, she reveals that she has generally had a satisfying sex life with her husband of 44 years. Initial discomfort with sexual intercourse

Box 31-5	Drugs That Frequently Interfere with Sexual Function

Drugs That Affect Neurotransmitters

- Anticholinergics (particularly affect the arousal phase)
- Selective serotonin reuptake inhibitors (can affect orgasms in both males and females); bupropion, duloxetine, mirtazapine, and nefazodone may have relatively fewer adverse sexual side effects
- Monoamine oxidase inhibitors
- Tricyclic antidepressants (e.g., clomipramine)
- Antihypertensives
- Peripheral sympatholytics (e.g., guanadrel)
- Central sympatholytics (e.g., clonidine)
- β-blockers
- Antipsychotics (via decreased dopamine inhibition of prolactin secretion)
- Metoclopramide

Drugs That Affect Androgens or Estrogens

- Cancer chemotherapy
- Cardiac glycosides (e.g., digoxin)
- Spironolactone
- Cimetidine, ranitidine
- Ketoconazole
- Luteinizing hormone-releasing hormone, agonists, antagonists
- Progestogens
- Estrogen analogs
- Alcohol, long-term use

Drugs That Cause Generalized Central Nervous System Depression

- Alcohol, short- or long-term use
- Antiepileptics (e.g., phenytoin, carbamazepine)
- Benzodiazepines (e.g., alprazolam, diazepam)

resolved after the birth of her first child. Then, a year ago, she began having more discomfort during intercourse. She describes the pain as an intense burning sensation at initiation of penetration. The pain usually resolves a few hours afterwards, and she has noted some spotty bleeding. She has increasingly avoided sexual activity because of the pain. She underwent menopause 19 years ago. She denies dysuria or vaginal discharge.

STUDY QUESTIONS

1. What are possible causes of Ms. Watson's pain?
2. What evaluation is indicated?
3. What treatment would you recommend?

Treatment of Dyspareunia

Estrogen to treat vaginal irritation and dryness comes in multiple forms: oral, transdermal, or vaginal (as a tablet, cream, or silastic ring). The dose needed to relieve vaginal symptoms may be less than that required to relieve significant vasomotor symptoms. Vaginal estrogen is absorbed systemically and therefore a progestin should be used concomitantly in women with a uterus. Selective estrogen receptor modulators (SERMs), such as lasoxiphene, which target estrogen receptors in the vagina, are under study. Several nonhormone water-based products are sold over the counter for vaginal lubrication and can often provide local relief without the potential side effects of hormones.

Treatment of Erectile Dysfunction

Therapeutic options for ED include (1) external vacuum tumescence devices, (2) oral pharmacotherapy, (3) intracorporeal or intraurethral pharmacotherapy, (4) penile prostheses, or (5) for hypogonadal men, testosterone.

EXTERNAL VACUUM TUMESCENCE DEVICES

External vacuum tumescence, or the vacuum erection device, produces an erection by creating a vacuum around the penis and causing increased cavernosal filling sufficient for erection. An elastic ring, placed at the base of the erect penis, inhibits venous drainage. The devices are effective in patients with a variety of etiologies of ED, but some couples may find the loss of spontaneity inhibiting. Others reject the device because of discomfort, discoloration, or cold temperature of the penis, or because the penis is hinged rather than firmly stabilized during a natural erection.

ORAL PHARMACOTHERAPY

In 1998, the Food and Drug Administration approved sildenafil (Viagra), an oral drug for the treatment of ED. Inhibition of PDE5 increases cGMP in the smooth muscle of the corpus cavernosum, causing prolonged vasodilation and a firmer, longer-lasting erection. There are now two other PDE5 inhibitors available: vardenafil (Levitra) and tadalafil (Cialis) (Table 31–1). PDE5 inhibitors have been shown to be effective in men with diabetes, hypertension, coronary artery disease, peripheral vascular disease, and spinal cord injury, as well as after coronary artery bypass surgery, transurethral prostatectomy (TURP), and radical prostatectomy. The poorer the blood supply, the more damaged the nerves (such as from surgery), and the more prolonged the dysfunction, the poorer the response. Unlike injection therapy, PDE5 inhibitors require sexual stimulation for an erection to occur.

Because PDE5 inhibition potentiates the hypotensive effects of nitrates, concomitant use (including recreational use) of nitrates of any kind is an absolute contraindication. The use of alpha adrenergic blockers (used in men for both hypertension and prostate hypertrophy) also increases the risk for hypotension and generally should be avoided. Relative contraindications include MI, stroke, or dysrhythmia within the past 6 months; poorly controlled hypertension or hypotension; uncompensated cardiac failure; unstable angina; a predisposition to priapism; and retinitis pigmentosa. PDE5 inhibitors do not appear to increase cardiac risk in men with table hypertension or coronary artery disease.[22–24] The most common side effects reported include headache, flushing, dyspepsia, and nasal congestion. The inhibition of phosphodiesterase 6 in the retina by sildenafil may cause altered color

Table 31–1	Currently Available PDE5 Inhibitors	
Generic Name (Brand Name)	**Characteristics**	**Side Effects**
Sildenafil (Viagra)	Take 60 minutes before intercourse on empty stomach; fatty food slows absorption; short duration (4–6 hours)	Headaches, flushing, dyspepsia, blue color distortion
Vardenafil (Levitra)	Take on empty stomach; fatty food slows absorption; onset and duration about the same as sildenafil	Headache, flushing, dyspepsia
Tadalafil (Cialis)	Longer effectiveness (up to 36 hours); may take with food	Headache, flushing, dyspepsia

vision—usually a blue tinge—or increased sensitivity to light in some men. Any association between non-arterial ischemic optic neuropathy and PDES inhibitors is uncertain.

Yohimbine is an oral alpha-2 adrenergic-receptor blocker that may improve erectile function better than placebo, particularly in psychogenic impotence, but most studies suggest little effect.[25,26] Studies remain ongoing for the use of melatonin, phentolamine, apomorphine, dopaminergic, and many other agents.[27]

Many nonprescription remedies for sexual dysfunction that combine a concoction of herbal ingredients and chemicals, like arginine, that claim to increase penile nitric oxide, are not scientifically tested but are widely advertised.

INTRACORPOREAL OR INTRAURETHRAL PHARMACOTHERAPY

Intracorporeal (IC) pharmacotherapy involves an injection into the corpora cavernosa of prostaglandin E_1, papaverine, phentolamine, or some combination of the three. While IC injections are often effective, the risks of prolonged erection (priapism) or penile fibrosis engender concern, although this is uncommon with prostaglandin use. Injection therapy may help men regain potency following neurovascular bundle (NVB)–sparing prostate surgery,[28] and some men who initially require injections may eventually be able to transition to oral PDE5 inhibitor therapy.

Prostaglandin E_1 (alprostadil) can also be administered intraurethrally as a small pellet. This method relies on absorption from the submucosal veins of the urethra that communicate between the corpus spongiosum and the corpora cavernosa. Use of this product may benefit men with penile prostheses by increasing glans engorgement and easing vaginal penetration.

PENILE PROSTHESES

Penile prostheses are devices that when inserted into the corpora cavernosa confer rigidity, either continuously as with the semirigid varieties, or on demand, as with the inflatable types. Although prostheses are very effective with high satisfaction rates, they are also expensive, require surgery, and can have significant complication rates. Thus, they should be used only after other therapies have failed.

TESTOSTERONE FOR HYPOGONADAL MEN

Finally, in hypogonadal men with ED, normalization of testosterone may improve libido and sexual functioning.[29] Measurement of early morning free (rather than total) testosterone may be a better measure of this androgen. Replacement may be by periodic injections,

skin patches, or topical gels. Because of their adverse effects on the liver, oral formulations are not recommended. Potential side effects of testosterone supplementation include breast tenderness, polycythemia, water retention, and acceleration of prostate cancer growth.

SUMMARY

Sexual function declines with age. Often sexual problems that could be relieved are not presented, and direct inquiry must be made. An understanding of the usual changes can help the maintenance of sexuality. Erectile dysfunction, dyspareunia, hypogonadism and other sexual problems are eminently treatable and should be addressed in the primary care setting.

References

1. Bretschneider JG, McCoy NL. Sexual interest and behavior in healthy 80- to 102-year-olds. Arch Sex Behav 17(2):109-29, 1988.
2. Monga M, Bettencourt R, Barrett-Connor E. Community-based study of erectile dysfunction and sildenafil use: the Rancho Bernardo study. Urology 59(5):753-7, 2002.
3. Morgentaler A. A 66-year-old man with sexual dysfunction. JAMA 291(24):2994-3003, 2004.
4. Diokno AC, Brown MB, Herzog AR. Sexual function in the elderly. Arch Intern Med 150(1):197-200, 1990.
5. Marsiglio W, Donnelly D. Sexual relations in later life: a national study of married persons. J Gerontol 46(6):S338-44, 1991.
6. Mulcahy JJ. Male Sexual Function: A Guide to Clinical Management. Totowa, NJ: Humana Press Inc, 2001.
7. Kaschak E, Tiefer L, eds. A New View of Women's Sexual Problems [Women and Therapy 24 (Nos. 1/2)]. New York: Haworth Press, 2001.
8. Maurice WL. Sexual Medicine in Primary Care. St. Louis, MO: Mosby, 1999.
9. Reamy K. Sexual counseling for the nontherapist. Clin Obstet Gynecol 27(3):781-8, 1984.
10. Manfredi R. HIV infection and advanced age: emerging epidemiological, clinical, and management issues. Ageing Res Rev 3(1):31-54, 2004.
11. Gebo KA, Moore RD. Treatment of HIV infection in the older patient. Expert Rev Anti Infect Ther 2(5):733-43, 2004.
12. Glatt AE, Zinner SH, McCormack WM. The prevalence of dyspareunia. Obstet Gynecol 75:433-436, 1990.
13. Feldman HA, Goldstein I, Hatzichristou DG, et al. Impotence and its medical and psychosocial correlates: results of the Massachusetts male aging study. J Urol 151(1) 54-61, 1994.
14. Tomlinson JM, Wright D. Impact of erectile dysfunction and its subsequent treatment with sildenafil: qualitative study. BMJ 328:1037-9, 2004.
15. Bodie JA, Beeman WW, Monga M. Psychogenic erectile dysfunction. Int J Psychiatry Med 33(3):273-93, 2003.
16. Feldman HA, Johannes CB, Derby CA, et al. Erectile dysfunction and coronary risk factors: prospective results from the Massachusetts male aging study. Prev Med 30(4):328-38, 2000.
17. Speel TG, van Langen H, Meuleman EJ. The risk of coronary heart disease in men with erectile dysfunction. Eur Urol 44(3):366-70, 2003.
18. Bacon CG, Mittleman MA, Kawachi I,, et al. Sexual function in men older than 50 years of age: results from the health professionals follow-up study. Ann Intern Med 139:161-8, 2003.
19. Derby CA, Mohr BA, Goldstein I, et al. Modifiable risk factors and erectile dysfunction: can lifestyle changes modify risk? Urology 56(2):302-6, 2000.
20. Esposito K, Giugliano F, Di Palo C, et al. Effect of lifestyle changes on erectile dysfunction in obese men. JAMA 291(24): 2978-84, 2004.
21. Bodie J, Lewis J, Schow D, et al. Laboratory evaluations of erectile dysfunction: an evidence based approach. J Urol 169(6):2262-4, 2003.
22. Marwick TH. Safe sex for men with coronary artery disease. Exercise, sildenafil and risk of cardiac events. JAMA 287:766-7, 2002.
23. Arruda-Olson AM, Mahoney DW, Nehra A, et al. Cardiovascular effects of sildenafil during exercise in men with known or probable coronary artery disease. A randomized crossover trial. JAMA 287:719-25, 2002.
24. Wysowski DK, Farinas E, Swartz L. Comparison of reported and expected deaths in sildenafil (Viagra) users. Am J Cardiol 89:1331-4, 2002.
25. Carey MP, Johnson BT. Effectiveness of yohimbine in the treatment of erectile disorder: four meta-analytic integrations. Arch Sex Behav 25(4):341-60, 1996.
26. Tam SW, Worcel M, Wyllie M. Yohimbine: a clinical review. Pharmacol Ther 91:215-43, 2001.

27. Burnett AL. Novel pharmacological approaches in the treatment of erectile dysfunction. World J Urol 19:57-66, 2001.
28. Gontero P, Kirby R. Proerectile pharmacological prophylaxis following nerve-sparing radical prostatectomy (NSRP). Prostate Cancer Prostatic Dis 7(3):223-6, 2004.
29. Rhoden EL, Morgentaler A. Risks of testosterone-replacement therapy and recommendations for monitoring. N Engl J Med 350:482-92, 2004.

Web Resources

1. Sexuality Information and Educational Council of the United States: www.siecus.org.
2. American Association of Sex Educators, Counselors and Therapists: www.aasect.org.
3. Center for Sexuality and Religion: www.ctrsr.org.
4. American Association for Marriage and Family Therapy: www.aafmt.org.

POSTTEST

1. A 76-year-old widower, who has just moved into an independent-living retirement village, comes to you proclaiming he is now "in heaven." He states there are five single women for every man, and he has a new date every night. His only regret is that he does not have the stamina he had when younger. You congratulate him and:
   a. Give him a prescription for a PDE5 inhibitor with multiple refills.
   b. Refer him to a urologist for a penile implant.
   c. Discuss STD risks and educate him about condom use.
   d. Tell him that vitamin E improves erections.

2. The wife of an 82-year-old man died 3 months ago. His only medical problem is hypertension, well controlled by medications. He tells you he has met another woman and he thinks he is in love again. However, he feels guilty because he still loves and misses his late wife. He also notes that when he has had "heavy petting" lately he was unable to attain a hard erection. He is able to get erections with masturbation, however. You tell him:
   a. His ED is all in his head and he needs to move on with his life.
   b. You will refer him to a urologist for a penile implant.
   c. You will refer him to a urologist for penile injections.
   d. His ED is psychogenic and you will refer him to a psychiatrist.
   e. His grief is normal, but a trial of PDE5 inhibitors may be worthwhile.

3. A 70-year-old man comes to your office for routine evaluation of his hypertension and diabetes mellitus. Just as you put your hand on the door knob to leave, he mentions all the TV advertisements proclaiming the new medicines available to make him "more of a man" and wants to know if he can try them. You tell him:
   a. That you do not have time to discuss it with him, or to review his current medications at that moment. He should make a follow-up appointment but you can give him a prescription for one that includes a discount coupon.
   b. To make a follow-up appointment so you can discuss that specific topic, and review in more detail his concerns as well as the risks and benefits of these medications.
   c. To go on the Internet and he can just try the cheapest one.
   d. That if old football coaches and players recommend it, so do you.

PRETEST ANSWERS

1. e
2. b
3. d

POSTTEST ANSWERS

1. c
2. e
3. b

CHAPTER 32
Elder Mistreatment and Neglect

Sonia R. Sehgal and Laura Mosqueda

- Describe the different types of abuse and neglect.
- Understand components of the history and physical exam that should raise suspicion of possible abuse.
- Discuss barriers to the identification of abuse.
- Describe initial assessment and management strategies.

OBJECTIVES

Upon completion of this chapter, the reader will be able to:

- Discuss the risk factors associated with elder mistreatment and neglect.

PRETEST

1. The national incidence of elder abuse is:
   a. Approximately 100,000
   b. Higher in the "old old," that is, people over the age of 80
   c. Likely to decline over the next 20 years

2. Some of the likely risk factors for being a victim of elder abuse include:
   a. Exhibiting combative behavior
   b. Being of low socioeconomic status
   c. Living with a family member
   d. a and c

3. Risk factors for being a perpetrator of elder abuse include:
   a. Depression
   b. Being a family member
   c. Being dependent on the older adult
   d. All of the above

Ms. Johnson

Ms. Johnson is an 86-year-old woman who comes to your office for a routine visit. She has been living in her own home by herself ever since her husband died 12 years ago. Despite the fact that she has Parkinson's disease, diabetes, and hypertension, she has remained independent. Over the past year, she has had some decline in her function, and is requiring meals-on-wheels and other services to remain at home. Her daughter Betsy recently moved from another state to live with her mother and provide assistance.

The physical exam reveals a pleasant woman who has a moderate amount of tremor at rest and who can ambulate slowly with the aid of a walker. You notice that Ms. Johnson seems withdrawn on this visit, and she tells you that it's been difficult to adjust to having a new person in the house even though she knows she needs help to stay there. The next visit is an urgent appointment because Ms. Johnson fell, and has multiple large bruises on her upper arms and forehead. Betsy brings her to see you, and tells you that "I just found Mom on the floor this morning." Ms. Johnson nods in agreement but says little else. No treatment is needed and she goes home.

Three weeks later another urgent appointment is made: Ms. Johnson has a dislocated shoulder and bruises on her upper chest wall. Again, her daughter says she fell. Despite Betsy's protests, you ask her to leave the exam room so that you may speak privately with Ms. Johnson. When you ask Ms. Johnson what happened, she breaks down in tears and reports that her daughter has been taking her money for years. Betsy moved in because she had no other place to live but promised that she would care for her mother in exchange for room and board. Once she was living there, Betsy asked her mother to sign over bank accounts. Initially, Betsy "just yelled at me and threatened to put me in a nursing home. But over the past month, Betsy became more aggressive and pushed me down several times. Last night she grabbed me and punched me because I would not sign the house over to her. I'm so ashamed.... I never thought my own daughter would do this to me."

STUDY QUESTIONS

1. Did you notice anything at the first visit that may lead you to worry about the possibility of abuse?

2. Do you think Ms. Johnson would have told you what happened if you did not ask her directly?

CASE DISCUSSION

The sad reality is that this is not an uncommon scenario. This primary care provider did the right thing: she was observant, noting that the patient was withdrawn and that the bruises were in unusual locations for a fall; she had the daughter leave the room so that Ms. Johnson could tell her story; she was reassuring but direct in asking Ms. Johnson what happened. This case also illustrates the common finding that victims of abuse are often subject to multiple types of mistreatment over a prolonged period of time. In this case, Ms. Johnson experienced financial, psychological, and physical abuse for many years.

Abuse and neglect of older adults is a common yet underreported problem that will be getting worse. While the number of older adults is increasing, the number of available caregivers is decreasing. This demographic trend of more vulnerable adults and fewer people to care for them combined with a national trend of decreasing social services is a harbinger of a new epidemic.

Translating the definition of abuse (Box 32–1)[2] to a diagnosis of abuse is not easy nor is it straightforward: It is often difficult to distinguish between injuries that occur through innocent mechanisms (e.g., falling) and injuries that occur as a result of abuse (e.g., being punched). While some acts of commission or omission are blatantly abusive, there is no simple method to tell when some acts, such as poor care, cross the line to become "abuse." But these are not good excuses to avoid making a diagnosis. Primary care providers are in a unique position to prevent, recognize, and respond to abuse. They are often the first to identify both victim and perpetrator and so must be mindful of the possibility and know how to respond. Interestingly, though, health care professionals, particularly physicians, are among the least likely to report suspicion of abuse to Adult Protective Services.[1]

> ● Clinicians in primary care are in a unique position to prevent, recognize, and respond to abuse. But health care professionals, particularly physicians, are among the least likely to report suspicion of abuse to Adult Protective Services.

INCIDENCE AND IMPACT

The 1996 National Elder Abuse Incidence Study estimated that 551,011 persons age 60 and over experienced mistreatment over a 1-year period.[1] Utilizing sentinels in the community, this study estimated that for every reported, substantiated case, at least four go unreported.[1] Furthermore, those aged 80 years and older were two to three times more likely to suffer elder mistreatment than their younger counterparts.[1] The types of elder mistreatment are shown in Fig. 32–1. Contrary to many people's preconceived notions, family members, particularly adult children

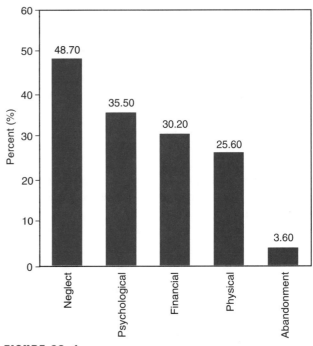

FIGURE 32–1

Types of elder mistreatment. Note: Total percent is greater than 100 because people are often victims of more than one type of abuse. (*Adapted from National Center on Elder Abuse. National Elder Abuse Incidence Study: final report. Washington, DC: Department of Health and Human Services Administration for Children and Families and Administration on Aging, September 1998.*)

| Box 32–1 | Elder Mistreatment: Definition |

- Intentional actions that cause harm or create a serious risk of harm (whether or not harm is intended) to a vulnerable elder by a caregiver or other person who stands in a trust relationship to the elder.
- Failure by a caregiver to satisfy the elder's basic needs to protect the elder from harm.

From Bonnie R, Wallace R. Elder Mistreatment: Abuse, Neglect and Exploitation in an Aging America. Washington, DC: National Academy Press, 2003.

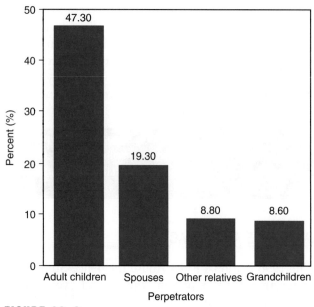

FIGURE 32–2

Breakdown of suspected perpetrators. Note: Only 16% of perpetrators are nonfamily members. *(Adapted from National Center on Elder Abuse. National Elder Abuse Incidence Study: final report. Washington, DC: Department of Health and Human Services Administration for Children and Families and Administration on Aging, September 1998.)*

and spouses, are the most common perpetrators of abusive acts (Fig. 32–2).[1]

In 2000, a 50-state survey found that 472,813 reports of elder mistreatment were received by Adult Protective Services. Of those reports received, more than 80% were investigated and almost 50% were substantiated, confirming that adults over 80 years of age were the most likely victims of abuse, excluding self-neglect.[3]

In 1996, it was estimated that between 1 and 2 million Americans aged 65 and older had been mistreated by an individual expected to provide care or protection.[1] With the aging of the Baby Boomers, the number of older adults is expected to almost double in size to comprise 20% of the U.S. population by 2030.[4] The pool of potential victims is growing at a rapid rate.

RISK FACTORS AND PATHOPHYSIOLOGY

Mr. Greenwood

Mr. Greenwood has been your patient for many years. You diagnosed him with Alzheimer's disease 3 years ago, and lately he has been quite agitated. He requires assistance with some ADLs, but gets upset when his daughter Camille tries to help. He

also follows her around the house and asks her the same questions repeatedly.

Camille brings him in for his appointments, and it is clear that she is unhappy and resentful. You ask how she is doing with her dad; she tells you "my father was never around when I was growing up. Now that he needs help he has come back into my life and is ruining it! I can't spend the time I want to with my own kids, and my husband is getting annoyed because the house isn't as organized as I used to have it." You smell alcohol on her breath when she was telling this to you. Although you have seen no evidence of abuse, you recognize that the potential exists.

STUDY QUESTIONS

1. What interventions might you implement to help calm this situation?
2. What issues might you discuss with Camille during this office visit?

CASE DISCUSSION

The primary care clinician is in an excellent position to prevent abuse if one recognizes the warning signs. The family cycle of violence, substance abuse on the part of the caregiver, anger and resentment of the daughter toward her father, and his increasing dependency on her are all warning signs. Interventions such as counseling, support groups, and day care programs may stop this from progressing to a violent situation.

Camille and her father have never had a good relationship, he is resistant to care, she is feeling overwhelmed and angry, she may be abusing alcohol, and her family is pressuring her to spend more time with them. Because you have recognized these as red flags (Box 32–2) for possible abuse, you intervene to prevent this situation from escalating into abuse. You ask Camille if she has ever hurt her father, and she tells you that she hasn't but that she is worried she might hit him when she gets upset and out of control. After empathizing with her situation and thanking her for her honesty, you explain how you will help her: You give Camille information about adult day care programs close to her home, support groups through the Alzheimer's Association, books on Alzheimer's disease, an appointment with a counselor, and information on assisted living facilities that specialize in caring for people who have dementia. You have them follow up with you in 1 week. As a result of your efforts, Mr. Greenwood starts attending the day care program 3 days a week, Camille understands more about the illness her father has, and she gets appropriate emotional support. When you see them again several months later, both Mr. Greenwood and his daughter are calmer and happier.

Elder mistreatment may be discovered during daily clinical practice, yet many health care providers do not recognize the potential or actual victims. Risk factor assessment is an important part of one's ability to identify potential victims and initiate treatment. Risk factors are found in the victim, perpetrator, and sociocultural environment in which they are embedded (see Box 32–2).

Patients with Alzheimer's disease living in a shared residence are at significantly increased risk of mistreatment.[5,6] By increasing the likelihood of interaction, a shared living situation can escalate from experiencing day-to-day annoyances to daily conflict and ultimately to mistreatment. While living alone places an older adult at less risk of being abused by others,[7] social isolation is dangerous because abuse may go unnoticed.

Simply having a dementing illness places a person at increased risk for mistreatment, particularly if the person with dementia displays disruptive behavior.[3] The estimated prevalence rate of abusive caregivers ranges from 5% to 14% in the dementia population, as compared to 1% to 3% in the general population.

Mental health problems such as depression are often present in perpetrators of abuse. Of note, in a study examining the care of Alzheimer's disease patients, caregiver depression was a strong predictor of physical abuse.[6,8] Physical abusers are more likely to be classified as depressed when compared to those

who abuse through neglect.[9] Alcohol and/or drug abuse among the perpetrators of elder mistreatment is also common.[10]

Furthermore, several studies have demonstrated that perpetrators are more likely to be dependent on the victim they are mistreating. Financial exploitation was estimated to affect 20% of victims of elder mistreatment as reported by the National Aging Resource Center on Elder Abuse in 2003.[11]

> ● Simply having a dementing illness places a person at increased risk for mistreatment, particularly if the person with dementia displays disruptive behavior.

DIFFERENTIAL DIAGNOSIS AND ASSESSMENT

Barriers to Diagnosis

Several barriers to diagnosis exist. Often the primary care provider is uncertain as to what constitutes abuse. In these times of short outpatient visits, detecting, questioning, and confronting abuse issues can be daunting. However, the primary care provider may be the only person with adequate contact to suspect and protect when abuse is present.

As most abuse occurs in the victim's home, it is easily hidden from health care providers and other witnesses. The victims often feel ashamed and embarrassed that they actually allowed it to happen, or that their "loved one" did this to them, or they may be fearful that they will be deemed incompetent and put in a nursing home. Some would rather be abused than be taken out of their home. Many abused older adults are depressed and find it difficult to confront their abuser or voice their concerns to health care workers. Many patients may aggressively hide their abuse, unlike patients seeking early detection for other medical disorders.

Dementia may interfere with an elderly person's ability to report abuse or to even understand that she or he is being abused. People with dementia are often dependent on their abuser for daily living, and may be socially isolated from third-party observers who may detect abuse.

While bruises and fractures can be clues to incidents of abuse, they can also be common findings in frail older adults as a result of falls and injury to delicate tissues. For this reason, it is important to understand the context in which these injuries occurred. In children, retinal hemorrhages and long bone fractures make up a constellation of findings that would trigger a provider to have an immediate suspicion of abuse. Unfortunately, such pathognomonic findings do not exist for abuse of the older adult. Awareness, suspicion,

---

Box 32-2	**Risk Factors for Elder Mistreatment**

Victim
- Advanced age
- Dependent for basic activities of daily living
- Dementia
- Combative behavior

Perpetrator
- Depression/mental illness
- Alcohol or drug dependence
- Financial dependence

and a comprehensive assessment are required to detect elder mistreatment.

Assessment

Abuse can span many years or present as a one-time, isolated incident. It is difficult to identify when events cross the line from inappropriate care to mistreatment because there is no clearly defined line. If a provider is unsure, it is prudent to make a report. Cases of abuse and neglect may be found during a routine visit at a primary care provider's office or a regular visit to a long-term care facility.

A thorough evaluation is indicated for patients who are thought to be victims of abuse. The patient should be examined alone, away from family members, as the victim may be embarrassed or may fear retaliation.[12] Direct questioning by the primary care provider in a nonthreatening manner should be conducted. Home environment and safety issues should be evaluated. Information regarding inciting factors, and frequency and type of abuse should be elicited. Factors suggestive of abuse include a delay in seeking treatment, confusing or unlikely causes of injury, or a past history of suspicious incidents.[13] A history of "doctor shopping" and caregiver avoidance of appointments should also raise suspicions of abuse.[14]

A complete physical examination should be performed on all patients suspected of abuse (Box 32–3). A full skin assessment should be undertaken. Areas hidden from plain sight should be examined, including soles of feet, inner thighs, axillae, and palms, with all areas of bruising, burns, tenderness, or abrasions doc-umented. Weight loss, hygiene, and a history of fractures should be noted. Sexual abuse cannot be overlooked, and a gynecological evaluation may be necessary. Assessment of patients suspected of any type of abuse warrants not only a physical but also a cognitive evaluation. Cognitive impairment as well as visual or auditory deficits can make an already challenging evaluation that much more difficult.

Care providers should be asked about their level of stress and their ability to function in their role of caregiver. Financial difficulties, anger, and resentment toward the patient should also be assessed. Caregiver burnout should be suspected when primary caregivers begin to complain about the patient, and blame the patient for situations that are out of their control.[15]

Confirmatory laboratory testing can be done to corroborate unusual findings. A complete blood count, blood urea nitrogen, creatinine, total protein, and albumin levels can help establish whether dehydration or malnutrition is present. Radiographs depicting old and new fractures can help suggest patterns of long-term abuse.

Contextual factors are often as important as the injury itself. For example, if a person presents with a stage IV pressure ulcer of his coccyx, the health care provider may know that this person is on hospice, and that all appropriate steps are being taken to prevent skin breakdown. However, if a patient who had been walking and talking 2 months ago suddenly appears in your office with the same wound, this is an unexpected finding that deserves careful questioning.

> ● Factors suggestive of abuse include a delay in seeking treatment, confusing or unlikely causes of injury, or a past history of suspicious incidents.

MANAGEMENT

The first step in management when elder mistreatment is suspected is an open conversation with the patient. If the patient understands his situation, he can take an active role in deciding about next steps. However, a patient who is depressed or demented may be incapable of meaningful participation in the planning process. Multidisciplinary teams consisting of social workers, physicians, and legal counsel are available in many communities when difficult management issues arise.

Most health care workers are mandated reporters of elder mistreatment and neglect in the 47 states that have a mandated reporting law. The definitions, requirements, and mandated reporters vary from state to state, so it is important for providers to be familiar with the laws in their state. Adult Protective Services (APS) is the agency responsible for taking and

---

Box 32-3 Possible Abuse Indicators

- Weight loss
- Dehydration
- Poor hygiene/elongated toenails
- Depression
- Inappropriate attire (e.g., not dressed warmly in cold weather)
- Abrasions/lacerations
- Hematomas
- Traumatic alopecia
- Bruises in unusual locations (e.g., breasts/genital area)
- Welts
- Burns
- Pressure ulcers
- Rectal/vaginal bleeding
- Signs of sexually transmitted diseases

investigating reports of abuse in community-dwelling older adults. In some states, they also investigate abuse in licensed facilities, and in others this is done by the state ombudsman. Police should be contacted in addition to APS in emergent situations. It is not a HIPPA violation to share medical information with police or APS when abuse is suspected.[16]

Careful documentation of physical findings such as bruises or abrasions is important. Photographs should be taken of unusual skin findings with a reference object in the visual field for an estimation of size. All lesions should have accurate documentation of their dimensions and locations. It is useful to describe the location of lesions in reference to two distinct fixed body parts; for example, a lesion on the upper back should have measurements to the lateral aspect of the shoulder and base of the neck. Diagrams are also helpful in charting locations of skin lesions. All facets of the history and physical exam can be used as evidence if a case goes to trial. For this reason, records should be legible and complete. Objective information should be recorded, including statements made by both the victim and perpetrator in addition to physical exam findings.

SCREENING

Most primary care providers and emergency room personnel do not screen routinely for elder abuse. However, in 1992 the American Medical Association encouraged physicians to "incorporate routine questions related to elder abuse and neglect into daily practice."[17] Current screening tools are limited, as several of them require accurate responses from victims, who may be cognitively or emotionally impaired, as well as from their caregivers. Fast and accurate tools need to be developed, but meanwhile, the provider can ask: "Are you afraid of anyone? Has anyone threatened you or harmed you?"

Prevention strategies can be employed during routine medical visits. At each visit, both the caregiver and patient should be questioned regarding stress in the living environment and observed for signs of feeling overwhelmed or discouraged. Respite services should be readily offered. Senior centers, adult day health care services, and other community programs may offer the caregiver and patient much needed time away from each other.

SUMMARY

Elder mistreatment is a national tragedy that has a serious impact on the health and happiness of elders and those who love them. Victims suffer from more illness and premature death. When all other risk factors are taken into account, elder abuse by itself imposes a threefold increase in the risk of death of community-dwelling older adults.[18] These patients have more psychiatric and physical disorders manifested by increased numbers of hospitalizations and emergency department visits.

Elder mistreatment and neglect are serious and complex issues that a primary care provider must face in clinical practice. A reasonable suspicion, identification of risk factors, and a multidisciplinary team approach will help victims and abusers obtain the treatment they need.

POSTTEST

1. Some of the barriers to detecting elder mistreatment include all except which one of the following:
   a. The tendency for many older adults to falsely claim they are being abused.
   b. The fear that one might be institutionalized if one admits to being abused.
   c. The shame that older adults feel if they have been a victim of abuse.
   d. The inability of a health care provider to make a determination regarding abuse if the victim is demented.

2. Physical manifestations of elder abuse often overlap with common age-related changes. Some physical findings that should lead a clinician to consider abuse rather than a common age-related change are:
   a. Bruises on the breasts
   b. Skin tears on the dorsal forearms
   c. Midtibial fracture in an older adult who has no history of falling
   d. a and c

3. Clues that may lead one to suspect abuse include:
   a. "Doctor shopping" by a caregiver
   b. Delay in seeking care for a stage IV pressure ulcer
   c. Malnutrition in a hospice patient
   d. a and b

References

1. National Center on Elder Abuse. National Elder Abuse Incidence Study: final report. Washington, DC: Department of Health and Human Services Administration for Children and Families and Administration on Aging, September 1998.
2. Bonnie R, Wallace R. Elder Mistreatment: Abuse, Neglect and Exploitation in an Aging America. Washington, DC: National Academy Press,; 2003.
3. National Center on Elder Abuse. A Response to Abuse of Vulnerable Adults: The 2000 Survey of State Adult Protective Services. Washington, DC: Department of Health and Human Services Administration for Children and Families and Administration on Aging, 2002.
4. Federal Interagency Forum on Aging-Related statistics. Key Indicators of Well-Being. Washington, DC: U.S. Government Printing Office, August 2000.
5. Pillemer K, Suitor JJ. Violence and violent feelings: what causes them among family givers? J Gerontol 47:S165-72, 1992.
6. Paveza GJ, Cohen D, Eisdorfer C, et al. Severe family violence and Alzheimer's disease: prevalence and risk factors. Gerontologist 32(4):493-7, 1992.
7. Pillemer K, Finkelhor D. The prevalence of elder abuse: a random sample survery. Gerontologist 28(1):51-7, 1988.
8. Coyne AC, Reichman WE, Berbig LJ. The relationship between dementia and elder abuse. Am J Psychiatry 150(4):642-6, 1993.
9. Reay AM, Browne KD. Risk factor characteristics in carers who physically abuse or neglect their elderly dependents. Aging Mental Health 5(1):56-62, 2001.
10. Homer AC, Gilleard C. Abuse of elderly people by their carers. BMJ 301(6765):1359-62, 1990.
11. Office of Community Oriented Policies Services. The Problem of Financial Crimes Against the Elderly. Washington, DC: U.S. Department of Justice, 2003.
12. Paris BE, Meier DE, Goldstein T, et al. Elder abuse and neglect: how to recognize warning signs and intervene. Geriatrics 50:47-51, 1995.
13. Swagerty D. Elder mistreatment identification and assessment. Clin Fam Pract 5(1):195-211, 2003.
14. Lachs MS, Fulmer T. Recognizing elder abuse and neglect. Clin Geriatr Med 9:665-75, 1993.
15. Lachs MS, Pillemer K. Abuse and neglect of elderly persons. N Engl J Med 332:437-43, 1998.
16. Campanelli R. In correspondence. Director. Washington, DC: Office for Civil Rights, Department of Health and Human Services. Reference number 04-23200. Received December 23, 2004.
17. American Medical Association (AMA). Amercan Medical Association Diagnostic and Treatment Guidelines on Elder Abuse and Neglect. Chicago: AMA, 1992.
18. Lachs MS, Williams C, O'Brien S, et al. Older adults: an 11-year longitudinal study of adult protective services use. Arch Intern Med 156:449-52, 1996.

Web Resources

1. National Center on Elder Abuse: www.elderabusecenter.org.
2. National Committee for the Prevention of Elder Abuse: www.preventelderabuse.org.
3. Continuing Medical Education, Elder Abuse and Neglect: http://www.ageworks.com/elderabuse.

PRETEST ANSWERS

1. b
2. d
3. d

POSTTEST ANSWERS

1. a
2. d
3. d

OBJECTIVES

Upon completion of this chapter, the reader will be able to:

- Identify risk factors and diagnostic criteria for alcoholism in older persons.
- Discuss screening instruments and laboratory tests used in the diagnosis of alcoholism and the effects of aging on their clinical use.
- Describe the mechanisms of initiating treatment and the types of treatment available.
- Discuss the relationship of alcohol dependency to other common syndromes of old age: dementia, depression, suicide, polypharmacy, falls, and multiple medical illnesses.

PRETEST

1. The diagnosis and treatment of alcohol dependency is best facilitated by using the model that defines alcoholism as a:
   a. Moral issue
   b. Psychological issue
   c. Disease
   d. Habit
   e. Response to social stresses

2. An 81-year-old woman is being evaluated for dementia. She describes no more than two drinks per day during the week and slightly more on the weekends. Which one of the following is true?
   a. At this level of intake, she does not have alcoholism.
   b. This quantity of use is safe.
   c. Quantity of use is a good screen for alcoholism.
   d. Alcoholism may be present if there are negative consequences.
   e. This report clearly defines how much ethanol is being ingested.

3. An 85-year-old man with depression reports himself to be a "social drinker." Which of the following is the best screening tool:
   a. Chart review for diagnosis of alcoholism
   b. Collaborative history and/or CAGE questionnaire
   c. Aspartame transferase (AST)/alanine transferase (ALT) and/or gamma glutamyl transferase (GGT)
   d. Quantity/frequency questions
   e. Minnesota Multiphasic Personality Inventory (MMPI)

James Beem, *Part 1*

James Beem is a 79-year-old seat-belted driver involved in a car crash. He has suffered a femur fracture, unilateral rib fractures, and a laceration of the left arm. He has been stabilized in the trauma bay and is currently in the surgical intensive care unit for monitoring. You have been asked to consult on hospital day 2 regarding his mental status (Mini-Mental Status Exam [MMSE] 17/30) and hypertension (BP 202/106, pulse 96). He has a past history of hypertension, glaucoma, cataracts, and hyperlipidemia.

STUDY QUESTIONS

1. Which of the many charted investigations do you seek first?
2. A family member is waiting to see you. What questions will you ask first?

PREVALENCE AND IMPACT

The diagnosis of alcoholism is often missed in older patients. Many of the classic clues are mistaken for age-related changes or diseases. The psychosocial factors that are often pivotal in moving younger alcoholics into treatment (spouse, job, and legal pressures such as being charged with driving while intoxicated) are less likely to occur in elders. Pharmacokinetic changes make the quantity of ethanol used a less reliable indicator of problems, falsely reassuring the health care professional. Clinicians must be alert to the significance of features such as falling, incontinence, poor social support, cognitive decline, depression, noncompliance, and others.

Alcoholism is difficult to diagnose, and yet it is one of the most remediable ailments of the elderly. Treatment modalities—developed over the past 50 years—are *particularly* effective in older patients.

Definition

Alcohol dependency is a medical syndrome. This is most important. It determines the types of treatment and professional responsibility for care.

Alcohol has been produced since 4000 to 6000 BC. Restrictions of consumption have been documented as far back as 1700 BC. Habitual drunkenness as a disease was first proposed in 276 AD by Domitius Ulpinus in Rome.

Early in the 20th century, alcoholism was defined in moralistic terms: treatment involved condemnation and punishment, and was in the scope of the religious and criminal justice systems. Although Benjamin Rush seriously reintroduced the concept of alcoholism as a disease in the early 1800s, it was not until the rise of Alcoholics Anonymous (AA) in the 1930s and the recognition of AA in 1956 by the American Medical Association that alcohol dependency became clearly categorized as a disease.[1] Alcoholism was thus moved from the legal system and placed in the purview of public health. The medical community then developed diagnostic criteria and prevalence and natural history data, and screening and treatment modalities were defined.

In the early 1950s, the definition by the World Health Organization (WHO) of alcoholism was paraphrased as "having problems from drinking and drinking anyway."[2] In 1975, the WHO redefined the drinking behaviors characteristic of alcohol-dependence syndrome: drink-seeking behaviors, increased tolerance of alcohol, repeated withdrawal symptoms, repeated relief or avoidance of withdrawal symptoms by further drinking, subjective awareness of a compulsion to drink, and reinstatement of the syndrome after abstinence.

In this chapter the terms *alcoholism, alcohol dependence,* and *alcohol addiction* are used synonymously. These terms imply development of tolerance, withdrawal reactions, loss of control of alcohol use, and psychosocial decline.[3] A practical classification scheme for elderly alcoholics identifies four patterns: (1) chronic, (2) intermittent, (3) late onset, and (4) reactive.[4] Reactive alcoholism as a term to imply impaired use after psychosocial stressors has not been a clinically useful term.

Prior studies must be interpreted carefully. Although some studies simply distinguished late from early onset in terms of the four-part classification, "chronic" and "intermittent" are almost always early onset, and reactive may be either late or early onset because the drinking is in response to a biopsychosocial stress. Two-thirds of older alcoholics fall in the chronic or intermittent class, and one-third are true late onset.[5]

> ● Only one-third of elderly alcoholics are truly "late onset."

Prevalence

Of the elderly, 5% to 10% are heavy alcohol users. It is estimated that there are a half million elderly alcoholics in the United States.[5] Alcoholism is the third most prevalent psychiatric disorder among elderly men (15%), surpassed only by dementia and anxiety disorders.[6] Elderly alcoholics often present to the health care system through associated diagnoses.[7] Older persons hospitalized for general medical and surgical procedures and institutionalized elderly demonstrate a prevalence of approximately 18% alcohol abuse.[3] One-third of older alcoholics are estimated to have begun their alcohol abuse *after* age 65.[5]

Patterns of alcohol use are affected by such experiences as the Industrial Revolution, the temperance movement, Prohibition, the Depression, and the two world wars. Alcohol use should be understood to be a habit, whereas alcoholism is a separate disease entity. These factors explain the apparent contradiction of elderly persons' decreased alcohol use, yet with no decline in alcoholism.

Table 33–1 summarizes the factors contributing to the low reported rates of alcoholism and to the increased impact of drinking in old age. Many of these factors arise from society's unwillingness to label older persons as alcoholics because of the continued stigma. The mistaken thought that older alcoholics are "untreatable" is prevalent and reduces detection.

> ● The mistaken thought that older alcoholics are "untreatable" is prevalent and reduces detection.

Impact

The older alcoholic is likely to drink only five to six times per week and only four to five drinks per occasion,[8] yet ethanol has greater pharmacologic impact as we age. Ethanol absorption is no different with increasing

Table 33–1 Factors Affecting Reported Rate and Impact of Alcoholism

Age-Related Factors	Other Factors Causing Low Reported Rates	Other Factors Increasing Impact
Increased biologic sensitivity (lower body water ratio, less efficient liver)	Institutionalized people excluded from community surveys	Institutionalized people not being diagnosed or treated
Under-diagnosis by health care providers	Less overall driving, so less driving while intoxicated	Coexisting conditions limit sensory input while driving
Cohort values and under-reporting	Cognitive impairment	Increased concomitant disease
Less socialization and less awareness by peers of drinking behaviors	Spontaneous remission	Increased prescription and nonprescription drug use
Less job or legal pressure to initiate treatment	Selective survival	
Family unwillingness to report	Ill health Financial constraints	

age. However, at an unchanged rate of ethanol intake, peak concentration is on average higher in the elderly. This is a result of the smaller volume of distribution because ethanol is distributed in body water, which is decreased in elderly persons.[4] The elderly patient is unlikely to be cross-addicted to other nonprescription drugs; however, the possibility of misuse of prescription drugs must be considered because it has been estimated to occur in over 10% of elders.

An important psychosocial change is the shrinking social support network. In one study, concern of a family member or friend was the most common factor motivating patients for admission to a treatment program.[9]

RISK FACTORS AND PATHOPHYSIOLOGY

Etiology

Alcoholism is best understood as a medical condition. In the past, attempts to treat alcoholism in a moral mode or in a model of personality disorder have been unsuccessful. The medical model removes patient blame and enables patients to be more participatory in recovery.

Evidence is very supportive that alcoholism is an inherited tendency: an increased number of direct relatives of alcoholic individuals have the disease. The genetic nature of the disease helps patients and families to understand and accept the diagnosis and allows them to be more active in their recovery. Ingestion of alcohol triggers the genetic tendency. There is increased endorphin production in response to alcohol intake. The full illness manifests as the inability to practice controlled usage. Approximately 8% of the American population is unable to ingest alcohol in a controlled-use, "social" pattern. Genetic predisposition is estimated to account for the 40% to 60% of patients with alcoholism.[10]

Changes in body fat to water ratio alter the pharmacokinetics of alcohol consumption in the elderly.

Clearance is decreased as a result of decreased liver blood flow and the decrease in liver mass, which results in higher blood alcohol concentration with similar alcohol ingestion. The same quantity of ingested alcohol in an older person leads to a higher blood alcohol concentration than it does in a younger person, because alcohol is water soluble and body water is relatively reduced in the elderly. These changes explain the paradox that older people appear to be drinking the same amount and yet are getting more negative effects from the alcohol.

DIFFERENTIAL DIAGNOSIS AND ASSESSMENT

Screening and Detection

Screening questionnaires have been shown to differentiate people suffering from alcoholism from people who are not, although such screening tests are less sensitive in older persons. Such questionnaires cover the quantity consumed, alcohol-related social or legal difficulties, alcohol-related health problems, symptoms of drunkenness or dependence, and self-recognition.[11,12] Certain questions on the CAGE questionnaire[13] and the Michigan Alcoholism Screening Test (MAST)[14,15] are significantly less likely to be answered in the affirmative if the subjects are elderly. Nonetheless, the CAGE questionnaire is a useful brief clinical screen (Box 33–1).[13]

Box 33–1   CAGE Questionnaire

- Have you ever felt you ought to *Cut* down your drinking?
- Have you ever been *Annoyed* by criticism of your drinking?
- Have you ever felt *Guilty* about your drinking?
- Have you ever felt the need for an *Eye* opener?

Source: Ewing J. Detecting alcoholism: the CAGE questionnaire. JAMA 1989;252:510, with permission.

The shorter 24-item MAST-G (Geriatric MAST) test is age-appropriate and therefore widely used.[16] An even shorter version (S-MAST-G, Fig. 33–1) has been developed for use in busy practices.[17] A systematic office assessment flow for alcoholism is summarized in Fig. 33–2.

Useful laboratory tests including a complete blood count (CBC), blood chemistries, liver function (LFTs), gamma glutamyl transferase (GGT), and blood alcohol level usually demonstrate some abnormality that may be attributable to alcohol use. Yet many of these tests are likely to be abnormal in a nonalcoholic older individual, limiting these tests' specificity. However, such tests can help reinforce the reality of the diagnosis, especially in patients or family members resistant to acceptance of the diagnosis. Blood alcohol levels, although more specific, lack adequate sensitivity as a screening tool. A number of clinical clues to alcoholism that are often misinterpreted in elders are summarized in Box 33–2.

The genetic nature of alcoholism renders the family history especially significant.

The most helpful clinical clue to the presence of alcoholism in an elderly person is often the presence of the disease in a child or grandchild. Families whose rituals and behaviors became distorted as a result of alcoholism are more likely to transmit the disease familially.[18]

⬤ The most helpful clinical clue to the presence of alcoholism in an elderly person is often the presence of the disease in a child or grandchild.

Alcoholism and Other Illnesses

The medical problems associated with alcoholism must be specifically sought: diseases of the esophagus, stomach, pancreas, or liver, as well as cognitive impairment, blackouts, and cerebellar dysfunction. Alcoholism has a significant effect on health; problem drinkers have poor overall health and significant mental health problems.[19]

Alcoholism is distinctly related to dementia; it is estimated that 10% of the instances of dementia in older persons are alcohol related. Cognition usually improves after treatment, but at the very least, progression can be aborted.

Depression is commonly the medical illness that is comorbid with alcohol abuse; alcohol is an easily available, nonprescription psychotropic. Although alcohol has mood-elevating effects in moderate doses,[4] it is primarily a central nervous system depressant. Of depressed people, 10% to 15% use it for self-medication.[20] One study found that over 50% of patients admitted for alcoholism treatment had symptoms of depression that persisted for at least 1 year after alcohol treatment.[21] Alcohol is also associated with suicide.

Short Michigan Alcoholism Screening Test Geriatric Version (S-MAST-G)	Yes (1)	No (0)
1. When talking with others, do you ever underestimate how much you drink?		
2. After a few drinks, have you sometimes not eaten, or been able to skip a meal, because you didn't feel hungry?		
3. Does having a few drinks help decrease your shakiness or tremors?		
4. Does alcohol sometimes make it hard for you to remember parts of the day or night?		
5. Do you usually take a drink to relax or calm your nerves?		
6. Do you drink to take your mind off your problems?		
7. Have you ever increased your drinking after experiencing a loss in your life?		
8. Has a doctor or nurse ever said they were worried or concerned about your drinking?		
9. Have you ever made rules to manage your drinking?		
10. When you feel lonely, does having a drink help?		
TOTAL S-MAST-G SCORE (1–10)		
SCORING: 2 or more "YES" responses indicate an alcohol problem.		

FIGURE 33–1

Short Michigan Alcoholism Screening Test-Geriatric Version (S-MAST-G). *(Redrawn from The Regents of the University of Michigan. Ann Arbor: University of Michigan Alcohol Research Center, 1991, with permission.)*

Flow diagram for alcoholism evaluation in context of new patient assessment or clinical suspicion

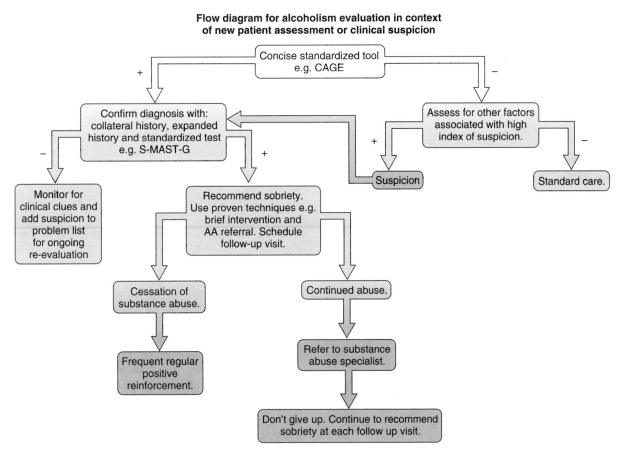

FIGURE 33–2

Flow diagram for alcoholism evaluation in context of new patient assessment or clinical suspicion.

Box 33–2   Alcoholism Clinical Clues Misattributed to Other Causes

Clues Misattributed to Common Problems of Old Age
- Dementia
- Confusion
- Memory loss
- Disorientation
- Falls
- Bruises
- Fractures
- Incontinence
- Malnutrition
- Polypharmacy
- Use of sedatives and anxiolytics
- Use of analgesics

Clues Misattributed Due to Age-Biased Views
- Treatment ineffectiveness
- Resistance to treatment
- Self-neglect

- Functional decline
- Sleep impairment
- Anxiety
- Postoperative problems.

Clues Misattributed to Coexisting Diseases Common in Older Persons
- Depression
- Hypertension
- Malnutrition
- Sleep disturbances
- Chronic fatigue
- Peripheral neuropathy
- Cerebellar degeneration
- Seizures
- Sexual dysfunction
- Repeated infections
- Cardiomyopathy

Conversely, factors associated with a diagnosis of depression include alcohol or substance abuse.[22]

Alcoholism has a definite relationship to falling. However, although there is a significant association of hip fracture with heavy alcohol consumption in younger persons, after age 65 the association is less strong.[23]

James Beem, *Part 2*

Mr. Beem has been initiated on a delirium tremens protocol and has responded well. He has been transferred to the floor. His tachycardia and hypertension have both improved. He reports a history of drinking. His cognition has improved, and he is resistant to the possibility that his alcohol consumption may be causing negative consequences. He insists that he drinks the same amount now as he did when he was younger.

STUDY QUESTION

1. How can you help him and his family understand this paradox?

MANAGEMENT

Treatment

The family is not only helpful in making the diagnosis but is the key element of treatment. In fact, using the family is the most significant advance in treatment and rehabilitation of the alcoholic patient (Box 33–3).

The effective approach to the patient and family is to avoid being judgmental and to emphasize the disease model and the need for further evaluation. It is important to initiate the treatment plan on the same day that the patient is confronted with the diagnosis. The physician can facilitate this by maintaining relationships with existing Alcoholics Anonymous (AA)

Box 33–3	**Principles of Treatment for Elderly Alcoholics**

- The family is the key to management
- Nonjudgmental, medical/disease approach
- Initiate plan same day patient is confronted
- Use Alcoholics Anonymous members
- Abstinence is the principle: controlled drinking is not recommended
- Replace drinking with people
- Group therapy
- Hospitalization for detoxification and/or delirium tremens

---

members who can be called upon to help. AA is appropriate for older patients; one-third of AA members are over 50 years old. The treatment plan must include family and friends. Legal commitment is occasionally necessary; recovery rates for such patients approximate those for persons who seek help voluntarily.[24] Recent evidence demonstrates that older persons respond to brief interventions in the primary care office with positive net results for such patients.[25]

Three significant *barriers to management* of elderly alcoholics have been defined: (1) physicians are less likely to identify elderly alcoholics; (2) if identified, the elderly patient is less likely to be referred; and (3) the elderly are less likely to be accepted into treatment programs.[26]

The first step in treatment is *recognition*. One study found that the diagnosis may be missed in three out of four elderly hospital patients with alcohol dependence.[3]

The essential principle of treatment is *abstinence*; controlled drinking is not recommended. Many successful modalities redirect the dependency from the alcohol onto others: "Replace drinking with people." Group therapy is the choice in most situations, including situations involving the elderly. Therapy may require more time in elders. Late- and early-onset alcoholism does not appear to differ substantially in terms of treatment. Use of disulfiram (Antabuse, an aversion therapy) is limited in the elderly because of its cardiovascular complications.

James Beem, *Part 3*

Mr. Beem is resistant to referral for more in-depth alcoholism assessment.

STUDY QUESTION

1. How will you help guide him into treatment?

Detoxification: Initial treatment may require hospitalization for control of drinking or detoxification.[27] Adverse functional and cognitive complications during alcohol withdrawal occur more frequently in elderly patients. Delirium tremens is a significant disease with a known mortality. Alcohol withdrawal states are just as common in the elderly; there is some evidence that initial withdrawal is more severe in elders.

Self-help: Self-help groups for family members (Alanon for spouses, Alateen for children, and ACOA for adult children of alcoholics) are important because a family-centered approach is universally recommended.

Efficacy: Evidence of effectiveness of alcohol treatment includes data from alcoholism treatment facilities which indicate that patients who seek or achieve reduced or moderate drinking tend to have consumed less alcohol, have fewer lifetime alcohol problems, and be more socially stable. Successful community-dwelling abstainers reported more drink-related problems and higher consumption than facility-based abstainers. They were also more likely to drink in order to reduce the negative effects of the alcoholism itself, whereas other drinkers drank for psychosocial reasons during evenings out and in family settings.[28] Thus, current debate focuses on the value of an elderly-specific milieu. Advantages could include the management of associated medical problems.

It is often thought that older alcoholics are more resistant to treatment; yet, using 6 months of sobriety as the definition of success, subjects over age 60 do at least as well as 20- to 60-year-old subjects.[18] Compliance in early-versus late-onset alcoholism treatment in elders is similar.[9]

Management of alcoholism involves effective treatment of individuals, controlled availability and advertising, and control by price and tax, as well as health and safety warning labels.[29]

James Beem, *Part 4*

Mr. Beem accepts referral to Alcoholic Anonymous (AA). He attends one meeting daily for the first 3 months. After 3 months, his MMSE is 29/30, and his BP is 138/82 on hydrochlorothiazide (HCTZ) 12.5 mg po qd. He has had no further trauma.

STUDY QUESTIONS

1. Is he likely to achieve sobriety in the long term?

2. How can you help him to do so?

SUMMARY

Although alcoholism is common and impairing in elders, and is under-recognized and under-treated by the health care system, elderly alcoholics are at least as treatable as (and probably more than) younger alcoholics.[30] Essentials of effective treatment include recognition and screening, involving the family, emphasizing that this is an inheritable medical illness, use of existing Alcoholics Anonymous members, absti-

nence (controlled drinking is not recommended), group therapy, and "replacing drinking with people." Many common problems of elders are worsened or often *caused* by alcoholism, a treatable but often overlooked medical condition.

References

1. Chafetz M. Alcoholism criteria: an important step. Am J Psychiatry 129:214, 1972.
2. Goodwin D. Commentary on defining alcoholism and taking stands. J Clin Psychiatry 43:394, 1982.
3. Beresford T, et al. Alcoholism and aging in the general hospital. Psychosomatics 29:61, 1988.
4. Scott R, Mitchell M. Aging, alcohol and the liver. J Am Geriatr Soc 36:255, 1988.
5. Blose I. The relationship of alcohol to aging and the elderly. Alcohol Clin Exp Res 2:17, 1978.
6. Myers J, et al. Six-month prevalence of psychiatric disorders in three communities: 1980 to 1982. Arch Gen Psychiatry 41:959, 1984.
7. Mulinga JD. Elderly people with alcohol-related problems: where do they go? Int J Geriatr Psychiatry 14(7):564, 1999.
8. Schuckit M. A clinical review of alcohol, alcoholism, and the elderly patient. J Clin Psychiatry 43:396, 1982.
9. Hurt R, et al. Alcoholism in elderly persons: medical aspects and prognosis of 216 inpatients. Mayo Clin Proc 63:753, 1988.
10. Enoch M, Goldman D. Problem drinking in alcoholism: diagnosis and treatment. Am Fam Phys 65:441, 2002.
11. Graham K. Identifying and measuring alcohol abuse among the elderly: serious problems with existing instrumentation. J Stud Alcohol 47:322, 1986.
12. Moran M, Naughton B, Hughes S. Screening elderly veterans for alcoholism. J Gen Intern Med 5:361, 1990.
13. Ewing J. Detecting alcoholism: the CAGE questionnaire. JAMA 252:510, 1989.
14. Willibring M, et al. Alcoholism screening in the elderly. J Am Geriatr Soc 35:864, 1987.
15. Dawson DA. Consumption indicators of alcohol dependence. Addiction 1994;89:345-50.
16. Blow FC, et al. The Michigan Alcoholism Screening Test-Geriatric Version (MAST-G): a new elderly-specific screening instrument. Alcohol Clin Exp Res 16(2):372, 1992.
17. Blow FC, Gillespie BW, Barry KL, et al. Brief screening for alcohol problems in elderly populations using the Short Michigan Alcoholism Screening Test—Geriatric Version (SMAST-G). Alcoholism Clin Exp Res 22(Suppl):131A, 1998.
18. Wolin S, Bennett L, Noonan D. Family rituals and the recurrence of alcoholism over generations. Am J Psychiatry 136:589, 1979.
19. Friedmann PD, et al. The effect of alcohol abuse on the health status of older adults seen in the emergency department. Am J Drug Alcohol Abuse 25(3):529, 1999.
20. Tobias C, et al. Alcoholism in the elderly. Postgrad Med 86:67, 1989.
21. Pottenger M, et al. The frequency and prevalence of depressive symptoms in the alcohol abuser. J Nerv Ment Dis 166:562, 1978.
22. Mulsant BH, Ganguli M. Epidemiology and diagnosis of depression in late life. J Clin Psychiatry 60(Suppl 20):9, 1999.
23. Felson D, et al. Alcohol consumption and hip fracture: the Framingham study. Am J Epidemiol 128:1102, 1988.
24. Haugland S. Alcoholism and other dependencies. Primary Care 16:411, 1989.
25. Fleming MF, et al. Benefit-cost analysis of brief physician advice with problem drinkers in primary care settings. Med Care 38(1):7, 2000.
26. Curtis J, et al. Characteristics, diagnosis and treatment of alcoholism in elderly patients. J Am Geriatr Soc 37:310, 1989.
27. Kraemer K, Conigliaro J, Saitz R. Managing alcohol withdrawal in the elderly. Drugs Aging 14(6):409, 1999.
28. Hermos J, et al. Predictors of reduction and cessation of drinking in community dwelling men: results from the normative aging study. J Stud Alcohol 49:363, 1989.
29. Prevention in perspective: a statement of the National Association of State Alcohol and Drug Abuse, Directors and the National Prevention Network, Washington, DC, 1989.
30. Council on Scientific Affairs, American Medical Association. Alcoholism in the elderly. JAMA 275(10):797, 1996.

POSTTEST

1. Alcoholism in older persons is associated with:
   a. Falls
   b. Hip fractures
   c. Osteoporosis
   d. Dementia
   e. All of the above

2. All of the following are patterns of alcoholism except:
   a. Resolved
   b. Chronic
   c. Late onset
   d. Reactive
   e. Intermittent

3. An 82-year-old man is involved in a car crash. Screening for alcoholism is best accomplished by:
   a. Blood alcohol level
   b. Liver enzymes AST/ALT
   c. GGT
   d. Questionnaire, for example, CAGE or S-MAST-G
   e. Physical exam

PRETEST ANSWERS

1. c
2. d
3. b

POSTTEST ANSWERS

1. e
2. a
3. d

The Older Adult Driver

Richard V. Sims and Karlene K. Ball

OBJECTIVES

Upon completion of this chapter, the reader will be able to:

- Describe the epidemiology and predictors of driving mishaps involving older adults.

- Discuss current and proposed techniques for assessing motor vehicle crash risk.

- Review the role of the primary care provider in driving competency evaluations.

PRETEST

1. What factor contributes most to the increased number of crashes involving older drivers?
   a. The lack of available alternative transportation
   b. The rapid absolute and relative growth of older-age cohorts
   c. The suboptimal driving skills of even healthy older adults
   d. Reductions in driving exposure by elders, who are aware of their impairments

2. Which of the following abilities is the most crucial for safe driving?
   a. Vision
   b. Cognition
   c. Balance
   d. Hearing
   e. Upper and lower extremity flexibility

3. Which one of the following driving conditions is most hazardous for older drivers?
   a. Turning left across traffic at an intersection
   b. Driving at night
   c. Merging into traffic on an interstate highway
   d. Driving on rural roads

Lawrence Smith, *Part 1*

Mr. Smith is a 91-year-old gentleman who was brought in by his family for assessment of driving safety. They can cite no particular problems with his driving, but are concerned about his advanced age and whether this activity is becoming "dangerous" for him. He has never had a motor vehicle crash, or been stopped by the police or issued a citation, but in recent years stopped driving at night.

Mr. Smith is fully independent in his self-care and instrumental activities of daily living, including medication self-administration, housework, shopping, and banking. He wears glasses for reading and for distance, and has had no apparent memory problems, falls, or urinary incontinence. Mr. Smith walks with a cane when outside his home. His medical history is remarkable for hypertension, osteoarthritis of the knees, atrial fibrillation, and a colostomy subsequent to a colon cancer, which was surgically removed 25 years ago. There is no history of alcohol or drug abuse, but the patient reported smoking during his military service.

His medications include warfarin, atenolol, low-dose hydrochlorothiazide, calcium, multivitamins, and acetaminophen, which are well tolerated. Mr. Smith takes occasional doses of diazepam for sleeplessness. A recent visit to the cardiologist confirmed well-controlled blood pressure and pulse, an enlarged heart, and a 2/6 murmur localized to the aortic area. Physical examination revealed a pulse of 64, irregularly irregular, blood pressure 136/70, normal hydration, and no signs of cardiopulmonary dysfunction.

With the patient wearing his glasses, visual acuity in the left eye was 20/30 and in the right 20/40. A distal colostomy was observed. Despite Heberden's nodes and signs of degenerative joint disease involving the right greater than left knees, there was no difficulty with joint instability, tenderness, or the range of motion of any joints. Neurological examination was normal except for some loss of vibration sense in the toes and absent ankle jerks. Folstein Mini-Mental Examination and 15-item Geriatric Depression Scale scores were 24 (the patient was educated through the ninth grade) and 3, respectively. A clock drawing was completed satisfactorily. The patient agreed to tapering and discontinuing the diazepam, substituting nonpharmacologic sleep aids and a referral to the local driving assessment clinic.

STUDY QUESTIONS

1. How much weight should be given to Mr. Smith's chronological age in the assessment of his driving safety?
2. What risk factors contribute to this patient's risk for motor vehicle crashes?

PREVALENCE AND IMPACT

Although seniors drive fewer total miles than younger drivers and are involved in fewer crashes per licensed driver, they are over-represented in crashes and fatalities per mile driven and are more likely relative to most other age groups to be killed or injured as a result of a collision.[1-3] Although motor vehicle accident rates for the overall population have declined 8.4% since 1980, they have increased 43% for drivers aged 65 years and older.[4] Vehicle crashes are also the leading cause of death caused by injury for persons 65 to 74 years of age; for even older individuals, crashes are the second-leading cause of traumatic death after falls. The rapid growth of older age cohorts, combined with the observation that the majority of seniors depend on automobiles to maintain mobility, predicts that increasing numbers of older adults will be driving in the future. From a public health point of view and that of individual seniors, the identification of potentially crash-prone drivers, many of whom may be eligible for remediation, will be an important priority in coming decades.

RISK FACTORS AND PATHOPHYSIOLOGY

Sooner or later, all older adults have declines in sensory, perceptual, cognitive, and physical function that challenge their independence and mobility. On-road driving studies suggest that healthy older adults possess equivalent or superior driving abilities compared with younger participants. Impaired individuals account for most older driver crashes, which typically occur when the driver is turning left against traffic, at intersections, during daylight hours, and under good road conditions.[5,6]

Driving is a complex task requiring intact function in several domains, including the cognitive, visual, auditory, and musculoskeletal systems.[7] Older individuals with age-associated medical conditions, such as diabetes, heart disease, stroke, epilepsy, dementia, and cataracts, are disproportionately represented in crash statistics.[8-16] However, medical diagnoses have proven to be insensitive indicators of vehicle crash risk, and emphasis has shifted in recent years to the functional implications of these conditions and to those caused, for example, by the effects of medications, such as long-acting benzodiazepines, sedating antihistamines, and alcohol.[10-21] Along these lines, Foley et al. reported that continued driving among older men with dementia was inversely proportional to the degree of cognitive impairment: whereas 78% of those with normal cognitive function continued to drive, 46% and 22% with very mild (Clinical Dementia Rating [CDR] scale score 0.5) and mild (CDR score 1.0) dementia, respectively, did so.[22] Thus, the functional consequences of dementia, rather than the diagnosis of dementia per se, should guide recommendations regarding driving cessation.[6,11,14,22] While considering age and medical diagnoses, this approach emphasizes the identification and, when possible, the amelioration of all variables affecting the overall functional state of the older person. Preliminary evidence indicating associations of adverse driving events with other mobility-related limitations, such as falling and walking less, attests to the degree to which these patients are impaired.[8,13,17]

Motor vehicle crash involvement appears to be caused by the effects of one or more interacting variables, some of which may be remediable and some not. The factors outlined in Box 34–1 appear to be associ-

---

Box 34–1 Deficits Associated with Older Driver Crashes

- Visual-cognitive: cataracts, glaucoma, decreased contrast sensitivity and visual acuity, useful field of view ≥40% reduction (impaired visual processing speed), difficulty with copying tasks, cognitive impairment
- Musculoskeletal: low back pain, more than three foot abnormalities, arthritis, bursitis
- Medication related: long-acting benzodiazepines and other hypnotics, narcotics, tricyclic antidepressants, alcohol, sedating antihistamines
- Psychiatric: depression, psychosis
- Physical function: difficulty walking ¼ mile, walking outdoors, or opening a jar; few blocks walked; falls
- Medical diagnosis: cardiopulmonary disease, diabetes, seizures, Alzheimer's disease, stroke, sleep apnea

ated with susceptibility to driving mishaps (e.g., being stopped by police, a moving violation, a motor vehicle crash, or driver license revocation) among older adult drivers.[6,8–21] For example, even mild cognitive deficits limit the ability of affected individuals to manage emergency maneuvers and to perform successfully on on-road and simulated driving tests.[6,10,14] Thus, a senior with moderately advanced Alzheimer's disease and visual impairments due to macular degeneration would be identified as crash prone and counseled to stop driving, given the progressive nature of both disorders. Another older adult, who has symptomatic cataracts, is taking long-acting benzodiazepines (e.g., diazepam), and is clinically depressed, may be at similarly high risk for a motor vehicle crash. However, in this instance, the patient's susceptibility to motor vehicle crashes could be reduced by surgical removal of the cataracts, tapering off the long-acting benzodiazepine (or substituting a short-acting agent with no active metabolites, like oxazepam), and initiating an antidepressant.

Among the factors listed in Box 34–1, intact visual and cognitive abilities are critically important to safe driving. It is likely that many other medical factors have their major effect by adversely affecting these domains (e.g., central nervous system–active medications, cataracts, stroke, and dementia). Poor performance on simple cognitive tests, such as the five-item recall, the Folstein Mini-Mental Status Examination, and design copying, have been associated with the occurrence of senior driver mishaps.[7,11,13,17] However, current driver screening practices, including static visual acuity measurements and traditional medical evaluations, do not reliably distinguish between safe and unsafe older drivers.[11,23–26] In an analysis of state policies on driver license renewal, Levy et al. reported that mandatory tests of visual acuity every 4 years for drivers aged 70 years and older reduced their risk for fatal vehicle crashes by only 7%.[25] Knowledge tests and on-road driving assessments contributed little additional benefit to the tests described above in the prevention of crash-related fatalities. A more recent review of state-level policy regulations on re-licensure of older drivers found that those who came into departments of motor vehicles had lower crash-related fatality rates than those who did not, suggesting that the former enjoyed better overall health than the latter. Nevertheless, vision and on-road driving tests did not improve on this result.[26]

> ● Even mild cognitive deficits limit the ability of affected individuals to manage emergency maneuvers and to perform successfully on on-road and simulated driving tests.

DIFFERENTIAL DIAGNOSIS AND ASSESSMENT

Primary care providers will find the recent joint publication of the American Medical Association and the National Highway Traffic Safety Administration, *Physicians Guide to Assessing and Counseling Older Drivers*, an invaluable resource in determining these regulations.[27] This guide can be found at The American Medical Association Website, as noted in the list of Web References. The assessment chapter of the guide recommends assessment of vision (visual acuity and visual fields), cognition (trail-making test part B, clock-drawing test), and function (rapid pace walk, range of motion, motor strength). The guide provides easy-to-use templates for documenting assessment, as well as patient and physician education materials.

In the research setting, a specific measure of visual processing speed and attention, The Useful Field of View (UFOV®) test, predicts driving competence, as well as falls and timed instrumental activities of daily living (e.g., finding a name in the telephone book). The test demonstrates high sensitivity (86.3%) and specificity (84.3%) in detecting older adult drivers who sustained state-recorded at-fault vehicle crashes in the previous 5 years.[6,28,29] In comparison to other neuropsychological measures, UFOV is the best predictor of crash incidence, and older drivers with at least a 40% reduction in the UFOV were 2.2 times (95% confidence interval of 1.2 to 4.1) more likely to be involved in a crash after 3 years of follow-up.[28–30] A recently completed meta-analysis of eight studies, in which speed of processing and objective driving measures (i.e., state-reported motor vehicle crashes and on-road and simulated driving performance) were compared, confirmed the robust relationship between poorer UFOV performance and negative driving outcomes.[31] This promising screening test is currently undergoing feasibility testing in three state departments of motor vehicles.

Lawrence Smith, *Part 2*

Mr. Smith returned 6 weeks after his initial visit and was clinically and physically unchanged. He described some temporary problems with sleeping, once his diazepam was stopped. The report from the driving assessment clinic was reviewed with the patient and his family: They found Mr. Smith's visual function, including static visual acuity and contrast sensitivity, to be acceptable. His UFOV test documented appropriate subtest and total UFOV times, and he passed an on-road driving evaluation without difficulty.

STUDY QUESTIONS

1. What recommendations should be made regarding Mr. Smith's continued driving?

MANAGEMENT

Role of Primary Care Clinician

How should the primary clinician determine when and if an older patient should be counseled to stop driving?

First of all, he or she should be familiar with regulatory requirements: Policies on driver license renewal vary by state for adults 70 years and older and whether health care providers are required to report impaired drivers to state agencies.[26] Clinicians will find the *Physicians Guide to Assessing and Counseling Older Drivers*[27] a resource in determining these regulations in each state. They should also be aware that most elders do not require intervention, because many of them voluntarily reduce or stop driving when they become physically impaired. Thus, senior drivers with sensory, motor, and/or cognitive limitations try to compensate by reducing the number of miles driven, their average speed, and exposure to potentially hazardous driving conditions, or by stopping driving altogether.[32–34] Female gender, low educational level, poor general health, visual and neurological impairments, arthritis, heart disease, and functional disabilities also correlate with driving cessation.[33,34] A laissez-faire strategy on the part of the clinician, however, is only partially successful, since seniors still experience three times the crash rate and crash-related mortality of middle-aged adults.[1–3] The clinician should also be prepared to manage the depression and loss of independence engendered by driving cessation.[35,36]

In many instances, the decision to counsel a senior to stop driving will be clear cut, as in the case of an individual with moderately advanced dementia or anyone with poorly controlled seizures, frequent hypoglycemia, active alcoholism, or legal blindness (i.e., binocular visual acuity less than 20/70). Alternatively, healthy or medically stable older adults, who are functionally competent, should be encouraged to continue driving for as long as they feel comfortable and capable of doing so. The difficulty for most practitioners is the elder whose crash risk is not obvious. This individual (or a family member) may complain of unsafe driving practices or a recent at-fault vehicle crash. Referrals to hospital- or community-based older driver programs, which provide objective assessments of driving competence and confidential feedback, can be very helpful in these cases.

What should a practitioner do about the unsafe elder who refuses to stop driving? For the cognitively intact individual, the clinician can appeal to reason and counsel the elder to avoid potentially hazardous situations (e.g., driving at night or during rush hour) and about alternative transportation options. Patience and sensitivity to concerns regarding isolation and loss of independence will serve to enhance eventual compliance with these recommendations. Demented individuals, who lack intact decision-making capacity, should be treated in a similar fashion, but may require intervention by caregivers (e.g., disabling the automobile), the courts, and state departments of motor vehicles.

> ● Patience and sensitivity to concerns regarding isolation and loss of independence will serve to enhance eventual compliance with these recommendations.

Model Programs for High-Risk Older Drivers

Some agencies have initiated multicomponent pilot programs to assess, counsel, and retrain older drivers, who either self-refer or are referred by their families, health care providers, the courts, or state departments of motor vehicles. Most such programs provide confidential evaluations, guidance about whether the senior is capable of continued driving, and options for retraining. The American Association of Retired Persons (AARP) and local areawide aging agencies may be resources for identifying formal driving assessment programs.

SUMMARY

Driving can be hazardous for the older driver, as well as others on the road and sidewalk. But driving is still essential for many if independence is to be maintained. Certain common issues (such as cognitive impairment) must be sought and assessed in an older individual who is still driving and the primary care clinician must be prepared, and know how, to stop the patient from driving, consistent with state laws, when necessary.

References

1. Evans J. Older driver involvement in fatal and severe traffic crashes. J Gerontol 43:S186-S193, 1988.
2. McCoy GF, et al. Injury to the elderly in road traffic accident. J Trauma 29:494-497, 1989.
3. Hu PS, Trumble DA, Foley DJ, et al. Crash risk of older drivers: a panel analysis. Accid Anal Prev 30 (5):569-581, 1998.
4. Barr RA. Recent changes in driving among older adults. Hum Factors 22:597-600, 1991.
5. Carr D, et al. The effect of age on driving skills. J Am Geriatr Soc 40(6):567-573, 1992.
6. Ball K, et al. Driving avoidance and functional impairment in older drivers. Accid Anal Prev 30(3):313-322, 1998.

7. Marottoli RA, Drickamer MA. Psychomotor mobility and the elderly driver. Clin Geriatr Med 9(2):403-411, 1993.
8. Koepsell TD, et al. Medical conditions and motor vehicle collision injuries in older drivers. J Am Geriatr Soc 42(7):695-700, 1994.
9. Hansotia P, Broste SK. The effect of epilepsy or diabetes mellitus on the risk of automobile accidents. N Engl J Med 324(1):22-26, 1991.
10. Fitten LJ, et al. Alzheimer and vascular dementias and driving: a prospective road and laboratory study. JAMA 273(17):1360-1365, 1995.
11. Johansson K, et al. Can a physician recognize an older driver with increased crash risk potential? J Am Geriatr Soc 44(10):1198-1204, 1996.
12. McGwin G, et al. Relations among chronic medical conditions, medications, and automobile crashes in the elderly: a population-based case-control study. Am J Epidemiol 152(5):424-431, 2000.
13. Sims RV, et al. An exploratory study of incident vehicle crashes among older drivers. J Gerontol A Biol Sci Med Sci 55(1):M22-M27, 2000.
14. Hunt L, et al. Driving performance in persons with mild senile dementia of the Alzheimer type. J Am Geriatr Soc 41(7):747-752, 1993.
15. Owsley C, et al. Impact of cataract extraction on motor vehicle crash involvement in older adults. JAMA 288(7):841-849, 2002.
16. Wallace RB, Retchin SM. A geriatric and gerontologic perspective on the effects of medical conditions on older drivers: discussion of Waller. Hum Factors 34(1):17-24, 1992.
17. Marottoli RA, et al. Predictors of automobile crashes and moving violations among elderly drivers. Ann Intern Med 121(11):842-846, 1994.
18. Leveille SG, et al. Psychoactive medications and injurious motor vehicle collisions involving older drivers. Epidemiology 5(6):591-598, 1994.
19. Foley DJ, Wallace RB, Eberhard J. Risk factors for motor vehicle crashes among older drivers in a rural community. J Am Geriatr Soc 43(8):776-781, 1995.
20. Hemmelgarn B, et al. Benzodiazepine use and the risk of motor vehicle crash in the elderly. JAMA 278(1):27-31, 1997.
21. Weiler JM, et al. Effects of fexofenadine, diphenhydramine and alcohol on driving performance. Ann Intern Med 132(5):354-363, 2000.
22. Foley DJ, et al. Driving cessation in older men with incident dementia. J Am Geriatr Soc 48(8):928-930, 2000.
23. Hakamies-Blomqvist L, Johansson K, Lundberg C. Medical screening of older drivers as a traffic safety measure: a comparative Finnish-Swedish evaluation study. J Am Geriatr Soc 44(6):650-653, 1996.
24. Ball K, Owsley C. Increasing mobility and reducing accidents of older drivers. In Schaie KW, Pietuicha M, eds. Mobility and Transportation in the Elderly. New York, Springer Publishing, 213-25, 2000.
25. Levy DT, Vernick JS, Howard KA. Relationship between driver's license renewal policies and fatal crashes involving drivers 70 years or older. JAMA 274(13):1026-1030, 1995.
26. Grabowski DC, Campbell CM, Morrisey MA. Elderly licensure laws and motor vehicle fatalities. JAMA 291(23):2840-2846, 2004.
27. Wang CC, Carr DB. Older driver safety: a report from the older drivers project. J Am Geriatr Soc 52(1):143-149, 2004.
28. Ball KK, et al. Visual attention problems as a predictor of vehicle crashes in older drivers. Invest Ophthalmol Vis Sci 34:3110-3123, 1993.
29. Owsley C, et al. Vision impairment, eye disease, and injurious motor vehicle crashes in the elderly. Ophthalmic Epidemiol 5(2):101-103, 1998.
30. Myers RS, et al. Relation of useful field of view and other screening tests to on-road driving performance. Percept Mot Skills 91(1):279-290, 2000.
31. Clay OJ, et al. Cumulative meta-analysis of the relationship between useful field of view and driving performance in older adults: current and future implications. Optom Vis Sci 82:724-731, 2005.
32. Stutts JC. Do older drivers with visual and cognitive impairments drive less? J Am Geriatr Soc 46(7):854-861, 1998.
33. Kington R, et al. Sociodemographic and health factors in driving patterns after 50 years of age. Am J Public Health 84(8):1327-1329, 1994.
34. Brayne C, et al. Very old drivers: findings from a population cohort of people aged 84 and over. Int J Epidemiol 29(4):704-709, 2000.
35. Ragland ER, Satariano WA, MacLeod KE. Driving cessation and increased depressive symptoms. J Gerontol A Biol Sci Med Sci 60(3):237-241, 2005.
36. Marottoli RA, et al. Consequences of driving cessation: decreased out-of-home activity levels. J Gerontol B Psychol Sci Soc Sci 55(6):S334-S340, 2000.

Web Resources

1. American Medical Assocation, Physician's Guide to Assessing and Counseling Older Drivers: www.ama-assn.org/ama/pub/category/10791.html.
2. Area Agency on Aging: www.agingcarefl.org/services/programs/gear.

POSTTEST

1. Which test has demonstrated very good sensitivity and specificity in distinguishing safe from crash-prone older drivers?
   a. Static visual acuity tests
   b. Knowledge tests
   c. Medical history and physical examinations
   d. Useful Field of View

2. Which medication class is not associated with simulated and on-road crash involvement?
   a. Alcohol
   b. Sedating antihistamines
   c. Narcotics
   d. Short-acting benzodiazepines
   e. Tricyclic antidepressants

3. Which approach should the clinician take in counseling an older driver, who may be worried about continued driving?
   a. Advise the patient to stop driving.
   b. Refer the individual to a local program designed to assess and counsel older adult drivers.
   c. Suggest that the patient reduce his or her exposure to unsafe conditions (e.g., driving at night).
   d. Perform a medical history and physical examination.

PRETEST ANSWERS

1. b
2. b
3. a

POSTTEST ANSWERS

1. d
2. d
3. b

Hypertension

Amrit Singh

OBJECTIVES

Upon completion of this chapter, the reader will be able to:

- Define hypertension and outline its prevalence and role as a risk factor in cardiovascular disease.
- Discuss the pathophysiology of hypertension.
- Discuss the difference between essential hypertension, secondary hypertension, and hypertensive urgency and emergency.
- Describe the appropriate evaluation of the elderly patient with hypertension.
- Discuss the evidence that treating hypertension, both systolic and diastolic, is beneficial in the elderly.
- Discuss goals for blood pressure reduction.
- Discuss pharmacologic and nonpharmacologic therapies for hypertension, including the tailoring of drugs to concomitant disease, when present.

PRETEST

1. You diagnose your 86-year-old patient, Ms. G, with hypertension. She asks you how common hypertension is in her age group. You respond by quoting the following statistic regarding prevalence of hypertension in older individuals:
   a. 15%
   b. 33%
   c. 50%
   d. 65%
   e. 80%

2. The most common change one might see in the blood vessels of an older patient like Ms. G is:
   a. Increased peripheral vascular resistance
   b. Decreased peripheral vascular resistance
   c. Increased response to β-adrenergic stimulation
   d. Increased response to the renin-angiotensin system

3. Mr. J comes to see you for an annual exam, and you notice that he has a systolic blood pressure of 160 mmHg and a diastolic blood pressure of 80 mmHg. What will you tell him about this blood pressure?
   a. "Nothing to worry about." (The diastolic blood pressure is normal.)
   b. "You have hypertension."
   c. "The blood pressure reading is concerning, and we need to follow this and get additional readings."
   d. "You need treatment with medications immediately to bring down your blood pressure."

4. You see Mr. J in your office several times and obtain the following blood pressure readings on three different occasions: 160/80 mmHg, 150/75 mmHg, and 165/80 mmHg. You diagnose him with isolated systolic hypertension. He asks you what risks isolated systolic hypertension pose to his health. You identify all of the following except:
   a. Stroke
   b. Myocardial infarction
   c. Congestive heart failure
   d. Left ventricular hypertrophy
   e. Hyperlipidemia

5. Ms. G fails to bring down her blood pressure adequately with lifestyle changes alone. You discuss and decide to initiate drug treatment, while also encouraging her to continue with lifestyle change. Which class of drugs is the best studied and most often-used first-line agent in treating hypertension in older patients?
   a. Beta-blockers
   b. Alpha-blockers
   c. Calcium-channel blockers
   d. Angiotensin-converting enzyme inhibitors
   e. Thiazide diuretics

6. What should Ms. G's goal blood pressure be?
   a. <160/90 mmHg
   b. <150/90 mmHg
   c. <140/90 mmHg
   d. Ten points lower than the starting systolic blood pressure

---

PREVALENCE AND IMPACT

Hypertension is one of the most common medical diagnoses in persons over the age of 65. Even though the disease is common, it is important to carefully diagnose a patient with hypertension because not every patient with an elevated blood pressure reading has hypertension. On the other hand, many patients with hypertension are either unaware of the diagnosis or are under-controlled.[1] Furthermore, the elderly constitute one of the populations with the lowest rate of blood pressure control.[2] Given the worldwide growth in the geriatric population and the association among age, hypertension, and cardiovascular death, an understanding of hypertension diagnosis and management is essential to effective geriatric care.

Hypertension management among geriatric patients has changed in the past 20 to 25 years. First, there is increasing evidence for the importance of isolated systolic hypertension and widened pulse pressure as predictors of cardiovascular morbidity and mortality. Second, individual studies and meta-analyses have shown consistent benefits of hypertension treatment in older patients, even octogenarians. Third, it is now acknowledged that many different classes of drugs are appropriate for hypertension treatment, and a rational approach to choosing agents involves the consideration of comorbid conditions and existing target organ damage.

Many elements of appropriate diagnosis and management of hypertension are the same for older as for younger patients: distinguishing essential from secondary hypertension, recognizing when hypertensive blood pressures pose an urgent problem to the health of the patient, recommending appropriate lifestyle changes, recognizing when to initiate medications, being familiar with the classes of drugs, and knowing the circumstances under which one class of drugs may be better suited to a patient than another class of drugs. In managing older persons, it is especially important to identify goals of treatment and to be aware of the benefits and risks one incurs when treating hypertension. It should also be acknowledged that choosing appropriate medication and deciding how aggressively to treat the older patient requires considerable clinical judgment from the primary care provider.

Sally Howard, *Part 1*

Ms. Sally Howard is a 78-year-old white woman who is new to your practice. She has just moved to the area and would like to initiate care with you. She has a history of breast cancer which was treated 10 years ago, with no recurrence to date, and mild urinary incontinence. She lives independently, and has no functional impairments. She is a former smoker, and does not drink. Her initial vital signs are as follows: height 5 feet 5 inches, weight 178 lb, and blood pressure 150/80 mmHg. She feels well and has no complaints.

Philip Garvin, *Part 1*

Mr. Philip Garvin is a 72-year-old black man with a long history of hypertension. He had a heart attack 3 months ago. Since discharge from the hospital, he has been taking the following medications: furosemide (Lasix), 40 mg/day; metoprolol (Lopressor), 25 mg twice daily; and doxazosin (Cardura), 2 mg per day. He is 6 feet tall, and weight and blood pressure readings for his last three office visits are as follows: 2 months ago, 190
pounds, 140/90 mmHg; 1 month ago, 195 pounds, 145/95 mmHg; and today, 198 pounds, 150/100 mmHg.

His blood pressure is essentially the same when measured after 2 minutes of standing. He reports that he is a little tired and somewhat short of breath. He has not had any chest pain. Although he quit smoking after his heart attack, he had been a one-pack-a-day smoker for 60 years.

Sadie Carter, *Part 1*

Ms. Sadie Carter is a 90-year-old black woman with a history of atherosclerotic cardiovascular disease manifested as an inferior myocardial infarction (MI) 10 years ago and a stroke 3 years ago that resulted in left hand weakness. She has had hypertension for at least 20 years. She takes hydrochlorothiazide, 25 mg/day. She is 5 feet tall, and her weight and blood pressure readings for her last three office visits are as follows: 2 months ago, 90 pounds, 170/90 mmHg; 1 month ago: 89 pounds, 172/86 mmHg; and today: 91 pounds, 164/88 mmHg.

After standing for 2 minutes, her blood pressure drops to 144/82 mmHg. She reports feeling a little dizzy at times, particularly after standing up, and feels a "little weak." She has not had any chest pain, shortness of breath, or recent episodes of numbness or weakness of any part of her body. She has never smoked, but she does use snuff occasionally.

STUDY QUESTIONS

1. Does Sally Howard have hypertension?
2. What should specifically be sought on physical examination of Philip Garvin and Sadie Carter?

> ● It should also be acknowledged that choosing appropriate medication and deciding how aggressively to treat the older patient require considerable clinical judgment from the primary care provider.

General Definition

Hypertension is defined across all age groups as a diastolic blood pressure reading of 90 mmHg or higher, or a systolic reading of 140 mmHg or higher. Because blood pressure readings can be variable, the diagnosis of hypertension requires at least three elevated blood

Table 35–1	Classification of Blood Pressures	
BP Classification	**SBP (mmHg)**	**DBP (mmHg)**
Normal	<120	and <80
Prehypertension	120–139	or 80–89
Stage 1 hypertension	140–159	or 90–99
Stage 2 hypertension	≥160	or ≥100

Source: Chobanian A, Bakris G, Black H, et al. The seventh report of the Joint National Committee on prevention, detection, evaluation and treatment of high blood pressure. JAMA 289:2560–72, 2003, with permission.

pressure readings taken over three separate occasions.[2] (See "Assessment of a New Case of Hypertension.")

Isolated systolic hypertension (ISH) is defined as a systolic BP of 140 mmHg or higher with a normal diastolic blood pressure.

Table 35–1 indicates blood pressure classifications, per the seventh report of the Joint National Committee on prevention, detection, evaluation, and treatment of high blood pressure.[2]

Prevalence

Estimates of the prevalence of hypertension differ somewhat because the definition of hypertension is not the same in every study. The Third National Health and Nutrition Examination Survey in the United States, completed in 1994, showed that hyper-

tension was present in 51% of all persons aged 60 to 69, 66% of persons aged 70 to 79, and 72% of persons aged 80 and older[3] (Fig. 35–1). More recent data suggest that 70% of individuals aged 75 and older in the United States have hypertension; the prevalence may even be higher (85%) in elderly women.[4,5]

Among elderly patients with hypertension, 60% to 87% have only elevated systolic blood pressures ("isolated systolic hypertension" [ISH]), making this type of hypertension the most common form in the geriatric population.[1,6,7] Systolic hypertension is more predictive of adverse outcomes in older individuals as compared to diastolic hypertension (see "Adverse Outcomes" below). Unfortunately, ISH is the least likely form of hypertension to be treated.[1,8,9]

Individuals with normal blood pressures at age 55 have a lifetime risk of 90% or greater for developing hypertension.[2,10] Unfortunately, currently only two-thirds of Americans are aware that they are hypertensive, and only one-third of those aware are under control; this percentage has not changed significantly in the past three decades.[2,11]

Adverse Outcomes

GENERAL RISKS OF HYPERTENSION

Framingham Study data (encompassing 36 years of follow-up) show a significantly higher age-adjusted

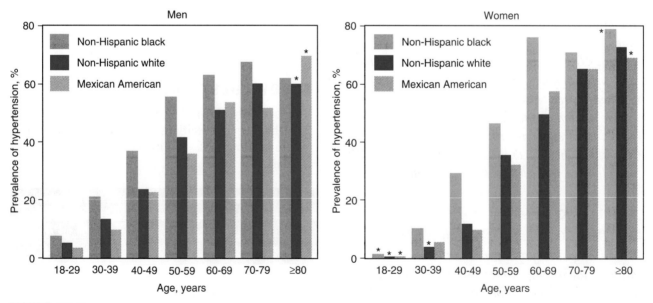

FIGURE 35–1

Prevalence of high blood pressure by age and race/ethnicity for men and women, U.S. population 18 years of age and older. *Estimate based on sample size not meeting minimum requirements of the National Health and Nutrition Examination Survey III design or relative standard error of measurement greater than 30%. (*Redrawn from Burt VL, Whelton P, Roccella EJ, et al. Prevalence of hypertension in the US adult population. Results. The Third National Health and Nutrition Examination Survey, 1988–1991. Hypertension 1995;25:305–13, with permission.*)

risk ratio for myocardial infarctions, sudden death, stroke, peripheral arterial disease, and heart failure among hypertensive participants aged 65 and older versus nonhypertensive elders.[6] The Joint National Committee on Prevention, Detection, Evaluation and Treatment of Hypertension (JNC), supported by population data and prospective cohort studies, indicates that the relationship of blood pressure to cardiovascular disease risk is "continuous, consistent, and independent of other risks."[2,12,13] For persons aged 40 to 70 years, starting at a blood pressure of 115/75 mmHg, there is a doubling in the risk of cardiovascular disease for each rise in systolic BP of 20 mmHg or diastolic BP of 10 mmHg.[2,14] This is particularly relevant to geriatric patients: the prevalence of hypertension is highest in this age group, age alone is a risk factor for cardiovascular events, and thus the association between blood pressure and cardiovascular events makes this population at high risk for hypertension-related morbidity and mortality. Hypertension is also linked to multiple medical issues affecting function and quality of life, including vascular dementia, erectile dysfunction and nephropathy.

> ● Hypertension is linked to multiple medical issues affecting function and quality of life, including vascular dementia, erectile dysfunction, nephropathy, and retinopathy.

ISOLATED SYSTOLIC HYPERTENSION

Between ages 50 and 60, systolic hypertension assumes a superior role over diastolic blood pressure as a predictor of adverse cardiovascular outcomes.[6,15–19] A meta-analysis of 61 prospective studies involving 1 million people of all ages demonstrated that systolic blood pressure was more predictive of strokes and cardiac events than diastolic blood pressure.[14] This finding was further corroborated in a meta-analysis of over 15,000 elderly patients involved in eight hypertension treatment trials.[20] The Cardiovascular Health Study demonstrated that for older individuals with a SBP higher than 169 mmHg, 5-year mortality increased by 2.4-fold.[21]

WIDENED PULSE PRESSURE

There is emerging evidence that pulse pressure (the difference between systolic and diastolic blood pressure) is a powerful and independent predictor of cardiovascular risk.[22–24] A meta-analysis of three large placebo-controlled trials of hypertension treatment in elderly individuals (European Working Party on High Blood Pressure in the Elderly Trial [EWPHE], Systolic Hypertension in Europe Trial [Syst-Eur], and Systolic Hypertension in China [Syst-China]) found that a 10-mmHg wider pulse pressure at baseline was

associated with a 20% increased risk for cardiovascular mortality.[25] Evidence also exists for the relatively greater benefit of hypertension treatment in older individuals with a wider pulse pressure versus a narrower pulse pressure: one meta-analysis has identified that for men aged 70 and older with hypertension, the number needed to treat (NNT) to prevent one cardiovascular death is 63 if the pulse pressure is 90 mmHg or wider, versus 119 if pulse pressure is less than 90 mmHg.[20]

> ● There is emerging evidence that pulse pressure (the difference between systolic and diastolic blood pressure) is a powerful and independent predictor of cardiovascular risk.

Rationale for Treatment

The benefit of treating hypertension in young individuals has never been questioned; however, historically there has been limited information regarding the benefits of treating older individuals, especially the very elderly (aged 80 and older). There has also been a lack of information regarding the benefits of treating isolated systolic hypertension.

This changed after 1990, with the publication of large-scale evaluations of hypertension treatment in older persons, including individuals aged 80 and older.[26–28] These studies showed clear reductions in morbidity and mortality among the treated subjects: stroke reduction of 30% to 36%, myocardial infarction reduction of 22% to 25%, and heart failure reduction of 39% to 54%. These trials also featured individuals with isolated systolic hypertension, and confirmed the benefits of treatment of ISH at levels around 160 mmHg.

Furthermore, the benefits of treatment occurred within 5 years of the start of most trials; indeed, in the Systolic Hypertension in the Elderly Persons (SHEP) trial, the divergence in stroke risk between treated and untreated individuals was evident within 2 years. This is particularly significant given the added years of life expectancy of 80- to 90-year-olds in the United States: at age 80, it is 8 years for men and 9 years for women, and at age 90, it is 4 years for men and 5 years for women.[29] Thus, these data suggest that hypertension treatment can be beneficial in very advanced ages.

There is one caveat to assuming that hypertension treatment benefits octo- and nona-genarians: the trials mentioned above included more individuals aged 65 to 79 than individuals aged 80 and older. No large-scale trials of hypertension treatment in octo- or nona-genarians have been completed as yet, although the Hypertension in the Very Elderly Trial (HYVET) is ongoing.[30] Therefore, for now, we must rely on secondary analyses of data from the existing trials. One such meta-analysis, published in 1999, reviewed the data from 1670 octogenarians involved in several of the randomized controlled trials of hypertension treatment noted above. This meta-analysis showed that hypertension treatment was associated with a 34% reduction in relative risk of stroke, 22% reduction in relative risk of cardiovascular events, and a 39% reduction in relative risk of heart failure. However, there was a nonsignificant 6% increase in all-cause mortality.[31] In contrast, two other meta-analyses reported a 34% to 36% reduction in stroke, a 19% to 25% reduction in coronary heart disease, and an 11% to 12% reduction in overall mortality in older treated hypertensive.[32,33] It is hoped that the results of the HYVET trial will more directly address this controversy regarding the benefits versus risks of hypertension treatment in the very elderly. For now, however, given the cardiovascular risks associated with age and with hypertension, and given the evidence of cardiovascular event reduction with hypertension treatment, limits on attempts at treatment should not be based upon age.

PATHOPHYSIOLOGY AND RISK FACTORS

Separating normal aging phenomena from changes associated with hypertension is difficult. The elasticity of large blood vessels normally decreases with age, and hypertension hastens this process. The difference in pathogenesis of diastolic versus systolic hypertension involves the type of vessel undergoing change: diastolic hypertension is associated with an increase in resistance of small peripheral vessels, while systolic hypertension is associated with an increase in large vessel resistance. As large vessel resistance increases, one sees a change in the timing of the arterial pressure wave, resulting in elevated systolic blood pressure and diminished diastolic pressure.[16,34] Ultimately, the decreased large vessel compliance produces an increase in afterload, leading to an increase in left ventricular mass (the latter being a compensatory mechanism, to allow the heart to maintain cardiac output against peripheral resistance). Additional changes include an increase in myocardial oxygen consumption, and a decrease in coronary perfusion pressure due to the drop in diastolic blood pressure.[34]

With age, blood vessels also become less responsive to β-adrenergic stimulation, which is necessary for vasodilation. On the other hand, alpha-adrenergic responsiveness remains unchanged. These changes also contribute to increased arterial resistance and to hypertension.[35]

The renin-angiotensin-aldosterone system (RAAS) affects blood pressure through control of angiotensin 2, which has been found to be responsible for sodium and volume retention, vasoconstriction, sympathetic activation, cell growth and proliferation, and possibly atherogenesis.[36] With age, plasma renin levels decline, and renin response to sodium depletion, diuretic administration, and upright posture declines as well. Therefore, although the RAAS is still important to blood pressure regulation, it may play less of a critical role in the development of hypertension in older adults than the vascular changes described above.

Finally, tobacco use, excessive alcohol intake, and excessive weight all contribute to elevations in blood pressure.

DIFFERENTIAL DIAGNOSIS AND ASSESSMENT

Definitions and Criteria

HYPERTENSION

Hypertension is defined as an average blood pressure of 140/90 mmHg or higher, based on at least three readings taken on three separate occasions over time.[2]

ESSENTIAL HYPERTENSION

Essential hypertension is not directly attributable to an underlying medical disorder. (The majority of the information in this chapter, and most specifically the information above regarding pathophysiology, refers to essential hypertension.)

SECONDARY HYPERTENSION

Secondary hypertension is attributable to an underlying medical disorder. See Box 35–1 for factors that suggest the presence of secondary hypertension, and Table 35–2 for etiologies and screening techniques. Hypertension due to secondary causes is less likely to be seen in elderly individuals. Therefore, when assessing accelerated or poorly controlled blood pressures, one should always evaluate for etiologies of poorly controlled (resistant) essential hypertension: poor compliance, inadequate drug prescribing, medications that raise blood pressures (decongestants, nonsteroidal anti-inflammatory agents, etc.), spuriously elevated

---

Box 35-1   Factors Suggesting Secondary Hypertension

- Sudden rise of diastolic blood pressure to >105 mmHg in a person known to be normotensive
- Diastolic blood pressure greater >100 mmHg or systolic blood pressure >160 mmHg on a rational three-drug therapy
- Accelerated hypertension (rapid worsening) in a person previously known to be hypertensive
- Acute decline in renal function after starting an ACE inhibitor
- Unexplained hypokalemia

Table 35–2	Causes and Screening Techniques for Secondary Hypertension	
Causes	**Tip-offs**	**Screening/Evaluation Methods**
Sleep apnea	Excessive daytime sleepiness, snoring, lack of refreshing sleep	Sleep study
Drugs (illicit or prescribed)[a]	See "Screening/Evaluation Methods"	Careful history taking Urine toxicology screen
Primary aldosteronism	Unexplained low potassium	Per endocrinology consult
Renal parenchymal disease	Elevated creatinine, abnormal urinalysis (hematuria, cell casts, proteinuria)	24-hour urine for protein and creatinine clearance, renal ultrasound, additional imaging studies per nephrology consult
Renovascular disease	Elevated creatinine, bruit, acute drop in renal function with use of ACE inhibitors	Gold standard: digital subtraction angiography Other: MRA, CTA, Doppler
Chronic steroid therapy	Cushingoid stigmata	Careful history taking
Cushing's syndrome	Cushingoid stigmata	24-hour urine for free cortisol
Pheochromocytoma	Episodic bursts of accelerated blood pressures	24-hour urine for metanephrines and/or urinary catecholamines
Coarctation of the aorta	Discrepancy in SBP and pulse between upper and lower extremities[b] Notching of the posterior third to eighth ribs on chest radiograph	MRI and/or echocardiogram[91]
Thyroid disease	Altered heart rate, weight changes, palpitations	Thyroid function tests
Parathyroid disease	Elevated calcium level	Parathyroid hormone levels
Polycythemia vera	Elevated red blood cell count	Bone marrow biopsy

[a]Nonsteroidal anti-inflammatory agents, cocaine, amphetamines, sympathomimetics, oral contraceptives, adrenal steroids, cyclosporine, erythropoietin, tacrolimus, licorice-containing products, ephedra, ma huang.

[b]Increased SBP in upper extremities, diminished or delayed femoral pulses, and low or unobtainable SBP in lower extremities.

blood pressures, increased volume expansion, and excessive sodium and/or alcohol intake.

HYPERTENSIVE URGENCY

Hypertensive urgency is markedly elevated blood pressure in the absence of acute target organ damage (Table 35–3). This requires treatment in the outpatient setting with oral medications to bring down the blood pressure.[2,37–39]

HYPERTENSIVE EMERGENCY

Hypertensive emergency is markedly elevated blood pressure in the presence of acute target organ damage (see Table 35–3), requiring emergency parenteral drug treatment to lower blood pressure in order to limit damage.[2,37–39] Blood pressure level is not a criterion for diagnosis of hypertensive urgency or emergency.

Assessment of a New Case of Hypertension

MAKING THE DIAGNOSIS

The diagnosis of hypertension is made when three separate blood pressure readings taken over three sep-arate occasions reveal a systolic blood pressure 140 mmHg or higher or a diastolic blood pressure 90 mmHg or higher.[2,40,41] Blood pressure measurements should be performed over a period of several months before establishing this diagnosis, unless one is dealing with hypertensive urgency or emergency. Some studies have shown significant variability in blood pressures between the first and subsequent office visits; this supports the idea of taking multiple readings over time to arrive at the correct diagnosis.[42,43]

Measurements taken outside the office should be encouraged, but it should be remembered that an average blood pressure self-measurement higher than 135/85 mmHg is considered abnormal.[2,41] In the setting of suspected "white coat hypertension" (blood pressures artificially elevated when taken in the presence of a physician, perhaps related to increased sympathetic drive associated with the visit), or in the setting of inconsistent office or home readings, ambulatory blood pressure monitoring can be done. Ambulatory readings also are generally lower than office readings, so an average awake blood pressure reading of higher than 135/85 mmHg or an average asleep blood pressure reading of higher than 120/75 mmHg would be considered hypertensive.[2,44]

Table 35–3	Target Organ Damage (Acute and Chronic) from Hypertension	
Organ System	**Acute Findings**	**Chronic Findings**
Heart	Unstable angina pectoris Acute myocardial infarction Acute left venticular failure Pulmonary edema	History of myocardial infarction or revascularization Left ventricular hypertrophy Congestive heart failure
Brain	Encephalopathy Intracranial hemorrhage Subarachnoid hemorrhage	History of stroke or transient ischemic attack
Kidneys	Acute renal insufficiency	Chronic renal insufficiency Proteinuria
Vasculature	Dissecting aortic aneurysm	Peripheral arterial disease
Eyes	Papilledema	Retinopathy

Furthermore, a blood pressure decrease of less than 10% to 20% during sleep would be concerning for an associated increased risk of cardiovascular events.[2,45]

> ● Measurements taken outside the office should be encouraged, but it should be remembered that an average blood pressure self-measurement of greater than 135/85 mmHg is considered abnormal.

BLOOD PRESSURE MEASUREMENT TECHNIQUE

Aneroid sphygmomanometers are most commonly used to measure blood pressures, but mercury sphygmomanometers seem to be the most accurate.[46] An appropriate cuff size is essential to an accurate reading: the bladder length should be at least 75% to 80% of the circumference of the upper arm, and the width should be 40% of the arm circumference.[2] Too small a cuff may produce an artificially elevated systolic blood pressure.

Blood pressure should be measured with the patient comfortably seated for at least 5 minutes, and with the arm at heart level. Talking should be avoided as that may raise blood pressure transiently. More than one reading should be done, and each should be separated by at least 1 to 2 minutes.[2,40,41,46,47] If two values in the same arm differ by more than 5 mmHg, subsequent readings should be taken until a reasonable average is achieved. The cuff should be inflated to 30 mmHg greater than the palpable systolic pressure, to avoid underestimating systolic blood pressure if an auscultatory gap is present.[46] *Auscultatory gaps* involve disappearance of the Korotkoff sounds transiently as the cuff is deflated below the true systolic blood pressure; these gaps can be found in elderly patients, may be associated with increase risk of cardiovascular disease, and can lead to underestimation of systolic blood pressures.[48] During deflation, the cuff should not be deflated faster than 2 to 3 mmHg per heartbeat.[26,41,49]

The blood pressure should also be measured in both arms, and in the event of a discrepancy, the arm with the higher pressure should be used for treatment decisions and for follow-up measurements.[41,46,47]

Smoking, ingesting caffeine, and exercising before blood pressure checks may affect the readings, so this should be considered when interpreting the readings.

BLOOD PRESSURE MEASUREMENT: ADDITIONAL CONSIDERATIONS

In the elderly, rigidly calcified or sclerosed blood vessels can lead to overestimation of blood pressure when measurements are made by a cuff.[50–52] This phenomenon is called pseudohypertension, and it generally involves a difference between measured and intra-arterial systemic and/or diastolic blood pressures of 10 mmHg or more.[50,51] It is thought that one may be able to check for this with the Osler's maneuver, in which the brachial or radial artery remains palpable (not pulsatile) when the cuff pressure exceeds the known systolic pressure.[51] However, Osler's maneuver is subject to poor inter- and intra-observer variability.[53,54] Furthermore, Osler's maneuver may not reliably detect pseudohypertension.[55] Nevertheless, if a patient is having difficulty tolerating medical treatment of hypertension (specifically, demonstrating orthostasis) despite a minimal drop in blood pressure, or if the blood pressure is excessively high in the absence of target organ damage, pseudohypertension should be considered.[50,56]

> **Sally Howard,** *Part 2*
>
> *Since you only have one documented blood pressure (150/80 mmHg in the office), you ask Ms. Howard to continue to check her blood pressure at home periodically, and to come into the office for a nurse check of her blood pressure once a month over the next 3 months.*

At the end of 3 months, you have the following readings: office blood pressures, 145/80 mmHg, 150/85 mmHg, and 142/78 mmHg; and home blood pressures, 140/82 mmHg, 145/80 mmHg, 135/78 mmHg, and 138/85 mmHg,

Ms. Howard's average systolic blood pressure, as measured in the office, is greater than 140 mmHg; it is greater than 135 mmHg, as measured at home. Thus, she meets the criteria for isolated systolic hypertension.

STUDY QUESTION

1. What will you look for on physical exam of this individual?

Initial Evaluation

Once a patient is diagnosed with hypertension, an assessment of contributing factors, target organ damage (see Table 35–3), and associated cardiovascular risk factors should be done.[2,40,41,46,47] Assessment of target organ damage and cardiovascular risk factors allows one to broaden the goal of treatment so that both blood pressure reduction *and* cardiovascular risk reduction are undertaken. Furthermore, knowledge of existing cardiac risk factors or target organ damage can direct the style of treatment (lifestyle change vs. lifestyle change plus medications), the choice of medications, and the goal blood pressure. Finally, an awareness of additional cardiovascular risk factors or existing hypertensive damage may be the tipping point for starting treatment of borderline elevated blood pressures.

> ● Once a patient is diagnosed with hypertension, an assessment of contributing factors, target organ damage, and associated cardiovascular risk factors should be done.

PAST MEDICAL HISTORY, FAMILY HISTORY, AND REVIEW OF SYSTEMS

The past medical/family history and the review of systems should target additional cardiovascular risk factors (diabetes, hyperlipidemia, family history of cardiovascular disease), past or present evidence of atherosclerotic disease (carotid and vertebrobasilar systems, retinal arterioles, coronary arteries, aorta, and peripheral vasculature), and renal and cardiovascular disease. A careful medication history, including over-the-counter and herbal preparations, should be taken. (See Table 35–2 for agents associated with elevated blood pressures.)

SOCIAL HISTORY

An assessment for drug use, alcohol, and tobacco use should be done. It also is important to query the patient about diet and exercise routines, support networks, and meal preparation abilities, as this information will be useful when counseling the patient about nonpharmacologic therapy.

PHYSICAL EXAM

The optic fundi should be examined for papilledema and for hypertensive retinopathy (arteriovenous nicking or arterial narrowing, hemorrhages, and exudates). Carotid, abdominal, and femoral arteries should be examined for bruits. The heart should be auscultated for murmurs or heaves, S3/S4, and/or a displaced point of maximal impulse. The lungs should be examined for evidence of pulmonary edema. The abdomen should be palpated for evidence of passive congestion of the liver (as may be seen with congestive heart failure), and for aneurysmal dilation of the aorta. The extremities should be examined for evidence of edema and for evidence of peripheral vascular disease (diminished pulses, atrophic changes, changes in color and temperature). The nervous system should be examined for focal neurological deficits, which could indicate prior strokes.

Patients who complain of postural dizziness, lightheadedness, or postural unsteadiness should be examined for orthostatic hypotension (see Chapter 20 on syncope for a detailed discussion of orthostatic hypotension).

Sally Howard, *Part 3*

On physical examination, Ms. Howard has a cataract obscuring the view of one eye, but normal vessels can be seen in the other eye. The cardiovascular exam is normal and the lung fields are clear. The abdominal examination is benign. She has two dorsalis pedis pulses and no peripheral edema.

Philip Garvin, *Part 2*

On physical examination, Mr. Garvin has moderate arteriovenous nicking in the fundi. The carotid arteries have normal upstrokes. He has bibasilar rales, and the heart examination is significant for an occasional irregular beat and a soft systolic murmur heard best in the aortic area. The liver is slightly enlarged, and he has 2+ peripheral edema. His peripheral pulses are only barely palpable.

Sadie Carter, *Part 2*

On physical examination, Ms. Carter has moderate arteriovenous nicking in the fundi. Her carotid arteries have normal upstrokes, but there is a soft sound on the left, which is probably a transmitted murmur rather than a bruit. Ms. Carter's lungs are clear and her heart examination reveals a regular rhythm with a systolic ejection murmur that is heard best over the aortic valve area. The liver is not enlarged and Ms. Carter has no peripheral edema. She has somewhat diminished pulses in her feet.

STUDY QUESTION

1. What laboratory and other investigations are appropriate in these three cases?

LABORATORY INVESTIGATION

The laboratory investigation should include an EKG, if one has not been done in the past 3 to 5 years, to assess for left ventricular hypertrophy and evidence of prior ischemic events (if the history is unclear), and to establish a baseline in the event of a future problem.[41,46,57,58] Blood urea nitrogen (BUN), creatinine, basic electrolytes, fasting lipid panel, and glucose should be measured.[40,41,46,47] Most expert committees recommend a urinalysis.[2,40,46,47] However, to assess for microalbuminuria or proteinuria, a urine microalbumin or 24-hour urine protein is more accurate. There is insufficient evidence to support obtaining a uric acid, complete blood count, or more detailed chemistries, although this may be reasonable in individual cases.[40,41,46,47] If secondary hypertension is suspected, additional labs may be appropriate (see Table 35–2). Finally, one can consider doing echocardiography to assess for left ventricular hypertrophy or for other cardiac structural problems, but ordering this routinely in all hypertensive patients is not recommended: there are no data from prospective trials evaluating outcomes and cost-effectiveness.[46]

Sally Howard, *Part 4*

Ms. Howard's lab work reveals a sodium of 138 mmol/L, potassium of 4.0 mEq/L, creatinine of 1.2 mg/dl, and fasting glucose of 90 mg/dl. Her lipid panel shows an LDL of 110 mg/dl, and her TSH and urine microalbumin are normal. An ECG shows evidence of left ventricular hypertrophy.

Philip Garvin, *Part 3*

Mr. Garvin has a sodium level of 140 mmol/L, potassium of 3.5 mEq/L, creatinine of 2.5 mg/dl, and glucose of 90 mg/dl. His LDL is 150 mg/dl. His urinalysis is normal (no protein). His ECG shows an old anteroseptal MI, unifocal premature ventricular contractions, and diffuse nonspecific ST and T wave changes. Due to his lung exam, you obtain a chest x-ray, which shows moderate cardiomegaly, fluid in the fissures, and small bilateral pleural effusions.

Sadie Carter, *Part 3*

Ms. Carter has a sodium level of 142 mmol/L, potassium of 3.0 mEq/L, and glucose of 72 mg/dl. Her LDL is 90 mg/dl, and her urinalysis shows 1+ protein, but a follow-up urine microalbumin is normal. Her hematocrit is 31%. Her ECG shows an old inferior MI and mildly flattened T waves.

STUDY QUESTION

1. How do these findings influence your management of these three cases?

Office Evaluation of the Chronic Hypertensive

BLOOD PRESSURE MEASUREMENTS

A patient with chronic hypertension can benefit from the same blood pressure measurement approach discussed under the initial assessment. If the patient complains of dizziness, lightheadedness, or postural unsteadiness, an evaluation for orthostatic hypotension should be conducted. This is particularly true when titrating medications, so as to avoid excessive drops in blood pressure.

For patients on blood pressure medications, the most reliable indicator of overall control is a blood pressure measurement taken before the next dose (i.e., at the expected low point of the drug effect). If this cannot be done in the office due to the timing of the office visit, additional outside-the-office measurements should be encouraged.

PERSISTENTLY ELEVATED BLOOD PRESSURES: RESISTANT HYPERTENSION

A patient with hypertension stubbornly above goal despite three or more medications may need specific exploration of factors that can account for the resistance: inadequate or ineffective therapy, excessive volume expansion, poor adherence to pharmacologic and/or nonpharmacologic treatment, medications or agents that raise blood pressures (decongestants, nonsteroidal anti-inflammatory agents, estrogen preparations, anabolic steroids, licorice-containing products, illicit drugs, alcohol, etc.), or artificially elevated blood pressures due to "white coat hypertension" or pseudohypertension (see "Blood Pressure Measurement: Additional Considerations"). Suboptimal therapy and poor compliance tend to be the most common causes of poorly controlled hypertension.[59–61] If "white coat hypertension" is suspected, it may be useful to have the patient get blood pressure readings taken outside the office, have in-office readings done by nurses or assistants only, and/or use ambulatory blood pressure monitoring (see "Making the Diagnosis" for information regarding normal ambulatory blood pressure measurements). Finally, some elderly patients will truly have secondary hypertension, and will need to be evaluated for this. See Table 35–2 for details.

CARDIOVASCULAR RISK REDUCTION

Cardiovascular risk assessment and reduction is a critical step in helping hypertensives remain healthy. The purpose of hypertension control is to reduce unfortunate cardiovascular outcomes (strokes, myocardial infarctions, etc.). Many hypertensives have additional modifiable cardiac risk factors (diabetes mellitus or impaired fasting glucose, hyperlipidemia, obesity, tobacco use, etc.), and the addition of hypertension to these risk factors compounds the risk of poor outcomes. Therefore, controlling blood pressure without addressing these issues constitutes suboptimal care. Concomitant risk factors (hyperlipidemia, diabetes, obesity) should be managed aggressively, tobacco cessation and moderation of alcohol intake should be encouraged, and periodic lipid and glucose testing should be done. Because cardiovascular disease may already be present in patients with hypertension, assessment for chest pain, shortness of breath, dyspnea on exertion, exercise intolerance, calf claudication, and/or other symptoms of cardiovascular disease should be done on a regular basis.

> ● Because cardiovascular disease may already be present in patients with hypertension, assessment for chest pain, shortness of breath, dyspnea on exertion, exercise intolerance, calf claudication, and/or other symptoms of cardiovascular disease should be done on a regular basis.

ADDITIONAL CARE

Patients on certain antihypertensives (thiazide diuretics, angiotensin converting enzyme [ACE] inhibitors, angiotensin receptor blockers [ARBs]) will need periodic electrolyte and renal function (BUN, creatinine) screening. All patients should be encouraged to monitor and reduce sodium intake, to exercise on a regular basis, and to maintain weight (unless underweight or nutritionally compromised).[2] Finally, but perhaps most importantly, adherence needs to be monitored. Adherence to hypertension drug therapy in the "real world" is lower than in published hypertension trials, and is determined by factors such as the occurrence of adverse effects, ease of the regimen, self-perceived efficacy, and cost.[62,63] Box 35–2 outlines some strategies for improving adherence.

Sally Howard, *Part 5*

Ms. Howard asks if you recommend that she begin to take medication for her blood pressure. She admits that she has not engaged in any physical activity or in dietary attempts to reduce her sodium intake. When you ask her about her willingness to engage in diet and exercise interventions for her hypertension, she indicates she is ready to do this, but she has many questions about exactly what she needs to do.

Box 35–2   Strategies to Improve Adherence to Medication Therapy

- Involve patient in education and treatment planning—elicit her or his perspective and concerns.
- Provide information regarding what to expect with current therapy (side effects, need to titrate or add meds, etc.).
- Use a once-daily dosing regimen, if possible.
- Assist with medication management (pill boxes, written instructions, calendars, etc.).
- Avoid expensive agents if cheaper but equivalently effective agents are available.
- Utilize drug company or pharmacy financial assistance programs, if appropriate, to overcome cost barriers.
- Utilize a nurse, pharmacist, or family member to help with medication monitoring.
- Be sensitive to patient's concerns regarding a particular medication, and prescribe an alternative if necessary.
- Once a two-agent medication regimen is established, consider finding a combination pill (if cost permits).

Philip Garvin, *Part 4*

Mr. Garvin has known coronary artery disease, suspected peripheral vascular disease, hyperlipidemia, and uncontrolled hypertension. Thus, you realize he is at high risk of further cardiovascular events if his risk factors are not modified. He is compliant with his medications, so his persistently elevated blood pressures prompt you to explore reasons for refractory hypertension. You discover that he has started eating out more often due to difficulties preparing meals, and seems now to be eating saltier foods. You also note that his volume expansion is contributing to his elevated blood pressures. You realize that his hyperlipidemia is also going unaddressed: his diet is not low in saturated fat, and you have never discussed with him his ideal LDL or the role of medications in bringing down the LDL.

Sadie Carter, *Part 4*

Ms. Carter's blood pressures are higher than ideal, but based on her complaints of dizziness and weakness with standing, you suspect she has orthostatic hypotension. The drop in her blood pressure with standing confirms this. She also has another potential complication of her treatment for hypertension: hypokalemia. Given that she is a frail-appearing 90-year-old, you are concerned about these adverse effects of hypertension treatment. Yet, you must balance these risks against the risk of untreated hypertension in a patient with established atherosclerotic disease.

STUDY QUESTION

1. What steps in hypertension management will you take for each of these individuals?

MANAGEMENT

Management of Hypertensive Urgency and Emergency

Hypertensive urgencies and emergencies (together, called *hypertensive crises*) may affect only 1% to 2% of the hypertensive population, but require immediate recognition and action.[38,39,64] The definition of hypertensive emergency and urgency is consistent throughout the literature (see "Definitions and Criteria" above). No specific blood pressure serves as a diagnostic criterion[2,37–39]; however, most patients with hypertensive emergency have a systolic blood pressure of 240 mmHg or higher and/or a diastolic blood pressure of 120 mmHg or higher.[37,39] Studies show great variability in choice of agents used to lower blood pressure during hypertensive crises, and there is no consistent data regarding a timetable for lowering pressures.[2,37–39] Furthermore, very elderly patients (age 80 and older) have been excluded from some studies of treatment strategies.[38] Therefore, with the exception of the concepts below, there is considerable room for clinical judgment in treating hypertensive crises.

Hypertensive emergencies require emergency room evaluation and initiation of treatment, followed by hospitalization (possibly in an intensive care unit, depending upon the medication chosen and the type of blood pressure monitoring required). The choice of agent used to lower blood pressures depends on the clinical situation and nature of target organ damage; see Table 35–4 for choices. One consideration is whether an underlying clinical condition is associated with a high renin state (e.g., renal artery stenosis, renal vasculitis, adrenergic crises such as pheochromocytoma), as hypertensive crises arising from those situations may respond well to ACE inhibitors.[37] In general, the goal of treatment is to lower the blood pressure quickly to limit target organ damage. There is no uniformly agreed upon blood pressure goal, but due to the possibility of impaired autoregulation of cerebral blood flow in older patients and in patients with cerebrovascular disease, it is important to avoid drastic lowering of blood pressure; drastic blood pressure lowering could provoke cerebral ischemia, or, by a similar mechanism, cardiac or renal ischemia. Therefore, a general rule of thumb is to reduce the mean blood pressure by no more than 20% to 25% within 2 hours, while monitoring the patient's clinical status. Some clinical practice guidelines further suggest that the blood pressure be reduced to 160/100 mmHg by 6 hours.[3,65,66] The frequency of blood pressure monitoring may range from every 30 minutes to continuous, and some patients will benefit from intra-arterial blood pressure monitoring. It should be noted that for hypertensive patients with acute stroke, these blood pressure lowering recommendations do not necessarily apply; rather, stroke-specific blood pressure management guidelines should be followed (for details, see Chapter 39 on cerebrovascular disease).

Hypertensive urgencies can often be managed in outpatient settings, and require administration of oral medication to lower blood pressure, followed by some monitoring of blood pressure response. See Table 35–4 for choices of agents, and information regarding

| Table 35–4 | Selected Agents for Hypertensive Urgencies and Emergencies |

Agent	Comments	Class or Mechanism	Onset of Action	Duration of Action	Dosage Range[a]
Oral					
Captopril	Adverse effects: angioedema, renal insufficiency	ACE inhibitor	15–30 minutes	4–6 hours	12.5–25 mg initially
Clonidine	Adverse effects: drowsiness	Centrally acting alpha-adrenergic agonist	30–60 minutes	4–6 hours	0.1 mg po, and then can repeat hourly
Prazosin	Adverse effects: syncope, reflex tachycardia	Alpha1-adrenergic receptor blocker	30–60 minutes	4–6 hours	1–2 mg
Labetalol	Avoid in bronchospastic disease Adverse effects: bradycardia	Alpha1- and Beta-adrenergic receptor blocker	30–120 minutes	3–6 hours	100–400 mg
Nifedipine	Not recommended by author due to unpredictable drops in blood pressure	Dihydropyridine calcium-channel blocker	15–30 minutes	3–6 hours	10–20 mg
Parenteral					
Nitroglycerin	Indications: acute coronary syndromes, pulmonary edema	Vasodilator	2–5 minutes	5–10 minutes	5–100 µg/min
Sodium nitroprusside	Indicated in most emergencies	Vasodilator	Immediate	2–3 minutes after infusion ends	0.25–10 µg/kg/min
Labetalol	Indicated for aortic dissection, hypertensive encephalopathy, acute coronary syndromes, intraoperative hypertension	Alpha1- and Beta-adrenergic receptor blocker	<5 minutes	3–6 hours	20–80 mg q 15 min. or 0.5–2 mg/min
Nicardipine	Indicated in hypertensive encephalopathy, stroke, subarachnoid hemorrhage, aortic dissection, post-op hypertension	Dihydropyridine calcium-channel blocker	1–5 minutes	1–5 minutes	10–15 mg/h
Fenoldopam	Indications: postoperative hypertension, pulmonary edema, renal failure	Selective postsynaptic dopaminergic receptor agonist	30–60 minutes	30–60 minutes	0.1–1.6 µg/kg/min
Enalaprilat	Indicated in congestive heart failure	Angiotensin-converting enzyme inhibitor	15 minutes	12–24 hours	0.625–1.25 mg q 6 hours
Phentolamine	Indications: pheochromocytoma, MAO inhibitor interactions	Alpha1-adrenergic receptor blocker	2–5 minutes	1–2 hours	1–5 mg q 6 hours
Diltiazem	Indication: atrial fibrillation	Nondihydropyridine calcium-channel blocker	2–5 minutes	6–12 hours	5–15 mg/h

[a]These doses are per the cited source. Please verify doses against package insert or published drug literature.

Source: Adapted from Mansoor G, Frishman W. Comprehensive management of hypertensive emergencies and urgencies. Heart Dis 4:358–71, 2002.

onset/duration of action. The rate of blood pressure lowering is slower than with hypertensive emergencies, and the goal blood pressure should be achieved in hours to days.[3,38,39]

Finally, patients presenting with hypertensive crises should be evaluated for secondary hypertension, as a significant portion will have this.[39,67]

Office Management of Chronic Hypertension

GOAL BLOOD PRESSURE REDUCTION

The goal for blood pressure reduction for elderly patients is the same as for younger patients: systolic BP of less than 140 mmHg and/or diastolic blood pressure less than 90 mmHg. However, the caveat is that this reduction should not occur at the expense of orthostasis (see "Initial Evaluation: Physical Exam" section), as orthostasis can produce serious injuries if a syncopal episode occurs.

- If a patient has diabetes mellitus, the goal blood pressure is less than 130/80 mmHg.[41,46]
- If a patient has proteinuria higher than 1 g/24 hours, the goal blood pressure is 125/75 mmHg or lower.[2,41,46]

For some individuals, treatment side effects, orthostasis, or extremely resistant hypertension may make a goal of a systolic blood pressure less than 140 mmHg and/or diastolic blood pressure less than 90 mmHg impossible to achieve. In this situation, it is useful to remember that a meta-analysis of 15,693 older patients with isolated systolic hypertension showed that just a 10-point reduction in systolic blood pressure, even if systolic blood pressure remained above 140 mmHg, was associated with a 30% reduction in strokes, 26% reduction in cardiovascular event-associated deaths, 23% reduction in myocardial infarctions, and 13% reduction in all-cause deaths.[20] Additionally, a review of 36 studies of hypertension in the elderly found that the strongest evidence for a treatment benefit occurred with an initial systolic blood pressure higher than 160 mmHg, and that there were weaker data to guide therapy if the systolic blood pressure was lower than this.[68]

J-CURVE HYPOTHESIS

One of the most controversial issues in treating hypertension in the elderly is whether there is a diastolic blood pressure below which coronary perfusion is compromised, therefore resulting in increased cardiovascular complications. This hypothesis stems from some clinical trials which have shown a J-shaped relationship between diastolic blood pressure and risk of coronary events.[69–74]

The validity of a "J-curve phenomenon" is, however, not well established. Some studies have failed to demonstrate this relationship,[26,75] and others have suggested that the increased risk of coronary events seen in people with lower diastolic blood pressures may actually be due to the presence of existing cardiac disease or chronic disease, for which low diastolic pressure is a proxy measure.[76,77] A meta-analysis of seven randomized clinical trials involving hypertension treatment of 40,233 patients found a J-shaped relationship between diastolic blood pressure and risk of total and cardiovascular deaths for both treated and untreated patients, suggesting that the increased death risk was not related to antihypertensive treatment but perhaps was related to underlying health conditions

causing low blood pressures.[78] In general, despite the unclear status of the J-curve phenomenon, it is advisable to monitor diastolic pressure reductions cautiously in patients with existing cardiovascular disease.

General Strategies

See the algorithm in Fig. 35–2 regarding when to initiate nonpharmacologic versus pharmacologic interventions.

NONPHARMACOLOGIC TECHNIQUES

When treating any hypertensive patient, it is important to emphasize the role of nonpharmacologic treatment, regardless of whether medications will be used. It may be helpful to enlist the spouse and a dietitian in an individual or group setting, to give assistance with lifestyle adjustments. Scheduling follow-up office visits to assess the effectiveness of nonpharmacologic interventions is important. If the provider gives less attention to nonpharmacologic measures than to compliance with medications, the patient will do the same. It should be noted that there is no evidence that lifestyle change alone reduces morbidity and mortality of hypertension, unlike studies using drug treatment. However, reductions in blood pressure can occur with lifestyle change, and can augment drug treatment if the latter is necessary.

Recommendations regarding the nonpharmacologic treatment of hypertension are given in Table 35–5. This table lists approximate reductions in blood pressure that can be expected with various lifestyle changes.

SMOKING AND ALCOHOL CESSATION

Smoking cessation is helpful to reduce the risk of cardiovascular events, and is certainly worth encouraging in the elderly patient with hypertension. Excessive alcohol consumption elevates the blood pressure of all

Table 35–5	Effects of Lifestyle Modification on Blood Pressure
Modification	**Approximate Reduction in Systolic Blood Pressure (Range)**
Weight loss	5–20 mmHg per 10 kg weight loss
DASH diet	8–14 mmHg
Sodium reduction	2–8 mmHg
Physical activity	4–9 mmHg
Moderation of alcohol intake	2–4 mmHg

Source: National Heart, Lung and Blood Institute. Available at: http://hin.nhlbi.nih.gov/nhbpep_slds/menu.htm.

patients, and the elderly should receive advice regarding the need for moderation (no more than two drinks per day in most men and no more than one drink per day in most women or in individuals with a low body weight).[2]

WEIGHT

Elderly patients with hypertension who are overweight (body mass index greater than 25 to 27) should be encouraged to lose weight to within 10% of their ideal body weight.[2,41,47] However, counseling elderly patients regarding dietary modification requires more understanding of their social situation, in that many have little control over food that is made available to them. Some elderly people depend on cafeterias, restaurants, or prepackaged meals (e.g., Meals on Wheels). Furthermore, many older patients may have limited financial resources to purchase fresh foods, which usually have fewer calories and less sodium than packaged or processed foods. Therefore, it is essential to spend some time talking with patients about their living and eating situation, before recommending dietary modifications for weight loss. It is also essential to understand that some older patients may have medical conditions and/or dental conditions that alter their caloric needs and their ability to eat and taste food normally. The key is that dietary advice regarding weight loss must be individualized to the person's circumstances.

PHYSICAL ACTIVITY

Most patients find it easier to lose weight if they also engage in some form of physical activity (optimally, aerobic exercise at least 30 minutes per day, most days of the week).[2] Consider the patient's total medical condition, including musculoskeletal and visual limitations and cardiovascular risk factors, before prescribing an exercise program. Walking is usually a safe activity for elderly patients, but in those with significant arthritis or other limitations in the lower extremities, swimming may be a better choice. Resistance exercise under supervision may also be useful in improving muscle mass, thus assisting with weight loss.

SODIUM RESTRICTION

Elderly hypertensives tend to be more salt-sensitive than younger hypertensives, and studies have shown that limiting sodium in the diet is effective in the elderly.[79-81] Many guidelines, including the JNC-7 guidelines, recommend limiting sodium to no more than 2.4 g of sodium or 6 g of sodium chloride per day. However, diets lower in sodium may be unpalatable, and may result in a decline in the patient's overall

nutritional status. In such cases, an acceptable option is the use of salt substitutes containing potassium chloride; however, care must be taken in patients who have impaired renal function or who are taking angiotensin-converting enzyme inhibitors, angiotensin receptor blockers, or potassium-sparing diuretics, as elevated potassium levels may result.

DIETARY APPROACHES TO STOPPING HYPERTENSION

The Dietary Approaches to Stopping Hypertension (DASH) diet is low in cholesterol and high in fiber, potassium, calcium, and magnesium. This diet has been featured in trials of nonpharmacologic therapy for hypertension, and the use of the diet has been found to be associated with reductions in systolic and diastolic blood pressure.[2,47,82-84] The composition of the DASH diet is as follows: 7 to 8 daily servings of grain products, 4 to 5 daily servings of vegetables and fruits, 2 to 3 daily servings of low- or non-fat dairy foods, less than 2 daily servings of meats, fish, or poultry, and 4 to 5 weekly servings of nuts, seeds, and legumes. This diet can be recommended to hypertensives to assist with blood pressure control, and it can be downloaded from www.nhlbi.nih.gov/health/public/heart/hbp/dash/ new_dash.pdf.

Sally Howard, *Part 6*

You counsel Ms. Howard that she is at least 20 pounds over her ideal body weight, and that losing these extra pounds will probably make her blood pressure easier to control. You explore her living situation and discover that she lives with her husband, cooks and prepares their meals, and is able to modify meal preparation and lifestyle. You note that weight loss will be easier if she also exercises, and suggest that she begin walking for at least half an hour three times a week at a pace that does not leave her winded. (Because she has no other cardiovascular risk factors and is already physically active, you do not insist on a supervised exercise program or on a pre-exercise stress test.) You also suggest that she start a low-sodium diet. You describe how to read food labels when shopping, you advocate for fresh or frozen vegetables over canned vegetables, and you caution her to read the sodium labels on prepared foods. In addition to giving Ms. Howard hand-outs on a 1500-calorie diet and low-sodium foods, you schedule an appointment for her with the dietitian next week.

You also schedule a return visit in 1 month, and then every 2 months afterwards for the next 6 months, so that you can assess her progress with these interventions. You encourage her to continue monitoring blood pressures at home, and to call you if questions or problems develop.

Philip Garvin, *Part 5*

Given that Mr. Garvin's diet seems high in sodium and thus may be a contributor to his refractory hypertension, you explore his lifestyle and then determine feasible dietary recommendations. Mr. Garvin lives alone, does not cook much anymore due to difficulty shopping and preparing food, and thus tends to eat out at a local cafeteria for lunch and dinner. You ascertain Mr. Garvin's food preferences, and using that information, you educate him about which foods have a higher-than-ideal sodium content. You instruct him to avoid those foods, and you provide concrete examples of foods he can purchase that are likely to have less sodium. You also include foods that are low in saturated fat in your recommendations, to help him address his hyperlipidemia.

Sadie Carter, *Part 5*

You advise Ms. Carter that her blood pressure medicine may be contributing to her weakness, dizziness, and hypokalemia, and that you would like to consider decreasing it. You explain that her blood pressure will still need treatment, however, and you decide to explore possible lifestyle interventions. You know that Ms. Carter lives with her daughter, who cooks for the family. The daughter has been concerned about Ms. Carter's low weight, and finds that if she intentionally seasons the food with salt, Ms. Carter finds the food more appetizing and thus eats better. You ask Ms. Carter and her daughter to visit the dietician to learn how to season food in ways that will be appetizing but that will not involve so much salt use. You also discuss the DASH diet with them, and give them sample recipes which you download from the National Heart, Lung, and Blood Institute website.

STUDY QUESTION

1. What recommendations will you make regarding the current anti-hypertensive drugs Mr. Garvin and Ms. Carter are taking?

Medications

WHEN AND WHY TO TREAT

Drug treatment for hypertension has been found to have a significant impact on cardiovascular morbidity and mortality among geriatric patients. Individual large-scale randomized, blinded, placebo-controlled trials of hypertension treatment in the elderly have shown reductions in stroke, coronary artery events, and other cardiovascular outcomes, generally with a systolic blood pressure reduction of as little as 11 to 14 mmHg and a diastolic BP reduction of 5 to 6 mmHg (Table 35–6).

The risk versus benefit of drug treatment for hypertension needs to be weighed carefully in frail older patients, and it is important to be aware of factors that may increase the risk of adverse drug reactions. For example, diminished baroreceptor activity and decreased intravascular volume can lead to orthostatic hypotension, and impaired cerebral autoregulation can produce cerebral ischemia with small drops in systolic pressure. There is a risk of dehydration, hyponatremia, hypokalemia, depression, and confusion related to the effects of certain blood pressure medications. Finally, decreased renal and hepatic function can cause drug accumulation, and polypharmacy can raise the risk of drug interactions.

See Figure 35–2 regarding when to initiate pharmacologic interventions. In general, patients with a systolic blood pressure of 140 mmHg or higher or a diastolic blood pressure of 90 mmHg or higher who are unable to bring down the blood pressure after 3 to 6 months of lifestyle change will require drug therapy.[2] Individuals with existing target organ damage or with cardiovascular comorbidities may need drug therapy at the outset, although lifestyle change must be emphasized as well. The JNC 7 recommends starting with one drug, usually a thiazide diuretic or beta-blocker. However, if the systolic blood pressure is 160 mmHg or higher or the diastolic blood pressure is 100 mmHg or higher, the JNC 7 recommends starting two drugs simultaneously to optimize blood pressure reduction. This recommendation should be individualized in the geriatric patient, as some frail older individuals may not tolerate the addition of two antihypertensive drugs simultaneously.

> ● Drug treatment for hypertension has been found to have a significant impact on the incidence of cardiovascular morbidity and mortality among elderly patients.

CLASSES OF MEDICATIONS

General properties of anti-hypertensive medications are described below. For some patients, there are compelling reasons to choose one agent over another, and

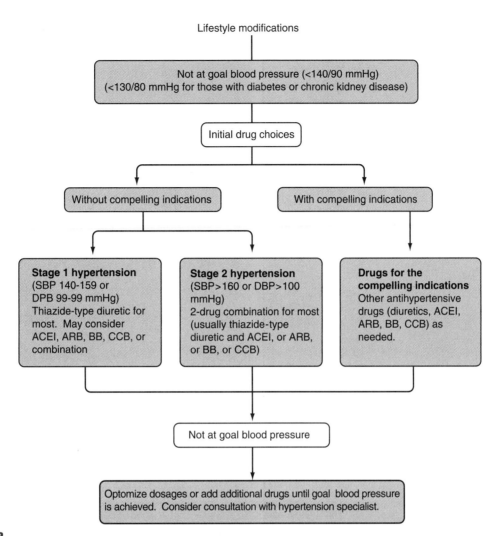

Lifestyle modifications

Not at goal blood pressure (<140/90 mmHg)
(<130/80 mmHg for those with diabetes or chronic kidney disease)

Initial drug choices

Without compelling indications

With compelling indications

Stage 1 hypertension
(SBP 140-159 or
DPB 99-99 mmHg)
Thiazide-type diuretic for
most. May consider
ACEI, ARB, BB, CCB, or
combination

Stage 2 hypertension
(SBP>160 or DBP>100
mmHg)
2-drug combination for most
(usually thiazide-type
diuretic and ACEI, or ARB,
or BB, or CCB)

**Drugs for the
compelling indications**
Other antihypertensive
drugs (diuretics, ACEI,
ARB, BB, CCB) as
needed.

Not at goal blood pressure

Optomize dosages or add additional drugs until goal blood pressure
is achieved. Consider consultation with hypertension specialist.

FIGURE 35–2

Algorithm for treatment of hypertension. *(Redrawn from National Heart, Lung, and Blood Institute. Available at: http://bin.nhlbi.nih.gov/nhbpep_slds/menu.htm.)*

Table 35–7 outlines these indications and medication choices. Table 35–8 provides an overview of recent head-to-head trials of classes of drugs used for hypertension treatment in the elderly.

DIURETICS

Thiazide diuretics are generally the best studied and the first-choice agents in hypertension treatment.[2,68] They have been shown to be effective in lowering both systolic and diastolic blood pressures, and also may be the most effective agents to reduce pulse pressure.[68] When thiazide diuretics have been compared with other agents in affecting cardiovascular outcomes, there have been conflicting findings (see Table 35–8, ANBP-2 vs. ALLHAT columns). The apparent differences in the results of these studies may be due to the differences in populations studied, and in the size and

power of the studies, with the ALLHAT study being much larger and having greater statistical power.[85,86]

Thiazide diuretics can be taken once daily and generally are quite inexpensive. However, they do have potential adverse effects: hypokalemia, hyponatremia, hyperuricemia (with an increased risk of gout), dehydration, and worsened urinary incontinence. Furthermore, they are generally not as effective if the creatinine clearance is less than 30 ml/min. Finally, high doses of thiazide diuretics (>25 mg/day of hydrochlorothiazide) are not recommended, as the adverse metabolic effects outweigh increases in effectiveness.

β-BLOCKERS

β-blockers have been available as antihypertensive agents for decades, and have been shown to reduce cardiovascular mortality, left ventricular hypertro-

Table 35–6	Large Randomized, Blinded, Placebo-Controlled Trials of Pharmacologic Hypertension Treatment in the Elderly						
	SHEP	**STOP HTN**	**MRC**	**Syst-Eur**	**Syst-China**	**STONE**	**EWPHE**
No. of patients	4736	1627	4396	4695	2394	1632	840
Mean age (years)	72	76	70	70	>60	66	72
Type of hypertension	Systolic	Systolic and/or diastolic	Systolic and/or diastolic	Systolic	Systolic	Systolic and/or diastolic	Systolic and/or diastolic
Treatment regimen	Thiazide diuretic ± B-blocker, reserpine	Thiazide diuretic ± B-blocker	Thiazide diuretic or B-blocker	Calcium channel blocker ± ACE inhibitor, thiazide diuretic	Calcium channel blocker ± ACE inhibitor, diuretic	Calcium channel blocker	Diuretic ± methyldopa
Relative Risk Reduction of:							
Stroke	36%[a]	47%[a]	25%[a,b]	42%[a]	38%[a]	—	36%
Coronary artery disease	27%[a]	13%	19%[b]	30%	—	—	20%
Congestive heart failure	49%[a]	51%[a]	Not reported	29%	—	—	22%
Other significant reductions	Coronary artery disease mortality	Major cardio-vascular events Total mortality		Vascular dementia	Cardiovascular mortality	Cardiovascular events	Fatal coronary events Cardiovascular mortality

[a]Statistically significant at $p<0.05$.

[b]This reduction was only noted in the thiazide arm.

SHEP, Systolic Hypertension in the Elderly Program[26]; STOP-HTN, Swedish Trial in Old Patients with Hypertension[27]; MRC, Medical Research Council[92]; Syst-Eur, Systolic Hypertension in Europe Trial[28]; Syst-China, Systolic Hypertension in China Trial[88]; STONE, Shanghai Trial of Nifedipine in the Elderly[93]; EWPHE, European Working Party on High Blood Pressure in the Elderly[74].

Source: Adapted from Harvey P, Woodward M. Management of hypertension in older people. Aust J Hosp Pharm 31:212–9, 2001, with permission.

Table 35–7	Recommended Antihypertensive Agents When Comorbid Conditions Are Present					
	Antihypertensive Drug Classes					
Comorbid Condition	**Diuretic**	**β-Blocker**	**Calcium Channel Blocker**	**ACE Inhibitor**	**Angiotensin Receptor Blocker**	**Alpha-1-Blocker**
Heart failure	+	+		+	+	
Prior myocardial infarction		+		+	+	
Prior stroke	+			+		
High risk for coronary artery disease	+	+	+	+	+	
Type II diabetes mellitus	+	+	+	+	+	
Chronic renal insufficiency				+	+	
Benign prostatic hypertrophy						+

+, Recommended.

Source: National Heart, Lung and Blood Institute. Available at: http://hin.nhlbi.nih.gov/nhbpep_slds/menu.htm.

Table 35–8	Head-to-Head Trials of Hypertension Treatment in the Elderly				
	ANBP-2	**ALLHAT**	**STOP-2**	**LIFE**	**INVEST**
No. patients	6,083	42,418	6,614		
Mean age (years)	76	67	76	70	66
Type of hypertension	Systolic and/ or diastolic	Systolic and/ or diastolic	Systolic and/ or diastolic	Systolic and/ or diastolic	Systolic and/ or diastolic
Treatment regimen	ACE inhibitor vs. thiazide diuretic	ACE inhibitor vs. thiazide diuretic vs. calcium channel blocker vs. alpha1-blocker[a]	ACE inhibitor or calcium channel blocker ("new drugs") vs. thiazide diuretic or B-blocker	Angiotensin receptor blocker vs. B-blocker ("old drugs")	ACE inhibitor and calcium channel blocker vs. thiazide diuretic and B-blocker
Median follow-up (years)	4	5	5	4	2
Reductions in stroke	No difference	Thiazide > ACE	No difference	ARB > BB	—
Reductions in cardiovascular events	ACE > diuretic (for men only, and p=0.05)	No difference	No difference between the newer drugs and older drugs, except ACE > CCB for MI	ARB > BB	No difference
Reductions in congestive heart failure	No difference	Thiazide = best	No difference between newer and older drugs, except ACE > CCB	—	—
Reductions in total mortality	ACE > diuretic (for men only, and p=0.05)	No difference	No difference	No difference	No difference

[a]Alpha1-blocker arm stopped early due to significantly higher incidence of major cardiovascular events.

ANBP-2, Second Australian National Blood Pressure study[85]; ALLHAT, The Antihypertensive and Lipid-Lowering Treatment to Prevent Heart Attack Trial[86]; STOP-2, Swedish Trial in Old Patients with Hypertension-2[94]; LIFE, Losartan Intervention for Endpoint Reduction in Hypertension[89]; INVEST, International Verapamil-Trandolapril study[95].

Source: Adapted from Dickerson L, Gibson M. Management of hypertension in older persons. Am Fam Phys 71(3):469–76, 2005, with permission.

phy, stroke, and heart failure. Typically, β-blockers have been classified as first-line agents for treatment of hypertension, alongside thiazide diuretics. However, at least one meta-analysis has shown a greater reduction in cardiovascular events and strokes with thiazide diuretics as compared to β-blockers.[87] Furthermore, no large-scale randomized controlled trials have assessed β-blockers as first-line therapy for isolated systolic hypertension. Since β-blockers are associated with decreased mortality after myocardial infarction, they are the best agents for hypertensive patients who have survived a myocardial infarction.

β-blockers increase peripheral vascular resistance, so these drugs may precipitate or worsen the symptoms of claudication in patients with peripheral vascular disease. They have a negative inotropic effect and should be used carefully in elderly patients with conduction abnormalities. Other potential side effects include exacerbation of reactive airway disease, central nervous system symptoms (including depression), and fatigue or poor exercise tolerance. Therefore, it is important to query patients about these issues when prescribing this class of medications, and it is important to choose the more cardiac-selective β-blockers (e.g., metoprolol and atenolol).

CALCIUM-CHANNEL BLOCKERS

Calcium-channel blockers decrease peripheral vascular resistance and, therefore, are theoretically ideal antihypertensive agents in the elderly. Long-acting dihydropyridine agents have been beneficial in the treatment of isolated systolic hypertension.[28,88] Because calcium channel blockers have no adverse effects on serum lipids and are less likely than β-blockers to cause fatigue, they are generally well tolerated. Most preparations of calcium channel blockers are available in sustained-release formulations, which can be taken once a day.

Calcium channel blockers do have side effects that are important for some patients. Verapamil and diltiazem can cause cardiac conduction defects and may impair myocardial contractility; thus, they should be avoided if a patient has an impaired ejection fraction. Nifedipine and amlodipine may cause peripheral edema. Calcium channel blockers are also associated with gingival hyperplasia (which may lead to problems with denture fit) and with constipation.

ANGIOTENSIN CONVERTING ENZYME INHIBITORS

The most common indication for ACE inhibitors in elderly hypertensives is the treatment of certain comorbid conditions (see Table 35–7). Thus, although older individuals generally have low renin activity, ACE inhibitors can act effectively as adjuncts to diuretic therapy for hypertension, and are preferential in the setting of diabetes, congestive heart failure, left ventricular hypertrophy, and renal insufficiency. However, there is much less evidence to support the use of these agents as first-line antihypertensives, as compared to thiazide diuretics.

ACE inhibitors have been associated with a persistent dry cough. They can increase the serum creatinine level, particularly in patients who are also receiving diuretics. In patients with bilateral renal artery stenosis, ACE inhibitors can lead to a precipitous drop in renal function. However, ACE inhibitors improve intrarenal blood flow and decrease proteinuria in patients with diabetes mellitus. They have been shown to prolong life in patients with congestive heart failure (CHF) by improving overall cardiac function, and they have been approved for use in post-myocardial infarction patients. Serum electrolytes, particularly potassium, should be monitored when prescribing these agents, as ACE inhibitor use in the setting of mild renal insufficiency or in combination with potassium-sparing drugs can lead to hyperkalemia.

> ● Although older individuals generally have low renin activity, ACE inhibitors can act effectively as adjuncts to diuretic therapy for hypertension, and are preferential in the setting of diabetes, congestive heart failure, left ventricular hypertrophy, and renal insufficiency.

ANGIOTENSIN RECEPTOR BLOCKERS

These agents have been less well-studied in the treatment of hypertension, by virtue of their newness. Due to their modulation of the renin-angiotensin-aldosterone system, they have similar benefits, indications, and precautions as the ACE inhibitors. They are more expensive than ACE inhibitors; however, they have the advantage of a lower incidence of cough. Only a few large trials have evaluated the efficacy of ARBs in treating hypertension in the elderly. The Losartan Intervention for Endpoint Reduction in Hypertension (LIFE) study showed that the ARB, losartan, had a significantly greater effect than a β-blocker on the endpoints of stroke reduction and of combined cardiovascular mortality, stroke, and myocardial infarction reduction in hypertensive elders.[89] The Valsartan Antihypertensive Long-term Use Evaluation (VALUE) trial assessed cardiac morbidity and mortality among 15,245 hypertensives aged 50 and older who received valsartan versus a calcium-channel blocker (amlodipine). The study found that amlodipine was associated with greater reductions in blood pressure, but that there was no significant difference in the two

treatment arms with regard to composite endpoint of cardiac morbidity and mortality.[90]

VASODILATORS

Vasodilators such as hydralazine directly lower peripheral vascular resistance, thus lowering blood pressure. They may be most useful in the treatment of hypertensive urgency. These agents are associated with reflex tachycardia and postural hypotension, but for patients who can tolerate them, they have the advantage of being inexpensive. However, typically these agents are used if the more standard agents above are contraindicated or not tolerated, or if a fourth agent needs to be added to a hypertensive regimen.

α-BLOCKERS

Agents that have α-adrenergic blocking activity (terazosin, doxazosin, etc.) also lower peripheral vascular resistance, and can be effective in lowering blood pressure in the elderly. However, these agents are frowned upon as first-line therapy for hypertension, in part because of their greater propensity to cause orthostatic hypotension (including first-dose syncope), and also because the ALLHAT study found an increased incidence of congestive heart failure in patients taking these drugs. α-blocking agents do have one very useful property: they decrease symptoms of prostatic outlet obstruction, and they may be useful for hypertensive men who have this problem.

CENTRALLY ACTING ALPHA 2-AGONISTS

These agents (e.g., methyldopa, clonidine) depress sympathetic outflow, thus lowering blood pressure. Oral clonidine is inexpensive, and can be effective in treatment of hypertensive urgency. However, when used as long-term antihypertensive agents, these agents have many disadvantages, including dry mouth, fatigue, sedation, depression, orthostatic hypotension, and rebound hypertension if doses are missed. In addition, these agents typically require a greater than once a day dosing schedule, and long-acting clonidine (in the form of a patch) is expensive. These agents are not generally recommended unless hypertension cannot be controlled with any of the above agents in combination.

Philip Garvin, *Part 6*

You advise Mr. Garvin that one of his medicines, doxazosin, could be exacerbating his congestive heart failure. Because he has had a heart attack and has CHF, you suggest that metoprolol be continued for now. However, you discontinue doxazosin because it is associated with higher rates of congestive heart failure. You suggest beginning an angiotensin-converting enzyme (ACE) inhibitor (benazepril), which will help with his congestive heart failure and with his blood pressure. You advise him that there is a chance that his kidney function may worsen with this medication and that you will want to recheck his creatinine and electrolytes within 1 week. Because the first dose of an ACE inhibitor can lower blood pressure in a person who is sodium depleted from a diuretic, you tell Mr. Garvin to discontinue his diuretic for 24 hours before starting the lowest dose of benazepril at bedtime.

Sadie Carter, *Part 6*

You advise Ms. Carter that you will reduce her dose of hydrochlorothiazide to 12.5 mg/day to reduce the drop in blood pressure when she stands. You also suspect that this change will help reduce the risk of hypokalemia. Because her standing blood pressure is adequately controlled on 25 mg/day, but may not be controlled on reduced dose of hydrochlorothiazide, you suggest that she have her neighbor (a retired nurse) measure her sitting and standing blood pressures several times over the next 2 to 3 weeks. Ms. Carter should then bring these values to her next office visit. If she is feeling better but her average home standing blood pressure is greater than 135/85 mmHg or her average office standing blood pressure is greater than 140/90 mmHg, you will discuss with her the risks and benefits of other drugs to lower her blood pressure.

SUMMARY

Hypertension (especially isolated systolic hypertension) is prevalent in the elderly, and is associated with increased cardiovascular morbidity and mortality. The JNC 7 guidelines, supported by population data and prospective cohort studies, indicate that the relationship of blood pressure to cardiovascular disease risk is "continuous, consistent, and independent of other risks." Blood pressure control is essential to reducing cardiovascular morbidity and mortality, and there is evidence that even octo- and nonagenarians can benefit from blood pressure reduction. It is essential that the diagnosis of hypertension be established properly, and that elderly patients with hypertension be assessed and treated for concomitant cardiovascular risk factors (hyperlipidemia, diabetes mellitus, etc.). The goal of hypertension treatment remains the same in young and old people (BP <140/90 mmHg), and lifestyle interventions (especially sodium reduction) are appropriate. However, many older persons will require pharmacologic treatment, particularly if the initial systolic blood pressure is 160 mmHg or higher. Thiazide diuretics are generally the first choice, although other agents may be used as first-line agents in certain clinical situations.

ACKNOWLEDGMENT

Minor portions of the hypertension chapter from the fourth edition of this text were retained in this chapter. The fourth-edition chapter was authored by Darlyne Menscer, MD.

POSTTEST

1. Mr. S is a 72-year-old white man who has a long history of chronic obstructive pulmonary disease, and now requires pharmacologic therapy for hypertension. The class of drugs that should be avoided when choosing an agent for him is:
    a. Central adrenergic inhibitors
    b. β-blockers
    c. Calcium-channel blockers
    d. ACE inhibitors
    e. Diuretics

2. Ms. M is an 82-year-old black woman who has had hypertension for many years. Recently she has developed congestive heart failure. The class of drugs that would be best for her antihypertensive therapy now is:
    a. Thiazide diuretics
    b. α-blockers
    c. ACE inhibitors
    d. Calcium-channel blockers

3. Mr. M is a 70-year-old white man who has had hypertension for years and now has type II diabetes mellitus. He is a retired physician and is worried about the new finding of diabetes mellitus. He wants to be treated with a drug that may limit the impact this condition, and his hypertension will have on his renal function. An agent from which of the following classes is most likely to be beneficial?
    a. α-blockers
    b. Diuretics
    c. Calcium-channel blockers
    d. Vasodilators
    e. ACE inhibitors

References

1. Franklin S, Jacobs M, Wong N, et al. Predominance of isolated systolic hypertension among middle-aged and elderly US hypertensives: analysis based on National Health and Nutrition Examination Survey (NHANES) III. Hypertension 37:869-74, 2001.
2. Chobanian A, Bakris G, Black H, et al. The seventh report of the Joint National Committee on prevention, detection, evaluation and treatment of high blood pressure. JAMA 289:2560-72, 2003.
3. The Sixth Report of the Joint National Committee on Prevention, Detection, Evaluation and Treatment of Hypertension. Arch Intern Med 157:2413-46, 1997.
4. Wolz M, Cutler J, Roccella E, et al. Statement from the National High Blood Pressure Education Program: prevalence of hypertension. Am J Hypertens 13:103-4, 2000.
5. National Center for Health Statistics. Health United States 2003. Available at: www.cdc.gov/nchs/. Accessed May 2, 2005.
6. Kannel W. Prevalence and implications of uncontrolled systolic hypertension. Drugs Aging 20(4):277-86, 2003.
7. Wilking S, Belanger A, Kannel W, et al. Determinants of isolated systolic hypertension. JAMA 260:3451-5, 1988.
8. Coppola W, Whincup P, Walker M, et al. Identification and management of stroke risk in older people: a national survey of current practice in primary care. J Hum Hypertens 11:185-91, 1997.
9. Fagard R, Van den Enden M. Treatment and blood pressure control in isolated systolic hypertension vs. diastolic hypertension in primary care. J Hum Hypertens 17:681-7, 2003.
10. Vasan R, Beiser A, Seshadri S, et al. Residual lifetime risk for developing hypertension in middle-aged women and men: the Framingham Heart Study. JAMA 287;1003-10, 2002.
11. Hajjar I, Kotchen T. Trends in prevalence, awareness, treatment, and control of hypertension in the United States, 1988-2000. JAMA 290:199-203, 2003.
12. Stamler J, Stamler R, Neaton J. Blood pressure, systolic and diastolic, and cardiovascular risks. US population data. Arch Intern Med 153:598-615, 1993.
13. Stokes J, Kannel W, Wolf P, et al. Blood pressure as a risk factor for cardiovascular disease. The Framingham Study-30 years of follow-up. Hypertension 13 (Suppl 5):113-8, 1989.
14. Lewington S, Clarke R, Qizilbasch N, et al. Age-specific relevance of usual blood pressure to vascular mortality: a meta-analysis of individual date for one million adults in 61 prospective studies. Lancet 360:1903-13, 2002.
15. Franklin S, Larson M, Khan S, et al. Does the relation of blood pressure to coronary heart disease change with aging? The Framingham Heart Study. Circulation 103:1245-9, 2001.
16. Staessen J, Wang J, Bianchi G, et al. Essential hypertension. Lancet 361:1629-41, 2003.
17. Staessen J, Wang J, Thijs L. Cardiovascular prevention and blood pressure reduction: a quantitative overview updated until 01 March 2003. J Hypertens 21:1055-76, 2003.
18. Elliott W. Management of hypertension in the very elderly patient. Hypertension 44:800-4, 2004.
19. Benetos A, Thomas F, Bean K, et al. Prognostic value of systolic and diastolic blood pressure in treated hypertensive men. Arch Intern Med 162:577-81, 2002.
20. Staessen J, Gasowski J, Wang J, et al. Risk of untreated and treated isolated systolic hypertension in the elderly: meta-analysis of outcome trials. Lancet 355:865-72, 2000.
21. Fried L, Kronmal R, Newman A, et al. Risk factors for 5-year mortality in older adults. The Cardiovascular Health Study. JAMA 279:585-92, 1998.
22. Darne' B, Girerd X, Safar M, et al. Pulsatile versus steady component of blood pressure: a cross-sectional analysis and a prospective analysis on cardiovascular mortality. Hypertension 13:392-400, 1989.
23. Benetos A, Safar M, Rudnicki A, et al. Pulse pressure: a predictor of long-term cardiovascular mortality in a French male population. Hypertension 30:1410-15, 1997.
24. Celis H, Fagard R, Staessen J, et al. Risk and benefit of treatment of isolated systolic hypertension in the elderly: evidence from the Systolic Hypertension in Europe Trial. Curr Opin Cardiol 16:342-8, 2001.
25. Blacher J, Staessen J, Girerd X, et al. Pulse pressure not mean pressure determines cardiovascular risk in older hypertensive patients. Arch Intern Med 160:1085-9, 2000.
26. SHEP Cooperative Research Group. Prevention of stroke by antihypertensive drug treatment in older persons with isolated systolic hypertension. Final results of the Systolic Hypertension in the Elderly Program (SHEP). JAMA 265:3255-64, 1991.
27. Dahlof B, Lindholm L, Hansson L, et al. Morbidity and mortality in the Swedish Trial in Old Patients with hypertension (STOP-Hypertension). Lancet 338:1281-5, 1991.
28. Staessen J, Fagard R, Thijs L, et al. Randomised double-blind comparison of placebo and active treatment for older Patients with isolated systolic hypertension. The Systolic Hypertension in Europe (Syst-Eur) Trial Investigators. Lancet 350:757-64, 1997.
29. National Vital Statistics Reports. 53(6):3, 2004.
30. Bulpitt C, Fletcher A, Beckett N, et al. Hypertension in the Very Elderly Trial (HYVET): protocol for the main trial. Drugs Aging 18(3):151-64, 2001.
31. Gueyffier F, Bulpitt C, Boissel J-P, et al. Antihypertensive drugs in very old people: a subgroup meta-analysis of randomized controlled trials. Lancet 353:793-6, 1999.
32. Insua JT, Sacks HS, Lau T-S, et al. Drug treatment of hypertension in the elderly: a meta-analysis. Ann Intern Med 121:355-62, 1994.
33. MacMahon S, Rodgers A. The effects of blood pressure reduction in older patients: an overview of five randomized controlled trials in elderly hypertensives. Clin Exp Hypertens 15:967-78, 1993.
34. Asmar, R: Benefits of blood pressure reduction in elderly patients. J Hypertens 21(Suppl 6):S25-30, 2003.
35. Grossman E, Messerli F. Angiotensin II receptor blockers for the older patient with hypertension. Clin Geriatr 11(1):38-50, 2003.
36. Nickenig G, Harrison D. The AT1-type angiotensin receptor in oxidative stress and atherogenesis. Part I: oxidative stress and atherogenesis. Circulation 105:393-6, 2002.
37. Blumenfeld J, Laragh J. Management of hypertensive crises: the scientific basis for treatment decisions. Am J Hypertens 14:1154-67, 2001.
38. Cherney D, Straus S. Management of patients with hypertensive urgencies and emergencies: a systematic review of the literature. J Gen Intern Med 17: 937-45, 2002.
39. Mansoor G, Frishman W. Comprehensive management of hypertensive emergencies and urgencies. Heart Disease 4:358-71, 2002.
40. Cardiovascular Steering Committee. Hypertension Diagnosis and Treatment. Bloomington, MN: Institute for Clinical Systems Improvement, January, 2002.
41. Hypertension in older people. A National Clinical Guideline. Scottish Intercollegiate Guidelines Network (SIGN), 2001. Available at: www.sign.ac.uk/guidelines/fulltext/49/index.html. Accessed May 24, 2005.
42. Watson R, Lumb R, Young M, et al. Variation in cuff blood pressure in untreated outpatients with mild hypertension: implications for initiating antihypertensive treatment. J Hypertens 5:207, 1987.
43. Perry H, Miller J. Difficulties in diagnosing hypertension: implications and alternatives. J Hypertens 10:887-96, 1992.
44. Pickering T. Recommendations for the use of home (self) and ambulatory blood pressure monitoring. Am J Hypertens 9:1-11, 1995.
45. Verdecchia P, Porcellati C, Schillaci G, et al. Ambulatory blood pressure. An independent predictor of prognosis in essential hypertension. Hypertension 24:793-801, 1994.
46. Feldman R, Campbell N, Larochelle P, et al. 1999 Canadian recommendations for the management of hypertension. CMAJ 161(Suppl 12):1-17, 1999.
47. The Hypertension Working Group. Diagnosis and Management of Hypertension in the Primary Care Setting. Washington, DC: Department of Veterans Affairs, May 1999.
48. Cavallini M, Roman M, Blank S, et al. Association of the auscultatory gap with vascular disease in hypertensive patients. Ann Intern Med 124:877, 1996.
49. Kaplan N, Rose B. Technique of blood pressure measurement in the diagnosis of hypertension. UpToDate Patient Information 13.1, December 20, 2004. Available at: patients.update.com.
50. Oster J, Masterson B. Pseudohypertension: a diagnostic dilemma. J Clin Hypertens 2(4):307-13, 1986.
51. Messerli F, Ventura H, Amodeo C. Osler's maneuver and pseudohypertension. N Engl J Med 312(24):1548-51, 1985.
52. Messerli F. Osler's maneuver, pseudohypertenion, and true hypertension in the elderly. Am J Med 80(5):906-10, 1986.
53. Prochazka A, Martel R. Osler's maneuver in outpatient veterans. J Clin Hypertens 3(4):554-8, 1987.
54. Hla K, Samsa G, Stoneking H, et al. Observer variability of Osler's maneuver in detection of pseudohypertension. J Clin Epidemiol 44(6):513-8, 1991.
55. Belmin J, Visintin J, Salvatore R, et al. Osler's maneuver: absence of usefulness for the detection of pseudohypertension in an elderly population. Am J Med 98(1):42-9, 1995.
56. Zuschke C, Pettyjohn F. Pseudohypertension. South Med J 88(12):1185-90, 1995.
57. National High Blood Pressure Education Program Working Group. National High Blood Pressure Education Program Working Group report on hypertension in the elderly. Hypertension 23:275-85, 1994.
58. World Health Organization. Hypertension Control. WHO technical report series. Geneva: WHO, 1996.
59. Yakovlevitch M, Black HR. Resistant hypertension in a tertiary care clinic. Arch Intern Med 151:1786, 1991.
60. Setaro JF, Black HR. Current concepts: refractory hypertension. N Engl J Med 327:543, 1992.
61. Berlowitz DR, Ash AS, Hickey EC, Friedman RH. Inadequate management of blood pressure in a hypertensive population. N Engl J Med 339:1957, 1998.
62. Bloom B. Continuation of initial antihypertensive medication after one year of therapy. Clin Ther 20:671-81, 1998.
63. Elliott W. Optimizing medication adherence in older persons with hypertension. Int Urol Nephrol 35:557-62, 2003.
64. Calhoun D, Oparil S. Treatment of hypertensive crises. N Engl J Med 323:1177-83, 1990.
65. Ramsay L, Williams B, Johnston G, et al. Guidelines for the management of hypertension: report of the Third Working Party of the British Hypertension Society. J Hum Hypertens 13:569-92, 1999.

66. Feldman R, Campbell N, Larochelle P, et al. 1999 Canadian recommendations for the management of hypertension. CMAJ 161(Suppl 12):1-17, 1999.

67. Houston M. Pathophysiology, clinical aspects, and treatment of hypertensive crises. Prog Cardiovasc Dis 2:99-48, 1989.

68. Chaudhry S, Krumholz H, Foody J. Systolic hypertension in older persons. JAMA 292(9):1074-80, 2004.

69. Fletcher A, Beevers D, Bulpitt C, et al. The relationship between a low treated blood pressure and IHD mortality: a report from the DHSS Hypertension Care Computing Project (DHCCP). J Hum Hypertens 2:11-5, 1988.

70. McCloskey L, Psaty B, Koepsell T, et al. Level of blood pressure and risk for myocardial infarction among treated hypertensive patients. Arch Intern Med 152:513-20, 1992.

71. Alderman M, Ooi W, Madhavan S, et al. Treatment-induced blood pressure reduction and the risk for myocardial infarction. JAMA 262:920-4, 1989.

72. Samuelsson O, Wilhelmsen L, Pennert K, et al. The J-shaped relationship between coronary heart disease and achieved blood pressure level in treated hypertension: further analyses of 12 years of follow-up of treated hypertensives in the Primary Prevention Trial in Gothenburg, Sweden. J Hypertens 8:547-55, 1990.

73. Cooper S, Hardy R, Labarthe D, et al. The relationship between degree of blood pressure reduction and mortality among hypertensives in the Hypertension Detection and Follow-Up Program. Am J Epidemiol 127: 387-403, 1988.

74. Staessen J, Bulpitt C, Clement D, et al. Relation between mortality and treated blood pressure in elderly patients with hypertension: report of the European Working Party on High Blood Pressure in the Elderly. BMJ 298:1552-6, 1989.

75. Hansson L. The BBB Study: the effect of intensified antihypertensive treatment on the level of blood pressure, side effects, mortality, and morbidity in "well treated" hypertensive patients. Behandla Blodtryck Battre. Blood Press 3(4):248-54, 1994.

76. Aromaa A. Blood pressure level, hypertension and five-year mortality in Finland. Acta Med Scand Suppl 646:43-50, 1981.

77. Lindholm L, Lanke J, Bengtsson B, et al. Both high and low blood pressures risk indicators of death in middle-aged males. Isotonic regression of blood pressure on age applied to data from a 13-year prospective study. Acta Med Scand 218(5):473-80, 1985.

78. Boutitie F, Gueyffier F, Pocock S, et al. J-shaped relationship between blood pressure and mortality in hypertensive patients: new insights from a meta-analysis of individual-patient data. Ann Intern Med 136:438-48, 2002.

79. Kumanyika K. Weight reduction and sodium restriction in the management of hypertension. Clin Geriatr Med 5:770, 1989.

80. Sander G. High blood pressure in the geriatric population: treatment considerations. Am J Geriatr Cardiol 11(4):223-32, 2002.

81. Whelton P, Appel L, Espeland M, et al. Sodium reduction and weight loss in the treatment of hypertension in older persons: a randomized controlled trial of non-pharmacologic interventions in the elderly (TONE). JAMA 279: 839-46, 1998.

82. Appel L, Moore T, Obarzanek E, et al. A clinical trial of the effects of dietary patterns on blood pressure: DASH Collaborative Research Groups. N Engl J Med 336:1117-24, 1997.

83. Labarthe D, Ayala C. Nondrug interventions in hypertension prevention and control. Cardiol Clin 20(2), 249-63, 2002.

84. Sacks F, Svetkey L, Vollmer W, et al. Effects on blood pressure of reduced dietary sodium and the dietary approaches to stop hypertension (DASH) diet. N Engl J Med 344:3-10, 2001.

85. Wing L, Reid C, Ryan P, et al. A comparison of outcomes with angiotensin-converting enzyme inhibitors and diuretics for hypertension in the elderly. N Engl J Med 348:583-92, 2003.

86. The ALLHAT Officers and Coordinators for the ALLHAT Collaborative Research Group: Major outcomes in high-risk hypertensive patients randomized to angiotensin-converting enzyme inhibitor or calcium channel blocker vs. diuretic. The Antihypertensive and Lipid-Lowering Treatment to Prevent Heart Attack Trial (ALLHAT). JAMA 288:2981-97, 2002.

87. Psaty B, Smith N, Siscovick D, et al. Health outcomes associated with antihypertensive therapies used as first-line agents. A systematic review and meta-analysis. JAMA 277:39-745, 1997.

88. Liu L, Wang J, Gong L, et al. Comparison of active treatment and placebo in older Chinese patients with isolated systolic hypertension. Systolic Hypertension in China (Syst-China) Collaborative Group. J Hypertens 16: 1823-9, 1998.

89. Dahlof B, Devereux R, Kieldsen S, et al. Cardiovascular morbidity and mortality in the Losartan Intervention for Endpoint reduction in hypertension study (LIFE): a randomized trial against atenolol. Lancet 359:995-1003, 2002.

90. Julius S, Kjeldsen S, Weber M, et al. Outcomes in hypertensive patients at high cardiovascular risk treated with regimens based on valsartan or amlodipine: the VALUE randomized trial. Lancet 363(9426):2022-31, 2004.

91. Teien DE, Wendel H, Bjornebrink J, et al. Evaluation of anatomical obstruction by Doppler echocardiogram and magnetic resonance imaging in patients with coarctation of the aorta. Br Heart J 69:352, 1993.

92. Peart S, Brennan P, Broughton P, et al. Medical Research Council trial of treatment of hypertension in older adults: principal results. BMJ 304:405-12, 1992.

93. Gong L, Zhange W, Zhu Y, et al. Shanghai trial of nifedipine in the elderly (STONE). J Hypertens 14:1237-45, 1996.

94. Hansson L, Lindholm L, Ekborn T, et al. Randomised trial of old and new antihypertensive drugs in elderly patients: cardiovascular mortality and morbidity the Swedish Trial in Old Patients with Hypertension-2 study. Lancet 354:1751-6, 1999.

95. Pepine C, Handberg E, Cooper-DeHoff R, et al. A calcium antagonist vs. a non-calcium antagonist hypertension treatment strategy for patients with coronary artery disease. JAMA 290:2805-16, 2003.

PRETEST ANSWERS

1. d
2. a
3. c
4. e
5. e
6. c

POSTTEST ANSWERS

1. b
2. c
3. e

Selected Clinical Problems of the Organ Systems

So we'll go no more a-roving
So late into the night,
Though the heart be still as loving,
And the moon be still as bright.

— GEORGE GORDON, LORD BYRON (1788–1824), *"So we'll go no more a-roving"*

Health is the primary duty of life

— OSCAR WILDE (1854–1900), *in The Importance of Being Earnest, Act One*

No gentleman ever takes exercise

— OSCAR WILDE (1854–1900), *in The Importance of Being Earnest, Act Two*

The wise, for cure, on exercise depend.
God never made his work for man to mend!

— JOHN DRYDEN (1631–1700)

Old people, on the whole, have fewer complaints than young; but those chronic diseases which do befall them generally never leave them

— HIPPOCRATES (c460–c357 BC), *in Aphorisms*

Sickness comes on horseback and departs on foot

— *Dutch proverb*

Mustn't grumble!

Universal response of old English ladies in the 60s and 70s, who had gone through the deprivations of the Second World War, to any doctor asking: "How are you?"

Is it not strange that desire should by so many years outlive performance?

— WILLIAM SHAKESPEARE (1564–1616), *in Henry IV*

The transformation of Dr Jekyll reads dangerously like an experiment out of "The Lancet".

— OSCAR WILDE (1854–1900), *in The Decay of Lying*

The older we grow, the greater become the ordeals

— JOHANN WOLFGANG VON GOETHE (1749–1832)

No skill or art is needed to grow old; the trick is to endure it.

— JOHANN WOLFGANG VON GOETHE (1749–1832)

I adore simple pleasures; they are the last refuge of the complex

— OSCAR WILDE (1854-1900), *in A Woman of No Importance*

I prefer to forget both pairs of glasses and pass my declining years saluting strange women and grandfather clocks.

— OGDEN NASH (1902–1971)

I smoke 10 to 15 cigars a day, at my age I have to hold on to something.

— GEORGE BURNS (1896–1996)

———

Coronary Artery Disease

Robert J. Luchi and Carlos A. Salazar

OBJECTIVES

Upon completion of this chapter, the reader will be able to:

- Appreciate the potential for the altered presentation of coronary artery disease (CAD) in older patients.

- Know and understand the main risk factors for CAD in older patients, and current strategies for risk factor reduction.

- Be up-to-date regarding assessment and treatment of the various clinical manifestations of CAD.

PRETEST

1. Important risk factors for CAD include all but which one of the following?
   a. Anemia
   b. Hypertension
   c. Diabetes mellitus
   d. Hyperlipidemia
   e. Age

2. The most common complications of acute myocardial infarction in the elderly include all but which one of the following?
   a. Atrial fibrillation
   b. External cardiac rupture
   c. Congestive heart failure
   d. Stroke
   e. Death

Ms. Watson, *Part 1*

Ms. Watson is an 80-year-old African-American woman who lives alone and is completely functional in activities of daily living (ADLs) and instrumental ADLs. She has the capacity to make decisions for herself. She always comes to your office accompanied by her daughter. You see her in your office now because of recent dyspnea and fatigue on walking to the bathroom of her home; this has occurred four times in the past week. The dyspnea is relieved by rest and is not accompanied by chest pain. Her medical history is positive for hypertension, diet-controlled type II diabetes mellitus, and degenerative joint disease of the knees and hip that is treated with acetaminophen. Her average blood pressure in your office has been in the range of 146/85. She has been fairly compliant with your treatment program of low-salt diet, triamterene-hydrochlorothiazide (37.5/25mg) daily, and amlodipine 5 mg/day.

Blood count, urinalysis, electrolytes, EKG, and CXR done 2 months ago in your office were normal. Physical examination shows the following: weight 10 lb over ideal weight; BP 150/82, pulse regular 52/minute, RR 16, no signs of CHF, an S4 gallop, good distal pulses, and good nutrition of the skin of the feet.

PREVALENCE AND IMPACT

CAD is so prevalent in older persons that it should be considered as a primary, contributing, or potentially complicating factor in many clinical scenarios encountered by primary care clinicians in their care of older patients.

A note about the evidence base in CAD: Caution should be exercised in interpreting the level of evidence for published articles regarding treatment, as well as guidelines published by various highly respected organizations. We recommend caution because very few (and sometimes no) older patients were included in the studies cited and guidelines often to not apply to older patients who have multiple interacting medical problems. We do not cite level of evidence for this reason. As always, the results of studies and guidelines offered should be noted, but their application to a specific older patient must be left to the clinician's judgment.

RISK FACTORS AND PATHOPHYSIOLOGY

Risk factors for CAD have been well defined[1,2] (Box 36–1). In older persons, the etiology of CAD is almost always atherosclerosis. Whether CAD produces angina pectoris, unstable angina pectoris, myocardial infarction or sudden death depends on the extent of the coronary obstruction by the following pathological features: atherosclerosis, propensity of the atherosclerotic plaque to incite platelet aggregation and clotting, and the degree to which the blood itself is prone to clot formation (hypercoagulable states).[3]

Box 36-1   Risk Factors for Coronary Artery Disease

Age

Gender (male/female disparity narrows with age)

Hypertension

Diabetes mellitus

Left ventricular hypertrophy on EKG

Hyperlipidemia

Smoking

Elevated homocysteine levels

Obesity

Metabolic syndrome

   Central obesity, blood pressure ≥130/85, insulin resistance, dyslipidemia (increased triglycerides, decreased HDL)

Sedentary lifestyle

Lipoprotein abnormalities without total cholesterol elevation

   Small dense LDL, increased lipoprotein a, increased postprandial VLDL and IDL

Note: Age is such a dominant risk factor that it alone, in the absence of other risk factors, should make one consider CAD. Atypical symptoms of angina pectoris are more common with increasing age. In cognitively impaired patients, anxiety or poorly described distress may be the presenting symptom.

Table 36-1   Presenting Symptoms of Angina Pectoris

	Classical	Atypical
Chest pain	Present	Absent
Pain radiating to jaw or arm	Often present	Absent
Sweating	Often present	Absent
Dyspnea	Often present	Often the only symptom
Fatigue	Often present	Often present; may be the only symptom
Symptoms related to exertion and relieved by rest	Present	Present

Note: It is important to do a multiple risk factor assessment using easily available programs. On the companion CD-ROM, see link to http://hin.nhlbi.nih.gov/atpiii/calculator.asp?usertype=pub. Programs such as these give an estimate of the risk of developing coronary artery disease based on Framingham data and offer guides to the physician for moderating or eliminating risk factors. We have also placed on the CD a table of the sensitivities and specificities of three types of echocardiographic stress testing (see Table "Sensitivity and Specificity of Exercise, Dobutamine and Dipyramidole Echocardiography").

DIFFERENTIAL DIAGNOSIS AND ASSESSMENT

Angina Pectoris

"Silent ischemia" in CAD is well described, but the clinical diagnosis of CAD requires an index symptom or symptoms. The index symptom of angina pectoris—as classically described—is chest pain. However, the older patient often does not have the chest pain typical of angina pectoris.[4] Commonly, it is dyspnea or fatigue—without chest pain—that is the index symptom of CAD in older patients, especially elderly patients with diabetes (Table 36–1).

The broader differential diagnosis of angina pectoris is outlined in Box 36–2. Initial tests when the clinical diagnosis is angina pectoris are listed in Box 36–3 along with notes on the rationale for ordering them.

Case Discussion

This patient has important risk factors for CAD: age, hypertension, and diabetes mellitus. Given this history of risk factors coupled with recent onset of exertional dyspnea on ordinary exertion, CAD must be considered as the most likely diagnosis. CHF is unlikely on the basis of physical examination, but you will get a CXR and order a BNP.

Underlying pulmonary disease as a cause of intermittent dyspnea is unlikely, and previous CXRs are normal. Pulmonary emboli may deserve consideration but are not your first concern in the overall setting. Anemia as a cause of dyspnea is unlikely, but you will do another blood count just to be sure.

Your first consideration should be CAD. One must rule out myocardial infarction (MI) because "silent" MIs are common in older persons with diabetes.

Box 36-2   Considerations in Differential Diagnosis of Chest Pain

- Ischemic cardiovascular disease
  Acute MI, unstable angina, and stable angina pectoris
- Nonischemic cardiovascular disease
  Dissecting or atherosclerotic aortic aneurysm, mitral valve prolapse, hypertrophic cardiomyopathy, pericarditis
- Gastrointestinal disorders
  Esophageal spasm, reflux, cholecystitis, peptic ulcer disease
- Musculoskeletal disorders
  Cervical disc disease, costochondritis, fibrositis
- Pulmonary diseases
  Pleuritis, pulmonary embolus, neoplasm, pulmonary hypertension
- Psychiatric
  Anxiety disorders and depression

Note: Dementia (often unrecognized) may prevent the patient from giving an accurate history.

Box 36-3 Studies to Consider in Patients Newly Diagnosed with Angina Pectoris

- To exclude associated acute myocardial infarction
  Troponin I
  Total CK and MBCK
- If dyspnea prominent symptom, to assess for CHF
  BNP
- If needed to exclude chest pain arising from GI tract
  Ultrasound of gallbladder
  Esophogram or UGD
- If statins are considered in treatment program
  LFTs
  CK
  Aldolase
- To confirm diagnosis and quantify risks of adverse CAD events
  CRP
  Exercise or pharmacologic stress test
  Coronary angiography

The patient's anginal equivalent (i.e., dyspnea) is not rapidly increasing nor severe and prolonged, excluding—on clinical grounds—unstable angina pectoris.

Ms. Watson, *Part 2*

She has stable vital signs and is in no distress now. She walks 100 ft in your office suite, which does not produce dyspnea or pain. There is no indication for hospitalization at this point.

Her new diagnosis is angina pectoris due to CAD. The prognosis is relatively good at the moment but guarded because patients with CAD may sustain unpredictable, sudden changes in the coronary circulation, leading to unstable angina, MI, or sudden death. You obtain permission from Ms. Watson to include her daughter in the discussion of diagnosis, prognosis, and treatment. You have previously determined that Ms. Watson has the capacity to make judgments for herself. You ask about treatment preferences. She wants to be resuscitated in case of a cardiac arrest but declines for the moment either stress testing or coronary angiography. In these circumstances, there is no immediate necessity for cardiac consultation.

CASE DISCUSSION

In addition to routine studies of blood and urine and a CXR, other tests are indicated. It is helpful—although not absolutely necessary—in this specific case to have the results back before the patient leaves your office. In other patients where there is more uncertainty about the diagnosis, you may want the laboratory tests back in 1 to 2 hours or have the patient sent to an emergency room. Blood count, urinalysis, and CXR are normal. The EKG is unchanged from previous tracings done in your office, showing RSR, LAD, and nonspecific ST-T changes in the lateral chest leads. Normal values for troponin I, CK, CRP, LFTs, and BNP are returned to your office in 2 hours. The homocysteine level will be sent to your office in the morning. You send the patient home having scheduled an RUQ ultrasound even though cholecystitis is not high on the list of differential diagnoses. Acute cholecystitis can rapidly lead to sepsis and death in diabetic patients. If stones were to be found in the gallbladder, you might consider cholcystectomy at some later time when Ms. Watson's cardiovascular status has been clarified. If the patient had not declined the possibility of stress testing, you would have ordered one. The techniques, sensitivities, and specificities of echocardiographic stress tests are on the CD-ROM.

Exercise. The patient should continue her usual activities to the extent that they do not produce dyspnea (or chest pain), but at this time, when information is still being obtained, a specific exercise program should not yet be prescribed.

Diet. The patient should be given an American Diabetes Association diet to slowly reduce her weight to ideal levels. The diet should also meet American Heart Association recommendations for total fat and cholesterol intake. You refer Ms. Watson and her daughter to a dietician.

Blood pressure meets Joint National Committee (JNC) criteria for hypertension stage 1 (see companion CD-ROM for link to JNC guidelines). You consider a beta blocker given the diagnosis of CAD, but her heart rate is 53/minute. You could increase the dose of amlodipine but the patient is diabetic. An ACE inhibitor added to or substituted for amlodipine is a better choice, since ACE inhibitors offer beneficial effects for the diabetic kidney and the heart compromised by CAD, in addition to reducing blood pressure.[5] *You add ramipril 2.5 mg daily and arrange for periodic checks on her electrolytes, BUN, and creatinine.*

Diabetes mellitus. *Weight loss and (eventually) exercise are good first steps. If the HbA$_1$C is not 6.0 or lower, an oral agent such as glipizide should be prescribed.*

Nitrates. *You should prescribe a long-acting nitrate (isosorbide mononitrate as Imdur 20 mg b.i.d) and nitroglycerin 0.4 mg sublingually after instructing the patient to sit or lie when taking the first several doses of nitroglycerin. You will have a visiting nurse monitor Ms. Watson's blood pressure and pulse at home to determine if this dose of isosorbide mononitrate causes postural or sustained hypotension.*

Statins. *Given the patient's diabetes, weight, and age, it is unlikely that her lipids will be too low to start a statin. Statins lower LDL, raise HDL, stabilize atherosclerotic plaques, and may even cause them to regress.*[6] *In addition, statins have a beneficial effect on endothelial function promoting coronary flow. You prescribe simvastatin 10 mg daily with the intent of going higher if necessary and if side effects permit.*

Aspirin. *Give 325 mg daily to help protect against untoward CV events in Ms. Watson such as heart attack and stroke. A smaller dose of ASA (100 mg/day) has been found to be effective in reducing risk of stroke, but not of adverse cardiovascular events in women.*[7]

You instruct the patient on what to do and whom to call if the pain is not controlled, and you arrange for an appointment in 1 week.

Ms. Watson, *Part 3*

She returns in 1 week. She has had only one mild episode of exertional dyspnea and it that was short-lived. She has no muscular aches or pain. She has been compliant with your suggestions with respect to diet and medications. Her BP is 138/76.

The results of the laboratory tests you ordered were as follows: BNP is 200 Pg/ml (5–100 Pg/ml); RUQ US is negative; total cholesterol is 200, LDL 111, and HDL 50 mg/dl; triglycerides 109 mg/dl; homocysteine 18 μmol/μ (5–15 μmol/l). Because of the elevated homocysteine level, you add 1 mg of folic acid to her regimen.

Ms. Watson, *Part 4*

Over the next year, Ms. Watson does well. Exertional dyspnea occurs on the average of once every 2 weeks, mostly with extended walking, but it is mild and short-lived. BP is 130/78. She fails to sustain a 5-lb weight loss. Hemoglobin A1C level is 5.8%. CPK and LFTs do not increase on the simvastatin. Electrolytes, BUN, and creatinine remain normal. Her lipid levels are total cholesterol 171, HDL 50, LDL 100 mg/dl, and triglycerides 72 mg/dl on simvastatin therapy. You consider further LDL reduction, but Ms. Watson does not tolerate higher doses of the simvastatin.[8]

Her daughter calls because her mother notices mild anterior chest discomfort while at rest and today her daughter noted that her mother was anxious, dyspneic, and diaphoretic for 15 minutes, and then recovered although she remains fatigued.

You are suspicious that these symptoms are the result of progression of her CAD—specifically that they represent unstable angina pectoris. Unstable angina is defined clinically by an increase in the frequency and/or severity of anginal symptoms on little or no exertion. Since unstable angina pectoris is a medical emergency, you advise the daughter to call 911. She elects to drive her mother to the emergency room where you will see her.

STUDY QUESTION

1. What tests should be ordered?

Diagnosis and Assessment of Unstable Angina

Unstable angina is a clinical diagnosis based on a significant change (instability) in the frequency or severity of the patient's angina. If the angina is new in onset, frequent, and precipitated by trivial exertion, one may also use this diagnosis. Unstable angina is a serious condition, frequently leading to death or MI if not promptly treated, and is almost always a reason to admit the patient to an intensive care unit.[9]

Changes in the pattern of angina may be caused by factors that increase the work of the heart such as hyperthyroidism, anemia, or high blood pressure. More frequently, unstable angina is due to a significant reduction in blood flow to the myocardium. Commonly, an existing atherosclerotic plaque will rupture, inducing thrombus formation in the artery, leading to a more critical obstruction of that artery.

The patient should be admitted to an ICU. Cardiology consultation is advisable. Laboratory studies include a CBC, basic metabolic panel, thyroid function studies, EKG, myocardial enzymes, and CXR. Treatment should always include aspirin, nitrates (given intravenously or orally), and beta-blocking drugs. After stabilization, an ACE inhibitor should be given to patients with diabetes mellitus. There is increasing body of opinion that in all patients with CAD, ACE inhibitors decrease the frequency of adverse cardiovascular events. Echocardiography and coronary arteriography are almost always indicated. Exercise stress testing is useful when the diagnosis of CAD is in doubt.

> ● Changes in the pattern of angina may be caused by factors that increase the work of the heart such as hyperthyroidism, anemia, or high blood pressure.

Ms. Watson, *Part 5*

You call the emergency department and order the following: troponin I, CK, MBCK, and an EKG, and ask for a cardiologist to see Ms. Watson in the ED with you. When Ms. Watson arrives in the ED her vital signs are BP 140/84, P 62, RR 20, and T 98.0. O_2 saturation is 99% on 2 liters nasal oxygen begun by the ED team. She is not symptomatic. Physical examination is unchanged as is the EKG. While waiting for the myocardial enzyme values to be returned, you order another 325-mg tablet of enteric-coated aspirin and an infusion of nitroglycerin 0.25 mg/kg/min, with instructions to reduce the infusion rate if the systolic blood pressure reaches 100 mmHg.

The cardiologist is delayed in responding to the consultation. You again ask for treatment preferences from Ms. Watson in the daughter's presence, having again established that Ms. Watson has the capacity to make medical decisions for herself. She still does not want a stress test or coronary angiography.

While the nitroglycerin drip is being started, Ms. Watson suddenly becomes pale, her heart rate increases from 62 to 96 while remaining regular, and her blood pressure is found to be 90/70. She is anxious, diaphoretic, and dyspneic. Inspiratory rales are now present at the bases of the lungs. The EKG now shows ST segment elevation in leads I, AVL, and V2-6.

Diagnosis and Assessment of Acute Myocardial Infarction

Unstable angina and MI are closely related. The distinction is that in the latter a significant portion of the myocardium dies. Thus, admission to an ICU and cardiac consultation are essential in most cases. Some patients may insist on home treatment of MI: home treatment of AMI is not optimal.

Diagnosis and assessment are carried out in large measure as for unstable angina. However, the clinician should exercise care in making the diagnosis of MI solely on the basis of a small and persistent elevation of troponin I (so-called "troponin leak").

> ● Unstable angina and MI are closely related; the distinction is that in the latter, a significant portion of the myocardium dies. Thus, admission to an ICU and cardiac consultation are essential in most cases.

Management of Angina Pectoris, Unstable Angina Pectoris, and Myocardial Infarction

Treatment of angina pectoris includes the prescription of exercises to increase skeletal muscle efficiency in using oxygen, slowing, stopping, or reversing atherosclerosis; medications to restore the balance between myocardial oxygen demand and supply; and medications that reduce cardiovascular morbidity and mortality in selected patients.

Cardiac oxygen demands should be reduced to the extent possible by treating elevated blood pressure and tachycardia, and reducing the patient's level of stress. Exercise, usually but not necessarily walking exercise, in a frequency and amount appropriate to the patient's cardiac and general health status, is recommended.

Unless there is a contraindication, aspirin (to prevent plaque-related thrombosis) is prescribed. Angina may be controlled with short- or long-acting nitrates alone or in combination, and beta-blocking drugs.

LDL cholesterol should be reduced to below 100mg/dl by diet alone or, more commonly, by diet and statins.

ACE inhibitors reduce cardiovascular morbidity and mortality in patients with CAD who have left ventricular dysfunction and those *without* left ventricular systolic dysfunction who have diabetes mellitus (HOPE trial). There is accumulating evidence that patients without either diabetes or left ventricular systolic dysfunction will also show reduction in death, MI, and stroke on ACE inhibitors.

The treatment plan for angina pectoris provides the basis for longer-term treatment of the other two clinical manifestations of coronary artery atherosclerotic disease. However, the initial treatment of unstable angina and acute MI poses different challenges for both the cardiologist and the primary care physician. In both conditions, time is of the essence: in unstable angina prompt treatment is essential to prevent myocardial infarction and death; in acute MI prompt treatment is essential to prevent death as well as limit infarct size.

The primary care physician has several responsibilities in the pre-hospital phase of each of these conditions: first, to educate the patient and family in the initial symptoms of each of these conditions and to ensure that they know how to contact the physician or an emergency medical service without delay; and second, to know the capabilities of the hospital(s) to which they may refer patients with unstable angina or MI.

The patient with unstable angina (UA) should be given an initial or an additional dose of aspirin and admitted to an ICU with cardiac consultation. Clopidogrel added to aspirin may have benefit but increases bleeding in patients who may require CABG. The decision to use clopidogrel (or glycoprotein IIb/IIIa antagonists) is best made after the patient's initial evaluation in hospital. Guidelines for in-hospital treatment are found at www.acc.org/ by clicking on "Clinical Statements/Guidelines."

Patients with acute myocardial infarction (AMI) at home should call an emergency medical service promptly. The patient should be taken by the emergency medical service to a hospital with the capability of performing angioplasty. If the patient cannot be admitted directly to a hospital with the capability of performing angioplasty, the patient should receive 1.5 M IU of streptokinase intravenously.

Ideal time goals for acute MI management:

- EMT on scene, 8 minutes
- If fibrinolysis, EMT to needle time, 30 minutes
- If angioplasty, EMT to balloon, 60 minutes

Contraindications to fibrinolysis and treatment guidelines for AMI are found at www.acc.org/ by clicking on "Clinical Statements/Guidelines."

Ms. Watson, *Part 6*

The diagnosis now is acute AMI with ST segment elevation. Ms. Watson is admitted to the cardiology care unit (CCU) under your care with the cardiologist as the primary consultant. She now will consider coronary angiography and whatever other therapy is indicated including thrombolytic therapy and percutaneous transluminal coronary angioplasty (PTCA), but still hesitates about accepting coronary artery bypass grafting. Ms. Watson is stabilized in the CCU, undergoes coronary angiography, and is found to have triple-vessel CAD. The proximal LAD has a critical stenosis, and a successful PTCA with stent placement is carried out. The patient leaves the hospital on a regimen of: 325 mg of enteric-coated aspirin, clopidogrel 75 mg/day, metoprolol 12.5/day (heart rate 50), simvastatin 10 mg/day, ramipril 2.5 mg/day, a low-salt AHA heart-healthy diet, 1 mg folic acid/day, and isosorbide mononitrate 30 mg/day.

The American College of Cardiology guidelines for treating acute MI with ST segment elevation in a patient such as Ms. Watson is not detailed here, but can be found by following this link located on the companion CD-ROM: www.acc.org/clinical/guidelines/stemi/Guideline1/index.htm#top.

ROLE OF PRIMARY CARE PHYSICIAN IN CARE OF PATIENT IN CCU

The primary care physician remains as the *advocate* for the patient and serves as an important *information link* between the care in the CCU and the patient and her family. The primary care physician: is the one who periodically assesses the patient for *capacity* to make medical decisions; continues to supervise *other aspects* of care, that is, other than those directly related to the AMI; recognizes the frequency with which CHF is caused in hospitalized elderly patients by vigorous IV fluid administration, and therefore *monitors IV* fluid orders of the cardiologist; is in the best position to recognize and treat *delirium*; assures that the patient is adequately *nourished*; and finally, when appropriate, *limits treatment* or transfers the patient to a palliative care unit.

Ms. Watson, *Part 7*

She is followed by you and the cardiologist and does well for the first 6 months. Her functional state gradually decreases, and you ask for a home health nurse to see her regularly. The home health visiting nurse is called by Ms. Watson's daughter because her mother wakes up one morning complaining of weakness, shortness of breath, and episodic sweating. The nurse advises them to take an aspirin 325 mg by mouth and call 911 so that she can be taken immediately to the ED for evaluation and treatment. However, Ms. Watson, who still has the capacity to make decisions, refuses to go to the hospital. The visiting nurse alerts you to the situation. You speak to both the patient and her daughter and confirm that Ms. Watson wishes to stay at home, even after you clearly explain the diagnostic possibilities and the risks of not going to the hospital. The nurse finds Ms. Watson to have mild chest pain, but no dyspnea or other clinical signs of congestive heart failure. She is lucid and fatigued, but firm in her decision to not go to the hospital. Blood pressure is 160/90 mmHg, HR 110, RR 22, and oxygen saturation 92%. Portable EKG shows ST elevation in leads II, III, and AVF.

STUDY QUESTIONS

1. What is the diagnosis now?
2. What will your orders be?

CASE DISCUSSION

The clinical picture corresponds to an acute inferior MI. If Ms. Watson had not declined the possibility of going to the emergency department, she would have been a suitable candidate to receive immediate reperfusion therapy with thrombolysis or percutaneous coronary intervention.

Ms. Watson, *Part 8*

You order oxygen 2 L by nasal cannula, and arrange for both formal and family caregivers to be with Ms. Watson 24 hours per day. Although you discuss the possibility of hospice care, Ms. Watson and her daughter wish to accept active treatment in the patient's home. You prescribe 1 to 2 mg morphine IM for pain control, and continue her beta blocker, aspirin, statin, and ACE inhibitor. Forty-eight hours after her acute MI, the charge nurse calls you to let you know that Ms. Watson's mental status has changed: she became transiently unresponsive and lost movement of the left arm and leg. Physical examination reveals an irregularly irregular heartbeat. Her daughter, to whom Ms. Watson had given durable power of attorney for health care decisions, now requests care for comfort only, and asks you to contact a hospice program.

STUDY QUESTIONS

1. What has happened?
2. How will this change the prognosis and care plan?

CASE DISCUSSION

Clearly Ms. Watson has developed a stroke that may be ischemic or embolic secondary to atrial fibrillation. Complications occur in roughly 0.1% of patients with acute MI, typically 2 to 7 days after the event. In the elderly, the most common complications are cardiac arrhythmias such as atrial fibrillation, congestive heart failure, stroke, and death. Ms. Watson is now no longer able to make decisions for herself. With hospice actively involved in Ms. Watson's care, you may elect to withdraw as the physician of record in favor of the hospice physician, or you may wish to maintain your role as physician of record and work collaboratively with the hospice physician and the hospice team.

Ms. Watson, *Part 9*

Ms. Watson is enrolled in home hospice care and dies peacefully at home in the presence of her daughter.

SUMMARY

Significant CAD, often subclinical but nonetheless pathological, is so common in the elderly that CAD must be considered as a primary, contributing, or possibly complicating factor in most clinical situations. Risk factors are dominated by age, but important contributing risk factors are diabetes, hypertension, and hyperlipidemia, while other factors play important but lesser roles. The primary care clinician plays a vital role in the early diagnosis of CAD, and therefore must be aware of the frequently atypical presentation of this common disorder in older persons. The primary care clinician and a team including nurse, nurse practitioner, dietician, physical therapist, cardiologist, cardiac surgeon, and social worker play important roles throughout all phases of treatment (including the CCU and SICU, and palliative and hospice care when appropriate). To play these roles effectively, the primary care clinician must know the capacity of the patient to make decisions and needs to express the patient's wishes to the other clinicians. If the patient lacks capacity to make decisions, the primary care clinician must if possible find the person to whom the capacity has been delegated.

POSTTEST

1. Lifestyle modifications useful in the treatment of CAD include all of the following *except*:
   a. Aerobic exercise
   b. Isometric exercise
   c. Reduction of stress
   d. Smoking cessation
   e. AHA heart-healthy diet

2. Sublingual nitroglycerin differs from isosorbide mononitrate given orally in which one of the following ways?
   a. Mechanism of relief of angina
   b. Effect on heart rate
   c. Duration of action
   d. Effect on postural blood pressure

3. Unstable angina differs from stable angina in having which one of the following features?
   a. More numerous atherosclerotic plaque
   b. Atherosclerotic plaque located more proximally in the coronary arteries
   c. Greater association with an elevated platelet count
   d. Greater frequency and severity of anginal attacks
   e. More common in the elderly female than the elderly male

References

1. Levy D. 50 Years of Discovery: Medical Milestones from the National Heart, Lung, and Blood Institute's Framingham Heart Study. Totowa, NJ: Humana Press, 2001.
2. Kannel WB. The Framingham Study: historical insight on the impact of cardiovascular risk factors in men versus women. J Gend Specif Med 5:27-37, 2002.
3. Fuster V, Topol EJ, and Nabel EG. Atherothrombosis and Coronary Artery Disease. 2nd ed. Philadelphia: Lippincott, 2005.
4. Tresch DD, Alla HR. Diagnosis and management of myocardial ischemia (angina) in the elderly patient. Am J Geriatr Cardiol 10:337-44, 2001.
5. Pitt B. The anti-ischemic potential of angiotensin-converting enzyme inhibition: insights from the heart outcomes prevention evaluation trial. Clin Cardiol 23(Suppl 4):9-14, 2000.
6. La Rosa JC, He J, Vupputuri S. Effect of statins on risk of coronary disease: a meta-analysis of randomized controlled trials. JAMA 282(24): 2340-6, 1999.
7. Ridker PM, Cook NR, Lee IM,, et al. A randomized trial of low-dose aspirin in the primary prevention of cardiovascular disease in women. N Engl J Med 352:1293-304, 2005.
8. La Rosa JC, et al. Intensive lipid lowering with atorvastatin in patients with stable coronary disease. N Engl J Med 352:1425-35, 2005.
9. Metules T, Bauer J. Unstable angina: is your care up to snuff? RN 68(2): 22-27, 2005.

Web Resources

American College of Cardiology guidelines for care of AMI: www.acc.org/clinical/guidelines/stemi/Guideline1/index.htm#top.

American Heart Association, Get with the Guidelines: www.americanheart.org/presenter.jhtml/identifier=3013965.

National Cholesterol Education Program: www.nhlbi.nih.gov/about/ncep/.

National High Blood Pressure Educational Guidelines, Seventh Report of the Joint National Committee: www.nhlbi.nih.gov/guidelines/hypertension/.

American Heart Association: www.americanheart.org/presenter.jhtml?identifier=1200000.

National Cholesterol Education Program: hin.nhlbi.nih.gov/atpiii/calculator.asp/usertype=prof.

Framingham Risk Score: www.nhlbi.nih.gov/about/framingham/riskabs.htm.

PRETEST ANSWERS

1. a.
2. b.
1. Answer a. The Framingham study clearly identifies hypertension, diabetes mellitus, age, and hyperlipidemia as risk factors for CAD but not anemia. Anemia can cause stress to the cardiovascular system and thereby may *provoke* angina, but per se, is not a risk factor for CAD.
2. Answer b. As noted in the text, while all are complications of acute MI, external cardiac rupture is not as common in the elderly as in younger people.

POSTTEST ANSWERS

1. b.
2. c.
3. d.
1. Answer b. While any type of exercise can help in reducing weight, it is aerobic exercise—not isometric exercise—that helps peripheral and muscle circulation respond to a given level of activity with less energy demand on the heart.
2. Answer c. Isosorbide mononitrate is a long-acting nitrate in contrast to sublingual nitroglycerin. Its effect on postural blood pressure, heart rate, and the mechanism by which it relieves angina pectoris are similar to those of nitroglycerin.
3. Answer d. Unstable angina is defined by acceleration in the frequency or worsening of the intensity of anginal pain. Otherwise, its pathophysiology and frequency in older men are roughly the same as in older women. The major reason that stable angina becomes unstable is that one or more atherosclerotic plaques show signs of rupture, platelet aggregation, and clot formation.

Congestive Heart Failure

Robert J. Luchi and George E. Taffet

OBJECTIVES

Upon completion of this chapter, the reader will be able to:

● Understand how the clinical features of congestive heart failure (CHF) are altered in the older patient and how brain natriuretic peptide (BNP) levels may aid in making the diagnosis of CHF.

● Appreciate that CHF may be caused by systolic dysfunction or diastolic dysfunction of the heart.

● Understand the important role of angiotensin-converting enzyme (ACE) inhibitors in the prevention and treatment of CHF associated with left ventricular systolic dysfunction.

● List and justify the important additional roles of angiotensin receptor blocker (ARBs) drugs, beta-receptor blocker drugs, spironolactone, nesiritide, and biventricular pacing in the treatment of CHF associated with left ventricular systolic dysfunction.

● Implement treatment strategies for treatment of CHF associated with normal left ventricular systolic function.

PRETEST

1. Atypical manifestations of congestive heart failure in the elderly are most frequently related to reduced perfusion of which of the following?
   a. Brain
   b. Heart
   c. Extremities
   d. Kidneys
   e. Lungs

2. In patients with congestive heart failure, the best indicator of left ventricular systolic function is
   a. Left ventricular ejection fraction
   b. Electrocardiogram
   c. Chest X-ray examination (CXR)
   d. Distended jugular veins
   e. Atrial fibrillation

3. In patients with congestive heart failure, ACE inhibitors are contraindicated when which one of the following is present?
   a. Creatinine clearance 45 ml/min
   b. Blood urea nitrogen (BUN) 32 mg/dl
   c. Blood pressure 105/60 mm Hg
   d. Serum potassium 5 mEq/l
   e. History of ACE inhibitor–induced angioedema

Betty Postle *(Part I)*

Mrs. Postle is an 83-year-old white woman who is new to you, brought in by an out-of-town daughter, who notes her mother's decreasing ability to take care of herself. Mr. Postle is now dyspneic with minimal exertion. Her caregiver had a recent motor vehicle accident, and both Mrs. Postle and her daughter are unclear about Mrs. Postle's medication regimen. On examination, her heart rate is 100 and blood pressure is 89/43 mm Hg. She has rales bilaterally extending halfway up the lung fields, jugular venous distention (JVD), and pedal edema. A II/VI pansystolic murmur is appreciated over her entire precordium with both an S3 and S4 gallop sounds. Chest X-ray (CXR) reveals cardiac enlargement, pulmonary venous vascular congestion (enlarged hila that appear indistinct because of perivascular edema), and increased prominence of the pulmonary veins draining the upper lobes (cephalization of flow). Hemoglobin is 13 g, white blood cell count is normal, and urinalysis shows 1+ protein without active sediment. Blood urea nitrogen (BUN) and creatinine are 30 mg/dl and 1.6 mg/dl, respectively. Serum albumin is 3.6 g/dl.

STUDY QUESTIONS

1. What is the significance of the S3? What about an S4?
2. What is the significance of the pedal edema?
3. How should treatment be initiated?
4. What further tests will guide optimal treatment? Why?
5. What factors precipitating congestive heart failure (CHF) should be ruled out?

RISK FACTORS AND PATHOPHYSIOLOGY

Asymptomatic left ventricular systolic dysfunction (ALVSD) frequently progresses to CHF. This progression can be retarded by angiotensin-converting enzyme (ACE) inhibitors.[1] ASLVD is a function of age. In community-based studies, almost all the young people with left ventricle systolic dysfunction (left ventricular ejection fraction [LVEF] greater than 30) are asymptomatic; in men over 65, half were asymptomatic, and in older women, only 27% were asymptomatic.[2] This may be because the symptoms of CHF are manifestations of compensatory mechanisms used to maintain cardiac output. Data for ages above 75 are not available.

Left ventricular systolic dysfunction causes CHF in the elderly patient in 50% to 60% of cases. In the remainder, LVEF is normal but evidence of impaired ventricular filling is present.[3] If significant valvular or pericardial disease is absent, CHF is then attributed to *diastolic dysfunction*. Normal LVEF, determined by echocardiography or nuclear techniques, is generally 50% or more. Significant left ventricular systolic dysfunction is defined as an LVEF less than 40%. There is no simple measure of diastolic function. CHF due to diastolic dysfunction may be so common in the elderly because aging itself results in a stiff, poorly relaxing left ventricle. Disease processes add to these aging effects.

CHF, a more advanced stage of *heart failure* (strictly defined as impairment in heart function leading to symptoms such as fatigue and dyspnea because of inadequate cardiac output), is defined as the presence of evidence of fluid retention manifested clinically by edema and congestion of the veins of the pulmonary and systemic circuits.

CHF is the most common reason for hospitalization in Medicare patients. Prevalence is typically between 10% and 20% in elderly cohorts. The incidence increases 10-fold from age 45 to age 85.[4] Five-year survival is less than 50% in both systolic and diastolic CHF.[5]

DIFFERENTIAL DIAGNOSIS AND ASSESSMENT

Diagnosis

Classically, the diagnosis of CHF is based on history, physical examination, and CXR.[6] Brain natriuretic peptide (BNP) testing has altered this approach. Diagnosis of CHF in the elderly may be difficult because the *history* is often atypical (Table 37-1), or unobtainable, or because the symptoms are minimized by the patient or attributed to age. One of the most common atypical

● BNP has revolutionized CHF diagnosis.

Table 37–1	Classic and Atypical Manifestations of Congestive Heart Failure in the Elderly	
Classic (Noncerebral)	**Atypical**	**Atypical (Cerebral)**
Dyspnea	Chronic cough	No history
Orthopnea	Insomnia	Falls
Paroxysmal nocturnal dyspnea	Weight loss	Anorexia
Peripheral edema	Nausea	Behavioral disturbances
Unexplained weight gain	Nocturia	Decreased functional status
Weakness	Syncope	
Poor exercise tolerance		
Abdominal pain		
Fatigue		

presentations is that of delirium, which is frequently superimposed on preexisting dementia.

Physical signs of CHF are often overlooked. JVD and hepatojugular reflux are excellent signs of "right-sided failure." S_3 gallop remains reliable but is often difficult to hear. In contrast, the S_4 is a common finding in otherwise healthy older patients. Crackles or rales on lung auscultation are nonspecific. Ankle edema may merely reflect inactivity or associated dependency of the legs.

A good-quality *CXR* may be difficult to obtain, especially in frail, older patients. Persistence until an adequate film is obtained pays rich diagnostic dividends. Consider performing the CXR examination with the patient sitting upright in the wheelchair. Key findings are an enlarged heart, enlarged hila with indistinct margins (perivascular edema), and prominent veins draining the upper lobes (cephalization of flow).

The measurement of *BNP* has revolutionized the diagnosis of CHF. BNP is specific to the ventricles, reflects stretch or tension of the left ventricle, and correlates well with the severity of CHF. BNP is elevated in both systolic and diastolic CHF. Patients presenting with dyspnea and normal BNP are unlikely to have CHF as the cause of their symptoms. BNP levels decrease as CHF patients improve, so monitoring BNP may be helpful. Healthy women have higher levels than do men, and BNP increases with age; thresholds used to discriminate normal from CHF may need age and sex adjustment. In addition, BNP is cleared by the kidneys, so renal function influences BNP. Various parts of the peptide have been assayed, but all appear to provide similar information.[7] BNP has beneficial effects: natriuresis, diuresis, vasodilation, and antagonism of endothelin, aldosterone, and renin. Nesiritide (recombinant human BNP) produces these effects when infused in decompensated patients despite their preexisting BNP elevations. Nesiritide may be less arrhythmogenic than is dobutamine, but experience in elderly patients is limited. BNP, for diagnosis and monitoring, is valuable in the elderly, whereas the use of nesiritide is still being defined.[7]

Precipitating Factors

Conditions increasing cardiovascular demand or interfering with compensatory mechanisms can precipitate CHF in otherwise compensated patients (Box 37-1). Frequent precipitating factors form the mnemonic DAMN IT:

*D*rugs—including withdrawal of ACE inhibitors, digitalis, or β-adrenergic antagonists, and the administration of steroids or nonsteroidal anti-inflammatory drugs (NSAIDs)

*A*rrhythmias—bradyarrhythmias, including heart block and tachyarrhythmias, especially atrial fibrillation

*M*yocardial ischemia—often presenting atypically (consider stress testing if suspicion is high)

*N*oncompliance—such as with diet, fluid restriction, or medications

*I*ntravenous fluid administration

Hyper*t*hyroidism (thyroid-stimulating hormone and free T$_4$ should be considered) (Box 37-2).

Pharmacological stress testing can be used if exercise testing is not obtainable. Once precipitants are treated, the ongoing CHF regimen may need to be modified.

> ● CHF precipitants: DAMN IT! Drugs, Arrhythmia, MI, Noncompliance, IV, Thyroid.

Box 37-1   Factors that Precipitate CHF

Anemia

Arrhythmias

Exacerbation of chronic obstructive pulmonary disease

Digoxin withdrawal

Drugs: cardiac depressants (e.g., antiarrhythmics, antineoplastics)

Hypoxia

Hyperthyroidism

Intravenous fluid overloads[a]

Infection

Myocardial infarction/ischemics

Dietary or medication noncompliance[b]

Pulmonary embolism

Renal insufficiency

Sepsis

[a]Most common precipitating cause in hospitalized patients.

[b]Most common precipitating cause outside hospital.

Box 37-2   Mnemonic of Frequent Precipitating Factors of Congest Heart Failure

Drugs

Withdrawal of angiotensin-converting enzyme inhibitors, digoxin, or β-adrenergic antagonists

Administration of steroids and nonsteroidal anti-inflammatory drugs

Arrhythmias

Bradyarrhythmias, including heart block

Tachyarrhythmias, especially atrial fibrillation

Myocardial ischemia

Often presents atypically; consider stress testing

Noncompliance

With diet, fluid restriction, or medications

Intravenous fluids

Thyroid: hyperthyroidism

Once the precipitants are treated, review the ongoing congestive heart failure regimen; it may need modification.

Betty Postle *(Part II)*

You find she has a long history of CHF due to coronary artery disease and hypertension. Current medications include an ACE inhibitor, furosemide, digoxin, spironolactone, low-dose beta-blocker, and nitrates. Her electrocardiogram (ECG) reveals sinus tachycardia and prolonged QRS duration. Her BNP is 3030 pg/ml. You control symptoms initially by prescribing a low-sodium diet and increasing her furosemide. As the edema clears, her "dry" weight is 105 pounds. The LVEF is 20%, confirming that CHF is caused by systolic dysfunction. You increase her ACE inhibitor, ramipril, to 2.5 mg twice a day.

STUDY QUESTIONS

1. Why should ACE inhibitors be used in this case?
2. What other medications or considerations should be made at this time?

TREATMENT

General measures include sodium restriction and appropriate exercise after acute symptoms have been controlled. Patient education and support groups help promote compliance. Prognosis should be discussed openly and completion of advanced directives regarding health care preferences encouraged.

Dietary *sodium intake* should be restricted to 3 g or less per day. The person preparing the patient's food should be instructed by a dietitian. Reduction in *alcohol* intake is recommended, and *smoking* is discouraged. Mild *aerobic exercise*, mainly walking or cycling, increases functional capacity and quality of life.

Repetition of the therapeutic program essentials is necessary for success. Information needs to be given concerning diet, drugs, prognosis, and safe level of activity.[5] This information is best given over several office visits.

There is little randomized clinical trial data directly relevant to very old patients. Extrapolation should be performed cautiously. Because each decision is a risk-benefit analysis, and the impact and likelihood of risks depend on the individual, it seems reasonable to take advantage of published data, but an actual evidence base upon which to make treatment decisions is not available.[8] The risk of medication use in the elderly is complicated by altered pharmacokinetics and by pharmacodynamics resulting from age- and disease-related changes in various organ systems.[6] The goals of treatment are increased quality of life and improved survival.

Loop diuretics (furosemide, bumetanide, torsemide, indapamide, ethacrynic acid) are used most frequently because glomerular filtration rate in the elderly is often less than 30 ml/min, rendering thiazides ineffective. The goal is gentle diuresis, avoiding hypotension and its consequences. Equivalent doses of loop diuretics are furosemide 40 mg, bumetanide 1 mg, and ethacrynic acid 50 mg. Whether given orally or intravenously, the first dose should be small because of the danger of an exaggerated "first dose diuresis." Usual maintenance dose is 20 to 40 mg furosemide daily, but 160 mg per day is not unusual. Bumetanide has a shorter duration of action. Ethacrynic acid is rarely used because of ototoxicity, but it is of use in patients allergic to furosemide and bumetanide. Major toxic effects include hypotension, hypokalemia, hyponatremia, and hypomagnesemia. Hypotension can be avoided by orthostatic blood pressure and BUN/creatinine monitoring and reduction of the diuretic dose at the first sign of volume depletion. Removing the last trace of peripheral edema or pleural effusion may decrease preload to the point at which cardiac output decreases. Serum magnesium and potassium should be measured routinely and replaced as indicated. The treatment of hyponatremia depends on the cause: sodium depletion from excessive diuresis calls for reduction in diuretic dose and lessening of sodium restriction;

hyponatremia secondary to relative retention of free water is treated by fluid restriction. Diuretic-related incontinence can be avoided by timing of diuretics or giving bumetanide. Other drugs with hypotensive effects can produce serious interactions. NSAIDs can completely inhibit the diuresis by their action on glomerular filtration rate. Potassium-sparing diuretics are useful, in combination with loop diuretics, to reduce potassium loss. Their major side effect is hyperkalemia, which can be additive to the hyperkalemia of ACE inhibitors (see below). When the patient is resistant to loop diuretics, metolazone may be added. A 2.5 mg test dose of metolazone is recommended to avoid profound volume depletion. Subsequently, 5 mg is given 1 hour by mouth before the loop diuretic.

ACE inhibitors improve survival and quality of life in patients with CHF with reduced LVEF. Side effects include hypotension, often precipitated by concurrent use of diuretics. ACE inhibitors should not be given to patients with volume depletion. It may be best to begin the inhibitors after the patient enters a stable state, after diuresis. Doses of ACE inhibitors should be started low and progressively raised while the physician monitors the patient closely. ACE inhibitors are frequently underprescribed, and reaping the benefits requires reaching target doses or at least the maximally tolerated dose.[9] Hyperkalemia and mild to severe angioedema occur, and cough is a symptom of mild airway edema. This may be a bradykinin effect because ACE inhibitors also inhibit kininase II, which breaks down bradykinin.[9] Other ACE inhibitor effects may also be bradykinin mediated.

● **ACE inhibitors: Don't underdose!**

Case Discussion

The calculated creatinine clearance for Mrs. Postle is below 40 ml/min. Because ramipril and the active metabolite ramiprilat are excreted in urine, correction for renal function is necessary. Therefore, the starting dose should be 1.25 mg twice a day, gradually increasing over time. Her renal function does not contraindicate a trial of ACE inhibitors, but electrolytes, BUN, and creatinine should be monitored regularly.

Aldosterone antagonists are used because the end result of activation of the renin-angiotensin system is aldosterone production by the adrenals. Aldosterone is a potent sodium- and water-retaining steroid with additional actions that are deleterious to the heart and blood vessels. Spironolactone and eplerenone are aldosterone antagonists with utility in moderate or severe CHF.[10] Spironolactone added to an ACE inhibitor improved functional status, reduced total death rate and death from cardiovascular causes, and reduced CHF hospitalizations. Although mean age was only 65 and just one-fourth were women, in older (age greater than 67) or female subgroups, spironolactone was still effective.

ACE inhibitors should eliminate aldosterone production, but they do not. The dose of ACE inhibitor may be insufficient or aldosterone can escape regulation with sustained ACE inhibitor treatment, so aldosterone production takes place in the absence of angiotensin II. Spironolactone also allows loop diuretic doses and potassium to be decreased. In the Randomized Aldactone Evaluation Study (RALES), hyperkalemia in patients treated with spironolactone was infrequent; subsequently, in "real world" application, it produced frequent life-threatening hyperkalemia. In older patients, especially those with renal impairment or diabetes, aggressive monitoring of potassium and careful patient selection is advised.

Digoxin's role has changed from a first-line drug in CHF treatment when a regular sinus rhythm is present to a second-line drug. Digoxin may improve quality of life and reduce hospitalizations in patients getting diuretics and ACE inhibitors. The dose of digoxin must be reduced when renal function is impaired, and the dose should be further reduced if renal functional impairment increases. Only serum digoxin levels obtained 12 to 24 hours after the dose are useful to evaluate if the dose of digoxin is acceptable.

Beta-blockers have beneficial effects on survival for patients with a history of myocardial infarction that may be additive to the effects of ACE inhibitors. Beta-receptor blocking agents also improve function, improve survival, and reduce hospitalizations for systolic CHF patients. Metoprolol or atenolol are the drugs commonly used. Carvedilol, which blocks both β- and α-adrenergic receptors, reduces rates of hospitalization and improves survival for patients with mild to moderate heart failure secondary to ischemic heart disease.[11] Carvedilol is known to reach 50% higher concentrations in the elderly.[11] Nebivolol, a β-adrenergic antagonist with nitric oxide–mediating effects, had modest efficacy in the Study of the Effects of Nebivolol Intervention on Outcomes and Rehospitalization in Seniors with Heart Failure (SENIORS), one of the few studies to feature typical elderly patients. Presently these investigators begin beta-receptor blocking therapy with metoprolol and reserve carvedilol (as a substitute for metoprolol) for those situations in which symptoms worsen in the face of maximal treatment. With all the beta-receptor antagonists, it may take 2 or 3 months of therapy before clinical benefit is noticeable.[9]

● Beta blockers help function and survival in CHF.

Betty Postle (*Part III*)

Mrs. Postle does well on a therapeutic program now including metoprolol 12.5 mg twice a day and digoxin 0.125 mg daily. Fourteen days after initiating this daily loading dose of digoxin, her serum digoxin level is 1.6 ng/ml and serum potassium is 3.7 mEq/l. She complains of a cough without sputum production. You discuss the possibility that cough may result from treatment with ACE inhibitors, but Mrs. Postle states that the cough is not that annoying and wishes to continue the ACE inhibitor. Two weeks later she calls to complain that the cough has become quite bothersome and asks if something can be done about it. Physical examination and CXR are negative.

STUDY QUESTIONS

1. What can be done about the cough without significantly impairing the therapeutic program?
2. What additional measures are indicated now to complete the therapeutic program and patient instruction?

Angiotensin II Receptor Blocking Drugs (ARBs) do not exhibit all of the actions of an ACE inhibitor (e.g. they do not inhibit kininase II), but they do improve the outcome in systolic CHF. In clinical trials, patients taking ARBs have much less cough; however, angioedema, although rare, may occur.[12] Those who develop angioedema on an ACE inhibitor are more likely (up to 10%) to develop angioedema with an ARB than is the general population.[13] ARBs share other side effects of ACE inhibitors, such as hyperkalemia, hypotension, and renal dysfunction, but in general ARBs are tolerated well. In African Americans the use of hydralazine and long-acting nitrates is clearly of benefit in study populations.

Betty Postle (*Part IV*)

You discontinue ramipril and substitute losartan 25 mg daily. She no longer has a cough. Her CHF remains controlled. You refer Mrs. Postle to a dietitian for counseling about a low-sodium diet. You add aspirin 81 mg and a statin for additional prophylaxis against ischemic cardiac or cerebral events. You prescribe a walking program of gradually increasing distance and time, with the exercise intensity not to produce dyspnea (patient unable to complete a sentence while exercising) or a heart rate greater than 100 beats per minute, and consider a referral to the invasive cardiologist and to a home health agency.

Biventricular pacing or cardiac resynchronization therapy (CRT) is a relatively new intervention for patients with systolic CHF and heterogeneity in the timing of cardiac activation: such patients may have wide QRS on ECG, or dyssynchrony on echocardiography or nuclear study. Conceptually, one can imagine a large left ventricle, activated in an uncoordinated fashion so that blood just sloshes around the ventricle instead of being ejected by a well-timed, homogeneously activated ventricle. CRT electrodes are placed in the right ventricular apex and in the coronary sinus. The delay between impulses is manipulated to optimally activate the ventricle to contract in a more coordinated fashion.

Some patients derive significant benefit from CRT, whereas 25% do not respond. Criteria for choosing between those likely to benefit and the nonresponders are still being defined. In addition to short-term benefit, CRT may remodel and improve the heart in the long term. Older patients, especially women, are underrepresented in published studies so data for decision making are inadequate. Nevertheless, for patients with dilated ventricles and dyssynchrony, CRT may be discussed (if only to be discounted).

Automatic Implantable Cardiac Defibrillators (AICDs) recognize arrhythmias and electrically terminate them. Sudden death is a very common cause of mortality in patients with heart failure. As the experience with anti-arrhythmic drugs was so discouraging, the research focus turned towards AICDs. A 25% decrease in mortality for CHF patients can be realized with AICDs. This benefit was similar in the oldest subgroup (those over 70). Perhaps the optimum in the very select subgroup in whom one should consider these expensive options would be the combined CRT-AICD device if there is dyssynchrony or the AICD alone if there is not. AICDs and CRTs will provide end-of-life challenges; these should be addressed beforehand, rather than in crisis.

Home care–based multidisciplinary efforts are effective in keeping patients out of the hospital and improving their quality of life.[14] Nurses, therapists, and pharmacists contribute to a team effort, supporting the patient in their regimen. Adjustments of diuretics or other medications can be made on a daily basis according to protocols.

Gladys Alden (Part I)

Mrs. Alden, a 73-year-old white woman, has mild hypertension, a myocardial infarction 1 year ago, and diabetes mellitus controlled with oral hypoglycemic agents. She presents with shortness of breath, nocturnal cough, and lower-extremity edema. Vital signs include blood pressure 150/80 mm Hg, pulse 92 and regular, resting rate 26,

and temperature 97°F. She has peripheral edema, JVD, positive hepatojugular reflux, bilateral basilar rales, S4, and a 2/6 systolic ejection murmur heard best at the base of the heart. ECG shows a regular sinus rhythm with evidence of an old anterior myocardial infarction.

You control symptoms of heart failure initially by means of a low-sodium diet and furosemide 40 mg daily. Potassium chloride mEq/day is added to counteract diuretic-related hypokalemia. As her edema clears, her "dry" weight is 105 pounds. You order an echocardiogram to determine if the CHF is due predominately to systolic dysfunction or diastolic dysfunction. The LVEF is 67% without evidence of pericardial or valvular disease, confirming that the CHF is primarily caused by diastolic dysfunction.

STUDY QUESTIONS

1. What factors in the history and examination would allow you to discriminate between CHF due to systolic dysfunction versus diastolic dysfunction?
2. What is her prognosis compared to a similar patient with systolic heart failure?

Diastolic Heart Failure

This is the more frequent type of heart failure in the elderly, in which cardiac contraction is maintained but filling is impaired. This may happen because of problems in active relaxation, passive stiffness of the ventricle, dyssynchrony of relaxation, or possibly coupling between the arterial tree and the ventricle. Thus, diastolic heart failure is probably just as heterogeneous as is systolic heart failure; some of the more promising interventions are directed outside the heart.[15]

The clinical signs and symptoms are, for the most part, identical to those of systolic CHF, and no historical features are unique to one or the other. For example, in our experience with older male veterans, past myocardial infarctions were equally common in both groups.[16] BNP levels may be lower for patients with diastolic CHF, although still clearly elevated.[17]

The mortality of diastolic CHF in the elderly is very high, almost as high as systolic CHF, and these outcomes are converging as advances are made in the management of systolic CHF while little progress is made in diastolic heart failure management. Also, in many older patients with systolic CHF, there is a significant component of diastolic dysfunction; interventions focused at diastolic CHF may thus help most such patients.

● Diastolic HF: As common as systolic HF in elderly.

Treatment of Diastolic CHF

The first line of treatment is decreasing the pulmonary congestion and venous pressures with diuretics. Because of the dependence of cardiac output on filling pressure, aggressive diuresis is very likely to result in hypotension or prerenal azotemia. Obviously, if myocardial ischemia is present, this should be addressed promptly; if hypertension is present, reducing afterload may improve cardiac function. Tachycardia will worsen or precipitate diastolic CHF because diastole (the time for ventricular filling) is disproportionately shortened. Reducing heart rate permits increased time for filling. If atrial fibrillation is present, then calcium channel antagonists or β-adrenergic antagonists may be used.

A few small, short-term studies of patients with diastolic CHF due to hypertension, ischemic disease, or both suggest calcium-channel blockers, ACE inhibitors, or angiotensin receptor blockers can improve exercise capacity modestly,[17] but overall the published data to direct management are very limited.

Gladys Alden (Part II)

You add an ACE inhibitor, ramipril, in a dose of 1.25 mg twice daily. No hypotension is noted at this dose. The dose of ramipril is then progressively increased to 2.5 mg twice a day. ACE inhibitors are also indicated in this diabetic patient as she has microalbuminuria. Mrs. Alden does well on a regimen including metoprolol 12.5 mg twice a day. Fourteen days later, her BUN is up to 62 and serum potassium is 5.7 mEq/l. She complains of weakness and lightheadedness when standing up. On physical examination, she has no edema.

As noted above, the tendency is to dry out patients with diastolic CHF, decreasing filling pressures and compromising cardiac output. It is likely that for Ms Alden to feel her best, she will need to have some pedal edema.

SUMMARY

Left ventricular systolic dysfunction, during its asymptomatic phase (ALVSD), can be slowed in its development into CHF by treatment with ACE inhibitors. CHF in elders is due to LVSD in more than one-half of patients. LVEF is normally more than 50%: significant LVSD exists if the LVEF is less than 40%. Heart failure (i.e., when there are symptoms due to poor cardiac output) often progresses to CHF (i.e., HF with evidence of fluid retention): CHF is the most common reason for hospitalization of Medicare patients. In both systolic and diastolic CHF, 5-year survival is less than 50%. Diagnosis of CHF has been revolutionized by BNP measurement: it is elevated in both systolic and diastolic CHF. Diastolic dysfunction is as common as is systolic dysfunction in elders. Precipitants of CHF are described by the mnemonic DAMN IT (clots, arrhythmias, myocardial ischemia, noncompliance, intravenous fluid, hyperthyroidism). Loop diuretics and ACE inhibitors are the main therapeutic agents for CHF, with aldosterone antagonists (e.g. spironolactone), digoxin, beta-blockers, and ARBs having significant roles. The place of pacing or CRT in therapy of older patients is not yet clarified.

POSTTEST

1. The *best* way to differentiate between patients with systolic CHF and diastolic CHF is by
   a. History
   b. Physical examination
   c. Echocardiography
   d. ECG
   e. Chest X-ray examination

2. Beneficial effects of converting atrial fibrillation with heart rate of 120 beats per minute to sinus rhythm with heart rate 80 beats per minute include all of the following except which one?
   a. Increased time for ventricular filling
   b. Restoration of atrial contributors to ventricular filling
   c. Decreased myocardial oxygen consumption
   d. Increased myocardial contractility
   e. Reduction in ventricular hypertrophy

3. Which one of the following would be inconsistent with the onset of CHF in an elderly patient?
   a. Dyspnea
   b. Worsening ability to self-care
   c. Anorexia
   d. Falls
   e. None of the above

References

1. The SOLVD Investigators. Effect of enalapril on mortality and the development of heart failure in asymptomatic patients with reduced left ventricular ejection fractions. N Engl J Med 1992;327:685-691.
2. McDonagh T, et al. Symptomatic and asymptomatic left-ventricular systolic dysfunction in an urban population. Lancet 1997;350:829-833.
3. Luchi R. Left ventricular function in hospitalized geriatric patients. J Am Geriatric Soc 1982;30:700-705.
4. Murphy NF, et al. National survey of the prevalence, incidence, primary care burden, and treatment of heart failure in Scotland. Heart 2004;90:1129-1136.
5. Varela-Roman A. et al. Heart failure in patients with preserved and deteriorated left ventricular ejection fraction. Heart. 2005;91:489-494.
6. Luchi R, Taffet G, Teasdale T. Congestive heart failure in the elderly. J Am Geriatr Soc 1991;39:810-825.
7. de Denus S, Pharand C, Williamson D. Brain natriuretic peptide in the management of heart failure: the versatile neurohormone. Chest 2004;125:652-668.
8. Yancy C. Heart failure therapy in special populations: the same or different? Rev Cardiovasc Med 2004;5(Suppl 1):S28-S35.
9. Yan A, Yan P, Liu P. Narrative review: pharmacotherapy for chronic heart failure: evidence from recent clinical trials. Ann Intern Med 2005;142:132-145.
10. Pitt B, et al. The effect of spironolactone on morbidity and mortality in patients with severe heart failure. N Engl J Med 1999;341:709-717.
11. Frishman W. Carvedilol. N Engl J Med 1998;339:1759-1765.
12. Brunner-La Rocca H, Vaddadi G, Esler M. Recent insight into therapy of congestive heart failure: focus on ACE inhibition and angiotensin-II antagonism. J Am Coll Cardiol 1999;33:1163-1173.
13. Cicardi M, et al. Angioedema associated with angiotensin-converting enzyme inhibitor use: outcome after switching to a different treatment. Arch Intern Med 2004;164:910-913.
14. Rich MW, et al. A multidisciplinary intervention to prevent the readmission of elderly patients with congestive heart failure. N Engl J Med 1995;333:1190-1195.
15. Little WC, et al. The effect of alagebrium chloride (ALT-711), a novel glucose cross-link breaker, in the treatment of elderly patients with diastolic heart failure. J Cardiac Fail 2005;11:191-195.
16. Taffet G, et al. Survival of elderly men with congestive heart failure. Age Ageing 1992;21:49-55.
17. Aurigemma G, Gaasch W. Diastolic heart failure. N Engl J Med 2004;351:1097-1105.

PRETEST ANSWERS

1. a
2. a
3. e

POSTTEST ANSWERS

1. c
2. c
3. e

Peripheral Arterial Disease

Vincent Marchello

OBJECTIVES

Upon completion of this chapter, the reader will be able to:

- Describe the major risk factors associated with the development of peripheral atherosclerotic occlusive disease.
- Describe the common patterns of lower-extremity atherosclerotic disease, its clinical presentations, and the characteristics of the patients who typically develop it.
- Describe the appropriate steps in making a diagnosis when lower-extremity arterial insufficiency is suspected.
- Describe a sequential approach to the management of lower-extremity arterial disease with mention of prevention, rehabilitation, and the uses and limitations of drug and surgical treatment.

PRETEST

1. Patients who have peripheral arterial occlusive disease are most likely to die of
   a. Peripheral vascular disease
   b. Renal failure
   c. Cardiovascular or cerebrovascular disease
   d. Diabetes mellitus

2. Which one of the following statements is false?
   a. Middle-aged men are twice as likely as are middle-aged women to suffer symptoms of lower-extremity arterial disease.
   b. Peripheral vascular symptoms often occur in the absence of significant coronary artery or cerebrovascular disease.
   c. Degenerative joint disease of the lumbar spine produces claudication pain on straight leg raising.
   d. Dangling the legs generally worsens venous stasis pain.

Albert Bern *(Part I)*

Mr. Bern is a 67-year-old retired waiter. He complains of burning calf pain that forces him to stop climbing after two flights of stairs. The pain is predictable and moderate and disappears after a brief rest. He was a heavy smoker until 2 years ago when he suffered a stroke with minimal sequelae. He has hypertension and hyperlipidemia.

Robert Ayrens *(Part I)*

Mr. Ayrens is a 76-year-old retired accountant. His type 2 diabetes mellitus has been poorly controlled for 20 years. His ankles are edematous and sore, and he has venous stasis and congestive heart failure (CHF). To help reduce the edema, you have prescribed custom-fit compression stockings. When he walks in the stockings, he experiences a new pain in the anterior tibial muscles and in the arches of both feet.

STUDY QUESTIONS

1. What modifiable risk factors for peripheral vascular disease do these two patients show?
2. What could be the mechanism for the new pain Mr. Ayrens is experiencing?
3. What is the differential diagnosis?
4. What should be emphasized in your history and clinical examination?

Symptoms of lower-extremity arterial insufficiency are common in old age. Associated ischemia often leads to suffering and disability and may lead to loss of limb or life. Assisting patients to reduce risk factors is the key to diagnosis and management must be skilled and proactive.

PREVALENCE AND IMPACT

Peripheral arterial disease (PAD) is a chronic occlusive disease that limits blood flow of the arterial circulation to the lower extremities caused by atherosclerosis. The disease may be asymptomatic at first, then it may progress to intermittent claudication, and eventually to severe ischemia in some cases. Although more than 50%

of those with PAD are asymptomatic, those with symptoms usually exhibit lower-extremity pain only with exercise (intermittent claudication). Signs and symptoms of severe ischemia include pain at rest, ulceration, and gangrene. This clinical presentation is related to the degree of ischemia, which causes a reduction in blood flow to skeletal muscle, tissue, and skin of the affected area.

The prevalence of PAD increases with age. In several epidemiologic studies, prevalence of PAD ranged from 13% to 32% in individuals 80 years of age.[1]

PATHOPHYSIOLOGY AND RISK FACTORS

Risk factors that predispose individuals to PAD are similar to those seen in atherosclerosis and coronary artery disease (CAD). They include cigarette smoking, hyperlipidemia, hypertension, diabetes mellitus, and a family history of CAD.[2] People with lower-extremity atherosclerosis often have significant atherosclerotic disease elsewhere as well, including CAD and cerebrovascular disease (CVD).

Atherosclerosis is a slowly evolving process of damage to the artery walls. It is first seen peripherally at the origins of major branches of the aorta and at their more distal bifurcations. The vessels may be under more stress from torsion, turbulent flow, and high pressure at these points than elsewhere. When stresses disrupt the endothelium, deeper tissues are exposed. Platelets adhere to this denuded vessel wall, forming small thrombi. The platelets then release factors that induce smooth muscle cells and macrophages to migrate to the area. These cells proliferate and lay down a lipid and connective tissue matrix. With further injury, these plaques thicken, stiffen, and develop cholesterol and calcific deposits. These complex atheromatous plaques further enlarge by mechanically injuring adjacent endothelium. Their surface may become rough and ragged, shedding thrombi and plaque fragments into the distal circulation.

Atherogenic risk factors work by amplifying vessel injury or disturbing healing. For example, elevated blood pressure tends to injure the endothelium, hyperlipidemia speeds up cholesterol plaque formation, and smoking promotes vessel spasm and platelet aggregation (along with many other harmful effects).

DIFFERENTIAL DIAGNOSIS

History

PAD typically presents with two characteristics of pain, intermittent claudication or ischemic rest pain. Ulceration and/or gangrene typically follow the latter presentation. The location for the claudication may involve the buttock and thigh area (iliac occlusive disease), calf (most commonly), or foot (rare). The patient's history should bring out the quality, intensity, and location of the limb discomfort and the pattern of how it develops and subsides. This serves to differentiate vascular disease from other causes of lower-limb pain. Degenerative joint disease of the lumbar spine can lead to stenosis of the spinal canal and impingement on the cauda equina and exiting nerve roots. This produces aching and burning pain of the buttock, thigh, and calf muscles when nerve compression is accentuated, such as during straight leg raising or prolonged standing. Because this condition is often misinterpreted as intermittent claudication, it has been referred to as *pseudoclaudication*. Venous stasis can cause aching of the calves and ankles. Although patients with pain from lower-extremity arterial disease (LEAD) while resting may find relief by dangling their legs, patients with venous disease report that this amplifies their symptoms. Patients with peripheral neuropathy often complain of dysesthesias or burning distal lower-extremity pains. As in severe arterial insufficiency, these pains may be more frequent at night. Dangling the feet typically does not help, but light foot exercise might.

Physical Examination

During the physical examination, signs of systemwide vascular disease should be carefully sought. Is there evidence of old cerebral infarct or myocardial damage? Is there evidence of retinal vascular changes, arcus senilis, carotid bruits, left ventricular hypertrophy, asymmetry of upper extremity pulses or blood pressure, aortic aneurysm, or abdominal or flank bruits? The pelvic girdle and lower extremities should be examined for muscle bulk and strength. The presence, symmetry, and quality of the femoral, popliteal, dorsalis pedis, and posterior tibialis pulses should be noted. The distal skin, hair, and nails need to be examined for the trophic changes of ischemia described previously.

INVESTIGATION

Individuals with PAD typically have reduced or nonpalpable pulses in the lower extremities. The measurement of the ankle brachial index (ABI), velocity wave form, and duplex ultrasonography are three noninvasive tests that can be used for diagnosis.

1. ABI—The systolic blood pressure measured at the ankle is compared with that measured in the arm. This is termed the *ABI*. Return of blood flow is measured with a handheld Doppler device as the cuff is slowly deflated. The normal index should be one or greater. In the active older individual who gives a classic history of exercise-induced claudication, the ratio is usually between 0.5 and one. In patients who have rest symptoms, it may be much lower than 0.5.

2. Velocity wave form—At the same time the ABI is being measured, the direction and velocity of blood flow through the lower-extremity arterial tree can be explored.[1] In a normal resting limb without arterial flow obstruction, a triphasic pattern of flow is audible with the handheld Doppler device. The phases correspond to main systolic forward flow, modest reverse flow, and then slower forward flow in late systole. At the arterial site of obstruction, an increase in the peak forward flow can be heard and flow reversal is lost. Just distal to the obstruction is an increased turbulence; more distally the forward velocity is decreased and the reverse component remains absent. It takes only a little practice to appreciate these flow velocity changes.

3. Duplex ultrasonography—This color-assisted test can detect stenoses and measure flow in a specific arterial segment for an accurate assessment of arterial circulation.

Magnetic resonance angiography (MRA) is another noninvasive test that can be useful in selected patients with severe PAD; it is used specifically to study tibial vessels before bypass surgery. Arteriography, an invasive test with higher risks than the tests discussed so far, is typically not performed unless surgery is being considered. MRA is a noninvasive imaging technique that is supplanting conventional angiography as the routine preoperative study in many instances because it appears to be at least as useful in delineating diseased vessels and is significantly safer.[3]

Albert Bern (Part II)

Mr. Bern is slim and vigorous. His blood pressure is 170/90 mm Hg, and his heart rate is 80 beats per minute with occasional ectopy. He has bilateral arcus senilis and early hypertensive retinal vascular changes. He has a right carotid bruit, a laterally displaced apical impulse, and an audible S_4. There are abdominal aortic and femoral bruits. His femoral pulses are equal and easily felt, but his popliteal pulse on the left and both dorsalis pedis pulses are diminished. Lower-extremity skin and musculature appear normal. The blood pressure measured at his ankle is abnormally low.

Robert Ayrens *(Part II)*

Mr. Ayrens becomes short of breath with minimal exertion. Bibasilar rales, an S_3, and symmetric ankle edema are present. The calves, ankles, and feet have thin, rubrous, shiny skin with no hair. The nails are thick and gnarled. The toes are

gaunt and have a violaceous hue that darkens toward the tips. Peripheral pulses are not palpable. During the capillary refill test that was described previously, return of color takes more than 30 seconds even when Mr. Ayrens dangles his feet.

STUDY QUESTIONS

1. What is your assessment of the severity of disease in these two patients?
2. Why has Mr. Ayrens suffered little pain?
3. What management would you recommend for both of these patients?

MANAGEMENT

Management of PAD begins with prevention by helping individuals reduce all modifiable risk factors early in life. Regular exercise has been shown to increase the distance a patient can walk before claudication emerges. This may be because of improvements in muscle efficiency, increases in collateral circulation, or both. Supervised exercise training is a well-documented treatment to relieve claudication and improve exercise performance.[4] Tobacco must be avoided, particularly in those who already have evidence of vascular disease. Smoking cessation decreases the progression of PAD to severe ischemia.[5] Careful attention to normalizing lipids with statin treatment,[6] blood pressure, and blood glucose is important in the effort to slow the disease progress. Unfortunately, patients who manifest PAD alone often do not receive as aggressive a level of medical management for risk factors as do those with CAD.

Once PAD is recognized, the patient must be helped to prevent complications. Poorly perfused tissue heals poorly, so the patient must avoid trauma, including extreme temperatures. Sturdy, well-fitting shoes must be worn at all times when the patient is up. The care of thickened and distorted toenails requires podiatric expertise. Poorly perfused feet, particularly those of a person with diabetes, are susceptible to fungal infections, interdigital maceration, and hard, scaly calluses. These sites are susceptible to smoldering and slowly deepening bacterial infections, which can threaten limb or even life. The patient must learn to inspect the feet daily for signs of trauma or infection and to keep the skin clean, soft, and free of callus and scaling.

Pharmacological Treatment

Pharmacological treatment for individuals with PAD should be directed at reducing cardiovascular morbidity and mortality by treating overall atherosclerosis and improving function by relieving intermittent claudication and severe lower-extremity ischemia. In addition to medications used to treat hypertension, hyperlipidemia, and diabetes, the pharmacologic treatment specific to PAD includes antiplatelet drugs and chelating agents. Antiplatelet therapy in individuals with PAD reduces the risk of CAD, myocardial infarction, stroke, and vascular death by 23%.[7] Medications in this category include aspirin, clopidogrel, and warfarin. Clopidogrel, (Plavix) an antagonist of adenosine diphosphate–induced platelet aggregation, provides a 24% relative risk reduction in the incidence of vascular death, myocardial infarction, and stroke compared with aspirin in patients with PAD.[8] Clopidogrel is an antiplatelet agent whose effectiveness in prevention of ischemic vascular events (e.g., stroke, myocardial infarction, and emergent LEAD) appears to be at least as great as aspirin but, unlike the older related agent ticlopidine (Ticlid), has no more side effects and perhaps less gastrointestinal bleeding than does aspirin. Chelating agents such as cilostazol have antiplatelet and vasodilating properties and have been shown by questionnaire to improve treadmill performance and functional status.[9] Pentoxifylline (Trental), the best-known such agent, decreases blood viscosity and increases peripheral perfusion by several mechanisms, including rendering the red blood cells more flexible in the microvasculature. Only some patients experience symptomatic improvement with pentoxifylline, and gains are modest. However, it appears to speed the healing of lower-extremity diabetic ulcers. Cilostazol (Pletal) is a newly approved potent inhibitor of platelet aggregation that also has vasodilation effects. Several large, double-blind studies have shown its significant benefit in reducing claudication symptoms.[9] However, cilostazol should not be used in patients with CHF. The major disadvantage of clopidogrel and cilostazol is their expense; each one typically costs the patient more than $100 a month.

Case Discussion

Mr. Bern has extensive vascular disease. If he continues to avoid tobacco and walk regularly, lowers lipids and other changeable risk factors, and takes proper care of his feet, worse peripheral disease may not develop. However, his existing cardiovascular and cerebrovascular problems are likely to produce further illness in the future. He should be on aspirin or another antiplatelet agent, as discussed below.

Mr. Ayrens has severe bilateral occlusive disease of the tibioperoneal vessels. Painful ischemia had not been evident because he does not walk much. The quality of the distal pulses is difficult to assess through edematous tissue. However, wearing the compression stockings further reduces the already low arterial pressure so that the need for increased muscle perfusion during walking cannot be met: claudication symptoms result. His CHF treatment needs optimizing, and his risk factors, particularly blood sugar, need aggressive management. He, too, should be on an antiplatelet agent, but not cilostazol (see below).

Surgery

Most elderly patients with lower-limb vascular disease never need surgery. Invasive therapies should be limited to patients with claudications who fail initial medical treatment, have severe disability as defined by validated questionnaires or treadmill testing, and have an appropriate anatomic lesion for bypass or angioplasty. Dilating a localized proximal stenosis, as in the common and external iliac arteries, by using percutaneous transluminal angioplasty (PTA) may be the procedure of choice. Improved stenting techniques have increased the immediate and long-term effectiveness of proximal angioplasty.[1] Angioplasty guidelines emphasize that more proximal lesions have better patency rates and durability than do more distal lesions.[9] The effectiveness of PTA decreases for lesions that are longer, more distal, or more stenotic. Management of frank occlusive disease at the femoropopliteal level and below is better with grafting than with PTA.[1] The better the distal flow, the more likely proximal angioplasty or grafting will remain patent. If disease is extensive in both proximal and distal vessels, surgery may not be possible.

SUMMARY

Managing PAD begins by reducing risk factors in everyone at any age, whether or not the person shows evidence of disease. Functional rehabilitation and prevention of complications, including routine foot self-care and podiatric care, are indicated in those with established disease. Unless contraindicated, patients with established atherosclerosis should receive antiplatelet therapy such as low-dose aspirin. Some will benefit from other drug therapy, and a few will eventually require angioplasty or surgery.

References

1. Ness J, Aronow WS, Ahn C. Risk factors for symptomatic peripheral arterial disease in older persons in an academic hospital based geriatrics practice. J Am Geriatr Soc 2000;48:312-314.
2. Stokes J III, Kannel WB, Wolf PA, et al. The relative importance of selected risk factors for various manifestations of cardiovascular disease among men and women from 35 to 64 years old: 30 year follow-up in the Framingham Study. Circulation 1987;75(6 pt 2):V65-V73.
3. Hiatt WR. Medical treatment of peripheral arterial disease and claudication. N Engl J Med 2001;344:1608-1621
4. Gardner AW, Poehlman ET. Exercise rehabilitation programs for the treatment of claudication pain: a meta-analysis. JAMA 1995;274:975-980.
5. Quick CRG, Cotton LT. The measured effect of stopping smoking on intermittent claudication. Br J Surg 1982;69(Suppl.):S24-S26.
6. Heart Protection Study Collaborative Group. MRC/BHF Heart Protection Study of cholesterol lowering with simvastatin in 20,536 high risk individuals: a randomized placebo-controlled trial. Lancet 2002;360:7-22.
7. Yusuf S, Sleight P, Pogue J, et al. Effects of an angiotensin-converting-enzyme inhibitor, ramipril, on cardiovascular events in high-risk patients: the Heart Outcomes Prevention Evaluation Study Investigators. N Engl J Med 2000;342:145-153.
8. CAPRIE Steering Committee. A randomized, blinded trial of clopidogrel versus aspirin in patients at risk of ischaemic events (CAPRIE). Lancet 1996;348:1329-1339.
9. Dawson DL, Cutler BS, Hiatt WR, et al. A comparison of cilostazol and pentoxifylline for treating intermittent claudication. Am J Med 2000;109: 523-530.

POSTTEST

1. Which one of the following statements is false?
   a. In many instances MRA is now the preoperative vascular study of choice instead of angiography.
   b. The proportion of women suffering symptomatic LEAD increases significantly after age 65.
   c. Dangling the feet may relieve ischemic pain but not neuropathic pain.
   d. An ABI of 1.0 or greater increases the likelihood of peripheral vascular disease.

2. Match the typical clinical presentation with the symptoms.
   a. 52-year-old male smoker with elevated lipids
   b. 75-year-old patient with a long history of poor control of diabetes
   c. 68-year-old hypertensive smoker of either sex
   I. Aching feet and anterior tibial muscles with exercise, fragile skin with nonhealing ulcers, and pain at night
   II. Aching or burning of the calves with exercise with significant coronary artery or cerebrovascular disease
   III. Poor sexual function and exercise-induced aching of the pelvic girdle and thighs

3. Most patients with identified LEAD will benefit from which of the following routine drug therapies?
   a. Pentoxifylline to reduce blood viscosity
   b. A peripheral vasodilator
   c. An antiplatelet agent such as aspirin
   d. A calcium channel blocker

PRETEST ANSWERS

1. c
2. d

POSTTEST ANSWERS

1. d
2. a, III; b, I; c, II
3. c

CHAPTER 39

Cerebrovascular Disease

Kyle R. Allen, William D. Smucker, Kathy Wright, and Janice Weinhardt

OBJECTIVES

Upon completion of this chapter, the reader will be able to:

- Identify stroke as a medical emergency and discuss how health professionals should advise and educate all patients and caregivers to seek medical attention immediately if they experience the signs or symptoms of a stroke.
- Identify the major modifiable and nonmodifiable risk factors for stroke and transient ischemic attacks.
- List the common signs and symptoms of stroke.
- Develop a primary care prevention and treatment plan for identification of patients at risk for stroke, including risk factor identification, goals for risk factor management, symptom recognition, and lifestyle modification.
- Describe the features of the most common types of strokes and presentations.
- Describe and outline an evidence-based management plan for patients in the acute stages of stroke or transient ischemic attack.
- Design and organize a comprehensive rehabilitation, follow-up, and management plan for post-stroke primary care and secondary prevention.

PRETEST

1. All of the following are true regarding treatment of stroke as a medical emergency, i.e., "brain attack," *except?*
   a. To receive intravenous thrombolytic therapy, stroke patients must present within 3 hours of stroke symptom onset.
   b. Patients over the age of 80 are at higher risk for adverse outcomes from thrombolytic therapy for stroke.
   c. Aspirin should be given to stroke patients who have received thrombolytic therapy within 24 hours to improve outcomes from thrombolysis.
   d. Older adults fail to recognize the symptoms of a stroke and thus present late for acute stroke treatment.

2. Which of the following are true regarding stroke risk factors?
   a. Age is the most important nonmodifiable risk factor for stroke.
   b. Hypertension is the single most important modifiable risk factor for stroke.
   c. Eating fruits and vegetables daily can reduce risk of stroke.
   d. Daily exercise can reduce risk of first or recurrent stroke.
   e. All of the above.

3. Which one of the following is false about use of antiplatelet medications for secondary prevention of stroke?
   a. Use of heparin has been shown to be effective in management of ischemic stroke patients.
   b. Clopidogrel with aspirin is an effective combination for stroke prevention.
   c. Aspirin plus extended-release dipyridamole is more effective than aspirin alone for stroke prevention, but cost and adverse effects may limit its benefit.
   d. For patients with first stroke or transient ischemic attack, aspirin 50 to 325 mg per day is recommended as first-line therapy for secondary prevention of stroke.

4. Which one of the following is true about the acute management of stroke?
   a. There is no evidence that stroke units improve outcomes as long as stroke patients are admitted to a medical unit with good general medical care.
   b. Blood pressure elevations should be treated once systolic reaches 150 mm Hg or diastolic reaches 100 mm Hg to preserve brain tissue and prevent poor stroke outcomes in the immediate post stroke period.
   c. Heparin should be used for treatment of moderate to severe hemispheric strokes.
   d. Aspirin at a dosage of 160 to 325 mg should be administered in the first 24 to 48 hours to decrease the likelihood of recurrent stroke, providing there are not contraindications to aspirin therapy.

PREVALENCE AND IMPACT

Stroke is the term used when parts of the brain experience cellular death as a result of the disruption of blood supply and oxygenation. More than 700,000 Americans suffer a stroke each year. Seventy-five percent of strokes occur in those over 65, with the peak incidence among those over age 80.[1] Stroke is the third leading cause of death and the leading cause of adult disability.[1] Strokes are called "brain attacks" to emphasize that they are emergencies requiring prompt evaluation and treatment to preserve brain function.

Strokes are associated with greater disability and mortality with increasing age. This is because of older adults' diminished physiologic, functional, and social reserves in combination with common secondary complications of stroke such as functional/cognitive impairment, falls, pneumonia, dysphagia, malnutrition, urinary incontinence, and depression. Together these may ultimately lead to higher rates of repeat hospitalization, longer lengths of hospital stay, poorer quality of life, increased costs, excessive caregiver strain, and premature institutionalization and/or death in the elderly.[2] Multiple risk factors for stroke exist (Box 39-1). It is possible to prevent a first or recurrent stroke by modifying stroke risk factors with lifestyle changes or medication.[3-6] The primary care clinician can play a pivotal role in primary prevention and secondary outcomes management for stroke victims

● It is possible to prevent a first or recurrent stroke by modifying stroke risk factors with lifestyle changes or medication.

PATHOPHYSIOLOGY

Stroke involves both the circulatory and the nervous system. Pathology of the heart and the arteries supplying the brain can lead to a sudden interruption in the local blood supply to the brain, resulting in brain cell dysfunction and death. The signs and symptoms caused by the disruption in blood supply depend on the location and function of the damaged brain cells.[3]

Strokes are classified as ischemic or hemorrhagic based on their underlying cause. This classification helps to guide both acute therapy and preventive interventions. About 85% of strokes in the elderly are ischemic. Ischemic strokes are further subclassified by whether the arterial occlusion is due to large-artery atherosclerosis, small-artery vascular occlusion, or cardioembolism. Hemorrhagic stroke involves rupture of a cerebral artery, which may be due to atherosclerosis, lipohyalinosis, amyloid angiopathy, aneurysm, arteriovenous malformation, trauma, or tumor. About 5% of strokes are due to unusual causes such as arteritis, cerebrovascular dissection, hypercoagulable states, endocarditis, sickle cell anemia, septic emboli, and drug use. Up to 20% of ischemic strokes cannot be categorized, and they are called *cryptogenic strokes*.

When signs and symptoms of a stroke completely resolve within 24 hours, the ischemic event is called a transient ischemic attack (TIA). Most TIAs last less than 3 hours. It is important to remember that even if symptoms resolve, a TIA is a *brain attack*. Up to 22% of patients hospitalized with a TIA will have infarction on their brain imaging study. After a TIA, the risk of a stroke within the next 10 days is 8%. For patients with a TIA, admission to a stroke unit (SU) is associated with improved survival and functional independence.[4]

● For patients with a TIA, admission to a SU is associated with improved survival and functional independence.

Martha Smith, *(Part 1)*

Mrs. Smith is a 68-year-old obese African American woman who lives in a two-story home with her developmentally disabled daughter. She provides primary care for her daughter and, as a result, does not

---

Box 39-1   Risk Factors for Stroke

Modifiable Risk Factors with Proven Preventive Efficacy

High blood pressure
Hyperlipidemia
Cigarette smoking
Inactivity
Obesity
Heavy alcohol use
Estrogen use
Atrial fibrillation
Carotid artery stenosis

Modifiable Risk Factors with Uncertain Preventive Efficacy

Diabetes mellitus
Sleep apnea

Non-Modifiable Risk Factors

Increased age
Previous stroke or transient ischemic attack
Male sex
Family history
Race (African American > Asian, Hispanic > Caucasian)
Family history of stroke or heart attack before age 60

follow up regularly for treatment of hypertension and diabetes. Over the past month, Mrs. Smith quit taking her blood pressure medication and diabetic medications because of the cost; she needed the extra money to care for her daughter. Her last blood pressure reading 6 months ago was 170/90 mm Hg. Her weight is 180 pounds, and her height is 5′ 2″ with calculated body mass index of 33. She is also smoking more because of the excessive stress in caring for her daughter. There are other children who have offered to help, but Mrs. Smith doesn't want to burden them.

STUDY QUESTIONS

1. What are Mrs. Smith's risk factors for a stroke?
2. Should she be on an antiplatelet medication? If so, what is the drug of choice?
3. What primary prevention interventions should be implemented?

DIFFERENTIAL DIAGNOSIS AND ASSESSMENT

One of the greatest barriers to improving stroke care is the recognition of stroke symptoms by the stroke patient, the caregivers, and even health care providers. Although older adults have the greatest risk for stroke, as a group they are the least likely to recognize stroke symptoms and report them. Acute stroke signs and symptoms may be subtle and can often be confused with other neurologic and medical conditions (e.g., Bell's palsy, hypoglycemia, vertigo). In addition, stroke does not cause pain or discomfort such as angina (with exception of headache with intracerebral hemorrhage); therefore, patients often do not perceive a need for emergent treatment. Education of the public, of patients with known risk for stroke, and of health care providers is essential for improved stroke recognition and will help raise awareness that stroke should be treated as a medical emergency ("time is brain").

Diagnostic tests are used to confirm the presence of a stroke, determine the presence of disease processes that cause symptoms of a stroke, and evaluate whether comorbid conditions exist that influence subsequent stroke management. Box 39-2 lists essential and optional testing for the patient presenting with acute stroke.

> ● Acute stroke signs and symptoms may be subtle and can often be confused with other neurologic and medical conditions. In addition, stroke usually does not cause pain or discomfort unlike angina; therefore, patients often do not perceive a need for emergent treatment.

Confirm the Diagnosis of Stroke

The diagnosis of a stroke is based primarily on history, physical examination, and exclusion of conditions that may mimic stroke. Strokes occur suddenly, usually over seconds or minutes. Exceptions to this rule are the stroke that develops during sleep, creating a new neurological deficit evident upon awakening, and the thrombotic stroke that produces a progressive neurological deficit that reaches maximum intensity over many hours. Additional elements of the history that favor the diagnosis of a stroke include a prior history of TIA, a history of stroke risk factors, evidence of atherosclerotic cardiovascular disease, and the presence of valvular heart disease or cardiac arrhythmia. Only a few conditions cause acute focal neurological deficits, and most of them can be detected with a focused history and a standard battery of diagnostic tests.

The computed tomography (CT) scan may not show any abnormalities in the first 48 hours of cerebral ischemia and infarction. One of the main uses of the initial CT scan of the brain is to detect cerebral hemorrhage. Cerebral hemorrhage is a medical emergency that requires neurosurgical consultation and

---

Box 39-2 **Diagnostic Tests for the Initial Evaluation of Possible Stroke**

Recommended	Optional (guided by history or physical findings)
Computed tomography (CT) of brain	Chest radiograph
Electrocardiogram	Carotid duplex ultrasound examination
Blood glucose	Magnetic resonance imaging (MRI) of the brain
Serum creatinine, urea, electrolytes	Magnetic resonance arteriography (MRA) of the brain
Complete blood count, including platelets	Liver function tests
Prothrombin time (PT) and partial thromboplastin time (PTT)	Serum ammonia level
Oxygen saturation (pulse oximetry)	Blood alcohol level
	Toxicology screen
	Electroencephalogram

monitoring in an intensive care unit. Detection of small lacunar infarctions and strokes in the cerebellum or brainstem may require magnetic resonance imaging (MRI) which is more sensitive for detecting these lesions.

Quantify Neurological Deficit

Clinicians who evaluate acute stroke should complete a focused neurological examination. Two commonly used tools are the Barthel Index and Modified Rankin Stroke Severity Scale.[7,8]

MANAGEMENT

Until the past decade, little could be done to "cure" an acute stroke, so little emphasis was placed on optimal acute and peri-acute stroke care principles. Because of newer treatments such as tissue plasminogen activator (tPA) and interventions that can limit the devastating aspects of stroke and preserve neurologic function, many acute hospitals and communities have started to reorganize stroke care delivery in an attempt to improve outcomes for stroke.

The management of acute stroke can be organized into discrete phases: prehospital, the acute emergency department (ED) evaluation, the first 48 hours of acute stroke care, the rehabilitation phase, and the chronic care or care coordination phase.

Prehospital and Emergency Medical Services Phase

Emergency medical services (EMS) personnel must have training to recognize stroke signs and symptoms. The paradigm of treating stroke as an emergency must be embraced by the EMS, and collaborative working relationships should be established between hospital and EMS providers.

> ● The paradigm of treating stroke as an emergency must be embraced by the EMS, and collaborative working relationships should be established between hospital and EMS providers.

Acute-Phase Emergency Department and First 48 Hours

Acute assessment and stabilization of a patient with signs and symptoms of an acute stroke should occur in the ED. The clinician should stabilize the patient, complete a diagnostic evaluation, confirm the diagnosis of acute stroke, determine the presence of a cerebral hemorrhage, quantify the neurological deficit, and determine eligibility for thrombolytic therapy.[5,6]

STABILIZE THE PATIENT

The clinician must assure that the patient's cardiac and pulmonary status is adequate to maintain optimum cerebral perfusion and oxygenation. A focused examination should asses the patient's vital signs and cardiac and pulmonary status, with attention to adequate airway, oxygenation, and blood pressure.

COMPLETE A DIAGNOSTIC EVALUATION

This is described in the Differential Diagnosis and Assessment section (see above).

DETERMINE ELIGIBILITY FOR THROMBOLYTIC THERAPY

The phrases *time is brain* and *brain attack* highlight the importance of assessing stroke patients rapidly and determining eligibility for thrombolytic therapy. Thrombolytic therapy restores cerebral perfusion and may reverse neurological loss if administered in the early hours of a stroke. Patients with an acute thrombotic stroke whose stroke symptoms have been present for less than 3 hours may be candidates for intravenous thrombolytic therapy.[3,9,10] Patients who awaken with stroke symptoms may be candidates for thrombolysis only if the diagnostic evaluation is completed within 3 hours from the time the patient went to sleep.

Intravenous recombinant tPa given within 3 hours of acute ischemic onset can reduce the rate of severe disability and death[3,6]; however, there is a significant rate of intracerebral hemorrhage associated with tPa (3% to 6% incidence).[10] This rate is higher in adults greater than age 80, although advancing age should not be used as the sole criterion to withhold tPA. One of the greatest single factors precluding the use of tPa in the eligible population is late presentation (i.e., more than 3 hours from symptom onset). Patients that present later than 3 hours but less than 6 hours may benefit from intra-arterial tPa.[3] However, intra-arterial tPa should be reserved only for carefully selected patients who will be cared for by experienced neurologists and neurointensivists.[3]

> ● The phrases *time is brain* and *brain attack* highlight the importance of assessing stroke patients rapidly and determining eligibility for thrombolytic therapy.

Martha Smith, *(Part 2)*

Mrs. Smith's sister called you and said Mrs. Smith has had episodes of blurred vision and left hand weakness over the past 2 days but refuses to seek treatment. On the third day, Mrs. Smith was transported to the ED because she was unable to use her left arm and had difficulty swallowing. On neurologic examination, she is alert and oriented ×3. She has a mild delay in answering questions secondary to expressive aphasia. Cranial nerves II through XII appear intact. She has left-sided weakness, with 4/5 in the upper extremity and 3/5 in the lower extremity. She has subjective difference in sensation to light touch on the left. The complete blood count is remarkable for hemoglobin of 11.1 and platelets of 128,000. Chemistry panel normal, with blood urea nitrogen (BUN) of 18, and creatinine of 1.0. Carotid ultrasound unremarkable. CT scan shows a punctate low density in the head of the caudate on the left, consistent with a remote lacunar infarct. There is a vague low density in the anterior limb of the internal capsule on the left, which is consistent with a punctate lacunar infarct of indeterminate age. There is also a vague low density in what is probably the left cerebral peduncle, again consistent with a small infarct of indeterminate age.

STUDY QUESTIONS

1. Is Mrs. Smith a candidate for tPA?
2. List the reasons why you would admit her to the hospital.

Hospital Phase

Patients with an acute ischemic stroke should be admitted to the hospital, preferably to a SU, for observation because up to 25% of these patients will experience a progression of their neurological deficit, a life-threatening complication, or death within the first 48 hours.[4,6] Similarly, patients with a TIA should be hospitalized because in the 10 days after symptom onset, they have a stroke rate of up to 8% and a death rate of up to 2%.[11] Too often TIAs are not treated as a medical emergency by primary care physicians.[4]

Consultation and collaborative care with a neurologist experienced in stroke care is prudent for several reasons: acute interventions that restore or preserve neurological function are continually evolving, the provisional diagnosis of TIA or stroke is frequently incorrect, and complications after stroke are common. Primary care physicians can play a valuable role by managing comorbid conditions, preventing acute complications of stroke, providing educational and emotional support, creating a plan to control stroke risk factors, and providing continuity of care as the patient moves from acute care to rehabilitation to outpatient care.

SUs have been shown to be the preferred model for management of acute stroke patients.[12] Multiple randomized controlled trials and meta-analyses of SU trials have demonstrated that SUs improve functional outcomes, decrease mortality, and decrease the need for long term institutionalization.[12,13] Standardized stroke orders that provide guidelines for management of blood pressure, blood sugars, dysphagia screening and management, deep venous thrombosis (DVT) prophylaxis, rehabilitation needs, nursing management, screening for depression, laboratory assessment, and appropriate medication treatment are recommended as part of SU organization.[12]

Common Post-stroke Complications

Numerous complications often accompany stroke, and evidence-based management of these complications is required to optimize stroke outcomes. Target blood pressures must be maintained after tPa administration to minimize the risk of intracerebral hemorrhage.[6] The elevation of blood pressure after ischemic stroke may be a physiologic response to increased cerebral perfusion pressure to preserve neurological tissue and minimize neuronal damage in the peri-infarct area known as the penumbra; thus guidelines must be followed in blood pressure management after ischemic stroke. Hyperglycemia and hypoglycemia can both adversely affect stroke outcomes by causing cell death in the penumbra.[14] Dysphagia must be screened for and managed to prevent aspiration pneumonia.[15,16] DVT can occur in 20% to 50% of stroke patients within the first 2 weeks after a stroke, and pulmonary embolus is the cause of 25% of deaths in the first month after stroke, so prevention is key.[17] Bladder dysfunction, which includes urinary retention (early complication) and urinary incontinence (later complication), occurs in 80% of acute stroke patients and latently in 25% of stroke survivors. Finally, pressure ulcers are a common complication of stroke. Please see Chapter 28 for a detailed description of the proper approach to diagnosis and treatment.

Martha Smith, *(Part 3)*

Mrs. Smith was admitted to an acute SU from the ED. She was evaluated as having a baseline function of 100% independence. At hospital admission she had persistent left-sided weakness and expressive aphasia. Fasting lipid panel showed total cholesterol 275, high-density lipoprotein 53.4, low-density lipoprotein 199, and triglycerides 113. Hemoglobin A1c was 11.0.

STUDY QUESTIONS

1. What interventions would you use to prevent aspiration pneumonia?
2. When should physical therapy and occupational therapy be initiated?

Medication Issues

The use of heparin has not been shown to be of benefit in acute stroke patients.[18] In fact, treatment with full therapeutic doses of parenteral anticoagulants is not recommended for any stroke subtype, including cardioembolic stroke, because they increase the risk of serious bleeding complications.[3]

Aspirin at dosages of 160 to 325 mg per day has been shown to be effective in preventing stroke and cerebrovascular events and should be given within 24 to 48 hours of acute stroke or TIA.[6] Other antiplatelet agents are not indicated in the first 48 hours.[6] Patients with an allergy to aspirin, those who received thrombolytic therapy within the past 24 hours, or those with other known contraindications should not receive aspirin.

Other antiplatelet agents effective for secondary prevention and recommended for patients with noncardioembolic ischemic stroke or TIA include aspirin plus extended release dipyridamole (ASA/ER-DP) and clopidogrel.[3] ASA/ER-DP given twice daily is an alternative to aspirin and may confer an additional secondary benefit; however, the cost prohibits it from being considered the first-line agent.[19] In addition, headache and nausea are side effects that may cause patients to discontinue the use of the medication, although these side effects are transient. Clopidogrel 75 mg a day is an alternative for patients who are allergic to aspirin, but it does not have any greater benefit than does aspirin alone for secondary prevention of stroke or TIA.[20] In addition, combining aspirin and clopidogrel is not superior to clopidogrel or aspirin alone and it significantly increases the risk of serious gastrointestinal bleeding.[21]

Warfarin is indicated for secondary stroke prevention for ischemic stroke and TIA patients with atrial fibrillation.[22] There is no clear benefit of using warfarin in noncardioembolic stroke.[3] Older adults are consistently undertreated with warfarin anticoagulation for atrial fibrillation.[23-25] This is of particular importance because cardioembolic stroke in older adults causes significant neurologic disability and functional impairment and is more lethal. The serious complications of stroke must be weighed against the calculation of risk for serious hemorrhage when warfarin therapy is used in older adults. Clinicians often overestimate the risk-to-benefit ratio. See Box 39-3 for amplification of these considerations.

Box 39-3   Determining Risk-to-Benefit Ratio of Warfarin Use

Assess benefit on quality of life

Assess stroke risk

Assess risk of bleeding complications and modify, for example, risk of falls

Modify lifestyle, medication, and treatment plan to reduce risk of bleeding

---

Advancing age and common age-associated comorbidities (e.g., gait problems, hypertension, heart disease, polypharmacy, renal insufficiency) increase the incidence of major hemorrhage with warfarin use. For primary prevention of stroke, warfarin is indicated for patients with nonvalvular atrial fibrillation and one high risk factor or more than one moderate risk factor (Table 39-1). Absolute contraindications to warfarin include bleeding diathesis, platelet count of less than 50,000, uncontrolled hypertension (more than 160/90 mm Hg), and noncompliance with medications or monitoring.[26] Relative contraindications include more than 2 ounces of alcohol per day and regular use of nonselective nonsteroidal anti-inflammatory drugs (NSAIDs) without cytoprotection.[26] Warfarin therapy can be safely used with gastric selective cyclooxygenase-2 NSAIDs, NSAIDs with gastric cytoprotection or proton pump inhibitor, or resolved peptic ulcer bleeding with *Helicobacter pylori* testing and treatment.[26]

Surgical Intervention

Carotid endarterectomy (CEA) has been shown to be beneficial for symptomatic patients with more than 70% stenosis without subtotal occlusion and is somewhat beneficial for those with occlusion of 50% to 69%. CEA is not indicated for occlusion less than 50%.[27] CEA for primary stroke prevention for patients with asymptomatic stenosis greater than 60% is controversial because of limited proven benefit. CEA should only be considered in patients who are

---

Table 39-1   Risk Factors for Stroke With Atrial Fibrillation

High	Moderate
Age >75	Age 65 to 75
Prior transient ischemic attack (TIA) or stroke	Diabetes mellitus
Hypertension	Coronary artery disease
Poor left ventricle function	

less than 75 years of age with a good life expectancy, greater than 70% stenosis, and low surgical risk.[28]

Rehabilitation and Secondary Stroke Prevention

Intensive rehabilitation should be considered for all stroke patients, although no specific rehabilitation method has been proven superior to others.[29,30] Stroke rehabilitation is an active process and begins on admission to the hospital. The rehabilitation process focuses on six key areas: (1) preventing, recognizing, and managing comorbid illness and medical complications; (2) training for maximum independence; (3) facilitating maximum psychosocial coping and adaptation by the patient and family; (4) preventing secondary disability by promoting community reintegration, including resumption of home, family, recreational, and vocational activities; (5) enhancing quality of life in view of residual disability; and (6) preventing recurrent stroke and other vascular conditions such as myocardial infarction that occur with increased frequency in patients with stroke.[29] To assure maximal success in rehabilitation patients must be medically stable, have moderate to severe functional disability, have the ability to learn new information, and be motivated. The setting for rehabilitation depends on several factors, including degree of impairment, involvement of care givers, physical endurance, and tolerance to therapy. See the chapter on rehabilitation for more detailed information.

Most recovery occurs by 11 weeks after stroke, with the best neurologic scores seen at 1 month by 80% of patients.[31] Stroke recovery can continue for up to 6 months. Several prognostic factors can help in organizing a rehabilitation plan. Poor recovery can be predicted by severity of initial stroke and impairment, progressive neurologic deficits in the immediate post stroke period (2 to 4 days), no motor return after 1 month, left- or right-sided neglect, poor cognition, dysphagia, incontinence of bowel or bladder, or coma at acute presentation.[31] Elevated temperature and blood glucose are also associated with poor neurologic outcomes. Diabetes is associated with higher mortality rates and longer rehabilitation needs.[32] Urinary incontinence has also been shown to be predictive of institutionalization and mortality, with the relative risk of death seven times greater than continent stroke patients.[32] Age is not an independent risk factor for neurologic recovery or mortality.

Prevention of complications of stroke during the acute period (e.g., pneumonia, DVT, pressure ulcers, constipation) will help patients maximize the attainment of their rehabilitation goals and minimize recovery time. A physiatrist should be consulted early in the acute stroke period to help guide the rehabilitation plan, set goals, and minimize post-stroke complications.

> ● Intensive rehabilitation should be considered for all stroke patients, although no specific rehabilitation method has been proven superior to others.

Martha Smith, (Part 4)

While in the rehabilitation unit, Mrs. Smith had disturbed sleep, poor appetite, and low motivation to participate in therapy. She also scored positive on a depression screen. The nurse aides complained about Mrs. Smith's frequent episodes of incontinence. A family meeting was held before discharge to arrange for equipment needs and caregiver support. Her family seems apprehensive about managing Mrs. Smith's insulin and diet. There also remains a concern about affording medications and caring for her developmentally disabled daughter. After 3 weeks Mrs. Smith was discharged to home. She will continue home therapy and then outpatient therapy over the next 6 months.

STUDY QUESTIONS

1. What secondary complications may affect Mrs. Smith's recovery? What interventions are appropriate?
2. How would you assess for caregiver stress? What resources are available to assist?

Secondary Prevention and Ongoing Monitoring

Traditionally stroke has been viewed as an "acute illness" when, in fact, it shares many of the characteristics of a "chronic illness." Similar to other chronic illnesses, stroke is associated with a high rate of recurrence or relapse, a set of typical poststroke complications, and a set of common comorbidities. The primary care clinician needs to use a similar evidence-based approach to poststroke care, just as secondary prevention has has been demonstrated to be beneficial for diabetes and heart failure.[33]

Of the 750,000 strokes per year, 200,000 of these are recurrent stroke. The cause of death in the first 30 days after a stroke is typically stroke related; however, over the next year 50% of all deaths will be from cardiovascular events such as myocardial infarction, sudden cardiac death, aortic aneurysm, or severe limb ischemia.

Table 39–2	Outpatient Treatment	
Risk factors for future stroke	**Treatment Targets**	**Preferred Treatments**
Hypertension	<140/90 mm Hg[36-39]	Angiotensin-converting enzyme inhibitors (especially in diabetes)
	<140/85 at 3 months after stroke[40]	Angiotensin receptor blockers (especially in diabetes)
	<130/80 at 1 year post stroke[40]	Thiazide diuretics
Atrial fibrillation (AF)	International ratio (INR) 2.5 (range 2.0 to normalization 3.0) in AF INR 3.0 (range 2.5 to 3.5) for patients with mechanical cardiac valves[3, 43]	Beta-blockers Warfarin
Hypercholesterolemia	LDL < 100	Statins for patients with transient ischemic attack or ischemic stroke
Diabetes	Glycated hemoglobin level < 7	Although the link between tight blood sugar control and stroke is unproven, most experts agree that blood sugar control is imperative to improve cardiovascular status in general
Cardio/peripheral vascular diseases	All transient ischemic attack and ischemic stroke patients should take an antiplatelet agent	Aspirin 160 to 325 mg/day Aspirin 325 mg + dipyridamole 200 mg twice per day to reduce the risk of recurrent stroke to 8.3% Clopidogrel 75 mg/day

During this 12-month period, 10% of deaths will be due to stroke-related issues and 5% to recurrent stroke.

Outpatient follow-up care should ensure that the patient achieves target goals for known risk factors for stroke and lifestyle modifications (Table 39-2).[34-36] Smoking cessation (level B),[16,38,39] physical activity (level A),[37] diet and weight control (level B),[16,35,39] reduction of salt and adequate potassium intake (level B), and avoidance of excess alcohol (level C) are all important lifestyle modifications necessary to reduce the risk of recurrent stroke. For instruction on influencing patients to change their lifestyles, see Chapter 5.

Assess and Monitor for Common Post-stroke Complications

The following conditions should be routinely screened and monitored for 6 months after the stroke, then annually: functional impairment (activities of daily living and instrumental activities of daily living, communication and speech, swallowing difficulties), depression, cognitive status, urinary and bowel incontinence, falls, osteoporosis, caregiver stress, adequacy of supports, access and ability to secure community resources (stroke support groups, exercise programs, educational classes), and sexual function.

Providing ongoing education regarding risk factor modification, warning signs and symptoms of recurrent stroke, and the appropriate action to take is an extremely important role for the primary care clinician. Stroke survivors often do not retain stroke education provided during the hospital stay and rehabilitation. Thus education should be provided and reinforced with the patient as well as the closest caregiver so they will be able to recognize stroke warning signs, take appropriate action, and implement lifestyle modifications.

SUMMARY

Stroke can be one of the most catastrophic illnesses, particularly for older adults. However, it is also one of the most preventable of all major illnesses.[38,39] The primary care physician has a significant role to play in the primary prevention, acute management, rehabilitation, and chronic care phases of stroke. By using an evidence-based approach to care, the primary care physician, partnering with the patient, can have a significant positive impact on quality of life, well-being, stroke prevention, and clinical outcomes.

References

1. American Heart Association. Heart Disease and Stroke Statistics, 2004 Update. Dallas, TX: American Heart Association. http://www.americanheart.org/presenter.jhtml?identifier=3000090.
2. Wolinsky F, Gurney J, Wan G, Bentley D. The sequelae of hospitalization for ischemic stroke among older adults. J Am Geriatr Soc 1998;46:577-582.

3. Albers GW, Amarenco P, Easton JD, Sacco RL, Teal P. Antithrombotic and thrombolytic therapy for ischemic stroke: the Seventh ACCP Conference on Antithrombotic and Thrombolytic Therapy. Chest 2004;126:483S-512S

4. Daffertshofer M, Mielke O, Pullwitt A, et al. Transient ischemic attacks are more than "ministrokes." Stroke 2004;35:2453-2458.

5. Smucker WD, DiSabato JA, Krishen AE. Systematic approach to diagnosis and initial management of stroke. Am Fam Physician 1995;52:225-234.

6. Adams HP, Adams RJ, Brott T, et al. Guidelines for the early management of patients with ischemic stroke. Stroke 2003;34:1056-1083.

7. Mahoney F, Barthel D. Functional evaluation: the Barthel index. MD Med J 1965;14:61-65.

8. Rankin L. Cerebral vascular accidents in patients over the age of 60. Scott Med J 1957;2:200-215.

9. NIHSS Training site. http://asa.trainingcampus.net/uas/modules/trees/index.asp.

10. The National Institute of Neurological Disorders, and Stroke t-PA Stroke Study Group. Tissue plasminogen activator for acute ischemic stroke. N Engl J Med. 1995;333:1581-1587.

11. Lisabeth LD, Ireland JK, Risser J, et al. Stroke risk after transient ischaemic attack in a population-based setting. Stroke 2004;35:1842-1846.

12. Stroke Unit Trialists' Collaboration. Organized inpatient (stroke unit) care for stroke (Cochrane Review). In The Cochrane Library, Issue 1. Chichester, UK: John Wiley and Sons, 2004.

13. Kwan J, Sandercock P. In-hospital care pathways for stroke (Cochrane Review). In The Cochrane Library, Issue 1. Chichester, UK: John Wiley and Sons, 2004.

14. Gray CS, Hildreth AJ, Alberti G, et al. Poststroke hyperglycemia natural history and immediate management. Stroke 2004;35:122-126.

15. Diagnosis and Treatment of Swallowing Disorders (Dysphagia) in Acute-Care Stroke Patients. Summary, Evidence Report/Technology Assessment, Number 8. Agency for Health Care Policy and Research, Rockville, MD, March 1999. http://www.ahrq.gov/clinic/epcsums/dysphsum.htm.

16. Royal College of Physician National Clinical Guidelines for Stroke, 2nd ed. London: Royal College of Physicians of London, June 2004. http://www.rcplondon.ac.uk/pubs/books/stroke/index.htm.

17. Geerts WH, Pineo GF, Heit JA, et al. Prevention of venous thromboembolism: the Seventh ACCP Conference on Antithrombotic and Thrombolytic Therapy. Chest 2004;126:338S-400S

18. Gubit et al: Anticoagulants for acute ischemic stroke. *Cochrane Database System Rev 2:* CD000024, 2000.

19. Diener HC, Cunha L, Forbes C, et al. European stroke prevention study, 2: dipyridamole and acetylsalicylic acid in the secondary prevention of stroke. J Neurol Sci 1996;143: 1-13.

20. CAPRIE Steering Committee. A randomized, blinded trial of clopidogrel versus aspirin in patients at risk of ischaemic events (CAPRIE). Lancet 1996;348:1329-1339.

21. Diener HC, Bogousslavsky J, Brass LM, MATCH investigators. Aspirin and clopidogrel compared with clopidogrel alone after recent ischaemic stroke or transient ischaemic attack in high-risk patients (MATCH): a randomized, double-blind, placebo-controlled trial. Lancet 2004;364:331-337.

22. Singer DE, Albers GW, Dalen JE, et al. Antithrombotic therapy in atrial fibrillation: the Seventh ACCP Conference on Antithrombotic and Thrombolytic Therapy. Chest 2004;126:429S-456S.

23. McCormick D, Gurwitz JH, Goldberg RJ, et al. Prevalence and quality of warfarin use for patients with atrial fibrillation in the long term care setting. Arch Intern Med 2001;161:2458-2463.

24. Whittle J, Wickenheiser L, Venditti LN. Is warfarin underused in the treatment of elderly persons with atrial fibrillation? Arch Intern Med 1997;157: 441-445.

25. Brophy MT, Snyder KE, Gaehde S, et al. Anticoagulant use for atrial fibrillation in the elderly. J Am Geriatr Soc 52;1151-1156.

26. Man-Son-Hing M, Laupacis A. Anticoagulant bleeding in older persons with atrial fibrillation: physicians fears often unfounded. Arch Intern Med 2003;163:1580-1586.

27. Rothwell PM, Eliasziw M Gutnikov SA, et al. Analysis of pooled data from the randomised controlled trials of endarterectomy for symptomatic carotid stenosis. Lancet 2003;361:107-116.

28. Halliday A, Mansfield A, Marro J, et al. Prevention of disabling and fatal strokes by successful carotid endarterectomy in patients without recent neurological symptoms: randomized controlled trial. Lancet 2004;363:1491-1502.

29. Gresham GE, Alexander D, Bishop DS, et al. Rehabilitation. Stroke 1997;28: 1522-1526.

30. AHRQ Post stroke rehabilitation guidelines. www.ncbi.nlm.nih.gov/books/bv.fcgi?rid=hstat6.chapter.27305.

31. Jorgensen HS, Nakayama H, Raaschou HO, Olsen TS. Stroke: neurologic and functional recovery, the Copenhagen Stroke Study. Phys Med Rehabil Clin N Am 1999;10:887-906.

32. Brittain KR, Peet SM, Potter JF, Castleden CM. Prevalence and management of urinary incontinence in stroke survivors. Age Ageing 1999;28: 509-511.

33. Rich M, Beckham V, Wittenberg C, et al. A multidisciplinary intervention to prevent the readmission of elderly patients with congestive heart failure. N Engl J Med 1995;333:1190-1195.

34. Muir KW. Secondary prevention for stroke and transient ischaemic attacks. BMJ 2004;328:297-298.

35. Hanley D, Gorelick P, Elliott WJ, et al. Determining the appropriateness of selected surgical and medical management options in recurrent stroke prevention: a guideline for primary care physicians from the National Stroke Association work group on recurrent stroke prevention. J Stroke Cerebrovasc Dis 2004;13:196-207.

36. Stroke Council. Statins after ischemic stroke and transient ischemic attack. Stroke 2004;35:1023.

37. Gordon NF, Gulanick M, Costa F, et al. Physical activity and exercise recommendations for stroke survivors: an American Heart Association Scientific Statement. Circulation 2004;109:2031-2041.

38. Pearson TA, Blair SN, Daniels SR, et al. AHA guidelines for primary prevention of cardiovascular disease and stroke: 2002 update. Circulation 2002;106:388-391.

39. Gorelick PB. Stroke prevention therapy beyond antithrombotics: unifying mechanisms in the ischemic stroke pathogenesis and implications for therapy. Stroke 2002;33:862-875.

Web Resources

1. www.americanheart.org.
2. www.stroke.org.
3. www.ninds.nih.gov.
4. www.strokeprotect.mednet.ucla.

POSTTEST

1. Which of the following is not a common poststroke complication that should be monitored?
    a. Depression
    b. Urinary incontinence
    c. Diarrhea
    d. Falls

2. Which of the following are true about warfarin anticoagulation and atrial fibrillation?
    a. The majority of older adults should not receive anticoagulation with warfarin because the risk of bleeding is too great.
    b. Physicians often overestimate the complications associated with anticoagulation.
    c. Atrial fibrillation is an uncommon cause of cardioembolic stroke in older adults.
    d. Strokes that result from cardioembolic sources such as atrial fibrillation tend to be more severe and have higher mortality rate.
    e. b and d
    f. a and b

3. All of the following are treatment and management considerations for acute stroke *except:*
    a. Hyperglycemia should be aggressively treated in the acute stroke period because elevated blood glucose has been associated with poor neurologic outcomes.
    b. For patients with major stroke with immobility, deep venous prophylaxis should be provided by use of heparin, pneumatic compression devices, or compression stockings.
    c. Indwelling urinary catheter should be used in incontinent patient with impaired mobility to prevent urinary tract infections.
    d. A swallowing evaluation should be performed at some point to reduce the risk of aspiration pneumonia.

4. A stroke that occurs in the middle cerebral artery territory will produce all of the following manifestations *except:*
    a. Visual field cut
    b. Aphasia
    c. Arm and leg weakness
    d. Arm and leg sensory loss
    e. Neglect

PRETEST ANSWERS

1. c
2. e
3. a
4. d

POSTTEST ANSWERS

1. c
2. e
3. c
4. a

OBJECTIVES

Upon completion of this chapter, the reader will be able to:

- Understand the changing epidemiology of adult diabetes mellitus (DM) and the impact it has on the elderly.
- Identify the risk factors for DM in older persons.

- Understand the continuum of the disease process in diabetes and how this affects the diagnostic criteria for DM.
- Be able to assess the elderly diabetic in a multisystem and multidisciplinary fashion, including the common geriatric syndromes
- Describe the roles and contraindications for pharmacologic and nonpharmacologic treatments of DM.

PRETEST

1. Which one of the following meet the American Diabetes Association (ADA) diagnostic criteria for diabetes mellitus?
   a. Fasting blood sugar (FBS) of 140 mg/dl on two separate occasions
   b. FBS of 126 mg/dl on two separate occasions
   c. 2-hour glucose of 200 mg/dl during a 2-hour 50 g glucose tolerance test
   d. HbA_1C of more than 7%

2. All of the following syndromes are more common in the diabetic elderly *except*:
   a. Polyarteritis
   b. Dementia
   c. Depression
   d. Polypharmacy
   e. Falls

3. In elderly patients with a life expectancy of less than 5 years or in patients in which the risk of intensive glycemic control does not outweigh the benefit, what is the goal HbA_1C?
   a. 7%
   b. 8%
   c. 9%
   d. 10%

4. In elderly patients who have had a stable HbA_1C at goal, how frequently should their HbA_1C be monitored?
   a. Every 3 months
   b. Every 6 months
   c. Every 9 months
   d. Every 12 months
   e. Every 24 months

Maria Sweetly, *Part 1*

Maria Sweetly is a 68-year-old Hispanic woman who presents to your office for hypertension follow-up and remarks that for 2 months she has had bilateral burning and numbness of her feet and that she has fallen recently at home, without injury. Medications include hydrochlorothiazide (HCTZ) 25 mg daily and metoprolol 50 mg twice a day. Her blood pressure is 144/88 mm Hg, pulse 60 beats per minute, weight 173 pounds, and body mass index 30; monofilament and light touch sensation is diminished in a stocking distribution, Achilles reflexes are +1, dorsalis pedis pulses are +1, and the remainder of the exam is unremarkable. Fasting serum glucose is 130 mg/dl, blood urea nitrogen (BUN) 19 mg/dl, and creatinine 1.2 mg/dl, and electrolytes are normal.

STUDY QUESTIONS

1. Can you name at least four of Mrs. Sweetly's risk factors for diabetes?
2. Can you make the diagnosis of diabetes at this time?
3. What additional laboratory tests would you order?

PREVALENCE AND IMPACT

Glucose tolerance and diagnosed diabetes mellitus (DM) increase in prevalence with age. In the past 20 years, the increase in DM in the elderly far outpaces all other age groups (Fig. 40-1). In 2002, the prevalence of cases of diagnosed DM in patients aged 65 to 74 (16.8%) was almost 14 times that in patients under 45 (1.2%).[1] This increase largely parallels the U.S. "obesity epidemic." The prevalence of DM is greater in nonwhites (Fig. 40-2). About 20 million people in

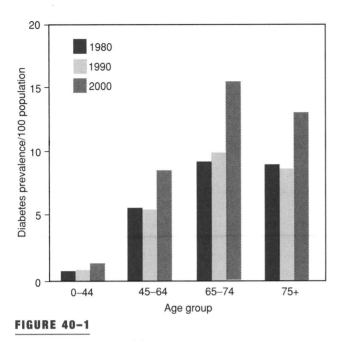

FIGURE 40–1

Increasing prevalence of diabetes.

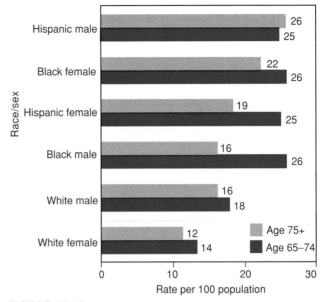

FIGURE 40–2

Race and sex and diabetes in older Americans, 2002.

the United States have prediabetes; most will develop type 2 DM within 10 years; according to the American Diabetes Association (ADA), DM in persons over the age of 65 is projected to increase by 56% between 2002 and 2020.[2]

Over half of direct medical expenditures on diabetes are for those persons over 65. One dollar in $10 spent on health care in the United States in 2002 was for diabetes. Nineteen percent of personal health care expenditures in the United States are for DM, although only 4.2% of the U.S. population are known to have diabetes. Adjusting for age, sex, and race/ethnicity, people with diabetes had medical expenditures 2.4 times higher than those without diabetes.[2]

The life expectancy at birth of people with diabetes was 64.7 and 70.7 years for men and women compared with 77.5 and 81.4 years without diabetes in a 2004 Ontario study.[3] A British study of persons over 85 found that only 32% of the remaining life of persons with diabetes was active, whereas it was 42% for those without diabetes.[4]

> ● Over half of direct medical expenditures on diabetes are for those persons over 65.

RISK FACTORS AND PATHOPHYSIOLOGY

There is a progressive continuum from the asymptomatic prediabetic state, with insulin resistance, through mild postprandial hyperglycemia and/or mild fasting hyperglycemia, to diagnosable type 2 diabetes (Table 40-1). Three basic metabolic defects characterize type 2 diabetes: insulin resistance, nonautoimmune β-cell dysfunction and inappropriately increased hepatic glucose production (HGP). The latter two may represent physiological phenotypes predisposed to diabetes.[5]

Adults from age 50 to 80 have no significant change in fasting glucose, whereas the postprandial blood glucose rises with age.[6] The progression from prediabetes begins with insulin resistance (resistance to the function of insulin of promoting the uptake of glucose by skeletal muscle and fat cells). At first, the pancreatic β cell compensates by secreting more insulin (compensatory hyperinsulinemia). These two changes, plus mild postprandial hyperglycemia characterize impaired glucose tolerance (IGT). Over time, the β cells begin to fail and insulin secretion declines. The inhibitory effect of insulin on HGP decreases and increased fasting hyperglycemia (IFG) develops. Further progression of DM involves absolute insulin deficiency, requiring insulin therapy.

DIFFERENTIAL DIAGNOSIS AND ASSESSMENT

Atypical or asymptomatic elders account in part for the up to 30% of undiagnosed elders with diabetes. They do *not* present with the "3 P's" (polyphagia, polydipsia, polyuria) (Table 40-2). The renal threshold for glucose increases with age, so glycosuria may not

Table 40–1	Risk Factors for Diabetes
Age	Age >65 increases risk of abnormal 2-hour postprandial glucose
Obesity	Body mass index >25 kg/m^2
Waist circumference	Men >102 cm, women >88 cm
Family history	First-degree relative
Race/ethnic population	Hispanic, black, Native American, Asian
History of gestational diabetes	Or having delivered a baby >9 pounds
Polycystic ovary syndrome (PCOS)	Elevated androgens, oligo/amenorrhea, and/or ovarian cysts
Dyslipidemia	HDL<35 mg/dl or triglycerides >250 mg/dl
Hypertension	BP ≥140/90 mm Hg
Vascular disease	History of MI, CVA, PVD
Endocrinopathies	Cushing's, acanthosis nigrans, acromegaly, pheochromocytoma, hyperthyroidism
Medications	Corticosteroids, thiazides, nicotinic acid, phenytoin
Diseases of exocrine pancreas	Pancreatitis, cystic fibrosis, neoplasia, hemochromatosis

HDL indicates high-density lipoprotein; BP, blood pressure; MI, myocardial infarction; CVA, cerebrovascular accident; and PVD, peripheral vascular disease.

From American Diabetes Association. Diagnosis and classification of diabetes mellitus. Mel Diabetes Care 2005;28:S37-S42.

occur.[7] Polydipsia can be absent; presentation in the elderly may be dehydration with altered thirst perception and delayed fluid supplementation. Polyuria can present as incontinence. More often, changes such as dry eyes, dry mouth, confusion, incontinence, or diabetic complications are the presentation.[8] Weight loss or hyperosmolar nonketotic coma (HONKC) are *occasional* presentations in the elderly. The common age-associated syndromes of persistent pain, urinary incontinence, cognitive impairment, depression, injurious falls, and polypharmacy are all increased in persons with diabetes, and so they are often the presenting problem. Conversely, all elderly diabetics should be screened for these common syndromes within 3 to 6 months of diagnosis.[9]

The laboratory diagnosis, similar to the pathophysiology, involves a continuum from prediabetes to the "diabetic threshold." The fasting blood glucose (FBS) is the preferred test to screen for prediabetes and diabetes (Table 40-3). It is easily available, and has a 95% confidence interval (±18%) when performed on fasting venous plasma glucose samples.[10] The elderly should be screened annually; however, up to 30% of the diabetic elderly have an FBS of less than 126 mg/dl yet have a 2-hour oral glucose tolerance test (OGTT) of more than 200 mg/dl.[11] The vast majority of those who meet the OGTT criteria for diabetes, but not the FBS criteria, will have an HbA$_1$C less than 7.0%, so the HbA$_1$C is still not recommended for diagnosis.[12]

Assessment of elderly diabetics is multisystemic and multidisciplinary, focusing on the complications: (1) macrovascular complications of coronary, carotid, and peripheral atherosclerosis (ask about transient neurologic symptoms, syncope, chest pain often atypical, exer-

Table 40–2	Differential Diagnosis of Elevated Blood Glucose
Venous Plasma Glucose	**Diagnosis**
FBS 100 to 125 mg/dl	IFG (impaired fasting glucose)
FBS ≥126 mg/dl on two separate occasions	Diabetes mellitus
2-Hour 140 to 199 mg/dl during 75 g OGTT	IGT (impaired glucose tolerance)
2-Hour ≥200 mg/dl during 75 g OGTT	Diabetes mellitus
Casual BS ≥200 mg/dl + diabetes symptoms	Diabetes mellitus

FBS indicates fasting blood sugar; IFG, impaired fasting glucose; OGTT, oral glucose tolerance test; IGT, impaired glucose tolerance; and BS, blood sugar.

From American Diabetes Association. Diagnosis and classification of diabetes mellitus. Mel Diabetes Care 2005;28:S37-S42.

Table 40–3	Fasting Blood Glucose as a Screening Test for Diabetes Mellitus		
Venous Plasma Blood Glucose	**Sensitivity**	**Specificity**	**+ Predictive Value**
FBS ≥126 mg/dl			
Age 50 to 64	60	99	60
Age 65 to 79	40	99	80

From Blunt BA, Barrett-Conner E, Wingard DL. Evaluation of fasting plasma glucose as screening test for NIDDM in older adults. Diabetes Care 1991;14:989-993.

tional dyspnea or fatigue, and claudication), and lipid profile and liver function tests and electrocardiogram are appropriate; (2) microvascular renal complications are assessed by urinalysis, urinary microalbumin, and serum creatinine; (3) retinal complications require an ophthalmologist for dilated retinal examination; (4) foot complications and vulnerability are best assessed by a podiatrist, especially in patients presenting with neuropathy or foot ulcers; (5) screening for mood and cognition should be considered annually (increased depression and dementia); (6) HbA$_1$C should be assessed at the time of diagnosis and every 3 to 6 months thereafter because average blood glucose levels and microvascular complications are significantly related.

All diabetics should be referred for teaching. Certified diabetic educators (CDEs) are nurses, pharmacists, or dietitians who have passed a comprehensive national examination and can instruct patients about nutrition, home glucose monitoring, recognition and prevention of hypoglycemia, and other complications. CDEs are central to the health care team; they develop great insight into their patients' functional capacity and compliance (most elderly diabetics require several drugs). Lastly, older persons with diabetes need annual assessment of pneumococcal and influenza immunization status.

Case Discussion

Maria Sweetly has multiple risk factors for DM, including age over 65, Hispanic descent, body mass index greater than 25, hypertension, and use of a thiazide diuretic. Her physical examination and history are compatible with peripheral neuropathy, and diabetes is a leading cause of peripheral neuropathy in the elderly. Other nondiabetic considerations that cause peripheral neuropathy are metabolic disorders (e.g., thyroid, azotemia, vitamin B$_{12}$ deficiency), alcohol and other toxins, iatrogenic illness (e.g., isoniazid, chemotherapy, HIV drugs), infections (e.g., HIV), and malignancy (e.g., bronchogenic carcinoma).[20] Although a single fasting plasma glucose of 130 exceeds the 126 mg/dl threshold for "diabetes," the World Health Organization and ADA require two fasting plasma glucose levels equal or exceeding 126 mg/dl in order to establish the diagnosis of DM. Additional laboratory tests to consider would be a lipid panel, HbA$_1$C, urinalysis, and urine microalbumin. Should the repeat FBS be less than 126 mg/dl, then a 75-g, 2-hour OGTT would be in order. A 2-hour value of 200 mg/dl or more

or a random (also called a casual) blood sugar of 200 mg/dl or more with diabetic symptoms would be sufficient to formally diagnose DM. Mrs. Sweetly has presented her diabetes with one of the six common geriatric syndromes seen in diabetics, namely, persistent pain. Diabetics should be screened for pain, cognitive decline, depression, injurious falls, urinary incontinence, and polypharmacy. Diabetes is also a recognized risk factor for osteoporosis.[22]

Maria Sweetly, *Part 2*

A repeat FBS was 127 mg/dl, and her HbA$_1$C was 8.9; total cholesterol was 205 mg/dl, triglycerides 250 mg/dl, high-density lipoprotein (HDL) 34 mg/dl, low-density lipoprotein (LDL) 121 mg/dl, and urine microalbumin 40 mg/L.

STUDY QUESTIONS

1. What treatment goals should you establish for her?
2. What changes would you make in her medications?

MANAGEMENT

Goals of therapy for an elderly patient with diabetes often differ from goals for younger people. Life expectancy, other medical conditions, and the patient's willingness and ability to comply with treatment are important factors. Elderly patients range from limited cognitive and/or physical functioning to others who are much more active. Patient goals should be documented and reassessed regularly.

Quality of life is an important issue in any elderly patient. Aggressive treatment plans may not be reasonable (complicated, costly, uncomfortable side effects).

Control of *cardiovascular risk factors* may induce greater reductions in morbidity and mortality than does hyperglycemia control. For example, the effects of blood pressure and lipid control can be seen after 2 to 3 years, whereas up to 8 years are needed before beneficial effects of glycemic control reduce long-term complications.[9]

Some *goals* for elderly diabetic patients include (1) prevention of hypoglycemia and hyperglycemia and associated symptoms; (2) decreased morbidity from microvascular and macrovascular complications; (3) maintenance or improvement in general health and quality of life; and (4) reduction or prevention of medication side effects.

● Quality of life is an important issue in any elderly patient; aggressive treatment plans may not be reasonable.

Nonpharmacologic Therapy

Diet—Medical nutrition therapy (MNT) must be individualized by patient size and energy requirements. Carbohydrate intake remains key to glycemic control. Extremely low carbohydrate diets (less than 130g per day) are not recommended as carbohydrates are important for energy, water-soluble vitamins and minerals, and fiber. In fact, 45% to 65% of daily calories should be carbohydrates. Moderate reduction in caloric intake in overweight patients results in weight loss of 1 to 2 pounds per week. Weight loss diets should supply a minimum 1,000 to 1,200 kcal/day for women and 1,200 to 1,600 kcal/day for men.[13]

Exercise—Physical activity improves insulin sensitivity, glycemic control, and selected risk factors for cardiovascular disease (hypertension, dyslipidemia), and decreases the risk of coronary artery disease. In elderly patients with decreased functionality, an evaluation screening for macro- and microvascular complications that may be worsened by physical activity should first be performed.[14]

Pharmacologic Therapy

Simple, inexpensive medication and monitoring regimens which maximize compliance are recommended, started at the lowest dose and titrated gradually to targets or side effects.

Sulfonylureas—First-generation agents include chlorpropamide (Diabinese), tolazamide (Tolinase), and tolbutamide (Tol-Tab) and (specifically, chlorpropamide) should be avoided (long half-life and increased hypoglycemia). Second-generation agents include glimepiride (Amaryl), glyburide (DiaBeta, Micronase), and glipizide (Glucotrol). Sulfonylureas stimulate insulin release from the pancreas, reduce glucose output from the liver, and increase insulin sensitivity peripherally. Patients should be educated about hypoglycemia, a dangerous side effect (diaphoresis, rapid heart rate, shaking, and nausea).

Biguanides—Metformin (Glucophage) is used as monotherapy in type 2 DM, or concomitantly with a sulfonylurea, insulin, or other oral agents. It decreases HGP and intestinal absorption of glucose, improving insulin sensitivity. As monotherapy, it typically does not cause hypoglycemia or long-term weight gain—the only oral diabetic agent to not do so. Older diabetic patients with reduced renal function (serum creatinine greater than 1.4mg/dl in women, or 1.5mg/dl in men) should not use metformin due to

risk of lactic acidosis. Older patients on metformin should have creatinine checks at least annually and with dose increases. Patients over 80 with reduced muscle mass should have creatinine clearance measured.[9] Maximum doses of metformin are not generally used in the elderly. Metformin should be discontinued in situations of potential hypoxemia (cardiovascular collapse, respiratory failure, acute myocardial infarction, septicemia), because lactic acidosis is a rare, potentially severe consequence. It should be avoided in impaired liver function, congestive heart failure, and metabolic acidosis and withheld before X-rays, and the renal function reevaluated after.

Thiazolidinediones—Pioglitazone (Actos) and rosiglitazone (Avandia) are indicated as monotherapy in type 2 diabetes as an adjunct to diet and exercise. They may be used with a sulfonylurea, metformin, or insulin. They lower glucose by improving target cell response to insulin, without increasing pancreatic insulin secretion; thus they require insulin for activity. When used as monotherapy, they generally do not cause hypoglycemia. Liver functions should be monitored; exercise caution with active liver disease. Class III or IV heart failure is a contraindication because of potential fluid retention.

Meglitinides—Repaglinide (Prandin) and nateglinide (Starlix) are indicated in type 2 diabetes as monotherapy when hyperglycemia cannot be managed by diet and exercise alone or in combination with metformin or a thiazolidinedione in patients whose hyperglycemia cannot be controlled by exercise, diet, or a single agent. There is no added benefit with sulfonylureas. They stimulate insulin release from the pancreas, reducing postprandial hyperglycemia.

Alpha-glucosidase inhibitors—Acarbose (Precose) and miglitol (Glyset) can be used as monotherapy, as an adjunct to diet and exercise or in combination with a sulfonylurea, metformin, or insulin. They reversibly inhibit intestinal alpha-glucosidases, resulting in delayed glucose absorption and lowering postprandial hyperglycemia. Flatulence and diarrhea are common; these side effects usually return to pretreatment levels with continued use. They are not recommended if the serum creatinine is more than 2 mg/dl and are contraindicated in diabetic ketoacidosis, cirrhosis, and many intestinal diseases.

Combination products—Combinations (of metformin and thiazolidimediones; metformin and sulfonylureas; and thiazolidimediones and sulfonylureas) may reduce patient "pill counts" and increase compliance.

Insulin—It is indicated for diabetes that has been unresponsive to treatment with diet and/or oral hypoglycemic agents, but initiation of insulin in elderly type 2 diabetes should involve a multidisciplinary team. It is often begun at a 10- to 15-unit dose, and as

Table 40–4	Pharmacokinetics of Common Insulin Preparations			
Class	Drug	Onset (hourrs)	Peak (hourrs)	Duration (hourrs)
Rapid acting	Humalog, Novolog, Apidra	0.25	0.5 to 3	2 to 5
Short acting	Humulin R, Novolin R	0.5 to 1	2 to 3	8 to 12
Intermediate acting	Humalog Mix 75/25, Humalog Mix 70/30	0.25	0.5 to 4	24
	Humulin 70/30, Novolin 70/30	0.5	4 to 8	24
	Humulin L, Novolin L	1 to 2.5	8 to 12	18 to 24
	Humulin N, Novolin N	1 to 1.5	4 to 12	24
Long acting	Humulin U	4 to 8	16 to 18	36
	Lantus	5	—	24+

glucose control is achieved, some of the patient's multiple oral diabetic medications can be withdrawn (see Table 40-4).

Case Discussion

The additional laboratory studies indeed confirm your suspicion of DM and suggest hyperlipidemia and the presence of her diabetes for at least 2 to 3 months. Mutual goal setting would be desirable, and because Mrs. Sweetly is otherwise healthy and presumably has good functional capacity, it would be reasonable to aim for blood pressures below 140/80 mm Hg or, if tolerated, below 130/80 mm Hg. A low-dose angiotensin-converting enzyme (ACE) inhibitor would be preferred because of her diabetes with microalbuminuria. There is no imperative to stop her HCTZ or beta-blocker, as multiple drug regimens are typically needed to achieve target blood pressure in diabetics. The theoretical problems with exacerbation of glucose intolerance with thiazides and the masking of hypoglycemic symptoms with beta-blockers are rarely clinically significant, especially in this patient's low doses. It is reasonable to set a goal of getting her HbA_1C down below 7%, and for her total cholesterol to be below 200, triglycerides below 150, HDL above 45, and LDL below 100. We can wait a few months to see if diet, exercise, and improved glycemic control are able to bring the lipids to goal before recommending lipid-lowering drugs, but it may be prudent to educate her that diabetics often require lipid-lowering agents to accomplish lipids low enough to prevent macrovascular complications such as myocardial infarction and stroke. Individualized MNT and diabetic education will be ordered, and self glucose testing can be recommended. Should this prove ineffective after several months, then oral agents would be indicated. Metformin is a good choice because it is typically associated with weight loss and is the only oral agent proven to prevent macrovascular complications.

Maria Sweetly, *Part 3*

Twelve weeks later she has substantial relief from her foot discomfort, and her blood pressure is 130/78 mm Hg on low-dose ACE inhibitor, HCTZ, and metoprolol. Her HbA_1C is 7.5 on metformin and glipizide, but she is having several symptomatic hypoglycemic episodes a week. This occurs despite FBSs in the 110 to 130 mg/dl range.

STUDY QUESTIONS

1. What changes in her therapy should be made?
2. What other measures can you recommend to reduce the macrovascular complications of coronary artery disease?

Long-Term Management Guidelines

Table 40-5 summarizes the quality and strength of evidence (see symbols IB etc. below).

Aspirin—Heart disease is the leading cause of diabetes-related deaths; patients with diabetes have a two to four times higher risk of heart disease–related death or stroke.[15] Studies show up to a 30% decrease in myocardial infarction and 20% in stroke in a wide variety of patients using aspirin.[16] It is recommended (in doses of 81 to 325 mg/day; IB)[9] for both primary and secondary prevention of cardiovascular events in older adults with diabetes who are without contraindications and on no other anticoagulant therapy.

Table 40–5 American Geriatrics Society Recommendations and Strength of Evidence: Diabetic Management

Indication	Comment	Evidence Level
Aspirin use	81 to 325 mg daily if no contraindications	IB
Smoking cessation	Assess willingness to quit; offer counseling and drug therapy interventions	IIA
HTN management	<140/80 mm Hg if tolerated	IA
	<130/80 mm Hg may provide additional benefit	IIA
	Gradual reduction in BP preferred	IIIA
	Interventions within 3 months when SBP is 140 to 160 or DBP 90 to 100; or within 1 month if BP >160/100 mm Hg	IIIB
	Test renal function and potassium levels within 1 to 2 weeks of initiation, with each dose increase and at least yearly in patients using ACE inhibitors	IIIA
	Test electrolytes within 12 weeks of initiation, with each dose increase and at least yearly in patients using thiazide or loop diuretics	IIIA
Glycemic control	A_1C <7% in patients with good functional status	IIIB
	A_1C <8% in patients with a life expectancy of less than 5 years or in situations when the risk of intensive glycemic control does not appear to outweigh the benefit	IIIB
	Patients who are stable at A_1C goal: check every 12 months	IIIB
	Patients not at A_1C goal: check every 6 months or as necessary	IIIB
	Self-monitoring of blood glucose schedule should be considered depending on functional and cognitive status, goals of care, A_1C and risk for hypoglycemia	IIIB
	Referral to diabetes educator or endocrinologist in patients with severe hypoglycemia	IIB
	Chlorpropamide should not be used	IIA
	Metformin should not be used in patients with creatinine ≥1.5 mg/dl in males and ≥1.4 mg/dl in females	IIB
	When metformin is used, check creatinine at least annually	IIB
Lipid Management	Correct lipid abnormalities if feasible	IA
	Recheck lipids every 2 years if LDL in ≤100 mg/dl	IIIB
	Recheck lipids annually if LDL 100 to 129 mg/dl and institute MNT and physical activity If not at goal in 6 months, institute drug therapy if feasible	IIIB
	Recheck lipids at least annually if LDL ≥130mg/dl. Drug therapy and lifestyle modifications should be instituted	IIIB
	Check LFTs within 12 weeks of initiation of niacin or a statin or if the dose is changed	IIIB
	Annual LFTs when taking a fibrate	IIIB
Eye care	New-onset DM: initial screening dilated-eye exam	IB
	Elderly patient with DM:	
	Dilated-eye exam annually in patients at high risk for eye disease	IIB
	Dilated-eye exam every 2 years in patients with lower risk of eye disease	IIB
Foot care	Comprehensive foot exam at least once a year or more frequently if specific foot conditions are present	IIIA
Nephropathy	Microalbumin test at diagnosis and annually thereafter in the absence of previously demonstrated macro- or microalbuminuria	IIIA
Diabetes education	Education about hypoglycemia should be given at diagnosis and periodically thereafter	IA
	Glucose monitoring technique should be routinely reviewed	IIIB
	Evaluate patient level of activity and educate on benefit of physical activity	IA
	Evaluate nutritional status and provide appropriate MNT	IA
	Education should be given when any new medication is prescribed (i.e., purpose, how to take, side effects, etc.)	IIIA
	Education should be provided about risk factors for foot ulcers	IB

HTN indicates hypertension; BP, blood pressure; SBP, systolic blood pressure; DBP, diastolic blood pressure; ACE, angiotensin-converting enzyme; LDL, low-density lipoprotein; MNT, medical nutrition therapy; LFT, liver function test; DM, diabetes mellitus.

Note: In this table, the following nomenclature is used for quality and strength of evidence

Quality of evidence

Level I Evidence from at least one properly designed randomized, controlled trial

Level II Evidence from at least one well-designed clinical trial without randomization, from cohort, from multiple time-series studies, or from dramatic results in uncontrolled experiments

Level III Evidence from respected authorities, based on clinical experience, descriptive studies, or reports of expert committee

Strength of evidence

A Good evidence to support the use of a recommendation; clinicians should do this all the time

B Moderate evidence to support the use of a recommendation; clinicians should do this most of the time

C Poor evidence to support or to reject the use of a recommendation; clinicians may or may not follow the recommendation

D Moderate evidence against the use of a recommendation; clinicians should not do this

E Good evidence against the use of a recommendation; clinicians should not do this

● Heart disease is the leading cause of diabetes-related deaths; patients with diabetes have a two to four times higher risk of heart disease–related death or stroke.

Smoking—This is the most important modifiable cause of premature death, associated with macrovascular, and microvascular complications.[16] Twelve percent of patients over age 65 smoke.[9] If an older patient with diabetes quits smoking, the risk may drop to presmoking levels so all diabetic patients who smoke should be assessed for willingness and offered counseling and pharmacological interventions as appropriate (IIA).[9]

Hypertension Management—This is associated with stroke, coronary artery disease, peripheral vascular disease, retinopathy, nephropathy, and potentially neuropathy. Blood pressure control in diabetes is very important. A goal of less than 140/80 mm Hg is recommended if tolerated; lowering to less than 130/80 mm Hg may have extra benefit (IIA). Gradual reduction is preferred (IIIA). Systolic pressure should initially be lowered by no more than 20 mm Hg; if this is well tolerated, further reduction is made. Patients with blood pressure greater than 160/100 mm Hg should be offered pharmacological and behavioral interventions within 1 month (IIIB); with BP of 140 to 160/90 to 100 mm Hg, intervention should be within 3 months.[9]

ACE inhibitors and angiotensin receptor blocking agents (ARBs) are preferred in diabetic hypertension because of their efficacy in lowering blood pressure and slowing the progression of proteinuria and nephropathy. Diabetes is not a barrier to the use of beta-blockers for hypertension and for cardioprotection in myocardial infarction or in hypertensive patients with diabetes with congestive heart failure. There is little evidence to justify withholding beta-blockers from diabetic patients because of metabolic concerns or fears of "masking" hypoglycemia.[17]

Because ACE inhibitor and ARB are associated with renal impairment and hyperkalemia, renal function and serum potassium should be tested within 1 to 2 weeks of starting the drugs, once a year, and at dose increases (IIIA).[9]

Thiazide diuretics have been associated with hypokalemia in the elderly; electrolytes should be checked within 1 to 2 weeks of starting, with dose increases, and once a year (IIIA).[9]

Self Monitoring of Blood Glucose—Frail, older patients with diabetes are more prone to hypoglycemia than are healthy older adults. Home self blood glucose monitoring should thus be considered; it has been shown to decrease the likelihood of hypoglycemia. Ability to self monitor depends on functional and cognitive status.

Patients with frequent or severe hypoglycemia may benefit from referral to a diabetes educator or endocrinologist, and should have more frequent contact with their primary clinician while therapy is being adjusted (IIB).[9] Hb A_1C goals should be individualized: with good functional status and a longer life expectancy, 7% or less is appropriate (IIIB). Short-term studies of adults 30 to 85 years who lowered their HbA_1C from 9.3% to 7.5% showed improved vitality, cognitive functioning, sleep, and depression.[18] A goal of 8% is appropriate with a life expectancy of less than 5 years or where the risk of hypoglycemia is a factor (IIIB).[9] Patients who have met their HbA1C goal and remain stable should be tested annually; before the HbAIC goal is met, it should be tested at least every 6 months (IIIB).[9]

Hyperlipidemia—Higher rates of cardiovascular disease in type 2 diabetes is in part due to lipid abnormalities.[10] Lowering LDL and triglycerides, and raising HDL, have been shown to reduce macrovascular disease and mortality in the diabetic population, especially in patients who have had a prior cardiovascular event.[10] Efforts should be made to correct lipid abnormalities after the patient's overall health status has been considered (IA).[9]

A lipid profile should be checked at least every 2 years in an older patient with DM and an LDL of 100 mg/dl or less, and at least annually in a patient with DM and an LDL between 100 and 129 mg/dl. MNT and increased physical activity are recommended at that time. If an LDL of less than 100 mg/dl is not achieved within 6 months, then drug therapy should be initiated (IIIB).[9] Lipid therapy should be checked at least annually for patients with an LDL of more than 130 mg/dl and drug therapy and lifestyle modifications should be initiated (IIIB).[9]

Goals for HDL and triglycerides in older patients are consistent with the ADA recommendations of HDL greater than 40 mg/dl and triglycerides less than 150 mg/dl. In patients with near normal LDL and low HDL or elevated triglycerides, fibrate therapy should be considered in addition to MNT.[9]

Eye Care—Diabetic retinopathy is the most frequent cause of new cases of blindness among adults age 20 to 74 years.[10] The incidence of retinopathy is associated with the glycemic control over the past 6 years and elevated blood pressure; progression of retinopathy is linked to older age, male sex, and hyperglycemia.[9] Early detection and treatment of diabetic retinopathy is paramount.

Elderly patients with new-onset diabetes should have an initial screening, dilated-eye examination performed by an eye-care specialist (IB)[9] and a dilated-eye examination annually if they are at high risk for eye disease, for example, those with symptoms of retinopathy, glaucoma, or cataracts, HbA_1C greater than 8%, type 1 DM, or blood pressure greater than 140/80 mm Hg. At lower risk, the dilated-eye examination can be every 2 years (IIB).[9]

Foot Care—Diabetic neuropathy is a microvascular complication of diabetes that can lead to foot ulcerations and even lower-limb amputation. Early recognition and management is key. At highest risk are persons with diabetes for more than 10 years, males, those with poor glycemic control, or those with cardiovascular, retinal, or renal complications.[10]

Patients should be educated on proper foot care and have a comprehensive foot examination at least once a year, more frequently if problems are already present (IIIA).[9]

Nephropathy—Diabetic nephropathy is the leading cause of end-stage renal disease; it occurs in 20% to 40% of patients with diabetes.[10] In the absence of previously demonstrated macro- or microalbuminuria, an annual microalbumin screening test should be performed (IIIA); it should also be done at the time of diagnosis of type 2 diabetes (IIIA).[9]

Blood pressure and glucose control will slow the progression of nephropathy. ACE inhibitors delay the progression from micro- to macroalbuminuria and can slow the decline in the glomerular filtration rate in patients with macroalbuminuria.[10]

Neuropathies—Peripheral neuropathy from diabetes affects up to 50% of older type 2 diabetic patients. Presentation is as an acute painful sensation, gradual onset numbness, or an asymptomatic foot ulcer. The monofilament pressure perception test, Achilles reflex, and 128-Hz tuning forks are useful in the physical diagnosis of this. Low-dose tricyclics, anticonvulsants, and lidocaine patches—but mostly improved glycemic control—are effective therapies. Podiatry consultation for footwear, physical therapy consultation for gait training, possible nerve stimulation, and even acupuncture modalities may be considered.[19] Peripheral neuropathy and orthostatic hypotension from autonomic neuropathy contribute to falling and to urinary incontinence.

Cognition—Hyperinsulinemia is directly related to declined memory-related cognitive scores; the risk of Alzheimer's dementia directly attributable to hyperinsulinemia or diabetes is as high as 39%.[20] However, whether glycemic control would lessen cognitive decline is speculative at present.

Diabetes Education—Elderly patients, as well as their caregivers, should complete comprehensive diabetes self-management education (DSME). It is a covered benefit under Medicare Part B.[10]

Patients should be advised that home self blood glucose monitoring, when appropriate, has been associated with improved glycemic control. Monitoring technique should be routinely reviewed as functional ability may change (IIIB).[9]

Education on medication use is vital; package inserts are often written in small print or on poor-quality paper. Language and health literacy may also be barriers to obtaining important information about medications. One study in older patients showed that 39% of patients stated that they could not read their medication labels, and 67% did not fully understand the labels.[9]

Physical activity combined with nutritional education can reduce weight and enhance blood pressure, lipids, and glycemic control.

Risk factors for foot ulcers and amputation should be provided (IB).[9] Older adults may have cognitive and visual impairment, which can limit their ability to properly evaluate their feet on a regular basis. Patient education on foot care in middle-age and older adults reduced rates of serious foot lesions and foot amputations. Recognition of hypo- and hyperglycemia symptoms significantly improves glycemic control and adherence to medication regimens.

> ● Language and health literacy may also be barriers to obtaining important information about medications.

Case Discussion

Mrs. Sweetly is having repeated hypoglycemia despite an ideal-looking fasting blood sugar and a HbA_1C that is still above 7%. Factors that predispose the elderly to hypoglycemia are poor or erratic nutritional intake, polypharmacy and noncompliance with medications, changes in mental status that impair the perception or response to hypoglycemia, and dependence or isolation that limits receipt of early treatment for hypoglycemia. Metformin as a sole agent should not be causing hypoglycemia, and thus the glipizide is the likely culprit if none of the factors above are involved. The glipizide should be discontinued, and a trial of another oral agent may be in order. More overall morbidity and mortality will be prevented by achieving the blood pressure and lipid targets, which have a greater impact on cardiovascular events, than does glycemic control, which is a more powerful influencer on microvascular complications. Keeping Mrs. Sweetly a nonsmoker and prescribing daily aspirin 81 mg are powerful componentsto her macrovascular complication prevention plan that are too often neglected.

SUMMARY

The elderly have an increased incidence of diabetes and should be screened yearly for DM with a fasting venous plasma glucose level. Diabetes presents atypically in the older individual. Upon diagnosis of diabetes or the pre-diabetes states of IFG and IGT, diabetic education, diet, exercise, and weight loss are appropriate interventions. Treatment goals for diabetes must often be balanced with the patient's expected lifespan and tolerance of side effects. Efforts to reduce diabetes-related mortality should be focused on macrovascular/cardiac complications with discontinuation of smoking, control of hypertension, and optimizing the lipid profile. Tight glycemic control has more impact on the microvascular complications. Elderly diabetics are at particular risk for the geriatric syndromes of persistent pain, urinary incontinence, cognitive impairment, depression, injurious falls, and polypharmacy and should be screened for these syndromes within 3 to 6 months of initial diagnosis and regularly thereafter. Our nationwide success in delivering quality care to diabetic adults by commonly accepted guidelines is currently less than 50%.[21] Only through multidisciplinary efforts, including the geriatrics clinician, diabetic educators, podiatrists, ophthalmologists, and pharmacists, will we truly optimize care of the elderly diabetic, reduce mortality, and preserve functional capacity.

POSTTEST

1. The preferred screening test for diabetes in the elderly is:
   a. OGTT every 3 years
   b. FBS every 3 to 5 years
   c. OGTT every year
   d. FBS every year

2. An elderly patient with diabetes should not use metformin if their serum creatinine is greater than:
   a. 0.9 mg/dl in females and 1.2 mg/dl in males
   b. 1.2 mg/dl in both males and females
   c. 1.4 mg/dl in females and 1.5 mg/dl in males
   d. 1.5 mg/dl in females and 2.0 mg/dl in males

3. The goal LDL in an elderly patient with diabetes is:
   a. Less than 100 mg/dl
   b. Less than 130 mg/dl
   c. Less than 160 mg/dl
   d. Less than 190 mg/dl

4. The *primary* mechanism of action of metformin is:
   a. Stimulation of insulin release from the pancreatic β cell
   b. Reversible inhibition of membrane-bound intestinal alpha-glucosidases, whichresults in delayed glucose absorption
   c. Decreased HGP (hepatic glucose production)
   d. Reduced target cell response to insulin

References

1. CDC National Center for Chronic Disease Prevention and Health Promotion: Diabetes Surveillance System, Data and Trends. http://www.cdc.gov/ diabetes/statistics/prev/national/figbyage.htm.
2. Hogan P, Dall T, Nikolov P: Economic costs of diabetes in the US in 2002. Diabetes Care 2003;26:917-932.
3. Manuel DG, Schultz SE. Health-related quality of life and health-adjusted life expectancy of people with diabetes in Ontario, Canada, 1996-1997. Diabetes Care 2004;27:407-414.
4. Jagger C, Goyder E, Clarke M, et al. Active life expectancy in people with and without diabetes. J Public Health Med 2003;25:42-46.
5. Meigs, JB, Muller DC, Nathan DM, et al. Baltimore Longitudinal Study of Aging: the natural history of progression from normal glucose tolerance to type 2 diabetes in the Baltimore Longitudinal Study of Aging. Diabetes 2003;52: 1475-1484.
6. Blunt BA, Barrett-Conner E, Wingard DL. Evaluation of fasting plasma glucose as screening test for NIDDM in older adults. Diabetes Care 1991;14:989-993.
7. Meneilly GS. Diabetes. In Oxford Textbook of Geriatric Medicine, 2 ed. (Evans JG, Williams TF, Beattie BL et al. eds.). New York: Oxford University Press, 2000.
8. Chau DL, Shumaker N, Plodkowski RA. Complications of type 2 diabetes in the elderly. Geriatric Times 2003;4.
9. California Healthcare Foundation/American Geriatrics Society Panel on Improving Care for Elders with Diabetes. Guidelines for improving the care of the older person with diabetes mellitus. J Am Geriatr Soc 2003;51:S265-S280.
10. Sachs DB, Bruns DE, Goldstein DE, et al. Guidelines and recommendations for laboratory analysis in the diagnosis and management of diabetes mellitus. Clin Chem 2002;48:436-472.
11. DECODE Study Group. Age- and sex-specific prevalences of diabetes and impaired glucose regulation in 13 European cohorts. Diabetes Care 2002; 26: 61-9.
12. American Diabetes Association. Diagnosis and classification of diabetes mellitus. Mel Diabetes Care 2005;28:S37-S42.
13. American Diabetes Association. Clinical practice recommendations: standards in medical care in diabetes. Diabetes Care 2005;28:S4-S36.
14. Zinman B, Ruderman N, Campaigne BN, et al. Physical activity/exercise and diabetes, Diabetes Care 2004;27:S58-S36.
15. American Diabetes Association. Diabetes for Seniors. http://diabetes.org/diabetes-statistics/seniors.
16. American Diabetes Association. Clinical practice recommendations. Diabetes Care 2004;27:S1-S143.
17. Shorr RI, Ray WA, Daugherty J, et al. Antihypertensives and the risk of serious hypoglycemia in older persons using insulin or sulfonureas. JAMA 1997;278:40-43.
18. Testa MA, Simonson DC. Health economic benefits and quality of life during improved glycemic control in patients with type 2 diabetes mellitus. JAMA 1998;280:1490-1496.
19. Boulton AJ. Management of diabetic peripheral neuropathy. Clin Diabetes 2005;23:9-15.

20. Luchsinger JA, Tang MX, Shea S, et al. Hyperinsulinemia and risk of Alzheimer disease, Neurology 2004;63:1187-1192.
21. McGlynn EA, Asch SM, Adams J, et al. The quality of health care delivered to adults in the United States. New Engl J Med 2003;348:2635-2645.
22. Brown SA, Sharpless JL. Osteoporosis: an underappreciated complication of diabetes. Clin Diabetes 2004;22:10-20.

Web Resources

1. CDC National Diabetes Education Program, http://www.cdc.gov/diabetes/ndep/.
2. American Diabetes Educators, http://www.diabeteseducator.org/.
3. American Diabetes Association http://www.diabetes.org/home.jsp.

PRETEST ANSWERS

1. b
2. a
3. b
4. d

POSTTEST ANSWERS

1. d
2. c
3. a
4. c

Thyroid Disorders

James W. Campbell

OBJECTIVES

Upon completion of this chapter, the reader will be able to:

- Describe the presentations of hypothyroidism in an elderly population.

- Describe the presentations of hyperthyroidism in an elderly population.
- Define the euthyroid sick syndrome.
- Understand the risks and benefits of thyroid replacement therapy in an elderly population.

PRETEST

1. The most common presenting feature of hyperthyroidism in the elderly is:
   a. Exophthalmus
   b. Atrial fibrillation
   c. Tremor
   d. Heat intolerance

2. Hyperthyroidism is diagnosed with which of the following:
   a. A decreased serum level of thyroid-stimulating hormone (TSH) and an elevated serum level of unbound thyroxine (free T_4)
   b. A normal serum level of TSH and an elevated serum level of unbound thyroxine (free T_4)
   c. A elevated serum level of TSH and a decreased serum level of unbound thyroxine (free T_4)
   d. A normal serum level of TSH and a decreased serum level of unbound thyroxine (free T_4)

3. Which one of the following is correct about subclinical hypothyroidism?
   a. A diagnosis can be made with a TSH less than 0.01 in the presence of a normal serum level of unbound thyroxine (free T_4).
   b. The medication of choice is levothyroxine.
   c. It is commonly associated with a multinodular goiter.
   d. If untreated, there is no increase in morbidity unless clinical hypothyroidism supervenes.

PREVALENCE AND IMPACT

Prevalence

Evidence of hyperthyroidism has a prevalence rate as high as 2.7%.[1] Hypothyroidism, including subclinical hypothyroidism, has a prevalence rate as high as 20% in the elderly population.[1] The reported prevalence of hypothyroidism is three times higher among women than men.[1] Abnormal TSH values are found in as many as 40% of acutely ill elderly patients.[2] It is important to note that there is a debate regarding clinical significance of elevations of thyroid-stimulating hormone (TSH) in the elderly population, particularly among the oldest old. Controversy exists about issues as critical as whether having mild thyroid dysfunction may actually have an improved mortality among older persons.

| ● Abnormal TSH does not mean thyroid disease. |

Mary Peterson, *Part 1*

Mary Peterson is an 84-year-old new patient to your office who presents for a complete evaluation. Initial history is remarkable for mild cognitive impairment, dysthymia, fatigue, and decline in instrumental activity of daily living (IADL) function. Physical examination is remarkable for slowing of deep tendon responses, bradycardia, and slowing of mobility as assessed by the "get up and go" test.

STUDY QUESTION

1. What would be appropriate initial screening laboratory test(s)?

Impact

Thyroid dysfunction, in particular hypothyroidism, may have significant impact on the high rate of mental illness, particularly depression, among elderly persons. Thyroid dysfunction is also significantly related to lipid abnormalities, and lipid levels should be checked in all patients with thyroid underactivity; as well, thyroid activity should be checked in all patients with elevated cholesterol levels.[3] Thyroid disorders are more likely to go undiagnosed in patients over the age of 65 than in younger populations.[3] Hypothyroidism has been associated with a general slowing of mental and physical function, cold intolerance, weight gain, constipation, effects on blood pressure, and anemia. Although hyperthyroidism is associated with irregular heart rhythms, congestive heart failure, weight loss, and muscular weakness, these symptoms are common findings in numerous geriatric syndromes.[4]

> ● Thyroid dysfunction *must* be sought when evaluating depression (and other mental illness) in elders.

RISK FACTORS AND PATHOPHYSIOLOGY

With age the thyroid gland atrophies, fibrosis occurs, and there is accompanied lymphocytic infiltration as well as increasing colloid nodular production. Production of thyroxin (T_4) decreases with age; however, triiodothyronine (T_3) levels remain unchanged. It is felt that the decrease in T_4 is a compensatory mechanism for the decreased use of the hormone by peripheral tissues and is not a manifestation of primary thyroid disease.[5] The body's decreased use of thyroid hormone is felt to be related to a decline in lean body mass, including the metabolically active muscle, skin, bone, and viscera.

Mary Peterson, *Part 2*

Ms. Peterson is screened for thyroid dysfunction with a serum TSH, and this reveals a TSH of 38 µIU/ml. This was confirmed by a low T_4.

STUDY QUESTIONS

1. Is this patient a clear candidate for thyroid placement?
2. Is this patient likely to have other identifiable symptoms of hypothyroidism on further review?

Hypothyroidism

The most common etiology of hypothyroidism is previous Hashimoto's disease (a cell-mediated autoimmune inflammatory process with the presence potentially of four different types of thyroid-directed antibodies), irradiation, surgical removal of the thyroid gland, or idiopathic hypothyroidism. Less com-

mon causes include pituitary and hypothalamic disorders leading to TSH deficiencies or iodine-induced hypothyroidism most commonly from medical agents, medications including amiodarone, potassium iodide, lithium, anti-thyroid drugs, or radio contrast agents.[5] Populations at high risk of thyroid dysfunction include people with high levels of radiation exposure, the elderly, and people with Down syndrome.[6] People with diabetes are also felt to be at high risk of hypothyroid dysfunction.

See "Mary Peterson, Part 3: Case Discussion."

Hyperthyroidism

Hyperthyroidism is most likely due to Grave's disease with multinodular or uninodular active nodular goiter. Grave's disease is an auto-immune disorder with antibody formation to the TSH receptor and/or thyroid follicular cells. This antibody has TSH-like activity. Other etiologies include granulomatous or lymphocytic thyroiditis, in which there is leakage of thyroglobulin from the follicles. There are also iatrogenic sources of hyperthyroidism, including that induced by iodine or the use of amiodarone or from the overingestion of thyroid repletion agents.[5]

Thyroid Nodules/Thyroid Cancer

Prevalence of thyroid nodules increases with age. Radiation is a risk factor for thyroid cancer. However, in the very old if that exposure was greater than 50 years ago, there is no indication of higher risk of cancer.[5] Papillary thyroid cancer is more common in older adults, as is anaplastic carcinoma, the most fatal histologic type of thyroid carcinoma. Thyroid cancer represents 1.5% of all cancers in women and 0.5% of all cancers in men.[1]

DIFFERENTIAL DIAGNOSIS AND ASSESSMENT

Barbara Simpson

Barbara Simpson is an 80-year-old woman evaluated in your office for mild dysthymia. She has a history of hypertension, glaucoma, and osteoarthritis. She has recently lost her husband of 46 years. As part of your evaluation, you check serum TSH, which is 9.7 µIU/ml. You order a T_4 test, which is at the lower end of the normal range.

STUDY QUESTIONS

1. Is Ms. Simpson suffering from hypothyroidism?
2. Would Ms. Simpson benefit from thyroid replacement?

CASE DISCUSSION

Ms. Simpson most likely is suffering from bereavement. The low-normal T_4 and the relatively mild elevation of TSH are consistent with subclinical hypothyroidism, and many of these patients do not progress to clinical hypothyroidism. Exposing her to thyroid replacement may not be beneficial.

Subclinical Hypothyroidism

The syndrome of subclinical hypothyroidism is a relevant differential from symptomatic hypothyroidism in the elderly. Debate is currently ongoing regarding the benefits or possible risks of treating subclinical hypothyroidism. Subclinical hypothyroidism is defined by a normal serum-free T_4 level combined with an elevation of the TSH level. The transition from subclinical to overt hypothyroidism is not inevitable and may only occur in 5% to 8% of the population with subclinical hypothyroidism on an annual basis.[1] Levels of TSH above 10 μIU/ml are considered to be clearly abnormal and those between 5 μIU/ml and 10 μIU/ml are considered to be of uncertain significance in the absence of any symptoms or signs of hypothyroidism.[1] Two recent studies have indicated potential detrimental effects of treatment of subclinical hypothyroidism by actually shortening survival.[7,8]

Hypothyroidism

There are a multitude of relatively nonspecific symptoms of hypothyroidism (Box 41-1). It is important to note that elderly patients have significantly fewer symptoms with hypothyroidism than do their younger counterparts. The complaints are often subtle and vague. Likewise, it is also important to be sensitive to the risk of attributing hypothyroidism symptomatology to an age-biased view of normal aging. Clearly a high index of suspicion for hypothyroidism is indicated in evaluation of the geriatric patient.

Screening of the Asymptomatic Patient

The current recommendation for screening asymptomatic well elderly persons includes recommendations of the American Academy of Family Physicians and the American Association of Clinical Endocrinologists to measure thyroid function "periodically in all older women." The Canadian Task Force on Periodic Health Examination recommends maintaining a high index of clinical suspicion for nonspecific symptoms presenting with hypothyroidism (Box 41-2). The

---

Box 41-1	**Symptoms of Hypothyroidism**
Probably less common in elders.[14]	↓ Libido
Fatigue[a]	↓ Appetite
Weakness[a]	Arthralgias
Depression[a]	Confusion
Dry skin[a]	Constipation[*]
Significantly less common in elders.	Brittle nails
Weight gain[b]	Loss of hair
Cold intolerance[b]	Easy bruisability
Muscle cramps[b]	Low back discomfort
Parasthesias[b]	

American College of Physicians recommends screening women over the age of 50 with one or more general symptoms that could be caused by thyroid disease. The American Thyroid Association recommends screening in elderly patients and all patients with autoimmune disease or with a strong family history of thyroid disease.[12] The American Thyroid Association recommends screening every 5 years for persons over the age of 35. The American College of Physicians in 1998 recommended screening in women over the age of 50. The U.S. Preventive Services Task Force did not find enough evidence to recommend screening in asymptomatic elderly women; however, they advised a high index of suspicion of low threshold for checking thyroid function in the at risk population. Care must be used in the screening of patients who are otherwise ill, as a substantial portion will have abnormal thyroid function in the absence of true thyroid disease owing to euthyroid sick syndrome.[9-11]

Regarding screening for thyroid cancer, at this time there is no clearly defined screening mechanism that

---

Box 41-2	**Clinical Conditions with Clear Indication for Thyroid Dysfunction Screening**

Depression

Down syndrome

Postpartum depression

Women with family history of autoimmune disease

Hyperlipidemia

increases the benefit by providing early detection with significant differential treatment outcomes. Palpation of the thyroid gland remains part of good clinical practice and routine examination, although there is not high-quality evidence to conclude that regular neck palpation could have a major effect on the natural history of this infrequent cancer.[1]

> ● Ill patients may have the euthyroid sick syndrome: abnormal thyroid function, but *not* true thyroid disease.

Oscar Madison

Oscar Madison is a long-term patient of yours and presents for his routine physical and well-adult care update in the fall. In addition to requesting his flu vaccination, he reports the following nonspecific symptoms; slowed mentation, diarrhea, and weight loss. His daughter reports as well he has decreased appetite. On examination he has a blood pressure of 142/86 mm Hg, pulse 88, respiratory 20, and temperature 37.0°F. Testing reveals a mini-mental state examination (MMSE) of 22/30 and a global deterioration scale (GDS) of 5/15. The physical examination is otherwise unremarkable. Your evaluation includes a TSH of 0.2 µIU/ml and an elevated T_4 on repeat examination; you suspect his thyroid gland may be enlarged without discrete nodule.

STUDY QUESTIONS

1. What further studies would you consider?
2. Are his clinical findings consistent with hyperthyroidism?

CASE DISCUSSION

These findings are consistent with apathetic hyperthyroidism. Mr. Madison may have coexistent depression and or mild dementia. However, in either case he would benefit from a more euthyroid state. Evaluation with a radioactive thyroid scan would be appropriate to rule out the possibility of a "hot nodule."

Hyperthyroidism

Prevalence in the elderly patient of overt hyperthyroidism is 0.2% to 2%, which is similar to that in the general population. Less than 25% of hyperthyroid

---

Box 41–3	Symptoms and Signs of Hyperthyroidism

This triad presents in more than 50%.[13]	Tremor
Tachycardia[a]	Atrial fibrillation
Fatigue	Anorexia
Weight loss	Nervousness

[a]Clinical suspicion should be raised at heart rates 90 or greater in older persons.

patients over the age of 65 present with typical symptoms.[5] Younger patients present with symptoms of tachycardia, goiter, and eye symptomology. Older patients are more likely to present with relative tachycardia, weight loss, and fatigue as primary symptoms. Diarrhea and sweating are also far less common presenting symptoms in older individuals. Likewise, a sense of agitation or anxiety is less commonly reported in older persons. It has been reported that the tremor is as likely to appear in both age groups (Box 41-3).

Elderly patients are likely to have both heart failure as well as the possibility of angina at time of presentation, and as many as 27% will present with atrial fibrillation.[1] Hyperthyroidism in the elderly can be complicated by depression, myopathy, and osteoporosis. But the most dangerous complication is clearly thyroid storm. The elder person with thyroid storm may be at greater risk for death from the fever, tachycardia, nausea, vomiting, mental status changes, and heart complications. Assessment is still best done initially with the serum TSH.

Felix Unger

Felix Unger is a 78-year-old man who was recently admitted to hospital for an acute right middle cerebral artery distribution cerebrovascular accident complicated by congestive heart failure and acute renal insufficiency. He was noted to have a slowing of cognition and was assessed with a TSH as well as other tests for reversible causes of functional decline.

STUDY QUESTIONS

1. If the TSH is elevated, can you conclude Mr. Unger has hypothyroidism?
2. How long would it be reasonable to wait after his episode of acute illness before reassessment of TSH?

CASE DISCUSSION

Mr. Unger has an acute medical illness, and his thyroid laboratory abnormalities may be secondary to a euthyroid sick state. Repeating the laboratory test after resolution of his acute illness in 2 to 4 weeks will help determine if there is genuine thyroid deficiency.

Euthyroid Sick Syndrome

Hypothyroidism should only be diagnosed in a patient with acute illness when there is an evaluation of T_4 and suppression of TSH, which does not normalize within 2 weeks after the resolution of the acute medical or psychiatric illness.[1]

MANAGEMENT

Mary Peterson, *Part 3*

Ms. Peterson agreed to initiation or replacement therapy and has no significant coronary artery disease.

STUDY QUESTION

1. What would be a reasonable starting dose of 1-T_4?

CASE DISCUSSION

Ms. Peterson has clinical hypothyroidism. TSH is the most appropriate screening test. As she has symptomatic hypothyroidism, she would benefit from replacement of thyroid hormone with low-dose Levo T_4. Once clinically suspected, more symptoms/signs attributable to hypothyroidism are likely to be appreciated.

Hypothyroidism

Overt hypothyroidism with symptoms is treated by careful repletion of thyroid hormone with synthetic thyroid. It is important to assess for the possibility of coronary artery disease. In situations of high risk for coronary artery disease and potential for long-standing hypothyroidism, a stress cardiac imaging study is appropriate before reinitiating a normal metabolic rate. As with other geriatric pharmacol-

ogy, starting low and going slow is clearly appropriate. A starting dose of 12.5 to 25 µg per day is appropriate. The dosage should be increased every 6 weeks. It is rare to require doses greater than 75 to 125 µg per day in an older person. Treatment goal is to restore T_4 to the normal range and TSH to the upper range of normal. These goals have to be tempered by coexisting cardiovascular disease. Over time, dosage may need to be decreased. Of particular note is the risk of over treatment leading to osteoporosis in women.

> ● With a high CAD risk and potentially long standing hypothyroidism, do a stress test *before* treatment; and always "start low, go slow."

Subclinical Hypothyroidism

As previously described, it is currently debated as to whether or not appropriate treatment should be instituted for levels between 5 and 10 without clear evidence of symptoms. Most important is to analyze and monitor for the appearance of true clinical hypothyroidism or an elevation into more clearly defined ranges of TSH. At this point in time, it does not appear that initially the treatment has a clearly proven benefit with subclinical hypothyroidism.

Hyperthyroidism

Cases owing to diffusely over-active thyroid or hyperfunctioning nodule or nodules are optimally treated with antithyroid medications propylthiouracil and methimazole. There is also a role for beta-blockade to improve symptomatic treatment, before the antithyroid medication restoring the patient to the euthyroid function. After a period of stabilization, radioactive iodine can be used for definitive treatment. After radioactive iodine treatment, the patient must be monitored for the appearance of hypothyroidism. In the case of possible underlying malignances, surgical options may be entertained. In the case of inflammatory disease, the etiology of hyperthyroidism tends to spontaneously resolve over weeks to months but may require temporizing symptomatic treatment for relief. This is accomplished with a cautious use of beta-blockade. Of note in severe cases of inflammation, there may be a period of hypothyroidism after the acute event that may temporarily require thyroid replacement.

POSTTEST

1. Which of the following is correct about thyroid disease in older adults?
   a. Hyperthyroidism is more common than hypothyroidism.
   b. Hypothyroidism is associated with weight loss in older adults.
   c. Elevated TSH levels are indicative of hypothyroidism and requires treatment even in the oldest old.
   d. Production of thyroxin (T_4) increases with age.

2. Which of the following statements about thyroid cancer are true?
   a. Radiation is a risk factor throughout the life span.
   b. Papillary thyroid cancer is more common in older adults.
   c. The prevalence of thyroid nodules decreases with age.
   d. Thyroid cancer represents 5% of all cancers in women.

3. If untreated, subclinical hyperthyroidism:
   a. May benefit those who are obese because weight loss can be expected.
   b. Can cause osteoporosis that is not prevented by estrogen-replacement therapy.
   c. May cause cardiac failure.
   d. Lowers the risk of abnormal cardiac rhythms.

REFERENCES

1. Canadian Task Force on Preventive Health Care. Screening for thyroid disorders/cancer. Can Med Assoc J 2003.
2. Finucane P, Rudra T, Church H, et al. Thyroid function tests in the elderly patients with and without an acute illness. Age Ageing 1989;18:398-402.
3. American Association of Clinical Endocrinologists. Thyroid through the ages: the senior years (Aging), 2001.
4. Thyroid Foundation of Canada. Thyroid disease in late life, 2000.
5. Thyroid disorders. In: The Merck Manual of Geriatrics.
6. Cornille A, Hueseman P. Thyroid hormones, symptoms, and treatment of hypothyroidism. Shawnee, KS: Association of Women for the Advancement of Research and Education (AWARE), 2004.
7. Gussekloo J, van Exel E, de Craen A, Meinders A, Frolich M, Westendorp R. Thyroid status, disability and cognitive function, and survival in old age. JAMA 2004;292:2591-2599.
8. Davenport J. Playing with fire. SAGE Crossroads, January 2005. http://www.sagecrossroads.org
9. Cavalieri RR. The effects of nonthyroid disease and drugs on thyroid function tests. Med Clin North Am 1991;75: 27-39.
10. Small M, Buchanan L, Evans R. Value of screening thyroid function in acute medical admissions to hospital. Clin Endocrinol 1990;32:185-191.
11. Drinka PJ, Nolten WE, Voeks S, et al. Misleading elevation of the free thyroxine index in nursing home residents. Arch Pathol Lab Med 1991;115:1208-1211.
12. U.S. Preventive Services Task Force. Guide to Clinical Preventive Services, 2nd ed. Washington, DC: U.S. Department of Health and Human Services, Disease Prevention and Health Promotion, 1996.
13. Trivalle C, Doucet J, Chassagne P, et al. Differences in the signs and symptoms of hyperthyroidism in older and younger patients. J Am Geriatric Soc 1996;44:50-53.

PRETEST ANSWERS

1. b
2. a
3. b

POSTTEST ANSWERS

1. b
2. b
3. c

CHAPTER

42

Osteoporosis

Bonny Neyhart

OBJECTIVES

Upon completion of this chapter, the reader will be able to:

- Differentiate primary and secondary osteoporosis and discuss the medical conditions and medications associated with secondary osteoporosis.
- Describe the screening laboratory tests that may reveal clinically unsuspected causes of osteoporosis.
- Appreciate the significance of fracture risk when developing a treatment plan for an individual with osteopenia.
- Interpret bone mineral density measurements in terms of fracture risk and the need for treatment of osteopenia.
- Discuss the role of exercise and supplementation with calcium and vitamin D in the prevention and treatment of osteoporosis.
- Describe the medications currently available for the treatment of osteoporosis, as well as their effectiveness in preventing fractures.
- Recognize the risk of osteoporosis in patients on long-term glucocorticoids and the need for early intervention.

PRETEST

1. A 67-year-old woman presents for her annual physical examination. She has no chronic medical conditions, worrisome symptoms, or findings on physical examination. With regard to bone health, which of the following is the best course of action?
   a. Recommend water aerobics and increased dietary calcium.
   b. Order a dual-energy X-ray absorptiometry (DXA) scan and recommend calcium and vitamin D supplements and a program of weight-bearing exercise.
   c. Recommend calcium and vitamin D supplements and order a DXA scan if she has risk factors for osteoporosis.
   d. Recommend calcium and vitamin D supplements and order a DXA scan only if she has abnormalities on her screening laboratory studies.

2. A 76-year-old man was recently started on high-dose corticosteroids for biopsy-proven giant-cell arteritis and symptoms of polymyalgia rheumatica. Which of the following is the most appropriate intervention to preserve bone integrity?
   a. Order a DXA scan
   b. Recommend calcium and vitamin D supplements.
   c. Recommend calcium and vitamin D supplements and begin bisphosphonate therapy.
   d. Recommend calcium and vitamin D supplements and begin a program of weight-bearing exercise.

3. You are taking over the practice of a retiring physician. On reviewing the medications of a 65-year-old woman who you are seeing for the first time, you note that she is taking estrogen and progestin. She is not certain why this was initially prescribed but believes that it had something to do with her bones. Which of the following statements reflects our current understanding regarding hormone replacement therapy (HRT)?
   a. HRT should be prescribed in the lowest possible dose for the shortest period of time for relief of symptoms associated with menopause.
   b. The benefits of long-term treatment with HRT are offset by the risks of therapy.
   c. Treatment with HRT confers an increased risk of breast cancer, heart attack, stroke, and blood clots in the lung.
   d. All of the above statements are correct.

Howard Connors, *Part 1*

Howard Connors is a 74-year-old widower who recently fractured his wrist after falling in his hotel room. When evaluated in the emergency department last week, he could not recall the specific circumstances of the fall and was noted to have a faint odor of alcohol on his breath. He is a life long tobacco smoker with "a touch of emphysema," which he treats with multiple prescription medications, including prednisone. He also suffers from a "sour stomach," which he treats with H_2-receptor antagonists. His haphazard medical care by multiple providers at a variety of public clinics has been going on for many years.

STUDY QUESTIONS

1. What elements of Mr. Connors' history increase his risk of osteoporosis?
2. What aspects of Mr. Connors' history increase his risk for future fractures?

CASE DISCUSSION

Mr. Connors risk of osteoporosis is increased given his chronic tobacco use, his probable chronic obstructive pulmonary disease (COPD), and his presumably lengthy treatment with prednisone. The history suggests alcohol abuse, which increases his risk of both osteoporosis and falls and thus his risk of fracture.

PREVALENCE AND IMPACT

Osteoporosis is an extremely common age-linked condition that is characterized by low bone mass, microarchitectural deterioration of the bones, decreased bone strength, and an increased risk of fracture. It is currently estimated that 20% of postmenopausal women in the United States have osteoporosis, and of these, 52% have low bone density at the hip. In practice, bone mineral density (BMD) screening of older women often leads to a diagnosis of osteoporosis that would otherwise be clinically inapparent. Low BMD in asymptomatic individuals is a predictor of fracture risk just as raised blood pressure portends increased stroke risk.

Half of postmenopausal women and 15% of white men over 50 will experience an osteoporotic fracture at some point. The most common fracture locations are the vertebrae (spine), proximal femur (hip), and distal radius (wrist). Most fractures cause pain, many produce lingering disability, and, in the case of hip fracture, can result in death. Osteoporosis exacts a psychological toll on individuals and their families, espe-

cially when the discomforts and limitations of fracture lead to depression and loss of independence. A major economic concern, osteoporosis-linked costs have increased in the United States from $3.8 billion in 1984 to a staggering $17 billion in 2001.[1,2]

> A major economic concern, osteoporosis-linked costs have increased in the United States from $3.8 billion in 1984 to a staggering $17 billion in 2001.

RISK FACTORS AND PATHOPHYSIOLOGY

Peak bone density is achieved between ages 25 to 30 years and is largely determined by genetic factors, although nutrition, physical activity, and health status during skeletal growth contribute as well. Maintenance of a healthy skeleton is achieved through the ongoing deposition of new bone and the removal or resorption of older bone. In both men and women, gradual bone loss begins in the fourth decade of life when the rate of new bone formation is outpaced by the rate of bone removal. Women undergo increased bone remodeling during menopause, which exaggerates the imbalance between bone formation and resorption, leading to reduced bone mass and disordered skeletal architecture. The bones become progressively more fragile over time, resulting in an increased vulnerability to fracture. Figure 42-1 illustrates the decreased bone mass and microarchitectural destruction associated with osteoporosis.

Primary osteoporosis occurs with normal aging, independent of disease or medication use. It is most commonly diagnosed in postmenopausal white women; risk factors for the development of osteoporosis should guide clinicians about screening middle-age women. Given the higher prevalence of osteoporosis in older women, there is consensus by both the National Osteoporosis Foundation and the U.S. Preventive Services Task Force (USPSTF) that *all*

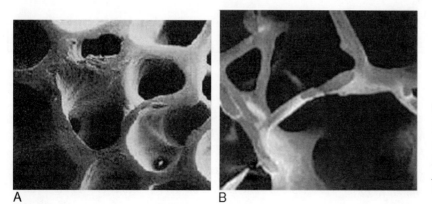

A   B

FIGURE 42–1

Micrographs of normal (*A*) versus osteoporotic (*B*) bone. (*From National Osteoporosis Foundation: Physicians guide to prevention and treatment of osteoporosis. http//www.nof.org.*)

Box 42-1   Medical Conditions Associated with Increased Osteoporosis Risk

Endocrine/Metabolic
- Cushing's syndrome
- Hemochromatosis
- Hyperthyroidism
- Hyperparathyroidism
- Hypogonadism
- Insulin-dependent diabetes

Gastrointestinal/Nutritional
- Gastrectomy
- Inadequate diet
- Inflammatory bowel disease
- Malabsorption syndromes
- Severe liver disease
- Weight loss

Hematologic
- Leukemia
- Lymphoma
- Multiple myeloma
- Pernicious anemia
- Thalassemia

Neurologic
- Multiple sclerosis
- Spinal cord transaction
- Stroke

Pulmonary
- Chronic obstructive pulmonary disease (COPD)

Rheumatologic
- Ankylosing spondylitis
- Rheumatoid arthritis

From National Osteoporosis Foundation. Physicians guide to prevention and treatment of osteoporosis. http//www.nof.org.

---

women aged 65 years and older should be routinely screened for osteoporosis.[1,4]

Secondary osteoporosis refers to bone loss caused by disease processes or medications. Secondary causes for osteoporosis are more commonly found in men than in postmenopausal women.[3] Boxes 42-1 and 42-2 list the conditions and medications associated with secondary osteoporosis; the most common etiologies in men are hypogonadism, glucocorticoid use, and alcoholism.[3]

Although decreased bone strength and a diagnosis of osteoporosis increase the likelihood of future fracture, other relevant risk factors for fracture are frequently overlooked: chief among these are the risk of falls or other trauma. Fall risk is increased in chronic diseases, especially those that affect the visual and neuromuscular systems; it is associated with medications such as sedative-hypnotics or drugs that are potentially hypotensive.

DIFFERENTIAL DIAGNOSIS AND ASSESSMENT

Medical History

Assessment of an older individual with suspected osteoporosis, whether because of fractures or low bone density, begins with a focused medical history; the goal is to exclude secondary causes of osteoporosis, as listed in Boxes 42-1 and 42-2. In men, up to 60% have a secondary cause for their osteoporosis.

Box 42-2   Drugs Associated with Reduced Bone Mass

- Anticonvulsants (phenobarbital, phenytoin)
- Corticosteroids
- Cytotoxic drugs
- Immunosuppressants
- Lithium
- Thyroxine in supraphysiologic doses
- Total parenteral nutrition

From National Osteoporosis Foundation. Physicians guide to prevention and treatment of osteoporosis. http//www.nof.org.

Cynthia Williams, *Part 1*

Cynthia Williams is a 67-year-old woman who is new to your practice who presents for a routine physical examination. She reports good health except back pain, takes no medications except acetaminophen, and is current with immunizations, mammography, pap smears, and colorectal cancer screening. Recent screening laboratory studies are normal. Her physical examination is notable for a height of 61 inches (a 3-inch decrease from her younger years), weight of 110 pounds, and a slight kyphosis of her thoracic spine.

STUDY QUESTIONS

1. Could Mrs. Williams' loss of height be caused by osteoporosis?

2. What other physical examination findings would support a diagnosis of osteoporosis?

3. What diagnostic studies should be ordered at this time?

CASE DISCUSSION

Mrs. Williams' loss of height could indeed be the result of osteoporosis-related vertebral compression fractures. Her thoracic kyphosis supports this diagnosis, and her low weight places her at increased risk for osteoporosis. We may presume that her intake of calcium and vitamin D is inadequate because she does not report taking any medications, although some patients do not mention their vitamins and supplements when asked about medications. A measurement of her wall–occiput distance would be an intriguing clinical exercise, as would measuring her rib–pelvis distance. Both of these clinical tools lack sensitivity and specificity for the diagnosis of osteoporosis and vertebral fracture. A dual-energy X-ray absorptiometry (DXA) or other technique for determining BMD is the most sensitive way to diagnose osteoporosis. A plain lateral radiograph of the spine can, however, reveal vertebral compression fractures and radiolucent bones late in the course of the disease.

Physical Examination

Low *body weight* correlates with low bone mass; in women, a weight of less than 51 kg is a fairly sensitive, although nonspecific, predictor of low bone mass.[5] However, being heavier does not exclude a diagnosis of osteoporosis. Loss of height, determined either by review of medical records or the patient's memory of their height at age 25, may reflect occult vertebral compression fractures. Because vertebral fractures affect height but not arm span, if arm span is significantly greater than height, occult vertebral compression fractures may be present. However, in a review of three studies of arm span–height difference, it was concluded that the arm span–height differential does not reliably correlate with vertebral fractures or low BMD.[5]

Thoracic kyphosis, sometimes referred to as "dowager's hump," can be the result of anterior compression fractures in the thoracic spine. A patient's self-report of a "humped back" was found in one study to correlate strongly with subsequently determined osteoporosis of the hip.[7] The degree of kyphosis can be measured as the wall–occiput distance; the patient stands with the back and heels against a wall, and the head held such that an imaginary line between the outer corner of the eye and the upper ear is parallel to the floor. The distance between the occipital prominence and the wall can be measured, but simple inability to touch the wall with the back of the head is a positive finding. A measurement greater than 7 cm correlates strongly with thoracic fracture; yet measurement of 0 cm does not exclude the diagnosis[6] (Fig. 42-2).

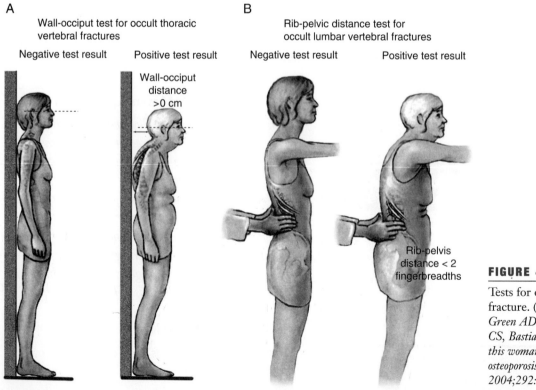

A

Wall-occiput test for occult thoracic vertebral fractures

Negative test result   Positive test result

Wall-occiput distance >0 cm

B

Rib-pelvic distance test for occult lumbar vertebral fractures

Negative test result   Positive test result

Rib-pelvis distance < 2 fingerbreadths

FIGURE 42–2

Tests for occult vertebral fracture. (*Redrawn from Green AD, Colon-Emeric CS, Bastian L, et al: Does this woman have osteoporosis? JAMA 2004;292:2890-2900.*)

Occult anterior lumbar fractures can be revealed by measuring the rib–pelvis distance. With the patient standing and their arms outstretched at a 90-degree angle, the examiner's fingers are placed in the gap between the inferior costal margin and the pelvis. The test is positive if the gap is less than two fingerbreadths at the midaxillary line (see Fig. 42-2).

Laboratory Testing

There is little consensus among the major medical organizations that have guidelines about the work-up of osteoporosis. This is largely because the exact prevalence of secondary causes is unknown and laboratory screening strategies therefore cannot be prioritized.[8] In a chart review study of women seen in an osteoporosis clinic, laboratory studies led to the finding of secondary causes in almost one-third of the patients; most of the secondary causes involved disordered calcium metabolism, vitamin D deficiency, exogenous hyperthyroidism, and Cushing's disease. The investigators calculated the diagnostic yield of five separate laboratory screening strategies that, if used in their patient population, would have led to a correct diagnosis 59% to 98% of the time. With one exception, improved diagnostic yield was related to the cost of testing (Table 42-1).[9] Further research is needed to tell if laboratory screenings are applicable to older men and woman seen in a primary care setting.

Bone Densitometry

BMD measurement can be used to establish or confirm a diagnosis of osteoporosis and to gauge the risk of future fracture. There is a continuous, inverse relationship between BMD and the risk of fracture; generally, the lower the BMD, the greater the fracture risk. A variety of densitometers are in clinical use, although the DXA scan is considered the gold standard because it is the test most extensively validated against fracture outcomes. A DXA scan takes less than 10 minutes, and radiation exposure is approximately one-tenth that of a standard chest X-ray.

Measurements of BMD by DXA are expressed as the T-score and the Z-score. The relationship between the patient's bone density and that of age- and sex-matched controls is reflected by the Z-score, whereas the T-score compares the patient's BMD with that of young adults of the same sex. The difference between the patient and the control is expressed in standard deviations (SDs) above or below the mean.

The World Health Organization (WHO) has established definitions for ranges of BMD in postmenopausal white women, summarized in Box 42-3.

Box 42-3 Established Bone Mass Definitions from the World Health Organization

- *Normal:* T-score −1.0 or greater
  (patient's BMD within 1 SD of young adult controls)
- *Low bone mass/osteopenia:* T-score between −1 and −2.5
  (patient's BMD is 1 to 2.5 SD below that of young adult controls)
- *Osteoporosis:* T-score at or below −2.5
  (patient's BMD is 2.5 SD below that of young adult controls)
- *Severe osteoporosis:* T-score less than −2.5 and patient has a history of fragility fracture/s

BMD indicates bone mineral density; SD, standard deviation.

From National Osteoporosis Foundation: Physicians guide to prevention and treatment of osteoporosis. Accessed 3/8/2005 at http//www.nof.org.

Table 42-1 Osteoporosis Screening Strategies, Diagnostic Yield, and Cost

Strategy	Urine Ca[a]	Serum Ca	PTH	TSH[b]	25(OH)D	Diagnostic Yield	Cost per Patient[c]
1	Yes	Only if abnormal urine Ca	Only if abnormal urine Ca	Yes	No	59%	$22
2	Yes	Yes	Only if abnormal urine or serum Ca	Yes	No	63%	$30
3	Yes	Yes	Yes	Yes	No	86%	$75
4	Yes	Yes	Yes	Yes	Yes	98%	$116
5	No	Yes	Yes	Yes	Yes	66%	$108

Ca indicates calcium; PTH, parathyroid hormone; TSH, thyroid-stimulating hormone; and 25(OH)D, 25-hydroxy vitamin D.

[a]24 hour urine calcium and creatinine.

[b]Only in women receiving thyroid hormone replacement therapy.

[c]Based on 1999 Medicare allowable charges in U.S. dollars.

From Tannenbaum C, Clark J, Schwartzman K, et al. Yield of laboratory testing to identify secondary contributors to osteoporosis in otherwise healthy women. J Clin Endocrinol Metab 2002;87:4431-4437.

Because DXA units are large and expensive, smaller and less costly units capable of measuring bone density at peripheral skeletal sites may be reasonable screening options. Peripheral DXA (pDXA) and single-energy X-ray absorptiometry (SXA) measure bone density in the wrist, finger, and heel. Ultrasound densitometry assesses the density of superficial bones such as the heel, tibia, and patella. Although ultrasound densitometry lacks the precision of DXA and SXA, it appears comparable for predicting fracture risk.

BMD testing should be done in all women 65 years and older regardless of risk factors and in those men suspected of having osteoporosis. Medicare covers biannual BMD testing in older women and in individuals with vertebral abnormalities, primary hyperparathyroidism, and patients receiving or planning to receive long-term glucocorticoid therapy.

Plain radiographs are useful for diagnosing suspected fractures, but they will not detect osteoporosis until roughly half the skeletal mass is lost!

> ● BMD measurement can be used to establish or confirm a diagnosis of osteoporosis and to gauge the risk of future fracture.

Howard Connors, *Part 2*

Physical examination reveals a thin, unkempt white man with several missing teeth and tobacco-stained nails. The diameter of his chest is increased, breath sounds are distant, and his nails are clubbed. There is a cast on the left forearm. He has epigastric tenderness and a tender, slightly enlarged liver. Laboratory studies are notable for an elevated hematocrit and gamma-glutamyl-transferase, his albumin is slightly decreased but his corrected calcium is normal.

Mr. Connors admits to binge drinking and poor nutrition and concedes that he is no longer able to care for himself. He agrees to enter a residential care facility where his alcohol intake and medication use will be monitored.

A subsequently obtained DXA scan revealed a T-score of −2.8 at the hip.

STUDY QUESTIONS

1. Does Mr. Connors have osteoporosis?
2. Which of his known medications contributes to osteoporosis and should be discontinued, if possible?
3. Should calcium and vitamin D be prescribed? Which of his known medicines would interfere with calcium absorption?

4. Are there any other medications for osteoporosis that should be prescribed at this time?

CASE DISCUSSION

Mr. Connors' T-score of −2.8 meets WHO criteria for the diagnosis of osteoporosis. The treatment of his COPD should be optimized and prednisone therapy eliminated, if possible. His use of H$_2$-receptor antagonists interferes with absorption of calcium, confounding what has likely been long-standing negative calcium balance, caused in part by inadequate calcium intake. Supplements should be prescribed to ensure a minimum daily calcium intake of 1200 mg, such as would be provided by taking 500 mg of elemental calcium twice or three times a day with meals. The recommended vitamin D intake is 800 IU per day. This may be provided as a separate daily supplement or in a combined calcium and vitamin D formulation. Mr. Connors' fracture history and proven osteoporosis make him a candidate for pharmacotherapy. Weekly treatment with either risedronate 35 mg or alendronate 70 mg should be initiated, after educating the patient about the risk of esophagitis and esophageal ulcers. Mr. Connor should be instructed to take the bisphosphonate with a large glass of water first thing in the morning after an overnight fast. He must not take any food, liquid, or other medications and remain upright for at least 30 minutes thereafter. Careful instructions are especially important given Mr. Conners' history of a "sour stomach".

Cynthia Williams, *Part 2*

Physical examination confirms a wall-occiput distance of 7 cm. Plain X-rays of the thoracic spine demonstrate several anterior vertebral compression fractures. On DXA, her vertebral T-score was −2.5 and her T-score at the hip was −2.0.

STUDY QUESTIONS

1. Assuming a negative history for secondary causes of osteoporosis, what screening laboratory studies would you consider ordering?
2. What is the recommended daily intake of vitamin D and calcium for Mrs. Williams? Can an adjustment to her diet accomplish this goal or will supplements probably be necessary?
3. Are there any other medications for osteoporosis that should be prescribed at this time?

CASE DISCUSSION

According to one study,[8,9] most clinically unsuspected secondary causes of osteoporosis can be revealed by obtaining four or five specific laboratory tests (Table 42.1). In women not taking thyroid supplements, the following studies are recommended by these investigators: serum calcium, 24-hour urine calcium and creatinine, and parathyroid hormone (86% sensitive, approximate cost $75). Adding a 25-hydroxy vitamin D level to these other laboratory tests increases both the sensitivity and cost (98% sensitive, approximate cost $116).

Supplements are usually required to achieve the recommended 1200 mg per day of elemental calcium and 800 IU per day of vitamin D.

In addition to ensuring adequate intake of calcium and vitamin D, bisphosphonate therapy is the most appropriate prescription for Ms. Williams. Alendronate and risedronate are the most effective agents for reducing the risk of vertebral and nonvertebral fractures in postmenopausal women with osteoporosis. The selective estrogen receptor modulator (SERM) raloxifene may be considered if Ms. Williams cannot tolerate weekly bisphosphonate therapy.

MANAGEMENT

Universal Recommendations

Several interventions to preserve bone integrity and reduce fracture risk are appropriate for the older population in general. All patients should be counseled to optimize their intake of calcium and vitamin D, maintain a regular exercise program, avoid tobacco and excessive alcohol, and reduce their risk of injury. Smoking cessation is appropriate advice for all patients; in patients with low BMD, there is a dose-dependent risk from smoking for osteoporosis and fracture. Identification and treatment of alcoholism is always clinically indicated, especially when secondary causes for osteoporosis are being sought. All patients should have their fall risk assessed, especially those with known osteopenia or osteoporosis.

EXERCISE

Regular weight-bearing exercise can decrease bone loss and may stabilize or improve BMD in older adults.[10] Walking correlates with greater bone mass in the elderly, but intervention studies have not demonstrated an increase in bone density or protection against bone loss. Several studies of progressive weight training in older men and women have shown significant increases in BMD. Other trials have failed to show an increase in bone mass but suggest that exercise slows the rate of bone loss.

The potential value of exercise in protecting older persons from falls must be recognized. Of the many risk factors for falls, muscle weakness is the condition most likely to benefit from progressive weight training. Indeed, there is epidemiologic evidence suggesting that being physically active can nearly halve the risk of hip fracture in older people.[11,12]

> ● The potential value of exercise in protecting older persons from falls must be recognized.

CALCIUM AND VITAMIN D

All patients should be counseled to optimize their intake of calcium and vitamin D. The recommended intake of elemental calcium for women and men over age 50 is 1200 mg per day.[1,15] Because the average American consumes less than 800 mg of calcium a day and because older individuals may consume as little as 400 mg per day, negative calcium balance is common in the elderly.[14] When intake is inadequate, circulating calcium levels are maintained by bone resorption. Older individuals often have medical conditions or medications that interfere with calcium absorption, for example, gastric achlorhydria, H_2-receptor antagonists, and proton pump inhibitors. Vitamin D deficiency impairs calcium absorption. Vitamin D deficiency is most common in institutionalized or homebound elders and in individuals living in northern latitudes, many of whom have limited exposure to sunlight. The National Osteoporosis Foundation recommends a daily vitamin D intake of 800 IU for *all* older men and women. Higher doses are needed in persons with malabsorption or rapid metabolism of vitamin D due to concomitant anticonvulsant drug therapy.

Many well-designed studies have demonstrated a small trend toward increased bone mass in calcium-treated individuals. However, trials designed to demonstrate that calcium supplementation leads to a decreased risk of fracture have yielded conflicting results.[16] One study showed a slight reduction in the risk of fracture among women older than 65 years taking both high oral intake of calcium and supplemental vitamin D.[14]

Calcium and vitamin D have no long-term data to establish anti-fracture efficacy, yet these supplements have been used in all trials of pharmaceutical treatment. Thus supplementation with calcium and vitamin D is considered standard treatment of osteoporosis.

Inadequate calcium intake can usually be assumed in older persons who are not taking dietary supplements. Calcium supplements are available in a variety of formulations in which the amount and absorption of calcium is variable; some include various amounts of vitamin D or other vitamins and trace elements. Our patients are therefore confronted with a confusing array of supplement products, some of which are intensely marketed and comparatively costly. Selection should be guided by the therapeutic goal of a daily elemental calcium intake of 1200 mg, through diet and supplements, along with 800 IU of vitamin D per day. Clinicians should periodically inspect the supplements their patients take.

Calcium supplements should be taken with food, so that intestinal transit time is increased and calcium absorption thereby maximized. Ideally, calcium supplements should be taken at the end of a meal. This instruction is especially important for individuals taking H_2-receptor antagonists and proton pump inhibitors. Supplements exceeding 500 mg of elemental calcium overwhelm absorptive capacity, thus dosing should be divided so that no more than 500 mg of elemental calcium is taken at any single meal.

Side effects of calcium supplements include constipation, bloating, and increased intestinal gas. These symptoms may improve with increased fluid intake. Troubling gastrointestinal symptoms are quite common with calcium carbonate; such symptoms generally resolve on changing to calcium citrate.

● Inadequate calcium intake can usually be assumed in older persons who are not taking dietary supplements.

Pharmacologic Therapy of Osteopenia and Osteoporosis

With the specific goal of reducing fracture risk, the National Osteoporosis Foundation[1] recommends initiating pharmacologic therapy under the clinical circumstances summarized in Box 42-4.

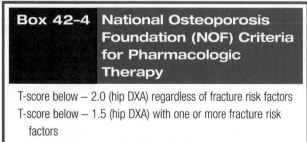

Box 42-4 **National Osteoporosis Foundation (NOF) Criteria for Pharmacologic Therapy**

T-score below − 2.0 (hip DXA) regardless of fracture risk factors

T-score below − 1.5 (hip DXA) with one or more fracture risk factors

Prior fragility fracture of the hip or vertebrae

DXA indicates dual-energy X-ray absorptiometry.

From National Osteoporosis Foundation: Physicians guide to prevention and treatment of osteoporosis. Accessed 3/8/2005 at http://www.nof.org.

The most clinically relevant measure of drug efficacy is reduction of fracture risk. There have been few head-to-head trials in which the efficacy of one medication has been directly compared with that of another. Comparisons in fracture risk reduction must therefore be interpreted cautiously.

BISPHOSPHONATES

Bisphosphonates suppress the resorptive phase of bone remodeling by inhibiting osteoclastic activity. Of medications currently approved by the Food and Drug Administration (FDA) for the prevention or treatment of osteoporosis, the bisphosphonates are the most effective drugs for reducing the risk of vertebral and nonvertebral fracture.[18]

The American College of Rheumatology recommends calcium and vitamin D *and* bisphosphonate therapy for patients in whom long-term glucocorticoid therapy is planned. This recommendation holds for adults of all ages, regardless of their T-score at baseline, who take prednisone in doses exceeding 5 mg per day (or another dose-equivalent glucocorticoid) for longer than 3 months. Both alendronate and risedronate are effective in the prevention and treatment of glucocorticoid-induced loss of bone density. In addition, based on an analysis of pooled data, risedronate 5 mg per day also appears to decrease the risk of vertebral fractures in this population.[19]

ALENDRONATE

This oral bisphosphonate can be dosed daily or weekly for the prevention or treatment of osteoporosis. Weekly dosing appears to be as effective as daily dosing and may be better tolerated.[15] Food and calcium reduce the absorption of this drug, so alendronate must be taken with water after an overnight fast and at least 30 minutes before any food, drink, or other medications are ingested. Adverse effects of alendronate include esophagitis and esophageal ulcers. To prevent these complications, patients are advised to swallow tablets with 6 to 8 ounces of water and remain upright for at least 30 minutes after dosing.

Alendronate has been shown to increase BMD and decrease the incidence of fractures of the hip, forearm and vertebrae.[17,18] The beneficial effects of alendronate persist for several years of treatment, but bone loss resumes when therapy is stopped.

RISEDRONATE

Similar to alendronate, this oral bisphosphonate can be dosed either daily or weekly, and both schedules appear equally effective. The adverse effects are similar to alendronate, and the same dosing precautions apply.

Risedronate increases BMD at the spine and hip and decreases both vertebral and nonvertebral fractures.

IBANDRONATE

This most recently FDA-approved oral bisphosphonate appears effective in reducing vertebral fractures in patients with osteoporosis, but long-term data regarding safety and efficacy are currently lacking. A potential advantage of this product is the option for once-monthly dosing, although fracture prevention efficacy of this formulation is unknown.

ETIDRONATE

The bisphosphonate etidronate lacks FDA approval for the prevention and treatment of osteoporosis but is used in Canada and Europe. Etidronate dosed at 400 mg per day for 2 weeks followed by 11 weeks of calcium 500 mg per day was shown in one study to increase BMD at the hip and lumbar spine and appeared to decrease vertebral fractures. Etidronate is generally thought to not produce the same adverse effects on the esophagus as do the other oral bisphosphonates.[15]

HORMONE THERAPY

The role of estrogen deprivation on the genesis of osteoporosis in women is well established, and prescription estrogen has been widely used for the prevention of postmenopausal osteoporosis. Estrogen is also effective in reducing the risk of vertebral and nonvertebral fractures in postmenopausal women. The positive effect on bone of combination estrogen/progestin therapy was confirmed by the Women's Health Initiative Randomized Controlled Trial, in which there were 34% fewer fractures among hormone-treated postmenopausal women. However, this antifracture benefit was offset by an increased risk of myocardial infarction, stroke, pulmonary emboli, and invasive breast cancer in the treatment group.[20] Research regarding the safety and effectiveness of estrogen therapy alone in women who have had a hysterectomy is currently underway. At present, short-term hormone therapy in the lowest effective dose is recommended only for the symptoms associated with menopause. For most women over 65, the risks of hormone therapy outweigh the known benefits of treatment (level of evidence = A).

SELECTIVE ESTROGEN RECEPTOR MODULATORS

The observation that tamoxifen users have a decreased risk of osteoporotic fractures stimulated the development of SERMs, in which the beneficial effects of estrogen are maximized and the risks eliminated or reduced. Raloxifene is the only SERM that is currently approved by the FDA for the prevention and treatment of osteoporosis in postmenopausal women. Raloxifene inhibits bone resorption and decreases bone turnover, as reflected by gains in BMD among treated women. Reduction in vertebral fracture risk of up to 55% has been demonstrated, but no reduction in hip or other nonvertebral fractures has been shown.[21]

One trial showed an impressive reduction in the risk of breast cancer in postmenopausal women taking raloxifene over 4 years, but this finding awaits confirmation. Raloxifene treatment is associated with decreases in total and low-density lipoprotein cholesterol. In one study of postmenopausal women with cardiovascular risk factors, those taking raloxifene had a lower risk of cardiac events, including unstable angina and myocardial infarction.[15] Additional research into the effect of raloxifene on the risk of breast cancer and heart disease is currently underway.

The main known risk of raloxifene is a twofold to threefold increased incidence of thromboembolic disease. Nuisance side effects include leg cramps and a slightly increased incidence of hot flashes. These side effects are seldom of sufficient severity to cause discontinuation of raloxifene.

Although tamoxifen is not FDA approved for the prevention or treatment of osteoporosis, women who are taking tamoxifen for breast cancer are also receiving treatment for osteoporosis.

> ● Raloxifene is the only SERM that is currently approved by the FDA for the prevention and treatment of osteoporosis in postmenopausal women.

CALCITONIN

Calcitonin decreases bone resorption and is recommended for use in osteoporotic women who are five or more years postmenopausal and cannot tolerate other medications. Given by nasal spray in a daily dose of 200 IU, studies have documented an increase in BMD and as much as a 33% decreased risk of vertebral fracture in women with established osteoporosis. The effect of calcitonin on sites other than the spine has been equivocal.

Calcitonin may also be effective as an analgesic for the pain associated with osteoporotic vertebral fractures. In over a dozen studies in which analgesic effectiveness was demonstrated, none included a comparison of calcitonin with commonly used analgesics. The clinical usefulness of calcitonin over nonspecific analgesics is therefore unknown, but calcitonin remains an attractive analgesic option for patients who cannot tolerate nonsteroidal anti-inflammatory drugs or narcotic medications.[22]

Table 42–2 Evaluation and Treatment of Osteoporosis		
Indication	Strategy	Level of Evidence for Effectiveness
Bone mineral density screening	All women older than 65 years with or without risk factors for osteoporosis	C
Reducing fracture risk in women with osteoporosis	Bisphosphonate therapy	A
Long-term glucocorticoid therapy in men and women regardless of T-score	Bisphosphonate therapy + calcium and vitamin D supplements	C

A indicates supported by one or more high-quality randomized trials; C, supported by one or more case series and/or poor-quality cohort and/or case-control studies.

Zizic TM. Pharmacologic prevention of osteoporotic fractures. Am Fam Physician 2004;70:1293-1300.

Intranasal administration of calcitonin can cause rhinitis and epistaxis. This side effect can be lessened in patients who alternate nostrils when administering this medication. Calcitonin is also available as an alternate-day injectable formulation. Subcutaneous calcitonin injection has not caused serious adverse effects, but flushing and nausea occur commonly.

RECOMBINANT HUMAN PARATHYROID HORMONE

The recombinant human parathyroid hormone teriparatide increases bone density by stimulating bone formation. In one well-designed clinical trial involving women with postmenopausal osteoporosis, teriparatide treatment led to significant increases in spine BMD and a reduction in vertebral fractures by 65% (20 µg injection) and 69% (40 µg injection) as compared with placebo. In addition, femoral neck BMD increased by up to 5%, and the incidence of nonvertebral fractures decreased by 35% and 40% in the 20 µg and 40 µg groups, respectively. In a separate study of men with hypogonadal and idiopathic osteoporosis, teriparatide therapy significantly increased lumbar spine BMD and led to a 50% decrease in the relative risk of new vertebral fractures.

Because teriparatide may exacerbate hypercalcemia, treatment is contraindicated in persons with pre-existing hypercalcemia and should be used cautiously in patients taking digoxin. An association between teriparatide therapy and osteosarcoma in rats eliminates the use of this drug in persons at increased risk for osteosarcoma, although a causative link in humans has not been noted to date. The most common adverse effects associated with teriparatide therapy are nausea, headache, dizziness, arthralgias, and leg cramps. The incidence of adverse effects is dose related.

Teriparatide is FDA approved for the treatment of postmenopausal women with osteoporosis who are at high risk for fracture and men with primary or hypogonadal osteoporosis who are at high risk for fracture. Treatment for longer than 24 months is not recommended as there is limited data regarding long-term safety and efficacy.[23]

Table 42-2 summarizes the strength of evidence for important aspects of the management of osteoporosis.

SUMMARY

With the growing average life expectancy of U.S. citizens, osteoporosis screening and treatment is becoming increasingly important. Bone density screening of all women over the age of 65 years is currently recommended. DXA is the gold standard method for determining BMD, although SXA and ultrasonography may be reasonable screening options. Clinical evaluation should be directed at identifying secondary causes of osteoporosis and reducing the risk of falls. Prudent laboratory screening may reveal pertinent and otherwise unsuspected secondary causes. All patients should be counseled to exercise, avoid tobacco, and optimize their intake of calcium and vitamin D. Bisphosphonate therapy has been shown to decrease the risk of fracture at both spinal and nonspinal sites. No studies demonstrate hip fracture risk reduction from treatment with either raloxifene or recombinant parathyroid hormone. When a diagnosis of osteoporosis has been made or prolonged glucocorticoid therapy is planned, bisphosphonates are the treatment of choice for both men and women.

References

1. National Osteoporosis Foundation. Physicians guide to prevention and treatment of osteoporosis. Washington, DC: National Osteoporosis Foundation. http//www.nof.org
2. Ray NF, Chan JK. Thamer M, Melton LJ 3rd. Medical expenditures for the treatment of osteoporotic fractures in the U.S. in 1995: report from the National Osteoporosis Foundation. J Bone Miner Res 1997;12:24-35.
3. NIH consensus development panel on osteoporosis prevention, diagnosis and therapy: osteoporosis prevention, diagnosis and therapy, JAMA 2001;285:785-795.
4. U. S. Preventive Services Task Force: Screening for osteoporosis in postmenopausal women: recommendations and rationale, Ann Intern Med 2002;137:526-528.
5. Green AD, Colon-Emeric CS, Bastian L, et al. Does this woman have osteoporosis? JAMA 2004;292:2890-2900.
6. Siminoski K, Lee K, Warshawski R. Accuracy of physical examination for detection of thoracic vertebral fractures. Bone Miner Res 2003;18(Suppl 2):S284-S282.
7. Kantor S, Ossa KS, Hoshaw-Woodard SL, et al. Height loss and osteoporosis of the hip, J Bone Densitom 2004;7:65-70.
8. Crandall C. Laboratory work-up for osteoporosis, Post Grad Med 2003;114:35-44.
9. Tannenbaum C, Clark J, Schwartzman K, et al. Yield of laboratory testing to identify secondary contributors to osteoporosis in otherwise healthy women. J Clin Endocrinol Metab 2002;87:4431-4437.

POSTTEST

1. You are seeing a 75-year-old man who sustained a wrist fracture when he fell while picking up the newspaper from the path outside his home. Which of the following medical conditions and medications increase the likelihood that this man has osteoporosis?
   a. Alcoholism
   b. Hyperthyroidism
   c. Hypogonadism
   d. Glucocorticoid therapy
   e. All of the above

2. You are reviewing the results of a screening DXA scan ordered on a healthy 67-year-old woman. Her T-score is − 2.8 at the spine and −2.6 at the hip. She walks daily and participates in a weight-bearing exercise program three times per week, in addition to taking an optimal dose of vitamin D and calcium supplements. Which of the following has been shown to be most effective for reducing the risk of vertebral and nonvertebral fractures in postmenopausal women with osteoporosis?
   a. Estrogen
   b. Raloxifene
   c. Risedronate and alendronate
   d. Calcitonin
   e. Recombinant parathyroid hormone

3. All patients should be advised to optimize their intake of calcium and vitamin D. Which one of the following statements regarding supplementation is correct?
   a. The recommended calcium intake for older men and women is 1000 mg/day.
   b. Calcium supplements should be taken on an empty stomach.
   c. H_2 antagonists and proton pump inhibitors interfere with calcium absorption.
   d. The recommended vitamin D intake for older men and women is 200 IU/day.
   e. All supplements contain the same amount of elemental calcium.

4. To optimize absorption and decrease adverse effects on the esophagus, patients taking oral bisphosphonates should be given which of the following instructions?
   a. Take bisphosphonate with a sip of water upon awakening and remain upright.
   b. Set your alarm clock 30 minutes before you have to get up. Take the bisphosphonate with a tall glass of water, and then press the snooze button for another half hour of sleep.
   c. Upon awakening, take bisphosphonate with a tall glass of orange juice and remain upright.
   d. After an overnight fast, take bisphosphonate first thing in the morning with a tall glass of water, remain upright and take nothing more by mouth for at least 30 minutes.

10. Snow CM, Shaw JM, Winters KM, et al. Long-term exercise using weighted vests prevents hip bone loss in post-menopausal women. J Gerontol A Biol Sci Med Sci 2000;55:M489-M491.
11. Kujala UM, Kaprio J, Kannus P, et al. Physical activity and osteoporotic hip fracture risk in men. Arch Intern Med 2000;160:705-708.
12. Rutherford OM. Is there a role for exercise in the prevention of osteoporotic fractures? Br J Sports Med 1999;33:378-386.
13. National Institute of Health Consensus Development Panel on Optimal Calcium Intake: Optimal calcium intake. JAMA 1994;272:1942-1948.
14. Dawson-Hughes B, Harris SS, Krall EA, et al. Effect of calcium and vitamin D supplementation on bone density in men and women 65 years of age or older. N Engl J Med 1997;337:670-676.
15. Drugs for prevention and treatment of osteoporosis: treatment guidelines. Med Lett 2002;1: 13-18.
16. Reid IR. The roles of calcium and vitamin D in the prevention of osteoporosis. Endocinol Metab Clin North Am 1998;27:389-398.
17. Nelson HD, Helfand M, Woolf SH, et al. Screening for postmenopausal osteoporosis: summary of the evidence. www.ahrq.gov/clinic/3rduspstf/osteoporosis/osteosumm1.htm.
18. Zizic TM. Pharmacologic prevention of osteoporotic fractures. Am Fam Physician 2004;70:1293-1300.
19. Wallach S, Cohen S, Reid DM, et al. Effects of risedronate treatment on bone density and vertebral fractures in patients on corticosteroid therapy. Calcif Tissue Int 2000;67:277-285.
20. Writing Group for the Women's Health Initiative Investigators. Risks and benefits of estrogen plus progestin in healthy postmenopausal women. JAMA 2002;288:321-333.
21. Ettinger B, Black DM, Mitlak BH, et al: Reduction in vertebral fracture risk in postmenopausal women with osteoporosis treated with raloxifene. JAMA 1999;282:637-645.
22. Blau LA, Hoens JD. Analgesic efficacy of calcitonin for vertebral fracture pain. Ann Pharmacother 2003;37:564-570.
23. Cappuzzo KA. Teriparatide for severe osteoporosis, Ann Pharmacother 2003;38:294-302.

Web Resources

1. National Osteoporosis Foundation. Physician's guide to prevention and treatment of osteoporosis. http://www.nof.org/_vti_bin/shtml.dll/physguide/index.htm.
2. Nelson HD, Helfand M, Woolf SH et, al. Screening for postmenopausal osteoporosis: summary of the evidence. http://www.ahrq.gov/clinic/3rduspstf/osteoporosis/osteosumm1.htm.

PRETEST ANSWERS

1. b
2. c
3. d

POSTTEST ANSWERS

1. d
2. c
3. c
4. d

CHAPTER
43

Arthritis and Related Disorders

Yuri Nakasato

- Recognize that arthritis in the elderly is different from that in the younger population.
- Characterize the different medications used in the elderly to treat musculoskeletal disorders.

OBJECTIVES

Upon completion of this chapter, the reader will be able to:

- Understand the differential diagnosis of common rheumatic conditions that affect the elderly population.

PRETEST

1. Which condition is the most prevalent in the elderly population?
   a. Osteoarthritis
   b. Giant-cell arteritis
   c. Polymyalgia rheumatica
   d. Rheumatoid arthritis
   e. Gout

2. An 80-year-old white female patient comes to your office worried about a repeated positive test of antinuclear antibodies (ANA) 1/80 with a speckled pattern. Her previous doctor diagnosed her with systemic lupus erythematosus (SLE). The patient is otherwise asymptomatic and functional, and her physical examination is normal. Which one of the following would be the best approach for this patient?
   a. Reassure the patient that lupus is treatable, and cure is the goal.
   b. Tell the patient that she is going to develop lupus in the next year or less.
   c. Repeat the ANA to see whether it has increased in titer in the last 2 weeks.
   d. Reassure the patient that her antinuclear antibodies do not have clinical significance.
   e. Instruct the patient to stay away from the sunlight as much as possible.

3. A 75-year-old Hispanic woman is admitted to the hospital because of atrial fibrillation and put on anticoagulation plus rate control medications. Her past medical history was important for rheumatoid arthritis (RA), and she was taking weekly methotrexate and daily folic acid. On the third day in the hospital, the patient developed significant right knee pain. Her last methotrexate dose was taken 6 days ago. Physical examination detected a red, swollen right knee. What would your next approach be?
   a. Restart methotrexate
   b. Start prednisone
   c. Request an arthrocentesis
   d. Order magnetic resonance imaging
   e. Start colchicine

Mrs. Montes, *Part 1*

Mrs. Montes, a 90-year-old Hispanic woman, presents to the office with nonspecific "multiple joint aches and pains." She was brought by three family members and is in a wheelchair. She has several comorbidities:

1. Diabetes
2. Hypertension
3. Hypercholesterolemia
4. Coronary artery disease (prior coronary artery bypass graft)
5. Congestive heart failure
6. Atrial fibrillation
7. Arthritis
8. Mild dementia

Mrs. Montes complains that the aches and pains are recent, but she cannot recall when they started. According to her family, 4 weeks ago she was able to do her basic activities of daily living (ADLs) and some of her instrumental ADLs. A week ago she started refusing to walk. She has early morning stiffness that lasts more than 1 hour. Her examination is notable for the presence of Heberden's and Bouchard's nodes.

STUDY QUESTIONS

1. What is the likely cause of Mrs. Montes' complaints?
2. What treatment should be offered?
3. What is the significance of the Heberden's and Bouchard's nodes on her physical examination?

PREVALENCE

Arthritis in the elderly is a common and prevalent condition that is acquiring more importance as the population ages. New models of care are proliferating to satisfy this demand through geriatric rheumatology or gerontorheumatology.[1–6]

The most common arthritic condition among the elderly is osteoarthritis (OA). It affects 12.1% of U.S. adults, or 20.7 million people (Table 43-1). Less frequently encountered forms of arthritis or rheumatic disorders that are prevalent among the elderly are rheumatoid arthritis (RA) (2.1 million cases in the United States), gout (2.1 million people), pseudogout (10,000 to 40,000 people ages 65 to 85), polymyalgia rheumatica (PMR; approximately 450,000 Americans, 90% of whom are more than 60 years old), and giant-cell arteritis (GCA; 110,000 Americans, 90% of whom are >60 years old)[6].

RISK FACTORS AND PATHOPHYSIOLOGY

Osteoarthritis

OA, although highly prevalent among the elderly, does not appear to be directly caused by the aging process. Predisposing factors include obesity, female sex, quadriceps weakness, major joint injury and/or instability, poor proprioception, heavy physical activity, and genetics. OA is manifest first by cartilage irregularity, followed by eburnation or ulceration of the cartilage surface and eventually by frank cartilage loss.

Rheumatoid Arthritis

RA incidence increases with age. Predisposing factors for the development of RA are unknown. There is inflammation of the synovium of the joints that extends to the cartilage (pannus formation) and then invades the adjacent bone causing erosions.

Gout and Pseudogout

Gout, an inflammatory reaction to monosodium urate (MSU) crystals, is associated with hyperuricemia. Other risk factors include diuretic use, renal disease, obesity, hypertension, and heavy alcohol use. Urate crystals are able to directly initiate and sustain intense intraarticular attacks of acute inflammation because of

their capacity to stimulate the release of numerous inflammatory mediators. Pseudogout, an inflammatory reaction to calcium pyrophosphate dehydrate (CPPD) crystals, has been associated with disorders of phosphate, magnesium, parathyroid and thyroid hormone, and hemochromatosis. Attacks may be provoked by trauma, acute diseases, or the stress of surgery.

Polymyalgia Rheumatica and Giant-Cell Arteritis

PMR and GCA are closely related entities. The precise localization of disease-initiating triggering of the immune system in PMR is unknown. GCA is a chronic, systemic vasculitis that affects the elastic membranes of the aorta and its extracranial branches, particularly the external carotid artery with its superficial temporal division.[17,18]

DIFFERENTIAL DIAGNOSIS AND ASSESSMENT

The differential diagnosis and assessment for arthritic conditions in the elderly is similar to that of younger individuals. Table 43-1 provides an extensive list of laboratory and X-ray studies to assist with assessment. A component of the assessment is determining whether the symptoms with which the patient presents are atypical manifestations of typical diseases, as indicated in Table 43-2. The highlights of the approach to common arthritic conditions in the elderly are discussed later.

Osteoarthritis

OA usually has an insidious onset and chronic course. It affects the distal interphalangeal (DIP) joints causing characteristic Heberden's nodes, and the proximal interphalangeal (PIP) joints causing Bouchard's nodes. In addition, there is frequent involvement of the hips, knees, back, and neck. OA is a progressive disorder that takes many years to cause significant disability. Unfortunately, there is no cure yet available. The development of Heberden and Bouchard nodes may take 1 or 2 years; they may be painful and soft at the beginning and later harden and calcify while the pain subsides. Two-thirds of patients above 65 years old have X-ray changes consistent with OA.[8] Laboratory studies reveal a negative antinuclear antibody (ANA) and rheumatoid factor (RA), and a normal erythrocyte sedimentation rate (ESR) and c-reactive protein (CRP). X-rays show osteophytes, with loss of articular space and subchondral sclerosis.

> ● Osteoarthritis usually has an insidious onset and chronic course.

Table 43–1 Differential Diagnosis of Prevalent Rheumatic Disorders in the Elderly[15]

Disorder	Prevalence etc.	Impact on Mortality	Pathophysiology and Risk Factors	Clinical Comparison	Laboratory	X-rays	Management
Osteoarthritis (OA)	12.1% of U.S. adults or [7] 20.7 million people.[8,9]	Prevalence of coronary artery disease (CAD) in patients with OA is 27%.[10]	Age predisposes and obesity, female sex, inheritance, quadriceps weakness, major joint injury/instability, poor proprioception, heavy physical activity.	Insidious and chronic. Affects DIPs, PIPs, CMCs, hips, knees, back, and neck. Heberden's nodes (DIPs), and Bouchard's nodes (PIPs) are prevalent.	ANA (−); RF (−) ESR normal; CRP normal.	Presence of osteophytes, loss of articular space, subchondral sclerosis.	See Table 43-5 —Canes, braces, thermotherapy, exercise, narcotics, and knee and hip replacement.
Younger-onset rheumatoid arthritis (YORA)	About 2.1 million in U.S.: 600,000 men and 1.5 million women. RA prevalence diminishes after menopause.	Prevalence of CAD is 50%. Cardiovascular mortality accounts for half of all deaths.[10,11]	HLA DR4 present in RF(+) patients and in some RF(−) patients.	Insidious and chronic. Affects MCPs, PIPs, wrists, knees, and shoulders. Compared to EORA, symptoms >distal.	ANA (+/−); RF (+): Anti-CCP (+)[12,13]; ESR high; CRP normal.	Loss of articular space, multiple erosions, juxtaar-ticular osteopenia, ulnar deviation.	See Table 43-6—Low dose steroids.
Elderly-onset rheumatoid arthritis (EORA; >60 years)	Unknown. Sex distribution 1:1.	No data.	HLA DR4 is present in RF(+) and less likely in RF(−) patients.	More acute and infectious-like. Symptoms: >proximal. Outcome: worse.	ANA (+/−); RF (+): As YORA 32-89%; ESR higher at onset.	As YORA	See Table 43-6—Low dose steroids.
Gout in elderly	U.S. prevalence is 2.1 million: 1.56 million men and 550,000 women. Most are men with onset at middle age. Elderly-onset gout is after age 60; sex distribution is 1:1. If onset after age 80, women are almost 100%.	Hyperuricemia may produce HTN.[14]	It is associated with diuretic use and renal disease. Other classical risk factors include obesity, hypertension, and heavy alcohol use (less common). Gout is an inflammatory reaction to MSU crystals.	Elderly-onset gout is still acute but more polyarticular, more likely to involve small joints and develop tophi more rapidly and in unusual locations.	ANA (−); RF (−); High serum uric acid. MSU (negative birefringent) on synovial fluid.	Overhanging edge, with erosions. Affects mainly the first MTP, but it is common in hands.	NSAIDs, colchicine, allopurinol, steroids PO or intraarticular. Diet low in red meats and seafood.[15]
Pseudogout in elderly	Age 65 to 75: 10,000 to 15,000. Age >80: 40,000 per 100,000 people.	Unknown	Inflammatory reaction to CPPD crystals. With intraarticular calcifications (chondrocalcinosis).	Affects mainly the elderly population, most commonly the knee. Concomitant OA.	CPPD crystals (positive birefringent on polarizing micro-scope) in synovial fluid.	Chondrocalcinosis in hands, pelvis, and knees mostly.	NSAIDs, Intra-articular steroids.
Younger-onset systemic lupus erythematosus (SLE)	SLE affects at least 239,000 Americans: 4,000 white men, 41,000 white women, 31,000 black men, and 163,000 black women.	Premature atheroscle-rosis. Interval between onset and diagnosis is 32.5 months. Survival 97% at 5 years and 90% at 10 years.	T-cell genetic susceptibility plus natural senescence, stress factors may tip the balance to clinical disease. Unspecified environmental stimuli, illness, and infection.	Insidious and chronic. Usually systemic affecting kidneys, brain, lungs, heart, blood, and skin. Renal failure a common fear.	ANA, dsDNA, Sm Ro/SSA (+); C3, C4: low; ESR: high; CRP: high; APS ab (+). Pancytopenia.	Pericarditis changes, pleural effusion. Jaccoud's arthropathy.	See Table 43-6— High-dose steroids for flares.

Disease	Prevalence	Prognosis	Etiology	Clinical Features	Labs	ANA/Diagnostics	Treatment
Late-onset SLE (>50 years)	Unknown.	Female to male (6.9:1) Compared with younger-onset SLE, more common in whites; 5-year survival rate is comparable to younger-onset SLE.	Genetic factors, nongenetic, environmental, and life-style factors.	Tend to be milder. Weight loss, muscular aches and pains, disturbances of cognition or affect. Arthritis and arthralgias of the hands and wrists, rash, Raynaud's phenomenon, vague central nervous system symptoms.	ANA (weakly +) (up to 36% of healthy elderly people have nonspecific low titers of ANA), AntidsDNA (+), AntiSm (+), AntiRo/SSA (+), C3, C4: low, ESR/CRP: high.	As younger-onset SLE.	As younger-onset SLE. Careful with side effects.
Polymyalgia rheumatica (PMR)	600 cases/100,000 90% are over 60 years. Total 450,000 Americans, most of whom are white.	Overall life expectancy is essentially identical to the general population.	Unknown. Synovitis with T-cell and macrophage infiltration.	At least 1 month of aching and morning stiffness in at least two of the following three areas: shoulders and upper arms, hips and thighs, neck, and torso.	ESR/CRP: high, RF (−), AntiCCP (−).	Negative	Steroids
Giant-cell arteritis (GCA)	200 cases/100,000 total 110,000 Americans	15% to 20% of patients with PMR will have GCA. 15% with GCA have visual loss.	Related to PMR.	Headache, jaw claudication, visual disturbances, scalp tenderness, fever, weight loss, fatigue.	ESR/CRP: high.	Negative unless patient develops a stroke.	Steroids; ASA to prevent strokes.[16]
Idiopathic inflammatory myopathies (IIM): polymyositis (PM), dermatomyositis (DM), and sporadic inclusion body myositis (S-IBM)	Unknown prevalence. S-IBM is the most common after age 50.	Starting after age 50 is associated with increased mortality. The frequency of malignancy in patients with PM-DM increases with age.	Consider hypothyroidism, hyperthyroidism, osteomalacia, amyloid myopathy, drug-induced, corticosteroids, alcohol, colchicine, lipid lowering agents.	The response to therapy and outcome of elderly patients with PM-DM is poorer than in younger adults. Weakness of limb-girdle and anterior neck flexors, progressive over weeks to months.	ESR/CRP: high, CK: high, Aldolase: high, AST/ALT: high, LDH: high, Anti-Jo antibodies + (PM-DM)	None. EMG/NCS usually positive. Muscle biopsy is the gold standard.	Steroids and DMARDs. Usually, S-IBM is unresponsive to treatment.

ANA indicates antinuclear antibodies; Anti-CCP, anti-cyclic citrullinated peptide; APS, antiphospholipid syndrome; APS antibodies, lupus anticoagulant and anticardiolipin antibodies; ALT, alanine aminotransferase; ASA, acetyl-salicylic acid; AST, aspartate aminotransferase; CAD, coronary artery disease; CK, creatinine kinase; CMC, carpometacarpal joints; CPPD, calcium pyrophosphate dehydrated; CRP, c-reactive protein; ds DNA, anti-double-stranded DNA; DIP, distal interphalangeal joints; EMG/NCS, electromyogram/nerve conduction studies; ESR, erythrocyte sedimentation rate; HLA, human lymphocyte antigen; HTN, hypertension; LDH, lactate dehydrogenase; MSU, monosodium urate crystals; NSAID, nonsteroidal anti-inflammatory drugs; PIP, proximal interphalangeal joints; RF, rheumatoid factor; and Sm: anti-Smith antibodies.

Table 43–2	Atypical Musculoskeletal Manifestations of Typical Diseases
Shoulder pain, costochondral pain	Acute myocardial infarction, pneumonia, intraabdominal bleeding, or perforation
Temporomandibular joint pain	Acute myocardial infarction
Hip pain	Pancreatitis, psoas muscle abscess or hematoma, hip fracture, hernia
Back or extremity pain	Bone metastasis, osteomyelitis, tumor, deep venous thrombosis
Myalgias	Rhabdomyolysis

Rheumatoid Arthritis

RA tends to have a more acute presentation in the elderly than in younger individuals, with more involvement of proximal joints. The diagnostic approach is similar to that of younger individuals, with a positive RF in 80% of cases, positive anti-cyclic citrullinated peptide (anti-CCP; sensitivity of 80% and specificity of 98% to 100%), high ESR, and CRP.[12] A positive ANA is usually seen in patients with RA. X-rays show loss of articular space, multiple erosions, juxtaarticular osteopenia, and ulnar deviation.

● RA tends to have a more acute presentation in the elderly than in younger individuals, with more involvement of proximal joints.

Gout

Gout in the elderly is acute, as in younger individuals, but tends to be more polyarticular and is more likely to involve small joints, particularly of the hands. It characteristically involves the metatarsal phalangeal joint (MTP). ANA and RF are negative, but uric acid is high. MSU crystals can be found in the synovial fluid. These are needle-shaped crystals that are bright yellow when parallel to the axis or negatively birefringent on a polarizing microscope. MSU crystals tend to be present inside the neutrophils in active inflammation owing to phagocytosis. X-rays show erosions that are usually slightly removed from the joint, which is atrophic and hypertrophic, leading to erosions with an "overhanging edge."

● Gout characteristically involves the MTP Joint.

Pseudogout

Pseudogout affects mainly the elderly population, primarily in the knee. It is often found accompanying OA. Its presence is confirmed by the finding of cal-

cium pyrophosphate crystals (CPPD) in the synovial fluid. The crystals are rod-shaped and blue when parallel to the axis or positively birefringent on a polarizing microscope. X-rays show chondrocalcinosis primarily in the hands, pelvis and knees.

● Pseudogout affects mainly the elderly population, primarily in the knee.

Polymyalgia Rheumatica and Giant-Cell Arteritis

PMR is a clinical diagnosis and usually presents with at least 1 month of aching and morning stiffness in at least two of the following three areas: shoulders and upper arms, hips and thighs, neck and torso. It characteristically is associated with very high ESR and CRP, with a negative RA and anti-CCP. X-ray studies are negative. GCA is related to PMR and often presents with headache, jaw claudication, visual disturbances, fever, weight loss, and fatigue. The involved temporal artery may be tender. GCA diagnosis is established by biopsy of the temporal arteries, or angiographic appearance of the large arteries (subclavian, axillary, or aorta). Most commonly visual failure is related to stenosis of a branch of the ophthalmic artery. The clinical presentation is sudden and painless.

Role of Arthrocentesis

Arthrocentesis looks for three things in the synovial fluid: cell count, crystals, and culture. The information obtained will suffice in the differential diagnosis of most arthritic conditions. Noninflammatory fluids tend to have less than 1000 white blood cells (WBC), whereas inflammatory fluids tend to have more than 2000 WBC. Fluids with more than 100,000 WBC are an indication of septic arthritis until proven otherwise. See Table 43-3 for greater detail regarding conditions that cause inflammatory versus noninflammatory arthritides. Carefully selecting the kind of needle for this procedure is important. For instance, ordinarily, an 18-gauge needle can be used safely in the knee. However, it is common practice to use a 20- or 21-gauge needle. If the patient is anticoagulated, a 22- or 25-gauge needle will minimize the risk of bleeding. There should be an attempt to obtain clean, blood-free fluid to avoid confusion in the analysis. As much fluid as possible should be drained with one needle-stick to minimize discomfort and pain. In anticoagulated patients, there is no need to stop anticoagulation if the procedure is properly done.

Table 43–3	Classification of Arthritic Conditions Based on Inflammation
Inflammatory	**Noninflammatory**
Rheumatoid arthritis	Ostearthritis
Polymyalgia rheumatica	Fibromyalgia or myofascial pain
Myositis or dermatomyositis	Soft-tissue disorders (e.g., tendonitis, bursitis)
Crystal arthropathies (gout and pseudogout)	Chronic low-back pain
	Diabetic cheiroarthropathy
Septic arthritis	Dupuytren's contracture
Spondyloarthropathies and seronegative oligoarthritis	Osteoporosis
Systemic lupus erythematosus, Sjögren's tissue disorders	Reflex sympathetic dystrophy (regional pain syndrome) and other connective
Vasculitis (giant-cell arteritis, and small-vessel vasculitis)	
Paraneoplastic syndrome	

● Arthrocentesis looks for three things in the synovial fluid: cell count, crystals, and culture.

Mrs. Montes, *Part 2*

You prescribed for Mrs. Montes acetaminophen up to 4 g a day. However, there was no subsequent improvement. Glucosamine and chondroitin were added with no further improvement. Mrs. Montes was anticoagulated with Coumadin because of atrial fibrillation, so traditional nonsteroidal anti-inflammatory drugs (NSAIDs) were contraindicated. Instead, cyclooxygenase (COX) 2 inhibitors were prescribed with mild improvement. The family discontinued the medications after being informed that COX-2 inhibitors could cause heart attacks.

On a return visit, Mrs. Montes' vital signs are stable. She is not willing to walk, but she can stand and walk with one-person assistance. There is swelling, redness, and warmth of both wrists. There is tenderness in the PIP joints and metacarpal phalangeal (MCP) joints. The right knee is swollen, red and painful. The rest of the physical examination is unremarkable.

STUDY QUESTION

1. What should be done to further manage Mrs. Montes' joint complaints?

CASE DISCUSSION

You conclude that 6 months ago the diagnosis of OA was correct. The local doctor followed proper evidence-based medicine guidelines, but the patient did not get significantly better. The fact that this patient had baseline OA does not preclude her from having an inflammatory condition such as gout or RA. Given the polyarticular distribution, the most common explanation for Mrs. Montes' problems would be RA. It could also be a polyarticular presentation of gout or a manifestation of septic arthritis.

The next step is a knee arthrocentesis. The arthrocentesis reveals 25 ml of turbid yellowish fluid that shows negatively birefringent crystals under the polarizing microscope. Concomitant studies include RF, ANA, ESR, CRP, blood cell count, comprehensive metabolic panel with uric acid, and X-rays of the hands, wrists, and knees. Given that Mrs. Montes does not appear acutely ill, you send her home on Tramadol for pain control and with instructions to the family to contact you if her symptoms worsen. You maintain concern about the possibility of a septic arthritis, given that elderly individuals can present with septic arthritis without a fever or the appearance of initially being acutely ill.

Subsequently laboratory results become available. The fluid is inflammatory at 40,000 WBC with no organisms in the Gram stain and negative culture. The RF is positive, ESR and CRP are high, anti-CCP is positive, and ANA is positive. The X-rays show periarticular osteopenia of the hands and no changes of the knees. The uric acid is normal. Thus, the patient is diagnosed with RA and launched on a course of low-dose steroids to take care of the acute flare. Subsequently she is tried on sulfasalazine and referred for rheumatological consult and treated with methotrexate.

The fact that this patient had uric acid crystals confounded the clinical picture. This patient may have had intercritical gout, given that it is uncommon to find gout and RA simultaneously. Additionally, having a normal uric acid was sufficient justification not to start treatment with allopurinol.

MANAGEMENT

General Considerations

In order to develop an appropriate management plan for an elderly individual, it is essential that an assessment be made of the impact of the musculoskeletal problem on the overall functional status of the patient.[19,20] There is little correlation between symptoms and x-rays. Patients may have moderate to severe x-ray findings consistent with arthritis but be asymptomatic and fully functional, or they may have absent or mild x-ray findings with severe pain and accompanying disability.[21,22] The approach to therapy will vary based upon whether the patient is robust, frail, demented, or at the end of life.[23] Patients with rheumatic disorders are more likely to die from cardiovascular problems than from the musculoskeletal condition.[10]

Once the patient's functional status and overall prognosis are determined, there needs to be an assessment of whether there is a cure, rehabilitation, or a need for aggressive palliative interventions in the rheumatic condition. The goal is to improve the patient's well-being and quality of life.

In many cases, the first line of therapy for arthritic conditions in the elderly is NSAIDs. Elderly patients with multiple comorbidities and who are anticoagulated are at higher risk of peptic ulcer disease and associated complications. If traditional NSAIDs or COX-2 inhibitors are to be used, then specific precautions should be taken (Table 43-4), otherwise other pain medications can be ordered until the etiology of the symptoms is determined and specific treatment is given.

The interdisciplinary team is important in the care of older individuals with arthritis. Physical therapists and occupational therapists can be key in training the patient to compensate for lost function, and to appropriately select and utilize assistive devices. Social workers are invaluable for their help in finding the best resources within the communities in which patients reside, particularly if the patient has a combination of problems, such as severe arthritis and dementia. Pharmacists help patients find the best way to combine prescribed medications and suggest ways to reduce cost and avoid interactions.

Table 43–4 Traditional Nonsteroidal Anti-Inflammatory Drugs (NSAIDs) and Cyclooxygenase (COX) 2 Inhibitors[24,25]
Traditional NSAIDs
Skip alcohol.
Take with food and water.
Watch for over-the-counter (OTC) NSAIDs adding to prescribed amount consumed.
Keep the dose minimal. Consider taking NSAID OTC medications, in which the dose is usually lower than the prescription dose.
Consider stopping the medication if the patient is dehydrated.
Elderly patients should be monitored for gastrointestinal and renal side effects. Serum creatinine should be checked periodically.
Consider combining NSAIDs with H_2-blockers, proton pump inhibitors (PPIs), or misoprostol (at least 800 µg units).
Salicylate levels should be measured in serum when more than 3,600 mg per day are consumed.
Nonacetylated salicylates lack the aspirin cardiovascular protective effect. However, they have less risk for peptic ulcers.
Combination of angiotensin-converting enzyme (ACE) inhibitors and NSAIDs could be nephrotoxic.
COX-2 Inhibitors
COX-2 inhibitors are no better at relieving pain than traditional NSAIDs.
Older patients are better off taking traditional NSAIDs because of the increased risk of cardiovascular events with COX-2 inhibitors.
COX-2 may increase blood pressure and edema and cause more renal failure than do traditional NSAIDs.
COX-2 has less gastrointestinal complications than do traditional NSAIDs.
COX-2 can be combined with aspirin, but the risks of gastrointestinal problems increases.
Monitoring of this medication is more important in the elderly population, and side effects and recommendations are similar to that of traditional NSAIDs.

⬤ The approach to therapy will vary based upon whether the patient is robust, frail, demented, or at the end of life; patients with rheumatic disorders are more likely to die from cardiovascular problems than from the musculoskeletal condition.

Osteoarthritis

Treatment options for OA, with the level of evidence that supports those options, are detailed in Table 43-5. The foundation for therapy is NSAIDs. The approach to the use of NSAIDs in presented in Table 43-4. Acetaminophen has not been found to be as effective, but serves as a reasonable alternative for those patients who cannot tolerate NSAIDs. Failing NSAIDs and/or acetaminophen, narcotic analgesics are reasonable next steps. Exercise, particularly guided by a trained thera-

pist, is essential for strengthening muscles around joints affected by OA, and relieving problems with pain and instability. Often physical and occupational therapists will recommend assistive devices, such as canes and braces. Ultimately, for patients who are not responsive to these interventions, knee and hip replacements are considerations.

Rheumatoid Arthritis

RA should be treated with one of the many disease-modifying antirheumatic drugs (DMARDs) outlined in Table 43-6. Baseline therapy starts with low-dose steroids at 7.5 mg of prednisone or its equivalent daily. If this dose is exceeded, prophylaxis for glucocorticoid-induced osteoporosis should be initiated, including calcium, vitamin D, and bisphosphonates.

Table 43–5   Treatment of Osteoarthritis[26, 27]

Treatment Method	Systematic Reviews	Level of Evidence
Acetaminophen (up to 4 gm/day)	The evidence to date suggests that nonsteroidal anti-inflammatory drug (NSAIDs) are superior to acetaminophen for improving knee and hip pain in people with osteoarthritis (OA) but have not been shown to be superior in improving function. In OA subjects with moderate-to-severe levels of pain, NSAIDs appear to be more effective than acetaminophen. At daily doses of less than 2000 mg/day, acetaminophen was not associated with an increased risk for upper gastrointestinal complications. Mean age of study subjects was less than 65 years old.	A for pain management but B when compared with NSAIDs
Nonaspirin, NSAIDs (traditional NSAIDs) for treating osteoarthritis of the knee and hip	No substantial evidence is available related to efficacy, to distinguish between equivalent recommended doses of NSAIDs.	C. See level of evidence compared with acetaminophen.
Viscosupplementation intraarticular (viscous hyaluronate acid injected directly in the knee)	A systematic review protocol is ongoing. Evidence is conflicting about its benefit compared to placebo. No studies in the sedentary elderly population who are interested in quality of life.	C
Glucosamine	It is effective and safe in OA. Long-term toxicity not known. There are no data about the many different preparations. There are no data yet available regarding its combination with chondroitin.	B
Plaquenil	A systematic protocol is ongoing. It may help with inflammatory osteoarthritis.	C
Thermotherapy	Cold packs seem to be better than hot packs when applied locally to the affected joint.	C
Electromagnetic fields	Electrical stimulation therapy may provide significant improvements for knee OA.	C
Herbal treatments	The evidence for avocado-soybean in the treatment of osteoarthritis is convincing. Mean age of study participants was less than 65.	C
Autologous cartilage implantation (ACI) for full-thickness articular cartilage defects of the knee	ACI must currently be considered a technology under investigation whose effectiveness is yet to be determined. No data on age of participants.	C
Exercise	Land-based therapeutic exercise was shown to reduce pain and improve physical function for people with OA of the knee. Insufficient data for OA of the hip.	A
Cyclooxygenase (COX) 2	COX-2 inhibitors reduce gastroscopically diagnosed ulcers compared with other NSAIDs, but the reduction in clinical effects was less marked, and COX-2 inhibitors may increase the risk of myocardial infarction.	B

Table 43–6	Disease-Modifying Antirheumatic Drugs (DMARDs)[28-30]		
Drug	**Price per Month**	**Usual Dose**	**Common Side Effects to Consider**
Azathioprine (Imuran)	$55	50 to 150 mg per day in 1 to 3 doses.	Myelosuppression, hepatotoxicity, lymphoproliferative disorders.
Methotrexate	$288 (with tablets)	7.5 to 20 mg per week in a single dose orally or subcutaneously. Start low and increase by 5 mg every 1 to 2 months until effects are achieved.	Myelosuppression, hepatic fibrosis, cirrhosis, pulmonary infiltrates or fibrosis.
Sulfasalazine (Azulfidine, Azulfidine EN-Tabs)	$30	500 to 3,000 mg per day in 2 to 4 doses.	Myelosuppression.
Leflunomide (Arava)	$60	10 to 20 mg per day in a single dose by mouth.	Hepatotoxicity, hair loss.
Hydroxychloroquine sulfate (Plaquenil)	$46.8	400 mg by mouth a day in two doses.	Macular damage.
Etanercept (Enbrel)	$1,400	25 mg subcutaneously twice a week, or 50 mg subcutaneously once a week. For psoriasis, 50 mg twice weekly.	Be clinically alert for tuberculosis, histoplasmosis, and other infections.
Infliximab (Remicade)	$2,000	3 to 10 mg/kg intravenously. Doses are given at 0, 2, 6, and then every 8 weeks. Usually taken with Methotrexate.	Same as for etanercept.
Adalimumab (Humira)	$1,433	40 mg subcutaneously every week or every 2 weeks. Usually taken with Methotrexate.	Same as for etanercept.
Anakinra (Kineret)	$1,105	100 mg subcutaneously once a day; 100 mg subcutaneously every other day for patients with severe kidney disease.	Same as for etanercept.

Hydroxychloroquine may be another intervention, started at the standard dose, with every 6-month to yearly follow-up with an ophthalmologist looking for reversible retinal deposits. Methotrexate can also help with control of inflammation. Finally, anti-tumor necrosis factor (anti-TNF) drugs can be added to the other DMARDs to get the maximum benefit of preventing subsequent erosions. However, before starting them, a tuberculosis skin test should be checked as these medications may put the patient at risk of developing tuberculosis, among other infections prevalent in the elderly. It is also important to make sure that RA patients are updated on their pneumococcal pneumonia and influenza vaccinations

The more complex DMARDs should probably be deferred to the judgment of a rheumatologist. It is very important that the patient with RA be actively involved in physical and occupational therapy, to preserve as much function as possible and to compensate for deformities that limit function. The physical and occupational therapists can be very helpful in determining appropriate assistive devices to compensate for diminished functional capacity.

Gout and Pseudogout

Gout is treated with NSAIDs and/or colchicine. Allopurinol should be initiated once the acute flare has been controlled. Oral or intra-articular steroids can be very helpful with a severe acute attack. Patients with gout should be instructed to consume a diet low in red meats and seafood. Pseudogout is treated with NSAIDs and, on occasion for severe attacks, with intraarticular steroids.

Polymyalgia Rheumatica and Giant-Cell Arteritis

PMR and GCA are treated with oral steroids. GCA patients should also be treated with low-dose aspirin to limit the likelihood of stroke (see Table 43-1).

SUMMARY

Working with a coordinated multidisciplinary team, the quality of life of older individuals with arthritis can be significantly improved. Getting the older individual with arthritis active and moving is essential. Exercise is known to minimize pain and improve function in individuals suffering from arthritis. Lifelong physical activity will maximize the well-known effects of exercise in patients with rheumatic disorders and will generally engage the individual in social activities. A well coordinated approach to arthritis in the elderly will help these patients achieve successful aging by modifying disability, maximizing physical and mental function, putting the patient into social activities, and ultimately changing the patient's course to help attainment of life potential.[31]

POSTTEST

1. A 90-year-old African American woman is found to have a uric acid of 13 mg/dl. She is currently asymptomatic and does not have any joint pain. She does have a history of osteoarthritis and congestive heart failure and is taking furosemide 80 mg. The best approach for this patient will be:
   a. Start colchicine
   b. Start allopurinol
   c. Start probenecid
   d. Reduce the furosemide dose
   e. Tell the patient that she has gout

2. A 90-year-old African American man presents to your office with complaints of pain in both knees. He tells you that he has had the problem for several years; he has morning stiffness for less than 1 hour a day and pain mostly in the hands and knees. On physical examination he has hard nodes on the distal interphalangeal (DIP) joints and no effusion on the knees, although they look bigger than normal. Laboratory work revealed a low titer–positive RF, while the ESR and c-reactive protein (CRP) were within normal limits. The rest of the physical examination was unremarkable.

The most likely diagnosis is:
   a. Osteoarthritis
   b. Rheumatoid arthritis
   c. Psoriatic arthritis
   d. Polymyalgia rheumatica
   e. Myositis

3. An 80-year-old non-Hispanic white was taking COX-2 inhibitors and heard on the news that it was bad for the heart. He was tolerating the medication, and his knee pain from osteoarthritis was well controlled. When he started having the pain 4 years ago, his primary care provider put him on the COX-2 inhibitor as a first option, and he has been taking the same medication since that time. He has a history of peptic ulcer disease and renal insufficiency. Which is the best option for this patient to try?
   a. Acetaminophen
   b. Traditional NSAIDs with food
   c. Traditional NSAIDs plus 200 µg of misoprostol
   d. COX-2 plus aspirin
   e. Traditional NSAIDs plus PPI (proton pump inhibitor)

References

1. Nakasato YR, Teasdale T, Iqbal A, Bernard MA. New outpatient geriatric rheumatology clinic: steps to implementation. The Gerontologist. 2004;44 (Special issue 1):350.
2. van Lankveld W, Franssen M, van Kessel M, van de Putte L. Gerontorheumatologic outpatient service. Arthritis Rheum 2004;51:299-301.
3. Boyer JT. Geriatric rheumatology. Arthritis Rheum 1993;36:1033-1035.
4. Van Lankveld W, Franssen M, Stenger A. Gerontorheumatology: the challenge to meet health-care demands for the elderly with musculoskeletal conditions. Rheumatology 2005;44:419-422.
5. [Issue on geriatric rheumatology]. Rheum Dis Clin North Am 26(3).
6. Primer on the Rheumatic Diseases, 11 ed. Atlanta: Arthritis Foundation, 1997.
7. Lawrence RC, Helmick CG, Arnett FC, et al. Estimates of the prevalence of arthritis and selected musculoskeletal disorders in the United States. Arthritis Rheum 1998;41:778-799.
8. Arthritis prevalence rising as baby boomers grow older [press release]. Bethesda, MD: National Institute of Arthritis and Musculoskeletal Conditions, 1998.
9. Felson DT, Naimark A, Anderson J, Kazis L, Castelli W, Meenan RA. The prevalence of knee osteoarthritis in the elderly: the Framingham Osteoarthritis Study. Arthritis Rheum 1987;30:914-918.
10. Straub RH, Schölmerich J, Cutolo M. The multiple facets of premature aging in rheumatoid arthritis. Arthritis Rheum 2003;48:2713-2721.
11. Kitas GD, Erb N. Tackling ischaemic heart disease in rheumatoid arthritis. Rheumatology 2003;42:607-613.
12. Lopez-Hoyos M, Ruiz de Alegria C, Blanco R, et al. Clinical utility of anti-CCP antibodies in the differential diagnosis of elderly-onset rheumatoid arthritis and polymyalgia rheumatica. Rheumatology 2004;43:655-657.
13. Rantapää-Dahlqvist S, de Jong BAW, Berglin E, et al. Antibodies against cyclic citrullinated peptide and IgA Rheumatoid factor predict the development of rheumatoid arthritis. Arthritis Rheum 2003;48:2741-2749.
14. Johnson RJ, Rideout BA. Uric acid and diet: insight into the epidemic of cardiovascular disease. N Engl J Med 2004;350:1071-1073.
15. Choi HK, Atkinson K, Karlson EW, Willett W, Curhan G. Purine-rich foods, dairy and protein intake and the risk of gout in men. N Engl J Med 2004;350:1093-1103.
16. Nesher G, Berkun Y, Mates M, Baras M, Rubinow A, Sonnenblick M. Low-dose aspirin and prevention of cranial ischemic complications in giant cell arteritis. Arthritis Rheum 2004;50:1332-1337.
17. Nordborg E, Nordborg C. Giant cell arteritis: epidemiological clues to its pathogenesis and an update on its treatment. Rheumatology 2003;42:413-412.
18. Weyand CM, Goronzy JJ. Giant cell arteritis and polymyalgia rheumatica. Ann Intern Med 2003;139:505-515.
19. Leveille SG. Musculoskeletal aging. Curr Opin Rheum 2004;16:114-118.
20. Fried LP, Ferrucci L, Darer J, Williamson JD, Anderson G. Untangling the concepts of disability, frailty, and comorbidity: implications for improved targeting and care. J Gerontol Med Sci 2004;59:255-263.
21. Loeser RA, Shakoor N. Aging or osteoarthritis: which is the problem? Rheum Dis Clin N Am 2003;29:653-673.
22. Gorevic PD. Osteoarthritis: a review of musculoskeletal aging and treatment issues in geriatric patients. Geriatrics 2004;59:28-32.
23. Beers MH, Berkow R. The Merck Manual of Geriatrics, 3 ed. Whitehouse Station: Merck Research Laboratories, 2000.
24. Dunkin MA, Siegfried D. Arthritis today's 2005: drug guide. Arthritis Today January/February 2005.
25. Adhiyaman V, Asghar M, Oke A, White AD, Shah IU. Nephrotoxicity in the elderly due to co-prescription of angiotensin converting enzyme inhibitors and nonsteroidal anti-inflammatory drugs. J R Soc Med 2001;94:512-4.
26. Cochrane Database Syst Rev. 2004;4.
27. Musculoskeletal disorders. In Clinical evidence. London: BMJ Publishing Group, 2004. www.clinicalevidence.com.
28. Olsen NJ, Stein M. New drugs for rheumatoid arthritis. N Engl J Med 2004;350:2167-2179.
29. American College of Rheumatology Ad Hoc Committee on Clinical Guidelines: Guidelines for monitoring drug therapy in rheumatoid arthritis. Arthritis Rheum 1996;39:723-731.
30. Walgreen prices of drugs. www.walgreen.com.
31. Kahn RL. On "successful aging and well-being: self-rated compared with Rowe and Kahn." The Gerontologist 2002;42:725-726.

Web Resources

1. http://www.niams.nih.gov/hi/index.htm (National Institute of Health).
2. http://www.arthritis.org/conditions/diseasecenter/default.asp (Arthritis Foundation).
3. http://www.rheumatology.org/ (American College of Rheumatology).

PRETEST ANSWERS

1. a
2. d
3. c

POSTTEST ANSWERS

1. d
2. a
3. a

Foot Problems

Arthur E. Helfand

OBJECTIVES

Upon completion of this chapter, the reader will be able to:

- Identify the primary systemic diseases associated with foot problems which are considered "risk factors" under Medicare
- Recognize primary changes in the aging foot
- Understand the important principles of podogeriatric assessment
- Identify some of the complicating foot problems in the older adult
- Recognize diabetic foot problems in the elderly
- Be knowledgeable about primary management procedures

PRETEST
1. True or False: All diabetic foot care is a covered service under Medicare without qualification?
2. True of False: All toenails with onychauxis are mycotic?
3. True or False: Pedal pulses are absent in all diabetic patients?
4. True or False: Paronychia usually requires systemic antibiotics as an important factor in management?

PREVALENCE AND IMPACT

Foot problems represent some of the most painful, distressing, and disabling afflictions associated with aging. As society considers the basic needs of the older population, it is recognized that health is but one of those needs and is not always the highest in priority. Given an ideal set of circumstances, there are two important catalytic factors in the older patient's ability to remain as a vital part of society. They are a keen mind and the ability to ambulate.

Disorders and diseases of the foot in the older patient are a significant health concern, both from a standpoint of prevalence and incidence.[1] The immobility that results from a local foot problem or as the result of complications of systemic diseases, such as diabetes mellitus, peripheral vascular diseases, lower-extremity arterial disease, and degenerative joint changes, can have a significant negative impact on the patient's ability to maintain a quality of life as a useful member of society.

RISK FACTORS AND PATHOPHYSIOLOGY

Medicare has indicated a number of diseases that present with neurologic and vascular insufficiency in older patients as special "at risk" diseases that may qualify patients to be covered, along with "class findings," for primary foot care. The special risk factors are noted in Box 44-1.

> The immobility that results from a local foot problem or as the result of complications of systemic diseases, such as diabetes mellitus, peripheral vascular diseases, lower-extremity arterial disease, and degenerative joint changes, can have a significant negative impact on the patient's ability to maintain quality of life as a useful member of society.

Many factors contribute to the development of foot problems in the elderly. They include the aging process itself and the presence of multiple chronic diseases. Other significant factors include the degree of ambulation, the duration of prior hospitalization, limitation of activity, prior institutionalization and episodes of social segregation, prior care, emotional adjustments to disease and life in general, multiple medications for multiple chronic diseases, and the complications and residuals associated with other risk diseases. The management of foot problems in the elderly patient requires a comprehensive and team approach to maximize the quality of care provided.

The skin is usually one of the first structures to demonstrate early change. There is usually a loss of hair below the knee and on the dorsum of the foot and toes. Atrophy then follows, with the skin appearing parchment-like and xerotic. Brownish pigmentations are common and related to the deposition of hemosiderin. Hyperkeratosis, when present, may be due to keratin dysfunction, a residual to repetitive pressure, atrophy of the subcutaneous soft tissue, and/or as space replacement as the body attempts to adjust to the changing stress placed on the foot.

The toenails undergo degenerative trophic changes (onychopathy), thickening, and/or longitudinal ridging (onychorrhexis) related to repeated micro-trauma, disease, and nutritional impairment. Deformities of the toenails become more pronounced and complicated

---

Box 44–1 Risk Factors for Foot Problems

- Peripheral vascular disease
- Diabetes mellitus
- Chronic venous insufficiency
- Malnutrition (general, pellagra)
- Peripheral neuropathies involving the feet
- Intractable edema - secondary to a specific disease (e.g., congestive heart failure, kidney disease, and hypothyroidism)
- Lymphedema - secondary to a specific disease (e.g., Milroy's disease, malignancy)
- Vitamin deficiency
- Alcoholism
- Malabsorption (celiac disease, tropical sprue)
- Raynaud's disease
- Amyloid neuropathy

- Amyotrophic Lateral Sclerosis (ALS)
- Arteritis of the feet
- Chronic induratedd cellulitis
- Buerger's disease (thromboangiitis obliterans)
- Pernicious anemia
- Multiple sclerosis
- Uremia (chronic renal disease)
- Traumatic injury
- Leprosy or neurosyphilis
- Drugs and toxins
- Hereditary sensory radicular neuropathy
- Angiokeratoma corporis diffusum (Fabry's)
- Carcinoma (anywhere)

---

by xerotic changes in the periungual nail folds as ony-chophosis (hyperkeratosis) and tinea unguium (ony-chomycosis). These conditions are usually long-standing, chronic, and very common in the elderly and, in the case of onychomycosis, present a constant focus of infection.

> ● Deformities of the toenails become more pronounced and complicated by xerotic changes in the periungual nail folds as onychophosis (hyperkeratosis) and tinea unguium (onychomycosis). These conditions are usually long-standing, chronic, and very common in the elderly and, in the case of onychomycosis, present a constant focus of infection.

There is a progressive loss of muscle mass and atrophy of tissue owing to disease, decreased function, and a lack of activity, which increases the susceptibility of the foot to injury; so that even minor trauma can result in a fracture and a marked limitation of activity.

Case Study

Mr. J. B. is a 70-year-old man with a history of mild congestive heart failure. Pedal pulses were present, and there were no clinical symptoms or signs of peripheral arterial disease. The patient presented with pain and a small hematoma on the dorsum of his left second toe. The patient indicates that he dropped a can on his foot but that he was wearing a soft slipper. The toe has continued to hurt, especially when walking. A mild hammertoe was noted, and the patient indicated that he has had arthritis for some time. What would be your primary consideration?

1. Fracture of the toe
2. Contusion

CASE DISCUSSION

Initial management would include radiographs to rule out a fracture. If there is a fracture in good position, a silicone mold can be fabricated to immobilize the toe with the possibility of a surgical or healing shoe. Without evidence of trauma, a silicone mold could still be employed for a shorter period to splint the joint, followed by the use of a silicone protective tube. The patient should be instructed to take special care when moving heavy objects from cabinets and to consider a leather opera-type slipper for extra protection.

DIAGNOSIS AND ASSESSMENT

The initial evaluation of the older patient should include a comprehensive assessment and risk stratification process. A comprehensive assessment enables practitioners to initiate a diagnostic and risk stratification procedure that includes multiple elements.[2] The Helfand index, a comprehensive assessment tool, can be used to assess both pathology and risk factors. These elements include demographics, history of present illness, and past medical history.[3] Current prescriptions and over-the-counter medications should be noted.

The dermatologic evaluation should include but is not limited to the following: hyperkeratosis, bacterial infection, ulceration, cyanosis, xerosis, tinea pedis, verruca, hematoma, rubor, discoloration, and preulcerative changes. The foot orthopedic assessment includes but is not limited to the following: hallux valgus, hallux rigidus–limitus, anterior imbalance, Morton's syndrome, digiti flexus (hammertoes), and bursitis.

The peripheral vascular evaluation should include but is not limited to the following: coldness, trophic changes, palpation of the dorsalis pedis and posterior tibial pulses, the history of night cramps and/or claudication, edema, atrophy, varicosities, atrophy, and other findings; amputation or partial amputation should be noted. The neurological evaluation should include but is not limited to the following: Achilles and superficial plantar reflexes, vibratory sense (pallesthesia), response to a loss of protective sensation, sharp and dull reaction, joint position, burning, and other findings.[4]

Identifying Complicating Foot Problems

The management of foot problems in the elderly patient requires the early recognition of their etiologic factors, the complaints and symptoms of the patient, physical signs, and the clinical manifestations of disease and degenerative change, which may be local in origin or a complication of a related systemic or functional disease.

Degenerative joint diseases as manifest in the elderly foot should be related to acute trauma, inflammation, metabolic change, repeated and chronic micro-trauma, strain, obesity, osteoporosis, and postmenopausal changes. These changes increase pain, limit motion, and reduce the ambulatory status of the patient.

The primary manifestations in the foot are noted but not limited to those listed in Box 44-2.

Diabetes and Foot care

The older diabetic patient presents a special problem in relation to foot health.[5] It has been projected that 50% to 75% of all amputations in the diabetic patient can be prevented by early intervention where pathology is noted, by improved health education, and by periodic evaluation before the onset of symptoms and pathology (secondary and tertiary prevention).[6,7] The elderly diabetic patient is a patient with all of the problems related to the disease itself. These include vascular impairment, the degenerative changes of aging, neuropathy, dermopathy, and marked atrophy and deformity related to both diabetes mellitus and aging. These factors are then complicated by the social restrictions related to these multiple pathologies.

> ● The older diabetic patient presents a special problem in relation to foot health. It has been projected that 50% to 75% of all amputations in the diabetic patient can be prevented by early intervention where pathology is noted, by improved health education, and by periodic evaluation prior to the onset of symptoms and pathology (secondary and tertiary prevention).

The elderly diabetic patient with neuropathy presents with insensitive feet, which will generally exhibit some degree of paresthesia, sensory impairment to pain and temperature, motor weakness, diminished or lost Achilles and patellar reflexes, decreased vibratory sense, a loss of proprioception, xerotic changes, anhidrosis, neurotrophic arthropathy, atrophy, neurotrophic ulcers, and the potential for a marked difference in size between two feet. There is a greater incidence for infection, necrosis, and gangrene. Vascular impairment adds pallor, a loss or decrease in the posterior tibial and dorsalis pedis pulse, dependent rubor, a decrease in the venous filling time, coolness of the skin, and trophic changes. Numbness and tingling as well as cramps and pain are demonstrated. There is usually a loss of the plantar metatarsal fat pad, which predisposes the patient to ulceration in relation to the existing bony deformities of the foot.

Hyperkeratotic lesions form as space replacements and provide a focus for ulceration owing to increased pressure on the soft tissues with an associated localized

---

Box 44–2   Primary Manifestations of Disease in the Foot

- Plantar fasciitis
- Spur formation
- Periostitis
- Decalcification
- Stress fractures
- Tendonitis
- Tenosynovitis
- Residual deformities
- Pes planus

- Pes cavus
- Hallux valgus
- Digiti flexus (Hammer Toes)
- Rotational digital deformities
- Joint swelling
- Increased pain
- Limitation of motion
- Reduced ambulatory status

avascularity from direct pressure and counter-pressure. Tendon contractures and claw toes (hammertoes) are common. A warm foot with pulsations in an elderly diabetic with neuropathy is not uncommon. When ulceration is present, the base is usually covered by keratosis that retards and many times prevents healing.[8] Necrosis and gangrene are related to infection with eventual occlusion and gangrene. Foot drop and a loss of position sense are usually present. Pretibial lesions are indicative of this change as well as microvascular infarction. Arthropathy gives rise to deformity, altered gait patterns, and a higher risk for ulceration and limb loss (Figure 44-1).

> ● Hyperkeratotic lesions in the diabetic patient form as space replacements and provide a focus for ulceration owing to increased pressure on the soft tissues with an associated localized avascularity from direct pressure and counter-pressure.

Radiographic findings in the foot in elderly diabetics usually demonstrate thin trabecular patterns, decalcification, joint position changes, osteophytic formation, osteolysis, deformities, and osteoporosis. Pruritus and cutaneous infections are more common in the diabetic. Dehydration, trophic changes, anhidrosis, xerosis, and fissures are predisposing factors to calcaneal ulceration. The most commonly demonstrated nail changes are noted but not limited those in Box 44-3.[9]

Case Study

Mrs. R. H. is a 75-year-old woman, living in her home with her husband. She has a history of Type 2 diabetes mellitus (NIDDM), with 12 years' since diagnosis. Her diabetes remains diet controlled with adequate control, as reported by her endocrinologist. She reports noticing a dark spot under her left great toe nail in recent months but with no pain. She presents with trophic changes and diminished pedal pulses.

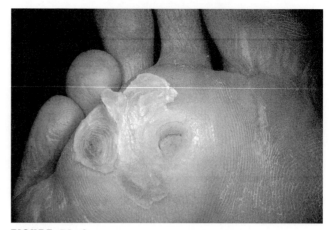

FIGURE 44–1

Diabetic ulcer, metatarsal pressure area, roofing with hyperkeratosis, subcallosal hematoma, atrophy of plantar fat pad, metatarsal prolapse, peripheral arterial disease, and xerosis.

Doppler studies detect both pedal pulses. Testing with a monofilament demonstrates a loss of sensation distal to the metatarsal shaft area. All toenails demonstrate onychorrhexis, and xerosis was noted. No other significant clinical findings were noted. What are your primary considerations given the patients lack of pain?

1. *Subungual heloma*
2. *Subungual ulceration*
3. *Subungual hematoma*
4. *Subungual exostosis*
5. *Subungual spur*
6. *Subungual melanoma*

CASE DISCUSSION

Initial management includes radiographs to rule out an exostosis or spur or other bony change. If the concern is related to a possible melanoma, biopsy should be completed with appropriate surgical referral. With a history of trauma, a subungual

---

Box 44-3   Common Toenail Changes

- Diabetic onychopathy (nutritional and vascular changes)
- Onychorrhexis (longitudinal striations)
- Onycholysis (shedding from the distal portion)
- Onychomadesis (shedding from the proximal portion)
- Subungual hemorrhage (bleeding in the nail bed)
- Onychophosis (keratosis)
- Onychauxis (thickening with hypertrophy)
- Onychogryphosis (thickening with gross deformity)
- Onychia (inflammation)

- Onychomycosis (fungal infection)
- Subungual ulceration (ulceration in the nail bed)
- Deformity
- Hypertrophy
- Incurvation or involution (onychodysplasia)
- Subungual hemorrhage (non-traumatic)
- Onycholysis (freeing from the distal segment)
- Onychomadesis (freeing from the proximal segment)
- Autoavulsion

hematoma should be considered. Without trauma, a subungual diabetic ulcer should be considered. If there is an enlargement of the dorsal aspect of the tip of the distal phalanx on X-ray, a subungual heloma should be considered. Appropriate management depends on the diagnosis. A silicone tube or lambs wool can then be employed to reduce pressure.

MANAGEMENT

The management of localized foot problems in the elderly requires a review of the etiologic considerations, the symptoms presented by the patient, the physical signs and clinical manifestations, and the appropriate diagnostic studies, including the use of weight-bearing and non-weight-bearing radiographs, vascular studies, etc. Complications, sequelae, relevant treatment, the prognosis, and the overall management of the elderly patient should reflect a reasonable approach that will reduce pain, improve the functional capacity of the patient, maintain that restored function, and provide for the comfort of the patient in his or her activities of daily living.[10–12]

Onychia

Onychia is an inflammation involving the posterior nail wall and nail bed. The onychial changes that occur in the elderly patient are the result of a new disease or are the residual of long-term disease, injury, and/or functional modification. It is usually precipitated by local trauma or pressure or by a complication of systemic diseases, such as diabetes mellitus, and is an early sign of a developing infection. Mild erythema, swelling, and pain are the most prevalent findings. Treatment should be directed to removing all pressure from the area and the use of tepid saline compresses for 15 minutes, three times per day. With systemic complications, systemic antibiotics should be instituted early along with radiographs and scans to detect bone change at its earliest sign. Lambs wool, tube foam, or shoe modification should also be considered to reduce pressure to the toe and nail. If the onychia is not treated early, paronychia may develop, with significant infection and abscess of the posterior nail wall. The infection progresses proximally, and deeper structures become involved. The potential for osteomyelitis is greater in the presence of diabetes mellitus and vascular insufficiency. Necrosis, gangrene, and the potential for amputation become reality. Management includes establishing drainage, culture and sensitivity, radiographs and scans as appropriate, the use of saline compresses, and appropriate systemic antibiotics.

Always advise against maceration of tissue. Early follow-up is essential as these conditions can result in significant problems in management (Fig. 44-2).

> ● Treatment of onychia should be directed toward removing all pressure from the area and the use of tepid saline compresses for 15 minutes, three times per day.

Deformities of the toenails are the result of repeated micro-trauma, degenerative changes, or disease. For example, the continued rubbing of the toenails over the years, against the inferior toe box of the shoe, is sufficient trauma to produce change. The initial thickening is termed onychauxis. Onychorrhexis with accentuation of normal ridging, trophic changes, and longitudinal striations is onychopathic when related to disease and/or nutritional etiology. When débridement is not completed on a periodic basis, the nail structure elongates, continues to thicken, and becomes deformed with shoe pressure. Onychogryphosis, or ram's horn nail, is usually complicated by fungal infection. The resultant disability can prevent the elderly from wearing shoes. Pain is usually associated with shoe pressure and the deformity. In addition, a traumatic avulsion of the nail is more frequent with this condition. The exaggerated curvature (onychodysplasia) may even penetrate the skin, with resultant infection and ulceration. Management should be directed toward periodic débridement of the onychial structures both in length and thickness, with as little trauma as possible. The degree of onycholysis (freeing of the nail from the anterior edge) and onychoschizia (splitting) help determine the level of débridement. With the excess pressure of deformity, the nail grooves tend to become onychophosed (keratotic). When this occurs, debridement and the use of mild keratolytics and emollients, such as Keralyt gel and 10% to 20%

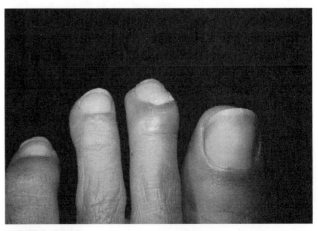

FIGURE 44-2

Onychia with early paronychia, second toe.

urea preparations, provide some measure of home care for the patient. With onycholysis, subungual debris and keratosis develop, which increases discomfort and may generate pain. However, the patient may not present complaints of pain and discomfort, and care should be provided with the deformity. In addition, with degenerative changes, the sense of pain may be lost, which tends to defer care by the patient until a complicating condition is presented (Fig. 44-3).

Onychomycosis

The most common nonbacterial infection of the toenails is onychomycosis. It is a chronic and communicable disease, and clinically it may appear as distal subungual, white superficial, proximal subungual, total dystrophic, and candida onychomycosis. In the superficial variety, the changes appear on the superior surface of the toenail and generally do not invade the deeper structures. In both the distal, proximal, and total dystrophic manifestations, the nail bed, as well as the nail plate, is infected. There is usually some degree of onycholysis (freeing of the nail from the distal edge) and subungual keratosis. In the elderly, owing to the long-standing chronic nature of this condition, the posterior nail wall and eponychium demonstrate xerotic changes and hypertrophy, as does the nail plate. Candida is most common in patients with some form of chronic mucocutaneous manifestation. Patients with AIDS may demonstrate subungual white onychomycosis (Fig. 44-4).

> ● The most common nonbacterial infection of the toenails is onychomycosis. It is a chronic and communicable disease, and clinically it may appear as distal subungual, white superficial, proximal subungual, total dystrophic, and candida onychomycosis.

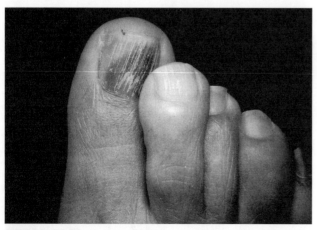

FIGURE 44-3

Subungual hematoma with superficial white onychomycosis, hallux, onychorrhexis, onychauxis, with early overlapping second toe.

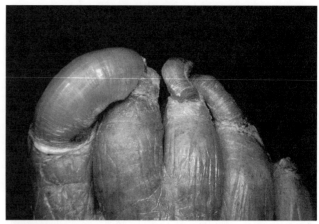

FIGURE 44-4

Onychogryphosis, onychomycosis, hammertoes, syndactyly, peripheral arterial disease, and xerosis.

The elderly patient usually presents with a chronic infection, involving one or more of the nail plates. The entire thickness of the nail plates is usually involved, with resultant hypertrophy and deformity. Pain is usually not a significant factor owing to the normal lessening of sensation in the elderly but can be present when the deformity becomes excessive and is related to external pressure. Mycotic onychia; auto-avulsion; subungual hemorrhage; a foul, musty odor; and degeneration of the nail plate are common findings. The most practical form of treatment in the elderly is one of management. Because of the chronicity of the condition and the fact that once the matrix of the nail is involved hypertrophy and deformity occur, the residuals cannot be reversed. In addition, multiple drug use for systemic diseases and vascular impairment limits systemic management. Periodic débridement, the use of 35% to 50% urea to aid in debridement, and the use of a topical fungicide in an alcoholic base to permit penetration provide a conservative approach to management. Systemic antifungals can also be employed as indicated. Onychomycosis must be viewed as a chronic infectious disease, deserving management as any other chronic condition such as hypertension and/or often mellitus (Fig. 44-5).

Ingrown Toenails

Ingrown toenails in the elderly are usually the end result of deformity and improper self-care. When the nail penetrates the skin, an abscess and infection result. If not managed early, periungual granulation tissue may form, which complicates treatment. Deformity and involution also provide a complicating factor. In the early stage, a segment of the nail can easily be removed using an English nail splitter and onychotomy, drainage established, saline compresses

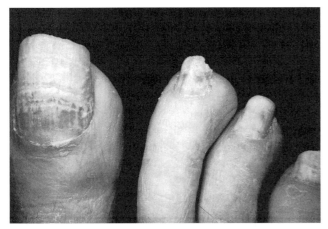

FIGURE 44-5

Onychomycosis, subungual and superficial white onychomycosis, onychauxis, onychodysplasia of hallux toenail, and Beau's lines.

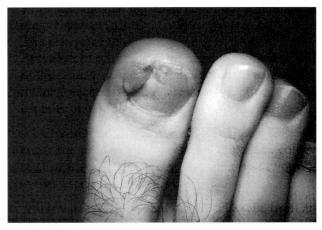

FIGURE 44-6

Onychocryptosis (ingrown toenail) with peri-ulcerative granulation tissue, and onychia.

employed for 15 minutes three times a day, and antibiotics used as indicated. Measures should be taken to prevent the problem in the future. When granulation tissue is present, excision, fulguration, desiccation, or the use of caustics such as silver nitrate (75%) and astringents are used to reduce the granulation tissue. In all cases, removal of the penetrating nail is primary. Partial excision of the nail plate and matrix can be completed by using regional anesthesia followed by chemical cautery of the matrix area with CP phenol, for example. With this procedure, post-operative management includes isopropyl alcohol compresses and topical steroid solutions, three times per day to healing. With aging, we also find changes in the nail plate, which when viewed distally appear C-shaped. This abnormal curvature is incurvation or involution. When present, the pressure of the nail plate on the nail bed and folds produces onychophosis (hyperkeratosis in the nail folds) and discomfort, with complaints similar to an ingrown toenail. The condition may precipitate pressure ulcerations and infection. When this condition is severe, early and total removal of the nail plate and matrix should be considered to avoid complications as the patient ages (Fig. 44-6).

Dryness and Xerosis

Dryness of the skin and xerosis are common problems in the older patient. The etiology is due to a lack of hydration and lubrication and, to some degree, is a part of the normal aging and degenerative process. There is usually some evidence of keratin dysfunction that can be associated with xerosis. Fissures develop as a result of dryness and, when present on the heel with associated stress, present a potential hazard for the development of ulceration. Initial management includes

the use of an emollient after hydration of the skin. Twenty percent urea is helpful to aid as a mild and safe keratolytic. A plastic or Styrofoam heel cup can be of assistance in minimizing trauma to the heel, thus reducing the potential for complications. Pruritus is a common complaint of the elderly and is usually more severe in the colder weather. It is related to dryness, scaliness, decreased skin secretions, keratin dysfunction, environmental changes, and defatting of the skin that is usually precipitated by the constant use of hot foot soaks. The patient will scratch with excoriations noted on examination. Chronic tinea, allergic, neurogenic, and/or emotional dermatoses should be considered as part of the differential diagnosis and treated accordingly. Management consists of hydration, lubrication, protection, topical steroids if indicated, and judicious use of antihistamines in minimal doses to control the itching, which is usually the primary complaint. Particular care should be taken in the male patient with a history of prostatic hypertrophy. If excoriations are infected, proper antibiotic therapy should be instituted.

> ● Initial management of fissures that are a result of dryness on the heel includes the use of an emollient after hydration of the skin. Twenty percent urea is helpful to aid as a mild and safe keratolytic. A plastic or Styrofoam heel cup can be of assistance in minimizing trauma to the heel, thus reducing the potential for complications.

Tinea Pedis

Tinea pedis in the elderly patient is many times an extension of onychomycosis, which serves as a focus of infection. It is more common in warmer weather, with the chronic keratotic type more common clinically in the elderly. Poor foot hygiene in many older patients and the inability to see their feet may motivate the patient to seek care only when the condition becomes clinically significant. The wide variety of topical medications available can usually control this condition. Solutions and/or creams (water washable or miscible) should be used when the patient is unable to easily remove an ointment base.

Hyperkeratotic Lesions

Common complaints of most elderly are the many forms of hyperkeratotic lesions, such as tyloma (callous) and heloma (corn) and their varieties, such as hard, soft, vascular, neurofibrous, seed, and subungual. Intractable keratoma, eccrine poroma, porokeratosis, and verruca must be differentiated from these keratotic lesions, although each may present initially as a hyperkeratotic area. The biomechanical and pathomechanical factors that help create these problems are those associated with stress, that is, compressive, tensile, and/or shearing. The loss of soft tissue as part of the aging process and atrophy of the plantar fat pad increase pain and limit ambulation. Contractures, gait changes, deformities, and the residuals of arthritis are all additional factors that need to be considered in management. The incompatibility of the foot type (inflare, straight, or outflare) to the shoe last is another factor to be considered. It is important to recognize that there is usually not one factor but a multiplicity of conditions, including skin tone and elasticity, which results in the development of keratotic lesions in the elderly. Their management is not routine, and the term "management" signifies a period of continuing care, as with any other chronic condition in the elderly to provide for ambulation and comfort (Fig. 44-7).

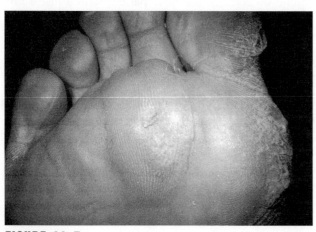

FIGURE 44–7

Hyperkeratosis (callus) related to pressure, xerosis, subkeratotic hematoma, hallux valgus, metatarsal prolapse, and anterior displacement of the plantar fat pad.

The common sites for the development of hyperkeratotic lesions (callous and corns) include but are not limited to dorsal or distal digital, plantar metatarsal heads, marginal calcaneal, and with deformities such as hammertoes, digital rotations, contractures, hallux valgus, bunion, and/or tailor's bunion. The above-noted deformities are precipitating factors to foot-to–shoe last incompatibilities that produce excessive pressure on segments of the foot. Management and treatment should be directed toward the functional needs of the patients and on their activity needs for daily living. Considerations include débridement, padding, emollients, shoe modifications, and last changes, orthoses, and surgical revision as indicated. Materials to provide soft-tissue replacement, weight dispersion, and weight diffusion are also indicated. It is also important to recognize that keratotic lesions of long-standing represent a hyperplastic and hypertrophic pathology and, even when weight bearing is removed, they tend to persist. In a sense, hyperkeratotic lesions are a form of body protection to pressure and are symptoms of an abnormal state. If permitted to persist, enlarge, and condense, they become primary irritants. With pressure such as weight bearing and ambulation, they produce local avascularity, which can precipitate ulceration and their resultant sequelae. Pressure ulcers in the foot usually begin with subkeratotic hemorrhage. Once debrided and managed properly, they usually heal but may be repetitive, unless adequate measures are instituted to reduce the pressure to the localized areas of ulceration. Even with all measures, the problem may persist owing to residual deformity and systemic diseases, such as diabetes mellitus. Thus management and monitoring are similar to any other chronic condition in the elderly and can have a significant impact on the social elements of society, for without ambulation the elderly patient is often institutionalized.

> ● The common sites for the development of hyperkeratotic lesions (callous and corns) include but are not limited to dorsal or distal digital, plantar metatarsal heads, marginal calcaneal, and deformities such as hammertoes, digitial rotations, contractures, hallux valgus, bunion, and/or tailor's bunion.

Foot Deformities

There are a variety of residual foot deformities that can be present in multiple combinations in the elderly. These include but are not limited to hallux valgus, hallux varus, splay foot, hallux flexus, digiti flexus (hammertoe), digiti quinti varus, overlapping toes, under-riding toes, prolapsed metatarsals, pes cavus, pes planus, pronation, hallux limitus, and hallux rigidus (Fig. 44-8).

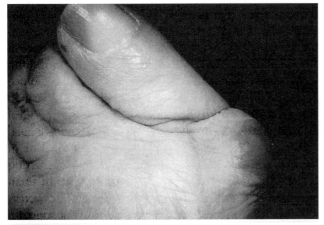

FIGURE 44–8

Hallux valgus, hammertoes, enlarged first metatarsal head, degenerative joint disease, rotational deformities, bursitis with inflammation.

Biomechanical and pathomechanical abnormalities create functional problems in relation to gait and obtaining adequate footwear. Treatment consists of both nonsurgical and surgical considerations. Age itself should not be the final determining factor in considering surgery. What is important is to determine what can be done to maintain quality of life for the patient. Consideration must also be given to the patient's ability to adapt to change in relation to ambulation, for to have an anatomically corrected joint and a patient that can not ambulate without pain defeats the treatment needs of the elderly (Fig. 44-9).

Conservative modalities include shoe last changes, shoe modifications, orthoses, digital braces, physical medicine, exercises, and mild analgesics for pain. The residuals of these deformities can produce inflammatory changes such as periarthritis, bursitis, myositis, synovitis, neuritis, tendonitis, sesamoiditis, and plantar myofascitis, for example, which need to be managed medically, physically, and mechanically to keep the patient ambulatory and pain free.

> ● Conservative modalities to treat biomechanical and pathomechanical abnormalities include shoe last changes, shoe modifications, orthoses, digital braces, physical medicine, exercises, and mild analgesics for pain.

SUMMARY

Much of the ability to remain ambulatory in the period of aging is directly related to foot health. To accomplish this aim, practitioners must think comprehensively and recognize that team care must be an essential part of geriatrics. Foot health education, such as programs developed by the "Feet First"[13] and "If the Shoe Fits,"[14] are available to both patients and professionals and should be employed as a part of all elderly patient education programs. With the high prevalence and incidence of foot problems in the elderly, much of their quality of life will depend on their ability to remain mentally alert and ambulatory.

References

1. Helfand AE. Public health and podiatric medicine. Baltimore, MD: Williams and Wilkins, 1987.
2. Helfand AE. Foot problems in older patients: a focused podogeriatric assessment study in ambulatory care. J Am Podiatr Med Assoc 2004;94:293-304.
3. Helfand AE. Public health strategies to develop a comprehensive chronic disease and podogeriatric assessment protocol. Natl Acad Prac Forum 1999;1:49-57.
4. Helfand AE. Clinical assessment of podogeriatric patients. Podiatr Manage February 2004, 145-152.
5. International Diabetes Federation. International consensus on the diabetic foot. Amsterdam, Netherlands: International Diabetes Federation, 2003.
6. American Diabetes Association. Preventive foot care in people with diabetes mellitus. Diabetes Care 2004;27(Suppl):S63-S64.
7. Helfand AE. Clinical podogeriatrics: assessment, education, and prevention. Clin Podiatr Med Surg 2003;20(3):xvii-xxiii.
8. Sanders L. Diabetic foot ulcers and amputations. Washington, DC: American Diabetes Association, 2001.
9. U.S. Department of Veterans Affairs, Veterans Health Administration. Clinical Guidelines for Management of Patients with Diabetes Mellitus, Washington, DC: Veterans Health Administration, 1997.
10. Helfand AE. Clinical podogeriatrics. Baltimore, MD: Williams and Wilkins, 1981.
11. Helfand AE. The geriatric patient and considerations of aging, Vol. 1 and Vol. II. Clin Podiatr Med Surg, 1993.
12. Robbins JM. Primary podiatric medicine. Philadelphia, PA: W.B. Saunders, 1994.
13. Helfand AE. Feet First. Harrisburg, PA: Pennsylvania Diabetes Academy, 1991.
14. Helfand AE. If The Shoe Fits. Harrisburg, PA: Pennsylvania Diabetes Academy, 1994.

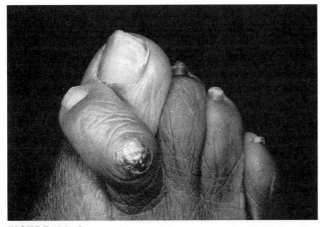

FIGURE 44–9

Hallux valgus, hammertoe, overlapping second toe, degenerative joint disease, xerosis, heloma durum, preulcerative keratosis, and subkeratotic hematoma.

POSTTEST

1. Which of the following systemic diseases is not considered as a risk factor for covered primary foot care under Medicare?
   a. Diabetes mellitus
   b. Peripheral arterial disease
   c. Alzheimer's disease
   d. Neuropathy associated with multiple sclerosis

2. True or False: The loss of protective sensation is a primary clinical finding in diabetic neuropathy.

3. True or False: Osteoporosis is not a common finding in the older foot.

4. True or False: Pretibial lesions in the older diabetic are an indication of microvascular infarction.

PRETEST ANSWERS

1. False
2. False
3. False
4. True

POSTTEST ANSWERS

1. c
2. True
3. False
4. True

OBJECTIVES

Upon completion of this chapter, the reader will be able to:

● Illustrate advances in chemoprevention of cancer.

● Summarize advances in the treatment of cancer.

● Provide examples of age-specific problems in cancer management.

● Apply geriatric assessment to decisions related to cancer management in older individuals.

● Study the interactions of geriatricians and oncologists in the management of the older cancer patient.

PRETEST

1. Which one of the following patients is a good candidate for cytotoxic chemotherapy?
   a. A 79-year-old woman with a 1.5-cm breast cancer that is negative for hormone receptors and negative axillary lymph nodes.
   b. An 86-year-old woman with breast cancer metastatic to the bone and to the lung that is no longer responsive to hormonal therapy. The patient has severe macular degeneration, is dependent for transfer and toileting, and has no symptoms related to cancer.
   c. A 72-year-old man with prostate cancer metastatic to the pelvic lymph nodes. The patient had an orchiectomy, and his prostate-specific antigen level dropped from 87 to 0.1 ng/ml. The patient is in excellent performance status, plays golf every day, and has no comorbid conditions.
   d. An 81-year-old woman admitted to the hospital with severe dehydration and renal failure. The patient was living alone and totally independent up to 2 weeks before admission. She has gastric outlet obstruction from gastric lymphoma.

2. Which of the following is true about raloxifene?
   a. It is a pure estrogen antagonist.
   b. It appears to prevent breast cancer.
   c. It prevents cerebrovascular diseases.
   d. It increases the risk of osteoporosis.
   e. It can be used in lieu of tamoxifen in the adjuvant treatment of breast cancer.

3. In which of the following patients is castration likely to prolong survival?
   a. A 78-year-old man with advanced dementia and prostate cancer metastatic to the bones.
   b. A 78-year-old man who had a radical prostatectomy 10 years earlier and now has a prostate-specific antigen level of 0.7 ng/ml (a year ago it was 0.1 ng/ml).
   c. A 78-year-old man who had radical prostatectomy 10 years earlier and who now has a prostate-specific antigen level of 4.5 ng/ml. A computed tomography scan of the pelvis shows an enlarged pelvic lymph node, and a bone scan is positive in the pelvic area.
   d. A 78-year-old man with prostate cancer limited to the prostate with a Gleason score of 6.

PREVALENCE AND IMPACT

Cancer is the second leading cause of death and a major cause of morbidity for persons age 65 and older.[1,2] Cancer control in older individuals includes prevention, individualized treatment plans, and terminal and palliative care. The primary care physician plays a key role in each stage of care. This chapter reviews the following recent information related to cancer management:

● Age-related changes in cancer biology
● Chemoprevention of cancer in the older person
● General principles of cancer management in the elderly
● Application of a comprehensive geriatric assessment (CGA) to the management of older individuals with cancer

● Age-specific issues in the management of specific cancers

RISK FACTORS AND PATHOPHYSIOLOGY

Cancer Biology and Aging

The behavior of some neoplasms changes with the age of the patient[3] as a result of two mechanisms (Table 45-1):

1. Older persons develop tumors that are different from younger persons. For example, acute myelogenous leukemia in older patients presents with a higher prevalence of chemotherapy-resistant cells.[4]
2. The older patient modulates tumor growth differently. For example, the concentration of interleukin (IL) 6 in the circulation increases with age.

Table 45–1	Age-Related Changes in the Behavior of Some Neoplasms	
Neoplasm	**Age-Related Change in Prognosis**	**Mechanism**
Acute myelogenous leukemia	Worse	Increased prevalence of multiple drug resistance Increased prevalence of stem cell leukemia
Large-cell non-Hodgkin's lymphoma	Worse	Increased circulating concentrations of interleukin-6
Breast cancer	More indolent	Increased prevalence of hormone-receptor–rich, well-differentiated, slowly proliferating tumors Reduced production of tumor growth factors from the tumor host
Non-small-cell lung cancer	More indolent	Unknown
Celomic ovarian cancer	Worse	Unknown

As IL-6 stimulates lymphoproliferation, the prognosis of non-Hodgkin's lymphoma (NHL) worsens with age.[5-8]

Two observations have clinical relevance:

1. Contrary to common expectations, cancer may become more aggressive with age.[9]
2. Age itself should not determine the treatment of cancer: 67% of older persons with acute myelogenous leukemia present with a disease that is difficult to treat, but 33% have a disease highly responsive to chemotherapy. Although 80% of older women have an indolent form of breast cancer, 20% of these patients have an aggressive disease that may benefit from adjuvant chemotherapy and radiotherapy.[10] The aggressiveness of the tumor is better judged from the tumor characteristics than from the age of the patient.

Chemoprevention of Cancer in the Older Person

Chemoprevention of cancer involves administration of substances that block or offset the late stages of carcinogenesis.[11] At least three groups of substances have demonstrated chemopreventative activity in humans:

1. *Hormonal agents.* Selective estrogen receptor modulators (SERMs), including tamoxifen and raloxifene, and aromatase inhibitors, including anastrozole, letrozole and exemestane may prevent breast cancer.[12-14] The 5-a reductase inhibitor, finasteride may prevent prostate cancer.[15]
2. *Retinoids* may prevent cancer of the upper airways in smokers.[11]
3. *Nonsteroidal anti-inflammatory* drugs may prevent death from cancer of the large bowel and of the breast.[16]

Recent studies indicate that the cholesterol-lowering drugs HMG-CoA reductase inhibitors may prevent different cancers, including cancers of the large bowel and of the breast.[17]

Although chemoprevention of cancer is a promising strategy of tumor control in the older person, the general use of chemoprevention cannot be recommended for the following reasons:

- No proof yet exists that chemoprevention reduces cancer-related morbidity and mortality. Of special concern is the case of finsteride,[15] which reduced the total incidence of prostate cancer but appeared to increase the risk of the most aggressive forms of the disease
- Medications used for chemoprevention may have serious complications. For example, tamoxifen has been associated with cerebrovascular accidents, deep vein thrombosis, and endometrial cancer. Recent report indicated that cyclooxygenase 2 inhibitors may also be associated with cardiovascular complications

DIFFERENTIAL DIAGNOSIS AND ASSESSMENT

Jane Thompson, *Part 1*

Jane Thompson, an 81-year-old woman, is brought to the hospital semicomatose by an ambulance. She was found lying on the floor of her apartment by her daughter, who had just come home from a 2-week vacation. Two weeks earlier, the mother was in excellent general health, with the exception of osteoarthritis. She was independent in her activities of daily living (ADLs) and in her instrumental ADLs (IADLs). She had lived alone for 12 years, since the death of her husband. On physical examination, the patient has a blood pressure of 60/0 mm Hg and a pulse rate 112, and she is visibly dehydrated. Her hemoglobin is 14.4, blood urea nitrogen (BUN) is 110, creatinine is 3.1, and albumin is 2.2. After fluid resuscitation in the emergency department, the patient becomes responsive but is still confused. She is unable to retain fluids in her stomach, and an esophagogastroscopy shows gastric outlet obstruction by a mass that is a large-cell lymphoma (LCL). By computed tomography (CT) scan the tumor appears unresectable. You initiate intravenous total parenteral nutrition (TPN) and call an oncologist for consultation.

STUDY QUESTIONS

1. Who will make decisions regarding how aggressive Ms. Thompson's medical care will be?
2. What options are available to provide nutritional support to Ms. Thompson?
3. What options are available to provide treatment for Ms. Thompson's tumor?

> ● Comprehensive geriatric assessment is an essential component of cancer treatment planning, to identify reversible comorbidity, to estimate life expectancy, and to assess the tolerance of the proposed treatment.

Assessment of the Older Cancer Patient

The National Cancer Center Network recognizes that some form of geriatric assessment may provide information essential to the treatment of persons 70 years old or older[26]:

The benefits of the geriatric assessment include

- Identification of reversible conditions that may interfere with cancer treatment: These include comorbidity, inadequate caregiver support, economic restrictions, insufficient access to care, depression, malnutrition, and polypharmacy.[32]
- Functional reserve and tolerance of chemotherapy: Patients who are dependent in IADLs, especially in the use of transportation, ability to take medications, and money management, are at increased risk for complications.[33] Underlying diseases and anemia may also reduce the tolerance of chemotherapy.
- Life expectancy.[34]
- Provision of a common language in the assessment of the older cancer patient; this common language is mostly needed to evaluate retrospective clinical experience and plan prospective clinical trials.

CGA represents a most fruitful ground of collaboration for the primary care physician and the oncology specialist. Based on the CGA, the primary care physician may establish the following:

1. Which patients may and may not benefit from an oncology referral.
2. Which patients may need further medical management before oncology referral.
3. Which patients may need special attention during oncologic care.
4. Which information the oncologist needs to know before instituting antineoplastic treatment.

Figure 45-1 shows the algorithm used by the Senior Adult Oncology program at the University of South Florida to establish the fitness of older patients to undergo cytotoxic chemotherapy. This may also be used by the primary care physician to establish the indication for referral.

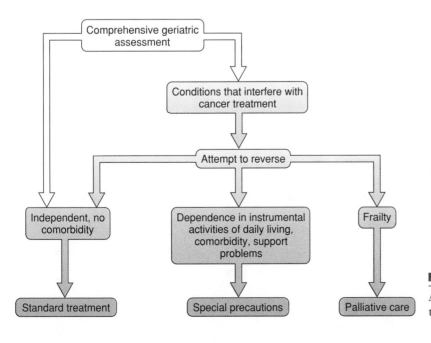

FIGURE 45-1

Approach to cancer treatment decisions in the elderly.

MANAGEMENT

Jane Thompson, *Part 2*

Ms. Thompson's three children believe that their mother would prefer only supportive care. You review the options for therapy with the oncologist, and after 3 days, the family agrees to limited therapy. The patient will be treated with cyclophosphamide, vincristine, doxorubicin, and prednisone (CHOP regimen) at reduced doses. The patient is sent home on TPN. After 20 days the patient returns to the oncologist's office able to eat on her own. She has also regained her independence. TPN is discontinued, and the patient receives six more courses of chemotherapy at full doses with G-CSF support (filgrastim, a hemopoietic growth factor). After 4 years she is still independent and in complete remission.

CASE DISCUSSION

The disease and the patient are two aspects of this case that are important.

The disease—LCL is highly responsive to chemotherapy. Although age is a poor prognostic factor, more than 50% of persons over the age of 60 experience a response to chemotherapy, and 30% are curable.

The patient—Although the patient had a poor performance status when she was brought to the hospital, she was totally independent 2 weeks before. Her poor condition was the result of an acute change that might have been reversed with aggressive fluid resuscitation and treatment of the gastric obstruction. Given their poor functional reserve, older individuals' general condition may deteriorate more quickly than that of younger individuals, in the presence of stress. To judge the fitness of older individuals for chemotherapy, their condition before stress rather than the changes resulting from stress should be considered.

> ● The fitness of an older patient to undergo chemotherapy should be judged from the patient's function *before* stress.

General Principles of Cancer Management

Cancer treatment involves local and systemic forms of treatment. Local treatment includes surgery and radiation therapy; systemic treatment includes cytotoxic chemotherapy, hormonal therapy, biologic therapy, and targeted therapy.

LOCAL THERAPY

Elective surgery is reasonably safe throughout the ninth decade of age.[18,19] The major differences in mortality between younger and older individuals are seen in emergency surgery of the gastrointestinal tract. Regular screening for cancer of the large bowel may substantially reduce the need for emergency surgery.

Several studies attest to the safety of radiation therapy in older patients, even those age 80 or older.[20,21] Radiation therapy is used in lieu of surgery for curative purposes, in patients who are poor surgical candidates, and for palliation of pain and obstruction. The combination of surgery and radiation therapy for cancer of the larynx, the anus, the esophagus, and small rectal tumors produces results comparable to surgery with the advantage of organ preservation.[22]

> ● The toxicity of chemotherapy in adults age 70 and over may be ameliorated by hemopoietic growth factors, erythropoietin, and adjustment of the doses to renal function.

SYSTEMIC THERAPY

The available systemic therapies for cancer are listed in Table 45-2.

Table 45–2 Systemic Antineoplastic Treatment

Type of Therapy	Agents
Hormonal therapy	Selective estrogen receptor modulators (SERMs) Aromatase inhibitors Progestins Luteinizing hormone-releasing hormone (LH-RH) analogs LH-RH antagonists Estrogens Androgens Androgen antagonists Adrenal antagonists Corticosteroids
Biologic therapy	Interferons Interleukin-2 Tumor vaccines
Cytotoxic chemotherapy	Alkylating agents Antimetabolites Antibiotics Plant derivatives
Targeted therapy	Monoclonal antibodies Immune-destruction of the tumor Carriers of cytotoxic material inside the tumor Inhibitors of the action of tumor growth factors Tyrosine kinase inhibitors Farnesyl transferase inhibitors Angiogenesis inhibitors

HORMONAL THERAPY

The aromatatase inhibitors have proven more effective than the older SERMs (tamoxifen and toremifene) in the management of breast cancer. For the majority of practitioners, these compounds are now the front-line treatment of choice, both in the adjuvant setting and in metastatic disease.[15,23] The aromatase inhibitors are active even in tumors that overexpress the HER2neu protein, for which SERMs are generally ineffective. The risk of endometrial cancer and cerebrovascular accidents is lower with aromatase inhibitors than with tamoxifen and toremifene. Of some concern, anastrozole has caused increased incidence of bone fractures, and letrozole has increase the levels of circulating low-density lipoprotein and has been associated with an excess of cardiovascular deaths in an European study. In face of osteopenia or osteoporosis, it appears prudent to administer bisphosphonates in concomitance with the aromatase inhibitors. A new SERM, fulvestrant (Faslodex), which is a pure estrogen antagonist, has recently become available. Its activity may be comparable to that of aromatase inhibitors. This agent is administered by intramuscular injections and appears to be indicated for patients who are not compliant with oral treatment. Progestins, whose activity is inferior to that of aromatase inhibitors, are used occasionally as third-line agents in metastatic breast cancer.

Luteinizing hormone-releasing hormone (LH-RH) analogs cause medical castration and are currently preferred in the management of prostate cancer.[21] The treatment with LH-RH analogs may be associated with the oral administration of androgen antagonists (bicalutamide, flutamide), during the first 2 weeks, to counteract the initial rise of testosterone after the first administration of the analogs. As single agents, the activity of androgen antagonists is inferior to medical castration. Adrenal suppressors include aminoglutethimide and ketoconazole at high doses and have some activity as second-line hormonal treatment of prostate cancer.

CYTOTOXIC CHEMOTHERAPY

Cytotoxic chemotherapy includes different groups of drugs that kill preferentially proliferating cells. Not surprisingly, the normal tissues with higher proliferation rate (bone marrow, mucosa) are the most vulnerable to chemotherapy. The growth fraction of most neoplasms (the proportion of proliferating cells to total cells) is higher than that of normal tissues. For this reason cytotoxic chemotherapy may destroy cancer while sparing the normal bodily tissues.[25] The most common toxicities of chemotherapy are listed in Table 45-3. Age is a risk factor for most of these complications.

Table 45–3 Chemotherapy-Related Toxicity in Older Individuals

Type of Toxicity	Agents Involved
Myelodepression	All agents, with the exception of vincristine, bleomycin, L-asparaginase, streptozotocin
Alopecia	Most agents with the exception of gemcitabine, oral fluorinated pyrimidine
Mucositis	Fluorinated pyrimidines (fluorouracil), methotrexate, anthracyclines (doxorubicin, daunorubicin, idarubicin, epirubicin)
Cardiotoxicity	Anthracyclines (doxorubicin, daunorubicin, idarubicin, epirubicin), mitomycin C
Peripheral neurotoxicity	Alkaloids (vincristine, vinblastine, vinorelbine), cisplatin, podophyllotoxins (etoposide, teniposide), taxanes (paclitaxel)
Central neurotoxicity	All agents (dementia), cytarabine in high doses (cerebellar toxicity)

● Anemia may worsen the toxicity of antineoplastic chemotherapy and cause fatigue that may precipitate functional dependence.

A number of provisions may ameliorate the toxicity of chemotherapy in older individuals including[26]:

- Adjustment of the dose to the renal function.
- Reduction of the dose—This strategy is ill advised in situations in which chemotherapy is administered for a cure, as the full dose improves the chances of achieving a cure.
- Support with hematopoietic growth factors—Pegfilgrastim prevents neutropenic infections in approximately 50% of cases and has largely replaced G-CSF because it can be administered once for each cycle of chemotherapy, whereas G-CSF requires daily administrations for 7 to 10 days. Epoetin A and darbepoetin A increase hemoglobin levels in approximately 75% of patients. Management of anemia during cytotoxic chemotherapy has two goals: prevention of fatigue and functional dependence, and prevention of chemotherapy-related toxicity. It is recommended to maintain hemoglobin levels of 12 gm/dl or higher. Concomitant administration of intravenous iron improves the response rate to erythropoietic growth factors.
- Cardiotoxicity may be improved by administration of anthracyclines as continuous infusions; concomitant administration of doxorubicin and dexrazoxane, which prevents the formation of free radicals in the myocardium; and administration of pegylated lyposomal doxorubicin "in lieu" of doxorubicin.

- Prevention and management of mucositis may include an oral solution of glutamine (AES12), a keratinocyte growth factor that reduces incidence and severity of mucositis from high-dose chemotherapy, and the substitution of intravenous fluorinated pyrimidines (fluorouracil and floxuridine) with capecitabine. Capecitabine is an oral prodrug activated into fluorouracil in the neoplastic tissue that minimizes the exposure of the normal mucosa to fluorouracil.

In addition to capecitabine and pegylated liposomal doxorubicin, a number of new drugs with a very favorable toxicity profile are useful in older individuals. These include taxanes in low weekly doses, vinorelbine, and gemcitabine.

Most of these recommendations have been endorsed by the National Cancer Center Network guidelines for the management of cancer in the elderly. In particular it is recommended that in individuals aged 65 and older, the dose of chemotherapy be adjusted to the glomerular filtration rate, G-CSF and pegfilgrastim be used routinely for chemotherapy of moderate toxicity, and hemoglobin levels be kept at 12 gm/dl or higher.

TARGETED THERAPY

New insights in cancer biology have allowed the development of substances that target specific components or specific metabolic processes of the tumor. Theoretically, targeted therapy would spare normal tissues. Monoclonal antibodies may target either tumor antigens or growth factors and growth factor receptors.[27,28] They may destroy the tumor by an immune mechanism, by carrying a cytotoxic substance within the tumor, or by interfering with the vital process of the tumor. Rituximab and alemtuzumab, target respectively the CD 20 and the CD 52 antigens and are effective in lymphoid malignancies. Trastuzumab (Herceptin) and cetuximab (Erbitux) target different components of the epithelial growth factor receptors and are effective in cancer of the breast and of the large bowel, respectively. Bevacizumab (Avastin) is a monoclonal antibody directed to the vascular endothelial growth factor and is effective in colorectal cancer. All monoclonal antibodies may cause anaphylactic reactions. Alemtuzumab may cause severe and prolonged myelosuppression and immune deficiency; trastuzumab may cause reversible heart failure, cetuximab acne-like reaction, and bevacizumab hypertension, bleeding, and visceral perforation. Rituximab and similar antibodies have been tagged with radioisotopes (radioimmunotherapy) to deliver high radiation doses to the tumor. Although highly effective, radioimmunotherapy may be associated with severe myelosuppression.

Angiogenesis inhibitors prevent the engraftment of metastases in distant organs by inhibiting formation of new tumor vessels. This group of drugs lacks the organ toxicity of cytotoxic chemotherapy. Thalidomide has substantial activity in multiple myeloma. Side effects include somnolence and constipation.[29] The monoclonal antibody bevacizumab also is antiangiogenic

Tyrosine kinase (TK) is a key enzyme of signal transduction. A number of small ATP-like molecules inhibit this enzyme and consequently tumor growth. Imatinib (Gleevec) inhibit the soluble TK and is very effective in chronic myelogenous leukemia (CML), in the forms of acute lymphoblastic leukemia (ALL) with Ph chromosome, in the stromal tumor of the stomach and in hypereosinophilia. Gefitinb (Iressa) and erlotinib (Tarceva), inhibit the TK associated with growth factor receptors and are effective in non-small-cell lung cancer.[30,31]

> ● Monoclonal antibodies and antiangiogenic factors represent an alternative to cytotoxic chemotherapy for older patients.

Breast Cancer

Mary Jones

In nursing facility, a nursing aide finds a 1.5-cm nodule on the right breast of your patient, Mary Jones, a 90-year-old woman. Ms. Jones is wheelchair bound because of osteoarthritis, has a Folstein mini-mental status of 20/30, and a history of congestive heart failure. You are aware that dependence in transportation, telephone use, and money management are risk factors for toxicity of cytotoxic chemotherapy.

After discussion with the patient's family and a medical oncologist, you recommend that a fine-needle aspiration biopsy be performed. The patient becomes agitated, and the procedure is aborted. The patient's son denies consent to the procedure after seeing his mother's reaction. The nodule is watched and measured every month and is found to be minimally enlarged in diameter 6 months later, when the patient dies after an acute respiratory infection.

The clinical history of breast cancer has been changed by the widespread use of screening mammography, by the advent of adjuvant treatment, and by the development of new drugs.[10]

CARCINOMA IN SITU

Approximately 20% of newly diagnosed breast cancers are in situ. This is an increase from 1% in 1970. The most common form is ductal carcinoma in situ, which is treated with total mastectomy or partial mastectomy and radiotherapy. Taking tamoxifen for 5 years may decrease the risk of local recurrence after partial mastectomy by 80%.[35]

LOCALIZED CARCINOMA OF THE BREAST

Localized carcinoma of the breast (stages I to IIIA) involves resectable breast cancer. The management includes the following:

- Total mastectomy or partial mastectomy and radiotherapy
- Axillary lymph node dissection
- Adjuvant treatment in selected cases

All mastectomy specimens should be tested for hormone receptors, proliferation rate, and HER2/neu antigens (the antigen for the epithelial growth factor receptor).[10]

Genomic profile may identify patients who benefit from adjuvant chemotherapy and allow all other patients to avoid the toxicity of chemotherapy. This approach is being tested in prospective clinical trials.

Several age-related issues have emerged in the management of localized breast cancer, including the following:

- The need for radiation therapy after partial mastectomy
- The need for axillary lymph node dissection
- The value of adjuvant chemotherapy

The goal of postoperative irradiation after partial mastectomy is prevention of local recurrence and breast preservation. Postoperative irradiation has no impact on freedom from distant metastases and overall survival. Irradiation of the breast has minimal complications in older women but is inconvenient and expensive. The risk of local recurrence after partial mastectomy declines with the age of the patient.[36] If a risk of local recurrence of 10% or less is acceptable to the patient, postoperative irradiation may be forgone in the older woman.

Axillary lymph node dissection is associated with substantial morbidity, including lymphedema and functional limitations. Lymph node mapping may obviate the need of this procedure in the majority of patients. After the injection of a radioactive tracer, it is possible to identify the so-called sentinel lymph node.[32] If this lymph node does not contain metastases, full axillary dissection is unnecessary.

Adjuvant treatment with aromatase inhibitors delay the recurrence of breast cancer more effectively than do SERMs in hormone receptor–rich tumor and is preferred by the majority of practitioners.[14] The benefits of adjuvant nonhormonal chemotherapy decline

with age and are not detectable after age 70. It is possible that older patients have been undertreated or that the chemotherapy is less effective in older individuals. In general, postmenopausal women with hormone receptor–rich tumors benefit minimally from adjuvant chemotherapy unless the tumor over expresses the HER2/neu antigen, in which case the chemotherapy containing an anthracycline may double the cure rate.[10]

METASTATIC CARCINOMA OF THE BREAST

The management of metastatic breast cancer depends on the characteristics of the tumor and the location of the metastases. Hormonal treatment is preferred for tumors that are rich in hormone receptors and in the absence of lymphangitic lung metastases, brain metastases, or extensive liver metastases. Cytotoxic chemotherapy is indicated for hormone receptor–rich tumors that have failed at least two forms of hormonal treatment or have produced lymphangitic lung metastases or liver metastases. Brain metastases may be managed with surgery or radiotherapy when they are single; multiple metastases generally require radiation therapy. Bone metastases involving weight-bearing bones such as the femur, the tibia, or the humerus should undergo surgical fixation to prevent pathologic fractures. It is important to remember that the patient's survival is predicated on the location of metastases (Table 45-4). In general, with metastatic disease, treatment has a limited impact on a patient's survival rate, and the risk and benefits should be carefully assessed in older women.[10]

Several forms of chemotherapy with limited toxicity are available. For patients with tumors that overexpress the HER2/neu antigen, a combination of Herceptin and weekly Taxol or Taxotere is the treatment of choice. For the other patients, weekly Taxol, Taxotere, or vinorelbine (Navelbine), oral capecitabine, or pegylated liposomal doxorubicin every 4 weeks are well tolerated and of similar efficacy. Of special interest to older patients are the bisphosphonates zalendronate or pamidronate. These drugs delay the development of pain and other bone complications in the presence of bony metastases. Of some concern, however, is the

Table 45–4	Median Survival of Patients with Breast Cancer According to the Location of Metastases
Location of Metastases	**Survival (Months)**
Liver (more than 30% of the organ)	3
Lung (lymphangitic)	3
Lung (nodular)	22
Skin	27
Bones	36+

increases incidence of jaw-bone necrosis after dental manipulation. These drugs should be discontinued at least a month before oral surgery, and therapy should not be reinstituted until the surgical wound have completely healed.

Case Discussion: Mary Jones

The recommendation of a biopsy for Mary Jones was reasonable because the procedure has negligible morbidity and might have provided valuable information related to the aggressiveness of the tumor and the need for surgical resection. The patient's reaction, however, and the denial of permission prevented the biopsy.

In a 90-year-old woman, a breast nodule should be considered cancer unless proved otherwise. Most likely the tumor was rich in hormone receptors because the prevalence of hormone receptor–rich tumors is higher than 80% in women of this age.

A number of approaches were reasonable in this case:

Local resection under local anesthesia—The benefit of this approach would have included prevention of local complications such as fungating, painful, and ulcerating masses.

Treatment with tamoxifen—This treatment had a 60% to 80% chance to obtain a response, including stabilizing the disease. The disadvantages include risk of deep vein thrombosis, which is increased for an older woman immobilized by arthritis.

Close observation—This approach was followed and was reasonable because the average life expectancy of this woman with severe dementia and func

tional impairment was probably less than 1 year. The median time for the tumor to reach a size capable of causing local complications was in excess of 3 years based on studies of medical treatment of local breast cancer, and close observation was possible thanks to the location of the disease.

Prostate Cancer

Prostate cancer is the most common cancer and the second most common cause of cancer death for American men.[24] The widespread use of prostate-specific antigen (PSA) for screening asymptomatic men has doubled the incidence of prostate cancer in the last decade. There is no conclusive evidence that screening has reduced the risk of death from prostate cancer, especially for men older than 65. The current staging and treatment of prostate cancer are summarized in Table 45-5.

Close observation for patients with localized disease is a reasonable approach for men age 70 or older with well-differentiated tumor (Gleason score of seven or less). In all other cases, some form of local treatment is reasonable. Brachytherapy (radiation by implant) is the form of treatment with fewer complications, but the experience with brachytherapy is still limited. Poor prognostic factors for localized disease include poorly differentiated tumor, involvement of the seminal vesicles, and a PSA level of 30 ng/ml.

Hormonal treatment is the mainstay of management of metastatic disease. It has been demonstrated that early hormonal treatment (upon diagnosis of metastases) is superior to delayed hormonal treatment (when symptoms develop).[37] It is unclear, however, whether hormonal treatment should be instituted as soon as the PSA rises after radical prostatectomy (D1.5-disease)

Table 45–5	Staging and Treatment of Prostate Cancer	
Stage	**Description**	**Treatment**
Local disease	A: Disease found at biopsy only	Observation
	B1: Palpable node involving one lobe	Radical prostatectomy or external beam irradiation or brachytherapy
	B2: Palpable node involving both lobes or greater than 1.5 cm in diameter	
Locally advanced disease	C	Radiation therapy in combination with hormonal therapy
Metastatic disease	D1: Involvement of pelvic lymph nodes	Lymph node dissection and adjuvant hormonal therapy
	D1.5: Rise of serum PSA after radical prostatectomy	Consider hormonal therapy if the doubling time of PSA is 10 months or less, if the recurrence occurs within two years of surgery, and if the original tumor had a Gleason score 8 or higher
	D2: Involvement of retroperitoneal lymph nodes and distal organs	Hormonal therapy
	D2.5: Rise of PSA	

PSA indicates prostatic-specific antigen.

because only one-third of these patients will develop clinical metastases within 10 years.[38]

A number of chemotherapy agents, including mitoxantrone, vinorelbine (Navelbine), and docetaxel, improve the bone pain of patients with metastatic prostate cancer. Of these docetaxel also prolongs the survival of patients with hormone-resistant disease.[39]

Palliation of bony metastases may be obtained with external beam irradiation; when multiple painful metastases are present, treatment with intravenous radioisotopes, including strontium 89 and samarium 153, is indicated. Strontium produces more prolonged responses but also more severe myelosuppression. Zoledronate may relieve the pain and delay the progression of bony metastases.

Cancer of the Large Bowel

Cancer of the large bowel is the second leading cause of cancer death in women and the third in men. The incidence of this neoplasm increases with age, at least until age 95. Cancer-related deaths may be reduced by regular screening involving yearly or biennial fecal occult blood after age 50 years[40] and serial endoscopic examinations.[41] Removal of adenomatous polyps also reduces cancer-related mortality, confirming that these polyps are premalignant lesions.[41]

The stages of cancer of the large bowel include the following:

- *Stage I*—The disease is limited to mucosa and submucosa
- *Stage II A*—Involvement of the muscularis propria
- *Stage IIB*—Involvement of the serosa
- *Stage III*—Involvement of regional lymph nodes
- *Stage IV*—Distant metastases

The clinical workup of cancer of the large bowel includes a full colonoscopy, a CT scan of the abdomen and pelvis, and a positron emission tomography (PET) scan. The serum carcinoembryonic antigen may be valuable when elevated before surgery because it implies a poorer prognosis. Also, sequential measurements of the carcinoembryonic antigen after surgery may allow detection of early local recurrences.

The treatment of stage I and IIA cancer with surgical resection results in a cure rate as high as 90%. Abdominal-perineal resections are performed rarely, even in the case of rectal cancer. Rectal cancers with a diameter of 2.5 cm that involve less than one-third of the rectal wall and with a depth of invasion that does not reach the serosa (by ultrasonography) may be managed with transanal resection followed by radiotherapy.[42]

Larger rectal cancers may be managed with preoperative chemo-radiation therapy that shrinks the tumor and allows an anterior resection in the majority of cases.[43]

Several studies have demonstrated the benefits of adjuvant treatment in stage III cancer and in some subsets of stage IIB cancer. Adjuvant treatment consists of a combination of fluorouracil and leucovorin administered over 6 months and, in the case of rectal cancer radiation therapy, should be added to chemotherapy to reduce the risk of local recurrences, unless radiotherapy had already been used preoperatively. The addition of oxaliplatin improves the cure rate of about 5% but is associated with significant toxicity, especially neurotoxicity and thrombocytopenia.[44]

In metastatic disease, the combination of fluorouracil, leucovorin, and irinotecan or oxaliplatin produces a response rate of approximately 40% with a median duration response of 8 months. The addition of bevacizumab (Avastin) or cetuximab (Erbitux) may further improve response and survival.[45]

In approximately 50% of patients, the only site of metastatic disease is the liver. When feasible, local management of liver metastases may prolong survival and may even result in cure. Surgical resection of liver metastases followed by infusional chemotherapy with floxuridine in the hepatic artery results in prolonged remission in approximately 40% of patients.[46] Thermoablation of metastases with ultrasound is an alternative to surgery suitable for older individuals at poor surgical risk.

All patients who have had a curative resection of cancer of the large bowel should undergo surveillance colonoscopy. The first examination is generally performed 1 year after surgery; the other examinations are performed at 3- to 5-year intervals. Yearly abdominal CT and periodic determinations of carcinoembryonic antigen for 5 years are also indicated.

Non-Hodgkin's Lymphoma

James Brown, *Part 1*

While examining James Brown, a 79-year-old man, you discover that he has enlarged lymph nodes in both axillae. After referral for biopsy, the pathologist confirms peripheral T-cell lymphoma (PTCL). CT scans of the chest and abdomen and bone marrow biopsy are negative for lymphoma. During the workup of the lymphoma, the patient consults an urologist for difficulty urinating. Circulating PSA is 82 ng/µl. Prostatic biopsy reveals a Gleason 8 (aggressive) prostatic adenocarcinoma. The patient's hemoglobin is 10.2, serum creatinine is 1.7, and BUN is 26. Serum erythropoietin levels are 3 µg/ml.

The patient is a widower who lives alone. His two children live in different states, but he has some close friends in the retirement center where he lives. He has his own apartment and prepares his own meals; he is independent in ADLs and IADLs and is cognitively intact. Although he denies symptoms of depression, a geriatric depression scale (GDS) reveals that the patient is severely depressed (his GDS score is 11/15).

The incidence of NHL in persons aged 60 years old or older has increased 80% since 1970. Currently, these neoplasms represent the sixth most common malignancy among older persons. One possible cause for this increase is exposure to agricultural pesticides.

A useful classification of NHL includes low-, intermediate-, and high-grade lymphomas. High-grade lymphomas are uncommon among older individuals. Age 60 or older represents a poor prognostic factor for both low- and intermediate-grade disease.[46,47] A possible reason for the poorer prognosis is that circulating levels of IL-6 increase with age, and IL-6 stimulates lymphoproliferation.[8] Another important age-related characteristic of NHL is increased incidence of extranodal lymphomas, including gastric, small-bowel, thyroidal, testicular, and central nervous system lymphomas.

The staging of lymphoma should involve bilateral bone marrow aspiration and biopsy, CT of the chest and abdomen, and a PET scan. The PET scan is useful for at least two reasons: to identify disease in unsuspected areas and to distinguish active neoplasm from scar tissue in patients with persistent radiographic masses after chemotherapy.

The primary therapeutic approach for NHL is systemic chemotherapy. In the case of low-grade disease, treatment should be instituted only in the presence of symptoms because the treatment in general is not curative. Oral alkylating agents and corticosteroids or fludarabine in combination with the monoclonal antibody rituximab are the most common forms of treatment used. In patients unwilling or unable to tolerate the toxicity of chemotherapy, rituximab as single agent may produce a 40% response rate. Repeated administrations of rituximab every 6 months for 2 years result in more prolonged remissions. Another important advance in the management of low-grade NHL is the development of monoclonal antibodies tagged with a radioisotope. Two of these preparations are available for clinical use in patients with disease refractory to chemotherapy and rituximab. In patients with gastric lymphoma developing in the context of *Helicobacter pylori* infection, eradication of the microorganism may cause regression of the lymphoma.

The treatment of large-cell NHL (the most common form of intermediate-grade lymphoma) involves a combination of an alkylating agent, an anthracycline, a glucocorticoid, and rituximab. The most popular of these combinations is R-CHOP (rituximab, cyclophosphamide, doxorubicin, vincristine, and prednisone). In early disease (stages I and II), three courses of R-CHOP followed by radiation therapy produce a cure rate of 60% to 80%.[49,50] In more advanced disease, six to eight courses of chemotherapy are administered with a cure rate of 60% to 80%. This form of chemotherapy should be followed by treatment with hemopoietic growth factors in patients age 70 years old or older in view of the high risk of myelotoxicity.[26]

James Brown, *Part 2*

The patient's daughters have come to visit Mr. Brown, and they participate in a number of consultations between you, the urologist, and the medical oncologist. You help the patient and family formulate the following treatment plan:

- *Treatment with CHOP (multidrug chemotherapy) will be immediately instituted for PTCL. The treatment will be administered every 3 weeks, the patient will receive G-CSF for 1 week, and you will administer weekly erythropoietin injections.*
- *Treatment with Paxil, 20 mg per day, will be immediately instituted.*
- *One of the daughters will spend the first week after chemotherapy in her father's house. If serious complications occur, the daughters will take turns spending 1 week after chemotherapy with their father.*
- *Treatment for the prostate cancer with LH-RH analog goserelin (Zoladex) and anastrozole (Casodex) will be instituted immediately.*
- *External-beam irradiation to the prostate will be administered after the patient has completed the chemotherapy for lymphoma.*

CASE DISCUSSION

Five years later Mr. Brown is free of lymphoma and has no urinary problems. His PSA level is 0.3 μg/ml. Mr. Brown's case allows examination of the following common problems related to cancer and age:

- *Multiple neoplasms are common in older individuals. The management should start with the neoplasm that most threatens the patient's life. Median survival of PTCL is approximately 18 months without treatment; that of prostate cancer stage C is approximately 5 years. Furthermore, prostate cancer may be kept under control with hormonal treatment while the patient receives chemotherapy. Concomitant administration of chemotherapy containing doxorubicin and radiation therapy to the pelvis may enhance the risk of radiation-induced cystitis and proctitis.*

- *Although the patient was functionally independent, he might have experienced severe neutropenia and infection while receiving chemotherapy. These complications need immediate attention. For patients older than 70 years old who are living alone or with inadequate caregiver (a spouse or a friend), it is important to arrange for timely and effective support if complications do develop.*

- *This case emphasizes the importance of a geriatric assessment in planning the treatment of older individuals. In this case, two elements that may have compromised the success of the treatment emerged from the geriatric assessment: the fact that the patient lived alone and the fact that the patient was severely depressed. Depression is associated with decreased life expectancy and may complicate the management of chemotherapy.*

- *Although it has not been conclusively proven that combined androgen blockade is superior to castration, in this case the addition of an antiandrogen to chemical castration was recommended. A spike in testosterone levels may follow the administration of LH-RH analogs in the first 2 weeks of treatment. This rise in testosterone may stimulate the growth of prostate cancer and precipitate urinary obstruction in a patient with urinary symptoms. The addition of an androgen antagonist (Casodex) will prevent this complication.*

- *The management of anemia in older individuals with cancer is important for the prevention of the complications of chemotherapy and the prevention of severe fatigue. It is important to establish the cause of anemia. In this patient with moderate renal insufficiency and low erythropoietin levels, the diagnosis of chronic anemia from renal insufficiency is likely.*

- *Anemia may enhance the toxicity of antineoplastic chemotherapy and cause fatigue that may precipitate functional dependence.*

SUMMARY

Cancer is the second leading cause of death and a major cause of morbidity for older adults. The behavior of some neoplasms changes with the age of the patient, and many cancers occur more commonly in older adults. Contrary to common expectations, cancer may become more aggressive with age. Age alone should not determine the treatment of cancer. Through a process of geriatric assessment, the primary care physician can determine patients who may or may not benefit from an oncology referral, who may need further medical management before oncology referral, and who may need special attention during oncologic care.

References

1. LaVecchia C et al. Cancer mortality in the elderly, 1969-1998: a worldwide approach. In Comprehensive geriatric oncology (Balducci L, Lyman GH, Ershler WB, Extermann M, eds.). London: Taylor & Francis, 2005.
2. Yancik RM, Ries LA. Cancer in older persons: magnitude of the problem and efforts to advance the aging/cancer research interface. In Comprehensive geriatric oncology (Balducci L, Lyman GH, Ershler WB, Extermann M, eds.). London: Taylor & Francis, 2005.
3. Balducci L, Extermann M. Cancer and aging: an evolving panorama. Hematol Oncol Clin 2000;14:1-16.
4. Willman CL. The prognostic significance of the expression and function of multidrug resistance transporter proteins in acute myeloid leukemia: studies of the Southwest Oncology Group Leukemia research program. Semin Hematol 1997;34(Suppl 5):25-33.
5. Burns EA, Goodwin JS. Immunological changes of aging. In Comprehensive geriatric oncology (Balducci L, Lyman GH, Ershler WB, Extermann M, eds.). London: Taylor & Francis, 2005.
6. Campisi J. Proliferative senescence and cancer. In Comprehensive geriatric oncology (Balducci L, Lyman GH, Ershler WB, Extermann M, eds.). London: Taylor & Francis, 2005.
7. Ershler WB. Interleukin 6: a cytokine for gerontologists. J Am Geriatr Soc 1993;41:176-181.
8. Preti HA, Cabanillas F, Talpaz M, Tucker SL, Seymour JF, Kurzrock R. Prognostic value of serum interleukin-6 in diffuse large-cell lymphoma. Ann Intern Med 1997;127:186-194.
9. Anisimov I. Biological interactions of aging and carcinogenesis. In Biological basis of geriatric oncology (Balducci L, Extermann M, eds.). New York: Springer, 2005.
10. Balducci L, Silliman RA, Diaz N. Breast cancer: an oncologic perspective. In Comprehensive geriatric oncology (Balducci L, Lyman GH, Ershler WB, Extermann M, eds.). London: Taylor & Francis, 2005.
11. Minton S, Shaw G. Chemoprevention of cancer in the older person. In Comprehensive geriatric oncology (Balducci L, Lyman GH, Ershler WB, eds.). London: Harwood Academic, 1998.
12. Ettinger B, et al. Raloxifene reduces the risk of incident vertebral fractures: 24 months interim analysis. Osteoporos Int 1998;3(Suppl):11.
13. Fisher B, Costantino JP, Wickerham DL, et al. Tamoxifen for the prevention of breast cancer: report of the National Surgical Adjuvant Breast and Bowel Project P-1 Study. J Natl Cancer Inst 1998;90:1371-1388.
14. Buzdar AU. The ATAC (Arimidex, Tamoxifen Alon or in Combination) trial: an update. Clin Breast Cancer 2004;5(Suppl 1):s6-s12.
15. Thompson IM, Goodman DJ, Tanger CM, et al: The influence of finasteride on the development of prostate cancer. N Engl J Med, 2003;349:215-224.
16. Stockbrugger RW. Nonsteroidal anti-inflammatory drugs (NSAIDs) in the prevention of colorectal cancer. Eur J Cancer Prev 1999;8(Suppl 11):S21.
17. Graaf MR, Richel DJ, van Noorden CJ, et al: Effects of statins and farnesyl-transferase inhibitors on the development and progression of cancer. Cancer Treat Rev 2004;30:609-641.
18. Kemeny MM, Busch-Devereaux E, Merriam LT, O'Hea BJ. Cancer surgery in the elderly. Hematol Oncol Clin North Am 2000;14:169-192.
19. Berger DH, Roslyn JJ. Cancer surgery in the elderly. Clin Geriatr Med 1997;13:119-141.
20. Zacharia B, Balducci L. Radiation therapy of the older patient. Hematol Oncol Clin North Am 2000;14:131-167.
21. Olmi P, et al. Radiotherapy in the elderly, The achievements of the Geriatric Radiation Oncology Group (GROG). In Comprehensive geriatric oncology (Balducci L, Lyman GH, Ershler WB, Extermann M, eds.). London: Taylor & Francis, 2005.
22. Balducci L, Trotti A. Organ preservation: an effective and safe form of cancer treatment, Clin Geriatr Med 1997;13:185-201.
23. Narashimamurthy J, Rao AR, Sastry GN. Aromatase inhibitors: a new paradigm in breast cancer treatment. Curr Med Chem Anti-Cancer Agents 2004;4:523-534.
24. Moon TD. Prostate cancer in the alderly. In Comprehensive geriatric oncology (Balducci L, Lyman GH, Ershler WB, Extermann M, eds.). London: Taylor & Francis, 2005.
25. Cova D, Balducci L. Cancer chemotherapy in the older patient. In Comprehensive geriatric oncology (Balducci L, Lyman GH, Ershler WB, Extermann M, eds.). London: Taylor & Francis, 2005.
26. Balducci L. Senior adult oncology clinical practice guidelines in oncology. J Natl Comp Canc Netw 2005;3:572–592.

27. Ross JS, Schenkein DP, Pietrusko R, et al. Targeted therapies for cancer, 2004. Am J Clin Pathol 2004;122:598-609.

28. Weiner GJ, Link BK. Antibody therapy of lymphoma. Adv Pharmacol 2004;51:229-253.

29. Singhal S, Mehta J, Desikan R, et al. Antitumor activity of thalidomide in refractory multiple myeloma, N Engl J Med 1999;341:1565-1571.

30. Silvestris N, Lorusso V. Extensive small cell lung cancer: standard and experimental treatment approaches in elderly patients. Ann Oncol 2006; 17:ii64-ii66.

31. Sawyer TK. Novel oncogenic protein kinase inhibitors for cancer therapy. Curr Med Chem Anitican Agents 2004;4:449-455.

32. Extermann M, Overcash J, Lyman GH, et al. Comorbidity and functional status are independent in older cancer patients. J Clin Oncol 1998;16: 1582-1587.

33. Monfardini S, Balducci L. A comprehensive geriatric assessment (CGA) is necessary for the study and the management of cancer in the elderly. Eur J Cancer 1999;35:1771.

34. Walter LC, Covinsky KY. Cancer screening in elderly patients: a framework for individual decision making. JAMA 2001;265:2987-2994.

35. Fisher B, Dignam J, Wolmark N, et al. Tamoxifen in the treatment of intra-ductal breast cancer: National Surgical Adjuvant Breast and Bowel Project B-24: randomized controlled trial, Lancet 1999;353:1993-2000.

36. Hughes KS, Schnaper LA, Berry D, et al. Lumpectomy plus tamoxifen with or without irradiation in women 70m years of age or older with early breast cancer. N Engl J Med 2004;351:971-977.

37. Messing EM, Manola J, Sarosdy M, Wilding G, Crawford ED, Trump D. Immediate hormonal treatment compared with observation after radical prostatectomy and pelvic lymphadenectomy in men with node-positive prostate cancer. N Engl J Med 1999;341:1781-1788.

38. Pound CR, Partin AW, Eisenberger MA, Chan DW, Pearson JD, Walsh PC. Natural history of progression after PSA elevation following radical prostatectomy. JAMA 1999;281:1591-1597.

39. Tannock IF, deWitt R, Berry WR, et al. Docetaxel plus prednisone or Mitoxantrone plus prednisone for advanced prostate cancer. N Engl J Med 2004;351:1502-1512.

40. Mandel JS, Church TR, Ederer F, Bond JH. Colorectal cancer mortality: effectiveness of biennial screening for fecal occult blood. J Natl Cancer Inst 1999;91:434-437.

41. Winawer SJ, Zauber AG, Ho MN, et al. Prevention of colorectal cancer by colonoscopic polypectomy. N Engl J Med 1993;329:1977-1981.

42. Marcet J, Yeatman T. Avoiding colostomy with conservative multimodality management of distal rectal cancer. Cancer Control 1996;3: 26-33.

43. Sauer R, Becker H, Hohenberger W, et al. Preoperative versus postoperative chemoradiotherapy for rectal cancer. N Engl J Med 2004;351:1731-1740.

44. Andre T, Boni C, Mounedij-Boudiaf L, et al. Oxaliplatin, fluorouracil, and leucovorin as adjuvant treatment for colon cancer. N Engl J Med 2004;350:2343-2351.

45. Hurwitx H, Fehrenbacher L, Novotny W, et al. Bevacizumab plus irinotecan, fluorouracil, and leucovorin for metastatic colorectal cancer. N Engl J Med 2004;350:2335-2342.

46. Kemeni MM. Chemotherapy after hepatic resection of colorectal metastases. Cancer Treat Res 1994;69:121.

46. Decaudin D, Lepage E, Brousse N, et al. Low-grade stage III-IV follicular lymphoma: multivariate analysis of prognostic factors in 484 patients, J Clin Oncol 1999;17:2499-505.

47. The International Non-Hodgkin's Lymphoma Prognostic Factors Project: A predictive model for aggressive non-Hodgkin's lymphoma. N Engl J Med 1993;329:987.

48. Miller TP, Dahlberg S, Cassady JR, et al. Chemotherapy alone compared with chemotherapy plus radiotherapy for localized intermediate- and high-grade non-Hodgkin's lymphoma, N Engl J Med 1998;339:21-26.

49. Coiffier B, Lepage E, Briere J, et al. CHOP chemotherapy plus ritux-imab compared with chop alone in elderly patients with diffuse large B-cell lymphoma. N Engl J Med 2004;346:235-242.

Web Resources

American Cancer Society. http://www.cancer.org/.

National Cancer Institute. http://www.nci.nih.gov/.

National Guideline Clearinghouse. http://www.guidelines.gov/.

POSTTEST

1. A 71-year-old woman has ductal carcinoma in situ of the left breast that was diagnosed with a mammogram. The tumor is 1.1 cm in diameter and has areas of necrosis. The patient underwent partial mastectomy. The patient has a history of thrombosis of the dural vein 10 years ago and is receiving anticoagulation with warfarin. The treatment of this patient should include which of the following?
   a. Radiotherapy
   b. Radiotherapy and tamoxifen
   c. Radiotherapy and raloxifene
   d. Radiotherapy and exemestane
   e. Lymph node dissection

2. Which of the following statements are true? Chemoprevention of breast cancer with tamoxifen:
   a. Is associated with increased risk of cerebrovascular disease.
   b. Reduces the death rate from breast cancer.
   c. Reduces the risk of colorectal cancer.
   d. Increases the risk of osteoporosis.
   e. Reduces the risk of deep vein thrombosis.

3. On admission to the nursing home, an 85-year-old woman was found to have a fungating mass on her right breast. The mass is 9 cm in diameter, partially ulcerated, and associated with edema of the arm and obvious pain. The patient has no children and had lived alone until recently, when a neighbor became concerned for what appeared to be a progressive loss of memory and neglect of the house. A nephew living in another city eventually came to take care of the situation and arranged for the admission. The patient appears confused and withdrawn; her appearance is disheveled, but she seems to be independent in her ADLs. The medical history is negative for any serious illnesses. She is a retired teacher, and until recently, she was able to drive her own car. She was married at 45 years old and has been a widow for 12 years. Which of the following is the best statement relating to the breast mass?
   a. Tamoxifen should be initiated immediately. If no response is seen in 3 months, the patient should receive chemotherapy.
   b. The mass should be biopsied to study hormone-receptor and HER2/neu antigen status.
   c. The patient should undergo surgery as initial treatment.
   d. The initial treatment should be radiation therapy.
   e. No treatment is indicated because the patient's average life expectancy is less than 1 year, and during this period of time the tumor is unlikely to cause local complications.

PRETEST ANSWERS

1. d
2. c
3. c

POSTTEST ANSWERS

1. a
2. a
3. b

CHAPTER 46

Chronic Obstructive Pulmonary Disease and Lower Respiratory Infections

David R. Mehr

OBJECTIVES

Upon completion of this chapter, the reader will be able to:

- Define strategies to prevent influenza in older adults and especially residents of long-term care facilities
- Diagnose and treat influenza in older adults.
- Appropriately treat acute bronchitis in older adults.
- Recognize that pneumonia has fewer symptoms at presentation in older adults
- Identify reasons to admit older adults with a lower respiratory infection to the hospital.
- Choose appropriate antibiotics for pneumonia.
- Choose appropriate management strategies for chronic obstructive pulmonary disease based on illness severity.
- Interpret results of purified protein derivative (PPD)testing in newly admitted nursing home residents and in residents tested during a tuberculosis outbreak.

P R E T E S T

1. Mrs. Johnson, an 82-year-old resident of a nursing home, develops chills, fever, and cough. A rapid influenza test reveals influenza A. An outbreak of influenza A is occurring in the local community. Which of the following is the best option for treating this patient and preventing further infection?
   a. Oseltamivir 75 mg daily for Mrs. Johnson and for other residents in the facility
   b. Amantadine 100 mg daily for Mrs. Johnson and for other residents in the facility
   c. Oseltamivir 75 mg twice daily for Mrs. Johnson and 75 mg daily for other residents in the facility
   d. Rimantadine 100 mg daily for Mrs. Johnson and for other residents in the facility
   e. Zanamivir 10 mg twice daily for the patient and amantadine 100 mg daily for other residents in the facility

2. A 75-year-old man presents to your office with complaints of cough and shortness of breath. He has been eating and drinking poorly for 2 days. His temperature is 38.4°C, pulse 90, and respirations 24. Lungs show coarse crackles at his left base, and a chest radiograph confirms an infiltrate. His pulse oximetry shows 88% oxygen saturation on room air. One month ago he finished a course of levofloxacin for prostatitis. In addition to admitting him to the hospital, which of the following antibiotic regimens will you start?
   a. Levofloxacin and azithromycin
   b. Clindamycin
   c. Cefotaxime and clindamycin
   d. Ceftriaxone and azithromycin
   e. Gatifloxacin

3. An 85-year-old nursing home resident with severe dementia is admitted to the hospital by your partner while you are out of town. On your return, she is slowly responding to treatment for pneumonia with levofloxacin. Which of the following would best guide future appropriate care?
   a. As she already has severe dementia, her prognosis is unchanged by this recent pneumonia episode.
   b. As aspiration is a likely cause of the pneumonia, a feeding tube should be considered.
   c. She probably has aspiration pneumonia and clindamycin should be added.
   d. In determining her 30-day mortality risk, the absence of an elevated white blood count would predict a poor prognosis.
   e. Average mortality in similar patients in 6 months is about 50%, and you should re-evaluate future care goals with her family.

Amanda Jones, *Part 1*

Your patient, Amanda Jones, is an 85-year-old woman who resides at Fairview Acres, a nursing home with 120 residents on two wings. She has Alzheimer's disease but is ambulatory and independent in most activities of daily living (ADLs). On December 1, she eats breakfast poorly and by mid-morning has developed a cough and fever to 38.5°C.

STUDY QUESTION

1. What conditions do you need to consider as part of her differential diagnosis?

PREVALENCE AND IMPACT

In those over age 65, chronic lower respiratory diseases, predominantly chronic obstructive pulmonary disease (COPD), represent the fourth leading cause of death, and influenza and pneumonia represent the fifth leading cause of death.[1] Although COPD is often thought of as a disease affecting middle-age people, in 2002, twice as many adults age 65 or older were discharged from acute-care hospitals for chronic bronchitis than were those aged 45 to 64, that is, 343,000 versus 161,000, respectively.[2] In that same year, pneumonia accounted for 776,000 hospital discharges. In the mid-1990s, hospitalizations from pneumonia among all adults cost $4 billion per year,[3] and COPD accounted for $18 billion per year in direct health care costs.[4]

Among nursing home residents, lower respiratory infections (LRIs), including bronchitis, pneumonia, and influenza, are also a leading cause of death,[5] and pneumonia is the immediate cause of death in 50% to 70% of those with dementia,[6-9] who constitute over half of the nursing home population. In a large study of Missouri nursing home residents who developed a LRI, 15% died and 27% were hospitalized within 30 days[10]; in those initially hospitalized, the average 30-day cost was $10,400.[11] Although there were only 15,075 reported cases of tuberculosis in the United States in 2002,[12] earlier studies suggested older adults make up one-fourth of cases, and the incidence is higher in nursing homes than in the community.[13]

> ● Pneumonia has both a higher incidence and a higher fatality rate in older adults.

RISK FACTORS AND PATHOPHYSIOLOGY

Influenza is a viral infection, which typically spreads through person-to-person exposure in community outbreaks. Because viral genes coding for antigenic determinants frequently mutate, new influenza variants often arise among circulating strains.[14] Therefore, prior infection or immunization does not always provide protection in future years. Coughing and sneezing are the primary means of transmission. Nonimmune individuals who are exposed to the virus develop inflammation of respiratory epithelium with necrosis of infected cells. Release of cytokines and inflammatory cell activation results in systemic symptoms.[15] The incubation period is 1 to 4 days, and adults are infective from 1 day before the onset of symptoms for approximately 5 days.[14] Children, who have the highest rates of infection, are infectious longer. Mortality is highest in those over 65.

Acute bronchitis is defined as an acute or subacute illness with cough lasting less than 3 weeks, often accompanied by other respiratory or general symptoms.[15] Respiratory viruses, including influenza, account for the majority of cases. However, *Bortadella pertussis*, *Mycoplasma pneumoniae*, and *Chlamydia pneumoniae* are occasional causes. The pathophysiology is essentially the same as with influenza, although with some viruses there are considerably fewer systemic symptoms.[15] The persistent cough is frequently associated with bronchial hyperreactivity. In the setting of COPD, colonization with bacterial respiratory pathogens is common, and it is unclear to what extent these are etiologically significant.[4]

Pneumonia has both a higher incidence and fatality in older adults. In two European community-based studies, increased age and chronic lung disease were risk factors for older adults to develop pneumonia[16]; the larger Finnish study also identified alcoholism, asthma, immunosuppression, heart disease, and institutionalization as risk factors. In nursing home residents, age, swallowing difficulty, inability to take oral medications, male sex, and immobility (defined as severe ADL impairment) were additional risk factors for pneumonia or other LRIs in a well-designed Canadian study.[17] Pneumonia often begins with aspiration of oropharyngeal contents, which may be trivial or more substantial. Massive aspiration of food contents may lead to chemical damage to lung, which may or may not be followed by infection. When infectious agents overwhelm local defenses, lung tissue fills with inflammatory exudate, which results in lobar or peribronchial consolidation or interstitial infiltrates.[18] Etiologic agents can include a variety of bacteria and viruses, but *Streptococcus pneumoniae* is the most prevalent both in community and long-term care settings.[16] Other relatively common pathogens likely include *Staphylococcus aureus*, *Haemophilus influenzae*, *Moraxella catarrhalis*, *Mycoplasma pneumoniae*, *Chlamydia pneumoniae*, aerobic Gram-negative bacteria, influenza virus, adenoviruses, and respiratory syncytial virus.[16,18] The importance of the atypical organisms (*Mycoplasma* and *Chlamydia* species) has varied across studies, but generally they are more important in younger adults. *Legionella* species are also a consideration, particularly in more severe infections. Older patients are frequently unable to produce adequate sputum, even where aggressive measures are undertaken to obtain specimens,[16,19] so etiologic studies have often suffered from limited data on many subjects. In addition, some frequently quoted studies have failed to adequately control for sputum quality.

In considering *tuberculosis*, it is important to distinguish between infection and disease. Infection results from the inhalation of airborne droplets containing *Mycobacterium tuberculosis* from a patient with active disease. Depending on the balance between an individual's defenses and the virulence of the bacteria, infection may or may not result in active disease.[12] Most healthy individuals can contain the infection with activation of macrophages. This quiescent state is termed a latent tuberculosis infection. However, some individuals will be unable to contain the infection or will later suffer reactivation. Cell-mediated immunity will still cause tissue destruction in these cases, but the result will be an enlarging cavity with erosion into bronchi and the production of highly infectious sputum.[12] Tuberculosis may reactivate years later, particularly with decline in immune function. This is the usual cause of illness in older adults, although spread within institutions has also been well documented. In addition to substantially higher risk with recent infection, a variety of conditions that can compromise immunity are related to developing active tuberculosis, including renal failure with hemodialysis, HIV infection, and immunosuppression associated with transplantation or chemotherapy.[20]

COPD is a disease state characterized by airflow limitation that is not fully reversible.[21] Tobacco smoke, occupational exposure to dusts and chemicals, and indoor or outdoor pollution are key risk factors. Undoubtedly there are genetic susceptibility factors also, but to date only the rare α_1-antitrypsin deficiency has been characterized. Chronic inflammation in the airways leads to mucous hypersecretion and airflow obstruction.[21] Destruction of lung tissue also eventually occurs, which exacerbates airflow obstruction because of collapse of small airways. Eventually, the capacity for gas exchange can be compromised leading to hypoxemia.

Amanda Jones, *Part 2*

Mrs. Jones has no history of smoking, pneumonia, COPD, or swallowing difficulty. You examine Mrs. Jones in the nursing home. She looks moderately ill.

She has a nonproductive cough. Lung sounds are clear except for some fine bibasilar crackles. For the past few weeks, you have been seeing younger community residents with influenza-like illnesses, but you had not previously heard of an outbreak of influenza among nursing home residents.

STUDY QUESTION

1. What will you do to confirm Mrs. Jones' diagnosis?

Robert Thompson, *Part 1*

Mr. Thompson is an 80-year-old retired carpenter. He lives with his 75-year-old wife in an assisted-living facility, which provides meals and cleaning services. He has some chronic shortness of breath and is relatively inactive. He has smoked one pack of cigarettes per day for the past 65 years. His wife brings him to see you on a Tuesday afternoon because she is concerned that he is just not himself. He has been restless and somewhat confused. When a friend stopped by, Mr. Thompson did not recognize him. He may be coughing more than usual. His weight is 72 kg, temperature is 36.5°C, pulse 92, respirations 24, and blood pressure 130/76 mm Hg seated. He exhibits suprasternal and intercostal retractions and appears somewhat anxious. Pulse oximetry shows 88% oxygen saturation.

STUDY QUESTIONS

1. What conditions could account for these acute changes?
2. What will you do next to evaluate Mr. Thompson?

> ● In community-acquired pneumonia (CAP), presenting symptoms in older adults are less prominent than in younger adults.

DIFFERENTIAL DIAGNOSIS AND ASSESSMENT

Influenza, Bronchitis, and Pneumonia

LRIs, including influenza, bronchitis, and pneumonia, may present with typical or atypical symptoms in older adults. Influenza is typically seen in the context of community outbreaks; however, even with influenza active nationally, a local outbreak may or may not be influenza. An English study found a wide variety of respiratory viruses circulating in nursing homes in one city while influenza was active nationally.[22] Typical influenza symptoms and signs include cough, fever, and severe malaise.[14] The cardinal symptom of bronchitis is persistent cough, but at the beginning of an acute illness when systemic symptoms, including fever, may be present, distinguishing bronchitis from pneumonia may not be simple.[15] Although experienced clinicians commonly look for atypical presentations of pneumonia in older adults, some respiratory signs or symptoms are usually present on careful evaluation. Nonetheless, it is important to remember that the presenting complaint may not refer to the respiratory system. Fever, new or increasing falls, decreased appetite or activity, or delirium may be the symptoms that bring a patient with pneumonia to medical attention.

For community-acquired pneumonia (CAP), presenting symptoms in older adults are less prominent than in younger adults. Fever is variably present and declines with age. Metlay and colleagues reported data from a large study of ambulatory and emergency department patients in three cities.[23] Very few of these patients were from nursing homes. They found that fever (at least 38°C) was present in 85% of adults age 18 to 44, but only 60% of those age 65 to 74 and 53% of those age 75 or more. The number of symptoms was also fewer, but at least 80% had cough. In a large study of LRI in nursing home residents (the Missouri LRI study),[10,24] 80% of residents with pneumonia had three or fewer symptoms; however, only 7.5% had no respiratory symptoms at all. Although fever was more common in those with pneumonia, only 44% whose chest radiograph showed possible or probable pneumonia had a temperature of 38°C or higher.

Depending on the patient's presentation, a variety of conditions might need to be considered. Where cough, dyspnea, and other respiratory symptoms are particularly prominent, other considerations include congestive heart failure, COPD, and pulmonary embolism. Where fever is a prominent symptom, other common and uncommon infections are possibilities, including infections of the skin, abdomen, and urinary tract. Where less specific symptoms, such as delirium, new or increased falls, or decreased eating are particularly prominent, a wide variety of conditions need to be considered, such as stroke, subdural hematoma, myocardial infarction, fluid and electrolyte disturbance, an adverse medication reaction, and acute intoxication.

> ● Although culture specimens are always desirable in treating infections, collecting adequate sputum specimens are frequently unsuccessful in older adults even with determined efforts.

The evaluation will thus need to be tailored to the specific presentation; however, a complete blood count, a chemistry panel that includes blood urea nitrogen (BUN) and creatinine, a chest radiograph, and pulse oximetry are usually useful for diagnosis (level of evidence = D) as well as prognosis (level of evidence = B) if pneumonia is present. Clinical findings generally are not sufficient to rule in or rule out pneumonia without a chest radiograph,[25] but one emergency department–based study found that where three vital signs were all normal (heart rate 100, temperature 37.8°C, respiratory rate 20), pneumonia was much less likely (negative likelihood ratio 0.18).[26] However, the mean age in this study was only 53.6, so the applicability of these results to very old adults who exhibit fewer symptoms is not clear.

Although culture specimens are always desirable in treating infections, collecting adequate sputum specimens are frequently unsuccessful in older adults even with determined efforts.[19] In those hospitalized for treatment of pneumonia, obtaining blood cultures is appropriate and recommended in several guidelines[27-29]; however, evidence of benefit is limited to select observational studies (level of evidence = B). Where a new outbreak of influenza is a major consideration, rapid diagnostic testing may be useful. Reported sensitivities range from 63% to 81% with specificities over 90%[30,31]; however, once influenza is known to be present in an area, physician judgment is as effective as diagnostic testing (level of evidence = B).[30]

Constance Newberry, *Part 1*

Mrs. Newberry is an 80-year-old woman newly admitted to Colonial Manor nursing home. She had previously lived alone since her husband died 12 years ago but has developed progressive Alzheimer's disease. Her family has decided on nursing home admission because she is no longer able to care for herself. On admission, you order two-step purified protein derivative (PPD) testing by the Mantoux method according to facility policy. The results are 5 mm of induration on the initial test and 12 mm on the second test.

STUDY QUESTIONS

1. What do these findings mean?
2. Does this patient have a new infection with tuberculosis?

Tuberculosis Case Finding

Tuberculosis most commonly appears in older adults as a reactivation of a prior infection that had been controlled by the patient's immune system. Presentation may be insidious with weight loss and fatigue or may be associated with cough.[13] Tuberculosis may also be discovered from a patient treated for pulmonary infiltrates, which do not respond to conventional antibiotic therapy.

The PPD skin test detects the presence of a cell-mediated immune response to a protein present in the cell wall of *M. tuberculosis* and other closely related species.[20] The only currently recommended method of administering PPD is the Mantoux method: intradermal injection of 0.1 ml of 5 tuberculin units. Results are based on a measurement of the area of induration at 48 to 72 hours after placement. The interpretation of a PPD test is shown in Table 46-1. An important distinction is the difference between a chronic positive response and a conversion from negative to positive. A conversion (defined as an increase in the reaction of 10 mm within 2 years) indicates a new infection with a much higher probability of going on to active disease.[20]

Data on the rate of PPD conversion to active infection are limited for older adults, but in a general mental hospital population, the rate of progression to active tuberculosis during the first year after a new conversion was 12.9 per 1000 patient-years.[20] In the same study, from 1 to 7 years after a new conversion, the rate was only 1.6 per 1000 patient-years. A reaction not known to be a new conversion usually indicates an old infection. Assuming that a chest radiograph does not show active disease or fibrotic scarring suggestive of a prior active infection, the probability of developing active disease is much smaller. An increased response to a second PPD test shortly after the first, the booster phenomenon,

should be considered the same as an established positive response.[13] This probably represents an amnestic response by the immune system. As with other positive tests, a chest radiograph is required to confirm the absence of active disease, but the response should be treated the same as an initial positive reaction. The American Geriatrics Society recommends that patients in nursing homes obtain two-step PPD testing in order to be prepared for the rare occurrence of an outbreak of tuberculosis.[32] Although logical and very helpful in managing an outbreak, this approach is based only on expert opinion (level of evidence = D).

> ● Clinical guidelines for COPD management stress the use of spirometry for diagnosis and classification of severity.

Chronic Obstructive Pulmonary Disease

COPD should be considered in the setting of chronic cough, sputum production, or dyspnea, particularly with a history of smoking or occupational exposure.[21] Although advanced cases can be suggested by physical and radiographic findings, the standard diagnostic test is a pulmonary function study. Whether a smoking history alone is sufficient to warrant testing is less clear. Other diagnostic considerations might include asthma (distinguished by reversible airflow limitation), congestive heart failure, bronchiectasis, and, on occasion, several other rarer conditions.[21] Chronic cough alone has multiple pulmonary and extrapulmonary causes; the latter include acid reflux, postnasal drip, and medications.[33]

Clinical guidelines for COPD management stress the use of spirometry for diagnosis and classification of severity. The Global Initiative for Chronic Obstructive Lung Disease (GOLD) published an extensive guideline in 2001,[21] which was updated in 2004.[33] Based on postbronchodilator results, if the ratio of forced expiratory volume in 1 second (FEV_1) to forced vital capacity (FVC) is less than 70%, then COPD is present.[33] Mild disease (stage 1) is characterized by FEV_1/FVC less than 70% and $FEV_1 \geq$ 80% predicted; moderate disease (stage 2) is characterized by 50% $\leq FEV_1 <$ 80% predicted; in severe disease (stage 3), 30% $\leq FEV_1 <$ 50% predicted; and in very severe disease (stage 4), FEV_1 is less than 30% predicted or FEV_1 is less than 50% predicted with chronic respiratory failure. Chronic respiratory failure is defined as partial pressure of oxygen less than 60 mm Hg or partial pressure of carbon dioxide greater than 50 mm Hg while breathing air at sea level.[33] The GOLD expert panel acknowledges that given the normal decline of lung function with aging, these guidelines may overstate the presence of COPD in older adults.

Table 46–1 | Criteria for Tuberculin Positivity in Older Adults by Risk Group

Risk Group	Tuberculin Reaction Size, mm
HIV-infected persons or persons receiving immunosuppressive therapy	≥5
Close contacts of tuberculosis patients	≥5
Persons with fibrotic lesions on chest radiography consistent with prior tuberculosis	≥5
Long-term care facility or other institutional residents and employees	≥10
Persons with high-risk medical conditions, including diabetes mellitus, some malignancies, injection drug use, end-stage renal disease, silicosis, and clinical situations associated with rapid weight loss	≥10
Low risk persons	≥15

Based on data from Centers for Disease Control and Prevention. Targeted tuberculin testing and treatment of latent tuberculosis infection: American Thoracic Society. MMWR Recomm Rep 2000;49(RR-6):1-51.

Once a diagnosis is made, assessing the history of occupational or other toxic exposures in addition to cigarette smoke is important. Measurement of arterial blood gases are indicated with more severe disease. In the event of an acute exacerbation, chest radiography (level of evidence = B) and arterial blood gas sampling are likely to provide helpful clinical information.[4]

Amanda Jones, *Part 3*

Mrs. Jones has a throat swab for a rapid influenza test. The result is positive for influenza A. You also discover that four other residents on the wing have influenza-like illnesses.

STUDY QUESTIONS

1. What treatment will you initiate for Mrs. Jones?
2. What other steps will you take to manage the influenza outbreak in the nursing home?

MANAGEMENT

Influenza

The most important step in managing influenza is prevention through the use of the influenza vaccine. Although the extent of protection from infection has been variable, particularly in adults over age 70, clear evidence links influenza vaccination to reductions in severe illness and mortality.[14] In the long-term care setting, immunization of facility staff may be even more important in preventing morbidity and mortality.[34]

In 2006, the Centers for Disease Control recommended oseltamivir and zanamivir as the preferred antiviral agents for both prophylaxis and treatment of influenza A and B.[35] Previously an adamantine (amantadine or rimantadine) had been recommended for prophylaxis of influenza A. The new recommendation was based on recent reports of circulating strains of influenza A exhibiting high-level adamantine resistance. Because of variable protection from infection by vaccination, prophylactic treatment with oseltamivir or zanamivir is a consideration when influenza is circulating in the community, particularly, in the event of nursing home outbreak.[35] All residents without contraindications should receive prophylaxis when there is an institutional outbreak. High-risk individuals who have a direct exposure to influenza, for example, by another person in the same household, or who have not been adequately vaccinated are also candidates for chemoprophylaxis. The prophylactic dosage of osteltamivir is 75 mg daily and for zanamivir 10 mg (two inhalations) daily; in both cases this is half the treatment dose. With severely impaired renal function (estimated creatinine clearance < 30 mL/min), oseltamivir dosage should be reduced. Zanamivir is not recommended for those with underlying airway disease, such as asthma. The duration of chemoprophylaxis is for the extent of the outbreak, especially in patients who have not received prior vaccination. For patients who receive vaccination at the beginning of an outbreak, chemoprophylaxis should be continued for at least 2 weeks to ensure time for the vaccination to take full effect.

When administered within 2 days of illness onset to otherwise healthy adults, zanamivir and oseltamivir can reduce the duration of uncomplicated influenza A and B illness by approximately 1 day, compared with placebo.[35] Data are limited regarding the effectiveness of antiviral agents for treatment of influenza among persons at high risk for serious complications of influenza.

Amanda Jones: Case Discussion

Cough and fever in an elderly nursing home resident suggest a LRI. This patient is also eating poorly, which is a nonspecific symptom associated with many acute illnesses in older adults. The additional information that influenza is present in the community immediately suggests that as a diagnosis. Fine crackles present in a patient's lungs may be significant but can also be a normal finding in an older adult. Because of the implications for the facility as well as the patient, some confirmation of the diagnosis is desirable. Once the diagnosis has been made, the patient could be treated with oseltamivir 75 mg twice daily for 5 days or zanamivir 10 mg (2 inhalations) twice daily for five days. Other residents in the facility should be treated with either oseltamivir or zanamivir (once daily in either case) to help control the outbreak. Chemoprophylaxis should continue at least through the peak of the community epidemic.

Robert Thompson, *Part 2*

Examining the lungs, you note some scattered wheezing throughout the lung fields and quiet breath sounds at the left base. Heart sounds are normal. There is no pedal edema. The patient is not oriented to time and is easily distracted. His short-term memory is poor. A complete blood count shows a white blood count of $15.0 \times 10^3/mm^3$.

Chemistries are normal except for a BUN of 28 mg/dl. Creatinine is 1.1 mg/dl. An electrocardiogram shows nonspecific ST and T-wave changes. Chest radiograph shows a left lower lobe infiltrate compatible with pneumonia. The diaphragms are somewhat flattened.

STUDY QUESTIONS

1. How will you treat Mr. Thompson's pneumonia?
2. What other diagnosis is likely?

> ● When assessing the severity of pneumonia in the nursing home, age is not an independent risk factor for mortality, but functional and nutritional status as well as a decline in mood in the past 90 days become important predictors.

Treatment of Bronchitis and Pneumonia

Consistent with most bronchitis being viral, there is little evidence that antibiotic treatment substantially improves acute bronchitis outcomes in healthy adults (level of evidence = A)[30,36]; however, very few older adults were included in these studies. There is some evidence that antibiotic treatment is beneficial in severe exacerbations of COPD.[4] A recent guideline supported by the Centers for Disease Control and Prevention (CDC), the Infectious Disease Society of America, the American Academy of Family Physicians, and the American College of Physicians recommends against antibiotic treatment for bronchitis in healthy community-dwelling adults but does not comment on frail older adults or those with significant comorbidities, such as congestive heart failure or COPD.[30] Among the predominantly frail older adults in the Missouri LRI Study who did not have pneumonia (and hence in most cases probably bronchitis), 30-day mortality was still 9%.[10] Treatment decisions must be individualized, but in more severe illness or where pneumonia is still a consideration even with a negative chest radiograph, antibiotic treatment may be appropriate. The same kind of regimens that are appropriate in pneumonia (see below) might be reasonable choices, but data are lacking to guide treatment. In several studies, inhaled bronchodilators, such as albuterol, appeared to offer some relief from cough symptoms in bronchitis,[30] although a Cochrane meta-analysis concluded that there was no benefit.[37]

In assessing treatment plans for CAP or nursing home–acquired pneumonia, two factors should always be considered: goals of care and risk of a poor outcome. Some individuals with pneumonia may be near the end of life from a chronic illness, such as dementia, a malignancy, congestive heart failure, or chronic obstructive lung disease. If the goal of care has become primarily comfort, then any decision about hospitalization or antibiotic treatment needs to be considered from the perspective of whether it will enhance comfort. However, a decision for palliative care requires discussion with the patient or the appropriate surrogate if the patient is not competent.

For the greater number of individuals in whom goals of care are not strictly palliative, a mortality risk-assessment tool may be quite helpful, particularly in identifying individuals appropriately treated outside the hospital. For patients with CAP, Fine's pneumonia severity index (Table 46-2) performs well. However, because the pneumonia severity index was designed for adults of all ages presenting to outpatient settings or emergency departments, very old individuals, particularly older nursing home residents, tend to be classified in the highest risk groups (classes IV and V). Nonetheless, patients with CAP who are class III or lower are often good candidates for treatment outside the hospital. A cluster-randomized trial of a clinical pathway for CAP patients presenting to emergency departments in Canada demonstrated that many with a class III or lower score on the pneumonia severity index could be treated safely outside the hospital.[38] As with all tools, judgment is required. Community-dwelling individuals might have other reasons for admission than illness severity alone, such as inadequate oxygen saturation, inadequate home support, or other active problems requiring inpatient care.

For nursing home residents with a LRI, the Missouri LRI Study risk score (Table 46-3) provides a tool that can assist with treatment decisions.[10] Lower-risk individuals (scores of six or less) are often good candidates for treatment within the nursing home. Even moderate risk patients (scores of seven to eight) may not benefit from hospitalization.[11] In the nursing home setting, where average age is very old and frailty is common, age is not an independent risk factor for mortality, but functional and nutritional status as well as a decline in mood in the past 90 days become important predictors.

> ● Older adults with severe dementia who are hospitalized with pneumonia have over 50% 6-month mortality despite aggressive hospital care.

In December 2003, the Infectious Disease Society of America released new suggested antibiotic guidelines for pneumonia.[28] Table 46-4 outlines recommended treatment for CAP and nursing home– acquired pneumonia in immunocompetent patients that do not require intensive care unit care. With increasing concerns about emerging antibiotic resistance, these

Table 46–2	Calculating the Pneumonia Severity Index (PSI) in Older Adults

Patient Characteristics	Points Assigned	Patient's Points
Demographic Factors		
Age		
Males (in years)	Age	
Females (in years)	Age −10	
Nursing home resident	+10	
Coexisting Conditions		
Neoplastic disease	+30	
Liver disease	+20	
Congestive heart failure	+10	
Cerebrovascular disease	+10	
Renal Disease	+10	
Physical exam findings		
Altered mental status	+20	
Respiratory rate ≥30/min.	+20	
Systolic BP <90 mmHg	+20	
Temperature <35° or ≥40°	+15	
Pulse ≥125/min	+10	
Laboratory findings		
pH <7.35	+30	
BUN ≥30 mg/dl	+20	
Sodium <130 mmol/L	+20	
Glucose ≥250 mg/dl	+10	
Hematocrit <30%	+10	
pO_2 <60mmHg or O_2 saturation <90%	+10	
Pleural effusion	+10	

TOTAL SCORE (sum all patient's points):

Risk Class (points)	Mortality (%) in Validation Studies
I*	0.1
II (≥ 70)	0.6
III (71–90)	0.9-2.8
IV (91–130)	8.2-9.3
V (> 130)	27.0-29.2

*Risk class 1 includes only those under 50 with no comorbidity, or abnormal physical findings.

Based on data from Fine MJ, et. al. A prediction rule to identify low-risk patients with community-acquired pneumonia. N Engl J Med 1997;336:243-250. Modified from material supplied by the author.

guidelines are noteworthy for the recommendation that where antibiotics were used in the last 3 months, a different regimen be used. In particular, resistance may emerge during fluoroquinolone therapy.[28]

For particularly frail older adults, during or after treatment for pneumonia in the hospital or nursing home, it may be appropriate to review treatment goals. For example, individuals with severe dementia who are hospitalized with pneumonia have over 50% 6-month mortality despite aggressive hospital care.[39] Such individuals with limited life expectancy might benefit from an approach focused on palliative care. Also, episodes of pneumonia should provide a reminder to review immunization status. Pneumococcal vaccination is recommended for all individuals over age 65, including those who received vaccination more than 5 years earlier who were younger than 65 at the time.[28] Although antibody titers wane, whether vaccination should be repeated in other individuals is not clear, and there is no recommendation for routine reimmunization from the CDC's Advisory Committee on Immunization Practices (ACIP).

Constance Newberry, *Part 2*

A chest radiograph is obtained and is negative. Because her reaction on the second step of PPD testing likely represents old infection, Mrs. Newberry does not receive any treatment for her latent tuberculosis infection. Six months later, another resident at Colonial Manor develops cough and weight loss and is found to have an apical infiltrate on chest radiograph compatible with active tuberculosis. Mrs. Newberry remains well except for her slowly progressive dementia.

STUDY QUESTION

1. How should you manage a case of active tuberculosis in a nursing home setting?

> ● The treatment of latent or active tuberculosis in nursing home residents is targeted at patients where there is evidence of active disease, a positive skin test represents a new conversion, or there is specific immune system compromise, such as immunosuppressive therapy or HIV infection.

Tuberculosis Management

Regardless of the setting, a patient with active tuberculosis requires temporary respiratory isolation while therapy is initiated. Several different regimens for treatment are available, but all require months of therapy and multiple medications. Details are beyond the scope of this chapter, but excellent references are readily available.[40]

A second treatment issue is whether to treat individuals with latent tuberculosis infection to prevent

Table 46–3	Missouri LRI Study Risk Score for Nursing Home-Acquired Pneumonia or Lower Respiratory Infection (LRI)		
Variable	**Value**	**Points Assigned**	**Patient Value**
Blood urea nitrogen (BUN; mg/dL)	16.0 or less	0	
	16.1 up to 27	1	
	27.1 up to 38	2	
	38.1 up to 49	3	
	49.1 up to 60	4	
	60.1 up to 71	5	
	More than 71.0	6	☐
White blood cell count (WBC; 10^9 cells/l)	14.0 or less	0	
	14.1 up to 24	1	
	More than 24.0	2	☐
Absolute lymphocyte count* (10^9 cells/L)	More than 0.8	0	
	0.8 or less	1	☐
Pulse (beats/minute)	72 or less	0	
	73 up to 102	1	
	103 up to 132	2	
	More than 132	3	☐
Gender	Female	0	
	Male	1	☐
Body mass index (kg/m²)†	31.0 or more	0	
	25.1 up to 31	1	
	19.1 up to 25	2	
	13.1 up to 19	3	
	13.0 or less	4	☐
Activities of daily living (ADLs)‡	0	0	
	1 or 2	1	
	3 or 4	2	☐
Mood deterioration over last 90 days	No	0	
	Yes	2	☐
Sum of item scores for resident			☐

To derive risk score, sum the assigned points. Risk of 30-day mortality is as follows:

1 to 4 points, 2.4%; 5 to 6 points, 6.9%; 7 to 8 points, 15.6%; 9 to 10 points, 34.5%; 11 to 17 points, 61.6%.

*To calculate absolute lymphocyte count, multiply WBC by percentage lymphocytes. For an individual with a WBC of 8×10^9/l and 15 percent lymphocytes, (8×10^9/L) × 0.15 = 1.2×10^9/l. This value would receive 0 points.

†BMI is calculated as weight in kilograms divided by the square of the height in meters (weight/height²). For a person weighing 145 pounds and 5′ 3″ tall, the calculation would be as follows: Divide weight in pounds by 2.2 to derive weight in kilograms (145 lb = 66 kg). Multiply height in inches by 2.54 to convert to cm, and then divide by 100 to convert to meters (63 in = 1.60 m). BMI = $66/1.60^2$ = 25.8 (rounding to one decimal point). This value would receive 1 point.

‡ADL scoring is based on four ADL variables: grooming, toileting, locomotion on the unit, and eating. Each is assigned a 0 if the resident is independent, requires supervision, or requires limited assistance; a 1 is assigned if the resident requires extensive assistance or is totally dependent. The four scores are summed to derive an ADL score of 0 to 4 which is assigned points as shown above.

reactivation. Although treatment is highly effective in reducing risk of developing active tuberculosis (level of evidence = A),[20] at minimum several months of treatment with potentially toxic drugs are required. Current CDC/American Thoracic Society recommendations emphasize targeting testing at higher-risk groups and generally discourage routine PPD testing unless there is a plan to treat a latent tuberculosis infection[20]; however, where there is a low risk of reactivation, the recommendations recommend weighing risks and benefits of treatment. Thus, healthy older adults living in the community should generally not

Table 46–4	Initial Empiric Therapy for Pneumonia in Older Adults
Setting	**Recommended Options**
Outpatient	
Previously healthy	
No recent antibiotic therapy	A macrolide (erythromycin, azithromycin, or clarithromycin) or doxycycline
Recent antibiotic therapy[a]	A respiratory fluoroquinolone[b] alone; an advanced macrolide (azithromycin or clarithromycin) plus high-dose amoxicillin (1 g orally three times day); or an advanced macrolide plus high-dose amoxicillin-clavulanate (2 g orally twice a day)
Comorbidities (COPD, diabetes, renal or congestive heart failure, or malignancy)	
No recent antibiotic therapy	An advanced macrolide or a respiratory fluoroquinolone
Recent antibiotic therapy	A respiratory fluoroquinolone alone or an advanced macrolide plus a β-lactam[c]
Suspected aspiration with infection	Amoxicillin-clavulanate or clindamycin
Influenza with bacterial superinfection	A β-lactam[c] or a respiratory fluoroquinolone
Nursing home	
Treatment in the nursing home	A respiratory fluoroquinolone alone or amoxicillin-clavulanate plus an advanced macrolide
Inpatient (not in an ICU)	
No recent antibiotic therapy	A respiratory fluoroquinolone alone or an advanced macrolide plus a β-lactam[d]
Recent antibiotic therapy	Same options as with no recent antibiotic therapy but recent use of a fluoroquinolone should dictate selection of a nonfluoroquinolone regimen, and vice versa.

COPD indicates chronic obstructive pulmonary disease; ICU, intensive care unit.

Note that specific doses may need to be adjusted based on estimated creatinine clearance, which on average decreases with age.

[a]Received antibiotic(s) for treatment of any infection within the past 3 months, excluding the current episode of infection. Recent use of a fluoroquinolone should dictate selection of a nonfluoroquinolone regimen, and vice versa.

[b]Moxifloxacin, gatifloxacin, levofloxacin, or gemifloxacin.

[c]High-dose amoxicillin, high-dose amoxicillin-clavulanate, cefpodoxime, cefprozil, or cefuroxime.

[d]Cefotaxime, ceftriaxone, ampicillin-sulbactam, or ertapenem.

Adapted from Mandell LA, Bartlett JG, Dowell SF, et al. Update of Practice Guidelines for the Management of Community-Acquired Pneumonia in Immunocompetent Adults. Clin Infect Dis 2003;37:1405-1433.

receive PPD screening unless potentially exposed to an active case. The CDC recommendations do not specifically address routine testing in the institutional setting except in terms of interpreting the results of a PPD skin test (see Table 46-1). However, given the relatively limited life expectancy of many older nursing home residents, nontreatment after a positive admission skin test would be reasonable in most instances. Exceptions would include where there is evidence of active disease, the positive skin test represents a new conversion, or there is specific immune system compromise, such as immunosuppressive therapy or HIV infection. Several regimens based on either isoniazid or rifampin are available for treating latent tuberculosis infection where this is deemed advisable.[20]

If a resident develops active tuberculosis in a nursing home or other long-term care facility, other residents and staff in the facility should receive PPD skin testing. In this setting, either a skin test conversion or a new reaction of 5 mm in size is considered a positive test and an indication for treatment. Where residents have received the two-step admission screening with PPD, interpretation of skin tests during an outbreak will be clearer, and unnecessary and potentially risky treatment may be avoided.

Constance Newberry: Case Discussion

Mrs. Newberry appropriately receives two-step PPD testing on nursing home admission according to the recommendations of the American Geriatric Society. She exhibits the booster phenomenon, which is an amnestic response to an old infection and not an indication of new conversion. When a case of active tuberculosis is diagnosed in another patient in

Mrs. Newberry's nursing home, this is very helpful information. Very old nursing home residents will usually not be candidates for treatment of latent tuberculosis unless they convert from a negative to a positive test or develop active disease. Staff members may be candidates for treatment of latent tuberculosis infection if they develop a positive test because of their much longer life expectancy.

Robert Thompson, *Part 3*

As his estimated creatinine clearance is more than 50 mL/min, Mr. Thompson receives treatment with levofloxacin 500 mg daily (oral after an initial intravenous dose). He also receives nebulized albuterol and ipratropium bromide in the hospital. After several days his delirium has cleared, and he is breathing more easily. His oxygen saturation at rest is 95% on room air. You note, however, that he continues to have dyspnea with exertion when walking in the hall.

STUDY QUESTIONS

1. What additional measures will you need to take before and after discharge?

⬤ Beyond smoking cessation, no treatments have been demonstrated to slow COPD disease progression.

COPD Management

Beyond diagnosis and monitoring of disease progression, management of COPD includes risk factor reduction, management of stable disease, and treatment of acute exacerbations.[21] Table 46-5, based on the revised GOLD guideline[33] and a guideline from the American College of Physicians,[4] outlines the evidence for specific interventions in each of these areas.

Risk factor reduction primarily concerns smoking cessation but may also include avoidance of occupational exposures or air pollution. Although only a small percentage of patients quit after brief physician counseling, the result is still important in reducing the risk of developing COPD and slowing its progression. More sustained counseling or social support interventions, particularly when combined with nicotine replacement or use of bupropion, can produce appreciable long-term quit rates (more than 20%).[33]

Beyond smoking cessation, no treatments have been demonstrated to slow disease progression; however, several treatments are beneficial.[33] Bronchodilators are effective in relieving symptoms and should be used as needed beginning with stage 1 disease. With stage 2 (moderate) and more advanced disease, long-acting bronchodilators may offer advantages, although they are more expensive.[33] Many therapies have received limited testing in older adults. For example, it is not known to what extent anticholinergic effects outside the respiratory tract might cause problems in older adults who use tiotropium, a long-acting anticholiner-

Table 46–5	Management of Chronic Obstructive Pulmonary Disease		
Indication	**Treatment Strategy**	**Level of Evidence for Effectiveness**	**Comments**
Risk factor	Physician counseling to stop smoking	A	Even brief counseling is somewhat effective
	Multicomponent programs to stop smoking	A	Structured programs and use of pharmacotherapy increase success
Management of stable COPD	Inhaled β_2 agonist or anticholinergic	A	Effective in symptom management
	Inhaled corticosteroids	A	In stage 3 or 4 disease with frequent exacerbations, exacerbations are reduced
	Oral corticosteroids	X	Equivocal benefit and harmful side effects
	Pulmonary rehabilitation	A	Improved exercise capacity and well being
	Home oxygen	A	For chronic hypoxemia
Management of acute exacerbations	Oral Antibiotics	A	Studies are old and improvement most evident with severe exacerbations
	Systemic corticosteroids	A	Improved spirometry and decreased relapse rate

A indicates supported by one or more high-quality randomized trials; B, supported by one or more high-quality nonrandomized cohort studies or low-quality RCTs; C, supported by one or more case series and/or poor-quality cohort and/or case-control studies; D, supported by expert opinion and/or extrapolation from studies in other populations or settings; X, evidence supports the treatment being ineffective or harmful.

gic bronchodilator. Pulmonary rehabilitation, including exercise training, leads to improved exercise capacity and sense of well being. However, effects wane if the patient does not continue to exercise after the conclusion of a formal program.[33] For patients with severe or very severe disease (stages 3 and 4) who also have frequent exacerbations, inhaled corticosteroids may reduce the frequency of exacerbations.[33] Oral corticosteroids are not recommended, except for acute exacerbations, because of their equivocal long-term benefit with substantial adverse side effects. Continuous home oxygen (at least 15 hours per day) prolongs life and reduces symptoms in advanced disease with decrease in oxygen saturation (usually 88% or less; 89% or less with evidence of pulmonary hypertension, congestive heart failure, or polycythemia).[33]

In managing acute exacerbations of COPD, in addition to bronchodilators and oxygen as needed, systemic corticosteroids can shorten recovery and reduce the risk of relapse.[4,33] In addition, in predominantly older studies, treatment with predominantly simple oral antibiotics (tetracyclines, amoxicillin, and trimethoprim-sulfamethoxazole) resulted in symptom improvement compared with controls. These effects were clearer in those with more severe exacerbations, which have been defined as the presence of increased dyspnea, increase in sputum volume, and increase in sputum purulence.[4] It is not known how broader spectrum agents (e.g., the fluoroquinolones) and the increased prevalence of antibiotic resistance affect these earlier findings. Where respiratory failure with hypercarbia is present, referral for noninvasive positive pressure ventilation may decrease the need for mechanical ventilation and possibly improve survival.[4,33]

Robert Thompson: Case Discussion

Mr. Thompson presents with an acute delirium, increased cough, increased respiratory rate, and decreased oxygen saturation. He has a long smoking history, so an exacerbation of COPD is a consideration as well. The absence of fever does not rule out pneumonia, and in fact, that is the diagnosis after further evaluation. He also has several clinical findings that raise a suspicion of COPD. In deciding on treatment, the first decision is to select the treatment setting. As an 80-year-old man with altered mental status and low oxygen saturation, he clearly fits into class IV of the pneumonia severity index, which suggests the need for

hospitalization. His poor oxygenation and delirium also suggest the need for hospitalization. A respiratory fluoroquinolone, such as levofloxacin is an appropriate choice for antibiotic therapy. His estimated creatinine clearance by the Cockcroft-Gault formula is (140 -80 years) × 72 kg/(72 kg × 1.1 mg/dl) = 54, so he does not need his dose of levofloxacin reduced.

After recovery from his pneumonia, he is still exhibiting some dyspnea. He needs to be evaluated to determine the severity of his COPD. In addition, smoking cessation counseling and probably pharmacotherapy will be very important. Other measures that will likely be appropriate depending on the severity of his COPD include pulmonary rehabilitation and treatment with bronchodilators.

SUMMARY

LRIs and COPD are prevalent and serious problems in older adults. Older adults with an LRI present with diverse symptoms, but at least one respiratory symptom is present in most cases on careful evaluation. Treatment depends on specific diagnosis, care goals, and illness severity. Mortality risk scores for CAP and nursing home–acquired LRI can assist with hospitalization decisions. Immunization of residents and staff of long-term care facilities as well as appropriate prophylaxis and treatment can reduce morbidity and mortality from influenza. Tuberculosis usually occurs in older adults by reactivation, and two-step PPD screening at nursing home admission can aid in controlling an outbreak of active disease if it occurs. COPD should be suspected in those with chronic cough, sputum production, or dyspnea and should be diagnosed with spirometry. Smoking cessation is the only intervention effective in slowing the progression of the disease, but other treatments based on disease severity can assist with controlling symptoms.

References

1. Anderson RN, Smith BL. Deaths: leading causes for 2002. Natl Vital Stat Rep 2005;53(17):1-89.
2. DeFrances CJ, Hall MJ. 2002 National Hospital Discharge Survey. Adv Data 2004;342:1-29.
3. Fine MJ, Auble TE, Yealy DM, et al. A prediction rule to identify low-risk patients with community-acquired pneumonia. N Engl J Med 1997;336: 243-250.
4. Bach PB, Brown C, Gelfand SE, McCrory DC, American College of Physicians-American Society of Internal Medicine, American College of Chest Physicians. Management of acute exacerbations of chronic obstructive pulmonary disease: a summary and appraisal of published evidence. Ann Intern Med 2001;134:600-620.
5. Gross JS, Neufeld RR, Libow LS, Gerber I, Rodstein M. Autopsy study of the elderly institutionalized patient: review of 234 autopsies. Arch Intern Med 1988;148:173-176.

6. Beard CM, Kokmen E, Sigler C, Smith GE, Petterson T, O'Brien PC. Cause of death in Alzheimer's disease. Ann Epidemiol 1996;6:195-200.

7. Burns A, Jacoby R, Luthert P, Levy R. Cause of death in Alzheimer's disease. Age Ageing 1990;19:341-344.

8. Molsa PK, Marttila RJ, Rinne UK. Survival and cause of death in Alzheimer's disease and multi-infarct dementia. Acta Neurol Scand 1986;74:103-107.

9. Thomas BM, Starr JM, Whalley LJ. Death certification in treated cases of presenile Alzheimer's disease and vascular dementia in Scotland. Age Ageing 1997;26:401-406.

10. Mehr DR, Binder EF, Kruse RL, et al. Predicting mortality from lower respiratory infection in nursing home residents: the Missouri LRI Study. JAMA 2001;2862427-2436.

11. Kruse RL, Mehr DR, Boles KE, et al. Does hospitalization impact survival after lower respiratory Infection in nursing home residents? Med Care 2004;42:860-870.

12. Raviglione MC, O'Brien RJ. Tuberculosis. In Harrison's Online (Kasper DL, Braunwald E, Fauci AS, et al., eds.). New York: McGraw-Hill; 2005. http://www.accessmedicine.com/content.aspx?aID=72477.

13. Yoshikawa TT, Norman DC. Approach to fever and infection in the nursing home. J Am Geriatr Soc 1996;44:74-82.

14. Harper SA, Fukuda K, Uyeki TM, Cox NJ, Bridges CB, Centers for Disease Control and Prevention (CDC) Advisory Committee on Immunization Practices (ACIP). Prevention and control of influenza: recommendations of the Advisory Committee on Immunization Practices (ACIP). Morbid Mortal Wkly Rep 2004;53(RR-6):1-40.

15. Gonzales R, Sande MA. Uncomplicated acute bronchitis. Ann Intern Med 2000;133:981-991.

16. Loeb M. Pneumonia in older persons. Clin Infect Dis 2003;37:1335-1339.

17. Loeb M, McGeer A, McArthur M, Walter S, Simor AE. Risk factors for pneumonia and other lower respiratory tract infections in elderly residents of long-term care facilities. Arch Intern Med 1999;159:2058-2064.

18. Marrie TJ. Pneumonia in the long-term-care facility. Infect Control Hosp Epidemiol 2002;23:159-164.

19. Marrie TJ, Durant H, Kwan C. Nursing home-acquired pneumonia: a case-control study. J Am Geriatr Soc 1986;34:697-702.

20. Centers for Disease Control and Prevention. Targeted tuberculin testing and treatment of latent tuberculosis infection: American Thoracic Society. MMWR Recomm Rep 2000;49(RR-6):1-51.

21. Pauwels RA, Buist AS, Calverley PM, Jenkins CR, Hurd SS, GOLD Scientific Committee. Global strategy for the diagnosis, management, and prevention of chronic obstructive pulmonary disease. Am J Respir Crit Care Med 2001;163:1256-1276.

22. Nicholson KG, Baker DJ, Farquhar A, Hurd D, Kent J, Smith SH. Acute upper respiratory tract viral illness and influenza immunization in homes for the elderly. Epidemiol Infect 1990;105:609-618.

23. Metlay JP, Schulz R, Li YH, et al. Influence of age on symptoms at presentation in patients with community-acquired pneumonia. Arch Intern Med 1997;157:1453-1459.

24. Mehr DR, Binder EF, Kruse RL, Zweig SC, Madsen R, D'Agostino RB. Clinical findings associated with radiographic pneumonia in nursing home residents. J Fam Pract 2001;50:931-937.

25. Metlay JP, Fine MJ. Testing strategies in the initial management of patients with community-acquired pneumonia. Ann Intern Med 2003;138:109-118.

26. Gennis P, Gallagher J, Falvo C, Baker S, Than W. Clinical criteria for the detection of pneumonia in adults: guidelines for ordering chest roentgenograms in the emergency department. J Emerg Med 1989;7:263-268.

27. Hutt E, Kramer AM. Evidence-based guidelines for management of nursing home-acquired pneumonia. J Fam Pract 2002;51:709-716.

28. Mandell LA, Bartlett JG, Dowell SF, File TM Jr., Musher DM, Whitney C. Update of practice guidelines for the management of community-acquired pneumonia in immunocompetent adults. Clin Infect Dis 2003;37:1405-1433.

29. Niederman MS, Mandell LA, Anzueto A, et al. Guidelines for the management of adults with community-acquired pneumonia: diagnosis, assessment of severity, antimicrobial therapy, and prevention. Am J Respir Crit Care Med 2001;163:1730-1754.

30. Gonzales R, Bartlett JG, Besser RE, et al. Principles of appropriate antibiotic use for treatment of uncomplicated acute bronchitis: background. Ann Intern Med 2001;134:521-529.

31. Rothberg MB, Bellantonio S, Rose DN. Management of influenza in adults older than 65 years of age: cost-effectiveness of rapid testing and antiviral therapy. Ann Intern Med 2003;139(5 Pt 1):321-329.

32. Two-step PPD testing for nursing home patients on admission: position statement. New York: The American Geriatrics Society, 2003. http://www.americangeriatrics.org/products/positionpapers/PPD-test.shtml.

33. GOLD Expert Panel. Global strategy for the diagnosis, management, and prevention of chronic obstructive pulmonary disease. Updated 2004. Global Initiative for Chronic Obstructive Lung Disease. National Heart, Lung, and Blood Institute. World Health Organization, 2004. http://www.goldcopd.org/goldwr2004clean.pdf.

34. Potter J, Stott DJ, Roberts MA, et al. Influenza vaccination of health care workers in long-term-care hospitals reduces the mortality of elderly patients. J Infect Dis 1997;175:1-6.

35. Smith NM, Bresee JS, Shay DK, Uyeki TM, Cox NJ, Strikas RA, Centers for Disease Control and Prevention (CDC) Advisory Committee on Immunization Practices (ACIP). Prevention and control of influenza: recommendations fo the Advisory Committee on Immunization Practices (ACIP). Morbid Mortal Wkly Rep 2006;55(Early Release):1-41.

36. Smucny J, Fahey T, Becker L, Glazier R. Antibiotics for acute bronchitis. Cochrane Database Syst Rev 2004;(4):CD000245.

37. Smucny J, Flynn C, Becker L, Glazier R. β_2-Agonists for acute bronchitis. Cochrane Database Syst Rev 2004;(1):CD001726.

38. Marrie TJ, Lau CY, Wheeler SL, Wong CJ, Vandervoort MK, Feagan BG. A controlled trial of a critical pathway for treatment of community-acquired pneumonia. JAMA 2000;283:749-755.

39. Morrison RS, Siu AL. Survival in end-stage dementia following acute illness. JAMA 2000;284:47-52.

40. Centers for Disease Control and Prevention. Treatment of tuberculosis. MMWR Recomm Rep 2003;52(RR-11):1-77.

Web Resources

GOLD Expert Panel. Global strategy for the diagnosis, management, and prevention of chronic obstructive pulmonary disease. Updated 2004. Global Initiative for Chronic Obstructive Lung Disease. National Heart, Lung, and Blood Institute. World Health Organization, 2004. http://www.goldcopd.org/goldwr2004clean.pdf.

Two-step PPD testing for nursing home patients on admission: position statement. New York: The American Geriatrics Society, 2003. http://www.americangeriatrics.org/products/positionpapers/PPD-test.shtml.

POSTTEST

1. A healthy 70-year-old woman living in the community has been repeatedly exposed to a handyman who is found to have active tuberculosis. The man, who was a Cambodian refugee, was actively coughing as he worked on several projects for the patient. Because of volunteer work, she had a PPD placed 2 years ago, which was read as showing 5 mm of induration. Which of the following is most correct about the interpretation of a new PPD placed after discovery of her tuberculosis exposure?
   a. If her reaction remains at 5 mm, she has no increase in risk of developing active tuberculosis.
   b. If her reaction increases to 15 mm, she should be regarded as a new converter and should be counseled about receiving treatment for latent tuberculosis infection.
   c. She should not receive treatment unless her reaction increases by 15 mm in size to 20 mm.
   d. She should only receive treatment if a chest radiograph shows a fibrotic lesion.
   e. The booster phenomenon means that her reaction will definitely increase in size.

2. A 75-year-old man living in the community has a 60 pack-year smoking history. He has a persistent cough and mild dyspnea. He has slightly quiet breath sounds and scattered wheezes. After bronchodilators, FEV_1/FVC is 65% of predicted and FEV_1 is 60% of predicted. Which of the following groups of treatments are most likely to be appropriate therapy for this patient?
   a. Smoking cessation counseling, a β_2-agonist bronchodilator, inhaled corticosteroids
   b. Smoking cessation counseling, pulmonary rehabilitation, short-acting bronchodilators only
   c. Pulmonary rehabilitation, short-acting bronchodilators, inhaled corticosteroids
   d. Smoking cessation counseling, a β_2-agonist bronchodilator
   e. Smoking cessation counseling, pulmonary rehabilitation, a β_2-agonist bronchodilator

3. A 70-year-old woman consults you because of slowly increasing shortness of breath. She has smoked one pack of cigarettes per day for 20 years. After pulmonary function testing, you diagnose moderate (stage 2) COPD. Which of the following treatments is most apt to alter the long-run course of her disease?
   a. Smoking cessation counseling and prescription of nicotine replacement therapy
   b. Pulmonary rehabilitation
   c. Oxygen therapy when her oxygen saturation has declined to 90%.
   d. Prescription of a tiotropium inhaler to be used daily
   e. Prescription of inhaled corticosteroids.

PRETEST ANSWERS

1. c
2. d
3. e

POSTTEST ANSWERS

1. b
2. e
3. a

Urinary Tract Infections

Charles P. Mouton, Kurt P. Merkelz, and
David V. Espino

OBJECTIVES

Upon completion of this chapter, the reader will be able to:

- Define the causes of urinary tract infections in the elderly.

- Discuss the diagnosis of complicated and uncomplicated urinary tract infection.

- Distinguish between catheterized and noncatheterized patients in terms of diagnosis, prevention, and treatment.

- Address the clinical significance of asymptomatic bacteriuria.

- Describe preventive techniques for urinary tract infection

PRETEST

1. Which one of the following predisposes older adults to urinary tract infections?
   a. Thiazide diuretic therapy
   b. Cardiovascular disease
   c. Cognitive impairment
   d. Selective serotonin uptake inhibitors

2. Which one of the following statements regarding the use of antibiotics in patients with indwelling catheters is false?
   a. Indwelling urinary catheters are the leading cause of nosocomial urinary tract infection.
   b. Indwelling urinary catheters are the most common predisposing factor in hospital-acquired, fatal, Gram-negative sepsis.
   c. After 1 month, virtually all patients with indwelling catheters have asymptomatic bacteriuria.
   d. Antibiotic treatment should be prescribed for patients with asymptomatic bacteriuria who have indwelling urinary catheters.

3. Which of the following statements regarding bacteriuria is (are) true?
   a. Declining physical functioning may be associated with bacteriuria in older adults in long-term care.
   b. Lack of a febrile response (temperature less than 101.2°F) rules out a significant bacteriuria.
   c. Long-term antibiotic treatment is required for recurrent asymptomatic bacteriuria.
   d. Irrigating in-dwelling catheter decreases the risk of bacteriuria.

PREVALENCE AND IMPACT

Lower urinary tract infection (UTI) is a common disease, especially in the elderly population. Table 47-1 compares UTI characteristics in older and younger patients. As many as 50% of women report having had at least one UTI in their lifetime.[1] UTI is the most common source of bacteremia in the elderly and is the most common cause of infection in nursing home residents, for men and women.[1] Community studies have shown prevalence rates of bacteriuria in the elderly to be 11% for community-based women, 18% for those living in congregate living arrangements, and 25% to 50% for those living in nursing home environments.[2,3] The prevalence of asymptomatic bacteriuria in patients older than 65 years of age ranges from 6% to 11% for ambulatory women and up to 50% for institutionalized elderly women.[2,3] The prevalence is lower in men.

Maria Alicea

Ms. Alicea is a 87-year-old woman who comes to see you after a recent bout with influenza because she has developed a problem with urinary urgency, increased urinary frequency, two episodes of urinary incontinence when she could not get to the bathroom on time, and had a sensation of suprapubic pressure for the past 4 days. A urinalysis done in your office shows 15 to 20 white blood cells per high-powered field. You begin treatment with double-strength trimethoprim-sulfamethoxazole twice daily, however, a urine culture shows no growth after 48 hours.

STUDY QUESTIONS

1. Should antibiotic treatment be continued?
2. Does the presence of pyuria change your treatment approach?

Table 47–1   Comparison of Urinary Tract Infections (UTIs) in Younger and Older Adults

Characteristic	Younger	Older Adults
Sex occurrence	Women-to-men ratio is 25 to 30:1	High in women and men; women-to-men ratio is 2 to 3:1
Etiologic organisms	*Escherichia coli* in most cases (uncomplicated UTI)	*E. coli, Proteus* species, *Klebsiella* species, *Enterococcus* species, staphylococci (chronic UTI)
Clinical findings	Dysuric syndrome, chills, fever, abdominal or flank pain, nausea	Most often asymptomatic change in function, dysuric syndrome, may present as sepsis
Diagnostic approach	Clinical finding and urinalysis in uncomplicated UTI may suffice	Urine culture required
Outcomes	High cure rate	Recurrences and treatment failure

Modified from Yoshikawa TT, Norman DC. Fever in the elderly. Infect Med 1998;15:704.

RISK FACTORS AND PATHOPHYSIOLOGY

Urine is normally sterile. However, when a potentially disease-producing organism is isolated from the urine, the term *uropathogen* is used. The vast majority of non-catheter-associated UTIs are caused by a single uropathogen, primarily enteric Gram-negative bacilli. The most common uropathogen is *Escherichia coli*, followed by *Klebsiella* and *Proteus*. *Serratia, Enterobacter, Enterococcus,* and *Pseudomonas aeruginosa* are common isolates in patients with indwelling urethral catheters or in patients receiving broad-spectrum antibiotics for other infections. Organisms such as *lactobacilli, alpha-hemolytic Streptococcus,* or anaerobes do not grow well in urine and are usually considered nonpathologic contaminants when isolated in urine.

Certain age-related factors place older adults at greater risk for UTI. Functional status and physical impairments, as well as genitourinary manipulation, anatomy, and function, predict how likely bacteriuria and UTI are to develop. In the nursing home population, risk factors for the development of UTI have been shown to be prior cerebrovascular accident, decreased functional status, decreased mental status, bladder instrumentation, and prior antibiotic treatment.[4] Other factors that predispose older adults to UTIs include use of urethral or condom catheters and neurogenic bladders with increased residual urine.

A number of anatomic and functional changes occur to the lower urinary tract with aging. In women, one of the most important age-related changes is the postmenopausal decline in estrogen leading to atrophy of supporting tissue, urethral weakness, and an increase in vaginal pH. These changes may increase susceptibility to UTI with a marked reduction in endogenous estrogen production. The vaginal epithelium becomes atrophied and dry and may become inflamed, contributing to symptoms of frequency, urgency, dysuria, and incon-

tinence. In men, prostatic hypertrophy can lead to large postvoid residuals and greater opportunities for bacteriuria and UTI. Other age-related changes include changes in concentrations of certain neurotransmitters, which may lead to disorders in micturition. Alterations in immune function may affect susceptibility to infection. Immobility, medications that affect bladder emptying such as anticholinergics, and poor perineal hygiene all may predispose the elderly patient to developing a UTI.

> ● Symptomatic and asymptomatic UTIs are more prevalent in older adults than in younger people.

DIFFERENTIAL DIAGNOSIS, ASSESSMENT, AND MANAGEMENT

Asymptomatic Bacteriuria

The clinical significance of asymptomatic bacteriuria in the elderly is unclear. Asymptomatic bacteriuria is characterized by greater than 10^5 colony-forming units/ml without dysuria, frequency, incontinence, pain, fever, or other signs of infection. Small numbers of white blood cells in the urine are common. The vast majority of elderly patients with bacteriuria are asymptomatic, and when questioned about symptoms of incontinence, frequency, or urgency, no significant differences have been found between bacteriuric and nonbacteriuric patients. The majority of data indicate that asymptomatic bacteriuria in the elderly does not lead to renal damage.[2] Bacteriuria clears spontaneously or occurs intermittently in the majority of patients. Organisms in the urethra or vagina often contaminate cultures obtained from clean-voided specimens. Therefore, repeat culture after 1 week is often performed to confirm the diagnosis. If the same organism grows in the second culture, asymptomatic bacteriuria can be presumed to be present.[5]

● Asymptomatic bacteriuria is not associated with increased morbidity or mortality in older adults, and there is no benefit from treatment attempts to eradicate asymptomatic bacteriuria.

Asymptomatic bacteriuria in the elderly is a benign condition that does not require treatment. Treatment reduces neither morbidity nor mortality but may increase the likelihood of drug-resistant microorganisms and adverse reactions to antibiotics. Exceptions to this principle are patients who are scheduled for a genitourinary procedure or who have obstructive uropathy, infectious stones, or a history of recurrent symptomatic infections.

Michael Thomas, *Part 1*

Mr. Michael Thomas is a 75-year-old man who comes to your office complaining of a 3-day history of painful urination, increased frequency, urgency, and incontinence. He has had no other symptoms, including no costovertebral angle tenderness. On examination, his temperature is 99.2°F (his usual temperature is 97.1°F). His blood pressure is 150/80 mm Hg, and his pulse is 78 and regular. He has 2+ prostatic enlargement on digital rectal examination. No other abnormalities are identified on physical examination.

STUDY QUESTIONS

1. What is the likely diagnosis?
2. What, if any, antibiotic would you start?

● Older adults with a UTI may present without genitourinary symptoms and may only manifest cognitive or functional changes.

Urinary Tract Infections

When bacteriuria becomes symptomatic, UTI occurs. Classic symptoms include fever, dysuria, urinary frequency, nocturia, and urgency. Other symptoms suggestive of a urinary infection include recent onset or worsening of urinary incontinence, functional decline, anorexia, nausea, vomiting, or mental confusion. Although it is often difficult to noninvasively obtain a clean-catch urine specimen from incontinent, cognitively impaired men and women, it is possible. Carefully cleaning the perineum and having the patient void into a disinfected collection device or "hat" for women and using condom catheters for men usually suffice. When functional impairment inhibits the suitable collection of a urine

specimen, in-and-out catheterization should be used. Rapid tests may be useful in determination of bacteriuria. The most reliable rapid test is the nitrate test, in which the conversion of nitrate to nitrite by bacteria in the urine is demonstrated by color change on dipstick analysis. This test has a high positive likelihood ratio of 25 and specificity of 98 but does not demonstrate bacteriuria caused by *Pseudomonas*, *Staphylococcus*, or *Enterococcus*, which are incapable of metabolizing nitrate.

Symptomatic infections should be promptly treated after a Gram stain and after appropriate cultures of the urine are obtained. Clinically unstable patients or patients who appear severely ill should be hospitalized and treated with parenteral antibiotics. If patients are able to receive treatment in a nursing home but require parenteral antibiotics, second- and third-generation cephalosporins may be administered intramuscularly. Noncatheterized patients who are able to receive treatment with oral agents can be treated with trimethoprim-sulfamethoxazole, amoxicillin, amoxicillin-clavulanic acid, second-generation cephalosporins, or fluoroquinolones. Duration of antibiotic therapy is generally 10 to 14 days in the elderly; shorter treatment regimens of 3 to 5 days are not satisfactory in the elderly patient. In the elderly patient, it may be difficult to evaluate reinfection from relapse. When possible, an attempt to distinguish between the two is useful because relapse may require further evaluation. Relapse in elderly patients may result from incomplete bladder emptying caused by diabetes mellitus, uterine prolapse, or prostatic hypertrophy. Box 47-1 lists the major causes associated with relapse. Genitourinary evaluation should include determination of renal function, quantitation of postvoid residuals, ultrasound and urologic evaluation, and determination if obstructive uropathy or other genitourinary abnormalities are present.

● In older adults, *Escherichia coli* continues to be a common urinary tract pathogen, but other Gram-negative bacilli and Gram-positive cocci become important uropathogens.

Box 47-1 Major Causes Associated with Relapse

- Anatomic abnormalities
- Genitourinary calculi
- Pyelonephritis
- Renal abscess
- Perinephric abscess
- Chronic bacterial prostatitis

Maria Alicea: Case Discussion

Both symptomatic and asymptomatic urinary infections increase with aging. In older patients, Escherichia coli remains a common pathogen, but other organisms such as Gram-negative bacilli and Gram-positive cocci also become important uropathogens. Transient immunosuppression can increase an older persons susceptibility to fungal UTIs. Older adults with a UTI may present without genitourinary symptoms and may manifest only mental status or functional changes. There is little evidence that asymptomatic bacteriuria by itself leads to negative long-term outcomes, and studies have consistently shown no benefit from treatment of asymptomatic bacteriuria.

Michael Thomas, *Part 2*

Mr. Thomas returns to your office 2 days after being started on ampicillin for bacterial cystitis. He is now complaining of fever, chills, confusion, and diarrhea. On physical examination, his temperature is 101.2°F, his blood pressure is 90/60 mm Hg, and his pulse is 98 and regular. He has slight abdominal tenderness but no costovertebral angle tenderness.

STUDY QUESTIONS

1. What is the most likely diagnosis in Mr. Thomas?
2. What are the antibiotic choices should you consider now?

> ● In patients with acute, uncomplicated pyelonephritis in which a Gram-negative rod is the suspected pathogen, start treatment with a second- or third-generation cephalosporin or a quinolone antibiotic.

Complicated Urinary Tract Infection

Distinction between uncomplicated and complicated UTIs is important because of the implications regarding pretreatment and posttreatment evaluation, type and duration of antimicrobial regimens, and extent of evaluation of the urinary tract. General symptoms of UTIs include dysuria, frequency, urgency, and abdominal or flank pain. Older adults, however, may not exhibit these symptoms and frequently may present with only mental status changes, especially in the long-term care setting. Factors suggesting severe or potentially severe UTI are listed in Box 47-2.[6]

Complicated UTI refers to infections that fail to resolve or recur within 2 weeks after standard therapy. These UTIs are associated with bacteremia or sepsis and are associated with periurethral abscess, obstructions, and pyelonephritis. Complicated UTIs occur in patients with structurally or functionally abnormal urinary tracts and may involve antibiotic-resistant pathogens. Structural complications that precipitate complicated UTI include intrinsic abnormalities such as renal stones, prostatic hypertrophy, neurogenic bladder, or the presence of external devices such as indwelling urethral catheters. Patients with a complicated UTI should be evaluated for structural and functional abnormalities with an ultrasound or intravenous pyelogram and voiding cystourethrogram. Patients with impaired renal function can be evaluated with a radionuclide renal scan or an ultrasound. Elderly men should be evaluated for prostatic enlargement. The presence of infected stones is associated with urease-producing bacteria, most frequently, *Proteus* species. Treatment consists of stone removal and culture-specific antibiotics. Once the stone is removed, the urine should be kept sterile by continuous antibiotic therapy for 1 month.[7] Periurethral abscess is an uncommon but life-threatening infection of the male urethra and periurethral tissue. Periurethral abscess is usually associated with the presence of Foley catheters. Symptoms include fever, positive urinalysis, scrotal/labial or penile swelling, and erythema. Therapy requires combination intravenous antibiotics with a cephalosporin and aminoglycoside for 10 to 14 days.

> ### Box 47–2 Factors Suggesting Severe or Potentially Severe Urinary Tract Infection
>
> - Male sex
> - Age over 60
> - Sepsis
> - Febrile urinary tract infection
> - History of urinary tract infection more than 7 days
> - Symptoms or signs of obstruction
> - Gross hematuria
> - History of stones
> - Recent exposure to antimicrobials
> - Recent hospitalization
> - Recent urinary tract catheterization or instrumentation
> - Concurrent diabetes or immunosuppression
> - Infection with resistant organisms.

Classic symptoms of acute pyelonephritis include dysuria associated with fever, chills, and costovertebral angle tenderness. *E. coli* is a less common cause of acute pyelonephritis in the elderly but is still responsible for approximately 60% of cases.[7] In more than 20% of patients, the predominant symptoms are not genitourinary but gastrointestinal or pulmonary. One-third of older patients do not show the usual febrile response and have no leukocytosis,[6] requiring a high index of suspicion and early radiologic examination. Treatment usually requires intravenous antibiotics with fluoroquinolones, cephalosporins, or aminoglycosides. Studies of oral fluoroquinolones have shown results comparable to standard intravenous antibiotic regimens,[8] allowing for elderly patients to avoid acute-care hospitalization in some circumstances. However, if urosepsis is suspected in a community-living older adult, early aggressive treatment with broad-spectrum antibiotics and hospitalization is generally indicated.

Michael Thomas: Case Discussion

In patients with presumed urosepsis in whom a Gram-negative rod is the likely pathogen, the patient should be treated with a second- or third-generation cephalosporin or a quinolone antibiotic. Aminoglycosides are effective and inexpensive, but their potential toxicity can usually be avoided.

Catheter-Associated Bacteriuria

Most patients with short-term indwelling catheters will be residents of acute care institutions. Most long-term indwelling catheters are used in patients in a nursing home setting. When necessary, the use of clean intermittent catheterization is preferred over the use of long-term indwelling catheters. Condom catheters may also be appropriate for some men, especially because condom catheters are more comfortable and have a lower incidence of bacteriuria than are indwelling catheters.[9] Bacteriuria is an inevitable event in patients requiring indwelling catheters, with virtually every patient developing colonization within 1 month of catheter placement.[10] Indwelling urinary catheters are the leading cause of nosocomial UTIs and the most common predisposing factor in hospital-acquired, fatal, Gram-negative sepsis. Interventions such as topical meatal antimicrobials, disinfectants added to the urinary drainage bag, antimicrobial coatings for catheters, and antimicrobial irrigations have not been shown to decrease the incidence of infection. Additional complications of long-term catheterization

include nonbacterial urethritis, nephrolithiasis, cystolithiasis, chronic renal inflammation, chronic pyelonephritis, bacteremia, and death. Although the high incidence of bacteriuria exists with the use of indwelling catheters, antibiotic prophylaxis is not recommended.[11] Prophylaxis may be associated with the development of antibiotic-resistant microbes. Because asymptomatic bacteriuria does not require treatment, there is no role for periodic urine cultures in the chronically catheterized patient.

Catheterized residents who have active UTI will generally not have genitourinary symptoms. In these patients, fever, cognitive impairment, functional changes, changes in appetite, tachypnea, tachycardia, and hypotension are more likely to be the presenting symptoms. When the patient with an indwelling catheter does develop symptoms of a UTI, a common practice is to insert a new catheter for collecting a urine sample for identification of the organism, although data doe not exist to support this practice. Urinary infections in patients with indwelling catheters are often polymicrobial and may include organisms such as *Pseudomonas*, *Proteus*, *Klebsiella*, and *Enterococci*. Among short-term catheterized patients, *E. coli* remains the most frequent bacteriuric species isolated.[9] When a UTI is suspected, empiric antibiotics should be started. Once the particular pathogen is identified, the antibiotic should be adjusted. Yeast may be isolated particularly when antibiotics are in use.[10] The selection of empiric antibiotics should be based on knowledge of common organisms in the care unit because the majority of the bacteria-causing, catheter-associated bacteriuria are from the patient's own colonic flora, including those recently acquired from a hospital environment. Because of the possibility of polymicrobial infection, appropriate empiric treatment should include a parenteral or oral regimen that is effective against both Gram-negative bacilli and *Enterococci*. Seriously ill or septic patients require a two-drug combination such as ampicillin and a third-generation cephalosporin (e.g., fluoroquinolone, aztreonam, or an aminoglycoside). Duration of antibiotic therapy is generally 10 to 14 days.

Candiduria may develop in catheterized patients, and its incidence is directly related to duration of catheterization.[10] Removal of the catheter results in the disappearance of candiduria in one-third of patients.[10] Patients in whom candiduria persists or who are symptomatic can be treated with oral fluconazole. Only two catheter hygiene principles are universally recommended to prevent infections in chronically catheterized patients. One is to keep the catheter system closed. Urine specimens can be obtained by needle and syringe without opening the catheter-collection tube. The second principle is to remove the catheter as soon as medically possible.[10]

Prevention

Some situations require antibiotic prophylaxis to prevent UTIs. Premenopausal and postmenopausal women with frequent recurrent UTIs, patients about to undergo urologic or gynecologic procedures, patients with spinal cord injury, and men with chronic bacterial prostatitis may benefit from antibiotic prophylaxis.[12] Other behaviors that may affect the risk for UTIs have been less thoroughly investigated and include increased fluid intake, increased voiding, and micturition after intercourse.[12] In women, local treatment with topical estrogens significantly reduces the pH of the vagina, reduces colonization with Gram-negative bacilli, and decreases the incidence of UTIs. Some research suggests that ingestion of commercially available cranberry juice or vitamin C in moderate amounts may be useful in preventing UTIs, mostly through its effects on urinary pH.[13]

SUMMARY

Both symptomatic and asymptomatic urinary infections increase with aging. In older patients, *E. coli* still plays a major role, but other organisms such as Gram-negative bacilli and Gram-positive cocci become important uropathogens. Older adults may present without genitourinary symptoms and may manifest only mental status changes. Men may have obstructive complaints. There is little evidence that asymptomatic bacteriuria by itself leads to potentially negative long-term outcomes, and repeated studies have consistently shown no benefit from treatment of asymptomatic bacteriuria. In patients with presumed urosepsis in whom a Gram-negative rod is presumed, a second- or third-generation cephalosporin or a quinolone antibiotic should be started. Aminoglycosides are effective and inexpensive, but their potential toxicity can usually be avoided.

References

1. Barnett BJ, Stephens DS. Urinary tract infection: an overview. Am J Med Sci 1997;314:245-249.
2. Nicolle LE. Asymptomatic bacteriuria in the elderly. Infect Dis Clin North Am 1997;11:647-662.
3. Hedin K, Petersson C, Wideback K, Kahlmeter G, Molstad S. Asymptomatic bacteriuria in a populations of elderly in municipal institutional care. Scand J Prim Health Care 2002;20:166-168.
4. Wood CA, Abrutyn E. Urinary tract infection in older adults. Clin Geriatr Med 1998;14:267-283.
5. Zilkoski MW, Smucker DR, Mayhew HE. Urinary tract infections in elderly patients. Postgrad Med 1988;84:191-194, 197-198, 201-206.
6. Pewitt EB, Schaeffer AJ. Urinary tract infection in urology. Infect Dis Clin North Am 1997;11:623-646.
7. Roberts JA. Management of pyelonephritis and upper urinary tract infections. Urol Clin North Am 1999;26:753-763.
8. McCue JD. Rationale for the use of oral fluoroquinolones as empiric treatment of nursing home infections. Arch Fam Med 1994;3:157-163.
9. Warren JW. Catheter-associated bacteriuria. Clin Geriatr Med 1992;8:805-819.
10. Warren JW. Catheter-associated urinary tract infections. Clin Geriatr Med 1997;11:609-622.
11. Sanjay S, Lipsky B. Preventing catheter-related bacteriuria: should we? Can we? How? Arch Intern Med 1999;159:800-808.
12. Stapleton A, Stamm WE. Prevention of urinary tract infection. Infect Dis Clin North Am 1997;11:719-733.
13. Jepson RG, Mihaljevic L, Craig J. Cranberries for preventing urinary tract infections. Cochrane Database Syst Rev 2005;2:1-30.

POSTTEST

1. The most appropriate treatment for a patient with a UTI in the presence of a bladder stone is?
   a. A trial of antibiotics for 14 days and then repeat urine culture to test for cure
   b. Surgically remove the stone
   c. Lifelong treatment with antibiotics for bacterial suppression
   d. Place indwelling catheter and perform daily bladder irrigations

2. Which of the following is (are) true regarding *asymptomatic* bacteriuria in older adults?
   a. There are no differences in the prevalence of incontinence or frequency, compared to those without bacteriuria.
   b. Bacteriuria requires at least one course of antibiotics to be resolved.
   c. At least one course of antibiotics reduces mortality due to bacteriuria.
   d. Antibiotics decrease the likelihood of the development of resistant micro-organism.

3. Which of the following is (are) true regarding catheter-associated UTI?
   a. Chronic indwelling catheterization has a lower rate of UTIs than intermittent catheterization.
   b. Bacteriuria is rare in patients with in-dwelling catheters.
   c. UTIs in the presence of indwelling catheters require long-term antibiotic treatment.
   d. Complications of chronic indwelling catheters include nephrolithiasis.

PRETEST ANSWERS

1. c
2. d
3. a

POSTTEST ANSWERS

1. b
2. a
3. d

The Acute Abdomen

Marcia L. McGory and Clifford Y. Ko

OBJECTIVES

Upon completion of this chapter, the reader will be able to:

- Appreciate the special problems of the increasing numbers of older patients undergoing emergency abdominal surgery.

- Characterize the medical and surgical causes of acute abdominal pain in the older patient.

- Explain the approach to an older patient with acute abdominal pain including history and physical examination, laboratory tests, and radiographic imaging.

- Discuss the rationale for the management options for an older patient with acute abdominal pain, including emergent operation, serial abdominal exams, observation, and nonoperative management.

PRETEST

1. Diagnosis of acute abdominal pain in the older patient is challenging for all of the following reasons EXCEPT:
   a. presentation with vague or non-specific symptoms
   b. lack of systemic signs (e.g. fever)
   c. older patients can be poor historians
   d. acute abdominal pain is uncommon in the older patient
   e. presence of multiple comorbid medical conditions

2. An older patient with an acute abdomen is at increased risk (compared to a younger patient) for which of the following:
   a. mortality
   b. morbidity
   c. misdiagnosis
   d. undergoing emergency surgery
   e. all of the above

Tom Jones *(Part 1)*

Mr. Jones presents to your primary care office complaining of vague abdominal pain since last night, after going out to dinner with his wife. He has not felt like eating and has had several episodes of small volume bilious emesis. He had one episode of diarrhea yesterday and continues to pass flatus. He is afebrile with normal vital signs.

STUDY QUESTIONS

1. What elements of the physical examination are essential?
2. What tests should be ordered in your office?

PREVALENCE AND IMPACT

The definition of an acute abdomen is "signs and symptoms of acute intraabdominal pathology requiring treatment by surgical intervention."[1] However, it should be noted that not all episodes of acute abdominal pain require surgery but rather prompt diagnosis and treatment.[2] Acute abdominal pain is a common chief complaint for older patients seen in the emergency department (ED),[3] and this population consumes a disproportionate amount of time and resources in the ED in comparison to younger patients.[4] In addition, approximately 50% of older patients presenting to an ED with abdominal pain will require hospital admission, and 30% to 40% of these patients will eventually require surgical intervention.[5]

Not only does acute abdominal pain in the older population impact the ED, but the aging population has also been predicted to have a significant impact on the field of general surgery. The amount of procedure-based workload in general surgery is expected to increase 13% by 2010 and 31% by 2020.[6] The aging population will significantly impact not only the number of procedures performed on older patients but also the percentage of emergency operations, because the risk of emergency surgery increases with age.[7] Previous research demonstrates significant variability in the percentage of emergency operations in the older population, ranging from 14% in a cohort of patients greater than 80 years of age who had noncardiac surgery at Veterans Affairs hospitals,[8] 56% in a cohort of octogenarians undergoing major abdominal surgery,[9] and 69-72% in two cohorts of nonagenarians.[10,11]

RISK FACTORS AND PATHOPHYSIOLOGY

The work-up of acute abdominal pain in the older patient is challenging for the following reasons: (1) older patients may present with vague or nonspecific symptoms that are not suggestive of a specific pathophysiologic process; (2) older patients often lack the systemic (e.g., fever) or clinical signs (e.g., right lower quadrant tenderness) suggestive of acute intraabdominal pathology; (3) older patients are poor historians, or there is often difficulty obtaining an accurate history owing to memory loss or dementia; (4) older patients may delay seeking treatment or be dependent on others to be sent to a hospital for evaluation (e.g., nursing home residents); and (5) presence of comorbid disease may alter both the clinical presentation as well as the diagnostic evaluation.[4,12-15]

Misdiagnosis of acute abdominal pain is common in the older patient for all of these reasons, so it is important to maintain a high index of suspicion.[16] Previous research has suggested a higher mortality for older patients with abdominal pain where the diagnosis occurred after admission to the hospital (19%) versus those patients with a correct preliminary diagnosis in the ED (8%).[17] Kizer et al. demonstrated that the sensitivity/specificity of a provisional ED diagnosis was lower for patients greater than 65 (82%/86%). In contrast, there was no difference in mortality based on agreement between the provisional ED diagnosis and the hospital discharge diagnosis, although there was a significant increase in disease-related morbidity.[14]

Age itself is a risk factor for some causes of an acute abdomen. Not only does the incidence of peptic ulcer disease increase with age, but in a series of 136 patients treated surgically for bleeding or perforated peptic ulcer, 80% of the deaths occurred in patients greater than 70 years of age.[18] In addition, it is estimated that 30% to 50% of older patients have underlying cholelithiasis, and 50% to 80% have colonic diverticulosis. The incidence of abdominal aortic aneurysm also increases with age and is present in an estimated 5% of men over the age of 65.[5] Advanced age also contributes to mild immunosuppression, which may make the diagnosis of an acute abdomen more difficult in an older patient. The decline in immune competence impairs the ability of the older patient to increase neutrophil production in response to infection, which explains why older patients with acute intraabdominal pathology may present with a normal white blood cell count.[19] A retrospective review of octogenarians with an acute abdomen demonstrated that 30% presented with temperature less than 37.5°C and a normal white blood cell count.[20] Comorbid medical disease such as diabetes mellitus, malignancy, or end-stage renal disease may also increase the degree of immunosuppression in an older patient.[5]

> ● Misdiagnosis of acute abdominal pain is challenging in the older patient – maintain a high index of suspicion.

DIFFERENTIAL DIAGNOSIS AND ASSESSMENT

The potential causes of acute abdominal pain in the older patient are numerous. One approach to classification of abdominal pain consists of determining which of the following four categories the cause of the pain falls into: (1) peritonitis, (2) bowel obstruction, (3) vascular catastrophe, or (4) nonspecific abdominal pain.[21] The differential diagnosis for both surgical and medical causes of acute abdominal pain in an older patient is shown in Table 48-1.

Several retrospective reviews have categorized the most common reasons for emergency abdominal surgery in the older patient. Arenal et al. performed a retrospective and prospective review of factors affecting mortality after emergency abdominal surgery in the older patient. The most common reasons for emergent exploration were intestinal obstruction (41%), peritonitis (29%), other etiology (21%), gastrointestinal (GI) bleeding (5%), and vascular mesenteric disorder (4%).[22] Zerbib et al. performed a retrospective review of 45 patients greater than 85 years of age who underwent emergency abdominal surgery. The most common causes of an acute abdomen were peritonitis secondary to cholecystitis or appendicitis (31%), small-bowel obstruction (SBO) (13%), mesenteric ischemia (13%), perforation secondary to diverticulitis or duodenal ulcer (13%), large-bowel obstruction secondary to sigmoid volvulus or obstructing colon cancer (11%), and other etiology.[23] Potts et al. performed a retrospective review of surgical abdomens in patients 80 years and older. The three most common diagnoses were acute cholecystitis (25%), hernia (21%), and bowel obstruction (16%).[20]

> ● In general, there are 4 main categories of a surgical acute abdomen: (1) peritonitis, (2) perforated viscus, (3) bowel obstruction, and (4) vascular

Tom Jones (Part 2)

The abdominal exam demonstrates no active bowel sounds, mild distension, and mild tenderness to palpation throughout the abdomen. The rectal examination reveals no impaction or tenderness, but the stool is heme positive. He is an 86-year-old man with a past medical history of chronic obstructive pulmonary disease (COPD) on home oxygen, coronary artery bypass graft for coronary artery disease, end-stage renal disease, and radical prostatectomy for prostate cancer. He was recently hospitalized for an exacerbation of COPD. During this hospitalization, he was started on hemodialysis; he was also discharged home on a steroid taper for the COPD.

Table 48–1	Differential Diagnosis of Acute Abdomen in the older patient

Surgical Causes of Acute Abdomen	Medical Causes of Acute Abdominal Pain
Peritonitis	**Cardiac**
Appendicitis	Myocardial infarction
Cholecystitis	**Pulmonary**
Diverticulitis	Empyema, pulmonary embolus
Perforated viscus	Pneumonia, pulmonary infarction
Diverticulitis	**Gastrointestinal**
Duodenal or gastric ulcer	Constipation, gastroenteritis, GERD, IBD
Large-bowel obstruction with perforation	Malignancy, peptic ulcer disease
Bowel obstruction	**Hepatobiliary**
Large—incarcerated hernia, malignancy, volvulus (cecal or sigmoid)	Ascending cholangitis
Small—adhesions, incarcerated hernia	Choledocholithiasis
	Cholelithiasis
Vascular	Other causes of acute pancreatitis
Aortic dissection	
Gastrointestinal hemorrhage	**Endocrine**
Mesenteric ischemia/infarction	Diabetic ketoacidosis
Ruptured or symptomatic AAA	**Genitourinary**
Other	Adnexal mass, cystitis
Gallstone pancreatitis	Pyelonephritis, renal calculi
	Other gynecologic pathology

GERD indicates gastroesophageal reflux disease; IBD, inflammatory bowel disease (e.g., Ulcerative colitis, Crohn's); and AAA, abdominal aortic aneurysm.

History and Physical Examination

Critical elements of the history and physical examination when evaluating an older patient with acute abdominal pain are outlined in Table 48-2. Careful attention must be paid to a thorough history and physical examination because the presentation of an older patient with an acute abdomen may be quite varied, ranging from mild abdominal pain to a change in mental status.[5] One distinction between medical and surgical causes of abdominal pain may be the temporal relation between the onset of pain and vomiting. Abdominal pain requiring an operation often precedes vomiting (e.g., acute appendicitis), whereas vomiting often precedes the abdominal pain secondary to a medical condition (e.g., gastroenteritis).[1]

Laboratory Testing

The initial diagnostic work-up of an older patient for an acute abdomen should include standard laboratory tests such as complete blood count with differential, electrolytes, and renal function. Liver function tests, as well as amylase and lipase, should be sent if the differential diagnosis includes hepatobiliary pathology or pancreatitis. A urinalysis and urine culture should be sent if the history and physical examination suggests a urologic cause (e.g., nephrolithiasis, pyelonephritis). Blood cultures may be useful when abdominal pain is associated with fever or there is a high index of suspicion for sepsis. Coagulation tests should be sent for any patient taking warfarin, as well as those with GI hemorrhage or known severe liver disease. Type and crossmatch should be sent for any patient with a

Table 48–2	Performing a History and Physical Examination in an Older Patient with Acute Abdominal Pain
Patient History	
Pain	Time of onset, location, radiation, quality, severity, palliating and provoking factors
GI function	Anorexia, nausea, vomiting, bowel habits, characterization of emesis (e.g., bilious, bloody) and stool (e.g., diarrhea versus constipation, presence of blood, melena), and last time the patient ate, passed flatus, or had a bowel movement
Associated symptoms	Generalized symptoms, including fever, chills, and fatigue, as well as organ-specific symptoms (e.g., chest pain, shortness of breath, cough with productive sputum, dysuria, hematuria)
Other medical problems	May elicit clues to the etiology of abdominal pain, especially prior history of diabetes and cardiac, pulmonary, or gastrointestinal disease
Surgical history	Ask about all previous operations (especially abdominal procedures)
Current medications	Ask about all current medications, especially NSAIDs (known association with gastrointestinal hemorrhage), warfarin (increased risk for bleeding or thrombotic/embolic event), steroids (immunosuppression), and beta-blockers (may blunt tachycardia).
Physical examination	
Vital signs	Monitor for tachycardia, hypotension; older patients are often normo- or hypothermic
Abdomen	*Inspect* for prior abdominal scars; *auscultate* for absence (e.g., ileus) or presence of bowel sounds (e.g., high pitched may be associated with bowel obstruction); *percuss* for presence of tympany (bowel obstruction) or pain (peritonitis); *palpate* for presence of mass (e.g., phlegmon, malignancy, abdominal aortic aneurysm if pulsatile); and *evaluate* for hernia in umbilicus, groin, and prior abdominal incisions
Rectal	Always do rectal to evaluate for tenderness, impaction, rectal mass, and presence of gross or occult fecal blood
Genitourinary	Assess for costovertebral angle tenderness; evaluate testicles/scrotum for presence of hernia; or do pelvic exam to assess for ovarian/uterine pathology

GI indicates gastrointestinal; NSAIDs, nonsteroidal anti-inflammatory drugs (e.g., ibuprofen, piroxicam).

source of active bleeding or a high likelihood of undergoing operative intervention with significant blood loss. Arterial blood gas or serum lactate may be useful when considering the diagnosis of mesenteric or bowel ischemia.

Radiographic Imaging

Radiographic imaging often provides useful information regarding the etiology of the acute abdominal pain. A chest X-ray could demonstrate pulmonary pathology as the source of the abdominal pain. Free air under the diaphragm is diagnostic for a perforated viscus, and will require an emergency exploratory laparotomy. An upright abdominal X-ray may demonstrate dilated loops of small or large intestine and/or air fluid levels, which could confirm small- or large-bowel obstruction. Other diagnostic findings on plain films include abnormal calcifications (e.g., 10% of gallstones, 90% of kidney stones, and 5% of appendicoliths are radio-opaque) and gas in the portal venous system (pneumobilia) or wall of the GI tract (pneumatosis intestinalis).[1]

Alternative radiographic images include ultrasound (US) and computed tomography (CT). Abdominal US can often be performed at the bedside and provides

information on the presence or absence of gallstones, abdominal aortic aneurysm, and hydronephrosis. A common radiologic investigation for an older patient complaining of abdominal pain in the ED is CT (90% of attending physicians in emergency medicine at a single residency program responded that it was their standard practice to order an abdominal CT scan for an older patient complaining of abdominal pain[24]). A prospective, observational, multicenter study assessed the use of abdominal CT in older ED patients with acute abdominal pain. Thirty-seven percent of older patients with acute abdominal pain were evaluated with abdominal CT scan, and of the patients receiving CT scans, 57% were diagnostic for the etiology of the pain, 31% had nonspecific findings, and 12% were read by a radiologist as normal. The diagnostic ability of CT was significantly higher for patients requiring urgent surgical intervention at 85% (versus 71% for patients requiring acute medical intervention and 34% for patients requiring no acute intervention). The most common diagnostic CT findings were SBO or ileus (18%), diverticulitis (18%), urolithiasis (10%), cholelithiasis or cholecystitis (10%), abdominal mass/neoplasm (8%), pyelonephritis (7%), and pancreatitis (6%).[13] Similarly, a prospective observational cohort study evaluated the ability of CT to change decision making in older patients presenting to the ED with acute abdominal pain. Abdominal CT altered the decision for admission in 26%, altered the decision for surgery in 12%, and altered the suspected diagnosis in 45% of cases.[24]

> ● Radiographic imaging options for work-up of an acute abdomen include chest X-ray, abdominal series, ultrasound, and computed tomography.

Tom Jones *(Part 3)*

Chest X-ray shows no evidence of pneumonia or free air, but there are several loops of dilated small bowel beneath the left hemidiaphragm. Laboratories are significant for a normal white blood cell count, hematocrit of 54%, and grossly abnormal electrolytes: sodium of 127 mmol/L, potassium of 6.5 mmol/L, chloride of 87 mmol/L, bicarbonate of 40, BUN of 85 mmol/L, and creatinine of 5.5 mg/dl. While you are discussing these results with the patient, he has an episode of large volume coffee-ground emesis. You repeat the vital signs: his pulse is now 120 with blood pressure of 70/40 mm Hg.

STUDY QUESTIONS

1. What are some potential causes of acute abdominal pain in this patient?
2. What is the most appropriate next step in this patient's management?

MANAGEMENT

Management of the older patient with an acute abdomen who appears seriously ill should initially follow the ABCs. First, the patient's *airway* and *breathing* should be assessed. If there is any concern about the adequacy of the airway or the ability of the patient to maintain oxygenation and ventilation, then the patient should be intubated. *Circulation* should be evaluated, including blood pressure, presence of active bleeding, and intravenous access. If peripheral intravenous access cannot easily be obtained, then a central line should be placed for fluid resuscitation with normal saline or lactated Ringer's. A surgical consultation should be obtained immediately for patients with a suspected diagnosis of ruptured abdominal aortic aneurysm, or mesenteric ischemia, or for the presence of free air on plain X-rays. In addition, if the diagnosis remains unclear after initial laboratories and X-rays, surgical consultation should be obtained.[5]

Tom Jones *(Part 4)*

The findings on X-ray suggest a SBO, which is likely complicated by GI hemorrhage (the coffee-ground emesis). Fluid resuscitation is initiated in your office, while awaiting transfer of the patient to the ED at the local hospital. On arrival he continues to have large volumes of coffee-ground emesis; the pulse is 110 with a systolic blood pressure of 90 mm Hg. A liter of normal saline is administered as a fluid bolus; nasogastric tube placement yields an additional 1500 ml of coffee-ground material.

STUDY QUESTION

1. What other specialties should be consulted in the care of this patient?

Preparing For Potential Surgery

All older patients with acute abdominal pain should be maintained on nothing by mouth until a decision is reached regarding (1) the need for urgent surgery, and (2) whether the probable etiology of the acute abdominal pain is medical or surgical. A nasogastric tube should be considered if there is a large volume of emesis and/or a diagnosis of bowel obstruction. A Foley catheter should be considered to monitor urine output, especially if a significant amount of volume resuscitation is required. Broad-spectrum antibiotics should be administered if there is evidence of peritonitis or perforation. Blood should be sent for type and screen/cross-match if blood transfusion *or* surgical intervention is anticipated.

Patient-Clinician Discussions

Postoperative complications for older patients undergoing emergency abdominal surgery are significant, with estimated rates of 30% to 68% morbidity and 5% to 31% mortality.[7,9-11,22,23,25] Given the known risks of perioperative morbidity and mortality in the older patient requiring emergency abdominal surgery, the surgeon should discuss the role of surgery with the patient and/or family members, the likelihood of complications and/or death, and the patient's preferences regarding cardiopulmonary resuscitation (CPR) and other life-sustaining measures. Before surgery, attempts must be made to discuss the patient's advance directive for medical decision making and to identify the surrogate decision maker. Previous research has demonstrated that clinicians often underestimate a patient's desire to withhold CPR.[26] The decision to withhold life-sustaining treatments increases with each decade of age by 19% for surgery, 15% for ventilator support, and 12% for dialysis.[27] Patient decisions to pursue aggressive treatments (such as surgery) are also influenced by the likely outcomes. For example, if the outcome was survival, but with severe functional or cognitive impairment, 74.4% and 88.8%, respectively, of participants would not choose to undergo treatment.[28] It is beneficial to quickly assess the patient's baseline functional status before surgery. A prospective cohort study demonstrated that seriously ill patients are more accurate in their estimates of future physical functioning than are either family members or physicians.[29] Also, a prognostic model for prediction of future functional status identified functional status 2 weeks before hospitalization as the single most important predictor of serious functional decline after hospitalization.[30]

> ● Physicians should document patient preferences regarding CPR and life-sustaining treatments *before* the patient undergoes surgery.

Tom Jones *(Part 5)*

A surgical consultation is obtained; a repeat abdominal series demonstrates severely dilated loops of small bowel with no air in the colon. Abdominal examiantion reveals tympany, and diffuse tenderness to percussion with guarding in the left lower quadrant. Given the presence of an upper GI bleed in addition to a likely complete SBO, the surgeon recommends aggressive fluid resuscitation, type and cross-match blood, and GI evaluation for upper endoscopy. A nephrology consultation for hemodialysis is needed, given the electrolyte abnormalities (especially the potassium of 6.5 mEq/dl) and the large volume of fluid resuscitation that will be needed (based on the patient's tachycardia, hypotension, and hemoconcentration; i.e., hematocrit of 54%). The patient's hemodynamic status and electrolytes are optimized, in anticipation of surgery. Upper endoscopy demonstrates a duodenal ulcer, which is not actively bleeding. A CT scan of the abdomen and pelvis obtained on hospital day 1 shows no passage of contrast into the large bowel. The patient is taken to the operating room for exploratory laparotomy and undergoes lysis of adhesions that have caused complete SBO: multiple adhesions are identified in the pelvis, related to the prior prostatectomy.

Nonoperative Management

If the patient does not require urgent operative intervention and a definitive diagnosis has not been reached, *observation* of the patient with serial abdominal examinations should be considered. Severe abdominal pain that lasts more than 6 hours increases the likelihood of surgical disease, whereas abdominal pain that improves with time decreases the probability of needing surgery.[1] Repeat laboratory tests and X-rays should be ordered for the following day to assess for changes in white blood cell count, degree of bowel obstruction, etc. Nonoperative management plays an important role in, for example, the conservative management of SBO, percutaneous drainage of an abscess from perforated appendicitis or diverticulitis, or colonic decompression of sigmoid volvulus.

> ● Not all patients with acute abdominal pain require emergency surgery; observation with serial abdominal examinations can play a role in nonoperative management.

SUMMARY

The population is aging, and increasing numbers of older patients are undergoing surgery. The risk for emergency abdominal surgery increases with age; some of the most common causes of acute abdomen in the older patient are cholecystitis and bowel obstruction. Diagnosis of an acute abdomen can be difficult, because older patients are less likely to present with fever, leukocytosis, severe abdominal pain, or other classic signs and symptoms of acute abdominal pathology. The approach to an older patient with acute abdominal pain should be methodical and include a thorough history and physical examination, laboratory data, and X-rays if indicated. Surgical consultation should always be obtained if the diagnosis is unclear. Stabilization should be attempted before surgery. The management options for an older patient with acute abdominal pain are varied and include urgent operation, observation with serial abdominal examinations, and nonoperative management. The patient's wishes regarding CPR and other life-sustaining interventions should be established early in the course of the illness. The risks and potential outcomes of surgical intervention must also be explained to the patient or surrogate.

References

1. Jones RS, Claridge JA. Acute abdomen. In Sabiston Textbook of Surgery (Townsend CM, ed.). London: Elsevier, 2004. http://www.intl.elsevier-health.com/e-books/pdf/903.pdf.
2. Silen W. Cope's early diagnosis of the acute abdomen, 20 ed. New York: Oxford University Press, 2000.
3. Ciccone A, Allegra JR, Cochrane DG, et al. Age-related differences in diagnoses within the elderly population. Am J Emerg Med 1998;16:43-48.
4. Caesar, R. Acute geriatric abdomen. In The textbook of primary and acute care medicine, part vi: gastrointestinal disease (Bosker G, ed.). Thomson American Health Consultants, 2004.
5. Bryan ED. Abdominal pain in elderly persons. www.emedicine.com. Accessed 3/21/06.
6. Etzioni DA, Liu JH, Maggard MA, et al. The aging population and its impact on the surgery workforce. Ann Surg 2003;238:170-177.
7. Pofahl WE, Pories WJ. Current status and future directions of geriatric general surgery. J Am Geriatr Soc 2003;51:S351-S354.
8. Hamel MB, Henderson WG, Khuri SF, et al. Surgical outcomes for patients aged 80 and older: morbidity and mortality from major noncardiac surgery. J Am Geriatr Soc 2005 53:424-429.
9. Abbas S, Booth M. Major abdominal surgery in octogenarians. N Z Med J 2003;116:U402
10. Rigberg D, Cole M, Hiyama D, et al. Surgery in the nineties. Am Surg 2000;66:813-816.
11. Blansfield JA, Clark SC, Hofmann MT, et al. Alimentary tract surgery in the nonagenarian: elective vs. emergent operations. J Gastrointest Surg 2004;8:539-542.
12. van Geloven AA, Biesheuvel TH, Luitse JS, et al. Hospital admissions of patients aged over 80 with acute abdominal complaints. Eur J Surg 2000;166:866-871.
13. Hustey FM, Meldon SW, Banet GA, et al. The use of abdominal computed tomography in older ED patients with acute abdominal pain. Am J Emerg Med 2005;23:259-265.
14. Kizer KW, Vassar MJ. Emergency department diagnosis of abdominal disorders in the elderly. Am J Emerg Med 1998;16:357-362.
15. Podnos YD, Jimenez JC, Wilson SE. Intra-abdominal sepsis in elderly persons. Clin Infect Dis 2002;35:62-68.
16. Kamin RA, Nowicki TA, Courtney DS, et al. Pearls and pitfalls in the emergency department evaluation of abdominal pain. Emerg Med Clin North Am 2003;21:61-72, vi.
17. Fenyo G. Acute abdominal disease in the elderly: experience from two series in Stockholm. Am J Surg 1982;143:751-754.
18. Bulut OB, Rasmussen C, Fischer A. Acute surgical treatment of complicated peptic ulcers with special reference to the elderly. World J Surg 1996;20:574-577.
19. Rosenthal, RA and Zenilman, ME. Surgery in the elderly. In Sabiston Textbook of Surgery (Townsend CM, ed.). London: Elsevier, 2004. http://www.textbookofsurgery.com
20. Potts FE 4th, Vukov LF. Utility of fever and leukocytosis in acute surgical abdomens in octogenarians and beyond. J Gerontol A Biol Sci Med Sci 1999;54:M55-M58.
21. Dang C, Aguilera P, Dang A, et al. Acute abdominal pain: four classifications can guide assessment and management. Geriatrics 2002;57:30-32, 35-36, 41-42.
22. Arenal JJ, Bengoechea-Beeby M. Mortality associated with emergency abdominal surgery in the elderly. Can J Surg 2003;46:111-116.
23. Zerbib P, Kulick JF, Lebuffe G, et al. Emergency major abdominal surgery in patients over 85 years of age. World J Surg 2005;29:820-825.
24. Esses D, Birnbaum A, Bijur P, et al. Ability of CT to alter decision making in elderly patients with acute abdominal pain. Am J Emerg Med 2004;22:270-272.
25. Marco CA, Schoenfeld CN, Keyl PM, et al. Abdominal pain in geriatric emergency patients: variables associated with adverse outcomes. Acad Emerg Med 1998;5:1163-1168.
26. Wenger NS, Phillips RS, Teno JM, et al. Physician understanding of patient resuscitation preferences: insights and clinical implications. J Am Geriatr Soc 2000;48:S44-S451.
27. Hamel MB, Teno JM, Goldman L, et al. Patient age and decisions to withhold life-sustaining treatments from seriously ill, hospitalized adults. SUPPORT Investigators. Study to Understand Prognoses and Preferences for Outcomes and Risks of Treatment. Ann Intern Med 1999;130:116-125.
28. Fried TR, Bradley EH, Towle VR, et al. Understanding the treatment preferences of seriously ill patients. N Engl J Med 2002;346:1061-1066.
29. Wu AW, Young Y, Dawson NV, et al. Estimates of future physical functioning by seriously ill hospitalized patients, their families, and their physicians. J Am Geriatr Soc 2002;50:230-237.
30. Wu AW, Damiano AM, Lynn J, et al. Predicting future functional status for seriously ill hospitalized adults. The SUPPORT prognostic model. Ann Intern Med 1995;122:342-350.

Web References

1. Bryan ED. Abdominal pain in elderly persons. www.emedicine.com. Accessed 3/21/06.
2. Jones RS, Claridge JA. Acute abdomen. In Sabiston Textbook of Surgery (Townsend CM, ed.). London: Elsevier, 2004. http://www.intl.elsevierhealth.com/e-books/pdf/903.pdf.

POSTTEST

1. All of the following are common causes of an acute abdomen in the older patient *except:*
   a. Acute cholecystitis
   b. Small-bowel obstruction
   c. Splenic infarction
   d. Perforated ulcer
   e. Appendicitis

2. The older patient with appendicitis will most likely present with which of the following:
   a. Vague or nonspecific abdominal pain
   b. Leukocytosis
   c. Fever
   d. Epigastric pain migrating to the right lower quadrant
   e. Emesis

3. The most basic work-up for an older patient with acute abdominal pain should include all of the following *except:*
   a. History and physical examination
   b. Complete blood count
   c. Electrolytes
   d. Chest X-ray
   e. CT of abdomen/pelvis

4. Immediate surgical consultation for an older patient should be obtained for all of the following *except:*
   a. Hypotension with a pulsatile abdominal mass
   b. Free air on chest X-ray
   c. Acute abdominal pain with hypotension or acidosis
   d. Nonspecific abdominal pain
   e. All of the above

5. Which one of the following items should be considered if you are preparing a patient for the operating room?
   a. Type and screen or type and cross
   b. Preoperative antibiotics
   c. Intravenous access with fluid resuscitation
   d. Nasogastric tube or Foley catheter
   e. All of the above

6. All of the following can be initially managed non-operatively *except:*
   a. Perforated diverticulitis with abscess
   b. Large-bowel obstruction with perforation
   c. Small-bowel obstruction
   d. Perforated appendicitis with abscess
   e. Sigmoid volvulus

PRETEST ANSWERS

1. d
2. e

POSTTEST ANSWERS

1. c
2. a
3. e
4. d
5. e
6. b

OBJECTIVES

Upon completion of this chapter, the reader will be able to:

- Describe the clinical anatomy, changes owing to aging, and function of the prostate.

- Know how to diagnose benign prostatic hyperplasia (BPH).

- Outline the treatment options for BPH.

- Implement recommendations for prostate cancer screening.

- Understand how to diagnose and treat prostatitis.

PRETEST

1. A 58-year-old African American (AA) male complains of nocturia (four to five times/night), hesitancy and incomplete emptying of the bladder. After taking a history and performing a physical examination including a digital rectal examination (DRE), you determine that he has lower urinary tract symptoms (LUTS) with an initial clinical diagnosis of benign prostatic hypertrophy. As per the 2003 American Urologic Association (AUA) practice guideline, which one of the following is *not* recommended as part of the initial evaluation?
   a. AUA symptom checklist for benign prostatic hyperplasia (BPH)
   b. Perform urine examination with a dipstick
   c. Obtain a serum creatinine
   d. Obtain a prostatic-specific antigen (PSA) test

2. A 75-year-old white man with a history of coronary artery disease, myocardial infarction, and severe congestive heart failure (New York Heart Association stage IV) comes in with inability to urinate for 14 hours. Which step is usually not recommended in this situation?
   a. Post void residual volume
   b. A urine dip-stick test
   c. DRE
   d. PSA test

3. You and your patient make a shared decision that trans urethral resection of the prostate (TURP) will be the best option to improve his LUTS and prevent further episodes of urinary retention. You educate the patient that the complications associated with all minimally invasive therapies for BPH are similar but a unique complication can occur post-TURP. This complication of TURP is:
   a. Postintervention urinary retention
   b. Irritative voiding symptoms for several weeks after intervention
   c. Postintervention hyponatremia
   d. Postintervention retrograde ejaculation

4. A weak test characteristic of PSA that limits its usefulness for prostate cancer screening is:
   a. Low sensitivity
   b. Low specificity
   c. High positive predictive value
   d. Low negative predictive value

This chapter reviews the natural history of benign prostatic hyperplasia (BPH), the impact of urinary flow obstruction on the bladder, the diagnostic algorithms for detecting BPH, and different treatment modalities, including surgical, nonsurgical, and complementary and alternative medicine (CAM). This chapter also provides updates on prostate cancer prevention and screening. Finally, the chapter discusses the diagnosis and management of the prostatitis syndromes.

John Baker, *Part 1*

Mr. John Baker is an AA male 68-year-old patient who comes to your office today complaining of per-sistent lower urinary tract symptoms (LUTS). He reports increased urinary frequency, hesitancy, sensation of incomplete voiding, a weak stream, and the need to strain. On physical examination, his prostate volume is around 40 ml, a prostatic-specific antigen (PSA) level is 1.9 ng/ml, and the American Urologic Association (AUA) score is 9. You explain that he has LUTS likely due to benign prostatic hypertrophy and that this may progress to cause urinary retention. He wants your opinion on what he should do to relieve his symptoms and prevent progression.

Adrian Sellers, *Part 1*

Mr. Adrian Sellers is a 75-year-old white man who is in moderately good health and independent in his activities of daily living. He has hypertension, dyslipidemia, coronary artery disease (a stent was placed 2 years ago), BPH, and osteoarthritis of knee. He is back in your office to follow-up on his recent annual physical examination. During this examination, you identified an increasing PSA level. Last year the level was 3.7 ng/ml, and this time it is 9 ng/l. His digital rectal examination (DRE) revealed a smooth prostate, and no hard nodule was found. His DRE was also normal last year.

You explain that you suspect prostate cancer and want to go through a shared decision process before taking the next step. Mr. Sellers understands the pros and cons of further tests and the treatment options. He agrees to proceed with the evaluation and possible intervention.

Juan Martinez, *Part 1*

Mr. Juan Martinez, a 58-year-old Hispanic man comes to your office with the complaint of increased urinary frequency and urgency for the past 2 days. He denies any chills or fever. He does not have any back pain. He denies any discharges or blood in the urine. He recently had sex with a new partner and denies having a previous history of sexually transmitted disease. His symptoms were mild initially, but over the past week, it has affected the quality of his life.

A physical examination including a DRE was performed after two tubes of were obtained, the first sample consists of the initial 5 to 10 ml of urine and second sample is a mid-stream sample. His DRE findings showed a slightly enlarged, nontender prostate (40 ml), and no nodules are felt. There is no costovertebral pain on percussion. The urine dipstick shows a positive leukocyte esterase but has a negative nitrite and no red blood cells. A clinical diagnosis of urinary tract infection (UTI) is made. Your differential diagnosis also includes Chlamydia infection so you send a DNA probe for Chlamydia along with the urine microscopic examination and culture. He is prescribed ciprofloxin, and you advise him to come back in 48 hours to go over the test results.

STUDY QUESTIONS

1. What would you recommend Mr. Baker to relieve his symptoms?
2. What would you do next to evaluate Mr. Sellers' increasing PSA levels?
3. List the underlying causes of Mr. Martinez's UTI.

● Benign prostatic hyperplasia is the major cause of lower urinary tract symptoms (LUTS) among older men.

PREVALENCE AND IMPACT

Prostate related diseases usually increase with age. Almost all patients with prostate-related disease eventually suffer from LUTS. In the U.S. general population, prevalence of LUTS gradually increases from 40 through 70 years of age. After 70 years of age, the prevalence of LUTS increases sharply. Among persons 40 years of age, 3% report nocturia three or more times, 6% report incomplete emptying, and 2% report hesitancy. In comparison, persons over 70 years of age report nocturia three or more times 21% of the time, incomplete emptying 23% of the time, and hesitancy 14% of the time.[1]

BPH is the major cause of LUTS. Other common prostatic diseases associated with LUTS include prostate cancer and prostatitis. Primary care physicians treat 49% of cases of BPH, a significant transition of care for BPH from urologists to the family medicine physicians and internists over the past decade.[2]

The incidence of BPH increases with age, whereas the prevalence increases as the proportion of the population in the older age groups increases. The exact prevalence of BPH is difficult to obtain owing to lack of consensus on the definition and lack of homogenous studies. The histopathological changes of BPH are rarely seen before age 40 years[3]; however by age 60 years, 50% of men will have histological changes of BPH, and by age 90 years 90% of men will show changes of BPH.[4]

● The widespread use of PSA testing has led to an increase in the detection of prostate cancer in patients who are asymptomatic and younger than 65 years of age.

Prostate cancer is the second leading cause of cancer deaths and is expected to cause 30,350 deaths in 2005. In the United States, lifetime risk of prostate cancer is 16% and the risk of dying from prostate cancer is 3%.[5] In 2005 an estimated 232,090 new cases of prostate cancer are expected in the United States. Risk factors for prostate cancer include age, ethnicity, and family history. Seventy percent of all prostate cancers occur in men 65 years of age and older. The highest rates of prostate cancer occur in black men. Hereditary factors account for about 5% to 10% of cases. The wide-spread use of PSA testing has led to an increase in the detection of prostate cancer in patients who are asymptomatic and younger than 65 years of age.[6] The American College of Surgeons National Cancer Database includes 54,000 registered prostate cancer patients. At the time of diagnosis, 70% had no symptoms and 98% had PSA level (greater than 4 ng/ml), independent of DRE results.[7] Most of the asymptomatic men (78%) were less than 60 years of age.

Since 1991, mortality rates of prostate cancer have been decreasing in the United States.[8] Although the decline in death rates has been observed in both whites and blacks, the death rate in blacks is considerably higher. Studies evaluating the association of PSA screening and the decline in prostate cancer mortality are inconclusive.[9]

Prostatitis syndrome is a cluster of disorders that are characterized by nonspecific symptoms in the lower urogenital tract and perineum. Prevalence rates for prostatitis range from 5% to 16%.[10] Prostatitis accounts for approximately 2 million visits to a physician a year in the United States. Approximately 1% of visits to family physicians are related to prostatitis, whereas 8% of all visits to urologist are for prostatitis.[11]

John Baker, *Part 2*

You explain to Mr. Baker that to relieve symptoms quickly an alpha-blocker (tamsulosin) needs to be started and to prevent progression a 5α-reductase inhibitor (finasteride) is recommended. Mr. Baker agrees but wants to know if there is any interaction with his other medications that include an angiotensin-converting enzyme (ACE) inhibitor (enalapril), a statin (pravastatin), and a phosphodiesterase inhibitor (sildenafil). You explain that there is a potential for developing hypotension when sildenafil (Viagra) and alpha-blockers are used simultaneously but if taken at least 4 hours apart he should be alright. You also add that the choice of a selective alpha$_{1A}$-blocker (tamsulosin) will help to minimize hypotension.

Adrian Sellers, *Part 2*

Mr. Sellers returns for the results of free PSA and a repeat PSA that you had ordered. His repeat PSA is 10 g/ml and free PSA is 1.5 ng/ml, which is less than 25% of total PSA. You explain that he has a high velocity in the PSA change and the free PSA is less than 25%, putting him in a high risk for prostate cancer, and you recommend he see an urologist for further evaluation. Mr. Sellers

understands the pros and cons of biopsy and the options for treatment.

Juan Martinez, *Part 2*

Mr. Martinez returns to your office 2 days later. He states his symptoms have become worse, and he now has a painful sensation when he urinates and he is tender just above his anal area. He also has chills and a fever of 102°F. Results of urine examination today shows 15 white blood cell (WBC)/high-power field, and his preliminary culture results include more than 100,000 colony forming units/ml with pending identification of bacteria. Because Mr. Martinez has constitutional symptoms, you admit him to the hospital for acute bacterial prostatitis and administer an intravenous third-generation cephalosporin. After 48 hours his fever subsides. His urine culture grows out Escherichia coli, sensitive to levofloxin. He is sent home with a 14-day prescription of oral levofloxacin.

STUDY QUESTIONS

1. How will you monitor if Mr Baker's symptoms are improving?
2. When should you order a free PSA?

RISK FACTORS AND PATHOPHYSIOLOGY

Anatomy and Physiology

The lower urinary tract includes the urinary bladder, prostate, and the urethra. The prostate weighs 1 g at birth and grows to an average size of 20 g by 20 years of age. No appreciable growth occurs again until approximately 45 years of age. Histologically, 50% to 80% of the prostate is made up of stromal tissue, mostly smooth muscle. The remaining 20% to 50% is made up of glandular tissues, primarily acinar glands, and ducts. The prostate has several identifiable areas that include the central zone, peripheral zone, transitional zone, and periurethral zone.[12] The peripheral zone, which is palpable by DRE, comprises 70% of the volume of the prostate and is the primary site for prostate cancer. The transitional zone, which is not palpable by DRE, comprises 15% of the gland and is the locus for benign hypertrophy.

The prostate is under the influence of a neurohormonal milieu. Adrenergic receptors are present in the smooth muscle of the prostate. The predominant type of adrenergic receptor is the α_1-receptor, which has been subclassified into three subtypes, α_{1A}, α_{1B}, and α_{1D}.[13] Stimulation of adrenergic receptors in urethral smooth muscle is much greater than stimulation of the smooth muscle of the bladder.[14] The α_{1A} adrenoreceptors are the sites where norepinephrine acts to maintain urethral tone and intraurethral pressure. In contrast, glandular tissue is under the influence of dihydrotesterone (DHT), which binds to receptors present in the cytoplasm, providing stimulus to grow from an early embryonic stage. The prostate has 5-alpha-reductase type I and II activity that converts testosterone, which has diffused into the prostate, to DHT.

The walnut-shaped prostate gland is located inferior to the urinary bladder and encircles the urethra. Excessive growth of the glandular tissue in the periurethral zone or stromal tissue in the transition zone can cause urinary symptoms. The growth of glandular tissue can be asymmetrical and can influence urinary flow accordingly. Inward growth is likely to cause urinary flow obstruction, whereas an outward growth is less likely to cause any urinary flow obstruction. Thus, the size of the prostate, which correlates with outward growth, may not correlate with urinary flow symptoms. Furthermore, increased tone of prostatic smooth muscle may cause symptoms of urinary flow obstruction without any prostate enlargement.

The process of voiding requires a coordinated action between the bladder and urethra. The prostate encircles a portion of the urethra. Parasympathetic nerves innervate the bladder. Stimulation of these nerves causes urinary bladder muscle contraction, which results in voiding. Sympathetic nerves innervate the bladder neck and prostate. Stimulation of these nerves causes closure of the bladder outlet. There is also a voluntary sphincter in the bladder neck supplied by the pudendal nerve, controlled by the higher cortical centers and diencephalons which thereby enables an individual to consciously control voiding. Urinary symptoms can be caused by anatomical changes of the prostate as well as dysfunction of the associated nerves, smooth muscle, or urethral sphincter. Both prostatic and nonprostatic diseases can affect the principle structures involved with voiding and result in lower urinary symptoms.

Lower Urinary Tract Dysfunction and Lower Urinary Tract Symptoms

Almost all diseases of the prostate eventually lead to lower urinary tract dysfunction (LUTD) and LUTS. LUTD includes those disorders that affect continence (stress incontinence, overflow incontinence, and urge incontinence), BPH, and male erectile dysfunction. Symptoms that are associated with LUTD are termed LUTS, but not all presentations of LUTS are due to LUTD, such as in the case of a UTI. To avoid confusion with terms used to define symptoms, signs, urodynamic observations, and conditions that are associated with LUTD, efforts were made to standardize the def-

initions.[15] LUTS is divided into three groups: storage, voiding, and postmicturition symptoms.

Storage symptoms include increased daytime frequency, nocturia (complaint of waking at night one or more times from sleep to void), urgency (complaint of sudden compelling desire to pass urine that is difficult to defer), urinary incontinence (complaint of any involuntary *leakage* of urine), enuresis (any involuntary *loss* of urine), and bladder sensation (defined by five categories: normal, increased, reduced, absent, and nonspecific).

The *voiding symptoms* are experienced during voiding phase. Voiding symptoms include a slow stream (perception of reduced urine flow), splitting or spraying (character of stream), intermittent stream (flow that starts and stops), hesitancy (difficulty in initiating micturition), straining (muscular effort used to initiate, maintain, or improve the urinary stream), and terminal dribble (prolonged final part of micturition, when flow has slowed to a trickle/dribble).

Finally, *postmicturition symptoms* are experienced immediately after micturition and include a feeling of incomplete emptying and postmicturition dribble (involuntary loss of urine immediately after completion of urinating and leaving the toilet in men and after rising from the toilet in women).

When a patient experiences LUTS, the differential diagnosis should include diseases that do not originate from the lower urinary tract area. For example, bladder outlet obstruction can occur in diabetic patients with associated diabetic neuropathy affecting the parasympathetic nerves of the bladder. Urgency can occur in patients with neurological disorders such as postcerebrovascular accidents, Parkinson's disease, multiple sclerosis, and spinal cord injuries.

BENIGN PROSTATIC HYPERPLASIA

Differential Diagnosis and Assessment

BPH is defined histologically as "a disease process characterized by stromal and epithelial cell hyperplasia beginning in the periurethral zone of the prostate."[16,17] Patients with BPH may experience LUTS, which may affect their quality of life. BPH is a progressive disease.[18] Without any intervention, BPH may cause long-term complications. Bladder outlet obstruction contributes to bladder wall hypertrophy, which results in an increase in bladder mass, which in turn may lead to irreversible bladder dysfunction and postvoid residual urine (PRV).[19,20] The bladder wall hypertrophy and increased mass can be reversed if the obstruction is relieved before there is irreversible bladder dysfunction.[21] Other serious complications include acute urinary retention (AUR), recurrent urinary infection, bladder stones, and ultimately renal dysfunction.

Diagnosis

The Agency for Health Care Research and Quality (AHRQ) BPH clinical practice guidelines from 1994 were updated in 2003.[22] An algorithm for the assessment and management of BPH is shown in Figure 49-1.

The updated guideline incorporated several minor updates, including the following:

1. PSA measurement is recommended in select patients.
2. Urine cytology is recommended as an option in men with predominantly irritative symptoms.
3. Other validated symptom assessment instruments are supplementary to the AUA symptom score.
4. Serum creatinine is no longer recommended on initial evaluation in the standard patient.

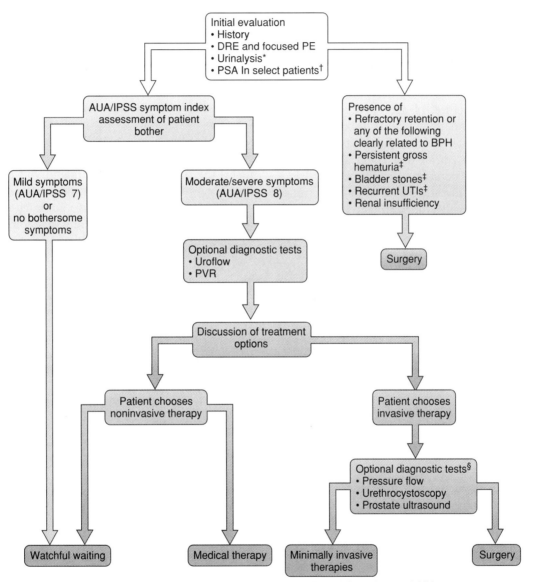

* In patients with clinically significant prostatic bleeding, a course of a 5 alpha-reductase inhibitor may be used. If bleeding persists, tissue ablative surgery is indicated.
† Patients with at least a 10-year life expectancy for whom knowledge of the presence of prostate cancer would change management or patients for whom the PSA measurement may change the management of voiding symptoms.
‡ After exhausting other therapeutic options as discussed in detail in the text.
§ Some diagnostic tests are used in predicting response to therapy. Pressure-flow studies are most useful in men prior to surgery.

AUA, American Urological Association; DRE, digital rectal exam; IPSS, International Prostate Symptom Score; PE, physical exam; PSA, prostate-specific antigen; PVR, postvoid residual urine; UTI, urinary tract infection.

FIGURE 49-1

Algorithm for evaluation and treatment of BPH. (Redrawn from American Urological Association. Copyright © 2003 American Urological Association Education and Research, Inc.)

5. Discussion of treatment options with the patient is recommended before pressure-flow testing is performed.

Initial Evaluation

In the initial evaluation of all patients with LUTS, the first step is to obtain a good medical history with careful attention to onset, duration, intensity, and aggravating or alleviating factors. Fluid intake and voiding patterns may also help to ascertain the cause of the patient's symptoms. A burning sensation when urinating accompanied with fever and chills should be assumed as a UTI until proven otherwise. Dysuria, with or without prostate enlargement, is associated with a wide variety of conditions. The differential diagnosis includes urethral stricture, bladder neck contracture, neurogenic bladder, and inflammatory disorders such as interstitial cystitis. The clinician should inquire about previous surgical procedures that could alter voiding functions and thereby confound the diagnosis of BPH. A review of comorbid diseases may identify other causes of LUTS and alter the plan for treatment. For example, if a patient suffers from orthostatic hypotension and is diagnosed with BPH, symptoms could be aggravated by prescribing an α-receptor blocker.

The AUA guideline recommends quantifying the symptoms of LUTS at the initial evaluation. Assessment tools such as the AUA symptom index (Table 49-1) provide a simple way to accomplish this task. The objective for obtaining a score is *not* to confirm a diagnosis of BPH but rather to quantify the symptom severity in order to guide management and evaluate the response to treatment. A score of seven is considered mild, and eight is considered moderate or severe. Scores derived from both assessment tools have been found to be sensitive enough to measure clinically important changes during treatment of BPH.[23]

Physical Examination

The initial physical examination should include a DRE and a focused neurological examination. DRE assesses the shape, size, and consistency of the prostate and may provided clues to prostate cancer. However, DRE, as a screening tool to detect prostate cancer, has marginal sensitivity (53%) and poor positive predictive value (18%).[24] Quantitatively the DRE usually underestimates the size of the prostate gland, but qualitatively, based on DRE, a prostate that is deemed enlarged usually is enlarged. The qualitative accuracy of the DRE has been corroborated by a study that compared clinical opinion and ultrasound of the prostate.[25]

Diagnostic Studies

Recommended diagnostic studies for the initial evaluation of LUTS include a urine analysis and PSA.

Table 49–1	American Urological Association Symptom Checklist for Benign Prostatic Hyperplasia					
	Never	**Less Than 1 Time in 5**	**Less Than Half the Time**	**About Half the Time**	**More Than Half the Time**	**Almost Always**
Over the past month, how often have you ...						
1. Felt that your bladder did not empty completely when you urinated?	0	1	2	3	4	5
2. Had to urinate again less than 2 hours after you finished urinating?	0	1	2	3	4	5
3. Had your urine flow stop ad start again several times when urinating?	0	1	2	3	4	5
4. Found it difficult to postpone urination?	0	1	2	3	4	5
5. Had a weak urinary stream?	0	1	2	3	4	5
6. Had to push or strain to begin urination?	0	1	2	3	4	5
	None	**1 Time**	**2 Times**	**3 Times**	**4 Times**	**5 or More Times**
Over the past month, how many times ...						
7. Did you typically get up to urinate from the time you went to bed at night until the time you got up in the morning?	0	1	2	3	4	5
TOTAL						

Total score is the sum of the seven circled items. Scores of 0 to 7 indicate absent or mild symptoms; 8 to 19, moderate symptoms; and 20+, severe symptoms.

Urine cytology is optional and should be restricted to patients who have predominately irritative symptoms or who are at increased risk for bladder cancer. The urine analysis can be done with a urine dipstick to screen for hematuria and infection. The measurement of PSA should be offered to patients who have a life expectancy of at least 10 years and who will benefit from a change in management to alleviate the voiding symptoms. Increases in PSA also can be used to predict prostate volume[26,27] and AUR.[28,29] Measurement of serum creatinine is *not* recommended in the initial evaluation of men with LUTS owing to BPH.

Additional tests should be considered if the patient has other medical problems, has other suspected causes for bladder dysfunction, or has failed medical treatment or if surgical intervention is planned. Urinary flow-rate and volume of PVR may help predict the response to surgery and severity of disease. Q_{max}, a measure of the urinary flow rate, may help determine if LUTS is secondary to BPH and can predict if the patient will benefit from surgery. A normal Q_{max} suggests that LUTS is *not* due to BPH. On the other hand, if Q_{max} is less than 10 ml per second, symptoms are likely owing to urodynamic obstruction and surgical intervention may prove beneficial.

Measuring PVR can assist with determining treatment outcome. Although a cut-off for PVR has not been established, some studies indicate that the presence of residual urine may predict a high failure rate for watchful waiting.[30] A large PVR, such as 350 ml, may indicate bladder dysfunction and portend a poor outcome from surgical intervention. A large PVR also may indicate that the disease is likely to progress. There are no long-term controlled studies of patients with elevated PVR who have minimal symptoms and do not have recurrent UTIs or renal insufficiency. Therefore, as quoted by the AUA guidelines, "No level of residual urine, in and of itself, mandates invasive therapy."

John Baker, *Part 3*

Three months later Mr. Baker returns to your office for a follow-up visit. His AUA score is now five, and his symptoms are not bothering him as much as before. He asks you if he could stop the finasteride. You answer that the prostate volume will decrease further if finasteride is continued and advice him not to stop it.

When Mr. Baker returns for his 6-month follow-up, his prostate volume decreased to 30 ml, and his symptoms have decreased further. You advise him to follow-up every year and to promptly come back to clinic if he has any signs of urinary retention.

STUDY QUESTIONS

1. If Mr. Baker cannot afford both finasteride and tamsulosin which one is better to continue for symptom relief?
2. What will your response be when Mr. Martinez asks if he will get completely well after taking the antibiotic?

● During the past decade, treatment for BPH has shifted dramatically from watchful waiting or surgery toward medical therapy with an emphasis on decreasing symptoms and increasing quality of life.

Management

Options for treatment depend on severity of LUTS, effect on quality of life, presence of complication, and the patient's wishes. In the past, treatments for BPH were mainly surgical interventions with the intention to reduce complications related to bladder outlet obstruction and the associated morbidity and mortality. During the past decade, treatment has shifted dramatically from watchful waiting or surgery toward medical therapy with an emphasis on decreasing symptoms and increasing quality of life. As a result of the success of medical intervention, fewer numbers of patients opt for watchful waiting and the frequency of traditional surgical interventions has decreased dramatically; however, urologists have offered a number of minimally invasive interventions that are discussed later in this chapter. The AUA recommends surgical intervention for patients with refractory retention or complications clearly related to BPH that are resistant to other therapeutic interventions such as persistent gross hematuria, bladder stones, recurrent UTIs, or renal insufficiency.

Medical Therapy

According to AUA guidelines, patients with mild symptoms of BPH (AUA symptom score of seven) who are not bothered by their symptoms can be managed by watchful waiting. The AUA guideline also advocates watchful waiting for patients with moderate to severe symptoms of BPH (AUA symptom score of eight) who are not bothered by their symptoms as long as there is no evidence of complications such as renal insufficiency, urinary retention, or recurrent infection. To relieve symptoms during watchful waiting, patients should be advised to decrease total fluid intake, decrease consumption of alcohol- and caffeine-containing beverages, limit the intake of salt and spices, and maintain time voiding schedules.[31] During watchful waiting, a yearly examination is required. Symptoms of LUTS should be reassessed quantitatively, and a DRE and urinalysis should be repeated. Prostate volume and PSA level are two predictors commonly used to assess the clinical progression of disease.[32] Results can be used to decide when to start medical treatment; however, prostate volume measured by DRE can be underestimated by 55% compared with a measurement carried out by transrectal ultrasound.[25] PSA, on the other hand, can be used as a surrogate for measuring the prostate size.[33] PSA levels above 1.5 ng/ml in men with mild symptoms of bladder outlet obstructions increase the risk of clinical progression.[34]

Two long-term studies have provided data that shows 5-alpha-reductase inhibitors can reduce incidence of clinical progression and AUR.[35] The consequence of watchful waiting can lead to bladder dysfunction that may not be reversible, even with surgical intervention. Studies on transurethral resection of the prostate (TURP) versus watchful waiting demonstrated that those who crossed over from watchful waiting to surgery because of bothersome symptoms experienced worse symptoms after surgery compared with those who had the surgery initially.[30,36] Furthermore, prostatectomy done when AUR occurs rather than when patient has LUTS is associated with an increase in mortality.[37] Interventions to alleviate LUTS are necessary in approximately 35% of 50-year-old men.[38] The best time to initiate medical interventions in patients with BPH and mild AUA symptom scores or moderate to severe AUA symptom scores who are not bothered by symptoms is still in debate. While awaiting further studies to answer this important question, clinicians should consider the benefits, side effects, and cost of medical intervention; discuss the risks and benefits with their patients; and make a shared decision.

The medical treatment can be categorized into α-adrenergic blockers, 5-alpha-reductase inhibitors, combination therapy, and phytotherapy.

α-ADRENERGIC BLOCKADE

LUTS due to BPH are attributed to smooth muscle tension in the prostatic stroma, urethra, and bladder neck mediated by α_1-receptors. Blockade of these receptors by alpha-blockers is the underlying mechanism that provides relief of symptoms. Alfuzosin, doxazosin, tamsulosin, and terazosin are the four alpha-blockers that are currently recommended by the AUA guidelines and deemed to have equal clinical effectiveness. There are slight differences in side effects and duration of action that may justify the use of one over the other but the efficacy of all four α-adrenergic blockers is comparable. All have warnings for orthostatic hypotension and carry a recommendation to rule out prostate cancer before initiating treatment. Rare cases of priapism have been reported. A comparison of these agents is provided in Table 49-2. Use of either prazosin or phenoxybenzamine, a nonselective alpha-blocker, is not recommended.

5-ALPHA-REDUCTASE INHIBITORS

DHT is essential for prostate growth as early as the embryonic stage of development. Prostate development is arrested if there is an absence of testosterone or an interruption in the conversion of testosterone to DHT by 5-alpha-reductase. This led to the development of 5-alpha-reductase inhibitors to arrest prostate growth, resulting in relief of obstruction of urinary flow produced by an enlarged prostate. Obstruction owing to causes other than prostatic enlargement is not affected by 5-alpha-reductase inhibitors. There are two 5-alpha-reductase inhibitors: (1) finasteride, which is selective for the type 2 isoenzyme of 5-alpha-reductase, and (2) dutasteride, which is selective but with a greater affinity for both type 1 and 2 isoenzymes. The efficacy compared with placebo is noted in patients with a prostate volume greater than 30 ml or PSA greater than 1.3 ng/ml. Improvement in symptoms has been shown to persist for at least 4 years in randomized clinical trials and 8 years in open label trials.[39,40] Both medications have similar efficacy and side effects; however, no long-term direct comparison studies have been done. Side effects include impotence, decreased libido, decreased volume of ejaculation, breast tenderness, and/or enlargement. Increases in testosterone levels and decreases in PSA levels have been observed. PSA levels decrease 40% to 50% over

Table 49-2	Alpha-Blockers Used for the Treatment of Benign Prostatic Hyperplasia			
	Supplied (mg)	**Dose/Titration (mg)**	**Max (mg)**	**Side Effects and Warning**
Doxazosin	1, 2, 4, 8	1 qd/double q 1-2 wk	8	Leukopenia/neutropenia
Alfuzosin	10 ER	10 qd	10	Increased by CYP3A4 Inhibitors
Tamsulosin	0.4	0.4 qd/double 1 to 2 wk	0.8	
Terazosin	1, 2, 5, 10	1 hs/slow increase every 4 to 6 weeks	20	Potentiated by blood pressure medications

3- to 24-month period; however, the free PSA to total PSA ratio is not altered. To interpret an isolated PSA level after 6 months of treatment with 5-alpha-reductase inhibitors, the PSA result should be doubled to compare with normal values.

On average, α_1-blockers decrease AUA symptom scores by five to seven points, increase urinary flow rate by 2 to 3ml/sec, and improve quality of life score compared with placebo. Finasteride is similar to alphablockers in improving the urinary flow rates. Alpha bockers alone were more effective than finasteride in reducing symptoms and improve flow. Combination of finasteride and alpha blockers did not show any added benefit compared to alpha blockers alone.[41,42] However, combination therapy is significantly superior to either therapy alone in decreasing the progression of LUTS, prostatic enlargement, and peak urinary flow rate.[43] The risk of symptomatic progression was reduced by 39%, 34%, and 67% by use of doxazosin, finasteride, and combination of the two, respectively. The combination of finasteride and doxazosin has been the best studied combination, but other alpha-blockers may produce similar results. Side effects with combination therapy reflect the combined side effects of each of the drugs when used independently.

PHYTOTHERAPY

The most common plant extract used for BPH symptom relief is *Serenoa repens*, derived from the berries of an American dwarf palm tree. Several mechanisms of action for *S. repens* have been proposed.[44] Phytotherapy is associated with a lower incidence of sexual dysfunction and ejaculatory disorders and appears to be suitable for mildly symptomatic patients with BPH. Phytotherapy may take more than 3 months to achieve an effect. Further trials are needed to determine if there is a reduction in urinary retention or surgery.

> ● Combination therapy with an α-adrenergic blocker and a 5-alpha-reductase inhibitor is significantly superior to either therapy alone in decreasing the progression of LUTS, prostatic enlargement, and peak urinary flow rate

Surgical Therapy

MINIMALLY INVASIVE THERAPIES

Several non-pharmacolgic interventions for treating urinary obstruction caused by BPH exist. There is a plethora of interventions encompassed under minimally invasive therapies (MITs). These include balloon dilatation (not recommended by AUA), insertion of permanent or temporary urethral stents, transurethral microwave thermotherapy (TUMT)

microwave therapy, transurethral needle ablation, electrovaporization, high-intensity focused ultrasound, and laser ablations. The MITs recommended in the AUA guideline, approved by the Food and Drug Administration and studied appropriately, are briefly described below.

The insertion of permanent or temporary metallic or polyurethane *urethral stents* can be placed in the prostatic urethra and maneuvered by fluoroscopic or endoscopic tools. Relief of obstruction is noted immediately. The use is limited by complication such as infection, encrustation, and chronic pain. The efficacy and benefit in relation to potentially safer and more effective procedures are not clear.[45] Thus, stents should be limited to patients who are too sick to undergo other procedures or to symptomatic, high-risk patients, particularly patients in either category with AUR.[46]

Transurethral needle ablation (TUNA) is carried out by the use of radiofrequency waves to heat and destroy prostatic tissue through two 18-gauge needles. This procedure is effective in patients with prostates measuring 60 g or less with predominantly lateral lobe enlargement.[47] Compared with TURP, the benefits of TUNA are less adverse events, preservation of sexual function, and cost-effectiveness for large prostate. In a comparative 5-year study, 14% in the TUNA group required further intervention, mostly TURP, versus 2% in the TURP group.[48] TURP seems to result in a better overall improvement, but TUNA is associated with less adverse events.[49]

Transurethral microwave thermotherapy (TUMT) has been demonstrated to result in 50% improvement in symptoms and urinary flow after 1 year: however, both tended to worsen after 4 years.[50,51] These data come from heterogeneous studies, and results should be interpreted cautiously. In a small study, costs associated with TURP were higher than those with TUMT even after taking into account the required reinterventions in TUMT.[52] Irritative voiding symptoms can be present for several weeks, and urinary retention is a common risk that requires intervention. Because unexpected procedure-related injuries have been noted with the use of TUMT, the use of TUMT should be carried out under general or spinal anesthesia following recommended safety measures.

Transurethral electrovaporization is a comparatively new procedure that uses roller ball electrodes and is similar to the standard TURP procedure. The instrument is passed over the prostatic tissue several times but using a higher wattage than used in TURP. The tissue is vaporized to the required depth. In a short-term follow-up study, transurethral electrovaporization and TURP were equivalent based on urinary flow rates, symptom scores, and quality of life.[53]

Postoperative irritative voiding symptoms, dysuria, and urinary retention requiring catheterization were higher in electrovaporization group. Sufficient large-scale studies are not available to comment on long-term outcomes.

Endoscopic laser therapy (ELT) for the treatment of BPH is gaining popularity. Outcomes with ELT interventions depend on type of laser used. Laser therapy (holmium laser) can enucleate the prostate and is deemed the best intervention for large prostates and will possibly be the treatment of choice in the future.

Visual laser ablation of prostate (VLAP) causes coagulation of the prostate tissue, which eventually necroses and sloughs, thereby relieving the obstruction. The AUA panel's meta-analysis found that 21% of patients required secondary catheterization after VLAP compared with 5% after TURP in single-arm studies. The postprocedure irritative voiding symptoms observed after VLAP may be more common compared with those of TURP.

Holmium laser enucleation of the prostate (HoLEP) has been performed over the past decade with reports of efficacy and safety similar to TURP.[54-56] Reduced perioperative morbidity, such as reduced blood loss, quicker catheter removal, and shorter hospital stay has been associated with HoLEP compared with TURP. There is a learning curve associated with the procedure for the urologist, and verifying the experience and record of the urologist maybe a prudent step to take before referring patients for HoLEP.

TRADITIONAL SURGICAL THERAPIES

TURP is carried out by endoscopically removing the inner portion of the prostate through the urethra. TURP has been the gold standard for surgical intervention, and all minimal invasive therapy is compared against the efficacy and adverse effects of TURP. The Veterans Affairs Cooperative Study[30] confirmed the effectiveness of TURP in patients with BPH needing surgical intervention. The study demonstrated similar risks for urinary incontinence and decline in sexual function compared with watchful waiting. The TURP syndrome, a dilutional hyponatremia caused by absorption into the bloodstream of the fluid used for irrigation after surgery, is a unique complication of TURP. Other complications include irritative voiding symptoms, excessive bleeding, hematuria, UTI, and bladder neck contracture.

Open prostatectomy (OP) is usually done when the prostate reaches 80 to 100 g in size and is associated with bladder stones or diverticula. During OP the inner core of the prostate, which contains the transition zone, is removed through a suprapubic or retropubic incision under general or regional anesthesia.

OP preserves the peripheral zone. OP is associated with higher morbidity owing to blood loss and longer recovery time; however, excellent results are obtained for urinary flow and irritative symptoms.

Adrian Sellers, *Part 3*

Mr. Sellers undergoes ultrasound directed biopsy of his prostate gland. The results reveal an adenocarcinoma in both lobes with a Gleason score of seven. Because of his PSA of 10, a CT scan of his pelvis and a bone scan is ordered. These tests document no regional lymph node or bone involvement. His TNO score is T2b, N0, M0, placing him in an intermediate risk group. Considering at his current age, he is just below a mean 10-year life expectancy and did not want radical prostatectomy; he agreed to undertake three-dimensional radiotherapy.

After radiation Mr. Sellers suffered form mild proctitis with limited rectal bleeding. He also had initially complained of urinary symptoms that subsided in 3 weeks. Follow-up in 3 months showed a PSA level at 1 ng/ml; at 6 months, 0.5 ng/ml. You explain that his PSA has reached a nadir and outcome will be good but close follow-up is required and advise him to have PSA testing every 6 months in the future.

STUDY QUESTIONS

1. How will you explain what does a Gleason score mean?
2. What are the three main options for treating Mr. Sellers prostate cancer?

● The U.S. Preventive Service Task Force states that there is good evidence that PSA use can detect early pathological stages of prostate cancer, but there are no conclusive studies that show interventions improve mortality rates.

PROSTATE CANCER

Differential Diagnosis and Assessment

Screening for prostate cancer continues to generate controversy and disagreement. The U.S. Preventive Service Task Force (USPSTF)[59] is neither for nor against the recommendation for routine screening owing to lack of evidence. The USPSTF agrees that there is good evidence that PSA use can detect early pathological stages of prostate cancer, but there are no conclusive studies that show interventions improve mortality rates. The American Cancer Society recommends annual PSA screening starting at the age of 50 years for average-risk asymptomatic men with life expectancy of 10 years.[58] The recommendation for not screening patients who have less than 10 years' life expectancy is based on a presumed slow progression of the disease. A shared-decision making process is recommended, which engages the clinician and patient in a discussion of the uncertain benefits and potential harm of screening. Such discussions can alter patients' decisions about PSA screening for prostate cancer.[57] Disagreement about screening decisions can arise when information is presented to both husband and wife, and clinicians may have to help in the decision-making process.[60]

PSA was introduced for clinical use in the 1980s, primarily to monitor the results of prostate cancer treatment. More recently PSA has been used to screen for occult prostate cancer; however, existing guidelines are not in agreement on correct use as a screening test. A major draw back to PSA as a screening test is lack of specificity. PSA is produced by the prostate epithelium and can be increased in patients with BPH as well as prostate cancer. Elevation of PSA is observed also with urinary retention and prostatitis and after vigorous prostate massage and ejaculation. Instrumentation such as the introduction of urinary catheters, cystoscopy, or prostate biopsy can increase PSA levels. Therefore, PSA tests should not be obtained for at least 6 weeks after instrumentation. On the other hand, finasteride, used to treat patients with BPH, can decrease PSA levels.

Another limitation of PSA as a screening test for prostate cancer is deciding on the level at which patients should undergo further diagnostic procedures such as ultrasound or biopsy. The currently recommended level of 4 ng/ml identifies patients who are assumed to be at increased risk for prostate cancer and should undergo further diagnostic studies; however, this level may miss early prostate cancer in certain age groups. A study reported in 2004 that prostate cancer can be commonly detected in patients whose PSA is lower than 4 ng/ml.[61] Some experts have recommended a threshold of 2.6 ng/ml in patients 60 years of age and younger for detecting prostate cancer.[62] The sensitivity and specificity at this level is 36% and 94%, respectively. Thus, lowering the PSA threshold may increase the chances of identifying more cases of prostate cancer, but it will also increase the false-positive rates and lead to unnecessary biopsies and potentially more harm. If PSA level is less than 2 ng/ml and there is a shared decision to continue monitoring, PSA maybe repeated every 2 years instead of every year without loss in overall specificity.[63]

The debate over PSA thresholds stimulated a search for other PSA-based criteria to screen for prostate cancer. Age- and race-specific PSA levels,

PSA velocity, PSA density, transition zone density, and PSA doubling time have been suggested as alternatives to improve the performance of PSA testing[7]. None of these alternative measures has been adopted owing to lack of practical application or failure to enhance the overall performance of the test.

Different serum forms of PSA have been another area of investigation to improve the specificity of PSA when the level is below 10 ng/ml. The most commonly used test is the free PSA. The ratio of free PSA to total PSA has been shown to discriminate between benign and malignant disease. Patients who have a free PSA that is 25% or less of the total PSA, when the total is between 4 and 10 ng/ml, are at an increased risk of prostate cancer.[64] Because of intraindividual variability in the PSA level, the PSA level should be repeated in 4 to 6 weeks if the initial value was greater than 4.0 ng/ml. Approximately 50% of patients will have normal levels when repeated.[65]

Recently, studies on the proenzyme of PSA, called pro-PSA, have found that pro-PSA may be a better marker of prostate cancer if the total PSA is between 2 and 10 ng/ml ranges.[66] A preliminary study found that only the ratio of pro-PSA to total PSA was able to discriminate benign from malignant disease.[67] If percentage of pro-PSA is used, 59% of the patients will not require further invasive work-up. In comparison, if percent free-PSA is used, only 33% of the patients will avoid further work-up.

Diagnostic work-ups for prostate cancer may include transrectal ultrasonogram, prostate biopsy, bone scan, and CT scan of pelvis. Once a patient is diagnosed with prostate cancer, risk stratification is required to a treatment strategy that will decrease the likelihood of progression. The PSA value, Gleason score, and clinical stage can help in classifying patients with prostate cancer into three risk categories. The Gleason score is based on the extent of histological differentiation from the normal gland and ranges from 2 to 10. The pathologist will ascertain scores for the two most common patterns, and the sum is reported. Higher scores are associated with a more aggressive type of cancer. The clinical staging is done by the TNM staging system (see Chapter 45, "Cancer").

Adrian Sellers, *Part 4*

Mr. Sellers does well for 4 years. However, when the PSA increases to 3.5 ng/ml, after discussion, the patient agrees to wait and not undergo any further testing. His PSA after another year rises to 8 ng/ml. At this point he agrees to start hormonal therapy to decrease the rate of progression. He starts on luteinizing hormone-releasing hormone

(LH-RH) given every 3 months by intramuscular injections. He is followed for another year and does well. He subsequently is admitted for an acute inferior myocardial infarction with severe hypotension and eventually can not be resuscitated.

Management

The three main treatment options for prostate cancer are watchful watching, radical prostatectomy, and radiotherapy. Hormonal ablation is an alternative option for certain stages of disease. Recently, chemotherapy has been used not only for palliative reasons but also for increasing survival. Radiotherapy includes external-beam radiation and local radioactive pellets placement (brachytherapy). Hormonal ablation includes LH-RH agonists with or without an anti-androgen and bilateral orchiectomy. Treatment of prostate cancer is a complex process based on age, comorbidity, and risk stratification and should take into account the patient's life expectancy and treatment preferences. The National Comprehensive Cancer Network (NCCN) guidelines for the management of prostate cancer[68] provide consensus recommendation by leading experts in prostate cancer that are evidence based (see Chapter 45, "Cancer").

PROSTATITIS

Differential Diagnosis and Assessment

The evaluation of a patient with suspected prostatitis should start with a thorough history, including a detailed sexual history and any previous diagnoses of prostatitis. The initial evaluation should thoroughly investigate the duration of symptoms; nature of any pain that may be present, including painful intercourse or ejaculation; symptoms associated with voiding; and impact on quality of life. The physical examination should focus on the abdomen, groin, genitalia, perineal area, and a DRE of the prostate.

The urine should be examined for blood, glucose, protein, WBC, and bacteria. The majority of patients with prostatitis will not have an infection or have WBCs in the urine; however, the clinician should look for a UTI during the initial evaluation of a patient who complains of pelvic pain or urinary symptoms.

To distinguish urethral and prostatic infection, Meares and Stamey[69] designed a test that is now used as the gold standard for diagnosing and following patients with the prostatitis syndrome. The process involves labeling four sterile tubes—VB1, VB2, EPS, and VB3—and collecting samples sequentially. The first specimen, VB1, is the first 5 to 10 ml of voided urine. The second specimen, VB2, is a midstream urine sample and reserved for culture. The third specimen, EPS, comes from expressed prostate secretions obtained by prostate massage. The final specimen, VB3, is the first voided urine after the prostate massage after collection of the EPS sample. Before collection of the split samples, patients should not have taken antibiotics for a month or ejaculated for at least 2 days. The patient should have a full bladder at the time the samples are collected. The presence of symptoms and 10 WBCs per high power field in the EPS sample is diagnosis of chronic prostatitis. Interpretations of the test results are presented in Table 49-3. A study by Nickel et al. cast some doubt regarding the clinical usefulness of the Meares test to distinguish chronic prostatitis.[70] Alternatively, the classification published by the Chronic Prostatitis Collaborative Research Network (CPCRN), which was sponsored by National Institute of Diabetes and Digestive and Kidney Disease, can be used to categorize the prostatitis syndromes (Table 49-4). To classify patients who are suspected of having prostatitis, using this taxonomy, the following information is required: (1) the clinical presentation of the patient, (2) presence or absence of white blood cells in expressed prostatic secretions (EPSs), and (3) bacteria in the EPSs.

Table 49–3	Interpretation of the Stamey Meares Test for Prostatitis				
Type of Prostatitis		**VB1**	**VB2**	**EPS**	**VB3**
Acute bacterial		+	+	Not done	Not done
Chronic bacterial		−	±	+	+
Chronic nonbacterial/CPPS inflammatory		−	±	−	+
Chronic nonbacterial/CPPS noninflammatory		−	−	−	−
Asymptomatic inflammatory		±	±	+	+

VB1 indicates no growth when negative and >100,000 colony forming units/ml when positive; VB2, <10 white blood cell (WBC)/high power field when negative and 10 to 20 WBC/high power field when positive; EPS, positive when significant bacteriuria in the postmassage specimen (any bacteria if the premassage urine is sterile or colony count per mL is at least 10 times greater than premassage count); and VB3, <10 WBC/high power field when negative and 10 to 20 WBC/high power field when positive.

Table 49–4	The Chronic Prostatitis Collaborative Research Network (CPCRN) Classifications

1. Acute bacterial prostatitis: acute infection of the prostate

2. Chronic bacterial prostatitis: recurrent infection of the prostate

3. Chronic nonbacterial prostatitis (CPPS) discomfort pain in the pelvic region ≥3 months with variable voiding and sexual symptoms, and no demonstrable infection
   3.1. Inflammatory CPPS: white blood cells in semen, EPS or VB3
   3.2. Non inflammatory CPPS: no white blood cells in semen, EPS or VB3

4. Asymptomatic inflammatory prostatitis: no subjective symptoms found, but white blood cells found in prostate secretions or prostate tissue during evaluation for other disorders.

Juan Martinez, *Part 3*

Mr. Martinez returns to your office 3 weeks after hospital discharge. He continues to complain of LUTS but denies fever or a burning sensation on urination. His BPH AUA score is nine. Clinically he appears to have symptomatic BPH. After discussion, a shared decision to start him on tamsulosin is made, which will possibly prevent the recurrence of a UTI owing to incomplete bladder emptying. He declines to undergo urodynamic testing for the time being. Over the next several months, his LUTS improves.

STUDY QUESTIONS

1. Which medications can prevent bacterial prostatitis?
2. How is chronic pelvic pain syndrome treated?

Management

ACUTE BACTERIAL PROSTATITIS

Antimicrobial therapy is essential in acute bacterial prostatitis. The clinical presentation and severity of the symptoms determine the route and type of antibiotic therapy. Patients who present with acute onset of symptoms; have constitutional symptoms such as chills, fever, low back pain, dysuria, or urinary obstruction; and an exquisitely tender prostate usually require parenteral antibiotics, which should be started as soon as urine and blood cultures are obtained. Prostatic massage in such cases is contraindicated. Hospitalization is frequently necessary. High doses of bactericidal antibiotics such as broad-spectrum penicillin derivatives, third-generation cephalosporins with or without an aminoglycoside, or a fluoroquinolone are required until the signs and symptoms of acute infection diminish. Thereafter, the antibiotic can be changed to an oral preparation and adminis-

tered for at least 4 weeks. In less severe cases, oral fluoroquinolones can be prescribed for 2 to 4 weeks. Treatment of sexual contacts is not required.

> ● The diagnosis of chronic bacterial prostatitis should be confirmed by culture and microscopy of expressed prostate secretions.

Chronic Bacterial Prostatitis

The diagnosis of chronic bacterial prostatitis (CBP) should be confirmed by culture and microscopy of EPS, as described by Meares and Stamey. Culturing the ejaculate can be misleading. The pathogens in CBP belong to the *Enterobacteriaceae*, predominantly *E. coli*, followed by others such as *Klebsiella* species, *Proteus mirabilis*, and less frequently *Enterococcus fecalis* and *Pseudomonas aeruginosa*. No definitive link to *Chlamydia*, mycoplasma, or ureaplasma species has been noted. Fluoroquinolones and macrolides are effective antibiotics because of their capacity to diffuse into prostate tissue. Lipid solubility, molecular size, and pKa of antibiotic determine diffusion capacity. Duration of treatment has been based on expert opinion, experience, and clinical trials. Authorities recommend 4 to 6 weeks of therapy with a fluoroquinolone after the initial diagnosis.[71] Occasionally CBP does not respond to antibiotic therapy and becomes a relapsing illness. In such cases, either low-dose suppressive antibiotic therapy or intermittent treatment with antibiotics for recurrent symptoms has been recommended.

Chronic Nonbacterial Prostatitis/Chronic Pelvic Pain Syndrome

Chronic pelvic pain syndrome (CPPS) is the least understood of the prostatitis syndromes. The exact etiology is still under investigation. Almost 90% of patients with symptoms of prostatitis have CPPS, which is difficult to cure. Treatment options are nonspecific and oriented toward minimizing symptoms and improving quality of life. The NIH chronic prostatitis symptom index helps clinicians monitor symptoms and helps tailor therapeutic interventions.[72] A thorough history of previous diagnostic studies and prior treatment should be obtained. Patients with CPPS usually have visited other clinicians and undergone various therapeutic interventions. If no pathological findings are noted, which is true for most of the cases of CPPS, treatment options should be based on the presence or absence of inflammation. A trial of antibiotic can be used if inflammation is present; however, there is no consensus of opinion for this approach.[73] The rationale for antibiotics is the supposition that infection can be present in deep-seated prostatic tissue, despite negative EPS cultures, and produces an inflammatory reaction. If empiric antibiotic therapy reduces pain and other associated symptoms, the antibiotics should be continued for 4 to 5 weeks. On the other hand, where there is no inflammation, antibiotics should not be used. Other interventions for pain relief have been tried. Some studies found that alpha-blockers, prescribed for 4 weeks, provide relief.[74,75] Nonsteroidal anti-inflammatory agents can be tried for pain relief, although a small study showed use of cyclooxygenase-2 inhibitors were not effective. Biofeedback therapy may also improve symptoms. In patients unresponsive to the above therapies, other causes of pelvic pain should be considered, including prostatic stones, bladder outlet obstruction, detrusor muscle dysfunction, and interstitial cystitis.

Asymptomatic Inflammatory Prostatitis

Asymptomatic inflammatory prostatitis is a diagnosis based on incidental findings. Patients are asymptomatic but show evidence of inflammation in tissue obtained from a prostatic biopsy or in the ejaculate collected for semen analysis. There is no indication for intervention for asymptomatic inflammatory prostatitis at the present time.

SUMMARY

LUTS associated with prostate gland disease are common in older men. BPH is the major cause of LUTS. Other common prostatic diseases associated with LUTS include prostate cancer and prostatitis. The treatment of BPH has shifted dramatically from watchful waiting or surgery toward medical therapy with an emphasis on decreasing symptoms and increasing quality of life. Screening for prostate cancer with the PSA test or modified PSA approaches continues to generate controversy and disagreement. A shared decision-making process is recommended when PSA testing is considered in older men. The use of antimicrobial therapy is essential in management of acute bacterial prostatitis. The CPCRN definitions can be used to categorize the chronic prostatitis syndromes and choose appropriate therapy.

POSTTEST

1. For a patient diagnosed with prostate cancer and with a life expectancy of less than 10 years, an option for intervention can include watchful waiting.
   a. True
   b. False

2. Chronic nonbacterial prostatitis treatments should be based on all *except*:
   a. Presence or absence of inflammation
   b. The AUA BPH scores
   c. The outcome of empiric antibacterial treatment
   d. Results of expressed prostatic secretion findings

3. The PSA level when screening for prostate cancer should be repeated in 4 to 6 weeks if the initial level is greater than 4 ng/ml owing to intra-individual variability.
   a. True
   b. False

4. In men, prostate cancer is the:
   a. Leading cause of cancer deaths.
   b. Second leading cause of cancer deaths.
   c. Third leading cause of cancer deaths.
   d. Fourth leading cause of cancer deaths.

References

1. Platz EA, Smit E, Curhan GC, Nyberg Jr. LM, Giovannucci, E. Prevalence of and racial/ethnic variation in lower urinary tract symptoms and noncancer prostate surgery. Urology 2002;59:877-883.
2. Bruskewitz R. Medical management of BPH in the U.S. Eur Urol 1999; 36(Suppl 3):7-13.
3. Berry SJ, Coffey DS, Walsh PC, Ewing LL. The development of human benign prostatic hyperplasia with age. J Urol 1984;132:474-479.
4. Barry MJ. Epidemiology and natural history of benign prostatic hyperplasia. Urol Clin N Am 1990;17:495-507.
5. Sakr WA, Grignon DJ. Prostate cancer: indicators of aggressiveness. Eur Urol 1997;32(Suppl 3):15-23.
6. Lowe FC, Gilbert SM, Kahane H. Evidence of increased prostate cancer detection in men aged 50 to 60: a review of 324,684 biopsies performed between 1995 and 2002. Urology 2003;62:1045-1049.
7. Miller DC, Hafez KS. Prostate carcinoma presentation, diagnosis and staging: an update from the National Cancer Data Base. Cancer 2003;98: 1169-1178.
8. Jemal A, Murray T, Samuels A. Cancer statistics. CA Cancer J Clin 2003;53: 5-26.
9. Chu KC, Tarone RE, Freeman HP. Trends in prostate cancer mortality among black men and white mend in the United States. Cancer 2003;97: 1507-1516.

10. Krieger JN, Riely DE, Cheah PY, Liong L, Yuen KH. Epidemiology of prostatitis: new evidence for a world-wide problem. World J Urol 2003;21:70-74.
11. Collins NM, Stafford RS, O'Leary MP, Barry MJ. How common is prostatitis. J Urol 1998;159:1224-1228.
12. McNeal JE. Normal histology of the prostate. Am J Surg Pathol 1988;12:619-633.
13. Hieble JP, Bylund DB, Clarke DE, Eikenburg DC, Langer SZ, Lekowitz RJ. International Union of Pharmacology, X: recommendation for nomenclature of alpha$_1$-adrenoreceptors:consensus update. Pharmacol Rev 1995;47:267-270.
14. de Groat WC, Yoshimura N. Pharmacology of the lower urinary tract. Ann Rev Pharmacol Toxicol 2001;41:691-721.
15. Abrams P, Cardozo L, Fall M, Griffiths D, Rosier P, Ulmsteen U. The standardization of terminology in lower urinary tract function: report from the standardization sub-committee of the international continence society. Urology 2003;21:37-49.
16. McNeal JE. Origin and evolution of benign prostatic enlargement. Invest Urol 1978;15:340-345.
17. Lee C, Cockett A, Cussenot K, Issacs W. Regulation of prostate growth. In Proceedings of the Fifth International Consultation on Benign Prostatic Hyperplasia, United Kingdom, 2001 (Chatelain C, Foo KT, Khoury S, McConell J, eds.). United Kingdom: Health Publications Ltd., 2001.
18. Emberton M, Andriole GL, deLa Rosette J. Benign prostatic hyperplasia: a progressive disease of aging men. Urology 2003;6:267-273.
19. Levin RM, Monson FC, Haugaard N. Genetic and cellular characteristics of bladder outlet obstruction. Urol Clin N Am 1995;22:263-283.
20. Levin RM, Levin SS, Zhao Y. Cellular and molecular aspects of bladder hypertrophy. Eur Urol 1997;32 (Suppl 1):15-21.
21. Kojima M, Innui E, Ochiai A. Reversible change of bladder hypertrophy due to benign prostatic hyperplasia after surgical relief of obstruction. J Urol 1997;158:89-93.
22. AUA Practice Guidelines Committee. AUA guidelines on management of benign prostatic hyperplasia (2003). J Urol 2003;170:530-547.
23. Barry MJ. Evaluation of symptoms and quality of life in men with benign prostatic hyperplasia. Urology 2001;58:25-32.
24. Mistry K, Cable G. Meta analysis of prostatic specific antigen and digital rectal examination as screening tests for prostate carcinoma. J Am Board Family Prac 2003;16:95-101.
25. Roehrborn CG, Girman CJ, Rhodes T, Hanson KA, Collins GN. Correlation between prostate size estimated by digital rectal examination and measured by transrectal ultrasound. Urology 1997;49:548.
26. Roehrborn CG, Boyle, P, Gould, A. L, Waldstreicher, J. Serum prostate-specific antigen as a predictor of prostate volume in men with benign prostatic hyperplasia. Urology 1999;53:581-589.
27. Wright EJ, Fang J, Metter EJ. Prostate specific antigen predicts the long-term risk of prostate enlargement: results from the Baltimore Longitudinal Study of Aging. J Urol 2002;167:2484-2487.
28. Roehrborn CG, McConell JD, Lieber M. Serum prostate specific antigen is a powerful predictor of acute urinary retention and the need for surgery in men with clinical benign prostatic hyperplasia. Urology 1999;53:473-480.
29. Marberger MJ, Anderson JT, Nickel JC. Prostate volume and serum prostate-specific antigen as predictors of acute urinary retention. Eur Urol 2000;38: 563-568.
30. Wasson JH, Reda DJ, Bruskewitz RC, Elinson J, Keller AM, Henderson WG. A comparison of transurethral surgery with watchful waiting for moderate symptoms of benign prostatic hyperplasia. The Veterans Affairs Cooperative Study Group on Transurethral Resection of the Prostate. New Engl J Med 1995;332:75.
31. Barry MJ, Cockett AT, Holtgrwe HL, McConell JD, Sihelink SA, Winfield HN. Relationship of symptoms of prostatism to commonly used physiological and anatomical measures of the severity of benign prostatic hyperplasia. J Urol 1993;150(2 Pt 1):351-358.
32. Fong YK, Milani S, Djavan B. Natural history and clinical predictors of clinical progression in benign prostatic hyperplasia. Curr Opin Urol 2005;15:35-38.
33. Mochtar CA, Kiemeney L, Van Riesmsdiijk M. Prostate-specific antigen as an estimator of prostate volume in management of patients with symptomatic benign prostatic hyperplasia. Eur Urol 2003;44:695-700.
34. Djavan B, Fong YK, Reissigl A. A longitudinal study of men with mild symptoms of bladder outlet obstruction treated with watchful waiting over 4 years. Urology 2004;64(6):1144-1140.
35. McConell JD, Roehrborn CG, Bautista OM. The long-term effect of doxazosin, finasteride, and combination on the clinical progression of benign prostatic hyperplasia. New Engl J Med 2003;349:2387-98.
36. Flanigan RC, Reda DJ, Wasson JH. 5-year outcome of surgical resection and watchful waiting for men with moderately symptomatic benign prostatic hyperplasia: a Department of Veterans Affairs Cooperative study. J Urol 1998;160:12-16.
37. Pickard R, Emberton M, Neal JC. The management of men with acute urinary retention. National Prostatectomy Audit Steering Group. Brit J Urol 1998;81:712-720.
38. Oesterling JE. Benign prostatic hyperplasia: medical and minimally invasive treatment options. New Engl J Med 1995;332:99-109.
39. Hudson PB, Boake R, Trachtenberg J, Romas NA, Rosenblatt S, Narayan, P. Efficacy of finasteride is maintained in patients with benign prostatic hyperplasia treated for 5 years: the North American Finasteride Study Group. Urology 1999;53:690.
40. Vaughan D, Imperato-McGinely J, McConell J, Matsumoto AM, Bracken B. Long term (7-8 year) experience with finasteride in men with benign prostatic hyperplasia. Urology 2002;60:1040.
41. Lepor H, Williford WO, Barry MJ, Brawer MK, Dixon CM, Gromely G. The efficacy of terazosin, finasteride, or both in benign prostatic hyperplasia. New Engl J Med 1996;335:533–539.
42. Kirby RS, Roehrborn C, Boyle P, Bartsch G, Jardin A, Cary MM. Efficacy and tolerability of doxazosin and finasteride. alone or combination, in treatment of symptomatic benign prostatic hyperplasia: the Prospective European Doxazosin and Combination Therapy (PREDICT) trial. Urology 2003; 61:119.
43. McConell JD. The long term effects of medical therapy on the progression of LUTS: results from the MTOPS trial. J Urol 2002;167:1042.
44. Fong YK, Milani S, Djavan B. Role of phytotherapy in men with lower urinary tract symptoms. Curr Opin Urol 2005;15:45-46.
45. Ogiste JS, Cooper K, Kaplan SA. Are stents still a useful therapy for benign prostatic hyperplasia? Curr Opin Urol 2003;13:51-57.
46. Lam JS, Volpe MA, Kaplan SA. Use of prostatic stents for the treatment of benign prostatic hyperplasia in high-risk patients. Curr Urol Rep 2001;2: 277-284.
47. Naslund MJ. Transurethral needle ablation of the prostate. Urology 1997; 50:167.
48. Hill B, Belville W, Bruskewitz R. Transurethral needle ablation versus transurethral resection of the prostate for treatment of symptomatic benign prostatic hyperplasia: 5 year results of a prospective, randomized, multicenter clinical trial. J Urol 2004;171:2336-2340.
49. Boyle P, Robertson C, Vaughan ED, Fitzpatrick JM. A meta analysis of trials of transurethral needle ablation for treating symptomatic benign prostatic hyperplasia. Brit J Urol 2004;94:83-88.
50. Trock BJ, Brotzman M, Utz WJ. Long term pooled analysis of multicenter studies cooled thermotherapy for benign prostatic hyperplasia results at three months through four years. Urology 2004;63:716-721.
51. Walmsley K, Kaplan SA. Transurethral microwave thermotherapy for benign prostate hyperplasia: separating truth from marketing hype. J Urol 2004;172(4 Pt 1):1249-1255.
52. Kobelt G, Spanberg A, Mattiasson A. The cost of feedback microwave thermotherapy compared with transurethral resection of the prostate for treating benign prostatic hyperplasia. Brit J Urol 2004;93:543-548.
53. Poulakis V, Dahm P, Witsch U. Transurethral electrovaporization vs transurethral resection for symptomatic prostatic obstruction: a meta analysis. Brit J Urol 2004;94:89-95.
54. Tan AH, Gilling PJ, Kennet KM. A randomized trial comparing holmium laser enucleation of the prostate with transurethral resection of the prostate for the treatment of bladder outlier obstruction secondary toe benign prostatic hyperplasia in large glands (40-200 grams). J Urol 2003;170:1270-1274.
55. Tooher R, Sutherland P, Costello A, Gilling P, Rees G, Maddern G. A systematic review of holmium laser prostatectomy for benign prostatic hyperplasia. J Urol 2004;171:1773-1781.
56. Westenberg A, Gilling P, Kennett K. Holmium laser resection of the prostate versus transurethral resection of the prostate: results of a randomized trial with 4 year minimum long-term follow-up. J Urol 2004;172: 616-619.
57. U.S. Preventive Services Task Force. Screening for prostate cancer: recommendations and rationale. 2002;137(11):915-916.
58. Smith RA. American Cancer Society Guidelines for the early detection of cancer. CA Cancer J Clin 2003;53:27-43.
59. Wolf AMD, Nasser JF, Wolf AM, Schorling JB., The impact of informed consent on patient interest in prostate-specific antigen screening. Arch Intern Med 1996;156(12):1333-1336.
60. Volk RJ, Cantor SB, Spann SJ., Preferences of husbands and wives for prostate cancer screening. Arch Family Med 1997;6:72-76.
61. Thompson IM, Pauler DK, Goodman PJ., Prevalence of prostate cancer among men with a prostate-specific antigen level ≤4.0 ng per milliliter. New Engl J Med 2004;350:2239-246.
62. Punglia RS, D'Amico AV, Catolona WJ. Effect of verification bias on screening for prostate cancer by measurement of prostate-specific antigen. New Engl J Med 2003;349:335-342.
63. Carter HB, Epstein JI, Cha DW, Fozard JL, Pearson J D. Recommended prostate-specific antigen testing intervals for the detection of curable prostate cancer. JAMA 1997;277:1456-1460.
64. Catalona WJ, Partin AW, Slawin KM. Use of the percentage of free prostate-specific antigen to enhance differentiation of prostate cancer from benign prostatic disease: a prospective multicenter clinical trial. JAMA 1998;279: 1542-1547.
65. Eastham JA, Riedel E, Scardino PT. Variation of serum prostate-specific antigen levels: an evaluation of year-to-year fluctuations. JAMA 2003;289:2695-2700.
66. Catolona WJ, Bartsch G, Rittenhouse HG. Serum pro prostate specific antigen improves cancer detection compared to free and complex prostate specific antigen in men with prostate specific antigen 2 to 4 ng/ml. J Urol 2003;170:2181-2185.
67. Sokol IJ, Chan DW, Mikolajczyk SD. Proenzyme PSA for the early detection of prostate specific antigen in the 2.5 to 4 ng/ml total PSA range: preliminary analysis. Urology 2003;61:274-276.
68. Scherr D, Swindle PW, Scardino PT. The national comprehensive cancer network guidelines for the management of prostate cancer. Urology 2003; 61(Suppl 2A):14-24.
69. Meares EM, Stamey TA. Bacteriological localization of patterns in bacterial prostatitis and urethritis. Invest Urol 1968;5:492-518.

70. Nickel JC, Alexander RB, Schaffer AJ. Leukocytes and bacteria in men with chronic prostatitis/chronic pelvic syndrome compared to asymptomatic controls. J Urol 2003;170:818-822.

71. Naber KG. Antibiotic treatment of chronic bacterial prostatitis. In Textbook of prostatitis (Nickel JC, ed.).Oxford: Isis Medical Media: Oxford, 1999.

72. Litwin MS, McNaughton-Collins M, Fowler Jr FJ, et al. The NIH Chronic Prostatitis Symptoms Index. J Urol 1999;162(2):369-375.

73. Naber KG, Bergman B, Bishop MC, Bjerklund TE. EAU guidelines on urinary and male genital tract infections. European Urol 2001;40:576–588.

74. Cheah PY, Liong ML, Yuen KH. Terazosin therapy for chronic prostatitis/chronic pelvic pain syndrome: A randomized, placebo controlled trial. J Urol 2003;169:592-596.

75. Nickel JC. The use of alpha$_1$-adrenoceptor antagonists in lower urinary tract symptoms: beyond benign prostatic hyperplasia. Urology 2003;62(Suppl 3A): 34-41.

Web Resources

American Urological Association Benign Prostatic Hypertrophy Clinical Guideline. http://www.auanet.org/guidelines/bph.cfm.

United States preventive Services Task Force Guideline on Prostate Cancer Screening. http://www.ahrq.gov/clinic/uspstf/uspsprca.htm.

Guideline for the management of prostatitis. London: Association for Genitourinary Medicine (AGUM), Medical Society for the Study of Venereal Disease (MSSVD), 2002. http://www.bashh.org/guidelines/2002/prostatitis_ 0601.pdf

PRETEST ANSWERS

1. c
2. d
3. c
4. b

POSTTEST ANSWERS

1. a
2. b
3. a
3. b

CHAPTER 50

Parkinson's Disease

Monica Stallworth and Richard King

OBJECTIVES

Upon completion of this chapter the reader will be able to:

- Define and recognize the clinical features that justify a clinical diagnosis of Parkinson's disease (PD)

- Describe the differences in clinical features and medication responsiveness of the illnesses from which PD must be differentiated

- Understand the role of levodopa in diagnosis and treatment and the indications for the use of adjunctive medications in PD in older persons

- Recognize and optimally manage the motor and non-motor complications of PD

PRETEST

1. Depletion of which of the following neurotransmitters is most strongly associated with Parkinson's disease?
   A. Norepinephrine
   B. Dopamine
   C. Glutamate
   D. Serotonin
   E. Gamma-aminobutyric acid

2. Which factor most helps to distinguish Parkinson's disease from other causes of parkinsonism?
   A. Bradykinesia
   B. Increased tone
   C. Postural instability
   D. Response to dopamine replacement

3. Your patient has difficulty with shaking and clumsiness of his left arm when reaching for objects. At rest, his arm does not shake. When asked to carry out with rapid alternating movements, he has difficulty with maintaining an even rhythm. This is most consistent with which type of disease?
   A. Parkinson's disease
   B. Essential tremor
   C. Cerebellar disease
   D. Chorea
   E. Dyskinesia

PREVALENCE AND IMPACT

Parkinson's disease (PD) is a progressive disorder that results in severe disability 10 to 15 years after its onset. It is the second most common neurodegenerative disorder after Alzheimer's disease (AD).

PD is characterized by rigidity, tremor, and bradykinesia; it is usually asymmetric and is usually receptive to dopaminergic treatment. Familial PD is described. Parkinson-plus syndromes refer to disorders that include parkinsonism with other clinical signs: they include dementia of Lewy body type (DLB), multiple system atrophy (MSA), progressive supranuclear palsy (PSP), and corticobasal degeneration.[1]

As in other industrialized countries, the prevalence is approximately 1% in persons over 65 in the United States, and rises to 3% in those over 85.[2] All ethnic origins can be affected, males somewhat more than females.[5]

RISK FACTORS AND PATHOPHYSIOLOGY

Role of Aging

Although the incidence of PD increases with age, and Lewy bodies are described in up to 16% of elderly asymptomatic people at autopsy,[9] PD is generally *not* considered a normal part of aging.

Genetic Predisposition

Most people with PD do not have a family history, but 15% do have a first-degree relative with PD, characteristically without a clear mode of inheritance.[4] Several genetic loci for PD are identified, although a common environmental etiology could explain familial patterns.[5]

Role of Environmental Exposure

Pesticides, rural environments, and well water have all been linked to PD.[6] In the early 1980s, a perthine analog, MPTP, was reported: the only environmental agent directly linked to levodopa-responsive parkinsonism. Cigarette smoking may lessen the risk![7]

Pathology

The underlying pathological change in PD is injury to the dopaminergic projections from the substantia nigra pars compacta to the caudate nucleus and putamen. Intraneuronal Lewy bodies and Lewy neurites are other pathological features of PD. Lewy bodies are often observed in the cortex, amygdala, locus ceruleus, vagal nucleus, and the peripheral autonomic nervous system[8]; this could explain some nonmotor features of PD. Aside from the few patients with PD from environmental exposure or a known gene mutation, the cause for PD is unidentified; it is almost certainly multiple factors acting in unison.

Brenda Wilmington *Part 1*

Mrs. Wilmington is a 79-year-old patient whom you have not seen for several years. She sees you because of difficulty walking and cognitive changes. She had several falls 18 months ago and now has difficulty working; she is a sculptor. On interview, she has difficulty answering detailed questions, and her memory is mildly impaired. On examination, cranial nerves are intact, yet she has a staring expression, with raised eyebrows and reduced blinking. Tone is increased in both legs, with cogwheeling in the left arm. There is no tremor. She walks stiffly, with a widened stance. She has reduced swing of the left arm and shuffles the left foot. With her eyes closed, she is unable to stand upright.

STUDY QUESTIONS:

1. How are her symptoms typical for a presentation of PD?
2. How are her symptoms atypical for PD?
3. Which medication should you prescribe?

DIFFERENTIAL DIAGNOSIS AND ASSESSMENT

Is It Parkinson's Disease?

Whereas autopsy is required to make the definitive diagnosis of PD, an accurate clinical diagnosis can usually be made. The diagnostic terms "clinically possible," "clinically probable," and "clinically definite" PD are recommended (Box 50-1).

Because levodopa provides most improvement in the motor manifestations, a definite response is regarded as a confirmatory test and is required for a diagnosis of clinically definite PD.[9]

Recognition and clinical diagnosis depend both on the classical features that Parkinson originally described, plus other features that, over the years, have been recognized to be associated with PD.

A clinical diagnosis of PD mandates two out of the three principal signs:

- Resting tremor
- Bradykinesia
- Rigidity

Supportive features include the following:

- Postural instability (often *not* present early)
- Expressionless face
- Speech problems (including hypophonia and dysarthria)

Box 50-1 Clinical Diagnostic Criteria for Idiopathic Parkinson's Disease

"Clinically possible"
One of:
- Asymmetric resting tremor
- Asymmetric rigidity
- Asymmetric bradykinesia

"Clinically probable"
Any two of:
- Asymmetric resting tremor
- Asymmetric rigidity
- Asymmetric bradykinesia

"Clinically definite"
- Criteria for clinically probable
- Definitive response to antiparkinsonian drugs

Exclusion criteria
- Exposure to drugs that can cause parkinsonism such as neuroleptics, some antiemetics, tetrabenazine, reserpine, flunarizine, and cinnarizine
- Cerebellar signs
- Corticospinal tract signs
- Eye movement abnormalities other than slight limitation of upward gaze
- Severe dysautonomia
- Early moderate to severe gait disturbance
- Dementia *early* in the disease
- History of encephalitis, recurrent head injury (such as seen in boxers), or family history of Parkinson's disease in two or more family members
- Evidence of severe subcortical white-matter disease, hydrocephalus, or other structural lesions on magnetic resonance imaging that may account for parkinsonism

From Calne DB, Snow BJ, Lee C. Criteria for diagnosing Parkinson's disease. Ann Neurol 1992;32(Suppl):S125–S127 and Ward CD, Gibb WR. Research diagnostic criteria for Parkinson's disease. Adv Neurol 1990;53:245–249.

- Abnormal gait: reduced arm swing, flexed posture, freezing, and festination
- Loss of fine-motor skills (such as writing, with micrographia)
- Reduced upward gaze, positive glabellar tap, and decreased blinking
- Excessive sweating and seborrheic skin.

However, parkinsonian features are frequently seen in older individuals without PD.

Although L-dopa responsiveness (see above) can help differentiate classical PD in most instances, an initial response to levodopa can occur in non-PD patients such as in Lewy body dementia (DLB) and multisystem atrophy. However, the *sustained* response to levodopa is confirmatory of PD, and it is the *motor* features that are most improved.

> ● Slow and rigid with a resting tremor: think Parkinson's, try levodopa

Other Clinical Features

Resting tremor, with a frequency of 3 to 5 Hz, is the first symptom in 70% of PD patients. Tremor is frequently asymmetric at onset and worsens with anxiety, with contralateral motor action, and with ambulation.

Muscular rigidity is resistance noted during passive joint movement in the normal range of motion of that joint. It may have a cogwheeling feature. It is often more prominent in the most tremulous extremity. Rigidity is increased by contralateral motor movement or a mental task.

Bradykinesia causes the most dysfunction in the initial stages of the illness. The patient is unable to perform fine-motor tasks effectively. Observing a patient suspected of having PD tying their shoelaces or writing a sentence can be helpful in diagnosis.

Postural instability onsets insidiously with progressively poor balance. It leads to increased fall risk. It can be demonstrated by testing for postural reflexes by pulling the patient forward (propulsion) or backward (retropulsion) to check for balance recovery.

Gait dysfunction is characterized as shuffling, slow walking, and by turning "en bloc."

Freezing is shown by difficulty initiating walking or by striking gait hesitation, on turning or on arriving at a real, or perceived, (Box 50-2) obstacle.

Autonomic dysfunction is common and causes bowel and bladder dysfunction and orthostatic hypotension.[10]

Dementia develops in about 40% of PD patients,[11] although in a study that followed patients until death, it was present in more over 80% in the end stage.[12] The combination of dementia and anti parkinsonian drugs can lead to *hallucinations and psychotic symptoms* in some.

Depression is common, affecting nearly half of patients.[13]

Box 50-2	Principles for Management of Parkinson's Disease in the Elderly

- Avoid (or stop) anticholinergics!
- Doses should start low and raise gradually.
- Lack of levodopa responsiveness may mean inaccurate diagnosis.
- Falls, decline in activities of daily living and aspiration are common problems, requiring a geriatrician and a multidisciplinary approach.
- Polypharmacy, poor compliance, and doctor shopping are all dangers.

Sensory symptoms in PD are quite varied and include pain.[14]

Disturbed sleep is common. Causes include nocturnal stiffness, nocturia, depression, restless legs syndrome, and REM (rapid eye movement) sleep behavior disorder.[15]

DIFFERENTIAL DIAGNOSIS

Essential tremor is the most common tremor and tends to be familial. It typically is first noted when it interferes with eating.[16] It tends to be bilateral but is frequently asymmetric. The frequency is higher (4 to 8 Hz) than in PD; in older patients the frequency is low in the range. In advanced cases, essential tremor can be present at rest and thus confused with PD; an older person may have both! If rigidity and bradykinesia are present, a trial of levodopa may be appropriate.

The following differential diagnoses are summarised in Table 50-1.

Drug-induced parkinsonism occurs after exposure to neuroleptics,[17] antiemetics, promotility agents, and some calcium-channel blockers. Symptoms are symmetric. It characteristically resolves when the drug is stopped, although resolution can take weeks or months.

Progressive Supranuclear Palsy (PSP) is a rare disorder. Onset is in the 50s. Approximately 4% of parkinsonian patients have PSP. It progresses rapidly and is characterized by oculomotor disturbance, speech and swallowing difficulties, imbalance with falls, and frontal dementia.[18] It is symmetric. Postural instability occurs early. Additional clinical manifestations include severe axial rigidity, absence of tremor, and a poor response to dopaminergic treatment. The defining characteristic is supranuclear gaze palsy, especially of downward gaze. Marked incapacity occurs within 3 to 5 years of onset, with death typically within 10 years.

Table 50–1	Distinguishing Parkinson's Disease from its Differential Diagnosis					
Disease	Bradykinesia and Rigidity	Tremor	Dementia	Other Features	L-dopa Responsiveness	Antipsychotic Sensitivity
Parkinson's disease	Yes Limb	Yes		More common in late onset	Yes	+
Drug-induced	Yes Limb	No			No	++
Progressive supranuclear palsy	Yes Axial	No	Yes, early	Loss of conjugate gaze (especially downward)	No	
Lewy body dementia	Yes Axial	No	Yes, early	Hallucinations	Yes, initially	+++
Vascular parkinsonism	Yes Limb	No	Yes, in some	Pyramidal signs	No	+
Multisystem atrophy	Yes	No	Yes	Pyramidal, cerebellar signs (OPCA) Dysautonomia	Yes, initially	

From Chan DKY. The art of treating Parkinson disease in the older patient. Aus Fam Physician 2003;32:927-931.

Multiple System Atrophy (MSA) involves the central, autonomic, and peripheral systems. The prominence and severity of autonomic dysfunction differentiates it from PD. The term multisystem atrophy includes a cluster of diseases previously regarded as separate entities: Shy-Drager syndrome, olivopontocerebellar atrophy, and striatonigral degeneration.[1] There is no response to levodopa. Presentation is with parkinsonism, cerebellar and autonomic dysfunction (orthostatic hypotension, bladder and bowel dysfunction, temperature dysregulation), and pyramidal dysfunction in various combinations. MSA-P (formerly called striatonigral degeneration) is characterized by symmetric parkinsonism without tremor and early, pronounced postural instability. MSA-C (formerly called olivopontocerebellar atrophy) manifests with cerebellar signs and parkinsonism. Corticospinal tract signs and respiratory stridor occur in all categories of MSA.

Dementia of Lewy Body Type (DLB) is a progressive dementia, which is often the primary, initial clinical feature, but occasionally the presentation more suggests an atypical depressive disorder. As the illness progresses, parkinsonian features develop, and in some cases, there are complex visual hallucinations, which are regarded as one of the "psychiatric" hallmarks of this particular dementia.[19] Unfortunately, there is marked sensitivity to the parkinsonian (extrapyramidal) side effects of neuroleptics (both the traditional and the "atypical" antipsychotics). Once a clinical diagnosis of DLB is established, these medications should not be used as it is probable that permanent neurological damage may occur. Resting tremor is rare. Frontal lobe disinhibited behaviors are often present. Sleep disorders can occur.

Dopaminergic treatment produces no improvement in motor manifestations. Cognition can be relatively improved on cholinesterase inhibitor (ChEI).[20]

Normal pressure hydrocephalus (NPH) is another progressive primary dementia, classically presenting with concurrent gait dysfunction, urinary incontinence, and progressive dementia. Often the gait is the initial presentation, with a wide-based, shuffling gait. Tremor is usually absent. Brain imaging shows ventricular dilatation, the hallmark of the hydrocephalic process. There is no therapeutic response to dopaminergic treatment; however, especially if diagnosed early, NPH can be *reversed* by a ventriculo-vascular shunt, a relatively simple surgical procedure. Even the dementia can reverse, if treated early.

Vascular parkinsonism has a similar etiology to vascular dementia (VaD); that is, multiple infarcts occur. The infarcts in vascular parkinsonism are in the basal ganglia and the subcortical white matter.[21] As in NPH, tremor is absent, and there is no therapeutic response to dopaminergic treatment. Vascular parkinsonism tends to be accompanied by dementia, pseudobulbar affect, urinary symptoms, and pyramidal signs. Brain imaging showing extensive small vessel disease is supportive, and treatment is mostly the management of the vascular risk factors.

MANAGEMENT

The *key therapeutic strategies* for PD (see Box 50-2) include the following:

- Increased dopaminergic stimulation
- Decreased cholinergic stimulation
- Decreased glutamatergic stimulation

Mild Symptoms

Because many patients have motor complications from long-term levodopa, considerable work in recent years has evolved other antiparkinsonian therapies, especially for younger patients. Newer dopaminergic agents include ropinirole or pramipexole. These agents are less effective, but the incidence of motor side effects is much lower; however, they have other side effects (leg edema, sleepiness, and confusion) and are even more expensive. They are best used in younger patients, who are better able to tolerate these side effects.

Late complications of PD usually start 5 years after initiation of levodopa. These are primarily motor fluctuations and dyskinesia. Comorbidities in older people contribute to unacceptable side effects.

Brenda Wilmington *Part 2*

A therapeutic trial of levodopa/carbidopa (Sinemet) is begun. She does not improve. Two months later, weakness develops in her left arm and leg. Her postural instability becomes more pronounced and her stride more abbreviated. Over the next 2 years, she becomes increasingly dependent on others. She moves into a nursing home at her assisted-living community. Urinary urge incontinence develops. While walking with the assistance of two, she has a shuffling, freezing gait, and her cervical spine has a more forward flexed posture.

STUDY QUESTIONS

1. She had been initially diagnosed as having PD; is this diagnosis now in doubt?
2. How does her lack of response change your thinking?
3. At what point would you refer her to a neurologist?

Brenda Wilmington *Part 3*

You refer her to a neurologist, who diagnoses her with multisystem atrophy (a Parkinson's-plus syndrome). Three and a half years after her illness had begun, she has lost her residual ability to rise, stand, and walk. She is able to exchange superficial pleasantries but cannot provide details about the changes in her condition. She continues to enjoy social encounters with her husband and follows puzzle games with interest.

Her bowel hygiene requires aggressive efforts. Nearly 5 years after her first fall, she dies in her sleep.

Levodopa

The decision to begin symptomatic therapy in PD is determined by the patient's choice and by functionality. If gait or functional independence is affected, it should be considered earlier. The progression of PD over the years is not uniform. Anticholinergics are commonly used in the younger population, but side effects limit their use in the elderly.

Levodopa is currently the most effective drug for the symptomatic treatment of idiopathic or Lewy body PD, especially for bradykinesia and rigidity. It is generally combined with a peripheral decarboxylase inhibitor, carbidopa in the United States, to block its conversion to dopamine in the systemic circulation and liver; this reduces the peripheral effects of nausea, vomiting, and orthostatic hypotension. This mixture—*Sinemet*—in the immediate release form is available in 10/100, 25/100, and 25/250 mg combinations (carbidopa/levodopa).

The starting dose is generally one-half tablet of Sinemet 25/100 mg three times daily, titrated upward over several weeks to 25/100 mg three times daily, as tolerated and according to the response. "Start low and go slow" is the rule, owing to adverse reactions, especially if dementia is present. There is a wide range of dose response in the elderly. The majority of those with idiopathic PD have a significant therapeutic response to moderate doses (400 to 600 mg/day). No response to 1000 to 1500 mg/day strongly implies that the diagnosis should be reviewed! Controlled-release Sinemet is less well absorbed, requiring doses up to 30% higher than the immediate release form; each tablet is typically less dramatic in effect than the immediate-release preparation, as the controlled-release form penetrates more slowly to the brain. Thus, therapy should start with an immediate release preparation, switching to controlled release when stabilized.

Sinemet should be *taken on an empty stomach* 1 hour before or after meals because of competitive absorption of other amino acids. This is more crucial in advanced disease with motor fluctuations. Unfortunately, initial *nausea* from levodopa is more likely on an empty stomach. So patients who become nauseous should take it with a snack or after meals. However, nausea is often because of *insufficient carbidopa*; manage this with supplemental carbidopa (Lodosyn) or with antiemetics such as trimethobenzamide (Tigan) before the Sinemet. Phenothiazine antiemetics and metoclopramide (Reglan) should be *avoided*; they can themselves cause drug-induced parkinsonism!

● Nausea on Sinemet? Try more carbidopa

Increasing the *duration* of the patient's responsiveness to levodopa can sometimes be achieved by taking the levodopa on an empty stomach, at least 30 minutes before meals or at least 45 minutes after meals. Increasing the levodopa dosage should also be tried if responsiveness drops. If these measures fail or cause unacceptable side effects, an adjunctive therapy should be tried (see below).

Neuroprotective Agents

Vitamin E, selegiline, and coenzyme Q10 have been studied as potential neuroprotective agents to slow disease progression. Vitamin E was not beneficial in a large multicenter trial of patients with early PD.[22] Selegiline, initially promoted as neuroprotective, is effective in delaying initiation of levodopa, but selegiline itself relieves motor symptoms. Whether selective monoamine oxidase B inhibitors are neuroprotective is an open question.

Motor Complications

Motor fluctuations and dyskinesia occur as the disease progresses. Such motor complications develop on average 5 years after therapy has been initiated, impacting about half of all patients. With advancing disease, the "wearing-off" effect is the most common type, but "delayed-on," "no-on," and "on-off" effects, as well as dyskinesias, occur.

Motor complications are a major cause of disability in advanced PD patients, so their alleviation is a major goal of patient management.

Adjunctive medications may reduce the frequency or duration of "off" periods, but none does so completely and each contributes its own side effects, which limit optimal dosing.

Surgery is another strategy to reduce "off" time; both pallidotomy and deep brain stimulation (DBS) of the globus pallidus or the subthalamic nucleus have been shown to be highly effective in this regard. However, surgery may be contraindicated in advanced elderly patients who could potentially most benefit from its effect on "off" time.

Motor fluctuations—After a number of years, the duration of responsiveness to levodopa becomes shorter, the "wearing off" reaction. Some patients react to "off" states with panic attacks, screaming, or even drenching sweats.[23] With disease progression, there is a tendency for the fluctuations to become increasingly less predictable. The "on-off" effect is the most unpredictable of these states.

Dyskinesias can, similar to periodic immobility, be induced by levodopa. They usually accompany the "on" state. The most common type is seen at the peak of the clinical effect of levodopa ("peak-dose" dyskinesias). The movements are typically choreiform or dystonic, and range from mild and of no consequence to severe and disabling. Most medical strategies for reducing "off" states can cause increased dyskinesias as a side effect; so a therapeutic balance must be found.

Adjunctive Medications

Adjuncts to levodopa have been shown to reduce the overall quantity of "off" time in patients with motor fluctuations. Other drugs without such an Food and Drug Administration–approved indication are also useful. With the exception of amantadine, these drugs have dopaminergic effects, with either longer half-lives or an ability to extend the half-life of levodopa, thus leading to more continuous dopaminergic stimulation. None of these completely relieve the "off" time problems.

Amantadine has been used for years as a treatment for early PD. More recently, it has been studied for its effects in fluctuating disease. Its most impressive effect in advanced PD is its efficacy against dyskinesias; one report shows a reduction in the severity of dyskinesias by 60%.[24] Problems that limit the wider use of amantadine in the elderly include edema of the legs, with a characteristic rash (livido reticularis), plus hallucinations and anticholinergic effects.

Dopamine agonists—Bromocriptine was the first of these to be used clinically. Others now available include cabergoline, pergolide, pramipexole, and ropinirole. They are useful in reducing "off" time because their half-lives are longer than that of levodopa: 27 hours for pergolide, 8 to 12 hours for pramipexole, and 6 hours for ropinirole. These drugs should be used cautiously. The dose is increased gradually over 4 to 8 weeks to an optimal level. If dyskinesia occurs, reduction of levodopa may be required. Motor score improvement is seen in around 20% to 35% of patients.[25] Because their antiparkinsonian efficacy is significantly less than that of levodopa, they work primarily by improving "off" episode disability. Dopamine agonists reduces total daily "off" time by about 2 hours, leaving still considerable "off" time. Adverse effects often limit their use: orthostatic hypotension, delirium, nausea, and vomiting.

MAO-B inhibitors—Selegiline is the only monoamine oxidase type B (MAO-B) inhibitor available in the United States. It is now approved as adjunctive therapy in fluctuating PD. It is believed to decrease the central catabolism of dopamine by blocking MAO-B.

COMT inhibitors—The enzyme catechol-*o*-methyl transferase (COMT) is key to the peripheral catabolism of levodopa. Blocking it with COMT inhibitors (entacapone or tolcapone) lengthens the plasma half-life of levodopa by 40% to 80%.[26] Adverse effects are diarrhea and dyskinesia. Tolcapone has liver toxicity, so monitoring of liver function is recommended.

Controlled-release levodopa—Unfortunately, these only slightly lengthen the duration of action of levodopa. The therapeutic effects are more unpredictable than those of immediate-release levodopa, especially important in older patients. Controlled-release levodopa reduces "off" time by 20% to 70%, increases the total daily dose of levodopa by about 20%, yet decreases the number of doses by 30%.[27]

Treatment of Dyskinesia

Chorea or choreodystonia are dyskinesias that occur as a peak dose effect of levodopa. Dopamine agonists sometimes help by allowing a reduction of levodopa dosage; COMT inhibitors tend to *worsen* dyskinesias. Amantadine, 100 to 300 mg per day, may reduce dyskinesia through the inhibition of glutamate-mediated neurotransmissions, but anticholinergic side effects can be problematic. Low-dose propranolol (20 mg three times per day) has some potential. For pure dystonia that does not respond to levodopa adjustment, anticholinergics may be helpful, but again, side effects need to be balanced against benefits. Surgery (pallidotomy or DBS—pallidal and substantial nigra) may be considered. However, in general, patients over 70 have less favorable outcomes owing to higher complication rates.

Management of Tremor

A mild resting tremor that does not impact function does not warrant treatment. When the tremor is severe or effecting function, levodopa is the first-line treatment in the frail elderly. However, rigidity and bradykinesia do not respond so well. Although anticholinergics such as benztropine and benzhexol may be useful in managing tremor, the risks of anticholinergic side effects (delirium, hallucinations, dry mouth, worsening prostatism, constipation, and blurred vision) usually outweigh the benefits; in patients with cognitive impairment, anticholinergics must be avoided.

Amantadine has no effect on tremor. Propranolol may reduce tremor amplitude in the anxious. Clozapine may be beneficial, but the mechanism is unclear and rare and severe side effects (agranulocytosis, myocarditis and cardiomyopathy) limit its use.

Box 50–3	**The 4Ds That Affect Treatment of Parkinson's Disease in Elderly**

Dementia—anticholinergics can worsen or precipitate delirium

Dysautonomia—postural hypotension (especially as most Parkinson's treatment tends to cause or exacerbate this)

Depression—common, coexists, needs to be treated

Dyskinesia and motor fluctuations—in late disease, difficult to treat

From Chan DKY. The art of treating Parkinson disease in the older patient. Aus Fam Physician 2003;32:927-931

Symptomatic Treatment of Motor Symptoms

Symptomatic treatment is begun when symptoms become bothersome or cause disability. Because dopamine agonist monotherapy rarely causes dyskinesia, treatment of early PD in younger and healthier patient generally *begins* with dopamine agonists; but because of their adverse effect profile in elderly people, levodopa is the preferred initial drug in the old and frail and is less expensive. It remains the most potent antiparkinson drug and is the backbone of treatment throughout much of the disease course. Most patients started on dopamine agonist therapy will need the addition of levodopa within 5 years. This drug is combined with carbidopa or benserazide to prevent peripheral conversion to dopamine by dopa-decarboxylase. Side-effects of levodopa are similar to those of dopamine agonists, except that somnolence, hallucinations, and leg edema are less common with levodopa than with dopamine agonists. Adding extra carbidopa or domperidone might reduce levodopa-induced nausea.

The primary cause of motor fluctuations is the short half-life of levodopa (90 to 120 min). Treatment for these fluctuations focuses on trying to improve absorption, altering timing of doses, and prolonging the effect of every dose. A high protein meal can reduce levodopa absorption and limit its ability to cross the blood-brain barrier. Spreading of protein intake throughout the day might help to reduce motor fluctuations. Prolongation of effects of every dose of levodopa can be achieved with controlled-release forms of levodopa but at the expense of making absorption somewhat more unpredictable. COMT inhibitors such as entacapone or tolcapone relieve end-of-dose wearing off by lengthening the half-life of circulating levodopa. Tolcapone is the most potent inhibitor, but small numbers of cases of fatal liver failure make it now unavailable in many countries. Dopamine agonists enhance effectiveness of levodopa and help to reduce off time.

Management of Nonmotor Symptoms

Autonomic dysfunction in patients with PD include orthostatic hypotension, constipation, urinary symptoms, and sexual dysfunction. Symptomatic orthostatic hypotension occurs in 15% to 20% of PD patients,[28] with potentially devastating results, such as falls. This may be from autonomic dysfunction but is also a side effect of many PD treatments. Reduction of the dose of antiparkinson drugs, enhancement of salt and fluid intake, and addition of fludrocortisone or midodrine are treatment options for hypotension. If systolic hypertension coexists, pindolol may be useful. Aggressive management of constipation entails escalation of water and fiber intake, addition of fiber supplements (e.g., psyllium), and use of stool softeners, suppositories, and enemas. Urinary urgency can be treated with peripheral anticholinergic drugs (oxybutynin and tolterodine) but is limited because of the side effects; adrenergic-blocking agents (prazosin and terazosin) unfortunately exacerbate hypotension.

Depression effects about 40% of PD patients.[29] Coexistent depression may significantly effect both the symptoms and rehabilitation efforts. An unblinded study has shown selective serotonin reuptake inhibitors (SSRIs) to be useful.[30,31] No head-to-head studies have been done to suggest one drug is superior to another in PD. Tricyclics can exacerbate orthostatic hypotension. In hypotensive patients, venlafaxine may be the drug of choice because it increases blood pressure. Lithium may worsen Parkinsonism.

Disorders of sleep in PD include daytime somnolence and sleep attacks, night-time awakenings attributable to overnight rigidity and bradykinesia, REM sleep behavior disorder, and restless legs or periodic limb movements. Daytime somnolence and sleep attacks have been linked to dopamine agonists and patients should be warned of these adverse effects. The prevalence has been estimated to be as high as 50%.[32] Elimination of the agonist or even use of a stimulant might be necessary. Patients and families should be warned about safety issues such as driving. Night-time awakenings and restless legs can be alleviated with a bedtime dose of long-acting levodopa or addition of entacapone. Low-dose clonazepam is very effective in treatment of REM sleep behavior disorder.

Psychosis is rare in untreated PD and is thought to be mostly drug-induced. Dopamine agonists are more likely to cause hallucinations than is levodopa. The first step in management is to discontinue the agonist or anticholinergic drug and to use the lowest levodopa dose possible. However, addition of an atypical neuroleptic is sometimes necessary. Two randomized, controlled trials have shown that clozapine is useful for symptoms such as visual hallucinations.[33,34] However, because of potentially fatal agranulocytosis, blood count must be measured every week or biweekly. Therefore, *quetiapine* (Seroquel) has become the most popular atypical neuroleptic in PD, in view of the absence of agranulocytosis and fewer extrapyramidal adverse effects than those of risperidone (Risperdal) and olanzapine (Zyprexa)-olanzapine can also cause agranulocytosis (less frequently than clozapine.). Findings of several open-label studies have suggested that dementia and psychosis in PD can be treated with ChEIs.

Dementia—Evidence is limited about this important aspect of treatment. One small randomized, controlled trial has shown that donepezil is useful in improving cognition in demented parkinsonian patients.[35] Another randomized trial has shown that rivastigmine is useful in dementia with Lewy bodies.[36] Cholinergic stimulation theoretically would be counterproductive in parkinsonism. Both anticholinergics and dopamine agonists should be avoided in patients with dementia because of the risk of increasing confusion. There is no evidence that one ChEI is superior to another in PD patients with dementia.

Surgical Treatment for Parkinson's Disease

There has been a resurgence of interest in surgical intervention in PD in the past few years, especially in patients who are poorly controlled with medication. With advancement in surgical technique and with new equipment being developed, surgical intervention should be considered when medical therapy is no longer effective.

There are two types of surgical treatment.

Ablative therapy, where parts of the brain (usually the globus pallidus) are surgically destroyed, is also known as a pallidotomy. The patient is usually awake during the procedure, so that the proper amount of tissue can be ablated to restore the balance between excitation and inhibition of movement. Pallidotomy is effective at reducing contralateral dyskinesias, as well as reducing symptoms such as bradykinesia. However, the procedure is not well tolerated in patients who have even a minor degree of cognitive impairment, or who are over 70 years old.

Deep brainstimulation (DBS) is the second type of surgery. Locations for placement of the stimulator include the globus pallidus, the subthalamic nucleus, or even the thalamus. DBS placement has the advantage of being adjustable as opposed to the permanent ablative treatment. The amount of energy sent through the device, as well as the rate at which the device operates, can be adjusted as the patient's symptoms progress. The procedure has similar benefits to ablative surgery in terms of reducing dyskinesia and bradykinesia but also may some additional benefit in terms of managing tremor (depending upon where the device is placed). DBS placement can have some complications, including bleeding and infection, hardware problems (such as dislocation of electrodes), or battery failure. The unit is expensive and requires considerable time to adjust parameters for optimal response.

SUMMARY

Levodopa therapy is the treatment of choice in elderly patients with PD. Doses should be started low and slowly titrated against motor response. Lack of levodopa response may mean a different diagnosis than PD. Dementia is more common in elderly patients with PD, and the use of anticholinergics is contraindicated owing to the risk of worsening confusion. Postural hypotension may limit the use of adjunctive therapy such as a dopamine agonists. Coexistent depression is common and needs to be addressed appropriately.

POSTTEST

1. Which of the following medications could worsen symptoms of Parkinson's disease?
   a. Sinemet
   b. Amantadine
   c. Haloperidol
   d. Entacapone
   e. Pramipexole

2. Mr. Smith is a 70-year-old man attends your office with a complaint of tremor of the mouth. He has a hard time putting his thoughts together enough to give you a good history. On examination, you notice that he has repetitive lip smacking and tongue thrusting, along with occasional twisting truncal movements. Tone is somewhat increased throughout his body. He has no tremor in his arms or legs. What is the likely cause of his movements?
   a. Side effect from chronic antipsychotic medication
   b. Early Parkinson's disease
   c. Cerebellar disease
   d. Parkinson's-plus syndrome
   e. Essential tremor

References

1. Mark MH. Lumping and splitting the Parkinson plus syndromes: dementia with Lewy bodies, multiple system atrophy, progressive supranuclear palsy, and cortical-basal ganglionic degeneration. Neurol Clin 2001; 19:607-627.
2. Rajput ML, Rajput AH. Epidemiology of parkinsonism. In Parkinson's disease: diagnosis and clinical management (Factor SA, Weiner WJ, eds.). New York: Demos, 2002.
3. Baldereschi M, Di Carlo A, Rocca WA, et al. Parkinson's disease and parkinsonism in a longitudinal study: two-fold higher incidence in men. Neurology 2000;55:1358-1363.
4. Payami H, Larsen K, Bernard S, Nutt J. Increased risk of Parkinson's disease in parents and siblings of patients. Ann Neurol 1994;36:659-661.
5. Calne S, Schoenberg B, Martin W, Uitti RJ, Spencer P, Calne DB. Familial Parkinson's disease: possible role of environmental factors. Can J Neurol Sci 1987;14:303-305.
6. Priyadarshi A, Khuder SA, Schaub EA, Priyadarshi SS. Environmental risk factors and Parkinson's disease: a metaanalysis. Environ Res 2001;86: 122-127.
7. Morens DM, Grandinetti A, Reed D, White LR, Ross GW. Cigarette smoking and protection from Parkinson's disease: false association or etiologic clue? Neurology 1995;45:1041-1051.
8. Wakabayashi K, Takahashi H. Neuropathology of autonomic nervous system in Parkinson's disease. Eur Neurol 1997;38(Suppl 2):2-7.
9. Gelb DJ, Oliver E, Gilman S. Diagnostic criteria for Parkinson disease. Arch Neurol 1999;56:33-39.
10. Jost WH. Autonomic dysfunctions in idiopathic Parkinson's disease. J Neurol 2003;250(Suppl 1):I28-I30.
11. Emre M. Dementia associated with Parkinson's disease. Lancet Neurol 2003;2:229-237.
12. Cedarbaum JM, McDowell FH. Sixteen-year follow-up of 100 patients begun on levodopa in 1968: emerging problems. Adv Neurol 1987;45:469-472.
13. McDonald WM, Richard IH, DeLong MR. Prevalence, etiology, and treatment of depression in Parkinson's disease. Biol Psychiatry 2003;54: 363-375.
14. Quinn NP, Koller WC, Lang AE, Marsden CD. Painful Parkinson's disease. Lancet 1986;1:1366-1369.
15. Stacy M. Sleep disorders in Parkinson's disease: epidemiology and management. Drugs Aging 2002;19:7337-39.
16. Jankovic J. Essential tremor: clinical characteristics. Neurology 2000;54 (Suppl 4):S21-S25.
17. Jimenez-Jimenez FJ, Garcia-Ruiz PJ, Molina JA. Drug-induced movement disorders. Drug Saf 1997;16:180-204.
18. Rajput A, Rajput AH. Progressive supranuclear palsy: clinical features, pathophysiology and management. Drugs Aging 2001;18:913-925.
19. McKeith IG. Clinical Lewy body syndromes. Ann N Y Acad Sci 2000;920:1-8.
20. McKeith I, Del Ser T, Spano P, et al. Efficacy of rivastigmine inn dementia with Lewy bodies: a randomised, double-blind, placebo controlled international study. Lancet 2000;356:2031-2036.
21. Foltynie T, Barker R, Brayne C. Vascular parkinsonism: a review of the precision and frequency of the diagnosis. Neuroepidemiology 2002;21:1-7.
22. Parkinson Study Group. Effects of tocopherol and deprenyl on the progression of disability in early Parkinson's disease. N Engl J Med 1993;328:176-183.

23. Riley DE, Lang AE. The spectrum of levodopa-related fluctuations in Parkinson's disease. Neurology. 1993;43:1459-1464.

24. Verhagen Metman L, Del Dotto P, van den Muncklof P, Fang J, Mouradian MM, Chase TN. Amantadine as treatment for dyskinesias and motor fluctuations in Parkinson's disease. Neurology. 1998;50:1323-1326.

25. Ahlskog J E. Medical treatment of later stage motor problems of Parkinson's disease. Mayo Clin Proc 1999;74:1239-1254.

26. Waters C. Catechol-o-methyltransferase (COMT) inhibitors. In Parkinson's disease: diagnosis and clinical management (Factor SA, Weiner WJ, eds.). New York: Demos, 2002.

27. Hutton JT, Morris JL, Elias J, Imke S, Roman G. A double-blind, crossover comparison of controlled-release carbidopa/levodopa (CR-4) and Sinemet in advanced Parkinson's disease. Neurology 1988;38(Suppl 1):329.

28. Senard J M, Rai S, Lapeyre-Mestre M, et al. Prevalence of orthostatic hypotension in Parkinson's disease. J Neurol Neurosurg Psychiatry 1997;63:584-589.

29. Oertel W H, Hoglinger G U, Ceracheni T, et al. Depression in Parkinson's disease: an update. Adv Neurol 2001;86:373-383.

30. Rampello L, Chiecho S, Raffaele R, et al. The SSRI, Citalopram, improves bradykinesia in patients with Parkinson's disease treated with L-dopa. Clin Neuropharmacol 2002;25:21-24.

31. McDonald WM, Richard IH, DeLong MR. Prevalence, etiology, and treatment of depression in Parkinson's disease. Biol Psychiatry 2003; 54:363-375.

32. Hobson D, Lang A, Wayne Matine W, et al. Excessive daytime sleepiness and sudden onset sleep in Parkinson disease: survey by the Canadian Movement Disorders Group. JAMA 2002;287:455-463.

33. Parkinson Study Group. Low dose clozapine for the treatment of drug induced psychosis in Parkinson's disease. N Engl J Med 1999;340:757-763.

34. The Parkinson Study Group. Low-dose clozapine for the treatment of drug-induced psychosis in Parkinson's disease. N Engl J Med 1999;340: 757-763.

35. Aarsland D, Laake K, Larsen J, et al. Donepezil for cognitive impairment in Parkinson's disease: a randomised controlled study. J Neurol Neurosurg Psychiatry 2002;72:708-712.

36. McKeith I, Del Ser T, Spano P, et al. Efficacy of rivastigmine in dementia with Lewy bodies: A randomised, double blind, placebo controlled international study. Lancet 2000; 356:2031-2036.

PRETEST ANSWERS

1. b
2. d
3. c

POSTTEST ANSWERS

1. c
2. a

CHAPTER 51 Oral Problems

Barbara J. Smith, Ingrid H. Valdez, and Douglas B. Berkey

OBJECTIVES

Upon completion of this chapter, the reader will be able to:

- List the major risk factors for oral cancer, its sites, and its public health significance.
- Explain the increased susceptibility of older adults to dental caries and periodontal disease.
- Discuss the clinical significance of mouth dryness and its causes.
- Report the reasons why denture wearers need follow-up care.
- Review the factors preventing older people from seeking dental care and name the indications for immediate referral to a dentist.
- Discuss the role of oral hygiene in controlling plaque and dental diseases.
- Relate the benefits of good oral health to systemic health and the relationship of medical conditions to oral health.
- Know the American Heart Association guidelines for antibiotic prophylaxis in cardiac patients at risk for infective endocarditis.

PRETEST

1. Which one of the following is an outcome associated with poor oral health?
   a. Bacteremias of dental or periodontal origin
   b. Difficulty chewing solid food
   c. Changes in speech
   d. Declining self-esteem
   e. All of the above

2. Which one of the following trends in oral health of Americans is false?
   a. More natural teeth are being retained in old age.
   b. Institutionalized patients generally have poor oral hygiene.
   c. Most patients over 65 are toothless.
   d. The peak incidence of oropharyngeal cancer is in elderly persons.

3. Which one of the following statements about infective endocarditis is false?
   a. Prophylactic antibiotic coverage can prevent most cases of infective endocarditis.
   b. Clindamycin is the drug of choice in the American Heart Association guidelines for antibiotic prophylaxis.
   c. Infective endocarditis is correlated with poor dental and periodontal health.
   d. Tooth brushing and chewing can cause transient bacteremias.

Just as oral health is an important component of general health, oral disease can be detrimental to systemic health, particularly in the medically compromised elderly. Nutrition and food selection are adversely affected by poor dentition or ill-fitting dental prostheses.[1] Patients with valvular heart disease are at risk for infective endocarditis because of bacteremia from dental treatment if not premedicated. Patients with diabetes mellitus must maintain good oral health to support appropriate dietary intake and to avoid infection. Cancer patients being prepared for chemotherapy or head and neck radiation therapy require evaluation and treatment by a dentist to avoid acute and chronic oral complications.

Oral health is an essential part of primary care. Oral health screening and appropriate referral will contribute to the elders' quality of life. Good oral health has numerous benefits to systemic health. Dental health influences chewing, speaking, and swallowing, as well as self-image and self-esteem.

Ruth Decker, *Part 1*

Ruth Decker, a 69-year-old black woman, returns to your office for follow-up. You have been treating her depression, hypertension, and osteoporosis for several years. Current medications are amitriptyline, enalapril, estrogen, and calcium. Today she says "my teeth keep breaking off" and "they've caused a sore on my tongue." She states that an ulcer has been present "for months it seems." She has smoked one pack of cigarettes daily for the last 50 years. You inspect her mouth and find a 0.5 × 0.5 cm ulcer on the left lateral border of the tongue. The lesion is posterior to the tooth-bearing area and does not appear to be associated with physical trauma.

STUDY QUESTIONS

1. How is the smoking history relevant to oral health?
2. What suspicions are raised by the oral ulcer?

CASE DISCUSSION

Both the frequency and duration of Ms. Decker's smoking place her at increased risk for oral cancer. Any long-standing ulcer in the mouth raises suspicion of malignancy. Immediate referral to an oral surgeon or general dentist is indicated.

Ruth Decker, *Part 2*

The soft tissues of the mouth appear dry, glossy, and friable; no other discrete lesions are noted. Scanty saliva is observed in the floor of the mouth. There are many chipped and broken teeth, as well as brown spots near the gum line on several teeth where the gums have receded.

STUDY QUESTIONS

1. What could be contributing to the fractures of her teeth?
2. What is the most likely cause for her dry mouth?
3. How does it relate to her dental condition?

OROPHARYNGEAL CANCER

Prevalence and Impact

The American Cancer Society estimates that oropharyngeal cancer is the seventh most common of all new cancers in the United States. Approximately 70% of oral and pharyngeal tumors occur in the oral cavity.[3] Mortality is high due to diagnostic delay and the aggressive dissemination of squamous cell carcinoma, approximately 50% at 5 years. Blacks have a lower survival rate than do whites for both oral and pharyngeal sites. Morbidity is high among survivors and includes the complications of surgery (disfigurement and loss of oropharyngeal function) and radiation (loss of teeth, severe xerostomia, vascular damage).

Oral cancer can be life-changing because of major oral functional impairments (e.g., tasting and chewing, swallowing, and speaking) as well as possible disfigurement from extensive surgery, yet only 14% of U.S. adults reported receiving oral cancer examinations.[4]

Risk Factors and Pathophysiology

Nearly all tumors are squamous cell carcinomas that spread via the lymphatic system. Advanced age is the number one risk factor associated with development of oral cancer, which peaks in the late 70s (Figure 51-1).[5] Most oropharyngeal cancers are associated with tobacco use (including both smoked and smokeless

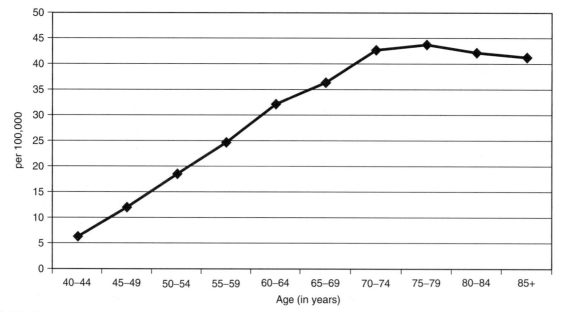

FIGURE 51-1

Age-specific incidence per 100,000 population of cancer of the oral cavity and pharynx (1998-2002) in the United States. About 70% of tumors occur in the oral cavity. Advanced age is the number one risk factor for oral cancer. Incidence increases with age, reaching 49.4 in persons 70-74 years old and declining slightly thereafter. Adapted from SEER Cancer Statistics Review; 1975-2002.

tobacco). Heavy smokers who are also heavy drinkers have a risk 15 to 20 times that of nonsmokers and nondrinkers.[3] Additional risk factors include certain viruses (e.g., human papillomavirus), black race, male gender, marijuana use, and low consumption of fruits and vegetables. Oral cancer carries an up to 20 times higher increased risk for a second primary cancer.[3]

Differential Diagnosis and Assessment

Early oral cancers are usually painless and often difficult to identify without a thorough assessment by a dental or medical professional. Oral cavity and pharyngeal cancers occur in anatomic sites that lend themselves to early diagnosis and treatment. Detection through periodic medical and dental examinations can significantly reduce the risk.

Unfortunately, many of the signs and symptoms of oral cancer are not present until later stages of the disease. These include:

- A mouth sore or lesion that fails to heal within 2 weeks or that bleeds easily
- A persistent white or red patch in the mouth
- A lump or thickening in the mouth, in the throat, or on the tongue
- Soreness in the mouth, in the throat, or on the tongue
- Difficulty chewing or swallowing food
- Difficulty moving the jaw or tongue
- Numbness of the tongue or other area of the mouth
- Swelling of the jaw that causes dentures to fit poorly or become uncomfortable

Biopsy is the most accurate method of diagnosing suspicious lesions. Excisional biopsy is usually performed on smaller lesions and multiple incisional biopsies may be indicated for larger diffuse lesions. When dealing with an area of significant mass, such as an enlarged lymph node, fine-needle aspiration cytology has found an increasing role. Cross-sectional imaging techniques which include computed tomography (CT) and magnetic resonance imaging (MRI) may help in the detection, characterization, local extension, lymphadenopathy, and/or metastasis of a mass.

Management

Treatment modalities depend on the stage of the cancer and usually incorporate surgery and radiation, with chemotherapy to decrease the possibility of a distant micrometastasis in localized cases or for those who have confirmed distant metastasis.

Oral cancer management is ideally multidisciplinary: surgeons, radiation oncologists, neuroradiologists, otolaryngologists, chemotherapy oncologists, dental practitioners (restorative and maxillofacial prosthodontists),

nutritionists, and rehabilitation and restorative specialists. Consider pain and symptom management, nutritional support, dental monitoring and care for radiation treatment effects, social services, and palliative care.

DENTAL CARIES

Prevalence and Impact

The proportion of Americans with natural teeth has grown over the past several decades. The average number of retained teeth has increased; this increases the potential for dental caries (tooth decay), which is common in this age group and the major cause of tooth loss. Dental cavities (caries) is the progressive destruction of tooth structure caused by acid metabolites of bacterial plaque (Figure 51-2). If untreated, caries can progress into the pulpal portion of the tooth, causing pain and a dental abscess, which may lead to bacteremia, facial/pharyngeal infection, septicemia, and brain abscess.

Nearly one-third of older adults have untreated dental caries; six out of 10 will experience a new coronal (that portion of the tooth covered by enamel) carious lesion within 3 years and average approximately one new carious surface *per* person *per* year.[6] Root caries is the most common type of tooth decay in the elderly. As the gum tissue (gingiva) recedes over the years, the tooth roots become exposed; this is termed recession. Over 86% of people over age 65 have moderate to severe recession. The roots are not protected by enamel and are prone to root caries. This type of decay progresses rapidly and will amputate the tooth at the gum line if untreated. Caries on tooth roots affect nearly 50% of those over the age of 75.[7]

> ● The quickest way to make many older patients feel better is to make their mouths more comfortable.

Risk Factors and Pathophysiology

Functional status is significant; institutionalized elderly may experience three times the prevalence of decayed teeth compared to community-living older adults.[8] This finding is likely related to medication induced dry mouth problems.

Functional status is significant; 25% of community-dwelling elders exhibit root caries, whereas 80% of institutionalized elderly do. This may be related to xerostomia in institutionalized elders, another risk factor for caries.

Differential Diagnosis and Assessment

Carious lesions in older adults are generally less symptomatic than in younger. Active surface lesions have a

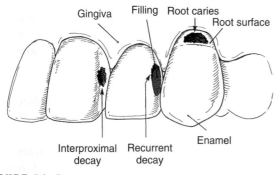

FIGURE 51-2

The most common form of dental caries in older adults is root caries: decay that attacks the portion of tooth not protected by enamel, that is, the root. Root caries may appear as a tan, orange, brown, or black discoloration in this area or as frank cavitation. Untreated root caries commonly amputates the tooth at the gumline. Recurrent caries develops adjacent to a filling at its margin. Interproximal caries occurs between teeth and may not be observed clinically.

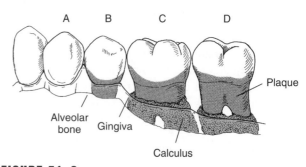

FIGURE 51-3

The periodontium consists of alveolar bone and gingiva, the anatomical foundation for sound teeth *(tooth A)*. This condition is maintained by thorough oral hygiene practices. When plaque bacteria accumulate on the teeth, gingivitis develops *(tooth B)*. The accumulation of plaque and calculus on teeth results in destruction of the periodontium known as periodontitis *(tooth C)*. Periodontitis is considered severe when over 50% of supporting bone has been lost *(tooth D)*.

yellowish brown color. Early root lesions are generally broad and shallow. Caries on coronal surfaces are typically associated with failing tooth restorations but can appear on a previously healthy portion of the tooth. Dental X-rays and transillumination are helpful in diagnosis.

Management

Timely treatment is very important. Dental amalgam, glass ionomer, and composite materials are used to conservatively restore the affected portions of the tooth. When affected areas are expansive, pins or other retentive approaches are used to enhance restoration longevity. When restoring more than half of the coronal portion of the tooth, full or partial coverage crowns (gold or porcelain) may be the best treatment.

PERIODONTAL DISEASE

Prevalence and Impact

Periodontal disease, or periodontitis, is a major cause of tooth loss in adults. It consists of a progressive destruction of the periodontium (gingiva and alveolar bone supporting the teeth), ranging from mild forms such as gingivitis to severe inflammatory disease that destroys the periodontal ligament and surrounding bone. Severe periodontal disease affects 14% of adults age 45 to 54; approximately 25% of older adults have loss of tooth-supporting structures because of advanced periodontal disease[9] (Figure 51-3).

Risk Factors and Pathophysiology

This chronic infection is caused by bacteria in dental plaque and calculus (mineralized plaque or tartar). The relationship between age and the prevalence and severity of periodontal disease is complex. Because periodontal disease is a progressive condition, its cumulative effects are often observed in older patients. It is characterized as episodic with frequent asymptomatic periods. Over 85% of dentate elderly individuals have some degree of periodontal disease. Poor oral hygiene, tobacco smoking, stress, osteopenia, osteoporosis, infrequent utilization of dental care, anaerobic pathogens, some medications (calcium channel blockers, immunomodulatory agents, anticonvulsants, others known to cause dry mouth), genetics, and salivary flow are important risk factors for periodontal disease.

Putative associations have been established between periodontal disease and various systemic conditions. Periodontal attachment loss is especially prevalent among diabetics. It has been assumed that diabetic patients are more prone to periodontal disease because they have a compromised ability to respond to infections. Periodontal disease may also exacerbate diabetes: severe periodontal disease at baseline is associated with increased risk of poor glycemic control two or more years later.[10] Clinicians should consider the periodontal status of diabetic patients having difficulty with glycemic control. Periodontal disease is modestly associated with diseases linked to atherosclerosis (e.g., cardiovascular disease, stroke, and peripheral vascular disease). The mouth may provide a significant nidus for respiratory pathogen colonization, leading to lower airway infection secondary to aspiration events in high risk patients.[11]

Differential Diagnosis and Assessment

Early disease is characterized by redness, bleeding, and edematous gingival tissues. As the disease progresses, alveolar bone and periodontal ligament destruction occurs, undermining supporting structures and resulting in tooth mobility. Periodontal pocket probing depths and radiographic imaging of alveolar bone support are important diagnostic components. Even in a person who is suffering from generalized periodontal disease, lesions are locally nested within an individual and usually act like an opportunistic infection. The entire oral cavity, including teeth, needs to be examined to determine the extent of periodontal disease.

Management

Treatment of periodontal disease is surgical as well as nonsurgical. Eradicating the microbial challenge in the mouth makes treatment difficult. The most important antimicrobial approach is promotion of oral hygiene by effective brushing, flossing, and tooth scaling by dental care providers. Other management strategies include more frequent dental visits, use of pharmacotherapeutics (e.g., chlorhexidine gluconate and Listerine), improved management of systemic diseases (e.g., diabetes, osteoporosis, immune system and connective tissue disorders), and locally applied and systemic antibiotics. Surgery is sometimes necessary to manage aggressive periodontal disease lesions as well as to improve bony architecture.

MOUTH DRYNESS

Prevalence and Impact

Xerostomia (the patient subjective complaint of mouth dryness) and hyposalivation (the objective reduction in salivary secretion) are correlated and prevalent problems in older adults. Prevalence has been estimated at 30% in persons over 65, and even higher with increasing age.[12] Adequate saliva is essential for maintaining oral and general health. Constant mouth dryness may reduce compliance with prescription medications; patients may alter dosage or stop the drug altogether. It may also restrict dietary choices and compromise nutrition by making chewing and swallowing uncomfortable, altering the taste sense, and disrupting food enjoyment. Lack of adequate salivation is associated with chronic esophagitis and gastroesophageal reflux disease.[13] In mouth dryness, the frequency and severity of dental caries are markedly increased: there is often rampant, rapidly progressive decay that is difficult to manage and more substantial periodontal disease. Also, the patient's ability to tolerate a denture is compromised by a lack of lubrication.

Risk Factors and Pathophysiology

Salivary flow does not decline with age; medical conditions and their treatment, rather than age, are associated with mouth dryness, which is most commonly associated with medications. Especially likely to cause mouth dryness are sedatives, antipsychotics, antidepressants, antihistamines, diuretics, and anticholinergics. Sjögren's syndrome (an autoimmune condition characterized by dry mouth and dry eyes) is the most common salivary gland disorder in the elderly leading to xerostomia. Reduced saliva may also be a result of patient dehydration, ductal obstructions (e.g., sialoliths or mucoceles), infections, tumors, and radiation therapy.

Differential Diagnosis and Assessment

The extra- and intra-oral mouth examination may yield various clinical signs. Dry, ulcerated, reddened, or furrowed lips and intraoral mucosa; generalized desiccated tissues with a lack of saliva pooling in the floor of the mouth; red, pale, or atrophic tissue appearance; and a fissured or inflamed tongue and the presence of halitosis may signal a dry mouth. Assessment can also be aided by palpating or "milking" the major salivary glands. An unexpected rise in dental caries and the presence of fungal infections may be sequelae of a dry mouth. The patient may also complain of xerostomia as well as having difficulty with swallowing, taste, speaking, and denture use.

Management

Preventive care is first in managing dry mouth; fluoride therapy, an antimicrobial mouth rinse, and reduction of refined carbohydrate consumption can mitigate the elevated risk of dental caries and periodontal disease. If a patient's medication is known to inhibit salivation, an alternative drug in the same class should be considered. Some have recommended modifying medication schedules so that the peak hyposalivary effect occurs during mealtime when there is a natural stimulus for salivation. Systemic salivary stimulants (pilocarpine and cevimeline) may be used, especially with Sjögren's syndrome, but should be avoided with glaucoma or pulmonary disease.

In many cases topical treatment using a "saliva substitute" may be helpful. Over-the-counter saliva substitutes such as Oral Balance gel (LaClede Products) and Saliva Substitute (Roxane Laboratory), and sugarless gum (BioTene sorbitol gum, LaClede Products) can help. Patients should avoid alcohol and caffeine because of diuretic effects.

● A dry mouth makes a patient feel ill: this can be treated, and it can often be prevented.

EDENTULOUSNESS

Prevalence and Impact

Although the proportion of Americans with natural teeth has grown steadily in recent years, edentulousness (toothlessness) remains a major health concern for U.S. elders. Edentulousness affects 28% of patients age 65 to 74, and 43% of patients over 75. More than half of the poor elderly have lost all their natural teeth. The presence of 21 or more natural teeth (a key determinant of function) is seen in only 41% of the 60 to 69 year olds and only 28% in the 80 plus group.[8] Many adverse outcomes include difficulty chewing solid food, undesirable dietary choices, trouble enunciating clearly, poor esthetics, and lowered self-esteem.

Up to 30% of denture wearers have oral lesions caused by the denture. Most lesions are inflammatory, infectious, or fibrous. As the fit and stability of dentures decrease, chewing efficiency is compromised. Regular dental care is essential for maintaining the functional benefits of dentures, and the health of the edentulous mouth.

Risk Factors and Pathophysiology

Dental caries and periodontal disease are the main determinants of tooth loss. Low-income individuals, and in particular low-income white adults, are most likely to be totally edentulous. Maintaining natural teeth is associated with exposure to community water fluoridation (particularly seen in the "baby boomer" population) and fluoride toothpaste, advances in dental technologies and treatment, changing patient and provider attitudes and treatment preferences, improved oral hygiene, and the regular use of dental services.

Differential Diagnosis and Assessment

A detailed intraoral examination should be performed to determine dentate status and utility of any prostheses. Dentures should be removed and tissues examined for oral mucosal lesions. Persons with *Candida*-associated denture stomatitis and angular cheilitis, traumatic ulcers, and denture irritation hyperplasia should be referred to the dental professional. Prostheses should be inspected to help determine functionality (retention, stability, and chewing capacity). Questions should be asked of the patient regarding his or her satisfaction with function and comfort.

Management

Complete dentures are the mainstay of treatment for restoring the edentulous mouth. Dentures are not fitted "for life"; they will get looser with time and need regular professional attention. The edentulous ridge (remaining alveolar bone) undergoes continuous resorption over the years, ultimately compromising the fit and stability of dentures. Only 13% of denture wearers seek annual dental care, and nearly half have not seen a dentist in 5 years.[5] Dental implant supported dentures may provide more functional capacity than less costly conventional dentures, but not every patient is an implant candidate.

William Cole, *Part 1*

Mr. Cole, an 86-year-old white male patient of yours, has had multiple health problems and hospitalizations over the past 20 years. He has survived prostate cancer, lung cancer, and chronic obstructive pulmonary disease (COPD). He has been clinically stable over the last few years, despite some difficulty maintaining his weight. At a routine follow-up visit, his wife reports, "he's not eating good" and "he has bad teeth."

STUDY QUESTIONS

1. What prevents an older patient from seeking dental care?
2. What should you do next?

LOW UTILIZATION OF DENTAL SERVICES

The elderly have the lowest dental services utilization rate of any age group. It is extremely common for an older patient not to have sought dental care for years. The primary reasons are that older persons do not perceive a need for dental care, dismiss oral problems as an inevitable part of aging, and do not have dental insurance. Only 15% of the elderly have any private dental insurance.[8] Unfortunately, Medicare does not reimburse for routine dental services; most state Medicaid programs provide limited coverage.

Older adults use medical services more frequently and repeatedly than dental services. Thus, it is primary care personnel who must screen for oral disease and make dental referrals. Primary care can be the link between the older patient and adequate dental care.

William Cole, *Part 2*

Mr. Cole has not seen a dentist since he first became ill. His wife states, "He's been in and out of the hospital so much, who has time to see the dentist?" Your screening examination reveals that all the upper teeth are decayed to the gum line, with some caries of the lower teeth as well. When questioned about this, Mr. Cole denies any symptoms related to the mouth but admits that "some foods" are difficult to chew.

STUDY QUESTIONS

1. Is the lack of symptoms consistent with the physical findings?
2. What can be done to improve dietary intake?

NEED FOR ORAL HEALTH SCREENING

Oral cancer screening reduces oral cancer mortality. The 50% survival rate among oral cancer patients has not improved significantly in the past 15 years. Early detection improves the prognosis; the 5-year survival for patients with distant metastasis at diagnosis is 18%, whereas the 5-year survival is 75% when disease is still localized at diagnosis. The American Cancer Society and American Dental Association recommend an oral examination annually for all elders. A panel of health care experts recently advocated routine oral examination by physicians for all individuals over age 65.[14] An annual examination is mandated by federal regulations for the institutionalized elderly.

Oral Health Screening

Screening for oral disease involves a few simple additions to routine examination technique. Questions on oral health are easily added to the review of systems (Table 51-1).

Older patients tend to have reduced symptoms: the presentation of oral disease may be altered, lessened, or delayed.

The screening examination includes extraoral and intraoral structures. The head and neck are inspected and palpated (Table 51-2). The oral soft tissues are inspected. The patient should remove dentures. Material such as food debris or denture adhesive can masquerade as a pathologic condition or obscure good vision, so the patient should rinse the mouth before the examination. Good lighting is essential. The highest risk locations for malignancy are the tongue and floor of mouth. To observe the lateral tongue, the clinician asks the patient to stick out the tongue. The clinician gently grasps the tip of the tongue with a gauze sponge and moves it laterally, with the mouth open wide. To observe the ventral tongue and floor of mouth, the clinician asks the patient to lift the tongue up to the roof of the mouth, with the mouth open wide. The remaining oral soft tissues are then inspected. Finally the teeth and gums are evaluated. Halitosis is often a sign of periodontal disease or poor oral hygiene. Findings that merit immediate referral to a dentist are summarized in Box 51-1.

Medical oral screening can miss occult disease of the jaws, periodontium, and dentition and includes chronic abscesses, periodontal disease, interproximal caries (decay between teeth) (see Figure 51-2), and root tips (necrotic teeth near the gum line). A thorough dental examination with X-ray is needed to rule these out.

Table 51-1 Oral Health Screening: History

To Assess	Ask About
Oral cancer risk	Age
	Smoking
	Drinking
	Sores in the mouth
Oral function	Trouble chewing
	Painful teeth
	Broken teeth
Self neglect	Last visit to a dentist
	Last time dentures were serviced
Dental caries	Cavities
	Food stuck between teeth
Periodontal disease	Bleeding gums
	Loose teeth
	Diabetic control
	Smoking
Xerostomia	Amount of saliva
	Mouth dryness when eating
	Medications, including those over the counter

Table 51-2 Oral Health Screening: Physical

Inspect	Look for
I. Masticatory muscles, including sternomastoid	Facial swelling
Salivary glands	Masses
	Lymphadenopathy
II. Lateral tongue	Masses
Ventral tongue	Erythroplasia (red lesion)
Floor mouth	Leukoplakia (white lesion)
Oropharynx	Erosion/ulceration
Palate	Dry, friable mucosa
Alveolar ridges	
Buccal mucosa	
Lips	
III. Dentition	Caries
Periodontium	Exposed roots/receding gums
	Fractured teeth
	Swollen gums
	Halitosis

Box 51-1	Reasons for Immediate Referral to a Dentist

- Tooth or gum pain
- Facial swelling/pus
- Mobile teeth
- Erythroplasia and/or leukoplakia
- Ulceration or erosion
- Foul odor

A patient with acute oral infection may seek emergency treatment from a primary care clinician. Dental infection may be characterized by pain in one specific tooth; the pain is typically unprovoked, continuous, and unremitting. Swelling may occur in the gingiva or vestibule or may progress to involve the fascial spaces. Medical management should include antibiotic therapy, pain control, and immediate referral to a dentist. Penicillin-V is generally considered the drug of choice for odontogenic infection. In the penicillin allergic patient, clindamycin is frequently the next drug utilized. Supportive care and hospitalization are needed in cases of advanced infection or debility.

Referral to a dentist has been emphasized here as the means of initiating individualized oral care for each patient, whether dentate or edentulous. A general dentist with interest and willingness to treat older patients is appropriate in most cases. The dental profession, as most health care fields, has become increasingly specialized. The primary care geriatrics team should be aware of these special interest areas. Geriatric dentists are emerging groups who have obtained additional training in geriatrics. Oral surgeons have extensive training in surgeries such as extractions, biopsies, and jaw reconstruction. Periodontists focus on the management of periodontitis, whereas endodontists restore the tooth with root canal therapy. Prosthodontists specialize in replacement of missing teeth. Hospital dentists and oral medicine specialists are often affiliated with medical centers and have training in the dental management of medically compromised patients.

PREVENTIVE AND LONG-TERM CARE

In recent decades, dental practice has changed dramatically with more emphasis on disease prevention and maintenance of the natural teeth. Dental research in the 1960s showed that dental caries and periodontitis are infectious diseases. These diseases can be prevented or controlled by eliminating dental plaque, (the complex of microorganisms that colonize the teeth and periodontium). Brushing and flossing are the chief methods of oral hygiene. Both procedures require an understanding of their purpose, as well as adequate eyesight and manual dexterity. These activities can be practiced by well-motivated, healthy elders. When cognition, vision, motivation, or dexterity is impaired, oral hygiene self-care declines and caregiver assistance is needed. The vast majority of nursing home residents, for example, have hard and soft deposits on their teeth, placing them at high risk for dental disease.

Chemotherapeutic adjuncts to mechanical plaque removal have an important role. Fluoride is effective in fortifying both enamel and root structure against decay. Prescription fluoride gels that are applied directly to the teeth are most effective. Antimicrobial agents such as chlorhexidine can also employed to reduce the oral microbial burden.

Long-term follow-up is recommended to maintain the oral health of both dentate and edentulous patients. The dentist typically establishes recall (reevaluation at intervals such as every 4 months, 6 months, or 1 year) for each patient based on the patient's condition.

William Cole, *Part 3*

Mr. Cole is referred to a general dentist, who finds that root caries has devastated his upper teeth. They are extracted, and a complete denture is fabricated. The lower teeth are preserved by routine fillings. Mr. Cole is placed on daily prescription fluoride therapy and scheduled for a 4-month recall. At follow-up, Mrs. Cole reports that her husband is eating a greater variety of solid foods than he has in years.

PREVENTING INFECTIVE ENDOCARDITIS

Infective endocarditis (IE) is a serious complication of dental treatment that may occur in susceptible patients. An increasing portion of patients with IE are aged 65 or older (55%).[15] Even with appropriate medical therapy, mortality ranges from 10% to 65%. A number of cardiac conditions place the patient at risk for endocarditis[16] (Table 51-3).

Invasive dental procedures and minor manipulations such as cleaning can result in transient bacteremia. Chewing and tooth brushing are associated with bacteremia. The frequency of such bacteremias is correlated to poor dental and periodontal health. In susceptible patients, blood-borne bacteria may lodge on damaged or abnormal heart valves or endocardium, resulting in bacterial endocarditis. *Streptococcus viridans* (alpha-hemolytic strep) is the most common cause of endocarditis after dental or medical procedures. Primary prevention is directed at this organism.

The clinician's goal is to prevent endocarditis from occurring in susceptible patients. To accomplish this, the clinician must

Table 51–3	Cardiac Conditions Associated with Endocarditis after Dental Procedures

Endocarditis Prophylaxis Recommended	Endocarditis Prophylaxis Not Recommended
High-Risk Category	**Negligible-Risk Category (No greater risk than the general population)**
Prosthetic heart valves	Isolated secundum atrial septal defect
Previous bacterial endocarditis	Surgical repair of atrial septal defect
Moderate-Risk Category	Previous coronary artery bypass graft surgery
Most other congenital cardiac malformations	Mitral valve prolapse without valvular regurgitation
Acquired valvular dysfunction (e.g., rheumatic heart disease, calcific aortic stenosis)	Physiologic, functional, or innocent heart murmurs
	Previous Kawasaki disease or rheumatic fever without valvular dysfunction
Hypertrophic cardiomyopathy (IHSS)	Cardiac pacemakers and implanted defibrillators
Mitral valve prolapse with valvular regurgitation	

Modified from Dajani AS, Taubert KA, Wilson W, et al. Prevention of bacterial endocarditis. Recommendations by the American Heart Association. JAMA 1997;277:1794-1801.

- Identify at-risk patients—Dentists often consult primary care providers to determine whether a patient is at increased risk owing to their cardiac status. Questions most often arise when the patient relates a history of a heart murmur (is it functional or organic?) or a history of rheumatic fever (is there evidence of rheumatic heart disease?). Patients who are at risk for IE should be informed about antibiotic prophylaxis for dental procedures.
- Use American Heart Association (AHA) guidelines for antibiotic prophylaxis (Box 51-2)[13]—This regimen involves one dose of oral amoxicillin before the procedure. Azithromycin or clindamycin is recommended for patients who are allergic to penicillins. If a patient is already taking penicillin for rheumatic fever or is taking penicillin for other reasons, azithromycin or clindamycin should be used for IE prophylaxis.
- Maintain good oral health to reduce the risk of bacteremia—Bacteremia of oral origin can be secondary to ordinary daily activities, particularly in those with poor oral health. Fewer than one in five cases of subacute bacterial endocarditis has, in fact, been associated with a dental or medical procedure. Patients should thus be encouraged to keep the mouth healthy through appropriate oral hygiene and dental follow-up visits. All at-risk patients should be referred to a dentist for counseling about the medical reasons for complying with dental recommendations.

Ruth Decker, *Part 3*

Ms. Decker is referred to an oral surgeon for evaluation of the tongue lesion. Excisional biopsy reveals a stage I localized squamous cell carcinoma with margins free of tumor. She also sees a general dentist who extracts the nonrestorable teeth, builds up the remaining teeth, and constructs partial dentures to replace the missing teeth. It is thought that the amitriptyline may be contributing to the patient's mouth dryness, so this is discontinued and she is given a trial of fluoxetine. On 6-month follow-up, Ms. Decker's depression is adequately controlled. She has regularly scheduled follow-up with her general dentist and oral surgeon.

PREVENTING LATE PROSTHETIC JOINT INFECTION

Artificial joints are vulnerable to bacterial colonization and infection from hematogenous seeding, especially in the first 2 years after joint replacement. Unlike IE, most prosthetic joint infections are caused by nonoral bacteria such as staphylococci. Thus, antibiotic prophylaxis is *not* routinely indicated for dental patients with total joint replacements.[17] Only those who are at increased risk are premedicated (Box 51-3). Use the identical AHA guidelines as for IE.

Box 51-2	American Heart Association-Recommended Prophylactic Regimen for Dental Procedures in Patient at Risk for Infective Endocarditis

Standard regimen:
- Amoxicillin, 2 g orally 1 hour before procedure

For penicillin-allergic patients:
- Clindamycin, 600 mg orally 1 hour before procedure
OR
- Azithromycin or Clarithromycin 500 mg orally 1 hour before procedure

Modified from Dajani AS, Taubert KA, Wilson W, et al. Prevention of bacterial endocarditis. Recommendations by the American Heart Association. JAMA 1997;277:1794-1801.

Box 51-3 Situations with Increased Risk of Hematogenous Total Joint Infection

- Rheumatoid arthritis
- Systemic lupus erythematosus
- Disease-, drug-, or radiation-induced immunosuppression
- Type 1 diabetes
- First 2 years after joint replacement
- Previous prosthetic joint infection
- Malnutrition
- Hemophilia

SUMMARY

Older adults exhibit a wide range of oral diseases and conditions, many of which can have a significant impact on systemic health. Because these conditions are among the most prevalent of chronic conditions experienced by older adults, the primary care physician must screen for dental problems and provide appropriate referral. Detecting oral cancer, mouth dryness, dental caries, and periodontal disease; preventing IE; and instituting a preventive approach to oral health in general are the major issues.

POSTTEST

1. Which one of the following is false concerning oropharyngeal cancer?
   a. It is most likely to occur in the aged.
   b. More tumors develop in the pharynx than in the oral cavity.
   c. Tobacco and alcohol are notable risk factors.
   d. Mouth dryness may be a complication of radiation treatment.

2. Which one of the following statements is true?
   a. Periodontal disease is generally an acute infection.
   b. Active dental caries is most frequently found on the enamel surfaces of the teeth.
   c. Dental caries is a common problem of the aged.
   d. Gingivitis is a very severe form of periodontal disease.

3. Which one of the following statements about mouth dryness is false?
   a. The clinical signs of mouth dryness include friable and glossy tissue.
   b. The most likely cause for dry mouth in the elderly is the physiological aging process.
   c. Xerostomia may lead to restricted dietary intake.
   d. Mouth dryness can lead to rapid and progressive dental decay.

4. Which one of the following statements is false?
   a. The vast majority of persons over 65 years old are totally edentulous.
   b. Alveolar bone resorption is a typical result of tooth extractions.
   c. Dental utilization rates for edentulous elderly are lower than utilization rates for those with teeth.
   d. Medical utilization rates exceed dental utilization rates for the elderly.

References

1. Ship JA, Duffy V, Jones JA, et al. Geriatric oral health and its impact on eating. J Am Geriatr Soc 1996;44:456-464.
2. American Cancer Society. Cancer facts and figures 2005. Atlanta, GA: American Cancer Society, 2005.
3. Swango PA: Cancers of the oral cavity and pharynx in the United States: an epidemiologic overview. J Public Health Dent 1996;56:309-318.
4. Centers for Disease Control and Prevention. National Health Interview Survey, 1998. Hyattsville, MD: National Center for Health Statistics, 1998
5. Ries LAG, Eisner MP, Kosary CL, et al. (eds): SEER Cancer Statistics Review, 1975-2002. Bethesda, MD: National Cancer Institute. http://seer.cancer.gov/csr/1975_2002/.
6. Griffin SO, Griffin PM, Swann, JL et al. New coronal caries in older adults: implications for prevention. J Dent Res 2005;84:715-720.
7. Griffin SO, Griffin PM, Swann, JL et al. Estimating rates of new root caries in older adults. J Dent Res 2004;83: 634-638.
8. Chalmers JM, Hodge C, Fuss JM, et al. The prevalence and experience of oral diseases in Adelaide nursing home residents. Aust Dent J 2002;47(2):123-30.
9. U.S Department of Health and Human Services. Oral health in America: a report of the Surgeon General. Rockville, MD: U.S. Department of Health and Human Services, National Institutes of Health, National Institute of Dental and Craniofacial Research, 2000.
10. Taylor GW, Burt BA, Becker MP, et al. Severe periodontitis and risk for poor glycemic control in patients with non-insulin-dependent diabetes mellitus. J Periodontol 1996;67:1085-1093.
11. Scannapieco F. Systemic effects of periodontal diseases. Dent Clin N Am 2005;49:533-550.
12. Ship JA, Pillemer SR, Baum BJ. Xerostomia and the Geriatric Patient. JAGS 2002;50:535-543.
13. Valdez IH, Fox PC. Interactions of the salivary and gastrointestinal systems, II: effects of salivary gland dysfunction on the gastrointestinal tract. Dig Dis 1991;9:210-218.
14. Sox HC. Preventive health services in adults. N Engl J Med 1994;330: 1589-1595.
15. Little JW, Falace DA, Miller CS, et al. Dental management of the medically compromised patient, 6 ed. St. Louis: Mosby, 2002.
16. Dajani AS, Taubert KA, Wilson W, et al. Prevention of bacterial endocarditis: recommendations by the American Heart Association. JAMA 1997;277: 1794-1801.
17. American Dental Association. American Academy of Orthopaedic Surgeons: advisory statement: antibiotic prophylaxis for dental patients with total joint replacements. J Am Dent Assoc 1997;128:1004.

Web Resources

http://www.oralcancerfoundation.org/treatment/pdf/guidelines.pdf.
http://www.cdc.gov/OralHealth/factsheets/adult-older.htm.
http://www.niapublications.org/engagepages/teeth.asp.

1. e
2. c
3. b

1. b
2. c
3. b
4. a

Skin Problems

Marlene J. Mash, Maria Fedor,
and Lucy Bonnington

OBJECTIVES

Upon completion of this chapter, the reader will be able to:

- Differentiate between chronologically aged and photo-aged skin.
- Describe and recognize the common benign dermatoses: solar lentigines, sebaceous hyperplasia, milia, acrochordons, seborrheic keratoses, Favre-Racouchot, xerosis and pruritus, erythema ab igne, seborrheic dermatitis, purpura, cherry hemangiomas, and venous lakes.
- Contrast the appearance of bullous pemphigoid, bullous erythema multiforme, allergic contact dermatitis, herpes zoster, and vesicular tinea pedis.
- Describe the appearance and management of the more common malignant skin neoplasms: actinic keratosis, basal cell carcinoma, squamous cell carcinoma, keratoacanthoma, and malignant melanoma.
- Arrange skin diseases by their color (flesh, white, brown, red, yellow, blue, and multicolored) to help classify the condition.

PRETEST

1. All of the following statements concerning skin changes in old age are true except:
   a. Seborrheic keratoses have a "stuck-on" appearance.
   b. Leathery, deeply furrowed skin is caused by sun exposure but not by chronologic aging.
   c. Sweat gland activity increases with age.
   d. Sebaceous glands increase in size but decrease in output with increasing age.

2. Multiple flat, scaly lesions, 2 mm to 1.5 cm in diameter, on sun-exposed areas of fair-skinned individuals are most likely:
   a. Benign
   b. Actinic keratoses
   c. Caused by xerosis
   d. Only cosmetically significant

Prevention remains the best treatment for every disease, including disorders of the skin. Both benign and malignant skin conditions can often be prevented by avoiding sun exposure or by using appropriate sunscreens. Understanding the difference between normally aged and photo-damaged skin not only helps clinicians convey the importance of these preventive measures but also helps the early detection of benign and malignant skin conditions. Early detection and appropriate management of these disorders reduce morbidity and are personally rewarding for both physicians and patients.

This chapter covers the recognition and treatment of the most common skin problems seen in the elderly population. Because a picture is worth a thousand words, color plates of pathologic skin changes found in the elderly patient are included. Physicians are encouraged to refine their diagnostic skills by using visual clues such as appearance and color (Table 52-1)

Walter O'Grady *(Part I)*

Mr. O'Grady is a 78-year-old, married, retired roofer who served on a battleship in the U.S. Navy in the South Pacific during World War II. His wife is concerned about a new growth on his ear. He has gout, which is well controlled on allopurinol (Zyloprim). He takes no other medications, drinks an occasional beer, and enjoys working in his vegetable garden. He has rarely worn sunscreen, despite his wife's urgings. On physical examination, Mr. O'Grady has a ruddy complexion, sparse and close-cropped gray hair, and blue eyes. The skin of his face and neck are furrowed and appear leathery and rough (Plate 1). He has many raised, rough, scaly patches less than 1 cm in diameter distributed over his scalp, forehead, temples, and cheeks. He has deep periocular and lateral temporal wrinkling, and thickening of the skin. A conical, skin-colored, bud-shaped lesion arising from his right helix measures 59 mm with 3 mm of elevation (Plate 2).

The dorsal aspects of Mr. O'Grady's forearms and hands show the same scaly patches seen on his face and scalp, but the upper arms are spared. Interspersed with these areas are multiple, blanchable telangiectasias. The skin beneath his undershirt is milky white and smooth, and his back and chest are dotted with multiple discrete, bright red papules varying in size from 3 to 5 mm in diameter. A few 1- to 2-cm, oval, brown, raised lesions appear "stuck on" to the skin on his upper back.

STUDY QUESTIONS

1. You suspect Mr. O'Grady has which of the following?
   a. Skin changes resulting from chronologic aging
   b. Skin changes resulting from photo-aging
   c. Actinic keratoses (AKs)
   d. Seborrheic keratoses
   e. Skin cancer
2. Which changes can be attributed to the patient's occupational history?
3. Which skin lesions require medical intervention?
4. Which lesions warrant surgical biopsy or excision?
5. What other disease processes would you include in your differential diagnosis?

PATHOPHYSIOLOGY

Normal Aging Versus Photo-aging of the Skin

At one time or another we have all observed how the sun-exposed skin of whites develops signs of premature aging. This prematurely aged look is really an acceleration of the normal aging process caused by cumulative exposure to the ultraviolet (UV) radiation present in sunlight. Deep wrinkling, irregular pigmentation, telangiectasias, yellowing, and a dry, leathery appearance of the sun-exposed areas of the skin are usually seen. In addition to causing a prematurely aged look, chronic sun exposure also increases an individual's risk of basal cell cancer, AKs, squamous cell cancer, and malignant melanoma. Many people in the United

Table 52–1	Common Skin Lesions in Old Age (Color and Type)				

Lesion	Type		Lesion	Type
Skin-colored			**Multicolored**	
Actinic keratoses	P		Malignant melanoma (brown)	M
Basal cell carcinoma	M		**Red**	
Dermal nevi	N		Cysts (inflamed or infected)	N
Epidermoid (sebaceous) cyst	N		Cherry hemangiomas	N
Lipomas	N		Erythema nodosum	N
Keratoacanthoma	N		Erythema ab igne	N
Molluscum contagiosum	N		Hypersensitivity reactions	N
Seborrheic keratoses	N		Erythema	N
Skin tags	N		Urticaria	N
Squamous cell carcinoma	M		Erythema multiforme	N
Warts	N		Toxic epidermal necrolysis	N
Brown			Vasculitis	N
Dermatofibroma	N		Insect bites	N
Compound nevus[a]	N		Seborrheic dermatitis	N
Dysplastic nevus	P		**White**	
Freckles	N		Milia	N
Junctional nevus	N		Pityriasis alba	N
Lentigines	N		Postinflammatory hypopigmentation	N
Blue			Tinea versicolor	N
Blue nevus	N		Vitiligo	N
Nodular malignant melanoma	M		**Yellow**	
Kaposi's sarcoma (red or brown)	M		Sebaceous hyperplasia	N
Venous lakes (bluish-red)	N		Xanthomas	N

M indicates malignant; N, nonmalignant; and P, premalignant.
[a]Biopsy if suspicious.

States still think that a suntan looks healthy, whether acquired on a beach or in a tanning salon. As a result, the incidence of all types of skin cancer has increased at an alarming rate. In contrast to the clinical features of the photo-aged skin (leathery appearance and deep wrinkles), chronologically aged skin has shallow, fine wrinkles and is finer in texture (see Table 52-2 and Plates 1–3).

Clinical Features of Elderly Skin

Clinically, it is difficult to make a distinction between the basic biologic effect of aging and the effect of photo-aging on the skin. Over the past decade, a considerable amount of research to define these two separable effects on the skin at the cellular level has been conducted.[1-3] Without question, the most damaging and cosmetically compromising effects on the skin have been found to be environmental and, more specifically, attributable to repeated sun exposure. Sun exposure far outweighs aging itself as a cause of pathologic and cosmetic changes in the skin in old age.

Walter O'Grady *(Part II)*

CASE DISCUSSION

Mr. O'Grady's skin changes are the result of both chronologic aging and photo-aging. The pronounced ruddiness of his complexion with scaly patches (AKs) and telangiectasias on his face and arms stem from the cumulative occupational sun exposure, beginning with his early service on a ship in the ocean and later his work as roofing contractor. Vegetable gardening since his retirement provides relaxation and continued exposure to UV radiation. The lesion on his left helix was removed by shaving it flat with a blade and electrodesiccating the base of the lesion. The pathology report from the excisional biopsy of the lesion on his ear confirms a hyperplastic solar keratosis. Mr. O'Grady's history of gout raised the question of a gouty tophus. Liquid nitrogen was applied to the multiple AKs covering his sun-exposed skin. The seborrheic keratoses (SKs) were not treated because they were not irritated and the patient was reluctant to have any nonessential surgery. Mr. O'Grady was counseled on the need for preventing further photo-damage to his skin and was asked to avoid the midday sun and to wear a wide-brimmed hat, long-sleeved shirt, and a sunscreen with a skin protection factor (SPF) of 20 while working in the garden. He made an appointment for another skin check in 6 months.

Frances West *(Part I)*

Mrs. Frances West is a 62-year-old housewife who enjoys playing golf and tennis with her husband and their friends several times a week. She is concerned about her appearance, specifically some "age spots" on her forehead and cheeks and "crow's feet" around her eyes; she says they make her look old. She washes her face with cold cream only, wears little makeup (preferring her "naturally" tan skin), but does use a sunscreen (SPF 8) when on the golf course or tennis court.

On physical examination Mrs. West has several 3-mm, yellow nodular lesions that appear to have a central pore or depression scattered over her cheeks and forehead. Multiple 1-mm white papules appear over the malar eminences and upper eyelids near the eyebrows.

Her neck is circled by small fleshy pedunculated growths, with one or two occurring bilaterally in the axillae. Her upper chest and shoulders are spotted with flat tan macules from 3 to 5 mm in diameter in the areas not covered by her tennis costume (Plate 3). A 1 × 1-cm, flat pigmented lesion with a variegated brown-red color and irregular border is on her right shin midway between her knee and ankle (Plate 4). Also noted are some superficial reticular varicosities over both thighs and lower legs, and the skin is somewhat dry and scaly to touch.

STUDY QUESTIONS

1. Which of Mrs. West's physical findings requires immediate evaluation?
2. Arrange the following potential interventions in the order you would perform them beginning with immediate:
   a. Sclerotherapy for venous varicosities of the legs
   b. Laser ablation of sebaceous hyperplasia of the face
   c. Excision of a malignant lesion of the lower leg
   d. Milia extraction
   e. Shave removals of acrochordons of the neck
   f. Punch biopsy of malignant lesion of the leg
   g. Skin care counseling
   h. Topical tretinoin for reversal of photo-aging
3. Which procedures are not indicated?

BENIGN DERMATOSES

Solar Lentigines

Solar lentigines ("brown spots" or "liver spots") are circumscribed, pigmented, nonmalignant macules (Plate 3). They are approximately 0.5 cm in diameter and induced by both natural and artificial sources of UV radiation. In rare cases and over a period of many years, lentigines develop into a melanoma (lentigo-maligna melanoma). These malignant lesions are usually larger than lentigines (ranging from 3 to 6 cm), and they are irregularly pigmented and irregularly shaped with irregular borders, whereas lentigines are usually circumscribed. If adequate treatment of a lentigo-maligna melanoma (i.e., complete surgical excision with adequate margins) is not provided, there is a 50% chance that the lesion will become invasive malignant melanoma and a 10% chance that it will metastasize (Plate 4).[2]

Milia

Milia are the 1-mm, white, epidermal cysts frequently seen on sun-damaged facial and periorbital skin. Patients sometimes need to be reassured that these cysts are not malignant and can be removed with a comedone or needle extractor for cosmetic reasons. Soap-free cleansers for the face are helpful in preventing the recurrence of milia. Patients should be advised to switch from their super-fatted soaps to one of the soap-free cleansers (e.g., Cetaphil or Ionil).

Seborrheic Keratosis

Brown-black, "stuck-on" lesions resembling barnacles, sometimes called *postage stamp lesions*, are common in the elderly and can appear anywhere on the body. They occur most frequently in the seborrheic areas (e.g., the back, chest, face, and inframammary areas) (Plate 5). SK has a hereditary predisposition and is not related to sun exposure. Most elderly patients have at least one SK, but multiple SKs are more common. Patients often feel that these lesions are cosmetically unacceptable. Superficial removal of the lesions can be accomplished by using a razor blade held parallel to the skin surface.[4] All specimens should be submitted for pathologic diagnosis.

Favre-Racouchot Syndrome

Favre-Racouchot syndrome encompasses a variety of primarily sun-induced skin changes, including nodular elastosis with cysts and comedones (Plate 6) and alterations in the superficial vascular system and pigmentation. Changes in the vascular system, such as friable, thin blood vessels, cause persistent erythema and telangiectasias. Irregular melanocyte distribution, with alteration in pigmentation, can be seen as multiple areas of hyperpigmentation, hypopigmentation, and scattered lentigines. Sebaceous hyperplasia can also be observed.

Erythema Ab Igne

"Redness from the fire" (Plate 7) is the clinical manifestation of the presence of melanin and hemosiderin in the dermis. Hyperpigmentation, hypopigmentation, telangiectasias, and atrophy of the skin can be observed. Acute or prolonged heat exposure is the direct cause of erythema ab igne, and patients should be warned about the danger of a severe burn when using heating pads or portable heaters to keep warm.

Seborrheic Dermatitis

Although seborrheic dermatitis is common in adolescence and young adulthood, it also affects the nursing home population, in general, and in-patients with Parkinson's disease in particular. Redness and scaling can be observed on the scalp, around the ears and the nose, in the eyebrows, and on the anterior chest. Medical treatment with topical ketoconazole (Nizoral) is usually effective in these patients. Prescription shampoos such as ketoconazole (Nizoral 2% shampoo) and chloroxine 2% (Capitrol shampoo) can also be helpful in the treatment of seborrheic dermatitis of the scalp.[5]

Purpura

With aging, thinning of the dermis leads to increased fragility of the dermal capillaries and blood vessels rupture easily with minimal trauma. The resultant extravasation of blood into the surrounding tissue, commonly seen on the dorsal forearm and hands, is referred to as *purpura* or *ecchymosis* (Plates 8 and 11). Patients with senile purpura should be reassured that they do not have a bleeding disorder and should be advised to protect their skin against trauma and friction. Long-sleeved shirts reduce shear and friction. Nursing home personnel should be advised that gentle handling of the patient is crucial in the prevention of bruising and skin tears. If a skin tear does occur, nonadherent dressings secured with tubular retention bandages should be used to prevent trauma of the surrounding skin.

Cherry Hemangiomas

Cherry hemangiomas are bright red papules, 1 to 5 mm in diameter, that may increase in number with advancing age. They are most commonly seen on the trunk, and their pathogenesis is unknown (Plate 9). These capillary hemangiomas do not appear to be related to sun exposure, and, except for cosmetic reasons, removal is unnecessary. Cherry hemangiomas respond to light electrodesiccation.

Venous Lakes

Benign venous angiomas, called *venous lakes*, occur most often on the lower lips or the ears of older persons. They are soft, compressible, flat, approximately 4 to 6 mm, and bluish red. Except for cosmetic reasons, treatment is usually unnecessary. However, if the lesion cannot be differentiated clinically from a melanoma, it should be removed for histologic examination.

Frances West *(Part II)*

CASE DISCUSSION

Changes in appearance that result from chronologic aging often motivate older people, women more often than men, to consult a dermatologist or plastic surgeon in the hopes of reversing some of the signs of aging.[6] Although Mrs. West's concerns about her skin are primarily cosmetic in nature, the pigmented lesion on her left leg demands evaluation before any cosmetic interventions are planned.

The lesion on Mrs. West's leg was excised with 5-mm margins and closed with a complex repair and adjacent tissue transfer. Because of its location over a bony prominence with moderate skin tension, extensive undermining of the area was necessary to achieve closure. The pathologist's report confirmed the diagnosis of malignant melanoma in situ with a depth of 2 mm, the lesion extending to one of the lateral margins. It was subsequently reexcised, and the margins were clear on reexcision. Mrs. West returned for follow-up visits for extraction of milia and laser removal of the sebaceous hyperplasia on her face and shave removals of the skin tags around her neck, which were benign. Mrs. West was encouraged to discontinue her cold cream facials and to use a soap-free cleanser and noncomedogenic moisturizer instead, as well as a sunscreen with an SPF of 20. A topical retinoid cream was prescribed for nightly use.

Mrs. West's history of malignant melanoma in situ warrants more frequent skin screenings, and she was asked to follow up in the office every 6 months. Staging of malignant melanoma is extremely important in determining the prognosis in this potentially fatal disease. Shave

removal of a dysplastic-appearing lesion is contraindicated because it interferes with the staging of the disease and leaves malignant cells at its base. Similarly, punch biopsy is not indicated. When a malignant melanoma is suspected, complete excision is the procedure of choice.

SUN-INDUCED SKIN CHANGES

Prevention

Photo-damage, not the normal aging process, has been estimated to account for 90% of age-associated cosmetic problems.[6] Clinicians need to educate patients about the relationship between sun exposure or exposure to UV light from other sources (e.g., tanning booths) and cosmetic problems and cancer. Clinicians should explain to patients that there is no safe tan and that, even if sun-induced skin changes have occurred, further damage can be prevented. Using a sunscreen with SPF 15 or higher helps protect the skin against further photo-damage. The relationship between SPF and degree of protection is not linear. An SPF 15 sunscreen will block 85% of UVB radiation, whereas UVB blockage is approximately 90% when an SPF 20 sunscreen is used. Above this SPF level the degree of added protection is minimal.

Ideally, a sunscreen protects against UVA and UVB radiation; product labels usually specify this. The patient should be taught to apply a sunscreen 30 minutes before going out into the sun, enabling it to bind to the skin, and to cover all exposed areas. The importance of reapplying the sunscreen every few hours as well as after swimming or perspiring should also be emphasized.

Treatment

Topical tretinoin (Retin-A) has received widespread attention for its role in treating sun-damaged skin, and controlled studies have shown it to be an effective treatment for many of the changes associated with photo-aged skin.[7] Topical tretinoin can be used as long-term therapy to reverse photo-damage. The major side effects of topical tretinoin use are skin dryness and increased sensitivity to sun exposure. Patients should be started at the lowest available concentration (0.025%) and should be instructed to apply the cream twice a week at first, gradually increasing the number of applications to twice a day. If the treatment is well tolerated, the tretinoin concentration can also be increased after several months. Patients who use tretinoin must be advised to avoid the sun and to use a sunscreen at all times.

Photo-damaged skin can be treated surgically by means of dermabrasion, chemical peels using trichloroacetic acid or glycolic and salicylic acids, or augmenting soft tissue using collagen injections. For additional information on surgical treatments, the reader is referred to the bibliography.[8,9]

John Decker *(Part I)*

Mr. John Decker, a 74-year-old retired bookkeeper, sees you in your office for evaluation of an intensely pruritic rash that came on suddenly after he was admitted to the residential care facility after a recent mild stroke. He has a history of aortic valvular disease, transient ischemic attacks, and hyperlipidemia. In addition, he relates a history of psoriasis that was treated with whirlpool baths. He is taking warfarin (Coumadin), atorvastatin (Zocor), and furosemide (Lasix), as well as eye drops for glaucoma. He complains that the itching prevents him from sleeping, and he cannot keep from scratching. The nurse's aide has been applying Lubriderm lotion to his chest and back twice a day without relief.

Physical examination reveals a frail-appearing elderly man with anxious facies and a barely audible voice. He has red-brown scaly lesions over both temples that appear irritated and crusted. His trunk is almost completely covered with a scarlet exanthem with sharply demarcated borders, faintly papular, sparing the horizontal skin fold areas over the abdomen (Plate 10). His forearms bear thin atrophic skin with excoriations and avulsions with large ecchymotic areas in a linear pattern (Plate11). The skin over the dorsum of his hands tents when pinched. His genital area has marginated erythema with central clearing and maceration of the skin involving the upper medial thighs; when asked, he complains that it too is pruritic.

STUDY QUESTIONS

1. What is the most likely cause of Mr. Decker's itchy red rash?
   a. Psoriasis flare
   b. Xerosis
   c. Drug reaction
   d. Tinea cruris
   e. Scabies
2. Which of his medications do you suspect could cause this eruption?
3. What other medication-related skin findings (if any) do you observe?
4. What procedure would you perform to confirm your diagnosis?
5. What measures can you take to relieve his pruritus while the workup is in progress?
6. What do you suspect the temporal lesions are?

PRURITUS AND XEROSIS

The most common cause of pruritus, a symptom that evokes scratching, is dry skin or xerosis.[10] Also known as asteatosis, "winter itch," or eczema craquelé, xerosis is common in the elderly (Table 52-2), and the unfortunate reference to "senile itch" implies that the condition is intrinsic to old age. Xerotic skin looks and feels dry, rough, and scaly. Changes are most pronounced over the anterior legs, the extensor aspects of the arms and forearms, and the dorsum of the hands. Chronic rubbing and scratching cause thickening, or lichenification, of the skin. Xerosis is usually more severe in the winter because low humidity, cold and windy weather, dry heat, and excessive bathing aggravate the condition. Severe cases (eczema craquelé) can result in superinfection and cellulitis. Before treatment of the dry skin is begun (or if xerosis treatment does not alleviate pruritus), it is important to rule out other potential causes of itching, such as contact allergy, medication or food allergies, scabies, metabolic diseases, diseases of the liver or biliary ducts, neoplasia, drug reactions, and psychogenic causes. Treatment of dry skin includes use of a humidifier and both patient and caregiver counseling. Patients should be advised to bathe or shower less frequently, to use warm instead of hot water when bathing, and to use mild and moisturizing soaps (e.g., Aveeno, Basis, or Dove) only. The patient should be instructed to lightly pat the skin dry and to apply a moisturizer (e.g., hydrophilic ointment, Vaseline, Eucerin, or Moisturel). Elderly patients should be discouraged from using bath oil because it makes the tub or shower slippery and hazardous, predisposing to falls. If hydrating the skin does not reduce skin dryness and alleviate the pruritus, Lac-Hydrin 5% or 12% moisturizer containing urea (a non-prescription item) has been found to be effective. If the skin is cracking or inflamed as in eczema craquelé, mid-potency to high-potency topical corticosteroids may be used acutely.

Table 52–2	Clinical Features of Elderly Skin	
Non–Sun-Damaged Skin	**Sun-Damaged Skin**
Shallow, fine wrinkles	Deep, coarse wrinkles (rhytides)
Animation lines of the face	Thickened, leathery, inelastic skin; yellowing discoloration; irregular pigmentation; comedones
"Frown lines"	
"Crow's feet"	
Loss of skin resiliency and elasticity	Clinically more apparent in photo-damaged skin
"Sagging" appearance	
Atrophy or thinning of skin from loss of collagen	Excessively dry skin, xerosis
	Telangiectasias, purpura, easy bruising more pronounced
Sebaceous gland hyperplasia	
Loss of hydration caused by reduced hyaluronic acid with moderate xerosis	Cutaneous neoplasms
	Actinic keratoses, basal cell cancer, squamous cell cancer
Thinning of vascular walls with propensity to easy bruising	
Smooth, unblemished surface	

John Decker *(Part II)*

CASE DISCUSSION

Although xerosis is certainly the most common cause of pruritus in the elderly population, it is not generally accompanied by the intense erythema with which Mr. Decker presents. Tinea cruris can produce erythema and itching, but the clinical picture differs from this dry confluent exanthem. The hallmarks of scabies, seen in nursing home populations, are linear excoriations and papules involving the intertriginous spaces and web spaces of the hands and feet.

Minimal trauma can produce the excoriations and tears in atrophic elderly skin. Scratching exacerbates the extravasation of blood into the superficial skin layers.

Because his move to the nursing care facility and changes in his medication predate the onset of Mr. Decker's generalized skin eruption, a drug-related eruption must be ruled out.[11] A punch biopsy from the margin of the exanthem on the abdominal wall was taken. Sutures were placed at the biopsy site for additional help with hemostasis because the patient was on warfarin (Coumadin). The pathologist's report suggested drug eruption with eosinophilia or the urticarial phase of bullous pemphigoid.

Mr. Decker's pruritus was treated with an oral antihistamine, hydroxyzine (Atarax) 25 mg, topical hydrophilic ointment with a mid-potency steroid hydrocortisone valerate (Westcort) 0.2%

added to the ointment, and an intramuscular injection of triamcinolone (Kenalog) 40 mg.

The most likely offending drugs simvastatin (Zocor) and furosemide (Lasix) were discontinued, ethacrynic acid was substituted for furosemide, and exanthem resolved over a 1-week period.

The irritated temporal dermatoses were excised by shave technique with electrodesiccation to the base of the lesion, and pathologic interpretation revealed squamous cell carcinoma (SCC).

Alice Fay Jackson *(Part I)*

Mrs. Jackson, a 58-year-old black elementary school teacher, complains of a 4-day history of skin sensitivity and aching of the area on the left side of her back extending to her axilla, which has prevented her from wearing her bra. Yesterday she noticed a patch of small painful blisters on her upper left abdomen (Plate 12). She has been applying calamine lotion to the area since the blisters appeared and taking ibuprofen (Motrin) without relief. She had an injection of cortisone a week ago in her family doctor's office to help relieve her back pain resulting from osteoarthritis. She sleeps with a heating pad under her back at night when her back pain flares.

Her prescribed medications include famotidine (Pepcid) for indigestion and hormone replacement therapy after a hysterectomy for uterine fibroids and menorrhagia.

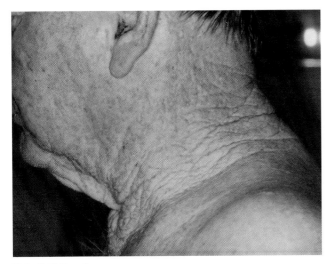

PLATE 1

Solar elastosis of the neck with thickened, furrowed appearance.

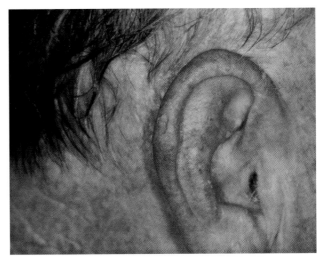

PLATE 2

Hyperplastic solar keratosis of the helix.

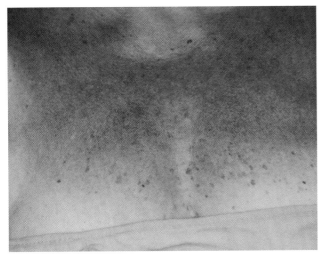

PLATE 3

Solar lentigines. Note the contrast between sun-exposed and covered areas.

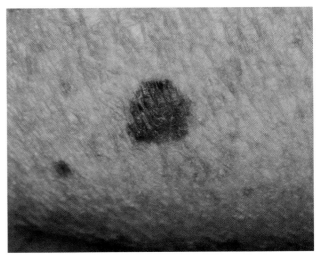

PLATE 4

Flat, irregular borders of malignant melanoma. Note that more than one color is present.

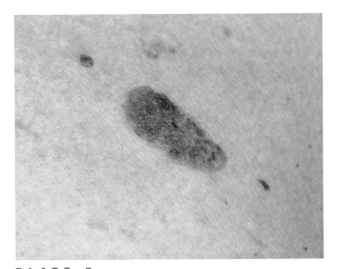

PLATE 5

Seborrheic keratosis may occur singly or cover large areas of skin.

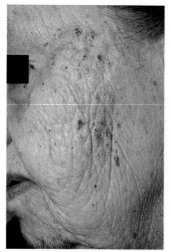

PLATE 6

Favre-Racouchot syndrome—the result of sun exposure.

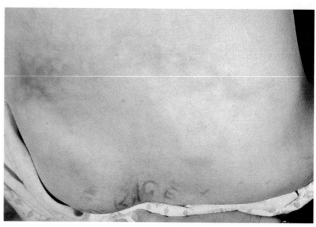

PLATE 7

Erythema ab igne, hemosiderin, and melanin deposition after thermal injury.

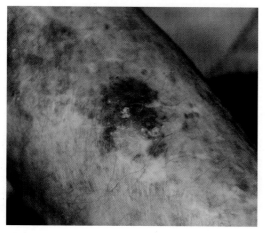

PLATE 8

Purpura in thinned skin of the forearm.

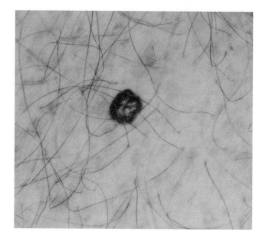

PLATE 9

Cherry hemangiomas are benign.

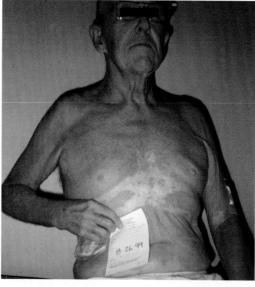

PLATE 10

Drug eruptions can present dramatically.

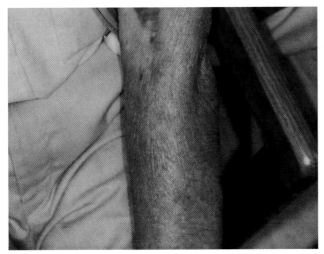

PLATE 11

Purpura can result from minimal trauma such as scratching.

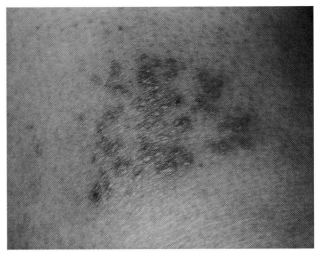

PLATE 12

Herpes zoster. Grouped vesicles on an erythematous base.

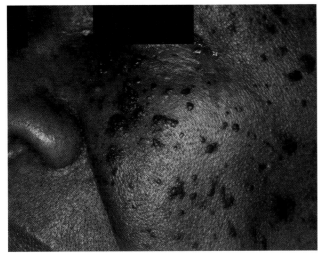

PLATE 13

Dermatosis papulosa nigra is a benign keratosis.

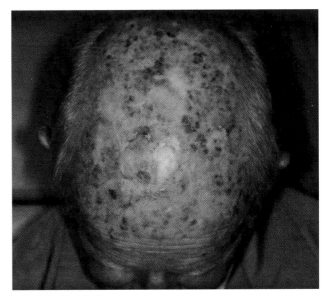

PLATE 14

Actinic keratosis, a premalignant sun-induced lesion.

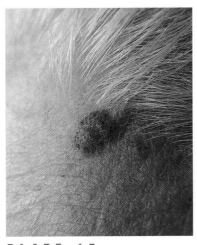

PLATE 15

Pigmented basal cell carcinoma.

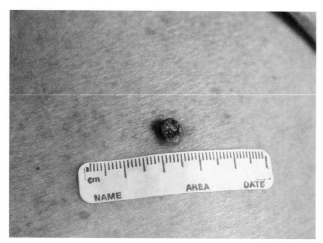

PLATE 16

Squamous cell carcinoma can arise from an actinic keratosis or develop in burn scars or chronic ulcers.

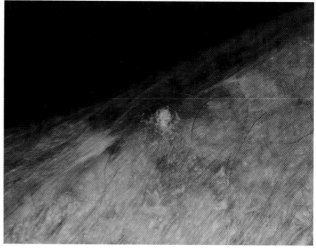

PLATE 17

Keratoacanthoma, a rapidly growing bud-shaped lesion.

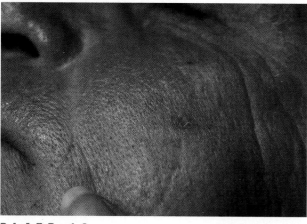

PLATE 18

Lentigo maligna.

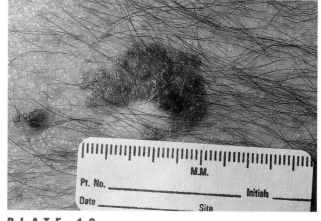

PLATE 19

Superficial spreading melanoma.

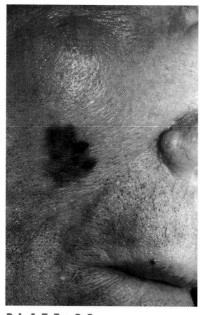

PLATE 20

Malignant melanoma.

On physical examination, you note some conjunctival pallor, but her skin is finely textured and relatively free of wrinkles. She has a sprinkling of 2-mm black papules across her nose and cheeks (Plate 13).

Erythematous papules and vesicles arising just lateral to her spine trace the T5 dermatome around to the anterior axillary line on the left, and the area is tender to palpation. Her sacral area appears hyperpigmented and mottled with a reticular erythematous pattern, fairly well demarcated in an oval shape approximately 8 × 10 cm.

STUDY QUESTIONS

1. What term describes the uncomfortable sensation that preceded Mrs. Jackson's rash?
2. What might have predisposed her to this outbreak?
3. Is there any significance to her being a school teacher?
4. Explain the significance of her lack of rhytides

BULLOUS DISORDERS

Bullous Pemphigoid

Bullous pemphigoid is a blistering disease characterized by the presence of tense bullae filled with straw-colored fluid arising from normal or red skin. Usually, bullae first appear on the distal extremities, followed by the groin and axillae. Eventually lesions become generalized and may include mucous membranes. Bullous pemphigoid is fairly common in the elderly and is the result of an autoimmune reaction in the epidermal basement membrane. If there is itching, it is usually severe. Diagnosis is made by biopsy with routine and direct immunofluorescence. The disease is self-limited but, if untreated, may last from a few months to several years with periodic remissions and exacerbations. Mortality is low, but patients are uncomfortable. Treatment with oral corticosteroids (40 to 60 mg/day) is usually effective. For mild disease, dapsone or tetracycline may be prescribed.

Allergic Contact Dermatitis

Vesicles and bullae occurring in the area of exposure to an allergen (e.g., poison ivy on the forearm) are classified as allergic contact dermatitis. There is usually, but not always, a pattern suggestive of external causation, such as lines from wearing a cap, ring, or necklace. If widespread, allergic contact dermatitis can be treated effectively with high-dose steroids (e.g., 40 to 60 mg) for 5 to 10 days. When symptoms are less severe, topical corticosteroids and lubrication are adequate treatment. Determining the cause of the reaction is important to prevent recurrence. Patch testing can help elucidate the causative agents in recurrent contact dermatitis.

Herpes Zoster

Herpes zoster, a self-limiting but uncomfortable condition, is a reactivation of the varicella-zoster virus (chickenpox) within the sensory neurons of the dorsal root ganglion. It typically appears as a grouped band of inflammatory vesicles and bullae in a pattern following a dermatome. Often patients will experience itching, tingling, or pain over the involved dermatome several days before the outbreak of the rash. These vesicles can occur anywhere on the skin but never cross the midline. Severe pain and a tingling sensation often precede the eruption. It is important to differentiate herpes zoster from herpes simplex. The latter does not occur in a dermatome pattern and is recurrent. Diagnosis is usually made after a careful history and inspection of the skin (Plate 12).

Treatment with acyclovir (Zovirax) 800 mg orally five times a day for 7 to 10 days has been found to reduce pain and facilitate healing. Valacyclovir (Valtrex) 1 g three times a day for 7 days and famciclovir (Famvir) 500 mg three times a day for 7 days are alternative therapies.[12] Both may reduce the duration of postherpetic neuralgia.[13] In immunocompromised patients, a workup for occult malignancy is warranted. In otherwise healthy adults, this is not generally necessary.

The use of corticosteroids to prevent postherpetic neuralgia is controversial. If corticosteroids are prescribed for this purpose, they should be started early in the course of the disease. Prednisone 60 mg is usually initiated and tapered over a 3-week period.

If the ophthalmic branch of the trigeminal nerve is involved, clinicians should be concerned about uveitis and corneal ulceration. In these instances, an immediate ophthalmologic consultation is warranted. Vesicles on the tip of the nose can serve as a marker for possible ophthalmic involvement.[14]

The pain of herpes zoster can be severe and difficult to treat. Analgesics, carbamazepine, and amitriptyline have been used with varying success. Topical capsaicin (Zostrix) can be recommended for postherpetic neuralgia, providing the lesions have healed. Application of topical capsaicin on open, active lesions is extremely painful and is therefore not advised.

Vesicular Tinea Pedis

Vesicular tinea pedis is an intensely inflammatory dermatophyte infection characterized by vesicles with surrounding erythema in the instep, toe webs, and soles of the feet. The diagnosis is confirmed by potassium hydroxide prep, but this can be falsely negative. Treatment with oral griseofulvin 500 mg twice a day or ketoconazole (Nizoral tablets) 200 mg daily is usually effective. Gram-negative infections, often present in chronically wet or macerated areas, must be treated with topical antifungals and appropriate antibiotics.

Erythema Multiforme Bullosum

Red, nonscaling papules and plaques with central bullae and oral membrane erosion are the clinical signs of erythema multiforme bullosum, also known as *Stevens-Johnson syndrome*. The distribution is typically generalized, including the palms, soles, and mouth. Erythema multiforme bullosum is a hypersensitivity reaction to, among others, a medication, bacteria, virus, or food. The condition can be life-threatening, especially if it causes toxic epidermal necrolysis. Prompt referral to a dermatologist and aggressive treatment (usually requiring hospitalization) are warranted.

Alice Fay Jackson (*Part II*)

CASE DISCUSSION

Mrs. Jackson sought treatment for dramatic symptoms of herpes zoster, most likely triggered by her steroid injection. The astute clinician must be alert for subtle signs of occult malignancy as well. Complicating the picture are signs of anemia of chronic blood loss resulting from leiomyomata of the uterus, and gastrointestinal bleeding resulting possibly from the use nonsteroidal anti-inflammatory drugs. The term dysesthesia is applied to the prodromal symptoms of herpes zoster. The patient perceived blisters to be a manifestation of rhus dermatitis, or poison ivy, and self-treated with calamine lotion, without relief.

It is possible that Mrs. Jackson's occupation as a teacher predisposed her to reactivation of varicella-zoster virus—the causative agent of chickenpox—because the virus is endemic in the elementary school population. The black papules are benign dermatoses that are found on the skin of blacks and people of Asian or Indian descent. These papules are called dermatosis papulosa nigra.

Mrs. Jackson's fine, unwrinkled skin reflects her avoidance of the sun and its damaging effects on the skin.

As Mrs. Jackson's primary care physician you should follow up her conjunctival pallor in light of her history of ibuprofen use, menorrhagia, and use of famotidine (Pepcid) for indigestion.

SKIN CANCER

Skin tumors can be classified as benign (see "Benign Dermatoses") or malignant. Malignant tumors are further categorized as nonmelanoma (e.g., AKs, basal cell carcinomas [BCCs], SCCs, and keratoacanthomas [KAs]) or melanoma.

Actinic Keratoses

AKs usually appear as multiple, flat or slightly elevated, rough, scaly macules or papules on a hyperemic base (Plate 14). They measure approximately 0.2 to 1.5 cm and occur on the sun-exposed areas (face and scalp, dorsum of arms and hands, neck, and trunk) of patients who are already genetically predisposed; hence, they are most commonly seen in fair-skinned individuals.

Curettage and application of liquid nitrogen are effective methods of removing a limited number of lesions. When many lesions are present, the treatment of choice is 1% fluorouracil cream applied to the more delicate areas (e.g., the face). The 2% and 5% creams have been found to be effective for less delicate areas (e.g., forearms and dorsum of the hands). The patient should be instructed to apply the cream daily to the affected areas until the lesions are inflamed, for 2 to 3 weeks. Without treatment approximately 5% to 10% of AKs progress to SCC.

Basal Cell Carcinomas

BCCs are the most common skin cancers. The incidence of BCCs to SCCs is 4:1. Most BCCs are classified as either nodular or ulcerative. BCCs often start as a small papule. As the papule slowly enlarges, a central depression, ringed by a pearly or waxy border with overlying telangiectatic vessels, is formed. BCCs are most often found on sun-exposed areas of the body, especially the face and neck. They are slow growing and rarely metastasize. However, they can invade the subcutaneous tissue and muscle layers and require extensive resection (Plate 15).

Squamous Cell Carcinoma

The clinical appearance of SCCs varies, but most appear as solitary, keratotic nodules with nondistinct borders on an erythematous base (Plate 16). SCCs can occur anywhere on the skin, including mucous membranes, but are most commonly found on sun-damaged skin and often arise from AKs. They can also develop in burn scars, radiation-damaged skin, lesions of hidradenitis suppurativa, and chronic wounds or ulcers. SCCs are usually slow growing but can metastasize, although rarely, to the regional lymph nodes (Table 52-3).

Treatment of Basal Cell Carcinoma and Squamous Cell Carcinoma

A variety of methods can be used to remove BCCs and SCCs, including curettage, electrodesiccation, excision, or radiation therapy. Primary care clinicians frequently remove lesions smaller than 0.5 cm by curettage, which allows histologic examination, or electrodesiccation, thus destroying the lesion but providing no specimen for pathologic interpretation. Patients with larger lesions are usually referred to a dermatologist for Mohs surgery, skin grafting, or a primary advancement flap.

Keratoacanthoma

A KA is a rapidly growing, bud-shaped, skin-colored to slightly reddish lesion that arises from a hair follicle (Plate 17). It is benign and occurs most often on exposed hair-bearing skin in people over 60 years of age. Sometimes the lesion becomes ulcerated. Sunlight exposure or artificial UV radiation and chemical carcinogens exposure (e.g., pitch or tar) has been found to be related to the development of KA. The lesion rapidly grows to approximately 10 to 25 mm followed by slow involution over 2 to 6 months. Occasionally, involution takes more than a year. For cosmetic and practical reasons, excision of the entire lesion is often recommended. Clinically and histologically, these lesions resemble a carcinoma, and complete excision helps confirm the diagnosis.

Malignant Melanoma

The importance of being able to evaluate any suspicious skin lesion has increased with the rising incidence of malignant melanoma in people of all ages. Early detection and prompt, aggressive treatment are essential for a cure. Widespread use of the ABCDE melanoma-recognition system, adapted by the American Cancer Society, has helped increase awareness. Patients should be taught to look for A, *asymmetry* of the lesion; B, *border* irregularity; C, *color* variation; D, *diameter* more than 0.6 cm; and the recently added E, *elevation* (Plates 18, 19, 20, and 4).

A flat lesion that becomes elevated should arouse suspicion. It is important, however, to tell patients that if their lesion meets only one of these criteria, they probably do not have a melanoma. If a patient is at risk for melanoma, concerned, or unsure about the ABCDEs, he or she are advised to make an appointment every 6 months or so because it is better to *always* (A), *be* (B) *checked* (C) by their *doctor* (D). Finally, health care professionals should be aware that only 20% of malignant melanomas arise on sun-exposed areas, so it is important to examine the entire body.[15, 16] Patients with a family history of malignant melanoma are encouraged to be examined yearly (Table 52-4).

Table 52–3	Key Features of Common Skin Malignancies		
	Actinic Keratoses	**Basal Cell Carcinoma**	**Squamous Cell Carcinoma**
Size	0.2 to 1.5 cm	0.5 to 1.5 cm	0.2 to 1.5 cm
Shape	Flat, slightly elevated	Nodule, ulcer	Nodule, ulcer
Color	Red or brown macule erythematous base	Pearly; may be pigmented	Erythematous base
Surface	Rough, scaly	Telangiectatic	Keratotic
Site	Sun-exposed skin	Sun-exposed skin, especially face and neck	Sun-exposed skin, mucous membranes, burn/radiation scars, chronic wounds or ulcers

Table 52–4	Lentigo Maligna Melanoma		
	Lentigo Maligna Melanoma	**Superficial Spreading Melanoma**	**Nodular Melanoma**
Shape	Irregular	Becomes more irregular as it grows	May be regular or irregular
Color	Dark or black on pale background	Dark brown or black; may be variegated	Dark brown or black; may be variegated
Surface	Nodular against a smooth background	Smooth, vertical growth occurs later	Nodular
Site	In preexisting lentigo maligna; usually facial	Sun-exposed areas	Most common on sun-exposed areas; can occur anywhere

Modified from Rose LC. Recognizing neoplastic skin lesions: a photo guide. Am Fam Physician 1998;58:873-884, 887-888.

Treatment of Malignant Melanoma

When a melanoma is suspected, a biopsy provides the definitive diagnosis. However, biopsy usually means excision of the entire lesion in the case of melanoma. Shaving the lesion prevents staging, which provides information about the depth of the lesion, whether it is limited to the dermis or has penetrated deeper into the subcutaneous tissue. The degree of penetration and spread determines the prognosis, and so a shave biopsy is not helpful. Similarly, a punch biopsy may not capture enough of the lesion to fully assess its pathogenicity. Excisional biopsy remains the most thorough tool for evaluation of a suspicious nevus. The growth and a border of normal surrounding skin and tissue, about 1 cm, are taken and sent for examination by the pathologist. Staging for the degree of vertical and horizontal spread determines the next step in treatment. Depending on the pathologist's report, the next steps are no further treatment, wide excision with skin grafting, regional lymph node biopsy or removal, or adjuvant chemotherapy. Radiation may be used to treat local recurrence of melanoma that is not amenable to surgical resection. There is a role for immunotherapy with interferon and interleukin-2, but these are still not first-line treatments.[17]

SUMMARY

Skin problems in the elderly are common. Patients with chronologically aged as well as photo-aged skin may seek the physician's care to help alleviate pain or itching, to voice their concerns related to a skin growth, or to ask advice on improving the appearance of their skin. Fortunately, the vast majority of skin problems in the elderly can be treated, greatly improving the patient's quality of life. After all, being older does not mean one has to be uncomfortable or itchy or live with unwanted skin lesions. In addition, physicians can play an important role in educating patients about the importance of sun protection to prevent any or further photo-damage. Because commonly encountered skin conditions in the elderly range from presenting a cosmetic concern or minor irritation to a stage IV melanoma with a 5-year survival rate of less than 50%, early recognition of the specific condition is crucial.[18] Understanding the appearance of chronologically aged and photo-aged skin (see Table 52-2) and the potential diagnostic value of the color of a lesion (see Table 52-1) helps clinicians guide their treatment plan.

POSTTEST

1. Which of the following statements concerning skin disease in old age is false?
   a. The most common cause of pruritus in the elderly is xerosis.
   b. Screening for malignancy should be considered in patients with herpes zoster.
   c. Actinic keratoses are not precancerous.
   d. Keratoacanthoma is not malignant.

2. Which of the following statements concerning skin disease in old age is false?
   a. Malignant melanomas can occur in non-sun-exposed areas.
   b. Squamous cell carcinoma is generally preceded by actinic keratoses.
   c. Asymmetry of a lesion is a good indication that it is not malignant.
   d. Basal cell carcinomas are four times more common than squamous cell carcinomas.

References

1. Fenske NA, Lober CW. Structural and functional changes of normal aging skin. J Am Acad Dermatol 1986;15:571-585.
2. Beacham BE. Common skin problems in the elderly. Am Fam Physician 1992;46:163-168.
3. Selamnowitz VJ, Rizer RL, Orentreich N. Aging of the skin and its appendices. In Handbook of the biology of aging (Finch CE, Hayflock L, eds.). New York: Van Nostrand Reinhold, 1977.
4. Shelly WB. The razor blade in dermatologic practice. Cutis 1975;16:843.
5. Jacobs PH. Seborrheic dermatitis: causes and management. Cutis 1988;41:182.
6. Gilchrest BA. Skin and aging process, Boca Raton, FL: CRC Press, 1984.
7. Kligman AM. Guidelines for the use of topical tretinoin (Retin-A) for photoaged skin. J Am Acad Dermatol 1989;21:650-654.
8. Alt TH. Technical aids for dermabrasion. J Dermatol Surg Oncol 1987; 13:638-648.
9. Elson ML. Soft tissue augmentation of periorbital fine lines and the orbital groove with Zyderm-I and fine gauge needles. J Dermatol Surg Oncol 1992; 18:779-782.
10. Denman ST. A review of pruritus. J Am Acad Dermatol 1986;14:375-392.
11. Sauer GC. Manual of skin diseases, 5 ed. Philadelphia: J.B. Lippincott, 1985.
12. Goldsmith LA. Adult and pediatric dermatology: a color guide to diagnosis and treatment, Philadelphia: F.A. Davis, 1997.
13. Alper BS, Lewis PR. Does treatment of acute herpes zoster prevent or shorten postherpetic neuralgia? J Fam Pract 2000;49:255-264.
14. Andreoli TE et al. Cecil essentials of medicine, 4 ed. Philadelphia: W.B. Saunders, 1997.
15. Rigel DS, Friedman RJ, Kopf AW, et al. Importance of complete cutaneous examination for the detection of malignant melanoma. J Am Acad Dermatol 1986;14:857-860.
16. Chiarello SE. The comprehensive skin examination: reasons for, facts, and methods. J Geriatr Dermatol 1994;2:99.
17. Johnson TM, Smith JW 2nd, Nelson BR, Chang A. Current therapy for cutaneous melanoma. J Am Acad Dermatol 1995;32:689-707.
18. National Cancer Institute. U.S. Department of Health and Human Services: Melanoma: research report. Bethesda, MD: National Institutes of Heallth. No 92-3020, February 1992.

SUGGESTED READINGS

1. Fitzpatrick TB et al. Dermatology in general medicine, New York: McGraw-Hill, 1993.
2. Young A, Newcomer VD, Kligman AM. Geriatric dermatology: color atlas and practitioner's guide, Philadelphia: Lea & Febiger, 1993.

PRETEST ANSWERS

1. c
2. b

POSTTEST ANSWERS

1. c
2. c

Page numbers followed by "f" denote figures; "t" denote tables; and "b denote boxes